# Internal Medicine

Jarrah Ali Al-Tubaikh

# Internal Medicine

An Illustrated Radiological Guide

**Second Edition**

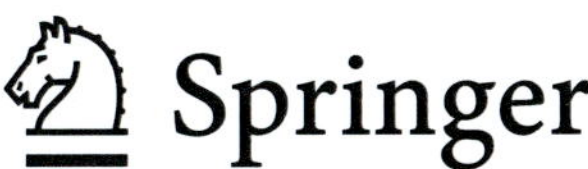

**Jarrah Ali Al-Tubaikh**
Department of Clinical Radiology
Amiri Hospital – Kuwait City
Kuwait City, Kuwait

All illustrations marked with ♟ were drawn by the author.

ISBN 978-3-319-39746-7        ISBN 978-3-319-39747-4    (eBook)
DOI 10.1007/978-3-319-39747-4

Library of Congress Control Number: 2016954639



Printed on acid-free paper

This Springer imprint is published by Springer Nature
The registered company is Springer International Publishing AG Switzerland

# Preface

It is a privilege to write another introduction to this book. When I wrote this book in Munich in 2010, I knew I was writing a book with an uncommon combination, linking internal medicine to radiology. I can still remember the comment of my mentor Prof. Maximillian Reiser after he saw the manuscript's content. He told me: "Why did you choose this layout and these disorders in particular?" I replied: "They are the most commonly encountered diseases daily in any busy medical department."

Over the years, I have noticed how the chapter's download numbers are increasing in Springer's official website. This reflects, to me at least, the continuous demand for such topics worldwide, especially among newly coming radiologists. They are the ones facing the fire daily in duties and emergency calls from physicians and surgeons around the clock. Moreover, radiology board teachings concentrate more and more over emergency cases, trauma cases, postoperative complications, and cancer screening and monitoring. I can assure you that almost 90 % of any radiologist's daily routine lies within one or more of the past four areas in radiology. Internal medicine disorders and complications are considered extracurriculum, and maybe special interest radiology.

Within the past 5 years since the publication of this book, I have noticed a skyrocketing increase in the radiological referrals through my work in two different hospitals. Sometimes, we get radiological referral for simple disorders that do not need radiological investigation, for example, more and more demands for ultrasound to exclude inguinal hernias, ultrasound for lipoma, CT for acute appendicitis suspicion, polytrauma PAN-CT, etc. As a radiologist, it is always nice to be needed; however, technology can be a double-edged sword, reducing the clinical experience of both the referring clinician and the radiologist. Many physicians, unfortunately, started to use radiology as a substitute for clinical examination and judgment. Although such a phenomenon is not necessarily widely found, it is there, no doubt about it.

I am pleased that the first edition of my book has helped many physicians I know to change their perspective toward radiological investigations. I have been contacted by many physicians here in Kuwait and outside of Kuwait who thank me for detailing what they should order and how to

investigate certain diseases. In the same fashion, many radiologists are pleased with the variety of images that detail the medical disorders and facilitate their detection.

Based on the past positive feedbacks, I aimed to expand the range of the book by including three more medical fields, which are not directly linked to internal medicine but however are important to know. The second edition of this book exposes the reader to occupational medicine and toxicology, which are uncommonly seen as cases of attempting suicide and accidental intoxications. The radiological literature is filled with different radiological signs reported by many researches detailing intoxications, which have become of great interest since the data are accumulating over the years.

Chiropractic and osteopathic medicine are two important fields that emerged more than a hundred years ago, and they are rarely, if ever, mentioned or taught in medical schools or board-certification programs, especially in specialties related to the orthopedics or the spine. Although they are not considered part of conventional medicine, both specialties have very solid neuroanatomical and neuropathophysiological basis. Chiropractic medicine in particular, founded by D. D. Palmar and perfected by B. J. Palmar, uses radiology as an essential part of its diagnostic techniques. Their radiographic imaging techniques are known as "spinography." Personally, I have been using their radiographic techniques in an extensive fashion to diagnose lower back pain and kinesiological disorders. Their radiological imaging techniques proved to be very valid and very accurate in diagnosing lower back pain, especially lumbar spine MRI with almost normal findings. Unfortunately, such radiological knowledge is very rarely encountered in commonly known radiological journals. I sincerely hope that the reader will find the chapter of chiropractic medicine imaging interesting and informative.

Lastly, a very new medical specialty is arising within the past 5 years: energy and quantum medicine. Although it started with the book *What Is Life?* (1944) by the Nobel Prize winner Austrian physicist Erwin Schrödinger, many new medical and biological researchers are now using quantum physics to define life, including Robert O. Becker, Jerry Tennant, Hans-Peter Dürr, Fritz-Albert Popp, Mae-Wan Ho, and so many others. Their works have now evolved to so many applications, emerging as unconventional therapies that use waves and frequencies to heal, such as pulsed electromagnetic field (PEMF) therapy, microcurrent therapy, phototherapy, and ultrasonic therapy. I have been personally using these devices for myself and my relatives and for special cases in the hospital, with a high success rate of controlling diseases and complications. I documented my findings on radiological images, imaging patients before and after such unconventional, energetic therapy to find out what has been changed in the disease status radiographically. I took the opportunity of publishing the second edition of this book to introduce the reader to a whole new world that uses therapies based on biophysics rather than biochemistry for conventional, pharmacological medicine uses.

In conclusion, I hope for the reader an interesting journey through the book, and I hope that this book can help someone somewhere in the world save a life.

**Jarrah Ali Al-Tubaikh, MD**
Kuwait City, Kuwait

# Contents

# Gastroenterology




© Springer International Publishing Switzerland 2017
J.A. Al-Tubaikh, *Internal Medicine*, DOI 10.1007/978-3-319-39747-4_1

## 1.1    **Liver Cirrhosis**

Liver cirrhosis is a term used to describe the histological development of regenerative hepatic nodules surrounded by fibrous bands in response to chronic liver injury.

Cirrhosis is an advanced, diffuse stage of liver injury, which is characterized by replacement of the normal liver parenchyma by collagenous scar (fibrosis). Cirrhosis is accompanied by diffuse distortion of the hepatic vasculature and architecture, resulting in vascular disturbance between the portal veins and the hepatic veins, plus porta hepatic fibrosis. The major cirrhosis consequences are hepatic function impairment, increased intrahepatic resistance (portal hypertension), and the development of hepatocellular carcinoma (HCC).

## Types of Liver Cirrhosis

— *Laennec's cirrhosis* is a type of micronodular liver cirrhosis that is seen in patients with malnutrition, alcoholism, or chronic liver steatosis.
— *Posthepatitic cirrhosis* is a micro- and/or macronodular liver cirrhosis commonly seen in patients with hepatitis C virus or uncommonly B virus.
— *Postnecrotic cirrhosis* is macronodular liver cirrhosis that can arise due to fulminating hepatitis infection or due to toxic liver injury.
— *Primary biliary cirrhosis (PBC) (vanishing bile duct syndrome)* is an autoimmune disease of unknown origin characterized by progressive intrahepatic bile duct, nonsuppurative inflammation, and destruction by T-cell lymphocytes, which leads later on to micronodular liver cirrhosis, hepatomegaly, with greenish-stain liver on gross examination due to bile retention. PBC occurs in middle-aged women in up to 90 % of cases. In symptomatic PBC, patients may complain of jaundice in the first 2–3 years, which develops later into portal hypertension and hepatosplenomegaly. In the asymptomatic PBC, the only symptom is abnormal serum hepatobiliary enzyme levels. PBC is classified pathologically into four main stages. *Florid duct stage (stage I PBC)* is characterized by vanishing intrahepatic duct and ductopenia due to destruction of the intrahepatic bile duct basement membrane and cellular bodies by lymphocytes. *Ductular proliferation stage (stage II)* is characterized by small bile ducts proliferation in an attempt to compensate the obstruction of the large bile ducts. The liver characteristically contains few large ducts and many small bile ducts. *Scarring (stage III)* is characterized by fibrosis and intrahepatic collagen deposition. *Hepatic cirrhosis (stage IV)* is characterized by architectural hepatic disruption and accumulation of the bile within the hepatocytes. The disease is diagnosed by liver biopsy, plus detecting antimitochondrial antibodies (AMA) in the serum.

— *Secondary biliary cirrhosis* arises due to extrahepatic obstruction of the biliary tree, causing bile stagnation within the liver. This type can be seen in cases of congenital bile duct atresia, chronic biliary stone obstruction, or pancreatic head carcinoma. The inflammation in the secondary biliary cirrhosis arises due to secondary infection of the bile, leading to neutrophilic acute inflammatory reaction. In contrast, PBC is a chronic, autoimmune disease with lymphatic and plasma cell inflammatory reaction.
— *Cirrhosis due to metabolic disease* is seen in glycogen storage diseases, α1-antitrypsin deficiency disease, hemochromatosis, and Wilson's disease. All the metabolic cirrhoses are micronodular except Wilson's disease (macronodular).
— *Cirrhosis due to circulatory disorders* is observed in patients with venous congestion due to right-sided heart failure, veno-occlusive disease due to herbal medicine, and Budd–Chiari syndrome. In congestive heart failure, chronic hepatic venous congestion may lead to intrahepatic hypertension, which results in sinusoidal congestion, pressure atrophy, and necrosis of pericentral parenchymal cells. Later, there is a collapse of the necrotic cells with perisinusoidal and periportal collagen deposition (fibrosis) extending to the central veins. These changes are known as "nutmeg liver" on postmortem liver examination.

Cirrhotic nodules are parenchymal nodules found in cirrhotic liver (seen in 25 % of imaging scans only), and they are divided into three main types:
— *Regenerative nodules* represent normal proliferation of liver parenchyma. The development of regenerative nodules can be explained pathologically by cellular repair mechanism known as "cell-to-cell and cell-to-matrix interaction." Cell-to-cell interaction describes the process of cellular inhibition when two cells touch each other (e.g., skin wound healing). Cell-to-matrix interaction describes the process of cellular proliferation inhibition when the regenerated cells touch the tissue matrix (connective tissue frame). In acute hepatitis, if the connective tissue matrix is preserved, then damage to the liver can be completely repaired without architectural distortion or residuals. In contrast, in chronic hepatitis, both the liver parenchyma and the connective tissue frame are damaged. This matrix damage results in random liver cell regeneration without cell-to-matrix cellular inhibition, which will result in regenerative liver nodule formation with fibrosis in between (liver cirrhosis). These nodules do not function normally because the relationship with the portal vein, hepatic artery, and bile ducts (porta hepatis) is lost.
— *Dysplastic nodules* are regenerative premalignant nodules.
— *HCC nodules* are nodules composed of neoplastic cells and are seen commonly in patients with cirrhosis due to hepatitis C virus.

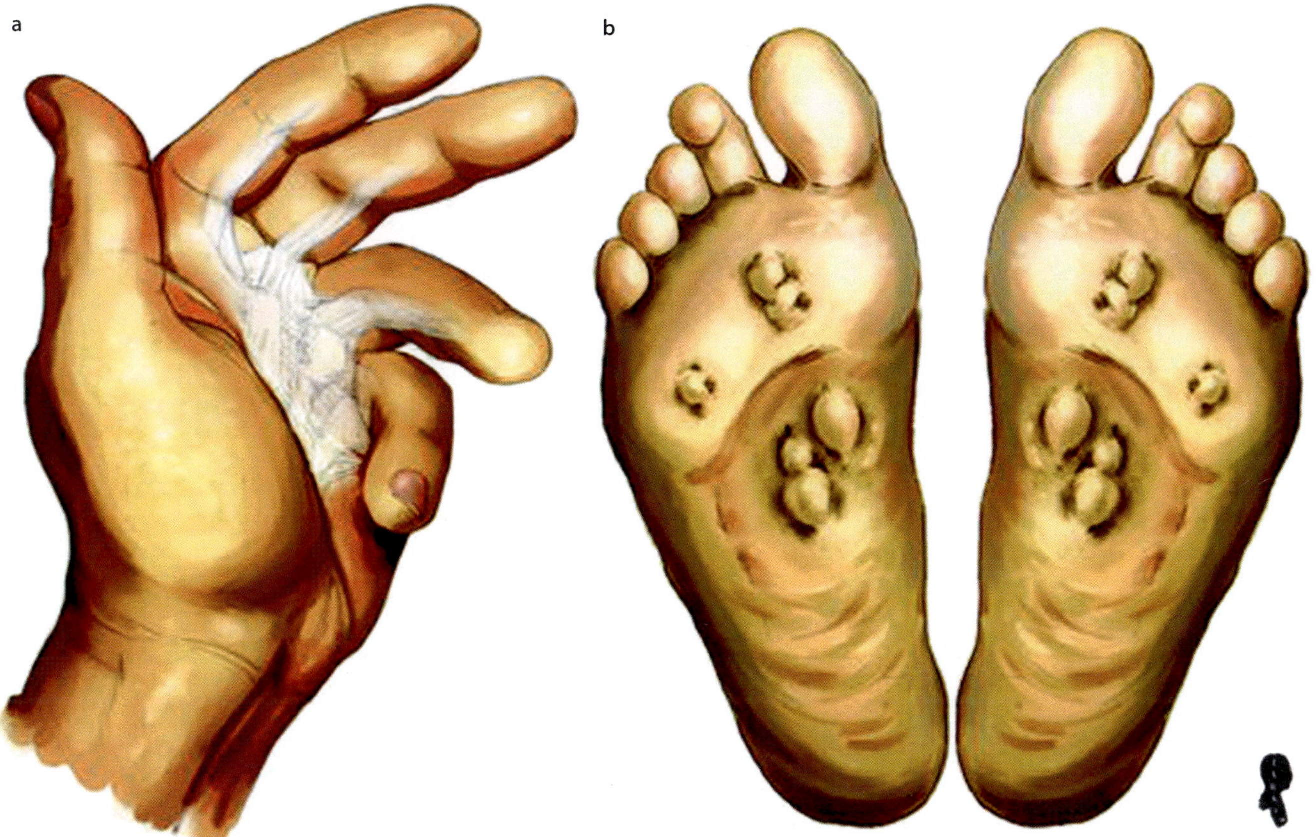

**Fig. 1.1.1** An illustration shows the clinical pathological picture of Dupuytren's contracture with illustrated thickening of the palmar aponeurosis (**a**) and bilateral plantar nodules representing the clinical manifestation of Ledderhose disease (**b**)

Patients with cirrhosis are asymptomatic, unless they develop signs of liver failure. Signs of liver failure include yellowish discoloration of the skin (jaundice), development of central arteriole dilatation with radiating vessels on the face (spider nevi), white nail bed due to hypoalbuminemia, painful proliferative arthropathy of long bones, gynecomastia and palmar erythema due to reduced estradiol degeneration by the liver, hypogonadism (mainly in cirrhosis due to alcoholism and hemochromatosis), anorexia and wasting (>50 % of patients), and diabetes mellitus type 2 (up to 30 % of patients). Some patients with liver cirrhosis may develop palmar fibromatosis.

*Fibromatosis* is a pathological condition characterized by local proliferation of fibroblasts which manifests clinically as soft-tissue thickening. Fibromatosis can affect the palmar aponeurosis (*Dupuytren's contracture*), causing limited hand extension and possibly bony erosions ( Fig. 1.1.1). Palmar fibromatosis that occurs in a bilateral fashion and is associated with bilateral plantar fibromatosis is called *Ledderhose disease* ( Fig. 1.1.1). Other forms of fibromatosis in the body include the male genital fibromatosis (*Peyronie's disease*) and fibromatosis of the dorsum of the interphalangeal joint (*Garrod's nodes*).

The development of portal hypertension can result in splenomegaly, ascites, and prominent paraumbilical veins (caput medusae). Multiple intra- and extrahepatic portosystemic collaterals develop to compensate the loss of the large portal venous flow that cannot be maintained longer due to increased intrahepatic venous pressure in portal hypertension. Intrahepatic portosystemic shunts occur when the portal vein communicates with the hepatic vein in or on the surface of the liver through a dilated venous system. In contrast, extrahepatic portosystemic shunts occur when the intrahepatic portal vein runs toward the outside of the liver communicating with the systemic veins. *Cruveilhier–Baumgarten syndrome* is a condition characterized by patent paraumbilical vein as a consequence of portal hypertension, which occurs as a part of portosystemic shunts. Paraesophageal and paragastric varices develop in patients with advanced liver cirrhosis and can cause life-threatening upper gastrointestinal (GI) bleeding.

*Hepatic encephalopathy* is a potentially reversible complication seen in advanced liver failure and cirrhosis characterized by motor, cognitive, and psychiatric central nervous system (CNS) dysfunction. Manifestations of hepatic encephalopathy include daytime deterioration (grade 1), disorientation in space (grade 2), or coma (grade 3).

Flapping tremor (asterixis) may be seen in patients with hepatic encephalopathy. The neurological manifestations of hepatic encephalopathy are due to inability of the liver to detoxify neurotoxins such as ammonia, phenols, short-chained fatty acids, and other toxic metabolites within the blood. These toxic metabolites cross the blood–brain barrier and deposits within the basal ganglia causing encephalopathy. Hepatic encephalopathy can be induced or exaggerated by sedation, high-protein diet, GI hemorrhage, and the use of diuretics.

*Hepatopulmonary syndrome* is an end-stage liver disease characterized by pulmonary failure, and it is seen in 15–20 % of cirrhosis patients. The diagnosis of hepatopulmonary syndrome requires the following three criteria: chronic liver disease, increased alveolar–arterial gradient on room air, and evidence of intrapulmonary vascular dilatation. Patients with hepatopulmonary syndrome present with liver cirrhosis with hypoxia (30 % of decompensated liver patients). This hypoxemia occurs due to pulmonary vascular dilatation and subsequent ventilation–perfusion mismatch due to decreased hepatic clearance or increased hepatic productions of circulating cytokines and chemical mediators (e.g., nitric oxide). Hypoxic respiratory failure can occur with cases of massive liver necrosis or fulminant hepatic failure.

*Hepatitis C virus-related arthritis* (*HCVrA*) may be seen in patients with liver cirrhosis due to hepatitis C virus. HCVrA affects 4 % of patients with HCV liver cirrhosis, and it has two forms: a frequent symmetrical polyarthritis affecting small joints similar to rheumatoid arthritis in a lesser form and an intermittent mono-/oligoarthritis that involves medium- and large-sized joints.

### Signs on Plain Radiographs

- *Hepatic hydrothorax* is defined as large pleural effusion in a cirrhotic liver disease patient in the absence of cardiac or pulmonary disease. Hepatic hydrothorax is seen in 10 % of patients. The pleural effusion can be right sided (67 %), left sided (17 %), or bilateral (17 %).
- Hepatopulmonary syndrome is visualized on plain chest radiographs as reticulonodular interstitial pattern located mainly at the lung bases (46–100 % of cases).
- Noncardiogenic pulmonary edema can be seen in 37 % in patients with fulminant hepatic failure.
- Esophageal varices may manifest on chest radiographs as focal lateral displacement of the mediastinum.
- On abdominal radiographs, ascites is detected as loss of the abdominal gases and the normal psoas shadows visualization. The abdomen structures are blurry due to the overlying fluid shadow (◘ Fig. 1.1.2).

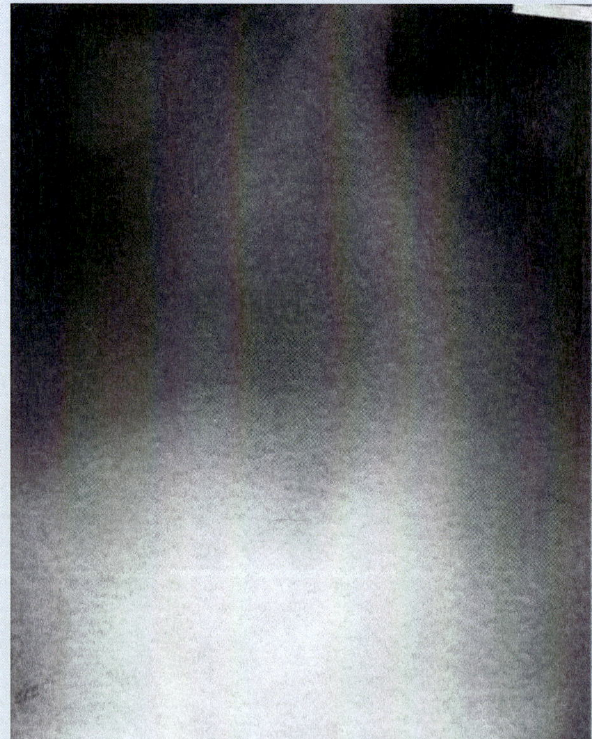

◘ **Fig. 1.1.2**    Plain abdominal radiograph in a patient with massive ascites shows complete blurry abdomen

## Signs on US

- Cirrhosis is detected as irregular nodular liver contour with inhomogeneous echo-texture. Liver right lobe atrophy with enlarged caudate lobe is a typical finding (caudate lobe/right lobe ratio >0.65) (■ Figs. 1.1.3 and 1.1.4).
- Mixed hypoechoic and hyperechoic texture of the liver parenchyma is detected when regenerative nodules are found.
- Signs of portal hypertension include splenomegaly (>12 cm), ascites, and dilated venous collaterals.

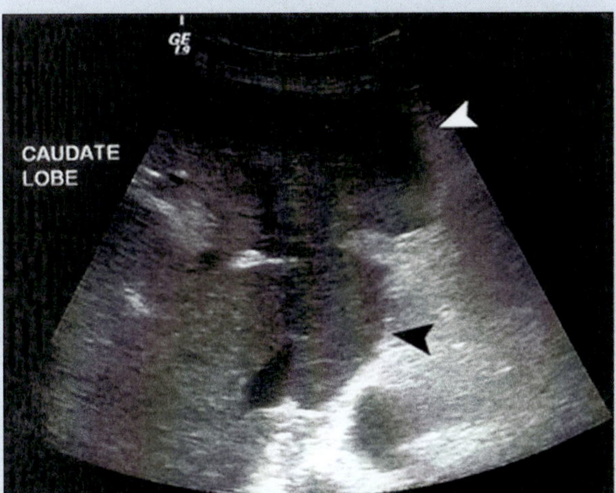


■ **Fig. 1.1.3** Transverse ultrasound image of a patient with liver cirrhosis shows atrophied left lobe (*white arrowhead*), with hypertrophied caudate lobe (*black arrowhead*)

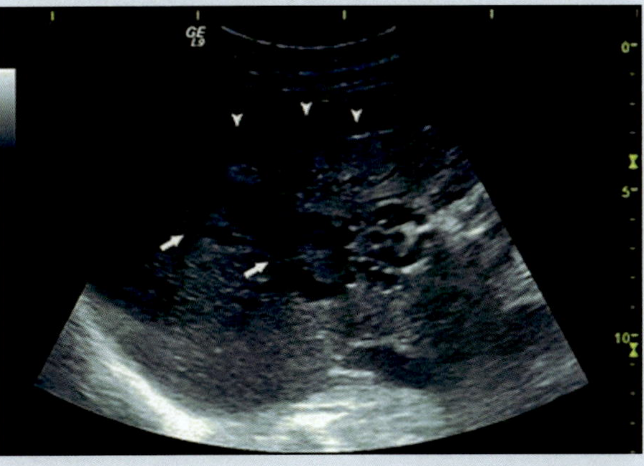


■ **Fig. 1.1.4** Transverse ultrasound image of a patient with liver cirrhosis due to hepatitis C virus shows irregular liver contour (*arrowheads*), with two intrahepatic liver hypoechoic masses, which were diagnosed on liver triphasic CT scan later as hepatocellular carcinoma (HCC) masses (*arrows*)

## Signs on Doppler Sonography

- *Hepatic veins*: hepatic veins join immediately the inferior vena cava, which is in direct communication with the left atrium. Due to the previous anatomical fact, the normal hepatic veins waveform is "triphasic," because it is affected by left atrial cardiac motion and Valsalva maneuver (■ Fig. 1.1.5). In patients with cirrhosis, the triphasic flow pattern is converted into biphasic and monophasic depending on the severity of cirrhosis.
- *Portal vein*: it supplies 70–80 % of the incoming blood to the liver, and the hepatic artery supplies only 20–30 %. The normal portal venous flow is always toward the liver (hepatopetal). The fasting mean velocity of normal portal vein is approximately 18 cm/s (range, 13–23 cm/s[3]), and the flow pattern is normally flat or monophasic (■ Fig. 1.1.6). Mildly pulsatile portal venous flow pattern can be seen normally in tall, thin patients (■ Fig. 1.1.7). Portal hypertension is detected as hepatic blood flow away from the liver (hepatofugal) due to increased intrahepatic venous flow resistance. Portal vein diameter (>13 mm) and splenic vein diameter (>10 mm) are other signs of portal hypertension. Hepatic vein thrombosis can be seen in patients with HCC, and it is visualized as partial or complete loss of flow signal within the portal vein.
- *Hepatic artery*: the normal hepatic artery in a fasting patient has a systolic velocity of approximately 30–40 cm/s and a diastolic velocity of 10–15 cm/s. The flow pattern normally is monophasic and has low resistance, with high diastolic flow (■ Fig. 1.1.8). The resistance index (RI), which is defined as the maximal systolic velocity minus the end-diastolic velocity divided by the maximal velocity, varies normally in a fasting patient from 0.55 to 0.81. There is increase in hepatic artery RI after mean or with age in a healthy person. The hepatic artery diastolic velocity is less than the peak portal vein velocity, and if the hepatic diastolic velocity is greater than the portal vein, one should suspect hepatic parenchymal disease. Also, the RI increases in patients with cirrhosis, and the after meal variation is absent (■ Fig. 1.1.9).
- *Cruveilhier–Baumgarten syndrome* is detected as a patent vein located at the umbilicus with typical monophasic venous flow (■ Fig. 1.1.10). The vein can be followed by the probe until identifying its relation to the intrahepatic portal veins passing through the ligamentum teres (■ Fig. 1.1.11).

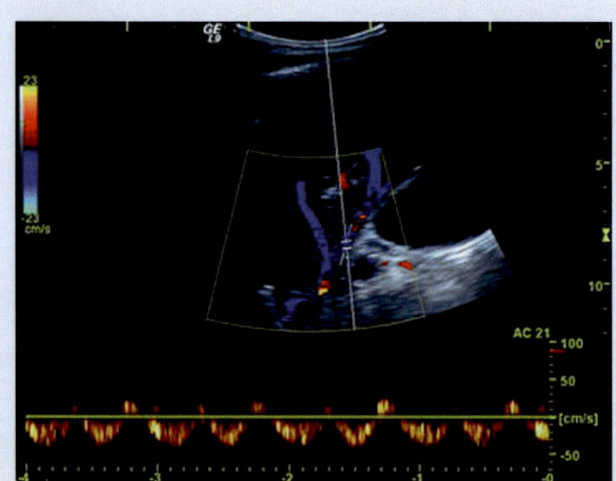

**Fig. 1.1.5** Color Doppler waveform spectrum of the hepatic veins shows the normal venous triphasic pattern

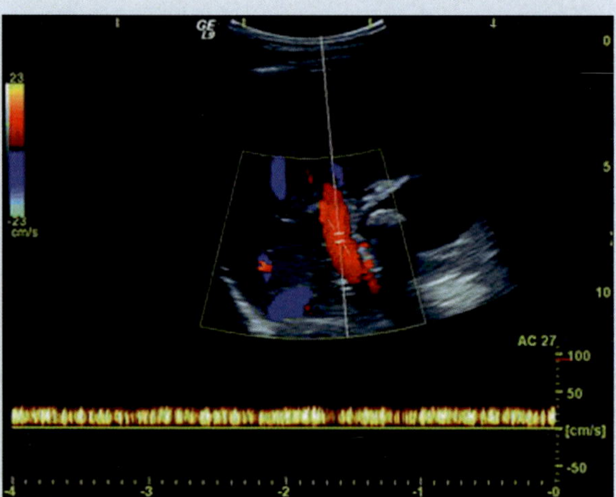

**Fig. 1.1.6** Color Doppler waveform spectrum of the portal vein shows the normal monophasic pattern

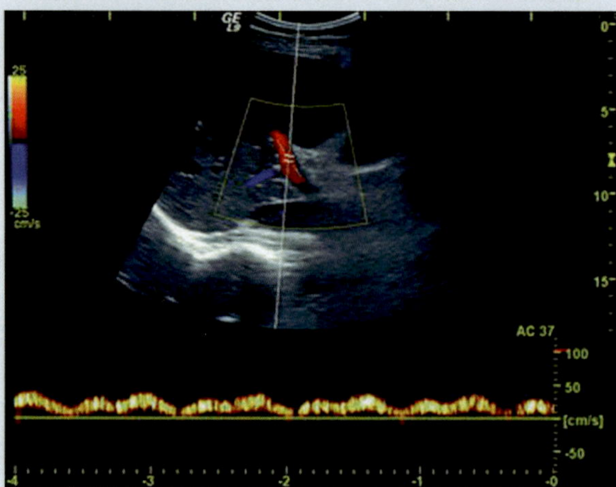

**Fig. 1.1.7** Color Doppler waveform spectrum of the portal vein shows the physiologic portal vein pulsation in athletic tall patient who came for a routine abdominal ultrasound checkup

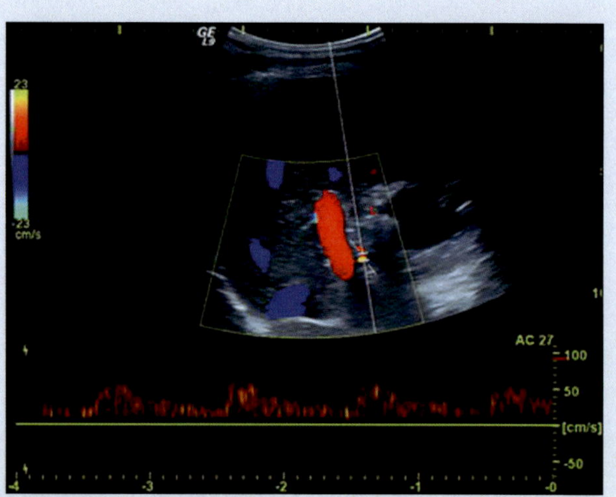

**Fig. 1.1.8** Color Doppler waveform spectrum of the hepatic artery shows the normal monophasic, low-resistance with high diastolic flow arterial pattern

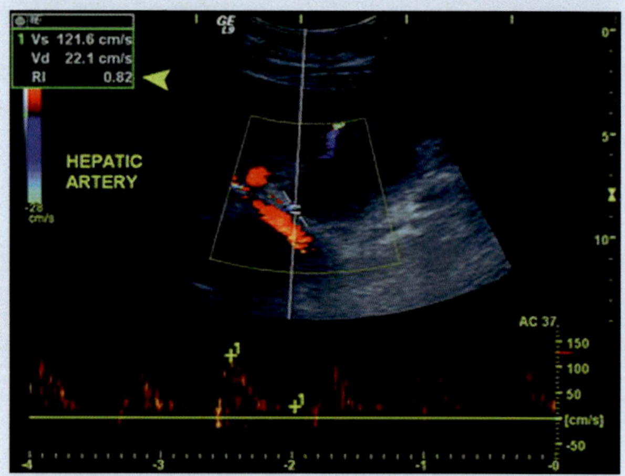

**Fig. 1.1.9** Hepatic artery color Doppler waveform spectrum in a patient with alcoholic liver cirrhosis shows high RI (*arrowhead*)

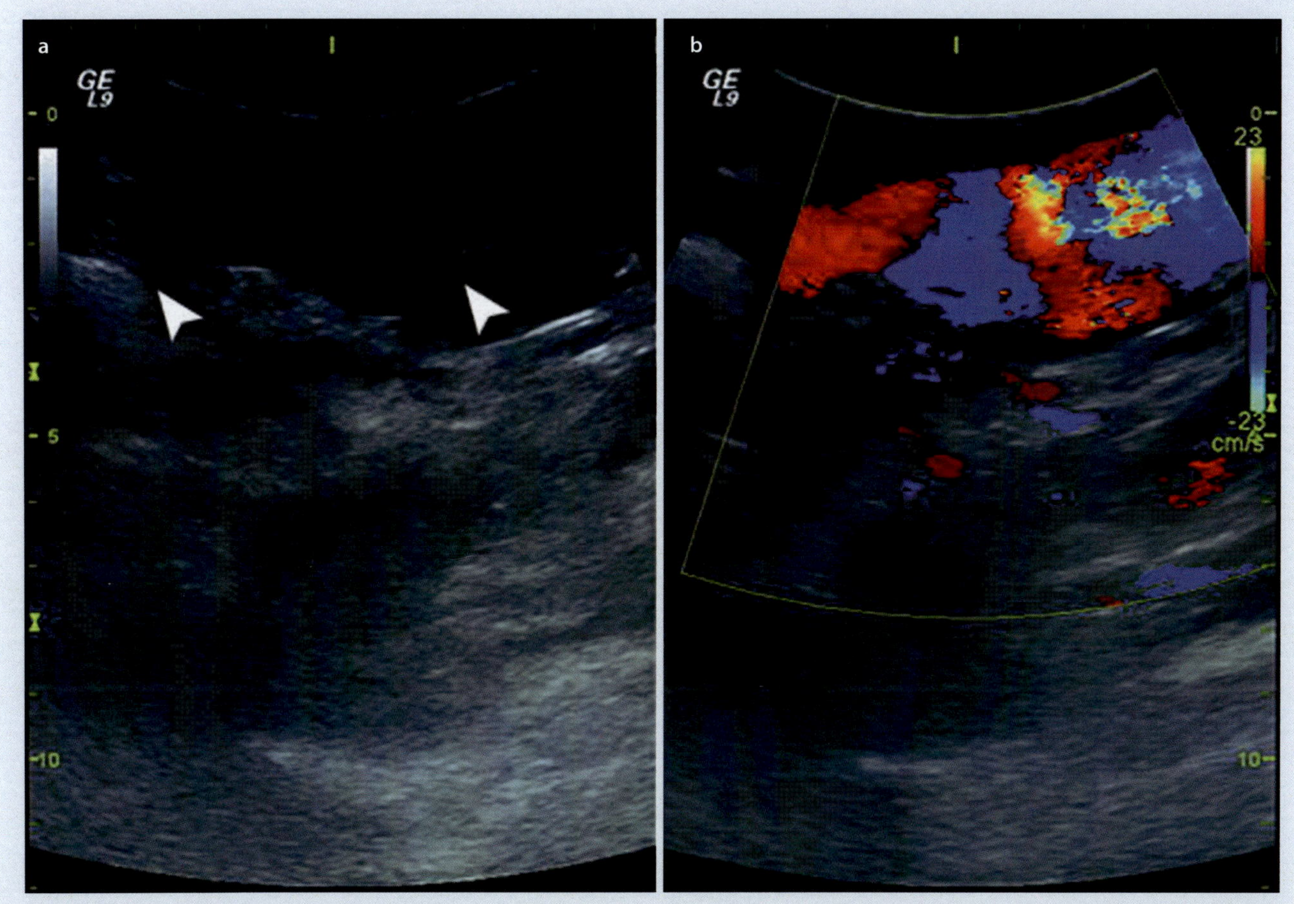

**Fig. 1.1.10** Color Doppler sonography image shows patent umbilical vein at the level of the umbilicus (*arrowheads*) in a patient with chronic liver cirrhosis and Cruveilhier–Baumgarten syndrome

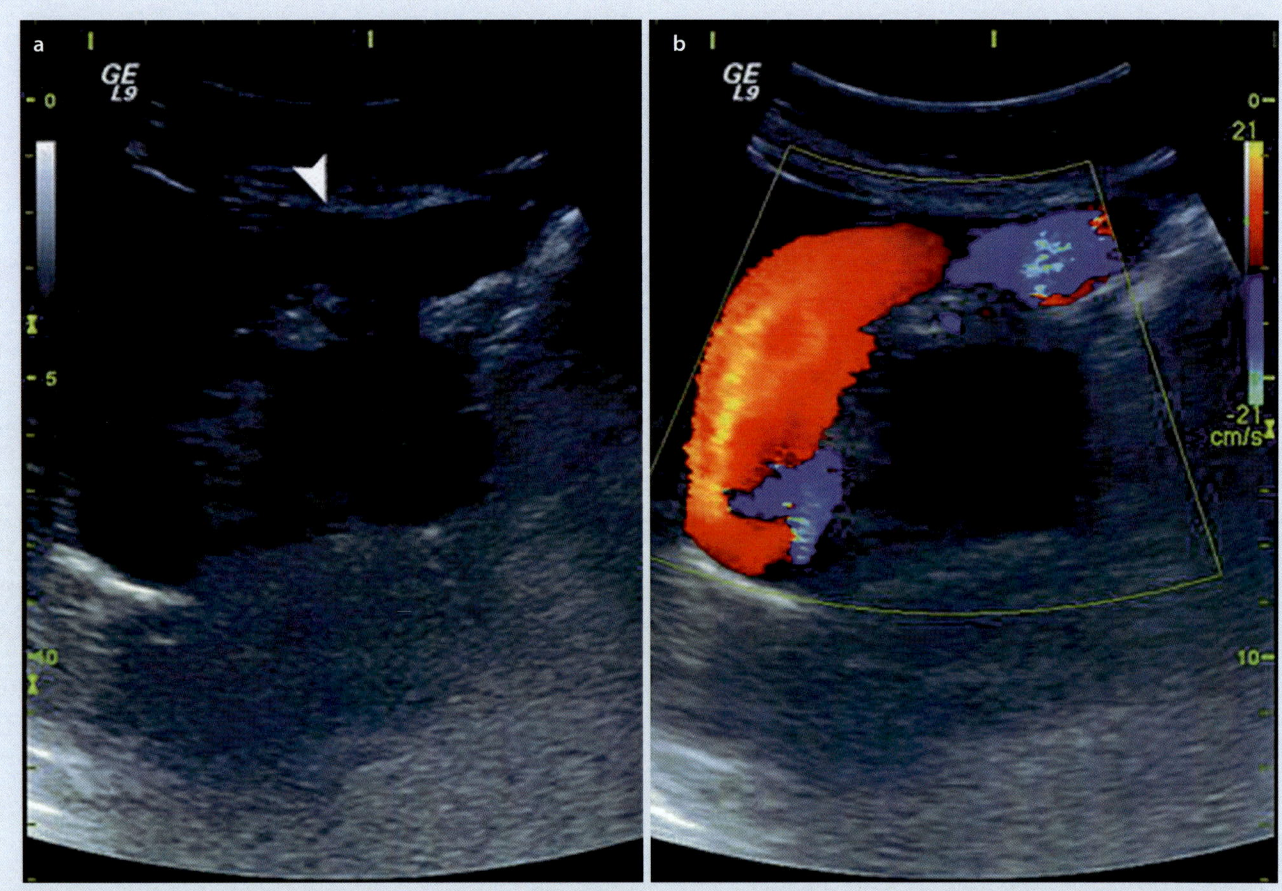

**◘ Fig. 1.1.11**    The same patient shows the connection of the patent umbilical vein to the dilated portal vein through the ligamentum teres (*arrowhead*)

### Signs on Barium Swallow
- Esophageal varices are visualized as serpiginous
  filling defects in the esophagus, usually located in the
  lower third (◘ Fig. 1.1.12).

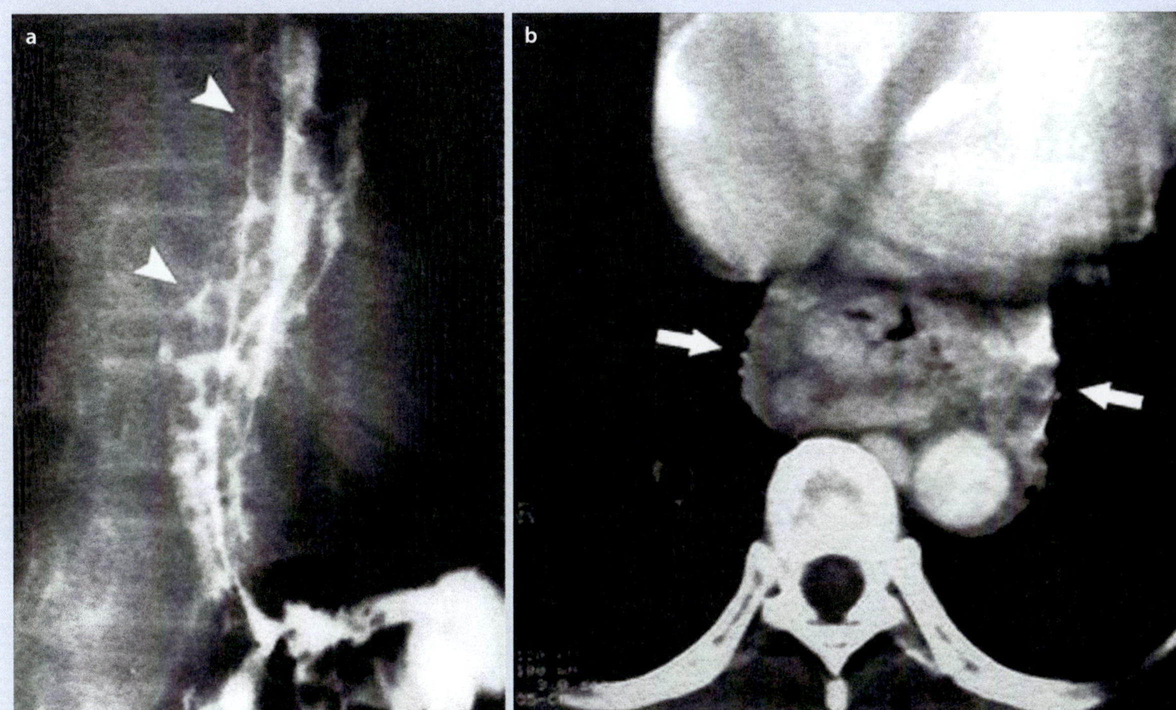

◘ **Fig. 1.1.12** Barium swallow (**a**) and axial thoracic-enhanced CT (**b**) images in two patients with esophageal varices. In (**a**), the varices
are visualized as serpiginous filling defects in the lower esophagus (*arrowheads*). In (**b**), esophageal varices are visualized as multiple
paraesophageal enhanced tubular densities adjacent to the esophageal wall (*arrows*)

### Signs on CT
- Cirrhotic liver appears small (<15 cm), with
  atrophied right lobe and enlarged caudate and left
  lobes. The liver contour is nodular and irregular
  due to parenchymal atrophy and nodular
  regeneration (◘ Fig. 1.1.13).
- *Regenerative nodules* are divided into
  micronodules (<3 mm in diameter) and
  macronodules (>3 mm in diameter). They do not
  enhance in arterial phase because they are
  supplied mainly by portal vein and enhance like a
  normal liver parenchyma. Occasionally, they may
  accumulate iron within them, which will make
  them seen in noncontrast scans as hyperdense
  nodules (*siderotic nodules*), which are typically
  seen in alcoholic liver cirrhosis.
- *Dysplastic nodules* are siderotic nodules larger than
  1 cm. They enhance homogeneously in both
  arterial and portal phases and are usually not seen
  in scans. Few nodules may show enhancement in
  the arterial phase and only differentiated from
  HCC by biopsy.
- *Hepatocellular nodule* is seen as a hypodense area
  in nonenhanced CT scan and shows enhancement
  in the arterial phase, which is the key to HCC
  diagnosis. Up to 50 % of nodules are not detected
  in the arterial phase because they behave as a
  normal liver parenchyma in the triphasic hepatic
  scan. The nodules become hypodense again in the
  portal venous phase of the scan (◘ Fig. 1.1.13).
- *Portal hypertension* can be detected if the portal
  vein diameter increases (>13 mm). Also,
  splenomegaly, dilated perisplenic collateral
  venous channels, and ascites may be found as
  signs of portal hypertension (◘ Fig. 1.1.14).
- *Esophageal varices* are seen as multiple, enhanced
  nodular or tubular densities inside the esophageal
  lumen (intraluminal varices) or adjacent to the
  esophageal wall (paraesophageal varices)
  (◘ Fig. 1.1.12).

- Enlarged porta hepatic lymph nodes might be seen in end-stage cirrhotic liver.
- *Cruveilhier–Baumgarten syndrome* is visualized as an abnormal vein that arises from the right or left intrahepatic portal vein and leaves the liver via ligamentum teres to attach itself to the umbilicus on the portal phase of contrast-enhanced liver CT (■ Fig. 1.1.15).
- On chest HRCT, *hepatopulmonary syndrome* is visualized as peripheral pulmonary arteriole dilatation with increased numbers of terminal branches extending to the pleura (■ Fig. 1.1.16).
- Liver venous hypertension due to congestive heart failure (nutmeg liver) may show characteristic reticulo-mosaic pattern of enhancement on postcontrast examinations (■ Fig. 1.1.17).

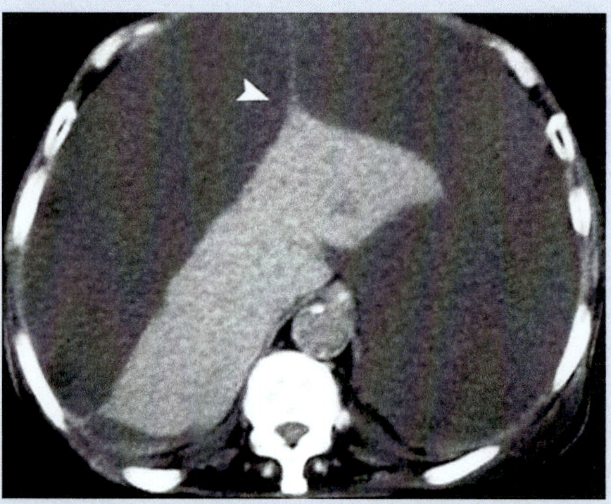

■ **Fig. 1.1.14**   Axial CT scan in a patient with liver cirrhosis shows massive ascites that nicely demonstrates ligamentum teres (*arrowhead*)

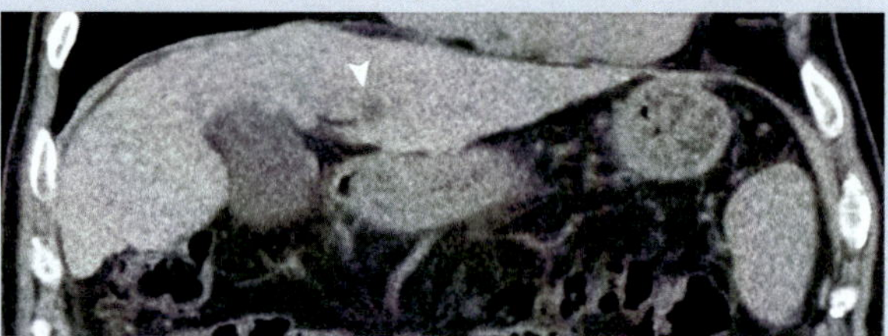

■ **Fig. 1.1.13**   Coronal nonenhanced CT image shows mildly shrunken liver due to cirrhosis with mild irregular contour and hypodense nodule in segment IVb (*arrowhead*), which was proven later to be HCC

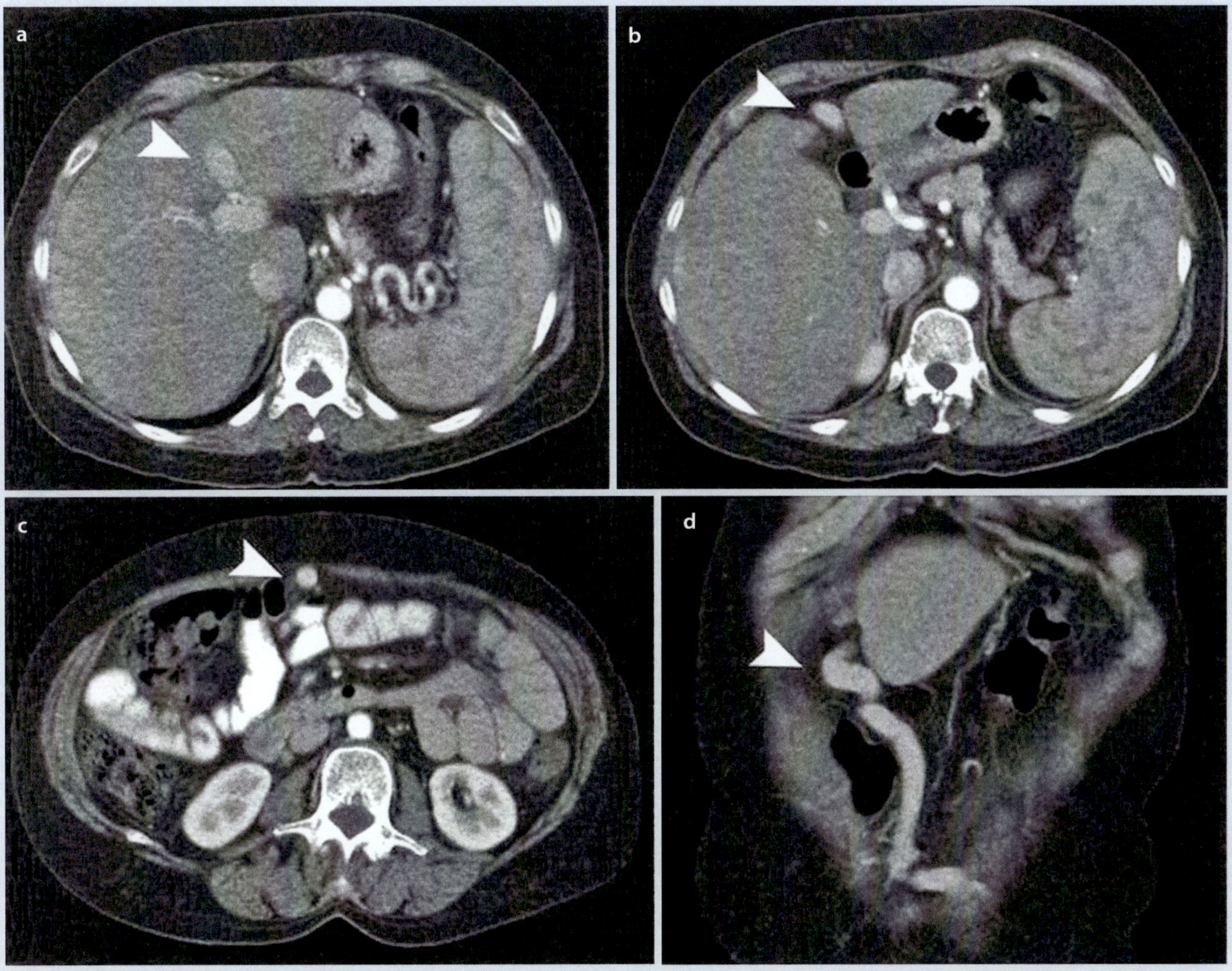

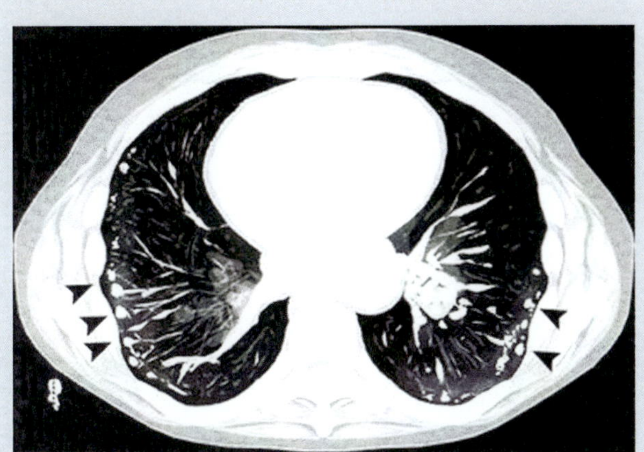

**Fig. 1.1.15** Sequential axial abdominal enhanced CT of a patient with liver cirrhosis shows patent umbilical vein arises from the left portal vein (**a**), runs through ligamentum teres (**b**), and joins the umbilicus (**c**). The course of the patent vein can be seen in the coronal image in (**d**)

**Fig. 1.1.16** Axial chest HRCT illustration shows multiple dilated peripheral pulmonary arterioles demonstrating hepatopulmonary syndrome in patients with liver cirrhosis

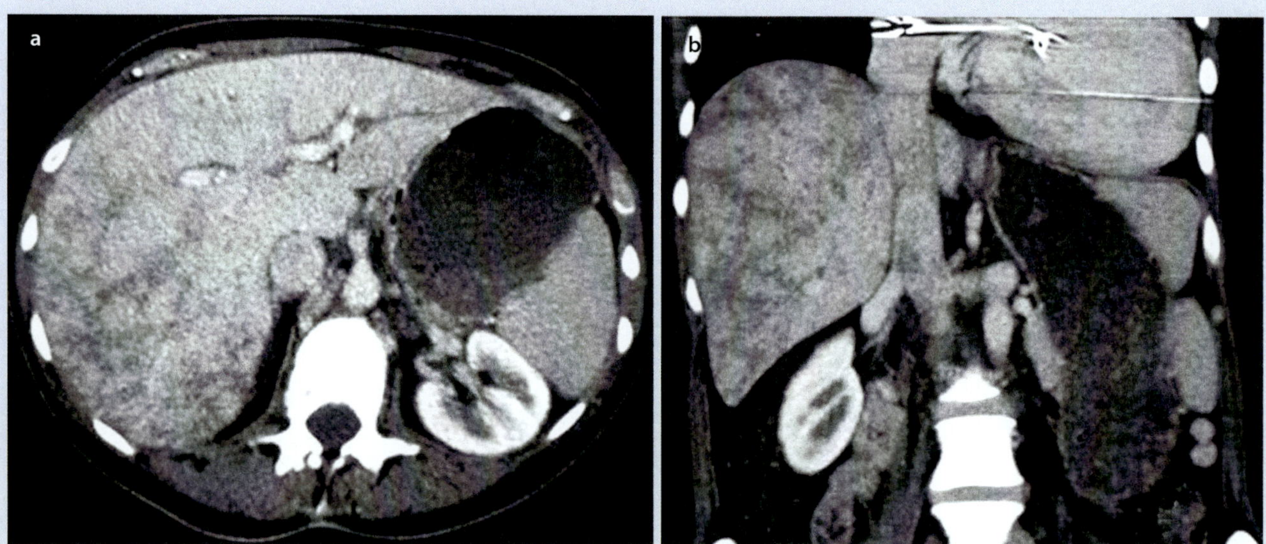



**Fig. 1.1.17**    Axial (**a**) and coronal (**b**) contrast-enhanced CT in a patient with right-sided heart failure due to tricuspid regurgitation shows the characteristic reticulo-mosaic pattern of enhancement of hepatic venous congestion

### Signs on MRI

- *Hepatic encephalopathy* has bilateral and symmetrical high-intensity signal on T1W images in the basal ganglia, especially in the globus pallidus (**Fig. 1.1.18**). The extent of the basal ganglia disease is related to the plasma level of ammonia. Cerebellar atrophy may be seen in advanced stages.
- Regenerated nodules with or without hemosiderin have low T2 signal intensity. In contrast, a hepatic carcinoma nodule appears hyperintense on T2W images and shows early arterial-phase contrast enhancement.
- In *PBC*, periportal hyperintensity signal on T2W images is observed in the initial stages of the disease (stages I and II), reflecting active periportal inflammation (**Fig. 1.1.19**). A *periorbital halo sign* may be seen as low-intensity signal centered around the portal venous branches on T2W images (**Fig. 1.1.19**). This sign is specific for the diagnosis of PBC. Lastly, a peripheral small wedge-shaped area may be seen in the early phases of liver contrast study, which represents arterial–portal shunting.
- Up to 50 % of uncompensated cirrhotic patients show dilated cisterna chyli, which is seen as high T2 signal intensity structure adjacent to the aorta, with delayed enhancement several minutes after gadolinium injection. This sign is detected on CT in 1.7 % of uncompensated cirrhotic patients.
- Plantar fibromatosis is visualized as bilateral infiltrative masses located at the deep aponeurosis adjacent to the plantar muscles in the medial aspect of the foot (**Fig. 1.1.20**). The masses typically show low T1 and T2 signal intensities due to the fibrous nature of the lesion. After contrast injection, enhancement of the masses can be seen in approximately 50 % of cases.

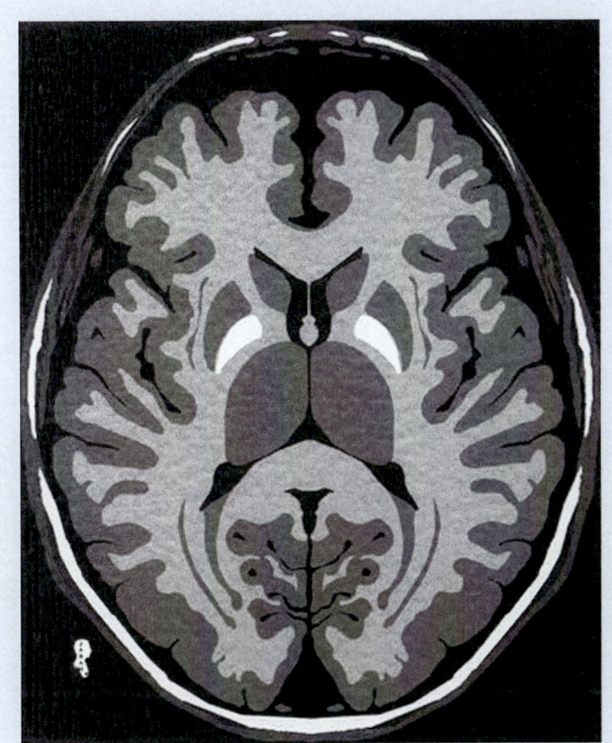

**Fig. 1.1.18** Axial T1W MR illustration shows bilateral symmetrical high density in the globus pallidus representing sign of hepatic encephalopathy

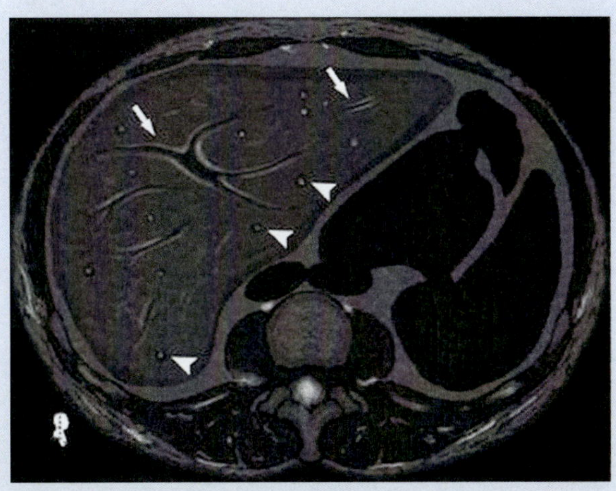

**Fig. 1.1.19** Axial T2W MR illustration of the liver demonstrates the periportal hyperintensity (*arrows*) and the periorbital halo sign (*arrowheads*)

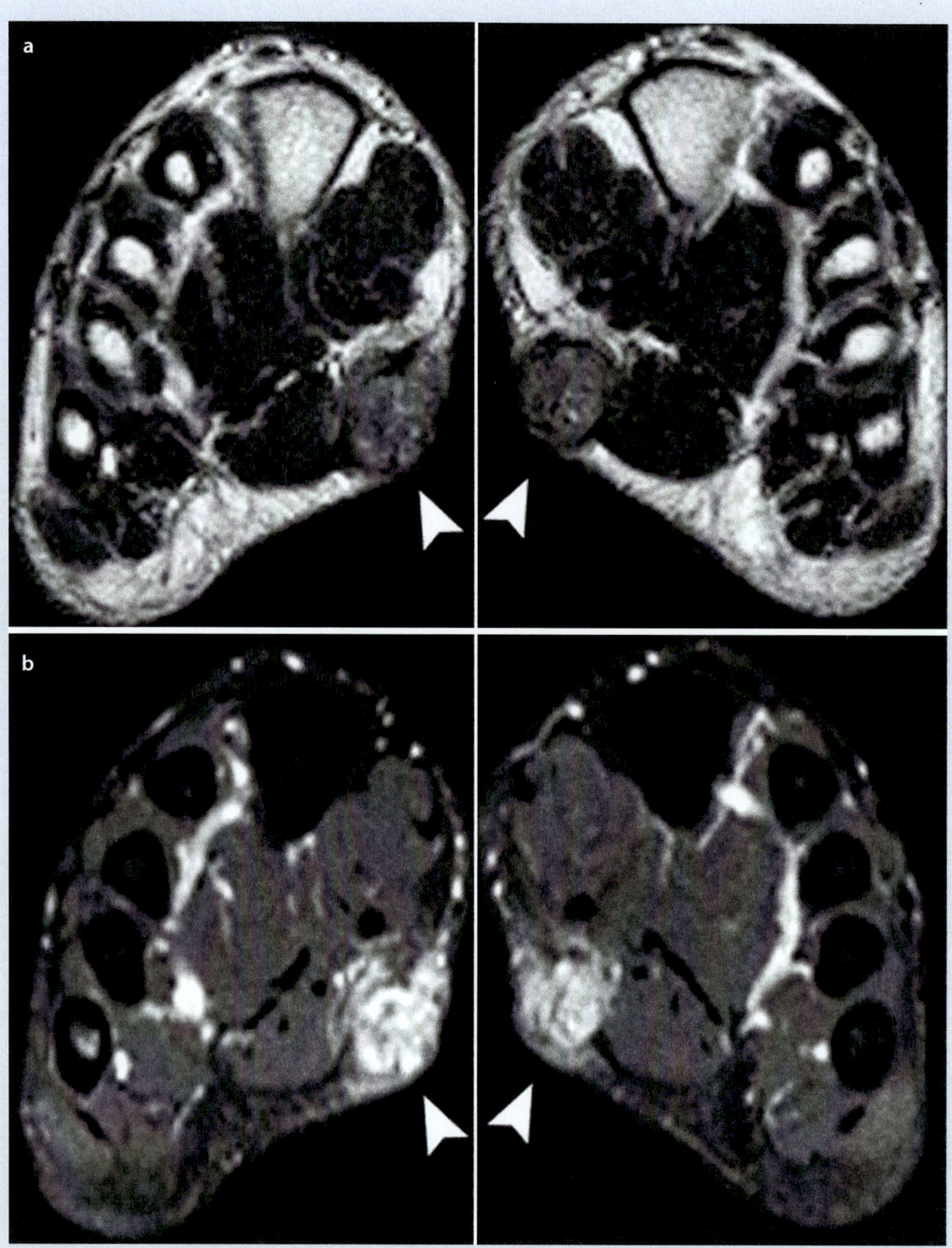

**Fig. 1.1.20**  Axial-oblique T2W (**a**) and T1W postcontrast MRI of the feet shows bilateral hypointense plantar masses (*arrowheads*) on image (**a**) diagnostic of Ledderhose disease (plantar fibromatosis). The masses show marked contrast enhancement after gadolinium injection (**b**)

## Further Reading


Ba-Ssalamah A, et al. Dedicated multi-detector CT of the esophagus: spectrum of diseases. Abdom Imaging. 2009; 34:3–18.

Bonekamp S, et al. Can imaging modalities diagnose and stage hepatic fibrosis and cirrhosis accurately? J Hepatol. 2009;50:17–35.

Chavhan GB, et al. Normal Doppler spectral-waves of major pediatric vessels: specific patterns. Radiographics. 2008; 28:691–706.

Colli A, et al. Severe liver fibrosis or cirrhosis: accuracy of US for detection – analysis of 300 cases. Radiology. 2003;227:89–94.

Ito K, et al. Imaging findings of unusual intra- and extrahepatic portosystemic collaterals. Clin Radiol. 2009;64:200–7.

Kobayashi S, et al. MRI findings of primary biliary cirrhosis: correlation with Scheuer histologic staging. Abdom Imaging. 2005;30:71–6.

Lim JH, et al. Regenerative nodules in liver cirrhosis: findings at CT during arterial portography and CT arteriography with histopathologic correlation. Radiology. 1999;210: 451–8.

Martinez-Noguera A, et al. Doppler in hepatic cirrhosis and chronic hepatitis. Semin Ultrasound CT MR. 2002;23:19–36.

Mauro MA, et al. Computed tomography of hepatic venous hypertension: the reticulated – mosaic pattern. Gastrointest Radiol. 1990;15:35–8.

Meyer CA, et al. Diseases of the hepatopulmonary axis. Radiographics. 2000;20:687–98.

Palazzi C, et al. Hepatitis C virus-related arthritis. Autoimmun Rev. 2008;8:48–51.

Schuppan D, et al. Liver cirrhosis. Lancet. 2008;371:838–51.

Sharma S, et al. MRI diagnosis of plantar fibromatosis – a rare anatomic location. Foot. 2003;13:219–22.

Verma SK, et al. Dilated cisternae chyli: a sign of uncompensated cirrhosis at MR imaging. Abdom Imaging. 2009;34: 211–6.

## 1.2    Fatty Liver Disease (Liver Steatosis)

Accumulation of lipid within cells is a pathologic process. Any type of lipid can accumulate within cells, such as cholesterol, triglycerides, and phospholipids. Fatty liver disease (steatosis) is characterized by accumulation of triglycerides within hepatocytes.

Normally, free fatty acids are taken up by the hepatocytes and then converted into cholesterol esters, triglycerides, ketone bodies, or phospholipids. Some of the lipids combine with apoproteins to form a specific type of lipoprotein called very-low-density lipoprotein (VLDL), which is then secreted into the blood. Liver steatosis can result from either excess delivery of free fatty acids into the liver (e.g., diabetes mellitus), increased formation of lipids within the liver (e.g., alcohol ingestion), hepatocytes disease (e.g., hepatitis), or decreased formation of VLDL by the liver (e.g., protein malnutrition).

## Types of Liver Steatosis

- *Diffuse fatty infiltration*: the liver is usually enlarged with uniform decrease in density in the liver scan.
- *Focal fatty infiltration*: there is an area of the liver that shows fatty infiltration while the rest of the liver is normal. It usually occurs in the same areas that are supplied by the third inflow systemic veins (porta hepatic, around ligamentum teres, and adjacent to gallbladder). It is seen most commonly in the left lobe of the liver.
- *Multiple fatty infiltrations*: there are scattered low-density areas within a normal density liver. This type can be easily mistaken with metastases on noncontrast-enhanced liver CT scan.
- *Focal sparring*: there are areas of normal liver parenchyma surrounded by large areas of low-density diffuse fatty infiltration. This type also may simulate neoplasms on noncontrast-enhanced liver CT scan.

**Signs on US**

- Fatty liver is visualized as highly echogenic liver. The high liver echogenicity can be compared to the echogenicity of the right renal cortex, which will show marked difference in echogenicity (◘ Fig. 1.2.1).
- Focal fatty infiltration is seen as a focal, highly echogenic area within a relatively isoechoic (normal) liver parenchyma (◘ Fig. 1.2.2).
- Focal sparring is seen as a focal area which is relatively hypoechoic (normal) within a highly echogenic liver.

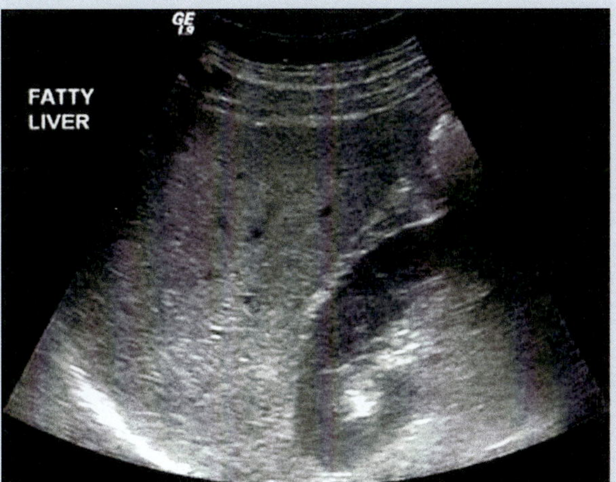


◘ **Fig. 1.2.1**    Transverse ultrasound image of the liver shows diffuse increase in liver echogenicity compared to the right renal cortex (liver steatosis)

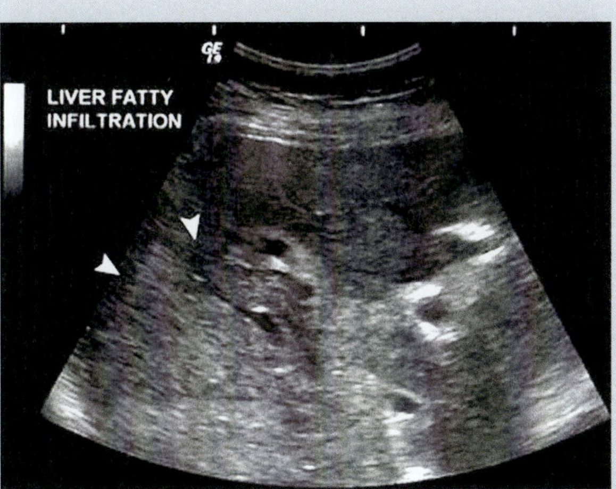


◘ **Fig. 1.2.2**    Transverse ultrasound image of the liver shows focal fatty infiltration involving segment VI and segment VII

### Signs on CT

- Hepatic steatosis is detected as diffuse or focal reduction of the liver normal density on noncontrast-enhanced scan (Fig. 1.2.3). The normal liver density is 8 HU (Hounsfield unit) above that of the spleen (60 HU). Fatty liver density is 10 HU below spleen density on noncontrast-enhanced scan (if the normal spleen is 52 HU, then the fatty liver is <42 HU).
- Focal fatty infiltration is seen as a hypodense area with nonspherical margins (metastases usually have round edge). The hypodense area or the mass does not show mass effect over the parenchyma around it and shows change over time (seen in films before the current scan or after few months' scan). The same criteria are applied to the focal sparring, but the mass will be isodense within a hypodense liver on noncontrast-enhanced scan.
- In both focal sparring and focal fatty infiltration, hepatic vessels course within the fatty infiltration or focal sparring undisturbed. In contrast, metastases or other hepatic lesions will be cutting off the hepatic vessels when they reach them.

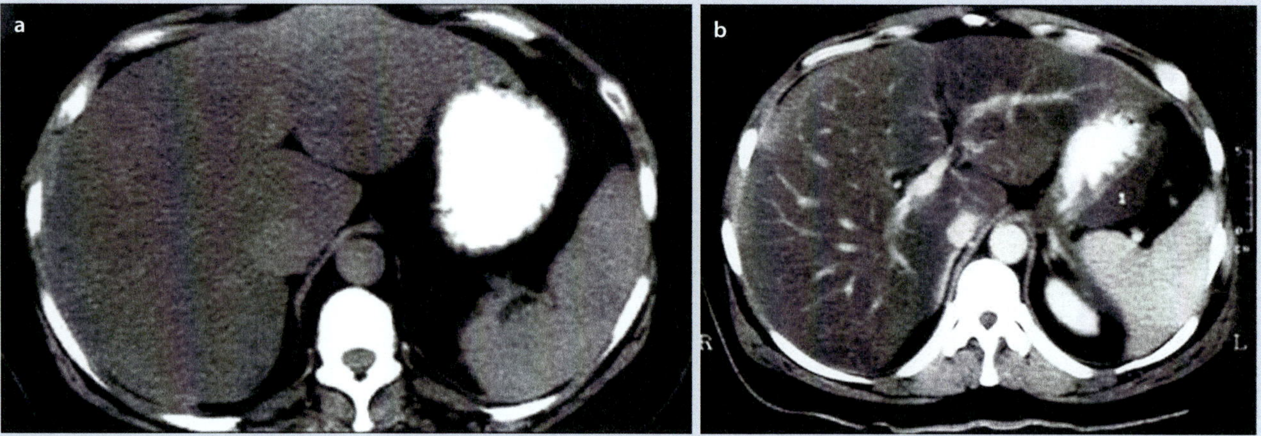

**Fig. 1.2.3**   Axial precontrast (**a**) and postcontrast (**b**) abdominal CT images show diffuse hepatic steatosis. Notice the density of the liver compared to the spleen in pre- and postcontrast images

### Signs on MRI

- Liver steatosis is diagnosed on MRI when the liver intensity drops to >30 % difference on both T1W in-phase and T1W out-of-phase images (Fig. 1.2.4).

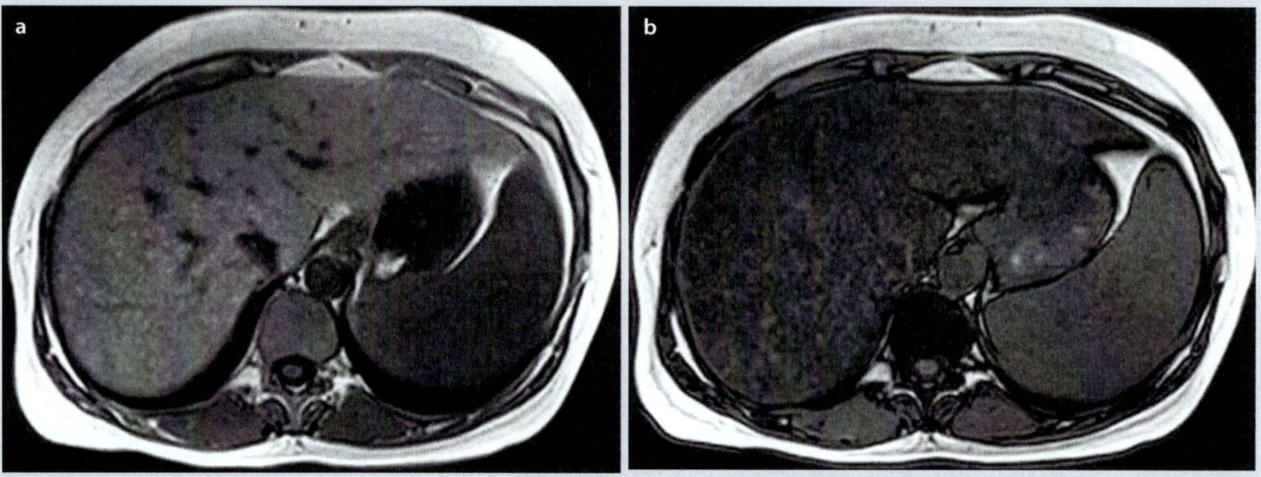

**Fig. 1.2.4**   Axial T1W in-phase (**a**) and T1W out-of-phase (**b**) MRI in a patient with liver steatosis shows drop in the liver signal intensity >44 % in the T1W out-of-phase image (**b**), diagnostic of hepatic steatosis

## Further Reading

Alpern MB, et al. Focal hepatic masses and fatty infiltration detected by enhanced dynamic CT. Radiology. 1986;158: 45–9.

Cassidy FH, et al. Fatty liver disease: MR imaging techniques for the detection and quantification of liver steatosis. Radiographics. 2009;29:231–60.

Karcaaltincaba M, et al. Imaging of hepatic steatosis and fatty sparing. Eur J Radiol. 2007;61:33–43.

Sabir N, et al. Correlation of abdominal fat accumulation and liver steatosis: Importance of ultrasonographic and anthropometric measurements. Eur J Ultrasound. 2001; 14:121–8.

Salmonson EC, et al. Focal periportal liver steatosis. Abdom Imaging. 1993;18:39–41.

Yates CH, et al. Focal fatty infiltration of the liver simulating metastastic disease. Radiology. 1986;159:83–4.

## 1.3 Recurrent Epigastric Pain

Epigastric pain is a term used to describe dull achy pain located at the area of the epigastrium beneath the xyphoid process. Epigastric pain is a very common complaint encountered in both medical and surgical casualty departments. Diagnosis often is established by proper history, examination, and laboratory investigations. This topic discusses some causes of recurrent epigastric pain, in which radiology can play an important role in establishing the underlying diagnosis.

## Gastroesophageal Reflux Disease

Gastroesophageal reflux disease (GERD) is a disease characterized by reduction of the lower esophageal sphincter pressure resulting in leaking of the stomach acidity into the lower third of the esophagus, causing esophagitis and epigastric pain.

The most common cause of GERD is hiatus hernia. Four types of hiatus hernias are known: sliding, paraesophageal, sliding and paraesophageal, and complete stomach herniation into the thorax.

Patients with GERD typically present with long-standing mild to moderate epigastric pain with burning sensation, usually postprandial. Severe cases of GERD may manifest due to propagation of gastric acidity to the upper esophagus. Symptoms like aspiration pneumonia, laryngitis, and teeth decay may be seen uncommonly due to advanced GERD. Medical treatments include antacids, histamine (H2) blockers, and proton pump inhibitors. Surgical management with gastric fundoplication is usually advised in cases where the medical therapy fails to control the symptoms.

Barium swallow is the most sensitive method to detect GERD and esophagitis. Esophagitis is defined as defects in the esophageal mucosa due to exposure to the gastric reflux acid and pepsin. *Barrett's esophagus* (BS) is a condition characterized by esophageal mucosal healing in a persistent acid environment. This healing process is characterized by metaplasia of the normal esophageal stratified squamous epithelium into columnar, gastric-like epithelium. Metaplasia is transformation of one cell type to another (e.g., cuboidal cell to columnar cell). BS has the potential for neoplastic transformation. Up to 50 % of patients with GERD show esophageal dysmotility disorders (EDM).

On barium swallow, sliding hiatus hernia is detected by identifying Schatzki ring. An esophageal ring is a short annular narrowing of the esophagus <1 cm in diameter. *Esophageal A ring* is a ring made up of smooth muscles that is seen at the tubulovestibular junction (muscular ring). *Esophageal B ring* (*Schatzki ring*) is an esophageal ring that is only visible radiologically when there is sliding hiatus hernia and is caused by propagation of the gastroesophageal junction above the diaphragm. *Esophageal C ring* is the normal abdominal retroperitoneal esophageal part (3 cm long) which makes a groove on the liver. In contrast to esophageal ring, *esophageal stricture* is defined as an esophageal segment with fixed narrowing. *Esophageal web* is an abnormal thick 1–2 mm diaphragm-like membrane that extends partially or completely around the esophageal lumen and always indents the esophagus anteriorly. The lower esophageal sphincter line where mucosal change is observed between the esophagus and the stomach on barium examination is sometimes referred to as the *Z-line*.

*Esophageal dysmotility disorders* are a group of diseases characterized by abnormal esophageal peristalsis seen on barium swallow. Types of EDM are tertiary contractions, corkscrew esophagus, esophageal achalasia, esophageal chalasia, and presbyesophagus.

*Tertiary esophageal contraction* is a nonpulsatile, uncoordinating contraction of the esophageal circular smooth muscles. The normal primary and secondary contractions of the esophagus help to push the food and fluids through the esophagus. This type of dysmotility is often seen with old age or GERD. *Corkscrew esophagus* is a term used to describe the same dysmotility as in tertiary contractions but arises posterior to the heart, causing pain in the retrocardiac region during swallowing. *Esophageal achalasia* is a disease characterized by contraction and narrowing of the esophagus due to a defect in the normal neuronal plexuses within the esophageal muscles, which results in failure of the smooth muscles to relax when the food arrives. Achalasia is commonly seen in the lower third of the esophagus. Achalasia can occur without prior cause (primary) or due to underlying pathology like Chagas' disease or malignancy (secondary). *Esophageal chalasia* is characterized by dilatation and widening of the gastroesophageal junction. *Presbyesophagus* is an asymptomatic condition characterized by failure of the primary peristaltic wave to pass completely through the esophagus, resulting in a combination of tertiary contractions, aperistalsis, and failure of the lower esophageal sphincter to contract (curling phenomenon).

Hiatus hernia can be congenitally seen in neonates and children. The most common congenital hiatal hernias are

Morgagni and Bochdalek's hernias. *Morgagni hernia* is stomach or bowel herniation into the thorax due to diaphragmatic defects that occurs in the anterior/inferior mediastinum. *Bochdalek's hernia* is stomach or bowel hernia into the thorax due to diaphragmatic defects that occurs in the inferior/posterior mediastinum.

## Differential Diagnoses and Related Diseases

- *Steakhouse syndrome* is a term used to describe acute food impaction of the esophagus, usually at its distal third. The most common cause of food impaction is esophageal webs. Patients often present to the emergency ward with acute esophageal food impaction, especially after meat ingestion, where the name came from. Patients present with intense retrosternal pain, which may be cardiac in origin, especially if the impacted food presses over the posterior cardiac border. Plain chest radiographs should be performed to exclude bony material impaction or signs of pulmonary aspiration.
- *Plummer–Vinson syndrome (Paterson–Kelly syndrome)* is a disease characterized by dysphagia, iron-deficiency anemia, and esophageal webs. Patients are commonly women (85 %), between 30 and 70 years of age. Upper aerodigestive tract carcinoma is seen in 4–16 % of cases, with almost all cases occurring at the postcricoid location.

### Signs on Chest Radiographs
- Hiatal hernia is diagnosed by finding the stomach bubble within the thorax, rather than under the left hemidiaphragm (◘ Fig. 1.3.1).
- Morgagni hernia is demonstrated as a mass, bowel loop, or stomach bubble lying in the inferior/anterior mediastinum on lateral radiographs (◘ Fig. 1.3.2). In contrast, Bochdalek's hernia is demonstrated as mass, bowel loop, or stomach bubble lying in the inferior/posterior mediastinum on lateral radiographs (◘ Fig. 1.3.3).
- In esophageal achalasia, there is paramediastinal shadow (widening of the mediastinum), with air–fluid level seen in the retrocardiac shadow (◘ Fig. 1.3.4).

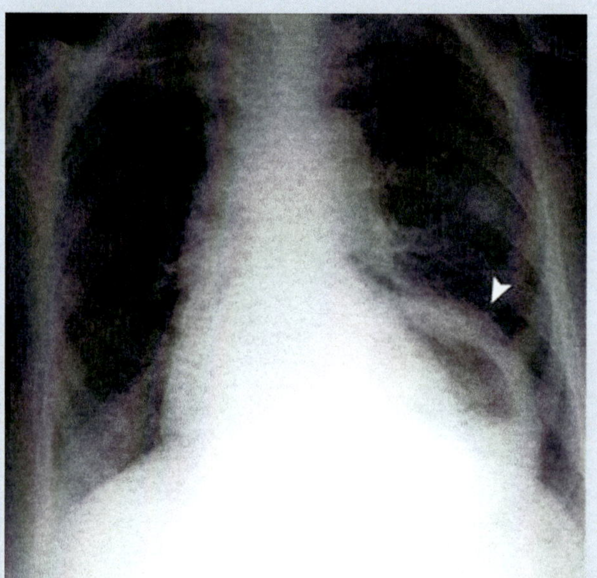

◘ **Fig. 1.3.1**   Posteroanterior plain chest radiograph shows herniated stomach into the thorax with the gastric bubble observed in the thorax (*arrowhead*)

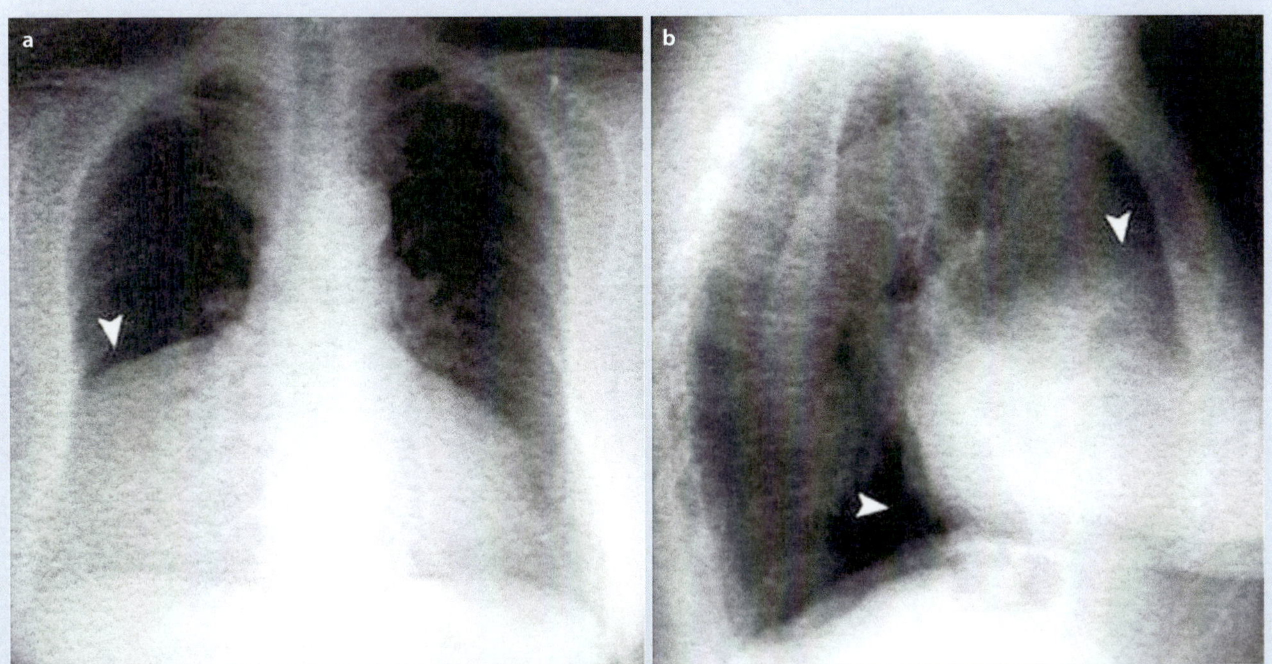

**Fig. 1.3.2** Posteroanterior (**a**) and lateral (**b**) plain chest radiographs show right mediastinal mass on (**a**), which is seen located within the anterior/inferior mediastinum on lateral radiographs (*arrows*). The patient is a child, and the mass was omental and bowel herniation due to an anterior congenital diaphragmatic defect (Morgagni hernia)

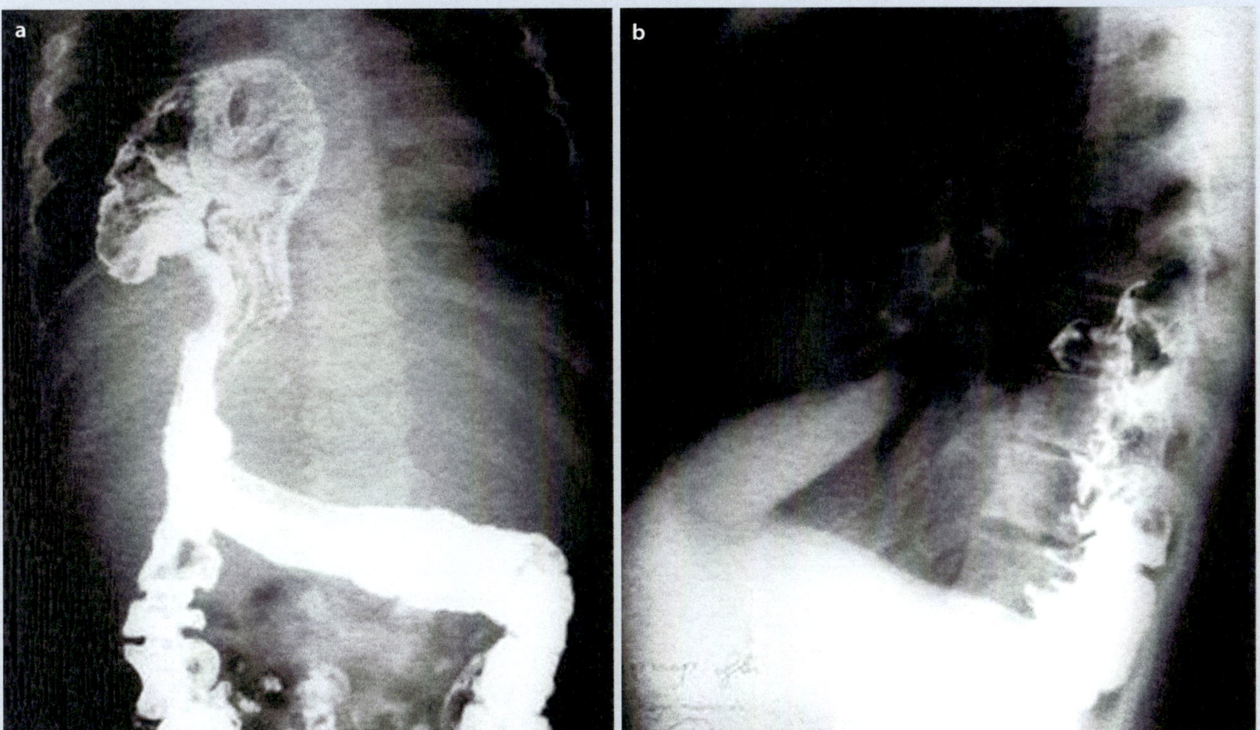

**Fig. 1.3.3** Posteroanterior (**a**) and lateral (**b**) barium enema radiographs in a baby with Bochdalek's hernia show herniation of part of the transverse colon through a posterior/inferior diaphragmatic defect (**b**)

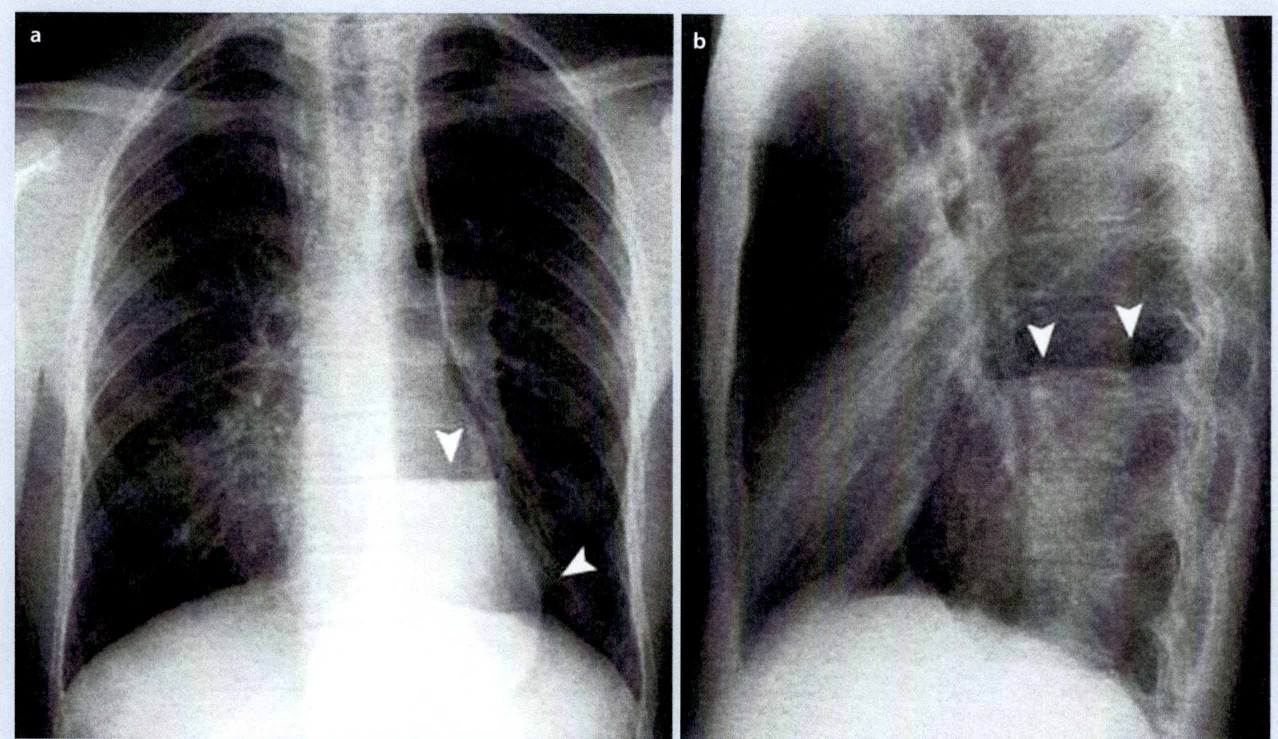

**Fig. 1.3.4** Posteroanterior (**a**) and lateral (**b**) plain chest radiographs in a patient with achalasia show mild widening of the mediastinum and air–fluid level behind the cardiac silhouette (*arrowheads*), representing fluid content within the dilated esophagus

### Signs on Barium Swallow

— In *esophagitis*, there is mucosal granularity, thickened mucosal folds due to edema, and linear ulcers seen as linear barium defects. Stricture formation is a sign of chronic ulceration (■ Fig. 1.3.5).

— Diagnosis of *hiatal hernia* depends upon identification of the gastroesophageal junction, which is typically located at the termination point of the converging gastric mucosa. Schatzki's ring is seen as a uniform round esophageal narrowing with a distended small pouch representing the herniated stomach above the diaphragm (■ Fig. 1.3.6). Herniation of the gastric fundus or body into the thorax is a definite sign of hiatus hernia. Esophageal webs are identified as incomplete esophageal narrowing located anteriorly.

— Barrett's esophagus is divided into two types: short-segment and long-segment BS. Short-segment BS is characterized by mucosal metaplasia <3 cm above the gastroesophageal junction, whereas long-segment BS is mucosal metaplasia >3 cm above the gastroesophageal junction. BS is classically suspected when multiple lower esophageal mucosal ulcerations, mid-esophageal stricture, and hiatal hernia are found. The explanation of such suspicion lies in the fact that the new gastric epithelium secretes acid, which causes regional ulcers and esophageal stricture later on. A reticular ringlike pattern of ulceration above the gastroesophageal junction, which mimics areae gastricae, is a relatively specific sign of BS (■ Fig. 1.3.7).

— In *tertiary contractures*, the esophagus wall is irregular with fine, multiple contractions that run in a wavy appearance (■ Fig. 1.3.8).

— In *achalasia*, there is narrowing of the distal esophagus with dilation of the esophagus proximal to the narrowing, giving the so-called mouse-tail appearance (■ Fig. 1.3.9).

— In *Plummer–Vinson syndrome*, anterior transverse linear esophageal filling defects (webs) with focal esophageal stenosis and poststenotic dilatation are typically found (■ Fig. 1.3.10).

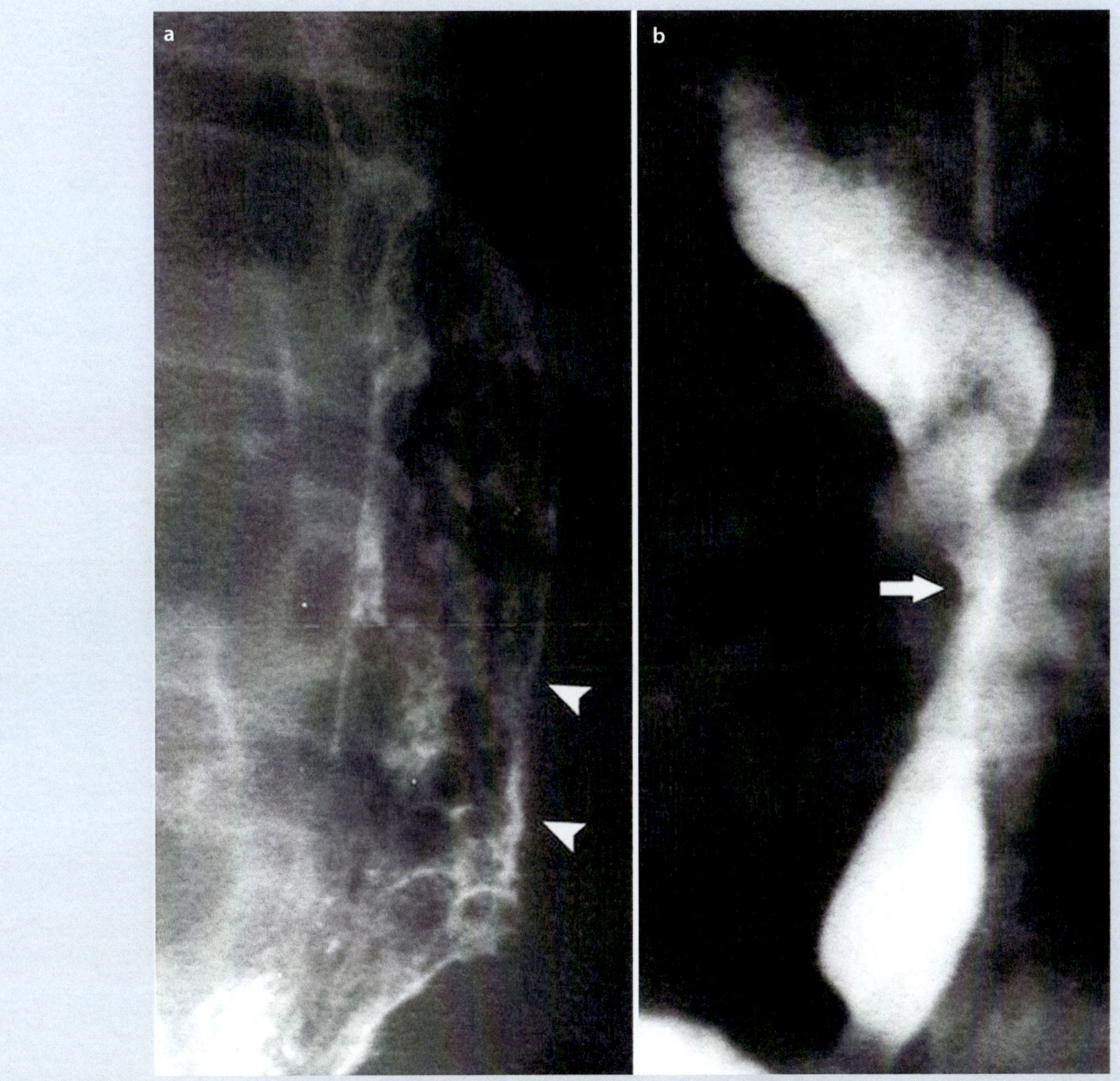

 **Fig. 1.3.5** Barium swallow examinations show patients with esophagitis. In patient (**a**), there is mucosal granularity with thickened mucosal folds (*arrowheads*). In patient (**b**), there is stricture seen at the distal end of the esophagus (*arrow*)

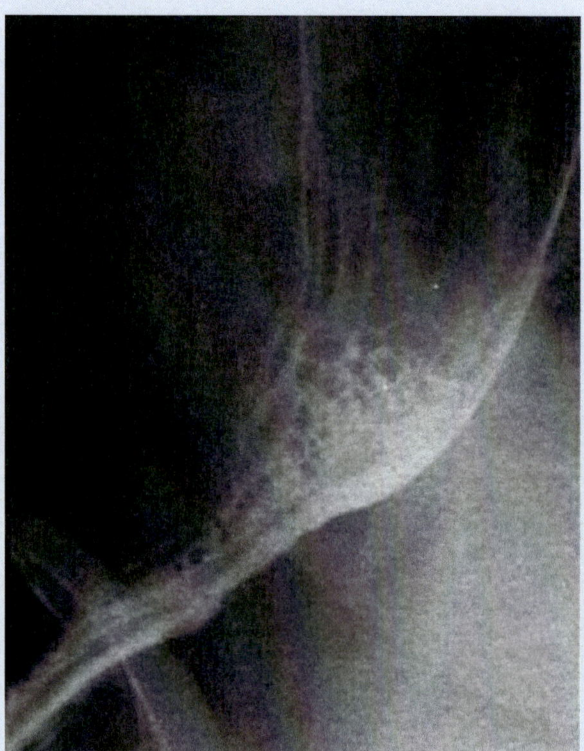

**Fig. 1.3.6** Barium swallow image at the distal third of the esophagus in a patient with hiatus hernia shows Schatzki's ring (*arrowheads*), with the herniated part of the stomach beneath it (*black arrow*)

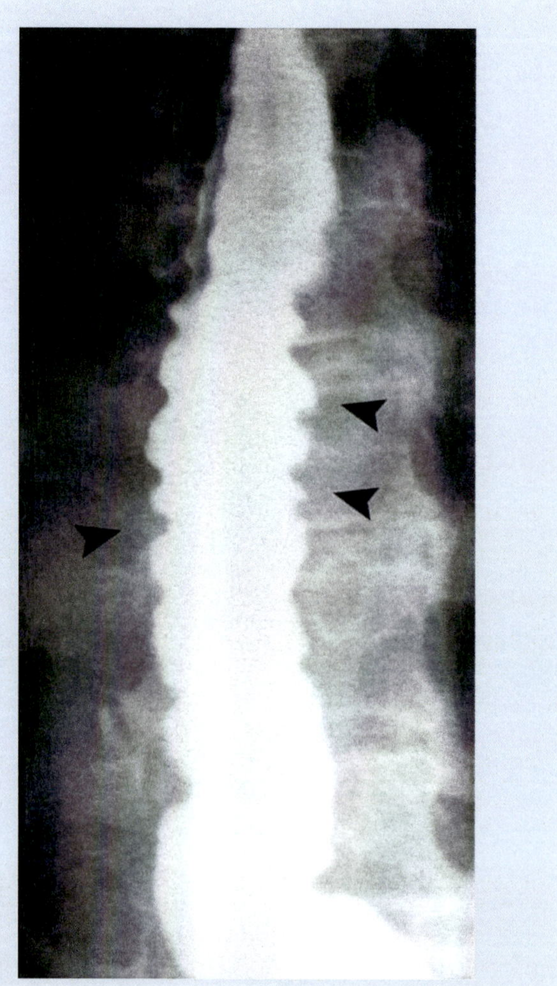

**Fig. 1.3.8** Barium swallow image shows the classical appearance of esophageal tertiary contractures as irregular, multiple contractions that run in a wavy appearance

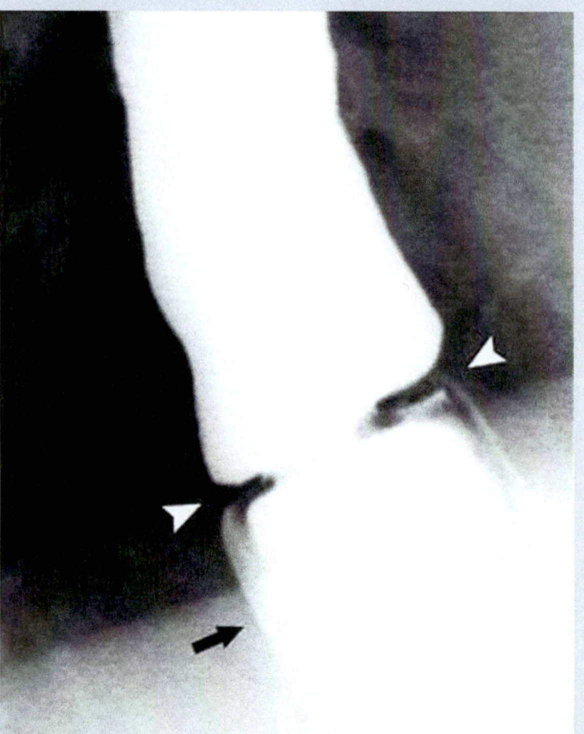

**Fig. 1.3.7** Barium swallow image at the gastroesophageal junction shows the specific pattern multiple ringlike ulcers and stricture of the esophagus >3 cm above the gastroesophageal junction (long-segment Barrett's esophagus (BS))

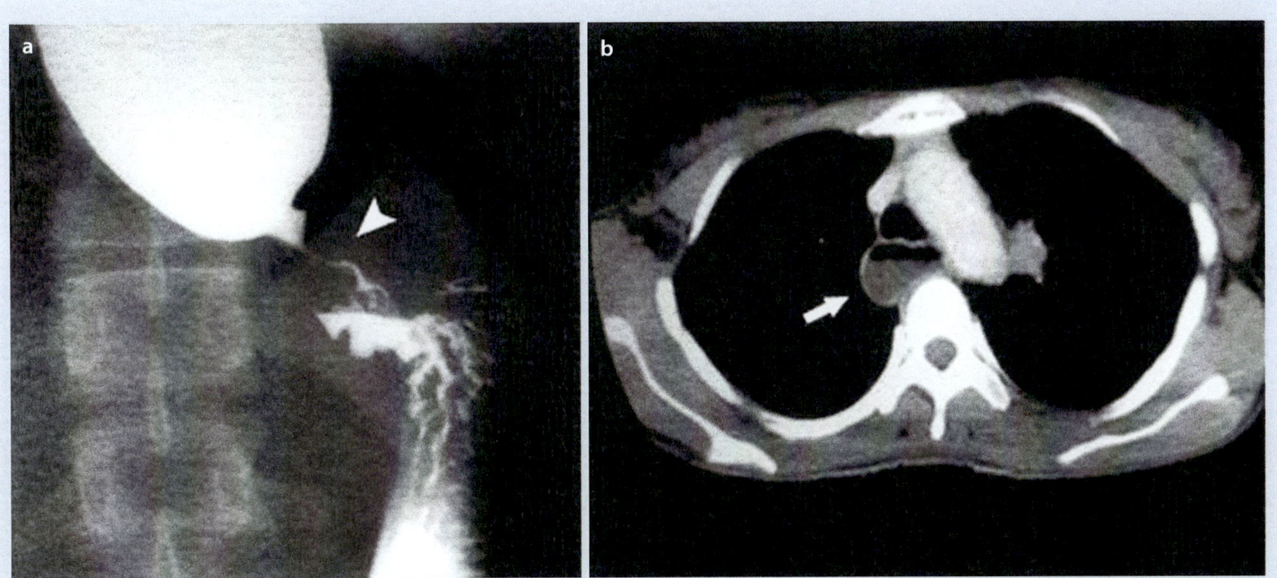

**Fig. 1.3.9** Barium swallow (**a**) and enhanced CT image (**b**) of two patients with achalasia shows the classical "mouse-tail" appearance in patient (**a**) (*arrowhead*) and prestenotic dilatation with fluid residual in patient (**b**) (*arrow*)

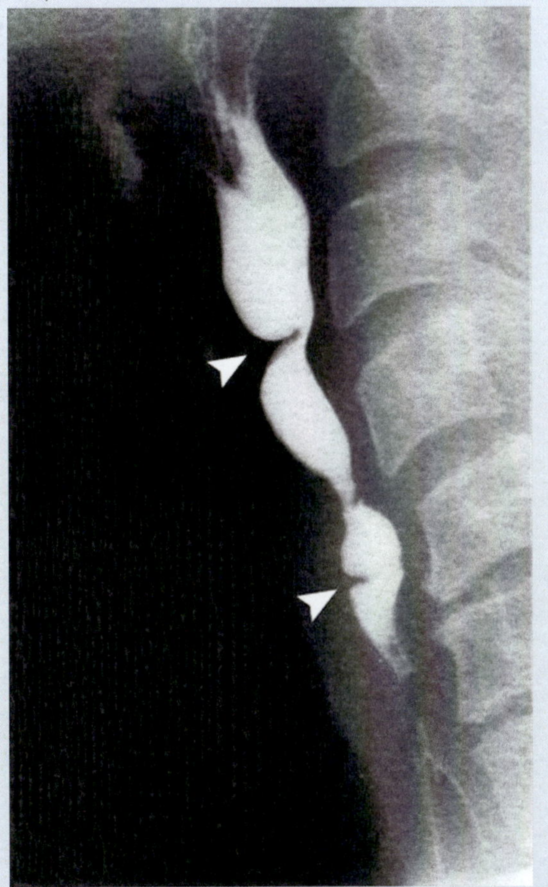

**Fig. 1.3.10** Lateral barium swallow image in a patient with Plummer–Vinson syndrome shows multiple anterior esophageal webs (*arrowheads*) with esophageal poststenotic dilatation

### Signs on CT
- Hiatus hernia is demonstrated by the stomach fundus or body lying within the posterior mediastinum (**Fig. 1.3.11**).
- Morgagni hernia is seen as the stomach or bowel within the anterior/inferior mediastinum, whereas Bochdalek's hernia is seen as the stomach or bowel within the posterior/inferior mediastinum.
- Esophagitis is visualized as uniform, circumferential wall thickening of the esophagus with a target sign formation.

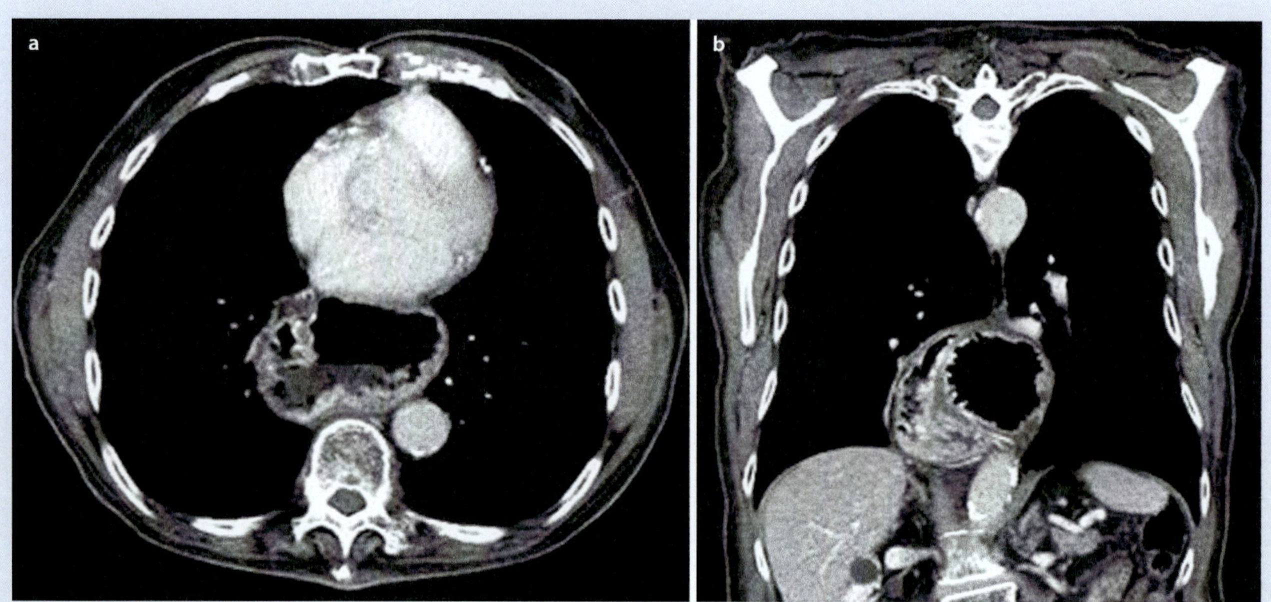



**Fig. 1.3.11**   Axial (**a**) and coronal (**b**) enhanced CT images show herniation of the stomach into the posterior mediastinum (*behind the heart and anterior to the vertebral column*) through the esophageal hiatus (hiatus hernia)

## Peptic Ulcer Disease

Peptic ulcer is a disease characterized by mucosal ulceration of the esophagus, stomach, or duodenum. *Erosion* is defined as an area of mucosal destruction that does not extend beyond the muscularis mucosae into the submucosa, whereas *ulcer* is defined as an area of mucosal destruction that extends beyond the muscularis mucosae into the submucosa or serosa (in perforation).

The gastric mucosa is divided into three types: cardiac mucosa, body-type (oxyntic) mucosa, and antral (pyloric) mucosa. The body-type mucosa contains parietal (oxyntic) cells that secrete hydrochloric acid and intrinsic factor and chief cells that produce lipase and the proteolytic enzymes pepsinogens I and II. The antral mucosa contains endocrinal cells that produce gastrin (G cells), somatostatin (D cells), histamine (ECL cells), and serotonin (enterochromaffin cells).

The main defensive mechanism against the harmful effects of the acid is the production of the mucus layer. Defects in the mucus layer result in gastritis and peptic ulceration.

Peptic ulcer initially starts as inflammation of the gastric mucosa (gastritis), which, when not properly treated, can progress into gastric ulcer. Causes of gastric ulcers include severe stress situations like burns (*Curling ulcer*), increased intracranial pressure (*Cushing ulcer*), alcoholism, cocaine abuse, nonsteroidal anti-inflammatory drug (NSAID) abuse, and bile salt reflux into the stomach in patients with gastroduodenostomy (Billroth I) and gastrojejunostomy (Billroth II).

Peptic ulcer disease and gastritis are linked to infection of the gastric or duodenal wall with *Helicobacter pylori*, a spiral-shaped gram-negative bacterium which is normally found in the gastric antrum. *H. pylori* gastritis is found in up to 80 % of patients with peptic ulcers.

*Zollinger–Ellison syndrome* (ZES) is a disease characterized by severe gastric ulcers due to parietal cell hyperplasia in the body and the fundus of the stomach, mostly due to gastrinomas (>80 %). Gastrinomas are gastrin-producing, non-B islet cell tumors that are commonly found within the gastrinoma triangle. The *gastrinoma triangle* is formed by a line joining the confluence of the cystic and common bile ducts superiorly, the junction of the second and third portion of the duodenum inferiorly, and the junction of the neck and body of the pancreas medially. Up to 25 % of gastrinoma cases are part of multiple endocrine neoplasia (MEN) syndrome type I, an autosomal dominant disorder with tumors of the parathyroid glands (87 %), pancreas (81 %), and pituitary gland (65 %). Ulcers are detected in the first part of the duodenum in 75 % of patients with ZES.

Radiological manifestations of gastric ulcer disease are defined according to the stage of the ulcer. There are signs of acute and chronic ulcers. The usual techniques to detect mucosal abnormalities are the double contrast barium meal and modern virtual gastroscopy. Virtual gastroscopy is a three-dimensional (3D) reconstruction rendering technique that uses multiplanar CT sections to reconstruct 3D images of the stomach interior that mimics the images seen in upper gastrointestinal endoscopy of the stomach.

## Signs on Plain Radiograph
- The sign of gastrointestinal or peptic ulcer perforation is usually diagnosed by the presence of free air under the diaphragm on erect abdominal or chest films (pneumoperitoneum) (◘ Fig. 1.3.12).

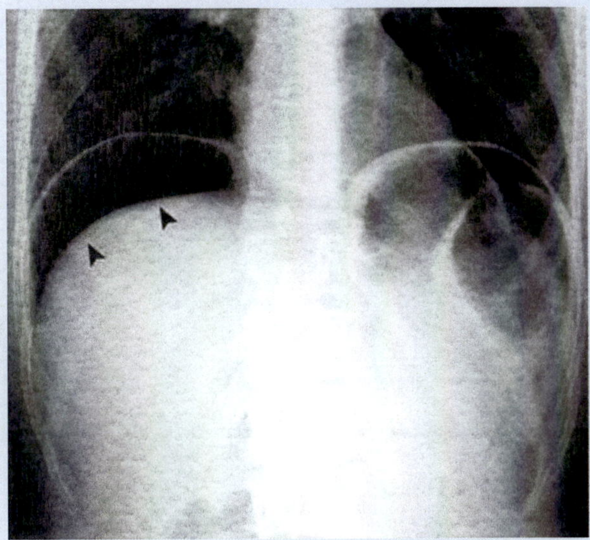

◘ **Fig. 1.3.12** Anteroposterior plain abdominal radiograph shows collection of air under the right diaphragm due to duodenal ulcer perforation (*arrowheads*)

## Signs on US
- In up to 30 % of cases, perforation of a peptic ulcer does not show free pneumoperitoneum but instead penetrate adjacent structures (confined perforation). In suspected cases of perforation, a sonogram of the epigastric region may show an extra-luminal inhomogeneous fluid collection seen within the subhepatic space. This fluid collection represents gastric contents leakage.
- The stomach wall is usually thickened, and the stomach is atonic, dilated, and maybe fluid filled due to gastric outlet obstruction.
- The presence of high echoic areas within the inhomogeneous fluid collection representing air is a pathognomonic finding of perforation.

## Signs of Acute Ulcer on Barium Meal
- *Ring sign*: the mucosal edge of the ulcer is covered with barium while the center is not.
- *Arc sign*: it occurs when the barium covers part of the ulcer's edge (◘ Fig. 1.3.13).
- *Smudge sign*: shallow smudge barium spot represents the area of mucosal ulceration (◘ Fig. 1.3.13).
- *Prominent area gastrica*: it is an area of columnar epithelium located in the stomach antrum, which is normally seen as 2–3 mm, sharply edged, polygonal radiolucencies on double barium meal. Prominent area gastrica suggests the possibility of *H. pylori* gastritis.
- In ZES, there are markedly thickened mucosal folds (Rugae), mainly found in the body and the fundus of the stomach.

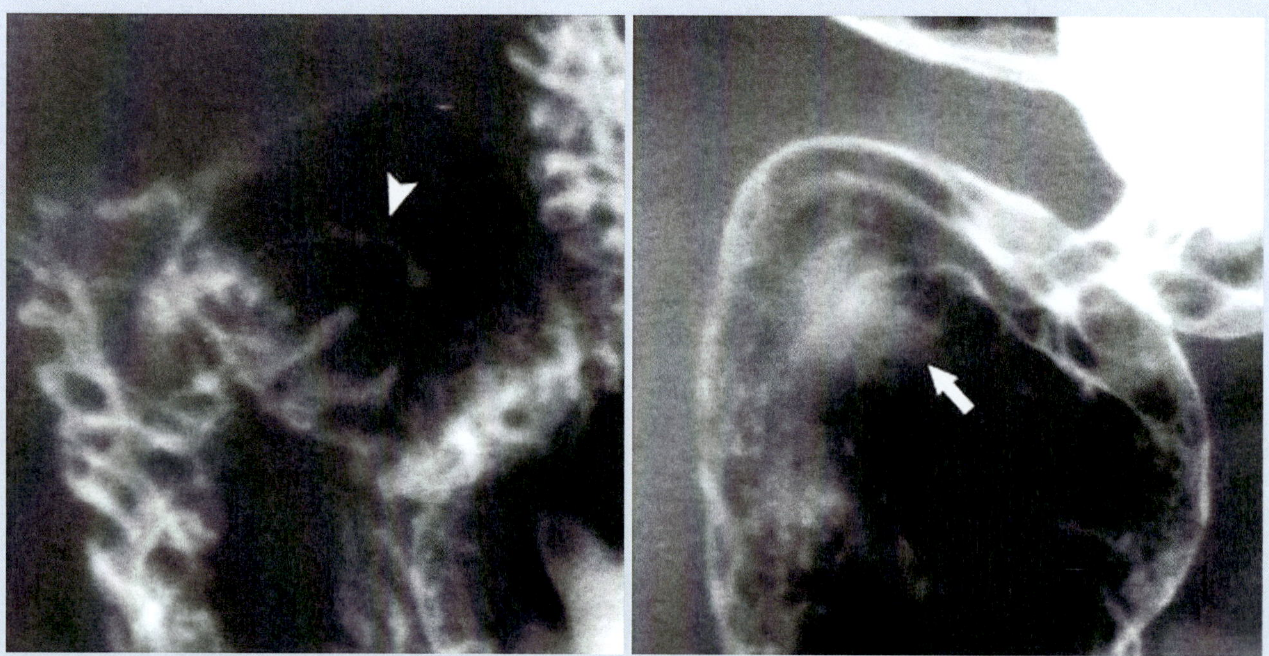



**Fig. 1.3.13** Barium meal images of the duodenum in two different patients show duodenal acute ulcer arc sign in patient (**a**) (*arrowhead*) and smudge sign in patient (**b**) (*arrow*)

## Signs of Chronic Ulcer on Barium Meal

- *Ulcer crater sign*: it is seen as a round area filled with barium, with gastric folds radiating from the crater due to fibrosis. This sign arises due to deep chronic ulcer's edge that mimics a volcano crater.
- *Incisura*: it is a fold in the greater curvature due to stricture of the mucosal folds around an ulcer. Incisura may be found as a normal finding in double contrast barium enema as an area of angulation of the lesser curvature (■ Fig. 1.3.14).
- *Meniscus sign*: the mucosa around the ulcer's crater makes a halo due to edema of the mucosa (■ Fig. 1.3.15).

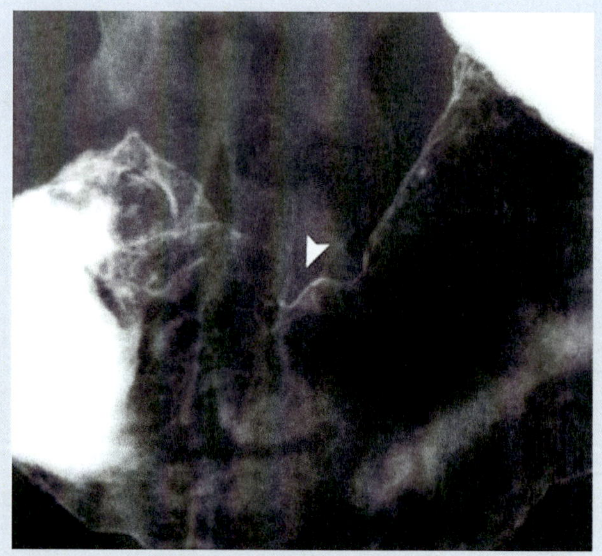

**Fig. 1.3.14** Barium meal image in a patient with normal examination shows the incisura (*arrowhead*)

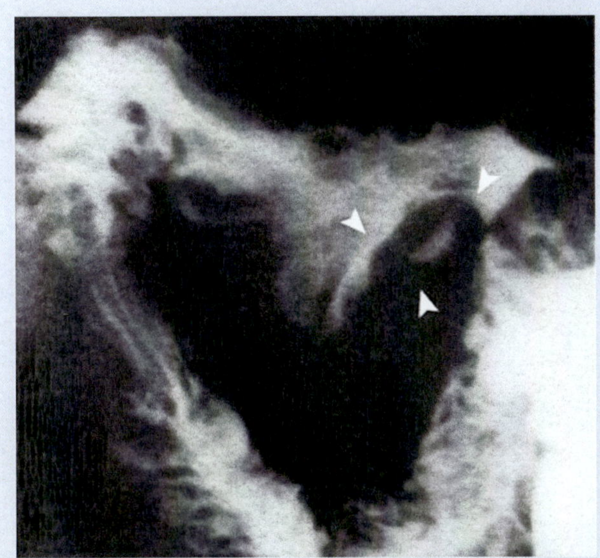

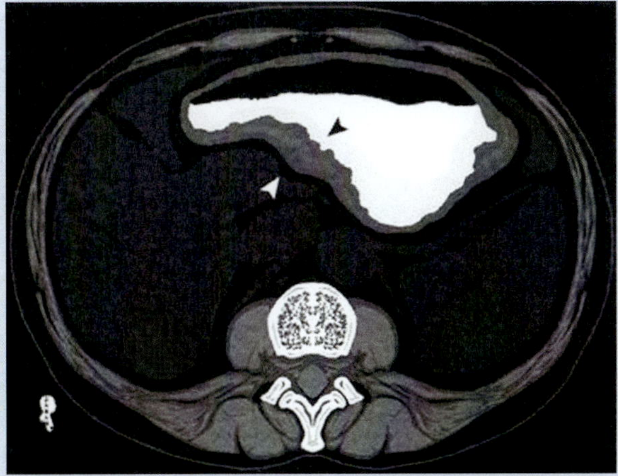

contrast injection, gastrinoma shows intense contrast enhancement in the arterial phase (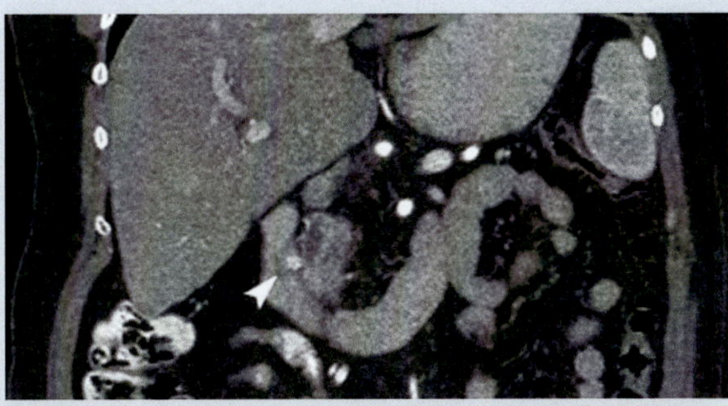 Fig. 1.3.17). Liver metastasis may be seen. On MRI, gastrinoma shows low T1 and high T2 signal intensities with marked contrast enhancement on the early arterial phase of the scan.

■ **Fig. 1.3.15**   Barium meal image of the duodenum in a patient with chronic duodenal ulcer shows the meniscus sign (*arrowheads*)

■ **Fig. 1.3.16**   Axial CT illustration demonstrates thickening of the stomach wall with nodularity as a sign of chronic gastritis (*arrowheads*)

### Signs on Virtual CT Gastroscopy
- The images can be viewed on multiplanar reformation (MPR) images or on 3D reconstructed images.
- In benign ulcers, there is thickening of the stomach wall with preservation of the wall stratification. Mild enhancement may be seen after contrast injection.
- In malignant ulcers, there is marked wall thickening, with strong enhancement more than the adjacent normal gastric wall after contrast injection.

■ **Fig. 1.3.17**   Coronal postcontrast CT image of a patient with Zollinger–Ellison syndrome (ZES) shows highly enhanced nodule located between the second part of the duodenum and the pancreatic head within the boundaries of the gastrinoma triangle representing gastrinoma (*arrowhead*)

### Signs on Conventional CT and MRI
- Gastritis and *H. pylori* infection is detected as a marked thickening and nodularity of the stomach wall, especially in chronic gastritis (■ Fig. 1.3.16). Biopsy of the nodules by endoscopy is important to exclude malignancy transformation. Up to 80 % of patients with stomach cancers that arise outside the cardia have positive antibodies against *H. pylori*.
- In ZES, there is a hypodense nodule with or without calcification often seen in the duodenum or the pancreas on nonenhanced images. After

## Superior Mesenteric Artery Syndrome (Wilkie's Syndrome)

Superior mesenteric artery syndrome (SMAS) is a disease characterized by compression of the third part of the duodenum by the superior mesenteric artery axis, causing recurrent, intermittent, or chronic duodenal obstruction.

The left renal vein, the uncinate process of the pancreas, and the third part of the duodenum pass in the space between

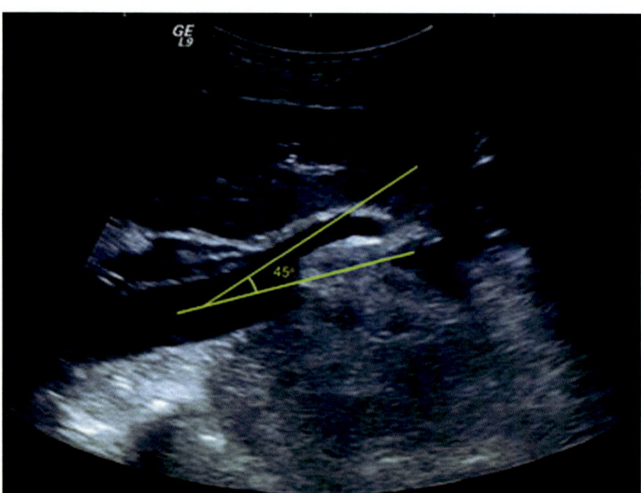

**Fig. 1.3.18** Sagittal ultrasound image shows the normal aorto-mesenteric angle

the retroperitoneal aorta and its branch, the superior mesenteric artery (SMA). The SMA can compress the left renal vein or the third part of the duodenum, a phenomenon known as "nutcracker phenomenon."

Compression of the third part of the duodenum by SMA is an uncommon clinical situation and has been attributed to loss of the retroperitoneal and mesenteric fat, exaggerated lumbar lordosis, abnormal high fixation of the ligament of Treitz, or an unusually low origin of the SMA. The theory of loss of the peritoneal fat as a predisposing factor for SMAS is strengthened by the fact that this syndrome is almost never observed in obese patients. SMAS has an incidence of 0.013–0.3 %.

The normal aorto-mesenteric angle is about 45° with the SMA-aorta distance of 10–28 mm (■ Fig. 1.3.18), where the third part of the duodenum passes across the aorta. Any condition that narrows the SMA-aorta distance or the aorto-mesenteric angle can produce SMAS.

Patients with SMAS typically present with postprandial epigastric pain, nausea, bilious vomiting, and abdominal distension. The pain is often relieved when the patient lies in the left lateral decubitus, prone, or knee–chest position. Acute presentation of the disease can be seen in patients who suffered a recent rapid weight loss (e.g., aesthetic regime).

### Signs on Doppler US
- The SMA shows high resistant waveform with low diastolic flow in a fasting patient because the intestine is not in vascular demand.
- In a fasting patient, SMA stenosis (>70 %) shows peak systolic velocity (PSV) >275 cm/s and end-diastolic velocity (EDV) >45 cm/s. Also, there is focal increase in velocity, with signs of turbulence. Turbulence within the SMA is observed as aliasing artifact with mosaic color flow.
- Reduced aorto-mesenteric angle (<45$_o$).

### Signs on Barium Meal
- Typically, the third part of the duodenum shows sudden, longitudinal filling defect in the middle, at the area where the duodenum passes below the SMA (pathognomonic) (■ Fig. 1.3.19).
- Dilatation of the first and second part of the duodenum with or without gastric dilatation is commonly seen.

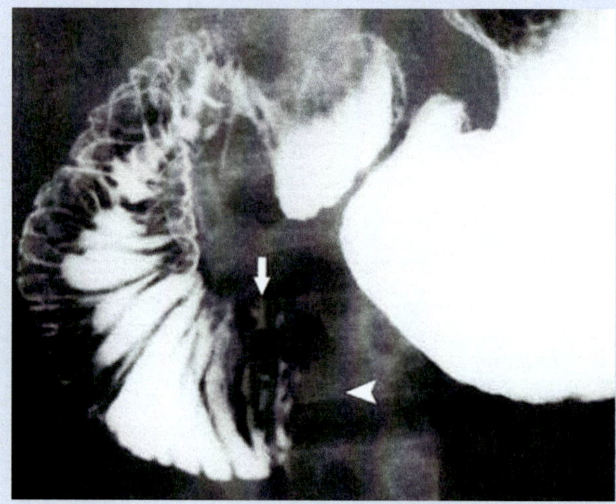

**Fig. 1.3.19** Barium meal image in a patient with superior mesenteric artery syndrome (SMAS) shows the classical barium signs. Notice the sudden barium filling cutoff of the third part of the duodenum (*arrowhead*) by the superior mesenteric artery (SMA) impression over the duodenum (*arrow*)

### Signs on CT
- The CT shows duodenal stenosis at the area where the duodenum passes beneath the SMA, with duodenal poststenotic dilatation (■ Fig. 1.3.20).

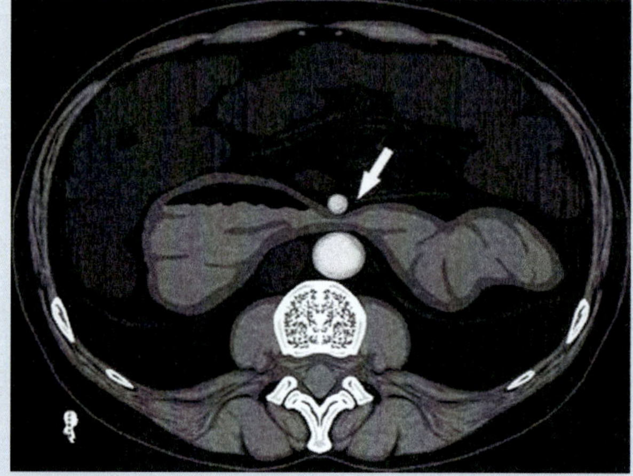

**Fig. 1.3.20** Axial CT illustration shows the typical appearance of superior mesenteric artery syndrome. The third part of the duodenum is compressed as it passes beneath the SMA (*arrow*)

# Median Arcuate Ligament Syndrome (Celiac Trunk Compression Syndrome/ Dunbar's Syndrome)

Median arcuate ligament syndrome (MALS) is a rare disease characterized by compression of the celiac trunk by the median arcuate ligament of the diaphragm at the level of the aortic hiatus. In most patients, the celiac artery is displaced cranially or the diaphragm is displaced caudally. The disease has an incidence of 2:100,000 patients and has high female incidence between 30 and 50 years of age.

Patients with MALS are classically young females (20–40 years) who are very thin presenting with recurrent, nonspecific epigastric pain due to intestinal ischemia and sympathetic–autonomic nerve plexi compression. The pain is often postprandial and may be accompanied by vomiting, nausea, and weight loss, making the clinical picture more like peptic ulcer disease or gastritis. Postprandial pain typically starts 30 min after eating and may last 1–4 h. The pain can be initiated by exercise and aggravated by deep expiration. Recurrent diarrhea is frequently seen and explained by the irritation of the celiac plexus. The symptoms appear most frequently in adults.

Clinically, in patients with MALS, an epigastric bruit or thrill may be heard by auscultation, due to the high blood velocity within the compressed celiac trunk.

Because of the rarity of this disease, assumption of MALS must be carried out after excluding all the common causes of epigastric pain like esophagitis, gastritis, and peptic ulcer disease by endoscopy.

MALS sometimes can be associated with cases of Takayasu arteritis due to inflammation of the celiac trunk.



**Signs on CT Angiography**
- The median arcuate ligament shows extrinsic compression of the celiac axis by a MAL (◘ Fig. 1.3.21).
- Pancreaticoduodenal artery aneurysm may occur in 3–18 % of cases of MALS.

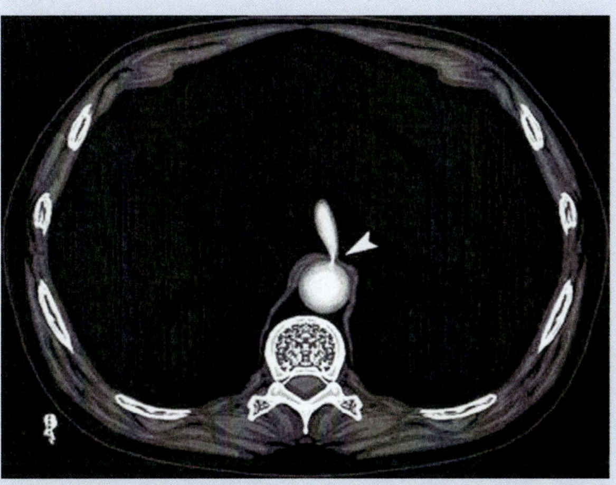

◘ **Fig. 1.3.21** Axial CT illustration shows the typical appearance of median arcuate ligament syndrome (MALS). The diaphragm compresses over the celiac trunk with arterial stenosis (*arrowhead*)

# Recurrent Abdominal Pain of Childhood

Recurrent abdominal pain of childhood is a common complain of school children (8–15 %). It is defined as abdominal or epigastric pain that occurs on at least three occasions within a period of at least 3 months. The pain may be severe and associated with pallor. It is mostly psychogenic in origin with no need for radiological diagnosis. Any other pain that does not match this definition should be investigated.

## Further Reading

Anderson SR, et al. Plummer-Vinson syndrome herald by postcricoid carcinoma. Am J Otolaryngol. 2007;28:22–4.

Ba-Ssalamah A, et al. Dedicated multi-detector CT of the esophagus: spectrum of diseases. Abdom Imaging. 2009; 34:3–18.

Bhattacharjee PK. Wilkie's syndrome: an uncommon cause of intestinal obstruction. Indian J Surg. 2008;70:83–5.

Bhattacharya D, et al. Superior mesenteric artery syndrome (Wilkie's syndrome) complicating recovery from posterior fossa surgery in a child – a rare phenomenon. Childs Nerv Syst. 2008;24:365–7.

Canon CL, et al. Surgical approach to gastroesophageal reflux disease: what the radiologist needs to know. Radiographics. 2005;25:1485–99.

Chen CY, et al. Differentiation of gastric ulcers with MDCT. Abdom Imaging. 2007;32:688–93.

Coulier B, et al. Gastric ulcer penetrating the anterior abdominal wall: ultrasound diagnosis. Abdom Imaging. 2003;28:248–51.

Ellison EC, et al. The Zollinger-Ellison syndrome: a comprehensive review of historical, scientific, and clinical considerations. Curr Probl Surg. 2009;46:13–106.

Fishman EK, et al. CT of the stomach: spectrum of disease. Radiographics. 1996;16:1035–54.

Foertsch T, et al. Celiac trunk compression syndrome requiring surgery in 3 adolescent patients. J Pediatr Surg. 2007;42:709–13.

Frangos SG, et al. Recurrent celiac trunk compression syndrome. Int J Angiol. 1999;8:150–3.

Hayes R. Abdominal pain: general imaging strategies. Eur Radiol. 2004;14:L123–37.

Iwazawa J, et al. Successful embolization of a ruptured pancreaticoduodenal artery aneurysm associated with the median arcuate ligament syndrome. Indian J Radiol Imaging. 2008;18:171–4.

Kim JH, et al. Imaging of various gastric lesions with 2D MPR and CT gastrography performed with multidetector CT. Radiographics. 2006;26:1101–18.

Kohler TR, et al. Pancreaticoduodenectomy and the celiac trunk compression syndrome. Ann Vasc Surg. 1990;4: 77–80.

Levine MS. Barrett esophagus: update for radiologists. Abdom Imaging. 2005;30:133–41.

Lippl F, et al. Superior mesenteric artery syndrome: diagnosis and treatment from the gastroenterologist's view. J Gastroenterol. 2002;37:640–3.

Makam R, et al. Laparoscopic management of superior mesenteric artery syndrome: a case report and review of the literature. J Minim Access Surg. 2008;3:80–2.

Okada M, et al. Radiographic findings of intractable gastric ulcers with H2-receptor antagonists. Abdom Imaging. 1996;21:133–41.

Ortiz C, et al. Familial superior mesenteric artery syndrome. Pediatr Radiol. 1990;20:588–9.

Payawal JH, et al. Superior mesenteric artery syndrome involving the duodenum and jejunum. Emerg Radiol. 2004;10:273–5.

Ranschaert E, et al. Confined gastric perforation: ultrasound and computed tomographic diagnosis. Abdom Imaging. 1993;18:318–9.

Reddy RR, et al. Superior mesenteric artery syndrome after correction of scoliosis – a case report. Indian J Orthop. 2005;39:59–61.

Rubesin SE, et al. Gastritis from NSAIDS to Helictobacter pylori. Abdom Imaging. 2005;30:142–59.

Santer R, et al. Computed tomography in superior mesenteric artery syndrome. Pediatr Radiol. 1991;21:154–5.

Stadler J, et al. The 'steakhouse syndrome.' Primary and definitive diagnosis and therapy. Surg Endosc. 1989;3: 195–8.

Sugiyama K, et al. Analysis of five cases of splanchnic artery aneurysm associated with celiac artery stenosis due to compression by the median arcuate ligament. Clin Radiol. 2007;62:688–93.

Thompson WM, et al. Unusual manifestations of peptic ulcer disease. Radiographics. 1981;1:1–16.

Vaziri K, et al. Laparoscopic treatment of celiac trunk compression syndrome: case series and review of current treatment modalities. J Gastrointest Surg. 2009;13:293–8. doi:10.1007/s11605-088-0702-9.

## 1.4    Inflammatory Bowel Diseases

Inflammatory bowel diseases (IBDs) are a group of diseases characterized by idiopathic chronic inflammation of the gastrointestinal (GI) tract, extraintestinal manifestations, and relapsing course. IBDs are divided into Crohn's disease, ulcerative colitis (UC), and indeterminate colitis (6%). Diagnosis of IBDs depends mainly on clinical presentation and biopsy-proved inflammatory changes in a sample taken by colonoscopy. Radiology offers multiple noninvasive methods to monitor the progression of the diseases and their complications through barium studies, CT of the bowel, and MR enteroclysis. Multiple radiographic signs are described in the literature describing different stages of IBDs. An understanding of the basic composition of the bowel wall is mandatory for the radiologist to understand the radiographic signs encountered while investigating IBDs in any radiological modality.

Bowels are hollow organs composed of circumferential wall and circular mucosal folds (plica circularis in intestines and haustrations in the colon). The basic layers of the entire GI tract are composed of the innermost layer (mucosa), inner layer (submucosa), middle layer (muscularis), and outer layer (adventitia and serosa). The mucosal layer of the intestine is composed of columnar epithelium with secretory activity and a thin layer of connective tissue, containing capillaries and lymphatics (Peyer's patches), and usually called "lamina propria." The lamina propria is separated from the submucosa by a thin layer of smooth muscles called the "muscularis mucosa." Beneath the muscularis mucosa lies the submucosa, which is a layer composed of loose areolar connective tissue containing the major lymphatic and vascular channels of the bowel wall. Also, glandular (crypts of Lieberkuhn) and neural structures (Meissner's plexus) lie within the submucosa. Below the submucosa lies the muscular wall or "muscularis propria," which is divided into an inner circumferential and an outer longitudinal layer. Between layers is the myenteric neural plexus of Auerbach. The outermost layer consists of loose connective tissue called the "adventitia," which is covered by a thin line of peritoneal layer called the "serosa." The normal bowel wall is 3 mm in thickness on radiographic examinations, and the mucosal folds are <3 mm in thickness.

## Crohn's Disease

Crohn's disease (CD) is a chronic, granulomatous, idiopathic IBD characterized by the development of multiple GI tract ulcers from the mouth to anus.

CD can affect any part of the GI tract. The most common sites for involvement are the terminal ileum and/or cecum (45 %), ileo-colonic (13 %), or colorectal (30 %) region. The disease can be subdivided according to its manifestation into three types: inflammatory, stricturing, and fistulating.

CD is rare before 8 years and after 50 years of age. Patients classically present with diarrhea and abdominal pain. Other symptoms include fever, weight loss, anorexia, and lethargy. Right iliac fossa pain, which occurs 30 min after a meal and reoccurs 3–4 h later, is a common symptom and suggests ileal disease. The right iliac fossa pain may be indistinguishable from the clinical picture of acute appendicitis. Recurrent CD after operation is common.

There is a positive association between CD and tobacco smoking. Also, nonsteroidal anti-inflammatory drugs (NSAIDs) have been reported to exacerbate or lead to reactivation of preexisting IBDs.

MR enteroclysis or barium studies are used to monitor manifestations of IBDs. Both barium studies and MR enteroclysis allow detection of subtle mucosal changes. Distension of the bowels by barium or any other contrast media used allows visualization and assessment of the mucosal folds and detection of ulcers or newly developed masses as intraluminal filling defects.

## Extraintestinal Manifestations of CD

— *Arthritis* in IBDs classically has two forms: one that is related to the disease activity and one that is independent of the disease activity. During an acute episode, a peripheral arthritis may develop in 13 % of patients. This type of arthritis resembles rheumatoid arthritis and should not be confused with arthritis in a patient with IBDs. The other form, which is independent from the disease activity, presents as radiographic sacroiliitis (10 %) or ankylosing spondylitis (3.7 %). Up to 15 % of patients may experience hip pain due to avascular necrosis of the femoral head. Psoas abscess may occur rarely.

— *Erythema nodosum (EN)* is an inflammation of the subcutaneous tissue (panniculitis). It is an immunological reaction that can be triggered by various causes like infections, malignancy, rheumatological disorders, and drugs. EN has an incidence of 1–5 per 100,000. EN typically presents as red, very painful, nonulcerated nodules of the lower extremities, especially over the shin. The lesions may cause difficulty in walking and usually subside after 2–6 weeks.

— *Pyoderma gangrenosum (PG)* is a nodule or pustule that breaks down centrally and forms an expanding ulcer with irregular outline, and a characteristic undermined bluish edge (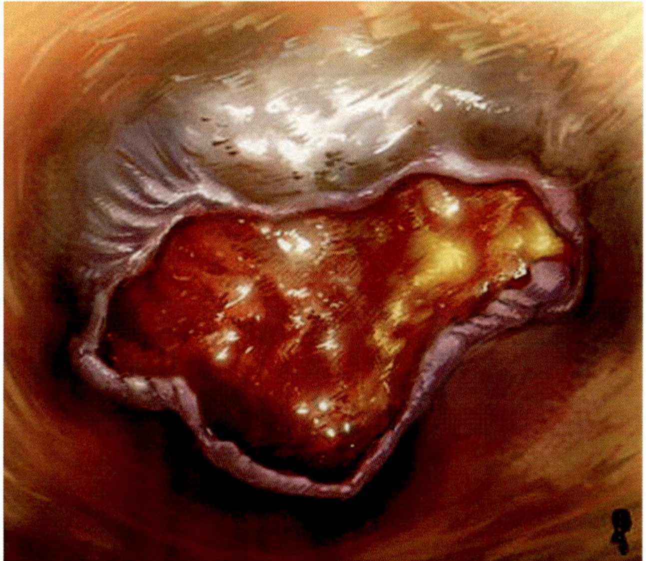 Fig. 1.4.1). PG is a form of noninfectious ulcer and can occur during or after the onset of IBDs. PG is often seen in IBDs, multiple myeloma, and leukemia.

— Sclerosing cholangitis.

— *Oxalate kidney stones and gallstones* mainly related to the bile stasis and disturbance in the liver–intestine bile cycle.

— *Osteoporosis* is common in patients with CD. This may be attributed to the disease activity, steroids use, and vitamin D malabsorption.

— *Fatty liver and amyloidosis* are changes commonly related to the disease activity. In contrast, sclerosing cholangitis develops in patients with IBDs independent from the diseases activity.

— *Aphthous stomatitis* is a condition in which aphthae are painful buccal ulcers with grayish central fibrinous membrane and erythematous halo (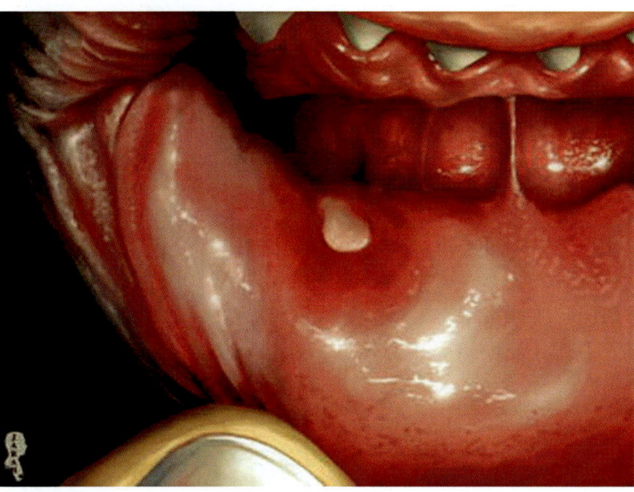 Fig. 1.4.2). They are commonly seen in the "movable buccal mucosa" like the tongue, cheeks, or gutter of the mouth. The pain often subsides within a few days, and the ulcer heals in a week. Aphthae ulcers are seen in around 10 % of patients with IBDs.

**Fig. 1.4.1** An illustration showing the clinical appearance of pyoderma gangrenosum

**Fig. 1.4.2** An illustration showing the clinical appearance of aphthous ulcer of the inner lip mucosal surface

### Signs on Barium (Enteroclysis) and Barium Enema

- The maximum diameter of the jejunum is 4.5 cm and the ileum is 3.5 cm on barium studies. The normal intestinal folds in a normally distended bowel loop are (<3 mm) in thickness. In IBDs, inflammation of the bowel wall affects the mucosal folds, resulting in thickening of the folds (>3 mm) due to edema or hemorrhage. This mucosal fold thickening is seen on barium studies and MR enteroclysis as an increase in distance between the mucosal folds (plica circularis). Segmental intestinal wall thickening with thickened mucosal folds is a common feature seen on CD.
- *Aphthous ulcer*: the earliest stage of the disease is characterized by lymphoid hyperplasia and lymphedema, which appears radiologically as aphthoid ulcers. Aphthous ulcer is an ulcer that starts as shallow ulceration of the mucosa and then tunnel deep within the intestinal wall as it progresses. CD ulcers characteristically violate the whole length of the intestinal wall, from the mucosal layer deep into the adventitia (mural ulcer). Barium will accumulate within the ulcer crater and is surrounded by a barium-free round halo made by mucosal edema (◘ Fig. 1.4.3). When barium enters deep within the intestinal wall due to transmural ulcer, small, white, rodlike lines are seen through the intestinal wall, which are called "rose-thorn ulcers."
- *Cobblestone appearance*: it is seen on barium (enteroclysis) as multiple filling defects grouped together due to aggregation of multiple ulcers in one place with severe edematous mucosa between them (◘ Fig. 1.4.4). The term cobblestone refers to street-like stones arrangement.

- *Multiple skip lesions*: they are seen as asymmetric distribution of ulceration along the small intestine.
- Narrowing of the lumen with poststenotic dilatation (*string sign*).
- *String ring of Kantor*: narrowing of the terminal ileum with thick wall separates it from the other loops.
- *Circumferential asymmetry of the bowel lumen*: part of the intestinal lumen will be straight without mucosal folds, while the other preserves its mucosal folds (◘ Fig. 1.4.5).In the colon, CD mainly affects the ascending color with relative sparing of the rectum (◘ Fig. 1.4.6).
- *Apple-core appearance*: this appearance is classic for circumferential mass within the bowel lumen. It can be seen due to carcinoma or hypertrophied polyps.

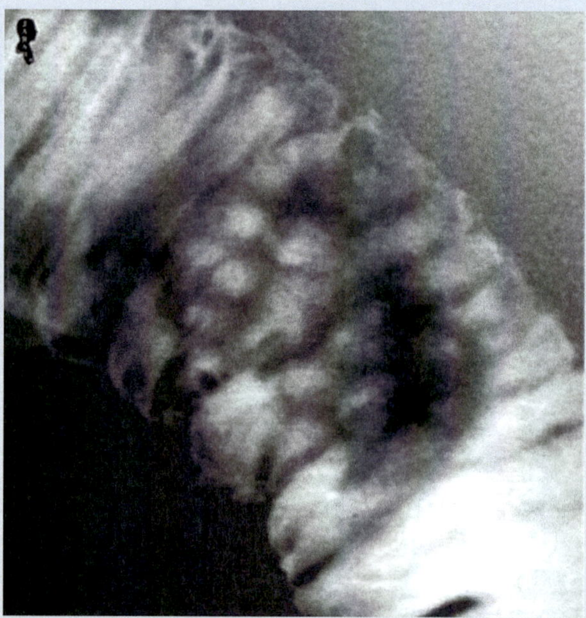

**Fig. 1.4.4** Barium (enteroclysis) illustration demonstrating the barium sign of cobblestone appearance

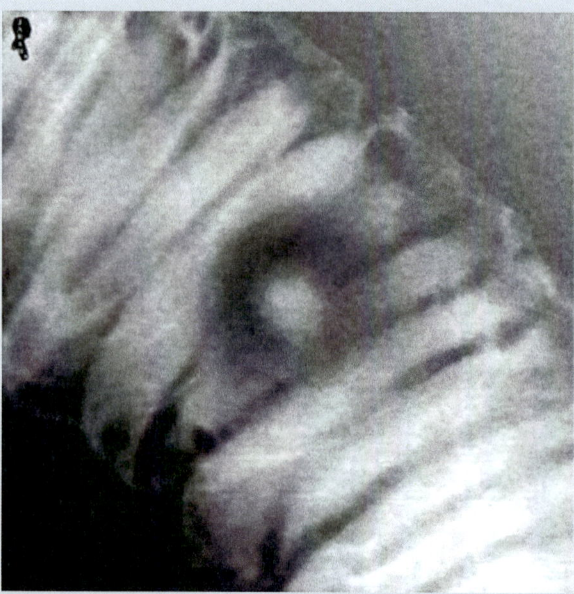

**Fig. 1.4.3** Barium (enteroclysis) illustration demonstrating the barium sign of aphthous ulcer

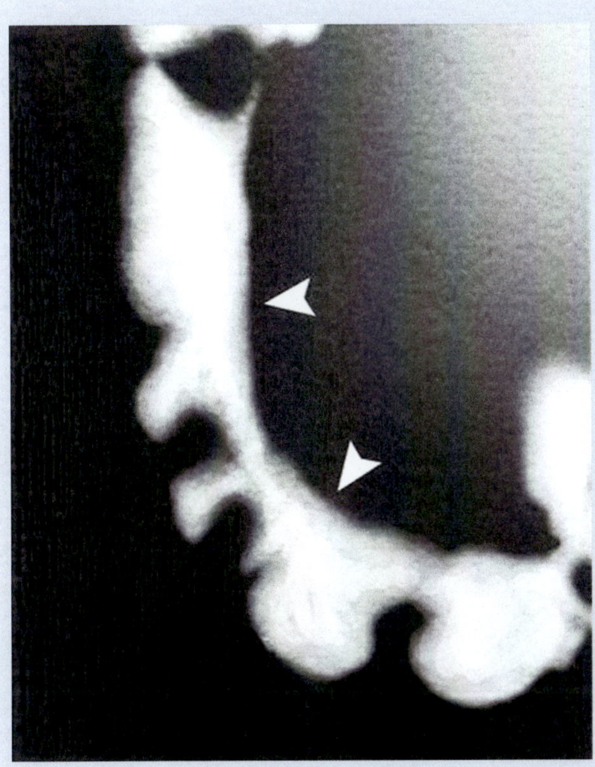

**Fig. 1.4.5** Barium (enteroclysis) illustration demonstrating the barium sign of circumferential asymmetry of the bowel lumen

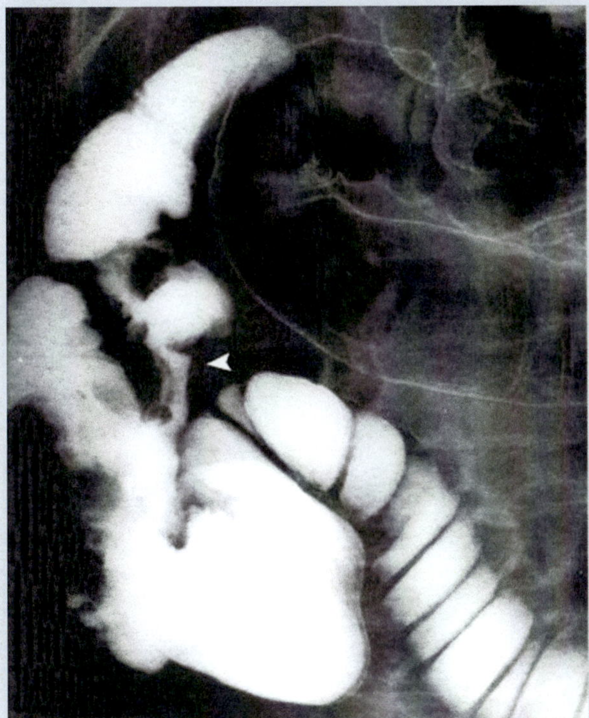

**Fig. 1.4.6** Barium enema image in a patient with Crohn's disease (CD) affecting the ascending colon resulting in stricture (*arrowhead*)

### Signs on US

- In active CD, ultrasound of the colon or the small intestine shows thickened intestinal wall on the B-mode sonography, mostly in the affected areas. The normal bowel wall thickness on US is equal to or less than 3 mm. Bowel wall thickness is considered pathological when it is >5 mm. Rectal wall thickness is considered normal up to 6 mm in thickness. Reactive lymphadenopathy may be found within the mesentery, which is identified as parallel hyperechogenic structures, about 1 cm thick.
- On PD, the inflamed thickened intestinal walls show high Doppler flow signal on both PD and color Doppler modes, reflecting the hyperemia of the active inflammation. This hypervascularization and abnormal Doppler signal within the wall is due to dilatation of small irregular vascular wall vessels <1 mm in diameter.

### Signs on CT

- After contrast enhancement, the bowel wall may show five different types of contrast enhancement patterns (Fig. 1.4.7). The first pattern is characterized by hyperdense (white) enhancement and is often seen in cases of bowel wall vascular dilatation or intramural injury with interstitial contrast leakage into the bowel wall, as in cases of ischemic "shock bowel." The second pattern is gray attenuation, where the wall shows little enhancement. This pattern is often seen in cases of neoplastic infiltration (e.g., lymphoma), especially when the wall thickness exceeds 3 cm. The third pattern is the water halo, where the bowel shows intraluminal water-density rings (commonly known as *target sign*). These rings represent edema within the submucosal layer, and they are commonly seen in inflammatory reactions and IBDs. The fourth pattern is the fat halo, which is characterized by deposition of fat within the submucosal layer (HU < −10). This sign is diagnostic of chronic CD. Also, this fat halo may present as a "normal variant" in the distal ileum and colon. The last sign is the black halo, where there is intramural black density that fails to enhance. This sign presents air within the bowel lumen (pneumatosis) and is commonly seen after intestinal infarction.
- *Bowel wall thickness*: this is one of the most common and early signs seen in CD. When the lumen is distended, normal bowel wall thickness is 1–2 mm; when the lumen is collapsed, normal thickness is 3–4 mm. Bowel wall thickness is diagnosed when the bowel wall thickness is >4 mm on distended bowel.

— *Creeping fat*: it refers to fibro-fatty proliferation seen in the mesentery around an inflamed bowel segment, which will cause separation of bowel loops (Fig. 1.4.8).
— *Comb sign* (*perienteric hypervascularity*): this sign is characterized by increased number of dilated mesenteric vessels around a thick bowel loop with intramural target sign (Fig. 1.4.9).
— *Abscess formation*: formation of an abscess is commonly seen in patients with intestinal fistulas, where the bacterial flora starts to invade the sterile peritoneal organs. Abscess is seen as a soft-tissue density lesion with thick wall and typical uniform ring enhancement after contrast injection. Air within the lesion is not a common sign but pathognomonic, reflecting gas-producing organism proliferation within the abscess. Abscess formation commonly occurs in the abdominal wall, psoas muscle, small bowel mesentery, and around the anus. The same picture is found on MRI.

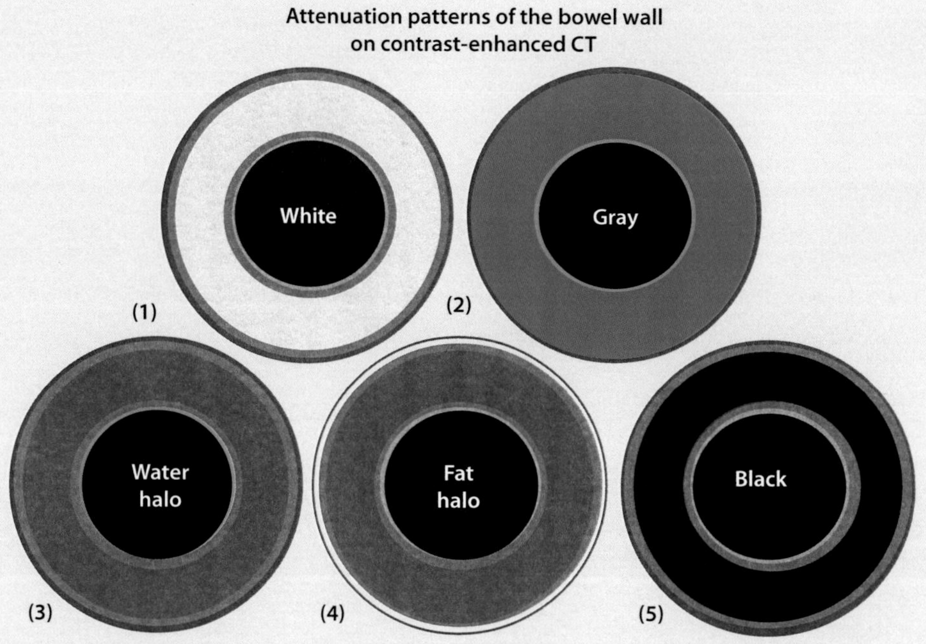


**Fig. 1.4.7**    An illustration demonstrating the five patterns of bowel wall attenuation: (*1*) hyperdense, (*2*) gray density, (*3*) water density, (*4*) fat density, and (*5*) black or air density

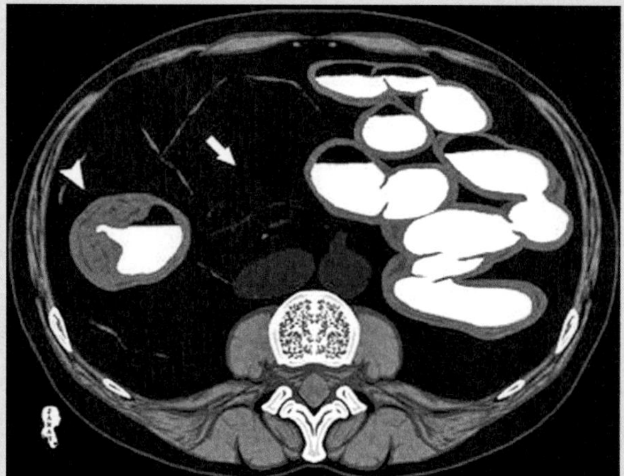

**Fig. 1.4.8**    Axial contrast-enhanced CT illustration demonstrates bowel wall thickening in CD (*arrow*), with surrounded creeping fatty proliferation that pushes the bowel loops to the left side of the abdomen (*arrow*)

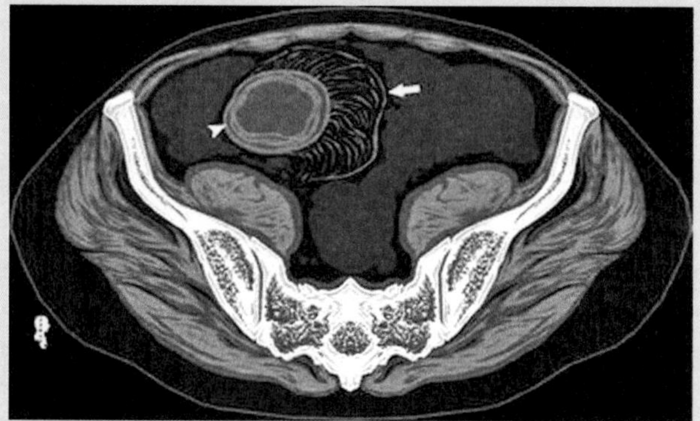

**Fig. 1.4.9**    Axial contrast-enhanced CT illustration demonstrates the bowel target sign in CD (*arrowhead*), with comb sign (*arrow*)

### Signs on MRI and MR Enteroclysis

— *Fistula formation*: the main advantages of MR examination over CT are lack of radiation and high soft-tissue details that make it ideal to detect fistulas. Fistula is an abnormal tract between two surfaces. In CD, fistulas are formed between the organs (e.g., vesicoenteric fistula) or between the internal organs and the skin surface (e.g., fistula-in-ano). Fistula-in-ano typically arises due to rectal crypts infection and abscess formation, which tunnels deep within the perineal tissues until it opens into the skin surface. Fistula-in-ano is identified as an abnormal longitudinal or linear tract that typically runs parallel to the rectum and opens into the skin surface. Thick granulation tissue line may be found surrounding the fistula in chronic cases. Active fistulas show signs of local inflammation and enhancement after gadolinium injection (◘ Fig. 1.4.10).

— Thickening of the ileocecal valve can be nicely demonstrated on coronal MR enteroclysis images (◘ Fig. 1.4.11).

— *Star sign*: this sign is observed in MR enteroclysis and represents multiple enteroenteric fistulae with wall-to-wall adhesions (◘ Fig. 1.4.12). The central attachment point between the intersected collapsed bowel loops will result in a starlike configuration.

— *Mucosal polyp formation* is seen in advanced stages of CD as signs of mucosal regeneration (◘ Fig. 1.4.13).

— *Mesenteric lymphadenopathy*: enlargement of the mesenteric lymph node is a common sign in CD (3–8 mm in size) (◘ Fig. 1.4.14). When the lymph nodes are >10 mm in size, carcinoma or lymphoma should be suspected.

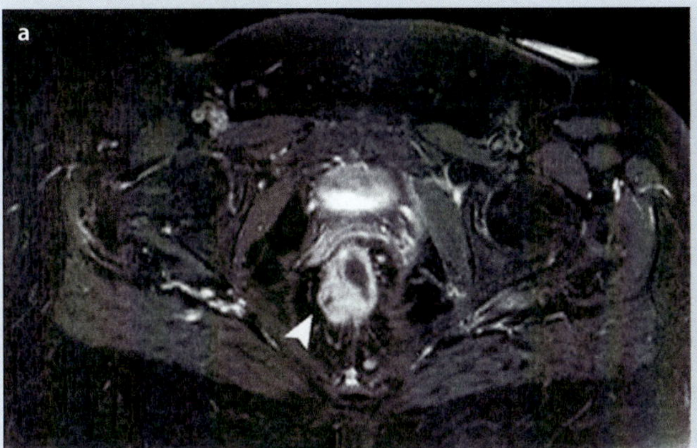
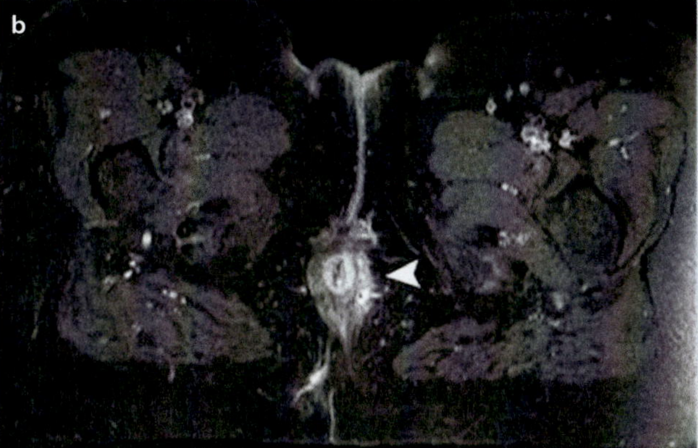

◘ **Fig. 1.4.10** Axial T1W postcontrasts with fat-saturation pelvic MRI in a patient with CD and fistula-in-ano seen as abnormal tract parallel to the anus in (**b**) and extends up to the rectum in (**a**) with contrast enhancement of the fistula wall (*arrowheads*)

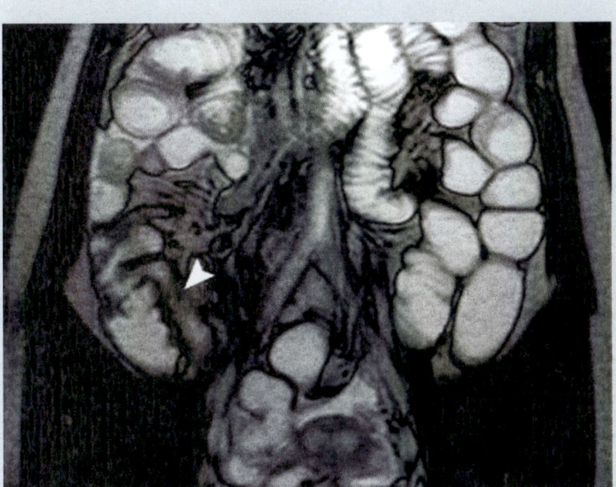

◘ **Fig. 1.4.11** Coronal MR enteroclysis image in a patient with CD shows thickening of the mucosa of the ileocecal valve (*arrowhead*)

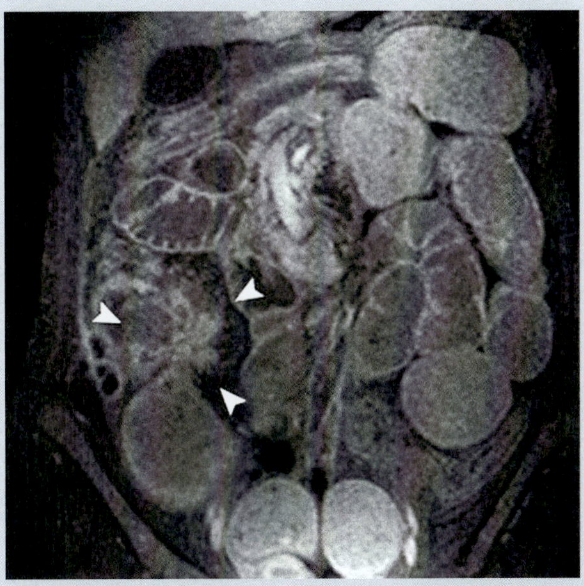

◘ **Fig. 1.4.12** Coronal MR enteroclysis image in a patient with CD shows the star sign (Courtesy of Dr. K. Herrmann, Klinikum Großhadern, Munich, Germany)

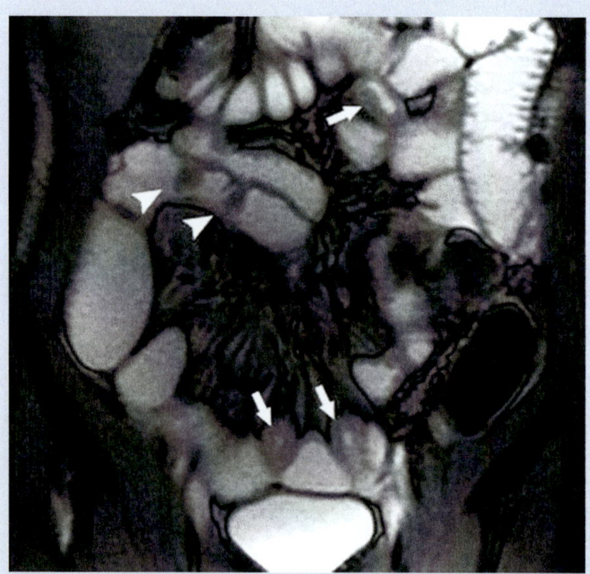

**Fig. 1.4.13** Coronal MR enteroclysis image in a patient with CD shows mucosal polyp formation (*arrowheads*) and bowel wall thickening (*arrows*)

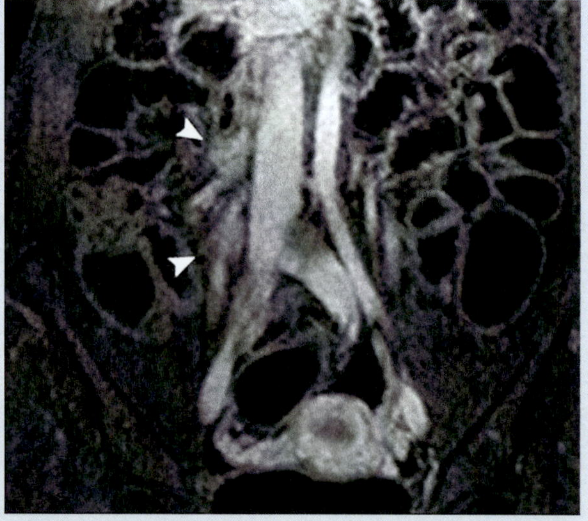

**Fig. 1.4.14** Coronal MR enteroclysis image in a patient with CD shows periaortic lymphadenopathy (*arrowheads*)

## Ulcerative Colitis

UC is a chronic inflammatory disease of unknown origin, characterized by rectal and colonic mucosal ulceration.

In contrast to CD, UC affects only the inner wall of the colon (superficial ulceration) and does not extend beyond the muscularis propria layer and affects the whole colon diffusely with no skip lesions. The rectum is involved in 95–100 % of cases. Patients commonly present with bloody diarrhea with mucus. Lower abdominal pain, tenesmus, and urgency are also common symptoms. *Backwash ileitis* refers to mucosal inflammation of the terminal ileum in patients with UC. *Fulminant UC* is a form of severe UC characterized by severe erosions that may lead to muscularis propria damage, causing loss of the haustra and colonic dilatation. Fulminant UC is seen in 15–20 % of cases.

CT is indicated in patients with UC when colonoscopy and barium enema are not possible, for example, in cases of sever inflammation, where the risk of perforation is high.

Both UC and CD carry the risk of malignant transformation. The risk of cancer in UC is 0.5–1 % after 10 years of universal colonic disease. Surveillance with CT or barium enema is recommended for chronic patients with UC to detect early colonic cancer that may present simulating strictures or infiltrative process.

## Extraintestinal Manifestations of UC

— *Arthritis*: it is the same as CD.
— *Sclerosing cholangitis*: sclerosing cholangitis can be seen in association with US in up to 70 % of patients with UC.
— *Central nervous system manifestations*: neurological manifestations of UC are rare and patient may present with seizures. On brain MRI, multiple, periventricular, intraspinal, and cerebellar hyperintense lesions may be seen (**Fig. 1.4.15**).
— *Pyostomatitis vegetans (PV)*: PV is a rare oral ulcerative lesion seen in UC patients and less frequently in patients with CD. PV is characterized by pustules (visible pus in a blister), erosions, and vegetative plaques which appear on the buccal and gingival mucosa forming a "snail-track" appearance. PV is a specific marker for IBDs (**Fig. 1.4.16**).

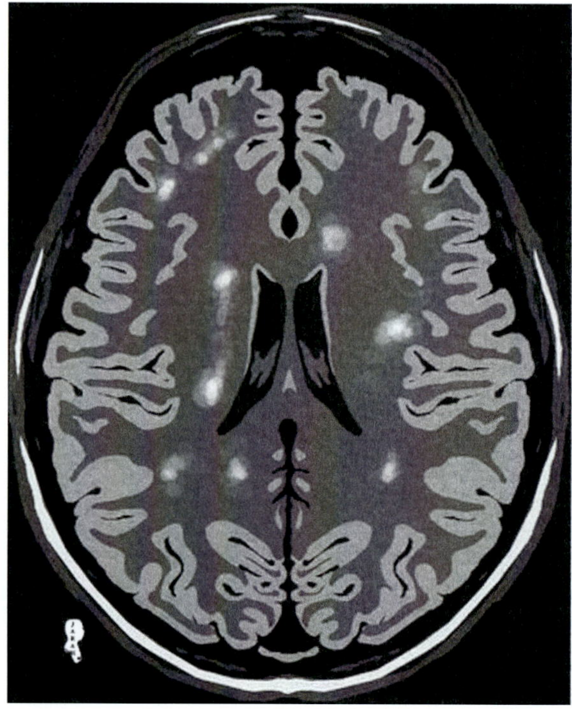

**Fig. 1.4.15** Axial FLAIR illustration demonstrates multiple T2 hyperintense signal intensity lesions in a patient with ulcerative colitis (UC)

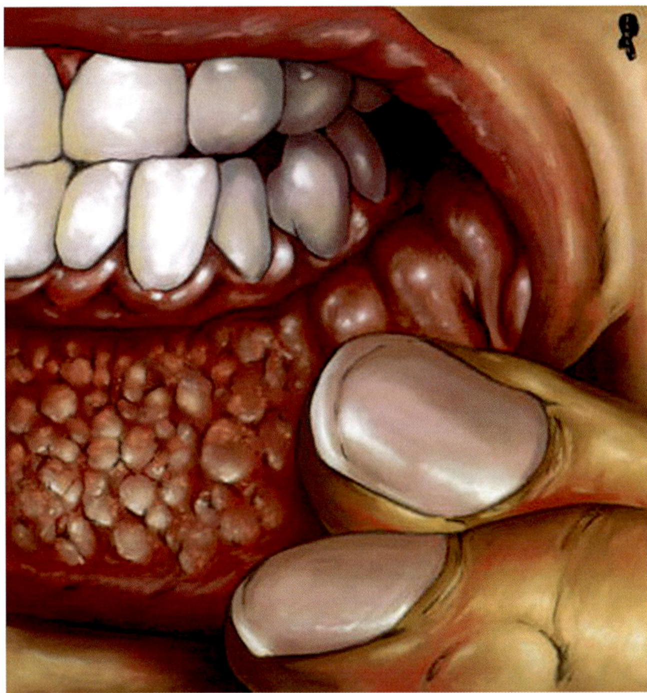

**Fig. 1.4.16** An illustration shows the clinical appearance of pyostomatitis vegetans (PV)

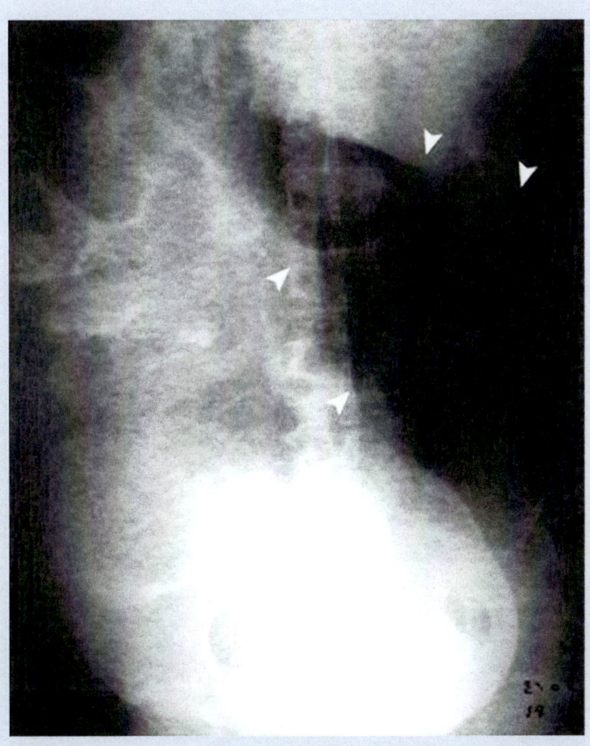

**Fig. 1.4.17** Plain abdominal radiograph shows toxic megacolon (*arrowheads*)

### Signs on Plain Radiograph
- Dilated colonic segments with no haustration (*adult toxic dilatation of the colon*)
- *Gasless abdomen*: due to chronic diarrhea
- *Absence of fecal materials*: because the bowel is not functioning well
- *Toxic megacolon*: abnormal distention of the colon with air (Fig. 1.4.17)

### Signs on Barium Enema
- *Collar-button ulcer*: it is a flask-shaped ulcer that is commonly seen in intermediate stage of UC. This type of ulcer is characterized by button-like shape barium appearance. This appearance is seen because UC causes erosions that extend until the muscularis propria, with some intact mucosal layer in between. The intact mucosal layer will have a mushroomlike shape. In barium enema, the barium will fill the erosion gaps between the intact mucosal layers, giving this collar-button appearance (Fig. 1.4.18). This sign is not specific for UC, as it can be seen in duodenal and gastric ulcers.
- *Pipe stem colon*: this refers to rigidity and narrowing of the colon due to longitudinal muscle spasm and hypertrophy (Fig. 1.4.19). This deformity is often seen in the mucosal regenerative stage of the disease.
- *Toxic megacolon*: toxic megacolon is one of the devastating complications of UC and is seen in <5 % of cases. Toxic megacolon is diagnosed when the bowel wall shows dilatation >6 cm. Up to 30 % of toxic megacolon develops during the first 3 months of the disease. Toxic megacolon is a contraindication for barium enema because of the risk of perforation during air inflation. A plain

radiograph should be done in any patient with UC planned for barium enema to exclude the presence of megacolon (■ Fig. 1.4.17).

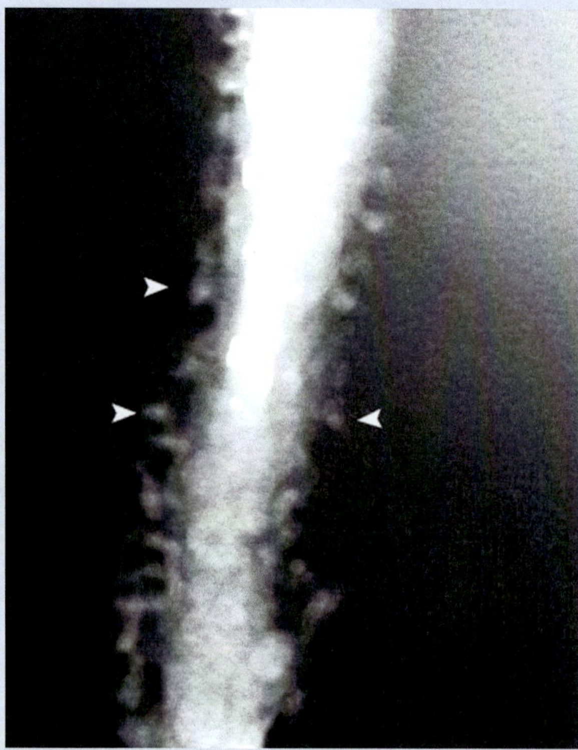

■ **Fig. 1.4.18**   Barium enema illustration demonstrates the barium sign of collar-button ulcer (*arrowheads*)

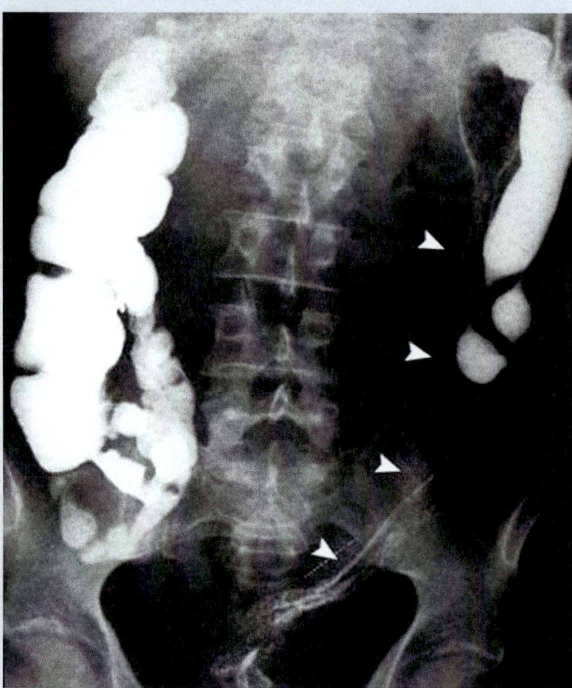

■ **Fig. 1.4.19**   Barium enema examination in a patient with chronic US shows marked stenosis and pipe-stem rigidity of the sigmoid colon and the rectum (*arrowheads*)

### Signs on CT

- The bowel wall thickness is diffuse and may affect the entire colon. In contrast, bowel wall thickness in CD may be eccentric and segmental with skip lesions.
- Perirectal fatty proliferation is seen as increased fatty tissues around the rectum (■ Fig. 1.4.20).

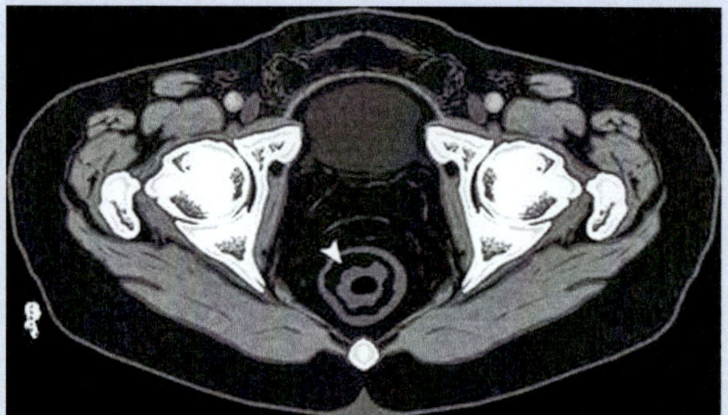

■ **Fig. 1.4.20**   Axial CT illustration demonstrates perirectal fatty proliferation with fatty infiltration of the rectal wall (*arrowhead*)

### Signs on Colonic MRI (MRI Is Used to Diagnose and Monitor UC when Endoscopy Cannot Be Performed for Whatever Reason)

- Hyperintensity and thickening of the colonic mucosa and submucosa on T1W and T2W images, caused by severe hemorrhagic changes.
- T1W post-Gd images show enhancement of the intestinal wall (■ Fig. 1.4.21). Postcontrast images can be used to monitor the severity and the activity of the disease; the stronger the signal, the higher the severity of the disease.
- Bowel wall thickening >10 mm with loss of the normal haustration may be seen.
- Increase in the perirectal fibro-fatty content with widening of the presacral space as a sign of long-standing disease.
- Wall stratification is seen in 60 % of cases as a hyperintense line on postcontrast T1W images located between two hypointense stripes (■ Fig. 1.4.22), representing edema and inflammation between the mucosa and the muscularis propria layers.

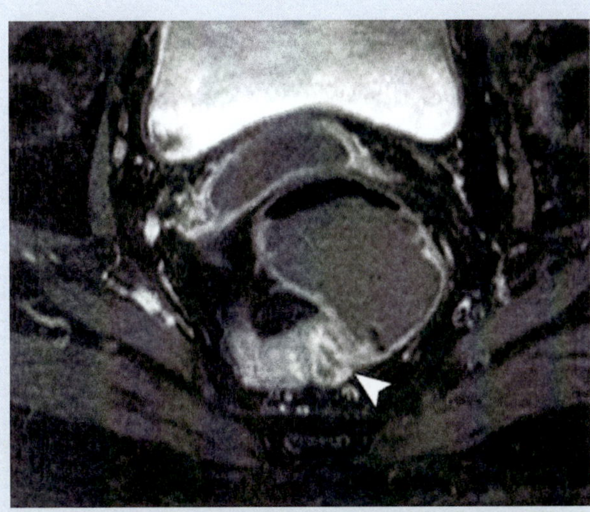

**Fig. 1.4.21** Axial T1W, fat-saturated, postcontrast MRI in a patient with UC shows focal rectosigmoidal bowel wall enhancement indicating acute inflammation (*arrowhead*)

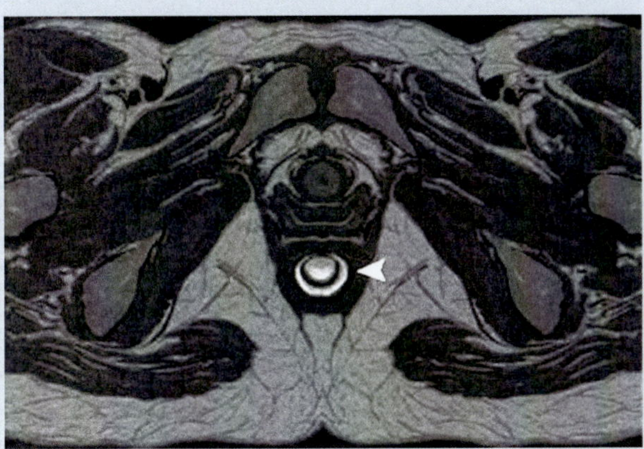

**Fig. 1.4.22** Axial T1W, fat-saturated, postcontrast MR illustration of a female pelvis demonstrates the rectal wall stratification

## Differences Between Ulcerative Colitis and Crohn's Disease

- CD commonly affects the ileum and the ascending colon and causes transmural (through the whole wall) inflammation. In contrast, UC affects the left colonic side and causes only inner mucosal layer erosions. Also, backwash ileitis is rare in CD.
- Enlarged mesenteric lymph nodes are commonly seen with CD.
- The rectum is involved in 95 % of cases in UC, while only 15–20 % of cases in CD.

## Differential Diagnoses and Related Diseases

*PAPA syndrome* is a rare, pediatric, autosomic dominant inherited auto-inflammatory disorder characterized by *pyogenic* aseptic *arthritis*, *PG*, and cystic *acne*. Patients present with recurrent destructive arthritis. The synovial fluid analysis shows purulent content with neutrophils accumulation, but cultures are invariably negative. The cystic acne is seen in the forehead, cheeks, nose, and chin. Humoral markers of inflammatory diseases, including antinuclear antibodies and erythrocyte sedimentation rate, can be negative. Up to 78 % of patients presented with at least one additional inflammatory disorder like IBD, monoclonal gammopathy, acne conglobata, or hidradenitis suppurativa.

### Further Reading

Al Roujayee A. Cutaneous manifestations of inflammatory bowel disease. Saudi J Gastroenterol. 2007;13:159–62.

Cammarota T, et al. US evaluation of patients affected by IBD: how to do it, methods and findings. Eur J Radiol. 2009;69:429–37.

Campa A, et al Management of a rare ulcerated erythema nodosum in a patient affected by crohn's disease and tuberculosis. J Plast Reconstr Aesthet Surg. 2008. doi:10.1016/j. bjps.2008.11.024.

Dekker BJ, et al. Prevalence of peripheral arthritis, sacroiliitis and ankylosing spondylitis in patients suffering from inflammatory bowel disease. Ann Rheum Dis. 1978;37:33–5.

Druschky A, et al. Severe neurological complications of ulcerative colitis. J Clin Neurosci. 2002;9:84–6.

Furukawa A, et al. Cross-sectional imaging in Crohn disease. Radiographics. 2004;24:689–702.

Giovagnoni A, et al. MR imaging of ulcerative colitis. Abdom Imaging. 1993;18:371–5.

Herrmann KA, et al. The "star-sign" in magnetic resonance enteroclysis: a characteristic finding of internal fistulae in Crohn's disease. Scand J Gastroenterol. 2006;41:239–41.

Horton KM, et al. CT evaluation of the colon: inflammatory diseases. Radiographics. 2000;20:399–418.

Javors BR, et al. Crohn's disease: less common radiographic manifestations. Radiographics. 1988;8:259–75.

Koulentaki M, et al. Ulcerative colitis associated with primary biliary cirrhosis. Dig Dis Sci. 1999;44:1953–6.

Lichtenstein JE, et al. The collar button. A radiographic-pathologic correlation. Gastrointest Radiol. 1979;4:79–84.

Maccioni F, et al. Ulcerative colitis: value of MR imaging. Abdom Imaging. 2005;30:584–92.

Maglinte DD, et al. Classification of small bowel Crohn's subtypes based on multimodality imaging. Radiol Clin North Am. 2003;41:285–303.

Neye H, et al. Evaluation of criteria for the activity of Crohn's disease by power Doppler sonography. Dig Dis. 2004;22:67–72.

Prassopoulos P, et al. MR enteroclysis imaging of Crohn disease. Radiographics. 2001;21:S161–72.

Roggeveen MJ, et al. Ulcerative colitis. Radiographics. 2006;26:947–51.

Sun MR, et al. Current techniques in imaging of fistula in ano: three dimensional endoanal ultrasound and magnetic resonance imaging. Semin Ultrasound CT MR. 2008;29:454–71.

Wittenberg J, et al. Algorithmic approach to CT diagnosis of the abnormal bowel wall. Radiographics. 2002;22:1093–9.

Yeon HB, et al. Pyogenic arthritis, pyoderma gangrenosum, and acne syndrome maps to chromosome 15q. Am J Hum Genet. 2000;66:1443–8.

## 1.5    Gastrointestinal Hemorrhage

Gastrointestinal (GI) bleeding is classically divided into upper and lower GI bleeding. Upper GI bleeding is defined as bleeding proximal to the ligament of Treitz, and lower GI bleeding is bleeding distal to the ligament of Treitz.

Causes of upper GI bleeding include erosions or ulcers, esophageal varices, Mallory–Weiss tear, and neoplasms. Lower GI bleeding causes include diverticulitis, ulcerative colitis, angiodysplasia, and neoplasms.

Patients with GI bleeding are often asymptomatic until blood loss exceeds 100 mL per day. Tachycardia and hypotension occur when bleeding exceeds 500 mL per day, and systemic shock develops when >15 % of the circulation blood volume is lost. Symptoms of upper GI bleeding include vomiting blood (hematemesis) and passing dark stool due to blood digestion (melena). Severe lower GI bleeding may present with passing fresh blood (hematochezia). In up to 75 % of upper GI bleeding cases and 80 % of lower GI bleeding cases, the bleeding will stop spontaneously with conservative treatment alone. In the remaining 20–25 % of cases, further intervention is required.

In recent years, the role of multidetector CT in detecting the source and the cause of bleeding has increased dramatically. CT angiography is commonly performed to detect the source of bleeding due to its fast scanning time and greater anatomical coverage. Disadvantages of CT angiography include radiation exposure and inability to perform intervention.

In the classical catheter angiography, bleeding rates as low as 0.5 mL/min can be detected with sensitivity of 63–90 % for upper GI bleeding and 40–86 % for lower GI bleeding. Conventional angiography specificity of up to 100 % is established for both. Active bleeding is detected by extravasation of the contrast material into the bowel lumen (pathognomonic sign). Indirect signs of bleeding include detection of aneurysms, arteriovenous fistula, neovascularity, and extravasation of the contrast material into confined space. CT angiography can detect active bleeding rate as low as 0.3 mL/min.

### Signs on CT Angiography

- Active GI bleeding is detected in the arterial phase of the scan when the contrast material is seen within the bowel lumen (91–274 HU). The extravasated contrast material may demonstrate jet-like, linear, swirled, or pooled configuration (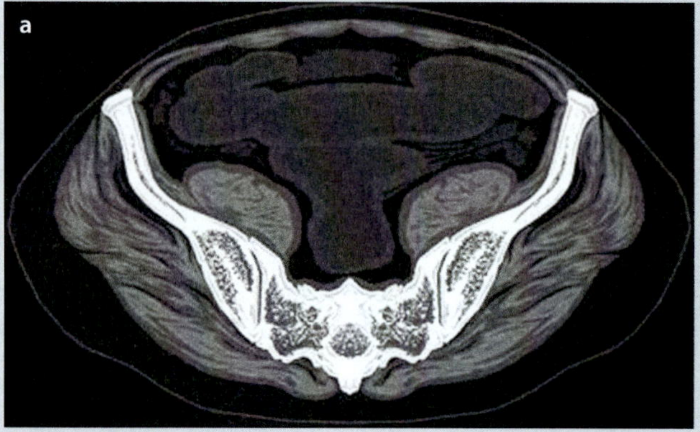 Fig. 1.5.1).
- The presence of hyperattenuated material within the bowel lumen in postcontrast images that was not seen in the precontrast images is diagnostic of acute GI bleeding (Fig. 1.5.1).
- For GI bleeding CTA, only intravenous contrast injection is used. CTA is performed without prior oral administration of water or contrast material. Water can dilute the extravasated contrast material, causing false-negative results.
- Clotted blood attenuation is 28–82 HU, which can be differentiated from active bleeding (>90 HU).

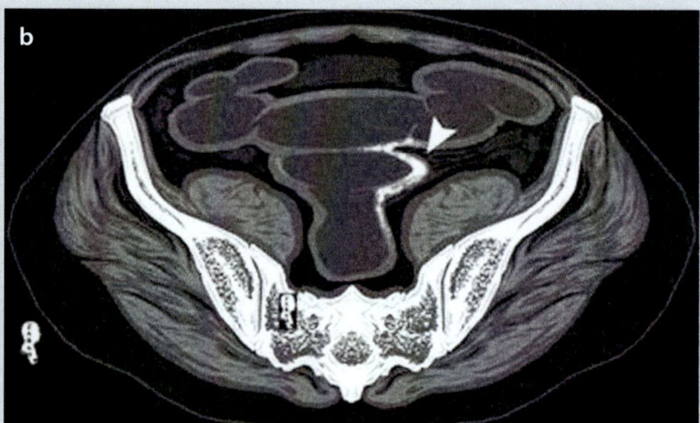

**Fig. 1.5.1**    Axial abdominal CTA illustration precontrast (**a**) and postcontrast (**b**). GI bleeding is detected in the arterial phase of the scan as an extravasation of the contrast material within the bowel lumen (*arrowhead*)

## Further Reading

Ernst O, et al. Helical CT in acute lower gastrointestinal bleeding. Eur Radiol. 2003;13:114–7.

Ha HK, et al. Radiologic features of vasculitis involving the gastrointestinal tract. Radiographics. 2000;20:779–94.

Jaeckle T, et al. Acute gastrointestinal bleeding: value of MDCT. Abdom Imaging. 2008;33:285–93.

Laing CJ, et al. Acute gastrointestinal bleeding: emerging role of multidetector CT angiography and review of current imaging techniques. Radiographics. 2007;27:1055–70.

Scheffel H, et al. Acute gastrointestinal bleeding: detection of source and etiology with multi-detector-row CT. Eur Radiol. 2007;17:1555–65.

Yamaguchi T, et al. Enhanced CT for initial localization of active lower gastrointestinal bleeding. Abdom Imaging. 2003;28:634–6.

Yoon W, et al. Acute gastrointestinal bleeding: contrast-enhanced MDCT. Abdom Imaging. 2006a;31:1–8.

Yoon W, et al. Acute massive gastrointestinal bleeding: detection and localization with arterial phase multi-detector row helical CT. Radiology. 2006b;239:160–7.

## 1.6  Pancreatitis

Pancreatitis is a disease characterized by inflammation of the pancreatic parenchyma, either in acute or chronic forms. Both acute and chronic pancreatitis have different etiologies and radiological manifestations, which should be addressed separately.

## Acute Pancreatitis

Patients with acute pancreatitis typically present with abdominal pain that can be epigastric or located in the right or less commonly left hypochondrial regions. The pain is described as stabbing and commonly radiating to the back. Patients with acute pancreatitis are partially relieved from the pain by leaning forward, decreasing the retroperitoneal pressure on the inflamed swollen pancreas. Laboratory investigations typically show highly elevated serum and urinary amylase and lipase levels.

The most common causes of acute pancreatitis are gallbladder stones, alcoholism, mumps, and hypercalcemia. Acute pancreatitis can be divided into two types according to severity: mild acute pancreatitis and severe acute pancreatitis. *Mild acute pancreatitis* is characterized by reversible inflammation and edema without pancreatic tissue necrosis. In contrast, *severe acute pancreatitis* has the same symptoms as mild pancreatitis but associated with parenchymal necrosis and hemorrhage. Radiological imaging has an important role in detecting and monitoring complications of acute pancreatitis which are:

(a) *Hemorrhagic pancreatitis*: it is a serious surgical emergency of acute pancreatitis that occurs due to erosion of the pancreatic vessels by the leaking pancreatic enzymes. It occurs 4 % of cases with mortality up to 50 %. Patients may present with discoloration of the flanks (*Grey Turner's sign*) and/or the umbilicus (*Cullen's sign*). Cullen's sign is a sign seen in cases of acute pancreatitis or ruptured ectopic pregnancy. The sign is characterized by the presence of fluid seen around the porta hepatic due to the spread of the inflammatory fluid from the subperitoneal space of the gastrohepatic and hepatoduodenal ligament through the Glisson sheath. The Glisson sheath is the part of the Glisson capsule that surrounds the intrahepatic portion of the hepatic portal system.

(b) *Necrotizing pancreatitis*: it is a pathologic condition characterized by diffuse of focal areas of nonviable pancreatic tissue due to inflammation. If the pancreatic fluid aspirated is sterile, then the condition is called *sterile pancreatic necrosis*, and abdominal scan should be repeated every 7–10 days to follow the evolution of the pancreatic necrosis.

(c) *Vascular thrombosis*: it can arise due to the inflammation around the vessels that will cause blood stasis. The superior mesenteric artery and the splenic vessels are the most common vessels affected by thrombosis due to acute pancreatitis.

(d) *Pancreatic pseudocyst*: it is a fluid-filled cystic mass confined by a fibrous capsule. It is called *pseudo* because its wall is not made of a true wall but a sac of granulation tissue. It occurs in 10 % of cases and maintains a communication with the pancreatic duct. Pseudocyst can be mistaken with cystic pancreatic tumor. Cystic pancreatic tumors, in contrast to pancreatic pseudocysts, have normal amylase level, while pseudocysts have high amylase level (typical scenario); also, the presence of carcinoembryonic antigen in the fluid of the cyst after aspiration to confirm cystic cancers (tumor marker). Fate of pancreatic pseudocyst will either (a) be resolved in 44 % spontaneously within 6 months or (b) develop a fibrous capsule after 6 weeks and then needs drainage.

(e) *Pancreatic abscess*: it is an infected necrotic tissue or fluid collection that occurs usually after 5 weeks with unhealed acute pancreatitis. It is a surgical emergence that occurs in 4 % of acute pancreatitis cases.

(f) *Pancreatic pseudoaneurysm*: it is a condition that occurs when an eroded blood vessel opens and bleeds into an adjacent pseudocyst. The pseudocyst will collect blood inside it forming what is called a pseudoaneurysm. The most common arteries involved are the pancreaticoduodenal artery and the gastroduodenal arteries.

(g) *Bowel ileus*: it can be focal affecting regional small bowel loops causing them to distend or diffuse affecting the entire intestine.

### *Differential* Diagnoses and Related Diseases

A. *Cholesterolosis (strawberry gallbladder)*: it is a rare condition with unknown characterized by deposition of lipid droplet saturated with cholesterol esters within the gallbladder wall submucosa. The disease can occur with or without the presence of gallbladder stones.

Cholesterolosis is associated with recurrent attacks of pancreatitis and acalculous cholecystitis.

B. *Juxtapapillary duodenal diverticulum*: it is defined as duodenal diverticulum located at peripapillary location. The diverticulum can be asymptomatic or predispose to choledocholithiasis, common bile duct dilatation, and pancreatitis.

### *Signs* on Plain Abdominal Radiograph

There are no reliable signs that can confirm or exclude acute pancreatitis in plain radiograph. However, one sign that can be highly suggestive of pancreatitis is the presence of significant gas within the duodenum due to adjacent inflammatory process ileus (*sentinel loop sign*).

### *Signs* on US

1. Normal ultrasound of the pancreas does not exclude acute pancreatitis. The typical sign of pancreatitis in ultrasound is thickening of the pancreas (head size >4.5 cm; neck, body, and tail >3 cm in thickness), associated with hypoechoic texture of the pancreas due to edema (◘ Fig. 1.6.1).
2. Demonstration of fluid collection in the peripancreatic region may be seen.
3. Assessment of splenic vein patency by Doppler sonography should be performed to exclude thrombosis.
4. Pancreatic pseudoaneurysm can be diagnosed by finding a mass with arterial flow within it (assessed by Doppler sonography).
5. In cholesterolosis, highly echogenic foci are detected within the gallbladder wall with posterior echogenic shadow that forms a comet-like appearance (highly specific) (◘ Fig. 1.6.2).

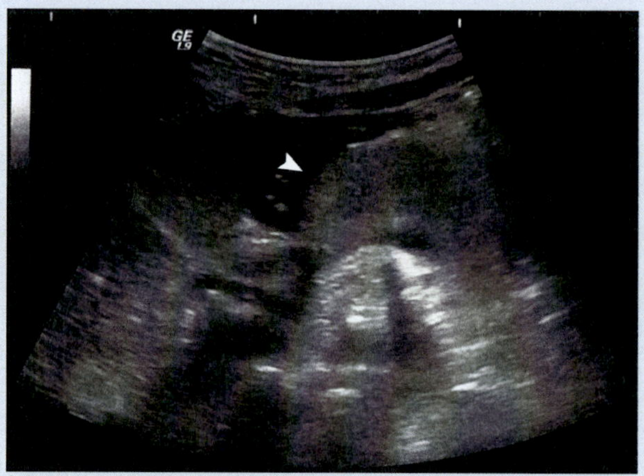

◘ **Fig. 1.6.1**   Ultrasound image of a patient with acute pancreatitis showing hypoechoic, edematous head of the pancreas (*arrowhead*)

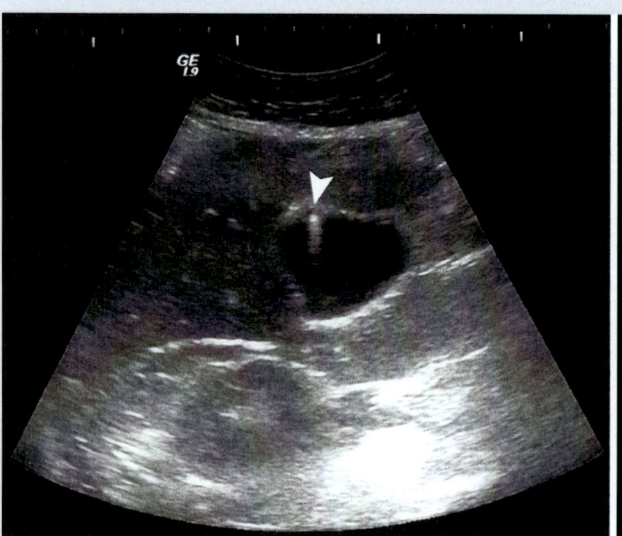 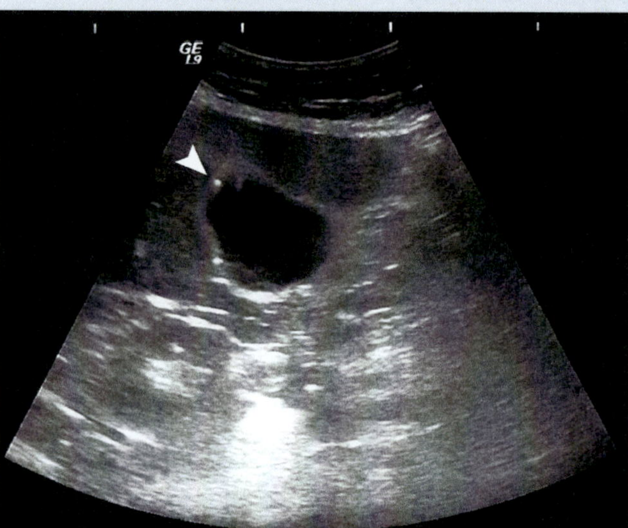

◘ **Fig. 1.6.2**   Ultrasound images showing cholesterolosis as hyperechoic foci within the gallbladder wall with "Comet-tail sign" (*arrowheads*)

### *Signs* on CT (Method of Choice for Diagnosis)

1. *Peripancreatic fluid*: because the pancreas has no capsule, the inflammatory fluid will roam free within the abdomen and will collect mainly in the lesser sac and the flanks first since the pancreas is retroperitoneal structures. The presence of free fluid within the lesser sac and the anterior pararenal space is diagnostic of acute pancreatitis (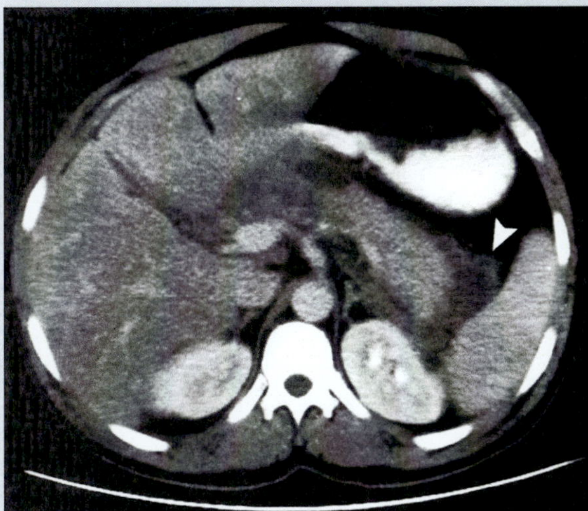 Fig. 1.6.3).
2. There is diffuse pancreatic swelling with blurring of its margin due to edema. Enlargement of the pancreas with reduction of its density and peripancreatic fluid collection in the lesser sac are the classical radiological triad of acute pancreatitis.
3. *Dirty peripancreatic fat sign*: due to inflammation and edema of the peripancreatic fat.
4. *Renal halo sign*: the kidney is separated from the fluid in the abdomen by the *Gerota's fascia* causing the perinephric fat to appear as a hypodense halo around it (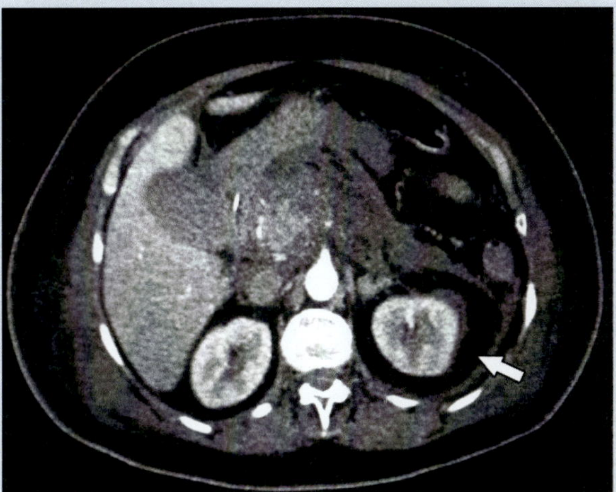 Fig. 1.6.4).
5. *Left-sided pleural effusion*: it may arise due to left phrenic nerve irritation and can be seen in 30 % of cases in chest radiographs.
6. In *hemorrhagic pancreatitis*, acute hyperdense blood will be seen in 5 % (HU > 80).
7. *Necrotizing pancreatitis* is diagnosed in CT by decrease density of the pancreatic tissue (<30 HU or less) and lack of enhancement after contrast injection. Sometimes, air can be demonstrated in the pancreatic body in CT confirming necrotizing pancreatitis (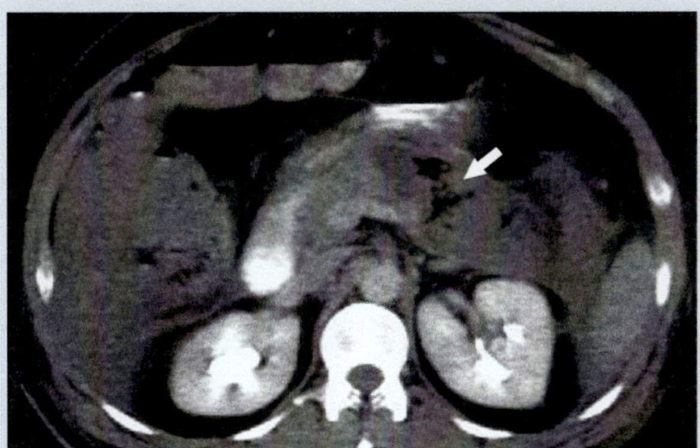 Fig. 1.6.5). If >90 % of the pancreatic width is necrotic, the gland is said to have undergone *central cavitary necrosis*.
8. *Vascular thrombosis* will be seen as lacking of vascular enhancement after contrast injection on CT.

9. *Pancreatic pseudocyst* is detected as unilocular pancreatic cyst full of fluid-density material without air with variable wall thickness (■ Fig. 1.6.6). The cyst material shows different attenuations according to the presence of necrotic material or hemorrhage. The cyst wall characteristically shows uniform enhancement after contrast administration. An important tool in differentiating pseudocyst from cystic neoplasms is evaluation of the lesion on serial exams. Up to 60 % of pseudocysts will resolve without intervention; besides the amylase levels are usually high in cases with pseudocysts.

In Siemens dual-source SOMATOM Definition Flash CT, a CT reconstruction technique known as *iodine window* can be used to differentiate pancreatic pseudocyst from pancreatic cystadenomas. In this technique, imaging using the two different CT

**■ Fig. 1.6.4** Axial abdominal, postcontrast CT image of a patient with acute pancreatitis showing fluid in the lesser sac that surrounds the left Gerota's fascia, showing the "halo sign" (*arrow*)

**■ Fig. 1.6.5** Axial abdominal, postcontrast CT image of a patient with acute pancreatitis affecting the body and tail showing severe edema and air within the pancreatic parenchyma, denoting necrosis; differential diagnosis includes "pancreatic abscess with gas formation" (*arrow*)

**■ Fig. 1.6.3** Axial abdominal, postcontrast CT image of a patient with acute pancreatitis showing fluid in the lesser sac (*arrowhead*)

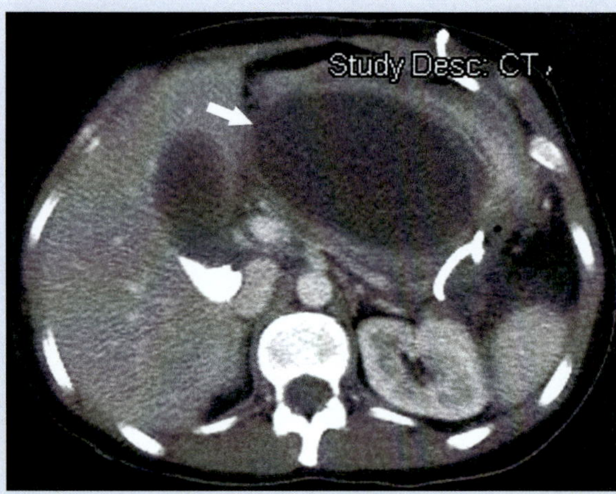

**Fig. 1.6.6**    Axial abdominal, postcontrast CT image of a patient with subacute pancreatitis that shows pseudocyst formation (*arrow*)

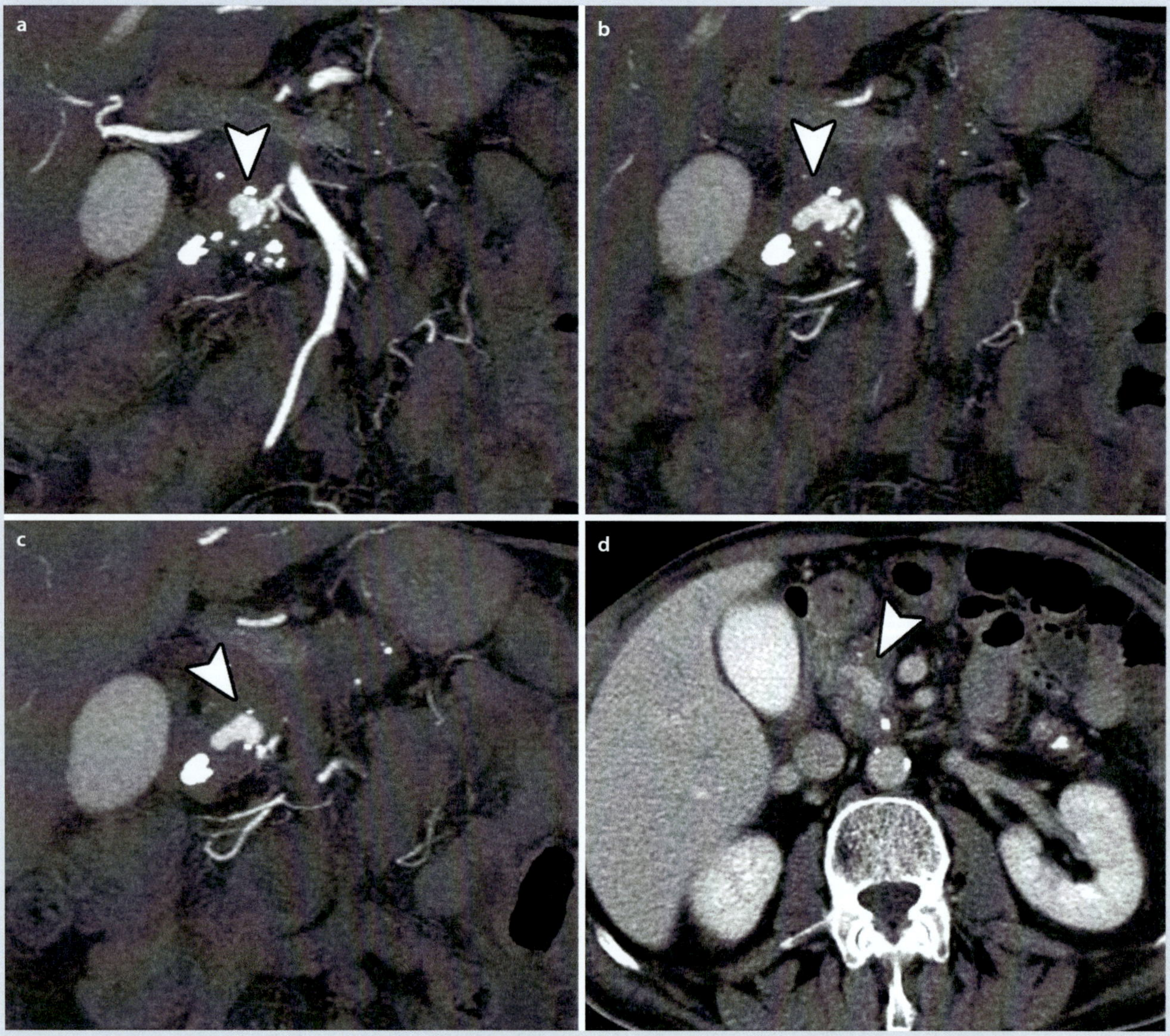

tubes voltage (e.g., at 80 kV and 120 kV) will show a slight difference in tissue attenuation that can be registered by the sensitive device. In the working station, the user can separate this slight difference in contrast enhancement and represent it as a digital, yellow hue layer over the plain CT images. Therefore, any small contrast uptake and enhancement can be represented as a yellow hue/color over the plain images. A pancreatic pseudocyst contains serous fluid; therefore, no enhancement should be noticed. In contrast, cystadenomas are cancerous cysts, so iodinated contrast enhancement will be seen *inside* the cyst, differentiating the cystadenoma from pseudocyst.

10. *Pancreatic pseudoaneurysm* is detected as a pancreatic pseudocyst with blood–fluid inside it. Rarely, true arterial aneurysm can arise from severe pancreatic inflammation ( Fig. 1.6.7).

**Fig. 1.6.7**    Sequential, coronal (**a–c**) and axial (**d**) abdominal, postcontrast CT images of a patient with acute pancreatitis who was discovered to have aneurysmal dilatation of the gastroduodenal artery at the site of inflammation in the pancreatic head (*arrowheads*) (Courtesy of Dr. Melvin D'Anastasi, Klinikum Großhadern (LMU), Munich, Germany)

11. *Pancreatic abscess* is seen as a cavity filled with air–fluid level, while the pseudocyst is a fluid-filled cavity without air. Gas is the only reliable sign for abscess diagnosis in CT (30–50 %) (Fig. 1.6.5).

12. *Juxtapapillary diverticulum* is typically found within a radius of 2–3 cm from papilla of Vater and is seen as a thin-walled pouch of intestinal dilatation that is filled with air or air–fluid level (Fig. 1.6.8). Differential diagnoses include pancreatic abscess.

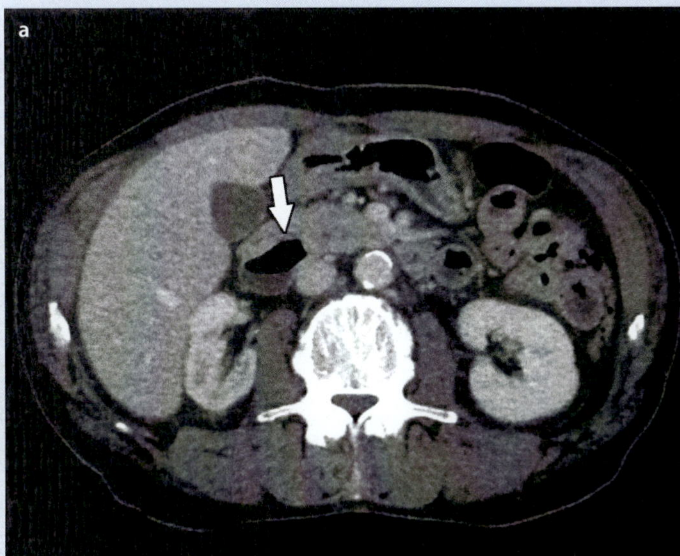

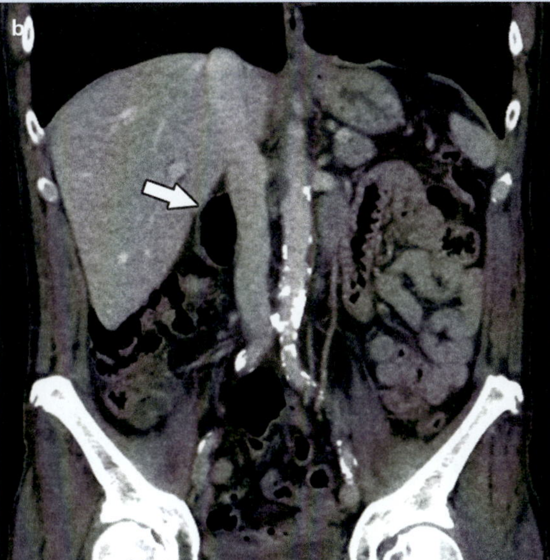


**Fig. 1.6.8** Axial (**a**) and coronal (**b**) abdominal, postcontrast CT images that show duodenal diverticulum (*arrows*)

## Chronic Pancreatitis

Chronic pancreatitis is defined as prolonged inflammation of the pancreas that is characterized by irreversible pancreatic damage with fibrosis, calcification, and loss of exocrine and/or endocrine functions. The most common cause is alcoholism (70 % of cases). Complications of chronic pancreatitis include pancreatic pseudocyst formation, diabetes mellitus, portal hypertension, and pleuropancreatic fistula. A *pleuropancreatic fistula* is a very rare complication of chronic pancreatitis characterized by pancreatic ductal disruption with leakage of pancreatic fluid not contained by the inflammatory response of the surrounding tissues in the retroperitoneum or the lesser sac. When the ductal disruption occurs posteriorly, the pancreatic fluid may track through the retroperitoneum via the aortic hiatus into the mediastinum and eventually into the pleural space, typically on the left side. Patients typically present with left-sided isolated pleural effusion. Up to 50 % of these patients may give a previous history of previous episodes of pancreatitis within the 12 months preceding this admission. Rare forms of chronic pancreatitis include:

(a) *Focal pancreatitis* is an acute pancreatitis that occurs on top of a chronic pancreatitis causing pancreatic head focal contour abnormality, common bile duct obstruction, and dilatation (biliary obstruction). It is a rare condition and occurs in 4 % of chronic pancreatitis cases. Focal pancreatitis is considered as carcinoma of the head of the pancreas when it is seen. It is diagnosed as focal pancreatitis when the biopsy returns negative for tumor cells and only inflammatory cells are found. Also, it can be suspected when pancreatic calcifications are found, which are not commonly seen in pancreatic tumors (except in endocrinal pancreatic tumors).

(b) *Hereditary pancreatitis* is a rare autosomal dominant cause of chronic pancreatitis characterized by recurrent attacks of acute pancreatitis, usually since infancy. Patients present with recurrent attacks of acute pancreatitis that will progress with time into chronic pancreatitis in 50 % of patients. Patients with hereditary pancreatitis have high risk of developing pancreatic carcinomas (50–60 times greater than normal population).

(c) *Autoimmune pancreatitis* (AIP) is a special form of chronic pancreatitis that can be primary or associated with other autoimmune disorders (e.g., Sjögren's syndrome).

AIP is characterized by (1) elevated serum levels of autoimmune antibodies (e.g., *high ANA titers*); (2) increased serum $\gamma$-globulin or IgG levels; (3) diffuse or focal enlargement of the pancreas on US, CT, or MRI that mimics carcinoma (*focal type*); (4) diffuse irregular narrowing of the main pancreatic duct; (5) fibrotic changes of the pancreas with lymphatic infiltration on histological examination; (6) obstructive jaundice due to stenosis of the common bile duct; (7) mild symptoms with the absence of acute attacks of pancreatitis; (8) association with other autoimmune disorders; and (9) good response to steroid therapy.

Patients with AIP often present with signs of obstructive jaundice, hypergammaglobulinemia, and type 2 diabetes mellitus (>50 % of patients). Diagnosis is established by detecting diffuse or focal narrowing of the main pancreatic duct with focal or diffuse pancreatic enlargement in radiological modalities, in association with other two criteria from the past nine criteria.

(d) *Groove pancreatitis*, also known as *paraduodenal pancreatitis with duodenal cystic dystrophy*, is a rare form of pancreatitis that arises from ectopic pancreatic tissues located in the groove between the pancreas and the duodenum. Patients with groove pancreatitis present with the same clinical history of the classical chronic pancreatitis (e.g., *alcoholism, recurrent pancreatitis attacks*). Peptic ulcer is markedly associated with groove pancreatitis.

Groove pancreatitis is commonly mistaken for pancreatic head carcinoma because of the radiological features and because it is usually associated with mild elevation in CA19-9 levels (*a marker for pancreatic carcinoma*). Diagnosis can be suggested radiologically; however, diagnosis has to be confirmed by biopsy, unless the radiological features and clinical history are so typical.

Two types of groove pancreatitis are distinguished histologically, "pure" and "segmental." Pure groove pancreatitis is characterized by scarring due to chronic inflammation that is located exclusively in the space between the pancreas and the duodenum. In contrast, the segmental groove pancreatitis is characterized by scarring of the pancreaticoduodenal groove with affection of the dorsocranial parts of the pancreas.

(e) *Idiopathic fibrosing pancreatitis (IFP)* is a rare form of chronic pancreatitis predominantly seen in childhood and adolescence with a male predominance. Two major forms of IFP have been described: the calcifying and the noncalcifying. The calcifying form is associated with hereditary or juvenile tropical pancreatitis. The noncalcifying or obstructive form is less common and causes pancreatic and biliary duct obstruction. IFP is a diagnosis that can only be made once other causes of chronic pancreatitis such as hereditary pancreatitis, cystic fibrosis, hypercalcemia, hyperlipidemia, sclerosing cholangitis, and congenital anomalies of the pancreatic and biliary trees are excluded. Histologically, IFP is characterized by diffuse fibrosis of the pancreatic parenchyma, with relative sparing of the islets of Langerhans and occasional sparing of pancreatic acini. Diagnosis can be suggested clinically especially if IFP is associated with other form of *multicentric fibrosis diseases* (e.g., *Riedel's thyroiditis*). Patients with IFP are typically children or adults presenting with abdominal pain, obstructive jaundice, passing dark urine, and pale stool, with normal amylase and lipase levels.

### *Signs* on Plain Radiograph

The presence of calcifications within the mid-abdomen at the region of the pancreas is highly specific for chronic pancreatitis (◨ Fig. 1.6.9).

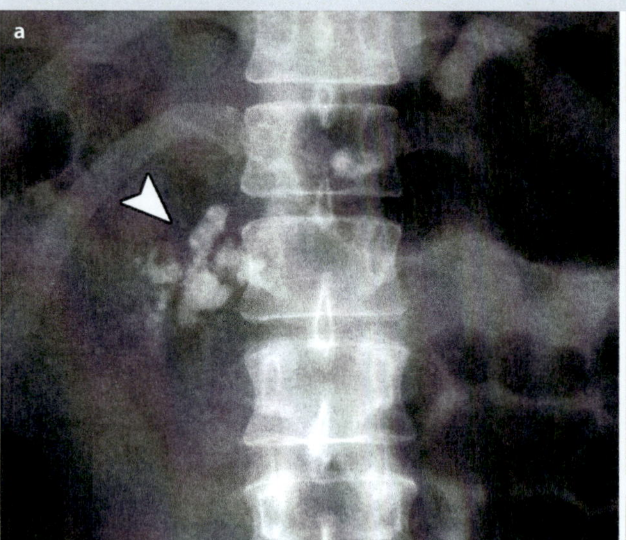
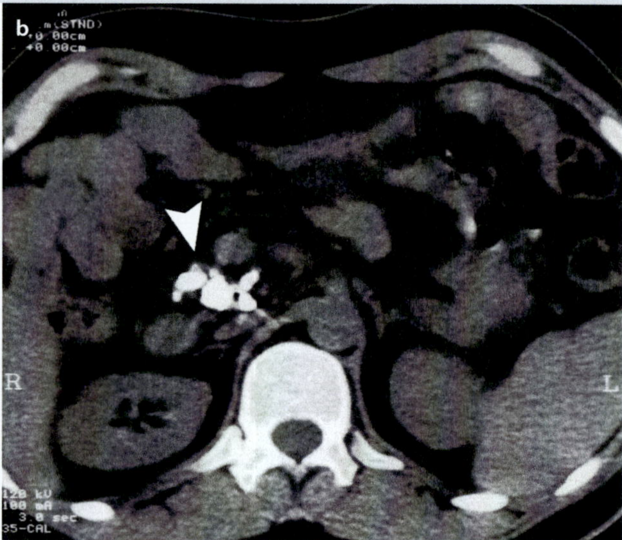

◨ **Fig. 1.6.9**   Plain abdominal radiograph (**a**) and plain axial CT image (**b**) of a patient with chronic pancreatitis showing dense calcification at the head of pancreas (*arrowheads*)

### Signs on US

1. There is irregular shape or contour of the pancreas with atrophic changes of the pancreas (more hyperechoic due to fat infiltration).
2. Pancreatic calcifications (*seen as hyperechoic clumps within the pancreas*).
3. Dilatation of the pancreatic duct is the most reliable sign (>2 mm in width) of chronic pancreatitis.
4. In autoimmune pancreatitis, there is diffuse or focal pancreatic enlargement with hypoechoic texture (sausage appearance), with complete compression of the pancreatic duct (of Wirsung).
5. In groove pancreatitis, there is a hypoechoic, band-like area typically seen between the pancreas and the duodenum (*represents the inflammation with edema*) and duodenal wall thickening with or without evidence of surrounding inflammation. The pancreatic head typically shows enlargement and hypoechoic texture due to inflammation and edema.

### Signs on CT

1. *Chronic pancreatitis*: stigmata in CT include the presence of pancreatic calcification (50 % of cases) ( Fig. 1.6.9), pancreatic atrophy due to chronic inflammation with fatty infiltration and fibrosis, and dilated pancreatic duct with multiple strictures giving beaded shape appearance ( Fig. 1.6.10).
2. *Autoimmune pancreatitis*: it is detected as focal or diffuse pancreatic enlargement with decreased pancreatic enhancement mimicking pancreatic adenocarcinoma. The lack of vascular invasion plus the history of associated autoimmune disease helps in establishing the diagnosis. However, definite diagnosis requires biopsy.
3. *Groove pancreatitis*: because of the chronic inflammation and the formation of scar tissue within the pancreaticoduodenal groove ( Fig. 1.6.11), groove pancreatitis is classically seen as a triad of a mass of soft tissue located between the pancreas head and duodenum with duodenal wall thickening, cystic changes of the second part of the duodenum's wall with or without air–fluid level, and dilatation of the proximal part of the common bile duct with or without intrahepatic biliary radical dilatation due to distal obstruction by the fibrous mass ( Fig. 1.6.12). The fibrous mass enhances after contrast injection. The enhancing fibrous mass, duodenal inflammation and cystic changes, and vascular sparing are features that may be useful in differentiating groove pancreatitis from pancreatic carcinoma. Moreover, groove pancreatitis shows patchy enhancement in the portal venous phase, with displacement of the

gastroduodenal artery leftward. In contrast pancreatic groove carcinoma often shows rim enhancement because the tumor cells are located more in the peripheral and the center may show necrosis, and the gastroduodenal artery is usually infiltrated by the mass or located within the mass rather than displaced.

4. *Idiopathic fibrosing pancreatitis*: there is typically pancreatic mass that mimics carcinoma, with dilated proximal common bile duct (CBD) due to distal CBD stenosis or obstruction and dilated intrahepatic biliary radicals (*mimicking pancreatic carcinoma*). The pancreatic duct usually is not seen.

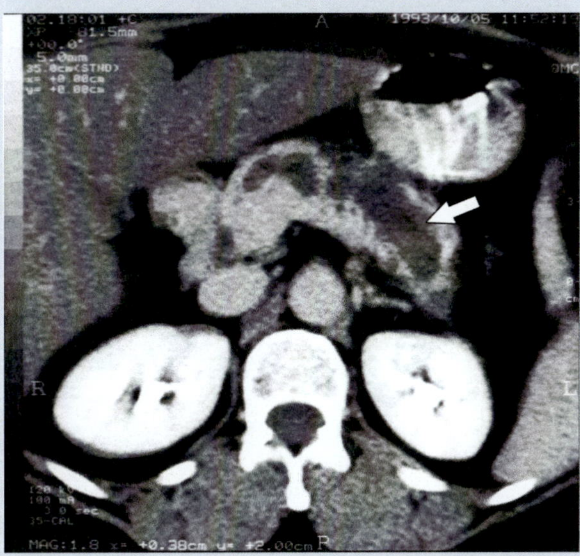

**Fig. 1.6.10** Axial abdominal, postcontrast CT image of a patient with chronic pancreatitis showing massive dilatation of the pancreatic duct (*arrowhead*)

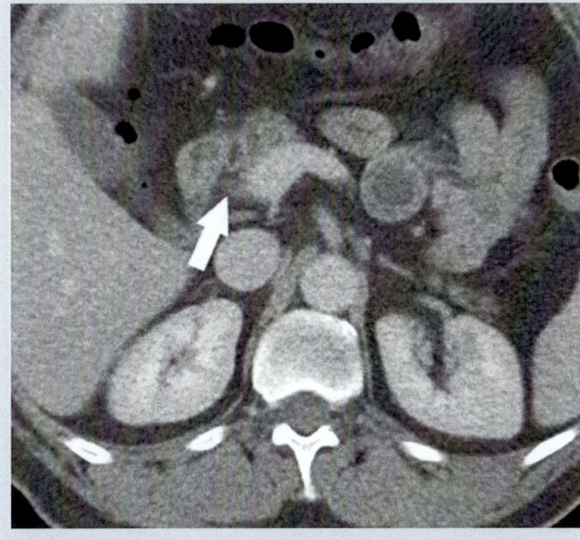

**Fig. 1.6.11** Axial abdominal, postcontrast CT image that demonstrates the pancreaticoduodenal grove location (*arrow*)

5. *Pleuropancreatic fistula*: it is seen as a fluid collection between the diaphragmatic crus and the posterior abdominal wall near the aorta, typically on the left side.

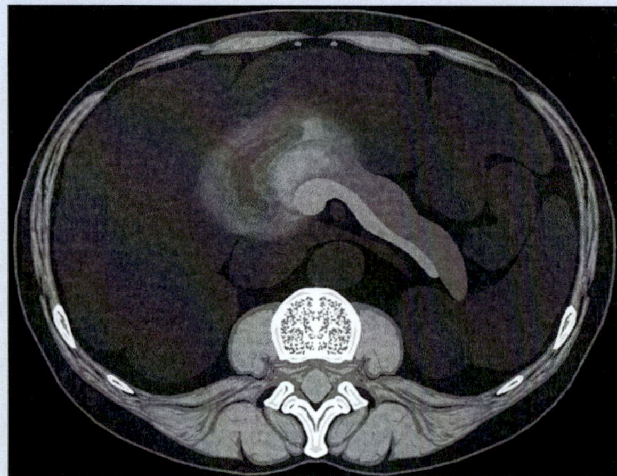

**Fig. 1.6.12**  Axial abdominal, postcontrast CT illustration that demonstrates the findings of groove pancreatitis

### *Signs* on MRCP
1. In groove pancreatitis, there is tapering or obstruction of the distal CBD with proximal CBD dilatation, with cystic dilatation (>1 cm in diameter) affecting the second part of the duodenum. If cystic dilatation is <1 cm in diameter, the duodenum appears thickened only.
2. A pleuropancreatic fistula is seen as a fluid signal fistula that arises from the pancreatic duct and ascends superiorly to the mediastinum on coronal MIP images.

### Selected References

Atkdnson GO, et al. Idiopathic fibrosing pancreatitis: a cause of obstructive jaundice in childhood. Pediatr Radiol. 1988;18:28–31.

Balci NC, et al. Juxtapapillary diverticulum. Findings on CT and MRI. J Clin Imaging. 2003;27:82–8.

Bollen TL, et al. Updates on acute pancreatitis: ultrasound, computed tomography, and magnetic resonance imaging features. Semin Ultrasound CT MR. 2007;28:371–83.

Delrue LJ, et al. Acute pancreatitis: radiologic scores in presenting severity and outcome. Abdom Imaging. 2010;35:349–61.

Harb R, et al. Idiopathic fibrosing pancreatitis in a 3-year-old girl: a case report and review of the literature. J Pediatr Surg. 2005;40:1335–40.

Ishigami K, et al. Differential diagnosis of groove pancreatic carcinoma vs. groove pancreatitis: usefulness of the portal venous phase. Eur J Radiol. 2010;47:e95–100.

Ju S, et al. Value of CT and clinical criteria in assessment of patients with acute pancreatitis. Eur J Radiol. 2006;57: 102–7.

Ketikoglou I, et al. Autoimmune pancreatitis. Dig Liver Dis. 2005;37:211–5.

Khan AZ, et al. Pleuropancreatic fistulae: specialist center management. J Gastrointest Surg. 2009;13:354–8.

Kimot WA, et al. Cholesterolosis in patients with chronic acalculous biliary pain. Br J Surg. 1994;81:112–5.

Macari M, et al. Duodenal diverticula mimicking cystic neoplasms of the pancreas: CT and MR imaging findings in seven patients. AJR Am J Roentgenol. 2003;180:195–9.

Schneider A, et al. Hereditary pancreatitis: a model for inflammatory diseases of the pancreas. Best Pract Res Clin Gastroenterol. 2002;16(3):347–63.

Sclabas G, et al. Juvenile idiopathic fibrosing pancreatitis. Dig Dis Sci. 2002;47(6):1230–5.

Segal D, et al. Acute necrotizing pancreatitis: role of CT-guided percutaneous catheter drainage. Abdom Imaging. 2007;32:351–61.

Siddiqi AJ, et al. Chronic pancreatitis: ultrasound, computed tomography, and magnetic resonance imaging features. Semin Ultrasound CT MR. 2007;28:384–94.

Whitcomb DC, et al. Hereditary pancreatitis: new insights, new directions. Baillieres Clin Gastroenterol. 1999;13(2):253–63.

## 1.7  Jaundice

Jaundice is a clinical condition characterized by yellowish discoloration of the skin and the conjunctival membrane over the sclera due to high serum bilirubin level (hyperbilirubinemia). Jaundice comes from the French word *jaune*, meaning yellow.

Mature red blood cells (RBCs) are renewed every 3 months (*life span of RBCs is approximately 120 days*). When RBCs die due to normal apoptosis or destructed due to hemolysis, the cellular content of the RBCs including hemoglobin is released into the bloodstream and engulfed by macrophages in the reticuloendothelial system (*liver, spleen, and bone marrow*). Macrophages degrade the hemoglobin into the globulin (protein) portion and the heme portion. The globulin is further degraded into amino acids and plays no portion in jaundice. The heme molecule is converted first into biliverdin, a green color pigment, by oxidation, and then into bilirubin, which is a yellow color pigment, by reduction.

The newly formed bilirubin is insoluble in water (unconjugated/indirect) and requires a special transport mechanism to reach the liver for further modification. Albumin molecules serve as a carrier for the unconjugated bilirubin to the liver by binding to unconjugated bilirubin creating a bilirubin–albumin complex in the intravascular compartment. This bilirubin–albumin complex retains the yellowish bilirubin pigment within the plasma. The albumin-binding capacity is reduced when the serum albumin is reduced (e.g., *hypoalbuminemia*), when albumin capacity is diminished by competition of other organic anion (e.g., *sulfonamides*, *salicylate*), and when albumin affinity is diminished by acidosis.

When the unconjugated bilirubin reaches the liver, the free bilirubin molecules are taken up by the hepatocytes and bind to special proteins within the hepatocytes called Y (ligandin) and Z proteins. These proteins are responsible for aggregating bilirubin molecules within the hepatocytes for conjugation. Ligandin is the preferential bilirubin-binding protein at low bilirubin concentration, whereas Z protein becomes more important binding protein as bilirubin concentration increases. Conjugation of bilirubin takes place within the endoplasmic reticulum, which is a process characterized by changing the chemical properties of bilirubin to be water soluble (conjugated) instead of lipid soluble (unconjugated). The bilirubin is converted to bilirubin glucuronide by the action of the enzyme uridine 5-diphosphateglucuronosyl transferase (UDPG-T).

The conjugated bilirubin is actively excreted by the hepatocytes to the biliary sinusoids in the liver, which in turn drain the bile into the biliary tree. A part of the conjugated bilirubin is stored in the gallbladder and a part enters the duodenum via ampulla of Vater. The conjugated bilirubin is converted to urobilinogen by the intestinal bacterial flora. A part of urobilinogen is reabsorbed by the intestine and enters the portal system back to the liver to complete the bilirubin intestinal–hepatic cycle, and the rest is excreted in the stool giving the stool its brown pigment. When the urobilinogen reaches the liver, it is further excreted from the body later via the kidneys into the urine. There is no intestinal absorption of conjugated bilirubin.

A group of disorders and rare hereditary syndromes results from disturbance of one or two steps in the bilirubin metabolism mechanism described above. Some of these conditions are benign and some are fatal as the following:

1. *Neonatal jaundice* is a term used to describe jaundice in neonates after birth that arises when the binding capacity of the albumin is exceeded. Also, the amount of Z protein in the liver after birth is comparable to that in the adult, but adult levels of ligandin are not attained until several weeks after birth. Both previous factors contribute to the development of the physiological jaundice in neonates. The condition is self-limited and lasts 8 days in normal births and approximately 14 days in premature births.

2. *Gilbert syndrome* is a rare disease characterized by isolated serum unconjugated hyperbilirubinemia (usually up to 6.0 mg/dL). The other liver serum biochemical tests are normal. The unconjugated hyperbilirubinemia can be precipitated by fatigue, alcohol consumption, stress situations, and diseases like influenza. The disease affects 1 % of the population. Gilbert syndrome is believed to be caused at least by the deficiency of ligandin and Z proteins in hepatocytes. The serum unconjugated hyperbilirubinemia is reduced by phenobarbital therapy.

3. *Crigler–Najjar syndrome* is a very rare disease characterized by complete or partial absence of the enzyme UDPG-T, which is responsible for bilirubin conjugation within hepatocytes. Neonates with Crigler–Najjar syndrome present with severe serum unconjugated hyperbilirubinemia that often leads to kernicterus. The disease is classified into type I and type II. Type I Crigler–Najjar syndrome is the most severe type and it is due to the complete absence of the enzyme UDPG-T action, and serum unconjugated hyperbilirubinemia is not responsive to phenobarbital therapy. In contrast, type II Crigler–Najjar syndrome arises due to partial absence of the enzyme UDPG-T action, and serum unconjugated hyperbilirubinemia is reduced by phenobarbital therapy. Type I Crigler–Najjar syndrome is inherited as autosomal recessive, whereas type II Crigler–Najjar syndrome is inherited as autosomal dominant.

4. *Lucey–Driscoll syndrome* is a rare disease characterized by serum unconjugated hyperbilirubinemia due to inhibition of the enzyme UDPG-T action in neonates due to serum factor coming from mother's breast milk. Infants become jaundiced when breastfed with their mother's milk but recover on withdrawal from breastfeeding.

5. *Dubin–Johnson syndrome* is a rare, autosomal recessive disease characterized by serum conjugated hyperbilirubinemia due to congenital abnormality in the active conjugated bilirubin excretion from the hepatocytes to the biliary canaliculi. The disease also is characterized by deposition of a melaninlike pigment within the liver causing the liver to be dark in gross examination. Patients' laboratory tests show conjugated hyperbilirubinemia plus mild elevation in liver enzymes. There are no purities or steatorrhea.

6. *Rotor syndrome* is a rare variant of Dubin–Johnson syndrome characterized by serum conjugated hyperbilirubinemia with the absence of purities or steatorrhea. Unlike Dubin–Johnson syndrome, there is no melaninlike pigment deposition within the liver.

Approximately 4 mg/kg of bilirubin is produced every day. The normal serum level of bilirubin is 0.5 mg/dL. Serum bilirubin level must exceed 1.5 mg/dL for the yellowish coloration to start visible on the patient. Jaundice itself is not a disease but rather a sign of an underlying condition. Conditions that predispose to jaundice can be categorized into three main categories:

1. *Prehepatic jaundice*: this type of jaundice arises due to increase rate of hemolysis with increased production of unconjugated bilirubin. Prehepatic jaundice is typically seen in hemolytic anemia, malaria, glucose-6-phosphate dehydrogenase deficiency, rat fever (leptospirosis), and hemolytic uremic syndrome. There is increased serum unconjugated bilirubin level with normal urinary color and bilirubin concentration, stool color, and serum liver enzymes.

2. *Hepatic jaundice*: this type of jaundice arises due to hepatocyte disease or liver enzyme failure. Hepatic jaundice is typically seen in hepatitis, hepatic failure, liver cirrhosis, Gilbert's syndrome, Crigler–Najjar syndrome, and Niemann–Pick disease type C. Laboratory investigations show abnormal liver enzyme profile and increased urinary urobilinogen level.
3. *Posthepatic jaundice*: this type of jaundice arises due to interruption to the drainage of the bile within the biliary tree. Posthepatic jaundice is typically seen in biliary gallstones (choledolithiasis), carcinoma of the pancreatic head, cholangiocarcinoma, biliary atresia, and Mirizzi syndrome. Laboratory investigations show hypercholesterolemia, abnormal liver enzyme profile, and increased urinary urobilinogen level. Patients may present with purities due to the neuronal irritation of the dermal nerve endings by the urobilinogen in the skin.

Radiological modalities can be used as tools to define the cause or asses complications of jaundice. The following discussed diseases show well-documented radiological signs that can be looked for in assessing a patient with jaundice.

## Kernicterus

Kernicterus is a pathological condition characterized by choreoathetoid cerebral palsy, hearing loss, and mental retardation due to bilirubin accumulation in the subthalamic nucleus, hippocampus, globus pallidus, putamen, cranial nerves (*especially III, IV, and VI*), and thalami.

Up to 50 % of patients with kernicterus die, while survivors develop bilirubin encephalopathy with the previous described manifestations. In the early form of the disease, symptoms may mimic sepsis, asphyxia, or hypoglycemia.

*Signs* **on MRI**
On T2W and FLAIR images, there is typically high signal intensity observed in the globus pallidus bilaterally (*the preferential site of bilirubin deposition in the brain*) (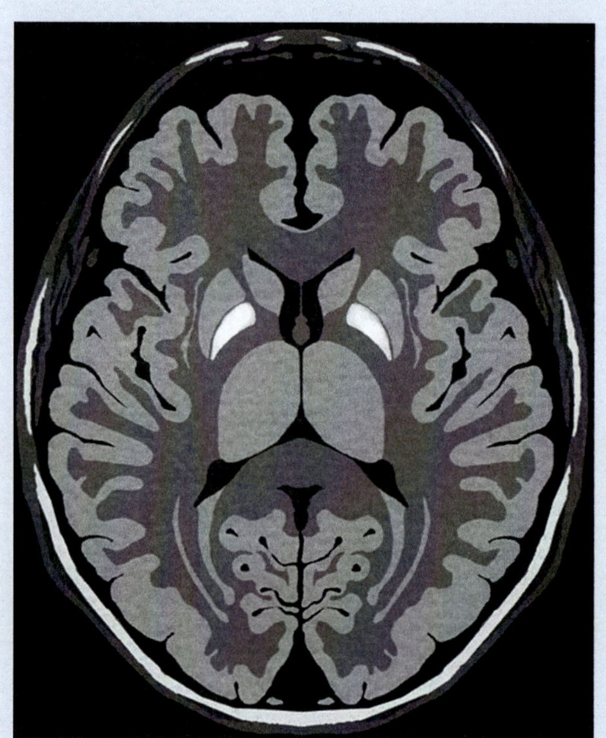 Fig. 1.7.1). Differential diagnosis of this MRI finding includes carbon monoxide poisoning, hypoglycemia, and hypoxia.

◻ **Fig. 1.7.1**    Axial, T2W MR illustration that demonstrates the brain findings in kernicterus. Differential diagnoses of such a sign include carbon monoxide poisoning, hypoglycemia, and hypoxia

## Obstructive Jaundice

Obstructive jaundice is a clinical condition characterized by systemic jaundice due to extrahepatic biliary duct drainage obstruction, with subsequent dilatation of the intrahepatic biliary tree radicals. The most common causes of obstructive jaundice are choledocholithiasis (bile ducts stones), pancreatitis, carcinoma of the ampulla of Vater, and choledochal cyst. Choledocholithiasis is found in approximately 15 % of patients undergoing cholecystectomy and usually results from migration of stones from the gallbladder to the CBD. Predisposing factors for choledocholithiasis include female sex, obesity, and older age.

### Signs on US

Cholestasis or intrahepatic biliary dilatation is diagnosed when the intrahepatic biliary radicals show dilatation (>2 mm in diameter) (◘ Figs. 1.7.2 and 1.7.3).

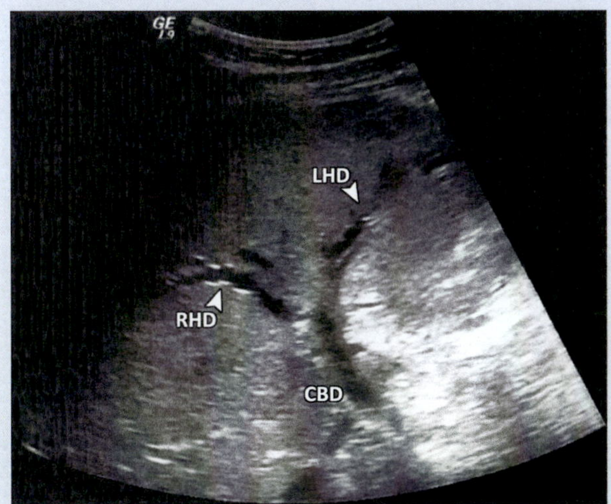


◘ **Fig. 1.7.2** Ultrasound liver image that shows dilatation of the main left hepatic duct (*LHD*) and right hepatic duct (*RHD*) (*arrowheads*) in a patient with obstructive jaundice

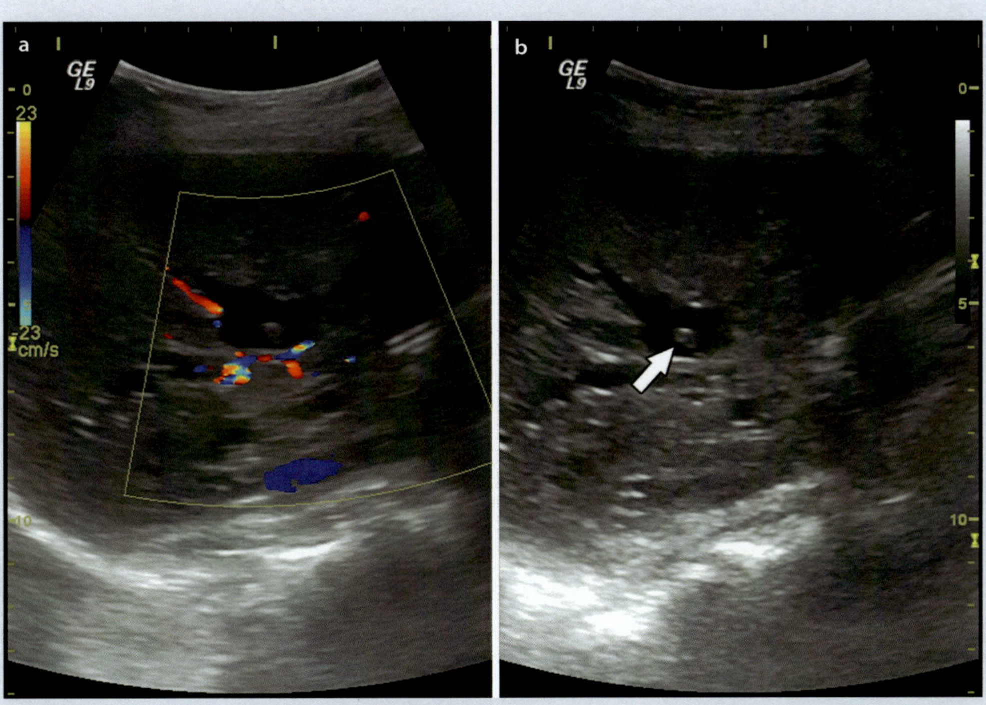


◘ **Fig. 1.7.3** B-Mode (**a**) and Doppler (**b**) ultrasound liver image of a patient with obstructive jaundice that shows dilatation of the intrahepatic biliary radicals and main duct with a biliary stone detected inside the intrahepatic bile duct (*arrow*)

### *Signs* on CT and MRI

1. The key radiological sign of obstructive jaundice is intrahepatic biliary plus extrahepatic biliary dilatation (■ Fig. 1.7.4).
2. The presence of gallbladder mild of calcium or stones further strengthens the diagnosis of obstructive jaundice due to choledocholithiasis (■ Fig. 1.7.4).
3. Signs of pancreatitis or carcinoma in the second part of duodenum may be detected.
4. Choledochal cyst is diagnosed by the presence of cystic lesion within the porta hepatis or within the CBD.

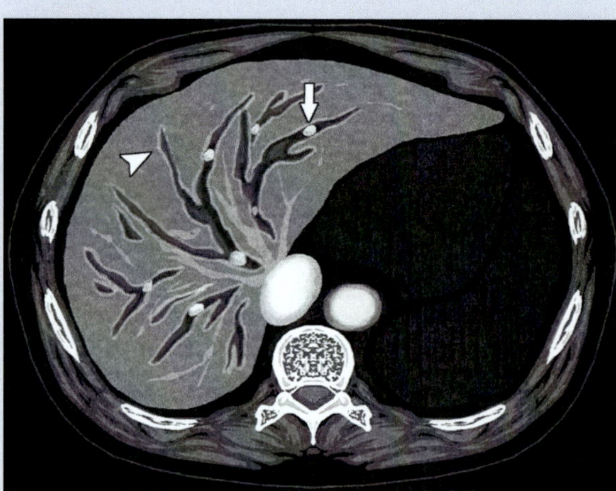

■ **Fig. 1.7.4**  Axial liver CT postcontrast illustration that demonstrates the findings in pyogenic cholangitis; the image illustrates dilatation of the internal biliary radicals with wall contrast enhancement (*arrowhead*) and the presence of biliary stones inside the dilated biliary ducts (*arrow*)

### *Signs* on MRCP

1. The CBD is dilated (>10 mm in diameter) with a filling defect inside the CBD representing stone if the cause of the obstructive jaundice is choledocholithiasis.
2. Choledochal cyst is detected as cystic dilatation of the CBD or the biliary radicals at the porta hepatis.

## Bile Plug Syndrome

Bile plug syndrome (BPS) is a disease characterized by extrahepatic biliary obstruction by inspissated pigmented bile sludge; BPS was first described in infants with maternal Rh and ABO blood group incompatibility, complicated by massive hemolysis. BPS can occur also in certain systemic conditions such as dehydration, hemolysis, and increased enterohepatic circulation in various intestinal diseases like Hirschsprung's disease, intestinal atresias, and stenoses.

BPS typically occurs in the absence of any anatomical abnormalities of the extrahepatic bile ducts. Newborns with BPS present with hepatomegaly, jaundice, and conjugated hyperbilirubinemia.

### *Signs* on US

BPS is commonly associated with enlarged gallbladder full of sludge observed in 20–30 % of ill newborns with jaundice and history of maternal Rh and ABO blood group incompatibility.

## Infectious Ascending Cholangitis

Infectious ascending cholangitis (IAC) is a condition characterized by inflammation of the extra- and intrahepatic bile duct dilatation due to infections, usually accompanied by the formation of infected, brown bile duct stones (choledocholithiasis). The main pathology in IAC is related to bile stasis, usually due to a stone, with superimposed infection

Patients with IAC typically present with right upper quadrant pain, fever, and jaundice (*Charcot's triad*), may be in association with confusion and hypotension (*Reynold's pentad*). Other symptoms include abdominal pain and discomfort and chills. IAC commonly affects male between 20 and 40 years of age. *Suppurative cholangitis* refers to the presence of pus within the biliary tree. Differentiation between suppurative and nonsuppurative cholangitis is crucial as the former requires urgent medical or surgical decompression. Discrimination can be established by CT.

*Oriental cholangitis*, also known as *recurrent pyogenic cholangitis*, is a rare disease characterized by recurrent or chronic infection of the bile ducts. The disease is usually found in Asian countries and arises due to parasitic infection with *Clonorchis sinensis* (Clonorchiasis).

### *Signs* on US

1. There is dilatation of the intrahepatic biliary ducts (>2 mm) (■ Fig. 1.7.2).
2. Stones may be found within the intrahepatic ducts (■ Fig. 1.7.3).
3. *Suppurative pyogenic cholangitis*: the CBD is dilated (>10 mm) and may show internal sludge, and the portal vein may show internal echoes due to thrombosis.

### *Signs* on CT and MRI

1. Typical imaging features of infectious ascending cholangitis include dilatation of the intra- and extrahepatic biliary ducts, thickening of the intrahepatic biliary radical walls with enhancement,

and the presence of stones within the biliary radicals ( Fig. 1.7.4). In the arterial phase of the liver scan, the liver may show heterogeneous parenchymal enhancement that may disappear in the portal or equilibrium phase; this heterogeneous enhancement is seen as patchy, nodular, geographical, or wedge-shaped parenchymal enhancement ( Fig. 1.7.5). This finding is often seen in suppurative cholangitis. The mechanism of this heterogeneous enhancement is related to the presence of arterioportal shunt, which can be also observed in other conditions like Budd–Chiari syndrome, hepatic congestion, acute cholecystitis, hepatic tumors, or hepatic abscesses.

2. In suppurative cholangitis, the duodenal papilla shows bulging into the second part of the duodenum and enhancement in a ringlike pattern (papillitis) due to the presence of pus within the CBD. This finding is characteristic to suppurative cholangitis and helps differentiating suppurative from nonsuppurative cholangitis.

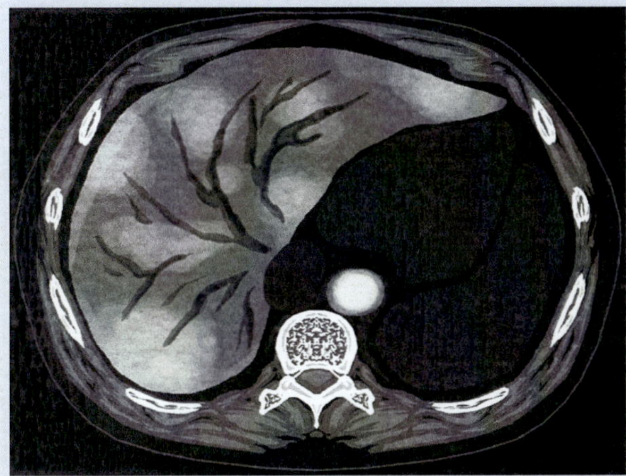

 Fig. 1.7.5 Axial liver CT arterial-phase, postcontrast illustration that demonstrates heterogeneous, patchy, nodular, geographical, or wedge-shaped liver parenchymal enhancement due to arterial shunting; this finding can be seen in pyogenic cholangitis among other differentials (*see text*)

## Choledochal Web

Choledochal web is defined as the presence of a mucosal web within the CBD that results in intermittent obstructive jaundice in neonates and children. Choledochal web is a rare cause of childhood intermittent jaundice. Obstructive jaundice may develop due to biliary sludge formation, mucus plugs, and choledocholithiasis.



## Selected References

Arai K, et al. Dynamic CT of acute cholangitis: early inhomogenous enhancement of the liver. AJR Am J Roentgenol. 2003;181:115–8.

Bader TR, et al. MR imaging findings of infectious cholangitis. Magn Reson Imaging. 2001;19:781–8.

Badley BWD. A physiological approach to jaundice. Clin Biochem. 1976;9(3):144–8.

Brown DM, et al. Bile plug syndrome: successful management with mucolytic agent. J Pediatr Surg. 1990;25:251–2.

Cebecauerova D, et al. Dual hereditary jaundice: simultaneous occurrence of mutations causing Gilbert's and Dubin-Johnson syndrome. Gastroenterology. 2005;129:315–20.

Germiller JA, et al. Early presentation of choledocal cyst transiently obstructed by an impissated bile plug. J Pediatr Surg. 1997;32:1522–5.

Hawes DA, et al. Imaging of the biliary sump syndrome. AJR Am J Roentgenol. 1992;158:315–9.

Kirks DR, et al. An imaging approach to persistent neonatal jaundice. AJR Am J Roentgenol. 1984;142:461–5.

Lee NK, et al. Discriminating of suppurative cholangitis from nonsuppurative cholangitis with computed tomography (CT). Eur J Radiol. 2009;69:528–35.

Mavrogiannis C, et al. Sump syndrome: endoscopic treatment and late recurrence. Am J Gastroenterol. 1999;94:972–5.

Mortelé KJ, et al. Usual and unusual causes of extrahepatic cholestasis: assessment with magnetic resonance cholangiography and fast MRI. Abdom Imaging. 2004;29:87–99.

Muhletaler CA, et al. Diagnosis of obstructive jaundice with nondilated bile duct. AJR Am J Roentgenol. 1980;134:1149–52.

Nazer H, et al. Crigler-Najjar syndrome in Saudi Arabia. Am J Med Genet. 1998;79:12–5.

Parekh HP, et al. Recurrent pyogenic cholangitis. Eur J Radiol Extra. 2003;47:121–3.

Shah Z, et al. MRI in kernicterus. Aust Radiol. 2003;47:55–7.

Shanser JD, et al. Computed tomographic diagnosis of obstructive jaundice in the absence of intrahepatic ductal dilatation. AJR Am J Roentgenol. 1978;131:389–92.

Sugama S, et al. Magnetic resonance imaging in three children with kernicterus. Pediatr Neurol. 2001;25:328–31.

Yonemitsu H, et al. Congenital extrahepatic portocaval shunt associated with hepatic hyperplastic nodules in a patient with Dubin-Johnson syndrome. Abdom Imaging. 2000;25:572–5.

## 1.8    Diarrhea and Malabsorption

Diarrhea is defined as passing loose stool >200 g/day. Chronic diarrhea is defined as diarrhea that persists >4 weeks, while severe diarrhea is defined as passing loose stool more than 6 times/day. Pathological diarrhea with serious cause is usually nocturnal, is associated with weight loss, contains bloody content, and is accompanied by fever. Lesions to the small intestine cause large volume watery diarrhea, whereas large intestine lesions cause small volume diarrhea with bloody or mucus contents.

*Malabsorption syndrome* is a term used to describe a group of disorders characterized by defective absorption of the main food elements (*carbohydrates, fat, and proteins*) from the small intestine, resulting in the passage of bulky, fatty, and foul-smell stool. Malabsorption syndrome can be due to:

1. *Sprue group*: including celiac disease and tropical sprue
2. *Constitutional diseases*: like Whipple's disease, scleroderma, and diabetes mellitus
3. *Small bowel diseases*: like intestinal lymphangiectasia
4. *Surgical operations*: like subtotal gastrectomy and small bowel resection

### Normal Anatomy

The cells of the small and the large intestine can be divided into three main functional cells:

1. *Absorptive epithelial cells* are composed of columnar epithelium that is found in the intestinal villi and absorb sodium, chloride, and nutrients. Generally, water absorption follows sodium absorption (up to 95 %).
2. *Secretory cells* are composed of goblet cells that are found in the intestinal crypts of Liberkühn and secrete chloride and bicarbonate in the intestine and chloride, bicarbonate, and potassium in the colon. Mucus is the largest component of colonic secretion by goblet cells, which protects the colonic epithelium from the fecal material.
3. *Enterochromaffin cells* are endocrine cells that secrete multiple neurotransmitters and endocrine peptides; they are found in the crypts of Liberkühn in the small intestine and colon. These cells are found in the small intestine only, not in the colon.

### Pathophysiology

Diarrhea is divided generally into two main types, watery and osmotic. *Watery diarrhea* arises due to increased chloride secretion, low sodium absorption, and increased intestinal motility. In contrast, *osmotic diarrhea* arises due to ingestion of osmotic, nonabsorbable material (e.g., *excess vitamin C intake diarrhea*) or the absence of brush-border enzyme required for digestion of food (e.g., *lactose intolerance*).

Three mechanisms of diarrhea have been described:

1. *Abnormal intestinal motility*: the enteric nervous system supplies the nervous supply to the smooth muscles in the intestinal and colonic walls. Inflammation of the neurons of the enteric system causes dysfunction of the intestinal wall's muscle movement, causing diarrhea or constipation. In intestinal inflammation, many inflammatory mediators such as *serotonin, acetylcholine, histamine, substance P, opioids*, and *dopamine* act like neurotransmitters for the enteric nervous system, augmenting the diarrhea effect by increasing intestinal motility.
2. *Decreased absorption*: any pathological condition that impedes the function of the absorptive cells in the small intestine will cause elevated water flux into the colon. When this water flux exceeds 4.5 l/day, diarrhea arises. Decreased absorption of sodium or other osmolar metabolites (e.g., *lactose*) can induce diarrhea by drawing the water from the blood in the intestinal walls into the lumen, increasing the water flux into the colon. Common osmolar agents that cause diarrhea include bile acids and their bacterial metabolites, gluten from wheat (celiac disease), and ascorbic acid (vitamin C).
3. *Increased secretion*: this mechanism involves increased secretion of chloride into the colonic lumen, which will cause drawing of water from the blood in the colonic wall into the colonic lumen, causing diarrhea. Any pathological condition that increases chloride secretion in the colon will cause "secretory diarrhea." Chloride secretion is increased by any pathological process that increases "cyclic nucleotides" (cAMP and cGMP) and/or "intracellular calcium" levels in the colonic cells, which will open the "cystic fibrosis transmembrane conductance regulator" (CFTR). Vasoactive intestinal peptide (VIP) is a molecule that works as a neurotransmitter causing increased chloride channel opening by raising cyclic AMP within the colonic and intestinal secretory cells; this form of diarrhea can be seen due to pancreatic neuroendocrine tumor (VIPoma).

### Common Causes of Diarrhea and Their Mechanism of Action

1. *Cholera*: cholera toxin also causes secretory diarrhea via raising cAMP in the secretory cells, like VIPoma.
2. *Celiac disease*: the gluten from the wheat is converted by the intestinal bacteria into a toxic metabolite called "gliadin." Gliadin causes inflammatory destruction of the intestinal villi, reducing absorption and causing osmotic diarrhea.
3. *Food allergy*: food allergy causes the release of histamine, which raises cAMP in secretory cells causing secretory diarrhea.
4. *Short bowel syndrome*: bile salts are absorbed in the terminal ileum and the ileocecal valve. Any disease that affects the terminal ileum (e.g., *Crohn's disease, tuberculosis, ileocecal valve syndrome*) will cause reduction of bile salt absorbance, causing bile salts to

enter the colon. In the colon, bile salts stimulate water and chloride secretion, resulting in osmotic diarrhea. Short bowel syndrome is a term used to describe symptoms related to dysfunctional terminal ileum (e.g., *bloating, diarrhea, fecal urgency, fecal incontinence*), with loss of bile salts in the colon.

5. *Infectious diarrhea*: infectious causes like bacteria (*Salmonella, E. coli, Shigella*), viruses (*Rotavirus*), and parasites (*E. histolytica, Giardia, Cryptosporidium*) all cause diarrhea by releasing enterotoxins, which causes inflammatory reaction releasing histamine, nitric oxide, and serotonin. The diarrhea in infection is a mixture between osmotic (*due to villi destruction*) and secretory (*due to raised cAMP*).

6. *Endocrine diarrhea*: many endocrine disorders cause diarrhea by secreting neurotransmitters such as VIP, serotonin, acetylcholine, substance P, and calcitonin, all of which cause secretory diarrhea. Also, some tumors cause diarrhea via secretion of the same neurotransmitters and hormones, for example, carcinoid tumors (*serotonin*), pancreatic neuroendocrine tumors (*VIP, gastrine*), and medullary thyroid carcinoma (*calcitonin*).

## Sprue

Sprue is a term used to describe diseases characterized pathologically by flattening, broadening, and coalescence of villi and sometimes complete loss of villi. Moreover, the lamina propria is infiltrated with lymphocytes, plasma cells, and eosinophils.

Sprue can be divided into tropical sprue and nontropical sprue, also known as celiac disease. *Tropical sprue* is a geographically localized form of malabsorption (*in some tropical areas*) that is characterized by folic acid deficiency; the disease responses dramatically to folic acid or antibiotics therapy. *Celiac disease*, on the other hand, is a disease characterized by autoimmune reaction that causes villi destruction after ingesting food that contains "gluten," like wheat, rye, oats, and barley.

Patients with sprue, like other malabsorption syndromes, present with steatorrhea, weight loss, and abdominal distension. The mucosal abnormalities in sprue tend to be more marked in the jejunum than in the ileum. Patients respond well to gluten-free diet. Celiac disease is seen in patients with type 1 diabetes mellitus, Down's syndrome, primary biliary cirrhosis, Sjögren's syndrome, and dermatitis herpetiformis (100 %).

*Ulcerative jejunoileitis* is an uncommon complication of celiac disease characterized by multiple benign ulcers of variable depth that is found predominantly in the jejunum, occasionally in the ileum, and rarely in the colon. Patients often present with fever, weight loss, abdominal pain, anorexia, and diarrhea.

Serological test to detect celiac disease includes detection of serum gliadin IgA antibodies (95 % sensitive) and endomysial antibodies (95 % sensitive and specific). The gold standard test for diagnosis of celiac disease is jejunal biopsy.

- ■ **Q: What Are the Main Differences Between Celiac Disease and Tropical Sprue?**

1. Tropical sprue is associated with folic acid deficiency, while celiac disease is associated with gluten-rich diet.
2. Tropical sprue patients respond well to folic acid and antibiotic therapy, while celiac disease patients respond well to gluten-free diet.
3. Both have the same radiological and histological features, so history and clinical background of the patient's recent travels are essential in differentiating the two conditions.

*Signs* **on US**

1. The signs more frequently recorded in celiac disease include fluid-distended small bowel loops, thickened valvulae conniventes, and increased small bowel peristalsis; this picture is the equivalent of the well-described *reversed jejunoileal fold pattern*.
2. There is increased caliber of the superior mesenteric artery in patients with celiac disease ranging from 8 to 11 mm, 2–3 cm distal to the artery origin.

*Signs* **on Barium Follow-Through**

1. *Dilatation*: there is significant dilatation of the small bowel loops, usually in the mid- and distal jejunum (*constant finding in sprue*).
2. *Segmentation*: this term applies to moderately large masses of separated barium associated with dilated bowel loops. Stringlike strands of barium may be found between the masses representing barium in collapsed bowel loops. Segmentation is best seen in the ileum in advanced cases.
3. *Hypersecretion*: this refers to large amount of fluids secreted into the intestinal lumen and causes barium dilution, which is seen as barium flocculation (*mostly a constant finding in sprue*).
4. *Transient time abnormalities*: transient time is the time required for the barium to traverse the small intestine and enter the cecum (*average 3 h in adults*). In sprue, the transient time is prolonged (3–5 h) or shortened (<30 min) depending on the disease activity.
5. *Moulage phenomenon*: it is a term used to describe the radiographic appearance of an intestinal lumen with complete destruction of the intestinal folds. The barium-filled lumen resembles a tube into which "wax" has been poured and allowed to harden.

### Signs on Abdominal CT

1. There may be *intussusception*, which is detected on axial view as "target sign" with crescent hypodense area inside it representing the mesentery. Enhancing mesenteric vessels within the mass is frequently seen (very characteristic).
2. *Ulcerative jejunoileitis* is an uncommon complication where patients present clinically with abdominal pain, weight loss, fever, and anorexia. There is thickening and ulceration of the jejunal and ileal mucosa.
3. *Cavitating lymph node syndrome* is a rare severe complication of celiac disease characterized clinically by weight loss, anorexia, and diarrhea. Mortality rate is up to 50 % due to sepsis. There is lymphadenopathy (2–7 cm in diameter) with characteristic fat–fluid level. Differential diagnosis includes lymphoma and bacterial infection (◘ Fig. 1.8.1).
4. *Malignancy* is detected on CT as a focal bowel wall thickening with lumen narrowing. Malignancies associated with celiac disease include lymphoma, adenocarcinoma, and squamous cell carcinoma.

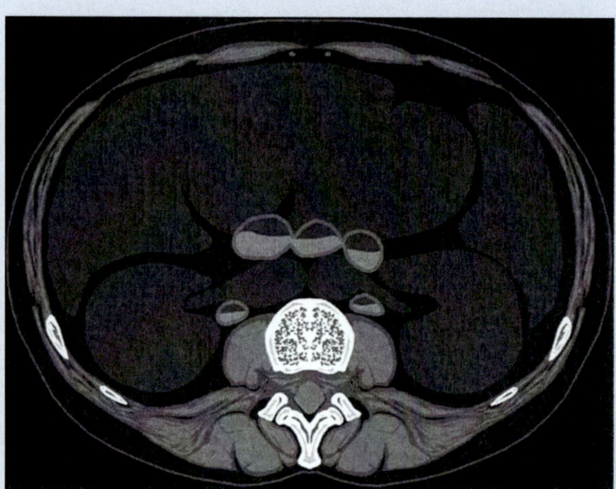

◘ **Fig. 1.8.1**  Axial abdomen CT illustration that demonstrates the cavitating lymph nodes seen in celiac disease, most commonly affecting the retroperitoneal and the mesenteric lymph nodes

### Signs on Neurological CT

Celiac disease patients may experience attacks of seizures (1.2–5 % of cases). When neurological manifestations of celiac disease appear, there are commonly bilateral cortico-subcortical occipital calcifications without contrast enhancement or brain atrophy (◘ Fig. 1.8.2).

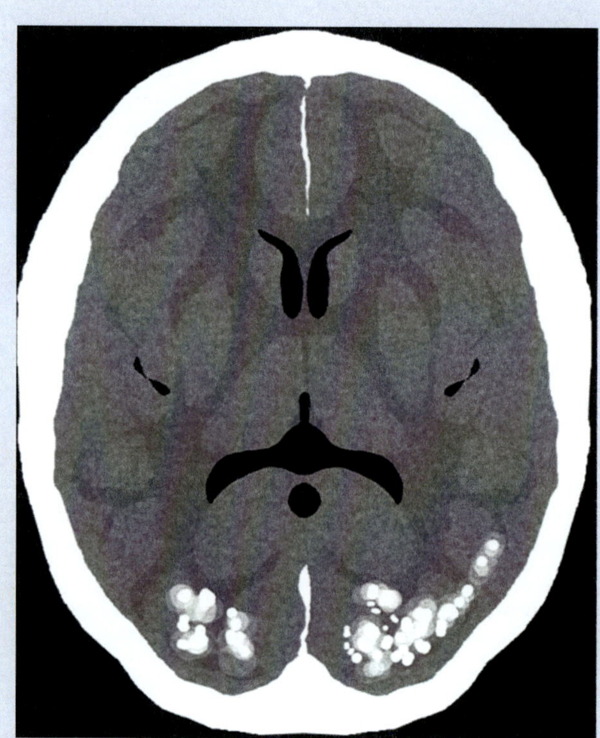

◘ **Fig. 1.8.2**  Axial brain CT illustration that demonstrates the rare sign of occipital calcification seen in neuro-celiac disease

#### ■ ■ Signs of Celiac Disease on MR Enteroclysis

1. *Fold pattern abnormalities*: the valvulae conniventes can appear *normal (most common)*, *squared end (rather than normal round shaped)*, *reversed jejunal folds (decreased folds in jejunum and increased in ileum)*, and *moulage sign (the absence of valvulae due to total atrophy)*.
2. In *reversed jejunal pattern*, jejunal folds are decreased if the number of folds <3-folds per inch, and ileal folds are increased if the number of folds >5 per inch.
3. Bowel wall thickening (>4 mm) is a common fining.
4. Mesenteric lymphadenopathy is found in 45 % of cases. When the lymphadenopathy is associated with thickening of bowel wall segments, lymphoma should be suspected (*the commonest malignancy in celiac disease*).
5. In *ulcerative jejunoileitis*, there is a circumferential thickening of bowel wall with a bilaminar configuration, bowel wall deep ulcers, and mucosal hyper-enhancement (*characteristic in patients with celiac disease*).

## Whipple's Disease (Intestinal Lipodystrophy)

Whipple's disease (WD) is a rare, multisystemic, infectious disease characterized by destruction of the intestinal villi and the lamina propria by macrophages that stain positive with periodic acid of Schiff (PAS) stain due to engulfed glycoprotein material.

WD is caused by slow-growing, intracellular, gram-positive bacterium called *Tropheryma whipplei*. Humans are the only known host for this infection. Diagnosis is confirmed by detecting these PAS stain-positive macrophages after intestinal biopsy.

Patients with WD clinically complain of steatorrhea, weight loss, abdominal distension and tenderness, skin pigmentation, lymphadenopathy (usually mesenteric), and intermittent, nondeforming, migratory arthritis (80 % of cases). Other manifestations include the eye, heart, and nervous system abnormalities. Neurological manifestations of WD include supranuclear gaze palsy, cognitive changes, ataxia, dementia, and seizures.

*Signs* **on Barium Follow-Through**

Unlike sprue, WD usually shows minimal signs of segmentation and dilatation in comparison to sprue. However, there is marked thickening of the mucosal folds, with maybe slightly nodular pattern on barium films (*most prominent radiological finding in WD*).

*Signs* **on MRI**

On brain T2W and FLAIR images, there may be areas of hyperintensities affecting both temporomesial regions, basal ganglia, thalami, internal capsule, the quadrigeminal plate, and around the third ventricle seen in patients with neuro-Whipple disease (■ Fig. 1.8.3).

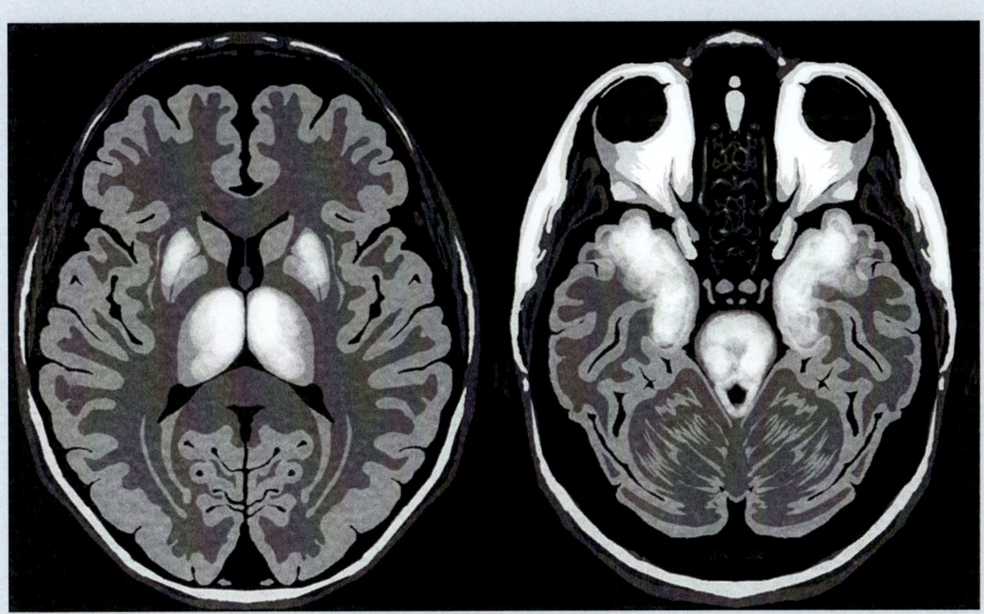

■ **Fig. 1.8.3** Axial brain T2W MR illustration that demonstrates the MR findings in patients with neuro-Whipple disease

## VIPoma (Werner–Morris Syndrome/ Pancreatic Cholera)

Vasoactive intestinal peptide-secreting tumor (VIPoma) is a disease characterized by *W*atery *D*iarrhea, *H*ypokalemia, and low or absence of gastric acid secretion or *A*chlorhydria (sometimes referred to also as *WDHA syndrome*), as classically defined in the medical literature.

Vasoactive intestinal peptide (VIP) induces smooth muscle relaxation of the gastrointestinal tract, stimulating water secretion into pancreatic juices and bile, inhibits gastric acid secretion, and inhibits absorption from the intestine. VIPoma may occur as part of multiple endocrine neoplasia type 1 (MEN 1) or may coexist with bronchogenic carcinoma.

Patients with VIPoma are usually 40 years old typically presenting with massive watery diarrhea with fecal fluid losses amounting to more than 10 l per day in some reported cases. The diarrhea has ranged from a few months to up to 15 years. Other features include weight loss, abdominal pain, nausea, and vomiting. Hypokalemia manifests during attack resulting in lethargy and marked muscular weakness.

Typically, most investigations are normal including upper GI endoscopy, barium enema studies, enteroclysis, stool culture for parasitic ova, and urinary 5-HIAA. Urinary levels of 5-hydroxyindole acetic acid (5-HIAA) are used to detect carcinoid tumors of the enterochromaffin cells of the small intestine. 5-HIAA determines the body's levels of serotonin.

Patients with renal failure may show falsely low levels of 5-HIAA. Serum potassium levels are usually low during the diarrheal attacks. Impaired glucose tolerance test has been observed in several patients with VIPoma and was attributed to a secondary effect of chronic hypokalemia. Hypercalcemia and acidosis are other laboratory features in VIPoma.

> *Signs* on CT and MRI
> 1. Up to 50 % of VIPoma have distant metastases at the time of presentation, usually to the liver and lungs.
> 2. The tumor is detected in the body or the tail of pancreas (75 %) or in the head of the pancreas (25 % of cases). On MRI, the tumor is detected with an intermediate signal on T1W images and high signal intensity on T2W images. Enhancement may be seen. Liver metastases are commonly detected (50 % of cases), which can assist in the diagnosis of VIPoma, taking into consideration the history, clinical presentation, and laboratory investigation of the patient.

## Selected Readings

Binder HJ. Causes of chronic diarrhea. N Engl J Med. 2006;355(3):236–9.

Buckle MJ, et al. Neurologically presenting Whipple disease: case report and review of the literature. J Clin Pathol. 2008;61:1140–1.

Buckley O, et al. The imaging of coeliac disease and its complications. Eur J Radiol. 2008;65:483–90.

Castiglione F, et al. Bowel sonography in adult celiac disease: diagnostic accuracy and ultrasonographic features. Abdom Imaging. 2007;32:73–7.

Gobbi G. Coeliac disease, epilepsy and cerebral calcifications. Brain Dev. 2005;27:189–200.

Kaiser L, et al. Infectious causes of chronic diarrhea. Best Pract Res Clin Gastroenterol. 2012;26(5):563–71.

Kunzelmann K, et al. Electrolyte transport in the mammalian colon: mechanisms and implications for disease. Physiol Rev. 2002;82(1):245–89.

Marshak RH, et al. Malabsorption syndrome. Semin Roentgenol. 1966;1(2):138–77.

Moser PP, et al. CT findings of increased splanchnic circulation in a case of celiac sprue. Abdom Imaging. 2004;29: 15–7.

Puget M, et al. Whipple's disease with muscle impairment. Muscle Nerve. 2006;34:794–8.

Sofka CM, et al. MR imaging of metastatic pancreatic VIPoma. Magn Reson Imaging. 1997;15(10):1205–8.

# Neurology




© Springer International Publishing Switzerland 2017
J.A. Al-Tubaikh, *Internal Medicine*, DOI 10.1007/978-3-319-39747-4_2

## 2.1 Stroke (Brain Infarction)

Stroke means the death of brain cells (infarction) due to ischemia or emboli.

The most common causes of stroke are atherosclerosis, embolic vascular occlusion, hypertension, and inflammatory vascular diseases (vasculitis). Patients present with sudden neurological deficits in the body according to the area of the brain affected. Up to 75 % of all cerebral infarctions occur due to middle cerebral artery occlusion. Occlusion of the posterior inferior cerebellar artery (PICA) causes infarction of the lateral medulla plus the inferior cerebellar peduncles (*Wallenberg's syndrome*).

- Imaging strokes involves the assessment of four Ps:
- *Parenchyma*: assess the area of stroke and excludes hemorrhage (checked by unenhanced CT).
- *Pipes*: assess the extra- and intracerebral blood vessels (carotid and vertebral arteries). Scanning for CTA should start from the head to the aortic arch.
- *Perfusion*: assess cerebral blood volume (CBV), cerebral blood flow (CBF), and mean transit time (MTT).
- *Penumbra*: the concept of penumbra in stroke refers to the salvageable brain tissue. When a vascular insult occurs, the infarcted tissue is surrounded by a region of stunned tissue due to reduction of the blood flow within the affected region. The identification of the penumbra helps the decision of using thrombolytics in acute stroke cases. On CT, the penumbra is assessed by showing parameters' mismatch, while on MR, it is assessed by showing diffusion/perfusion mismatch. Penumbra = MTT minus CBV.

Thrombolytics are not given to stroke patients beyond 3 h from the start of the symptoms due to the risk of hemorrhage. Hemorrhage is an absolute contraindication for thrombolytic therapy. Stroke is evaluated on unenhanced CT, CT angiography, and CT perfusion study.

*Hemorrhagic infarction* is usually caused by hypertension or embolic occlusion. Hemorrhagic infarctions arise due to two mechanisms:

- *Venous thrombosis*: the high flowing arterial blood is obstructed by a blocked vein, which raises the intracapillary pressure causing them to rupture and bleed.
- *Arterial embolism*: the embolus blocks the artery, and in some times a small hole develops within the embolus making blood gush into the capillaries with high speed and pressure, causing them to rupture and bleed.

*Lacunar infarctions (cerebral microangiopathy)* are infarctions less than 1 cm in size and occur due to occlusion of the penetrating arterioles of the brain parenchyma. Usually, they are seen in the basal ganglia, the thalamus, and the internal capsule. Lacunar infarctions are commonly seen in diabetic patients.

## Differential Diagnoses and Related Diseases

*Pusher syndrome* is a very specific disease of postural orientation, commonly affecting poststroke hemiparetic patients. In the pusher syndrome, patients use their nonparetic arm and/or leg to actively push from the nonparalyzed side toward the paralyzed, which results in loss of balance and falling toward the paralyzed side (◘ Fig. 2.1.1). These patients also resist any attempt to correct their tilted body posture toward the vertical upright position. Pusher syndrome can be seen in up to 10 % of patients with hemiparesis due to strokes. Pusher syndrome may be also arising due to brain trauma or tumors.

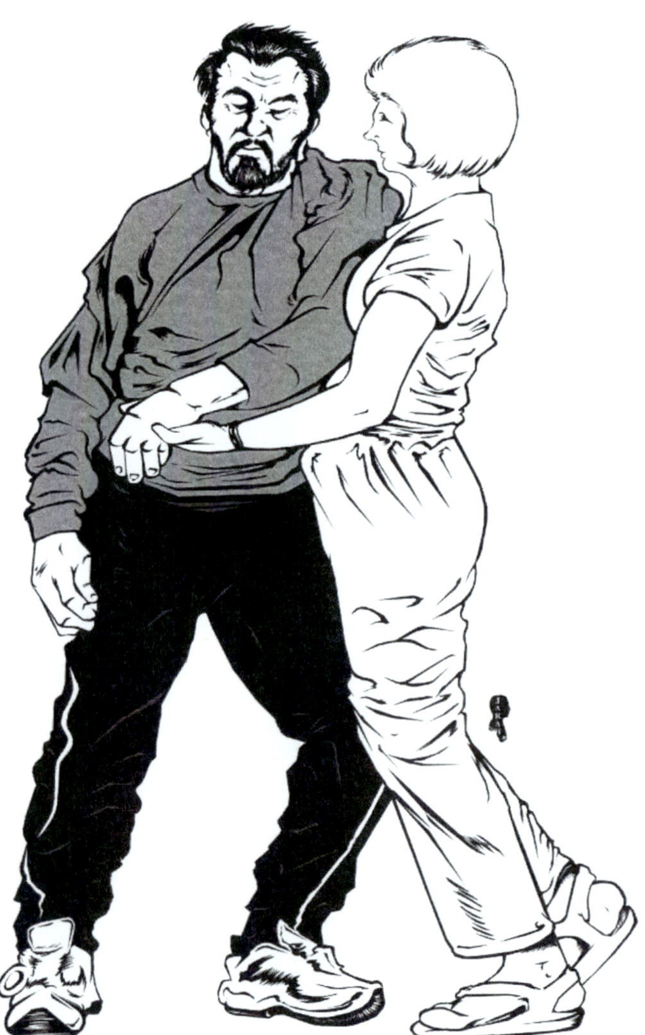

◘ Fig. 2.1.1 An illustration demonstrates pusher syndrome; the patient is actively pushing and extending his right side (nonparalytic side) toward the left side (paralytic side), which is assisted by the nurse

### Signs on CT

— *Hyperacute stage* (the first 3–6 h): unenhanced CT usually is normal. It must be repeated after this period within 24–48 h.

— *Acute stage* (from 6 to 24 h): nonenhanced CT shows a wedge-shaped hypodense area surrounded by edema that may cause mass effect on the ventricles with effacement of the cerebral sulci (◘ Fig. 2.1.2a).

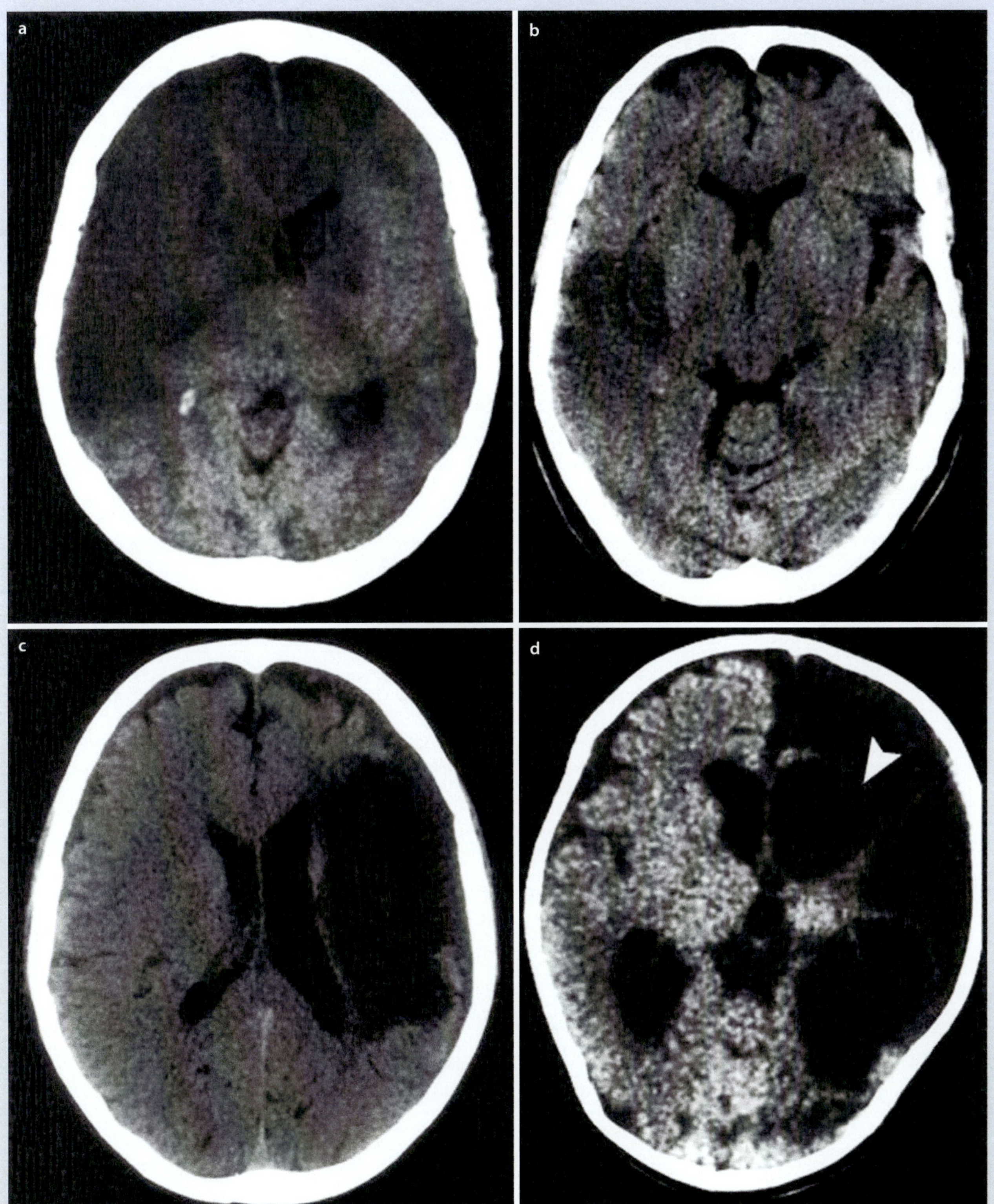

◘ **Fig. 2.1.2**   Multiple axial CT of the brain with different stages of infarction: (**a**) acute infarction, (**b**) subacute infarction, (**c**) chronic infarction with gliosis, and (**d**) chronic infarction with formation of porencephalic cyst (*arrowhead*)

The hypodense lesion follows a vascular territory (Fig. 2.1.3). Cytotoxic edema starts after 30 min from the stroke attack, and vasogenic edema starts from 4 to 6 h postattack. Each increase in 1 % of parenchymal edema reduces the Hounsfield unit (HU) by 2.5 HU.

- *Subacute stage* (days to weeks): there is a hypodense lesion without edema (Fig. 2.1.2b). Edema resolves and the mass effect decreases at 7–10 days postattack.
- *Chronic stage* (more than 3 months postattack): the tissues around the lesion will lose their volume (gliosis), which will cause negative pressure upon the adjacent ventricles, causing their dilatation (*evacuee dilatation*) (Fig. 2.1.2c). When the evacuee dilatation is massive, the negative pressure causes the ventricle to open into the infarction, creating a porencephalic cyst (Fig. 2.1.2d). *Porencephalic cyst* is a cerebrospinal fluid cyst that is communicating with the ventricles.
- *Hyperdense vessel sign*: on nonenhanced CT, a thrombosed vessel may appear as a hyperdense structure due to the thrombus within it. Normal blood measures 40–60 HU and is normally not seen on nonenhanced CT, while thrombosed blood measures 77–80 HU and can appear on nonenhanced CT. The thrombosed blood vessels are usually asymmetric, and bilateral symmetrical hyperdense vessel is unlikely to be thrombosis.
- *Obscuration of the lentiform nucleus*: hypoattenuation and obscuration of the lentiform nucleus due to cytotoxic edema are another signs of acute infarction.
- *Insular ribbon sign*: it refers to hypoattenuation of the insular region with loss of the gray–white matter definition.
- *HU window alteration*: the standard HU window setting is 80 HU widths and 20 HU center. If no abnormality in attenuation is seen in the image, lower the window to 8 HU widths and 32 HU center. The last settings increase the sensitivity for detection of hypodense areas.*Luxury perfusion*: When you inject contrast into an acute infarction, you'll get contrast diffusion as multiple lines into the gyri (Fig. 2.1.4). This sign appears within the first 3 days of the attack. It is best recalled by Elster's rule of 3 (as early as 3 days, maximum at 3 days to 3 weeks and gone by 3 months).
- *Hemorrhagic infarction* is seen as an area of hyperdense blood within the brain parenchyma surrounded by hypodense area of cytotoxic edema.
- *Lacunar infarction* is seen as a small (<2 cm), hypodense area within the brain parenchyma with no mass effect (Fig. 2.1.5).
- Disruption of the normal circle of Willis branches is classically detected in stroke (Fig. 2.1.6).

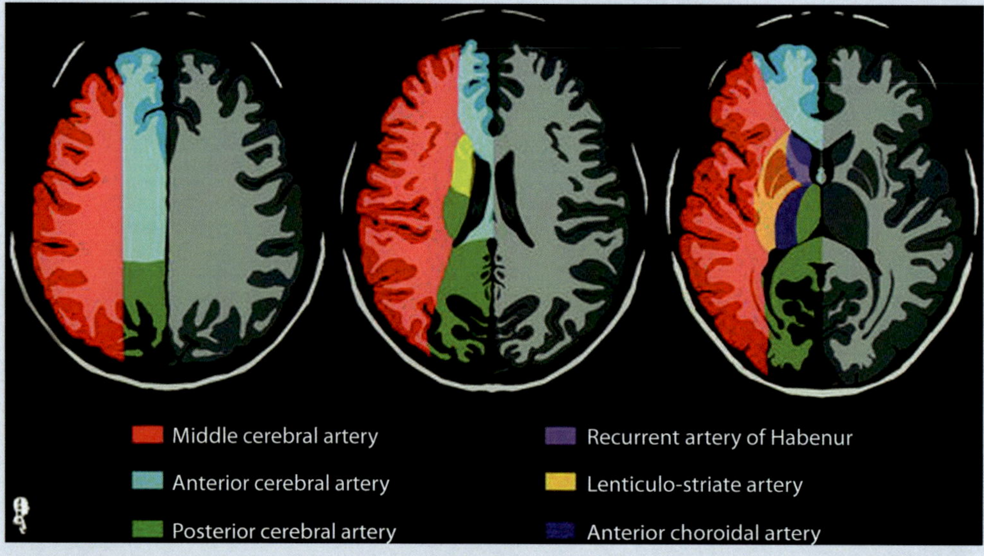


**Fig. 2.1.3**  Sequential axial brain MR illustrations demonstrate different vascular territories of the brain parenchyma

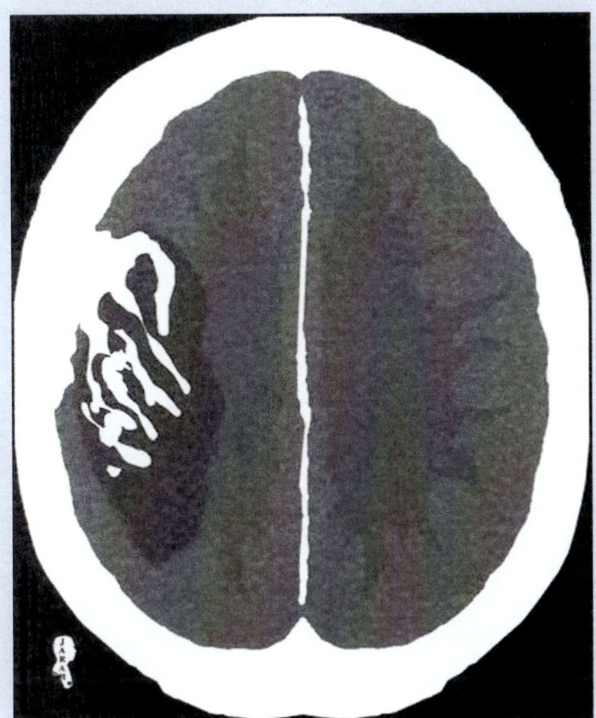

**Fig. 2.1.4** Axial brain CT illustration demonstrates infarction within the vascular region of the middle cerebral artery with multiple enhanced lines inside it representing luxury perfusion

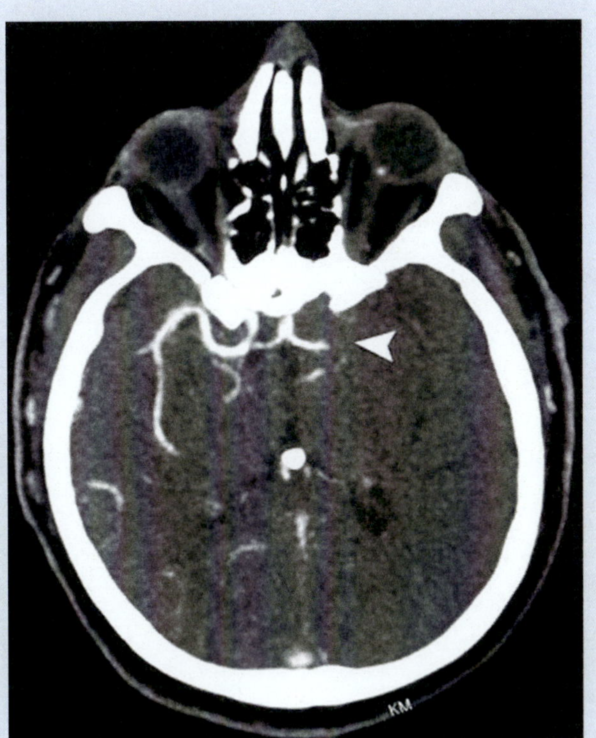

**Fig. 2.1.6** Axial brain CTA image of a patient with left brain infarction shows blockage of the left middle cerebral artery (M1) segment (*arrowhead*)

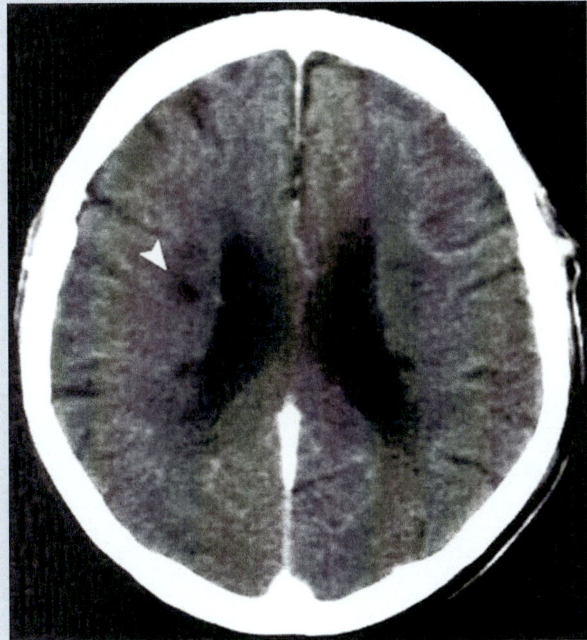

**Fig. 2.1.5** Axial brain CT image shows acute lacunar infarction in the right centrum semiovale with small ring of cytotoxic edema around it (*arrowhead*)

### Signs on MRI and DWI
- *Hyperattenuated vessel sign*: it is seen on T2* images as hyperintense vessel (like on unenhanced CT images).
- *T2* images*: they are very sensitive to detect hemorrhage and microhemorrhages. Hemorrhage is seen as areas of abnormal blooming, while hemosiderin is seen as areas of low signal intensities.
- *DWI*: areas of infarction are seen as areas of high signal intensity due to water motion impedance (cytotoxic edema), usually 30 min from the start of the attack (**Fig. 2.1.7**). On the ADC map, the areas of high signal intensity on DWI show low signal intensity. Chronic infarction shows low signal intensity on DWI and high signal intensity on ACD maps. The two must be assessed together to diagnose chronic infarction. DWI is accurate in detecting brain stem and lacunar infarctions.
- *MR spectroscopy* in infarction shows high lactate and low *N*-acetyl aspartate, choline, and creatine (present up to 5 weeks postattack).

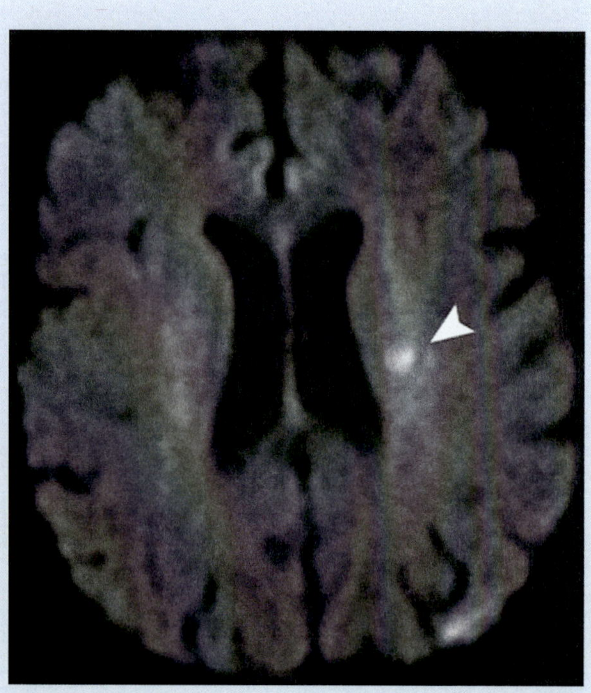

**Fig. 2.1.7**    Axial brain DWI shows acute lacunar infarction in the left paraventricular area (*arrowhead*)

## Further Reading


de Lucas EM, et al. CT protocol for acute stroke: tips and tricks for general radiologists. Radiographics. 2008;28:1673–87.

Johannsen L, et al. "Pusher syndrome" following cortical lesions that spare the thalamus. J Neurol. 2006;253: 455–63.

Karnath H-O. Pusher syndrome – a frequent but little-known disturbance of body orientation reception. J Neurol. 2007;254:414–24.

Mullins ME. The hyperdense cerebral artery sign on CT scan. Semin Ultrasound CT MR. 2005;26:394–403.

Shetty SK, et al. CT perfusion in acute stroke. Neuroimaging Clin N Am. 2005;15:481–501.

Srinivasan A, et al. State-of-the-art imaging of acute stroke. RadioGraph. 2006;26:S75–95.

Vu D, et al. Non-contrast CT in acute stroke. Semin Ultrasound CT MR. 2005;26:380–6.


## 2.2    Stroke Diseases and Syndromes

Stroke can be a symptom rather than an actual disease. Some systemic diseases present in the form of stroke. Other diseases or syndromes are associated with stroke as one of their diagnostic criteria. Some syndromes or diseases arise due to stroke in a certain area of the brain. This topic discusses some of the known and uncommon causes, syndromes, and diseases of stroke.

### Moyamoya Disease (Progressive Occlusive Arteritis)

Moyamoya disease is characterized by a progressive occlusion of arteries of the circle of Willis due to intimal wall thickening of the distal internal carotid artery and its proximal anterior cerebral artery branch bilaterally, with the formation of abnormal collateral networks that develop adjacent to the stenotic vessel. These collaterals give the shape of a puff of smoke, which is called "moyamoya" in Japanese.

Moyamoya disease is a rare disease worldwide but with high incidence in Japanese. Occlusion usually occurs in both hemispheres, but unilateral occlusion can occur. The disease can be seen in association with sickle cell disease and neurofibromatosis.

The disease peaks in the first decade and dips in the fourth decade. Patients present in young age with recurrent strokes, headaches, and behavioral disturbance. The disease can be suspected in a young adult presenting with stroke, with no predisposing factors. Diagnosis is essentially established by angiography or MR angiography.

> **Signs on CT, MRI, and MR Angiography**
> - Large network of collaterals in the basal ganglia and brain stem fed by the internal carotid artery, the basilar artery, and the anterior cerebral artery giving the appearance of a puff of smoke (pathognomonic) (Fig. 2.2.1).
> - On T1W images, there are multiple hypointense, flow void lesions located in the basal ganglia representing the abnormal collateral networks (Fig. 2.2.2).

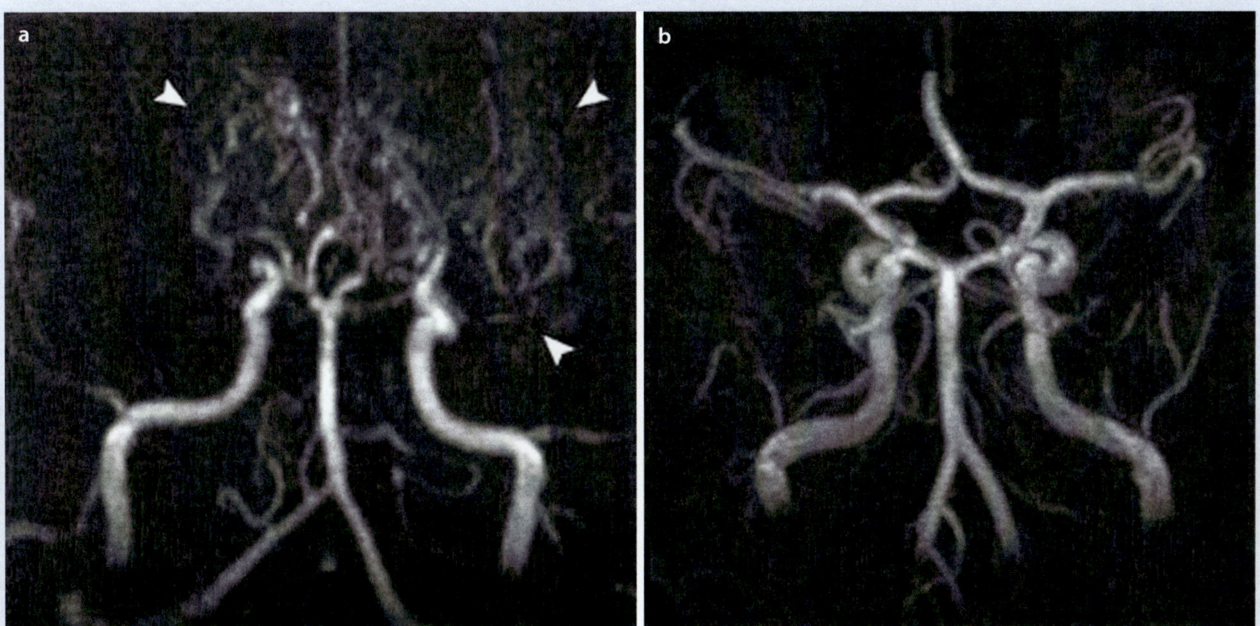

**Fig. 2.2.1** MR angiography of a patient with moyamoya disease (**a**) and MR angiography in a normal healthy patient (**b**) for comparison. In (**a**), there is irregular arterial collateral formation in the region of the anterior cerebral arteries bilaterally in figure (**a**) (*arrowheads*), with complete disappearance of the middle cerebral artery (MCA) (M1 segment). Compare the image in (**a**) with the normal MRI appearance of the circle of Willis in (**b**)

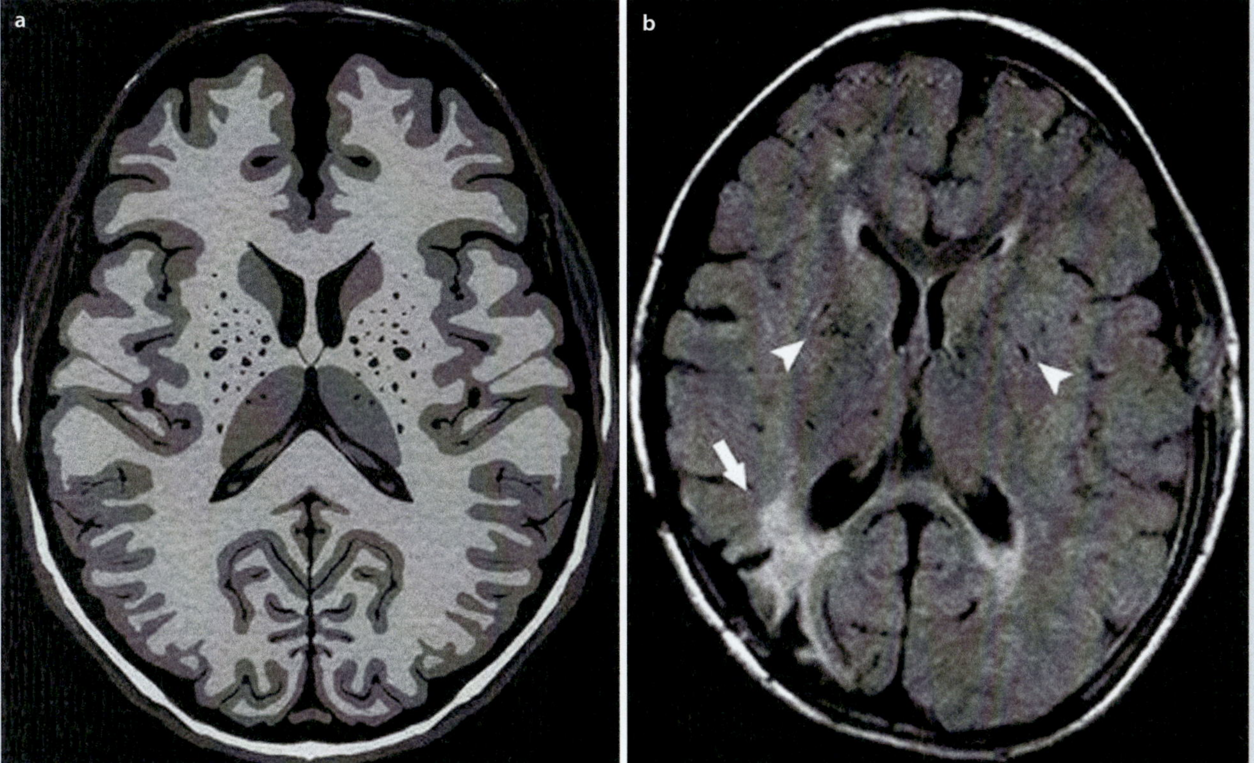

**Fig. 2.2.2** Axial T1W brain MR illustration (**a**) with axial FLAIR MRI (**b**) of a patient with moyamoya disease shows multiple flow void signal intensities in the region of the basal ganglia bilaterally representing the abnormal collateral formation (*arrowheads*). Leukoencephalopathy at the region of the posterior horns of the lateral ventricles (**b**) can be seen (*arrow*) affecting the right side more than the left side

## Cerebral Amyloid Angiopathy

Cerebral amyloid angiopathy (CAA) is a disease that occurs due to deposition of a protein (AB peptide) or amyloid substance in the arteriolar wall of the cerebral vessels, causing weakening and fragility of blood vessel walls. Later, intracerebral bleeding develops due to spontaneous blood vessel rupture.

In CAA, amyloid proteins replace the contractile element of the arteriolar muscle layer, leading to increased fragility of the walls. CAA is not a part of systemic amyloidosis, and it is the most common cause of spontaneous, nontraumatic intracranial bleeding in nonhypertensive elderly patients.

CAA should be suspected when an elderly patient (60 years) presents with unexplained spontaneous intracranial bleeding that is lobar and located very superficial in the cortex. It is responsible for up to 20 % of nontraumatic brain hemorrhage and hemorrhagic infarction and up to 30 % of lobar bleeding.

CAA can be associated with Alzheimer's disease, with dementia occurring in up to 40 % of cases. Dementia in CAA patients occurs and progresses much faster than dementia in patients with Alzheimer's disease. Diagnosis of CAA is usually done by clinical history and the radiological features of the CT or the MRI.

### Signs on CT and MRI

- Acute intracranial bleeding area (lobar hemorrhage) is seen as high-density area on CT images or with high T1/T2 signal intensities on MRI that is located in the superficial cortex and the subcortical white matter (◘ Figs. 2.2.3 and 2.2.4), with a distribution different from those resulting from hypertensive bleeding (usually deep within the brain). Bleeding due to CAA is characteristically multiple, spares the basal ganglia and brain stem, and is located at the corticomedullary junction.
- On MRI, multiple chronic microhemorrhages are seen as signal void, a few millimeters in size hypointense lesions in the deep white and the subcortical white matter on T2* images (◘ Fig. 2.2.3).
- CAA affects commonly the frontal and the parietal lobes. Up to 10–50 % of cases bleed in more than one lobe.

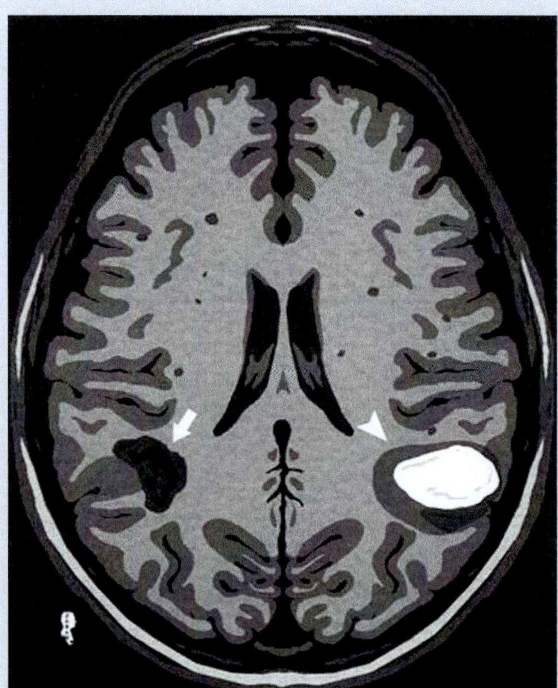

◘ **Fig. 2.2.3**  Axial T1W brain MR illustration demonstrates cerebral amyloid angiopathy (CAA). There is corticomedullary bleeding in the left parieto-occipital area surrounded by cytotoxic edema (*arrowhead*). Multiple areas of hypointense signal intensities scattered within the white matter representing chronic microhemorrhages. An area of low signal intensity is seen in the right parieto-occipital area representing gliosis (*arrow*)

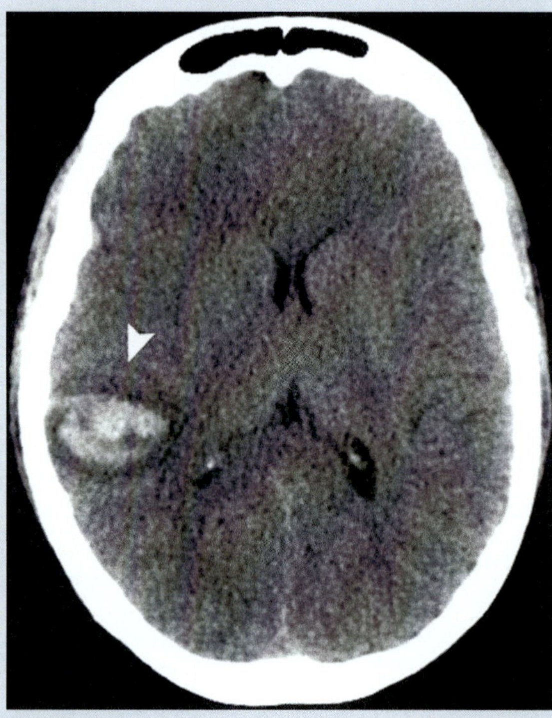

◘ **Fig. 2.2.4**  Axial brain nonenhanced CT in a patient with intracranial bleeding due to CAA shows an area of bleeding in the right temporo-occipital region involving the cortices and the corticomedullary junction with a rim of cytotoxic edema (*arrowhead*)

## CADASIL (Cerebral Autosomal Dominant Arteriopathy with Subcortical Infarcts and Leukodystrophy)

CADASIL is the most common form of familial strokes with progressive dementia due to vasculopathy of the deep perforating arteries of the cerebral white matter. Patient with CADASIL presents with multiple attacks of strokes beginning usually between 40 and 60 years of life. Patients typically have no risk factors for stroke. Psychiatric symptoms occur in 30 % of cases (e.g., depression).

### Diagnostic Criteria for CADASIL

- Young age (<50 years)
- Two of the following clinical findings: stroke-like episodes with permanent neurological defects, migrainous headache, major mood disturbance, or subcortical dementia
- No risk factors for stroke
- Positive family history for such stroke attacks
- On MRI, white matter changes without cortical infarcts

### Signs on MRI

- Extensive white matter lesions and basal ganglia abnormalities in the absence of cortical infarcts typically seen in the temporal lobes and the extreme and external capsule (◨ Fig. 2.2.5). The lesions do not enhance after contrast injection.
- Widening of the periventricular spaces (*Virchow–Robin spaces*) (◨ Fig. 2.2.6).
- MR angiography is typically normal (no vascular lesion).

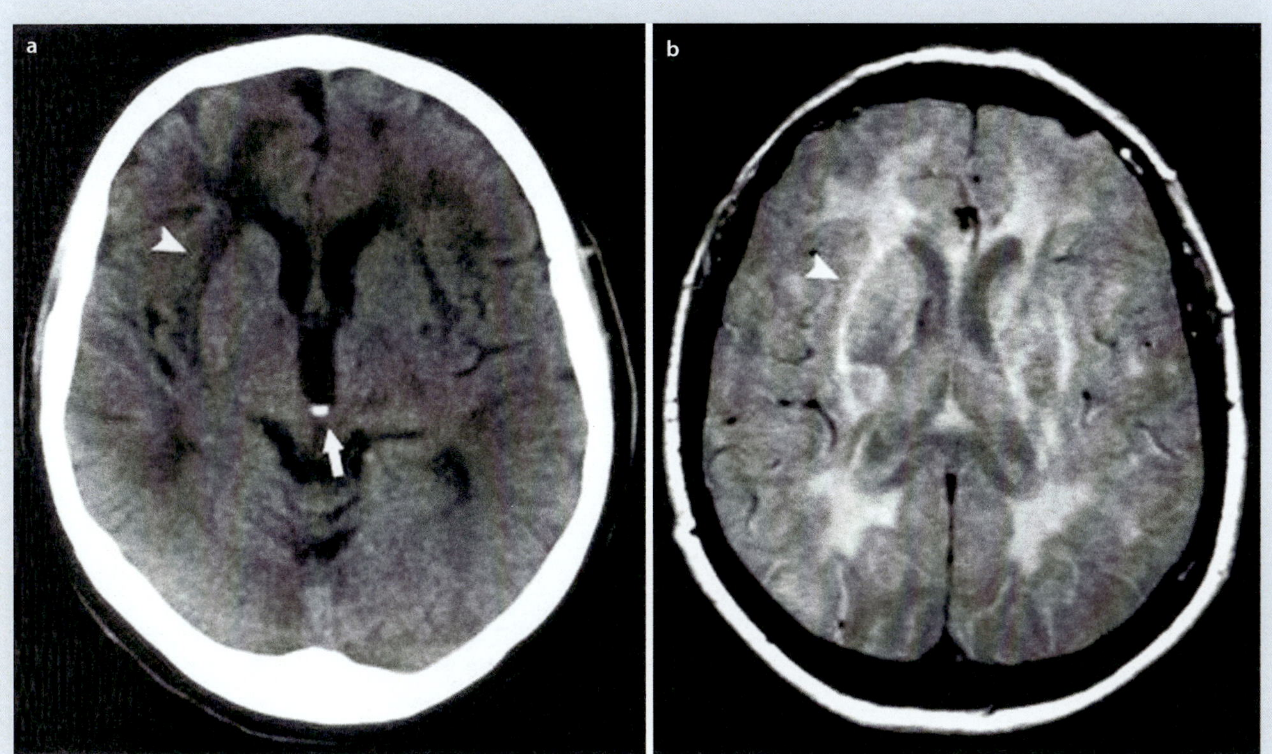

◨ **Fig. 2.2.5** Axial nonenhanced brain CT (**a**) and axial FLAIR MRI (**b**) of a patient with cerebral autosomal dominant arteriopathy with subcortical infarcts and leukodystrophy (CADASIL) show bilateral diffuse white matter lesions with affection of the right external capsule (*arrowheads*). Pineal calcification can be seen as a secondary finding (*arrow*)

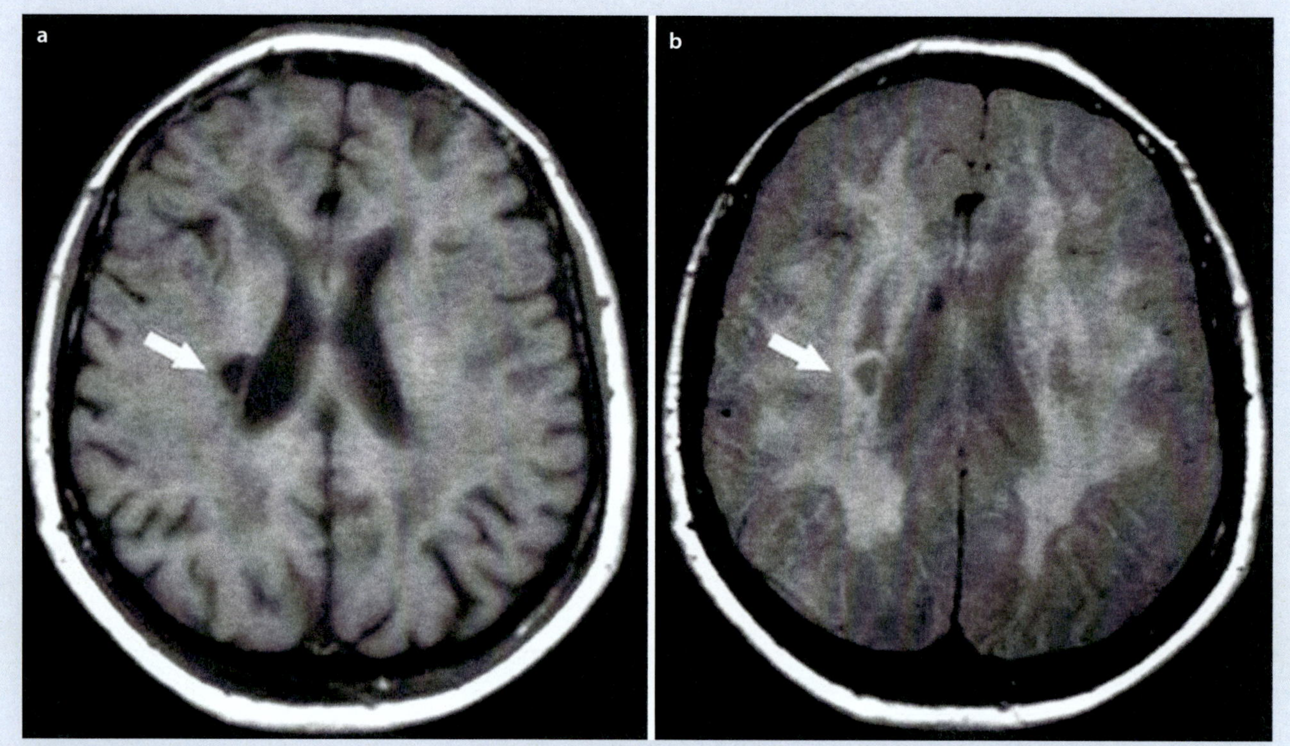



**◼ Fig. 2.2.6**   Axial T1W (**a**) and FLAIR (**b**) brain MRI of another patient with CADASIL shows bilateral diffuse white matter lesions (leukoencephalopathy) with dilated right Virchow–Robin space (*arrowhead*)

## MELAS (Mitochondrial Myopathy, Encephalopathy, Lactic Acidosis, and Stroke-Like Episodes)

MELAS is a mitochondrial disease characterized by episodes of infarction-like cerebral injuries causing hemiparesis or hemiplegia, hearing loss, or cortical blindness. The disease is characterized by elevated serum levels of lactic acid (lactic acidosis).

MELAS starts during early infancy or between the ages of 2 and 5 years. The child presents with vomiting, seizures, failure to thrive, and infarction-like injuries that can occur anywhere in the brain. Interestingly, angiography reveals no vascular occlusion or vascular disease. The infarction-like episodes are due to abnormal physiology rather than abnormal anatomy or vascular occlusion.

### Signs on CT and MRI
- There are hypodense, asymmetric areas on CT located mainly in the occipitotemporal areas representing infarction that does not follow a vascular territory (◼ Fig. 2.2.7). The same area shows low T1/high T2 signal intensities. Diffuse brain atrophy can be seen.
- On CT, bilateral basal ganglia calcification may be seen due to old infarctions (◼ Fig. 2.2.7).
- MR angiography is typically normal (excluding vasculitis or moyamoya).
- High lactic acidosis peak in MR spectroscopy.

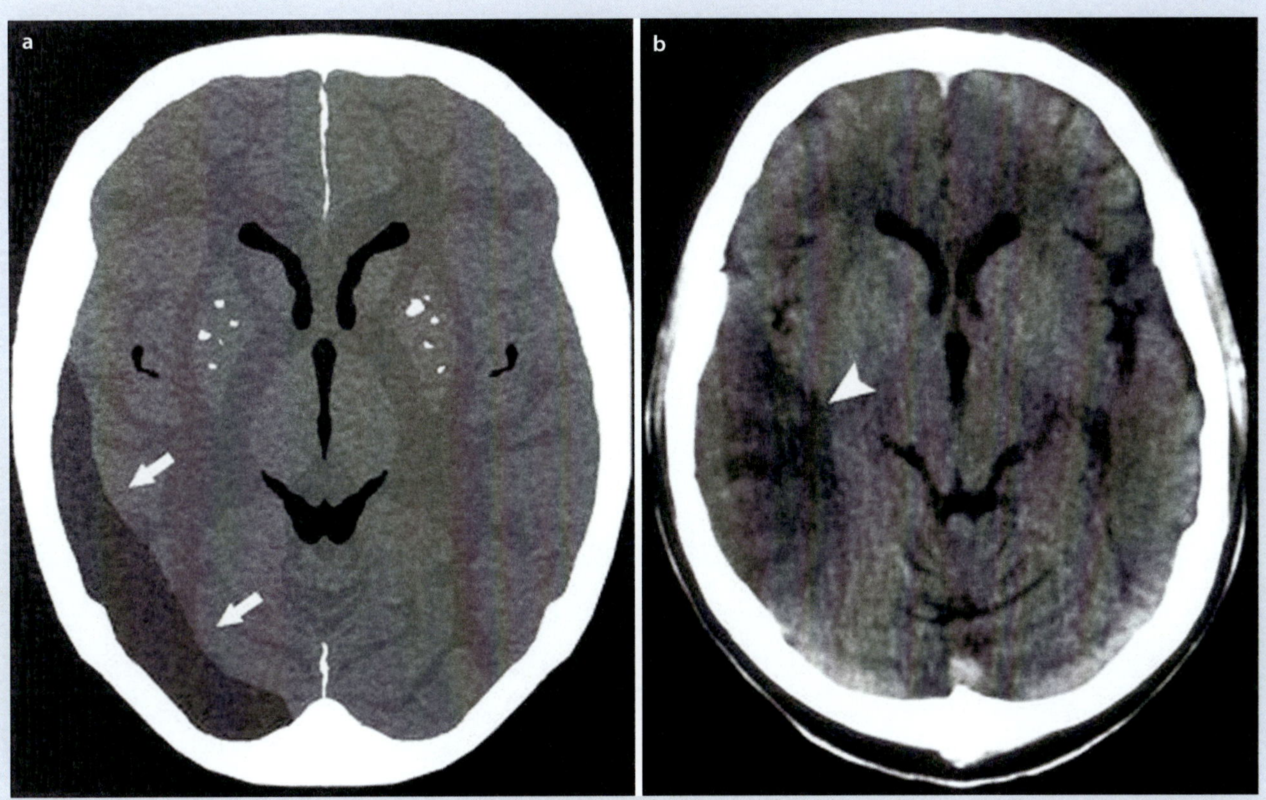

**◘ Fig. 2.2.7** Axial nonenhanced brain CT illustration (**a**) and image (**b**) of a patient with mitochondrial myopathy, encephalopathy, lactic acidosis, and stroke-like episodes (MELAS) demonstrate the radiological features of MELAS. In (**a**), there is a hypodense lesion in the right temporoparietal region that does not follow a vascular territory (*arrows*) with bilateral basal ganglia calcifications, as typical signs of MELAS. In (**b**), a young patient diagnosed with MELAS shows hypodense lesions in the right temporal area representing infarction (*arrowhead*)

## Cortical Laminar Necrosis

Cortical laminar necrosis (CLN) is a disease characterized by destruction of different layers of the cerebral cortex, most prominently the third cortical layer.

On histopathological examination, CLN shows brain infarction of the cortical neuronal elements and the blood vessels (pan-necrosis) without hemorrhage or calcification. CLN has been reported in patients with Reye's syndrome.

*Reye's syndrome* is a rare condition characterized by acute noninflammatory encephalopathy and fatty degeneration of the viscera, commonly the liver. It commonly affects children between 2 months and 15 years of age. The classical clinical presentation is a child presenting with vomiting, headache, convulsions, and signs of encephalopathy, associated with hepatic dysfunction and elevated liver enzymes. Liver biopsy classically shows fatty infiltration. A liver biopsy can help to rule out other conditions that may be affecting the liver and causing liver dysfunction.

The explanation of Reye's syndrome pathology is linked to hepatic and neuronal mitochondrial dysfunction triggered by certain toxins or infections. The most common causes of Reye's syndrome are reaction to salicylate (aspirin) or infections like influenza B and chicken pox (varicella-zoster virus infection). Chicken pox encephalitis can lead to the development of Reye's syndrome among other cerebral complications.

**Signs on MRI**
- Typically, CLN lesions show hyperintense curvilinear lines along the cortical gyri and convolutions on both T1W and FLAIR images (◘ Fig. 2.2.8), usually seen from 1 month to 1 year after the ischemic event.
- CLN lesions show contrast enhancement after contrast injection, classically 2 weeks after the initial attack.
- In Reye's syndrome, the brain shows diffuse or focal ischemia in a laminar pattern similar to CLN. Multiple abnormal white matter lesions with heterogeneous signal intensities may be found reflecting different stages of Wallerian degeneration. The latter finding is commonly seen in chronic stage of the disease. *Wallerian degeneration* is a type of neurological degeneration that is seen after an axonal injury. The distal and the proximal segments of the damaged axon with its myelin are fragmented until the first node of Ranvier.

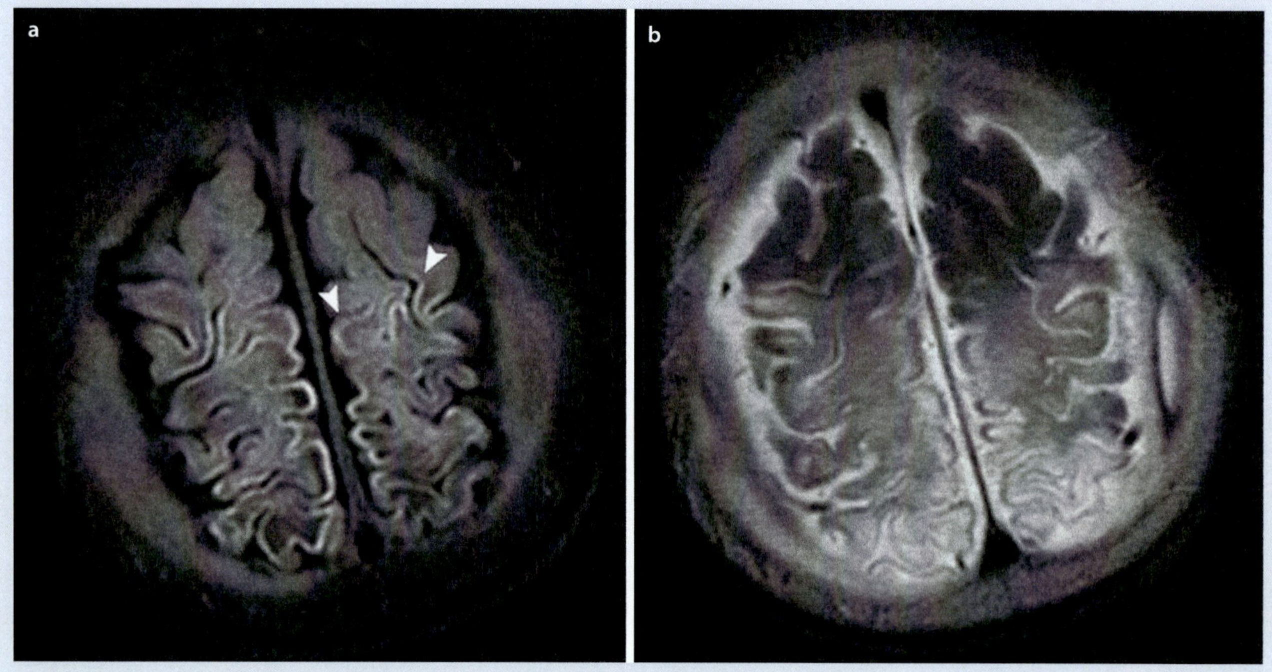

**Fig. 2.2.8**   Axial T1W (**a**) and T2W (**b**) brain MRI in a 7-year-old child with chicken pox encephalitis shows cortical laminar necrosis (CLN). Notice the curvilinear hyperintense signal intensity lines that follow the convolutions of the gyri on both hemispheres (*arrowheads*), with diffuse white matter lesions seen on T2W images

## Man-in-the-Barrel Syndrome

Man-in-the-barrel syndrome (MIBS) is a rare disease characterized by paralysis of both arms while the cranial nerves and motor functions of the legs are functioning, giving the patient appearance of a man being confined to a barrel.

MIBS is caused by bilateral ischemia or infarction involving the border-zone areas between the anterior cerebral artery and the middle cerebral artery (MCA) (watershed zones) at the level of the motor cortex of the arm. Spinal cord disease paralyzing both brachial plexus can cause this disease, but it is extremely rare.

The most common cause of MIBS is systemic hypotension following cardiac surgeries or cardiac arrest. MIBS association with pontine myelinolysis, head trauma, and cerebral metastasis has been reported.

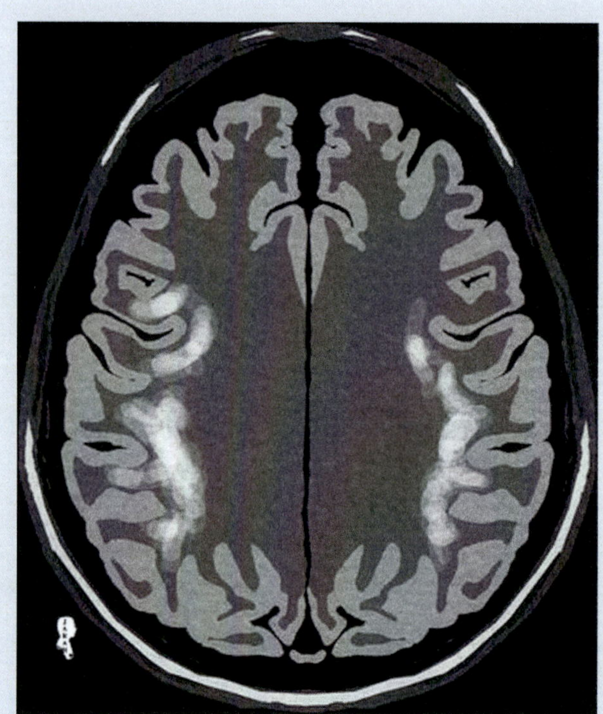

**Fig. 2.2.9**   Axial brain FLAIR MR illustration shows the radiological findings in patients with man-in-the-barrel syndrome (MIBS)

**Signs on CT and MRI**
- CT can be normal.
- MRI typically shows bilateral low T1 and high T2 signal intensities in the parietotemporal, sensorimotor cortical areas of the arm and hand in the brain (**Fig. 2.2.9**).

## Locked-In Syndrome

Locked-in syndrome (LIS) is a rare disease characterized by normal wakefulness and cognition, anarthria, quadriplegia, and gaze paralysis, caused by ventral pontine infarction.

Patients with LIS are fully conscious, yet they experience almost complete motor paralysis. Typically, patients are able to communicate via vertical gaze movement and blinking. LIS is classically caused by infarction or hemorrhage involving the pontine perforating arteries arising from the basilar artery. Other causes of LIS include Guillain–Barré syndrome, West Nile encephalitis, and amyotrophic lateral sclerosis.

> **Signs on CT and MRI**
> Brain scan typically shows infarction or hemorrhage involving the ventral pontine region or the cerebral peduncles.

## Brain Stem Infarction Syndromes

The brain stem holds nuclei of the cranial nerves. The midbrain contains the nuclei of the cranial nerves 3 and 4. The pons contains the nuclei of the cranial nerves 5–8, and the medulla contains the nuclei of the cranial nerves 9–12. Infarction within the brain stem can result in cranial nerve palsies among other complications. Different syndromes may arise according to the infarcted region within the brain stem. A summary of the most common disorders arising due to brain stem infarction is presented below:

— *Millard–Gubler syndrome*: unilateral hemiplegia or hemiparesis with contralateral lower motor neuron facial (CN 7) paralysis due to hemorrhage, tumor, or infarction of the pons.
— *Claude syndrome*: unilateral oculomotor (CN 3) nerve palsy with contralateral hemiataxia due to paramedial midbrain infarction (Fig. 2.2.10).
— *Benedikt syndrome*: unilateral oculomotor (CN 3) nerve palsy with contralateral limb tremor or paralysis. It can be caused by pontine infarction due to posterior cerebral artery occlusion.
— *Weber syndrome*: unilateral oculomotor (CN 3) nerve palsy with contralateral hemiplegia due to midbrain infarction.
— *Avellis syndrome*: hemiparalysis of the larynx and soft palate on the same side due to infarction of the nucleus ambiguous in the medulla oblongata (central) or a mass lesion around the jugular foramen (peripheral) involves the glossopharyngeal and the vagus nerves (CN 9 + 10) (Fig. 2.2.11).
— *Foix–Chavany–Marie syndrome*: pseudobulbar palsy (CN 9–12) due to bilateral cortical infarction in the territory of the MCA.
— *Babinski–Nageotte syndrome*: ipsilateral Horner's syndrome; facial loss of pain and temperature; cerebellar hemiataxia, with paresis of the larynx and pharynx; and contralateral hemiparesis and loss of pain and temperature. The disease arises due to unilateral infarction of the medulla oblongata involving the spinal trigeminal tract and nucleus, nucleus ambiguous, lateral spinothalamic tract, sympathetic fibers, corticospinal tract, and afferent spinocerebellar tract (Fig. 2.2.11).
— *Cestan–Chenais syndrome*: has same clinical presentation as Babinski–Nageotte syndrome and arises due to unilateral infarction of the medulla oblongata involving the spinal trigeminal tract and nucleus, nucleus ambiguous, lateral spinothalamic tract, sympathetic fibers, and corticospinal tract (Fig. 2.2.11).
— *Lateral medullary (Wallenberg) syndrome*: ipsilateral Horner's syndrome; facial loss of pain and temperature; cerebellar hemiataxia, with paresis of the larynx and pharynx; and contralateral loss of body pain and temperature. It arises due to unilateral infarction of the medulla oblongata involving the spinal trigeminal tract and nucleus, nucleus ambiguous, lateral spinothalamic tract, sympathetic fibers, afferent spinocerebellar tracts, and vestibular nuclei (Figs. 2.2.11 and 2.2.12).
— *Dejerine syndrome*: ipsilateral tongue weakness with contralateral hemiparesis and face sparing hemihypesthesia. It arises due to unilateral infarction of the medulla oblongata involving the hypoglossal nucleus or fibers, corticospinal tract, and spinal medial lemniscus (Fig. 2.2.11).
— *Reinhold (hemimedullary) syndrome*: ipsilateral Horner's syndrome; facial loss of pain and temperature; cerebellar

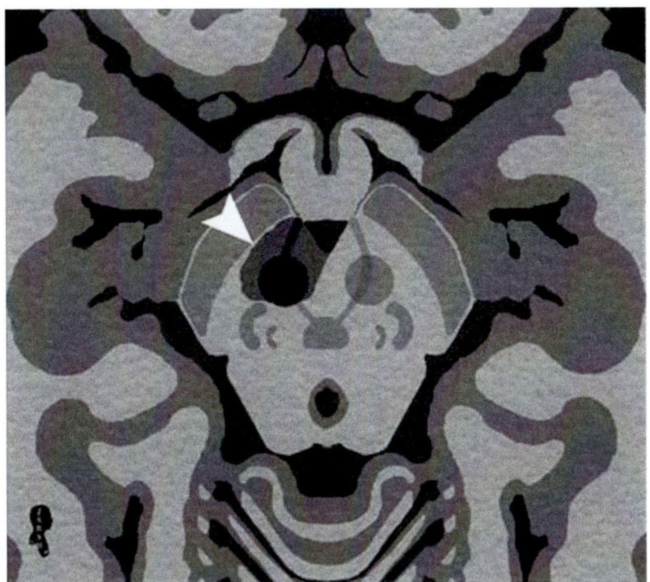



**Fig. 2.2.10**   Axial T1W brain stem MR illustration at the level of the pone demonstrates the typical infarction region causing Claude syndrome (*arrowhead*)

hemiataxia, with paresis of the larynx and pharynx; and contralateral hemiparesis and face sparing hemihypesthesia. It arises due to unilateral infarction of the medulla oblongata involving the spinal trigeminal tract and nucleus, nucleus ambiguous, afferent spinocerebellar tracts, sympathetic fibers, hypoglossal nucleus or fibers, corticospinal tract, and spinal medial lemniscus (◻ Fig. 2.2.11).

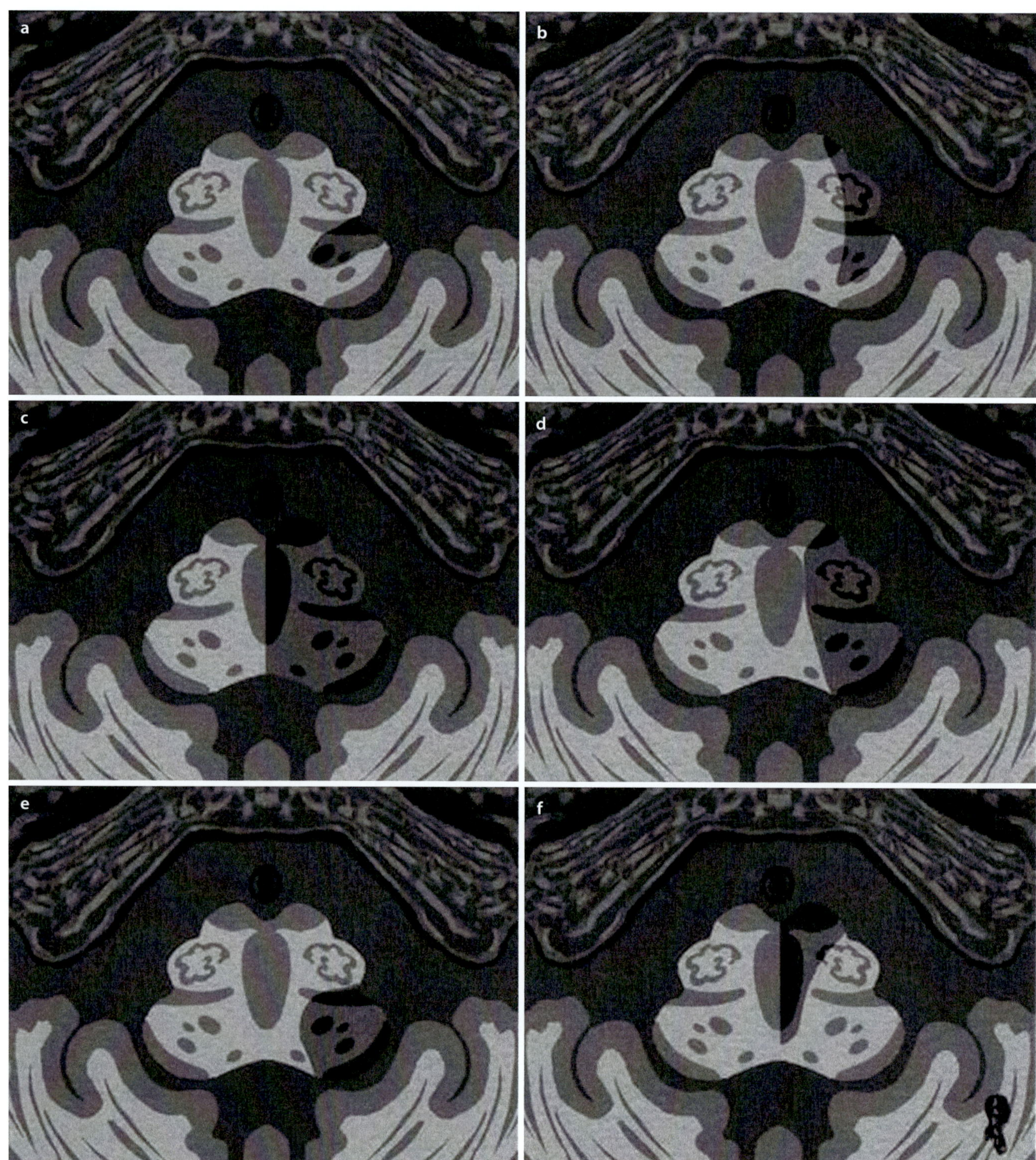

◻ **Fig. 2.2.11**    Axial T1W brain stem MR illustration at the level of the medulla demonstrates different kinds of diseases according to the area of medullary infarction: (**a**) Avellis syndrome, (**b**) Cestan–Chenais syndrome, (**c**) Reinhold (hemimedullary) syndrome, (**d**) Babinski–Nageotte syndrome, (**e**) Wallenberg syndrome, and (**f**) Dejerine syndrome

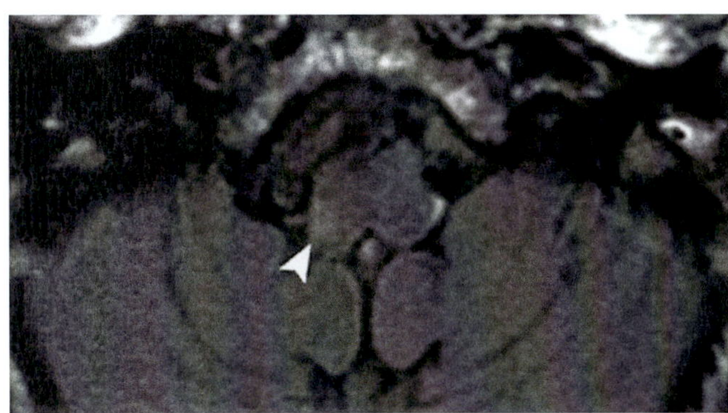

**Fig. 2.2.12** Axial FLAIR image in the region of the medulla in a patient with Wallenberg syndrome (*arrowhead*) shows hyperintense signal intensity lesion in the lateral portion of the right medulla oblongata (*arrowhead*)

## Subclavian Steal Syndrome

Subclavian steal syndrome (SSS) is a disease characterized by subclavian stenosis or occlusion at the segment between its origin from the aortic arch and the origin of the vertebral artery. This stenosis or occlusion causes reverse blood diversion (stealing) from the basivertebral arteries through the vertebral artery at the same side of subclavian occlusion to supply the ipsilateral arm (blood flow from the head and neck to supply the arm, rather than flow normally from the aortic arch toward the head via the vertebral artery).

Most patients with SSS are asymptomatic. However, symptomatic patients present with brain stem ischemia or stroke at rest or after exercise due to increased arm blood demand. Also, patients often complain from dizziness, cerebral dysfunction, and drop attacks when the disease is severe. Symptoms in the affected arm ranged between decrease pulses, coldness to claudications.

SSS doesn't appear when the stenosed subclavian artery is accompanied by vertebral artery arising separately from the aortic arch (6 % of population). Angiography is the gold standard to establish the diagnosis of SSS.

*Coronary-subclavian steal syndrome (CSS)* is a disease seen in patients with previous history of coronary artery bypass graft surgery (CABG). The internal thoracic (mammary) artery, which is a branch of the subclavian artery, is commonly used as a graft for the left anterior descending artery (LAD). Severe stenosis of the subclavian artery that compromised the arm blood supply causes the blood flow to reverse in direction. The blood is withdrawn (stolen) from the coronary arteries via the internal thoracic artery graft to supply the arm. Patients typically present with exertional angina precipitated or exacerbated by arm exercise. Diagnostic keys of CSS include history of CABG (mandatory), difference in blood pressure between the two arms >20 mmHg, and angina produced by activity of the affected arm, while activity of the contralateral normal arm produces no symptoms.

### Signs on Angiography

Stenosis of the subclavian artery is seen in arch aortography. After injecting the contrast within the normal vertebral artery, the contrast is seen flowing within the contralateral vertebral artery via the vertebrobasilar system in a retrograde pattern to supply the arm when the patient is asked to exercise his arm (**Fig. 2.2.13**).

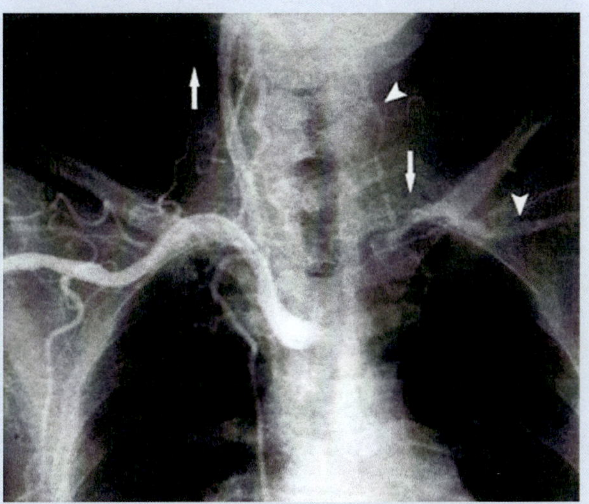

**Fig. 2.2.13** Selective right subclavian artery angiogram shows retrograde flow in the left vertebral artery to supply the left arm via the brachial artery (*arrowheads*). The direction of the contrast flow is demonstrated by the *arrows*

### Signs on Doppler Sonography

- The earliest manifestation of stealing phenomenon is a transient sharp deceleration of blood flow after the first systolic peak. This deceleration is observed as a systolic peak with a median notch, creating two systolic peaks of the vertebral artery with stealing phenomenon. The nadir of the notch becomes progressively lower until it reaches and crosses the baseline.
- On rest, the vertebral artery flow shows double peak systolic waveform with a median notch. The waveform is classified according to the velocity of the nadir into a nadir velocity greater than that of end diastole (type 1), a nadir velocity equal to the level of end diastole (type 2), a nadir velocity that reaches the baseline (type 3), and a nadir velocity that crosses the baseline (type 4).
- After asking the patient to exercise his ipsilateral arm or applying brachial artery blood pressure cuff and then deflating it to induce the stealing phenomenon, the arterial flow waveform of the vertebral artery is reversed, and it is seen below the baseline, confirming the reversal blood flow.

> **Signs on MRI**
> In axial sections of 2D time-of-flight sequence, the vertebral artery with stealing phenomenon shows flow void signal compared to the contralateral vertebral artery and both internal carotid arteries (*localizer sign*), which indicates reversal of flow.

## Further Reading


Benito-Leon J, et al. "Man-in-the-barrel" syndrome: MRI and SPECT imaging. Eur J Radiol. 1997;24:260–2.

Cuisset T, et al. Coronary-subclavian steal syndrome: an usual cause of refractory unstable angina. Int J Cardiol. 2008;127:e181–2.

Deleu D, et al. "Man-in-the-barrel" syndrome as delayed manifestation of extrapontine and central pontine myelinolysis: beneficial effect of intravenous immunoglobulin. J Neurol Sci. 2005a;237:103–6.

Elting JW, et al. Predicting outcome drome coma: man-in-the-barrel syndrome as potential pitfall. Clin Neurol Neurosurg. 2000;102:23–5.

Ferrari G, et al. Foix-Chavany-Marie syndrome: CT study and clinical report of three cases. Neuroradiology. 1979;18:41–2.

Girija AS, et al. Neurological complications of chickenpox. Ann Indian Acad Neurol. 2007;10:240–6.

Hoffmann HJ. Moyamoya disease and syndrome. Clin Neurol Neurosurg. 1997;99 Suppl 2:S39–44.

Holz A, et al. Moyamoya disease in a patient with hereditary spherocytosis. Pediatr Radiol. 1998;28:95–7.

Hsu C-Y, et al. Moyamoya disease: the clue from computer tomography. J Emerg Med. 2004;26:339–42.

Hurwitz ES, et al. A cluster of cases of Reye syndrome associated with chickenpox. Pediatrics. 1982;70:901–6.

Kaneko A, et al. Color-coded Doppler imaging of the subclavian steal syndrome. Intern Med. 1998;37:259–64.

Kim I-O, et al. Mitochondrial myopathy-encephalopathylactic acidosis and strokelike episodes (MELAS) syndrome: CT and MR findings in seven children. AJR Am J Roentgenol. 1996;166:641–5.

Kinoshita T, et al. Reye's syndrome with cortical laminar necrosis: MRI. Neuroradiology. 1996;38:269–72.

Kliewer MA, et al. Vertebral artery Doppler waveform changes indicating subclavian steal physiology. AJR Am J Roentgenol. 2000;174:815–9.

Komiyama M, et al. Serial MR observation of cortical laminar necrosis caused by brain infarction. Neuroradiology. 1998;40:771–7.

Krasnianski M, et al. Babinski-Nageotte's syndrome and Hemimedullary (Reinhold's) syndrome are clinically and morphologically distinct conditions. J Neurol. 2003;250:938–42.

Krasnianski M, et al. Between Wallenberg syndrome and hemimedullary lesion. Cestan-Chenais and Babinski-Nageotte syndromes in medullary infarctions. J Neurol. 2006;253:1442–6.

Luxenberg EL, et al. Locked-in syndrome from rosto-caudal herniation. J Clin Neurosci. 2009;16:333–4.

Marquardt F, et al. The coronary-subclavian-vertebral steal syndrome (CSVSS). Clin Res Cardiol. 2006;95:48–53.

Masuzawa H, et al. Pontine gliomas causing locked-in syndrome. Childs Nerv Syst. 1993;9:256–9.

Prasad BKD, et al. Cerebral amyloid angiopathy. Ind J Radiol Imag. 2006;16:745–7.

Roldan-Valadez E, et al. Imaging diagnosis of subclavian steal syndrome secondary to Takayasu arteritis affecting a left-side subclavian artery. Arch Med Res. 2003;34:433–8.

Sheehy N, et al. Contrast-enhanced MR angiography of subclavian steal syndrome: value of the 2D time-to-flight "localizer" sign. AJR Am J Roentgenol. 2005;185:1069–73.

Trattnig S, et al. Colour Doppler imaging of partial subclavian steal syndrome. Neuroradiology. 1993;35:293–5.

Van Son JAM, et al. Diagnosis and management of the coronary-subclavian steal syndrome. Eur J Cardiothorac Surg. 1998;3:565–7.

Yamada I, et al. Moyamoya disease: diagnostic accuracy of MRI. Neuroradiology. 1995;37:356–61.

Zakaria T, et al. Locked-in syndrome resulting from bilateral cerebral peduncles infarctions. Neurology. 2006;67:1889.


## 2.3    Intracranial Hemorrhage

Intracranial hemorrhage is a condition characterized by the presence of free blood within the cranium. The free blood can be collected in the epidural space, subdural space, subarachnoid space, intrabrain parenchyma, or intraventricular spaces.

Intracranial hemorrhage can be caused by head trauma, anticoagulants use, ruptured aneurysms, vascular malformations, and hypertension. The most common areas of intracranial hemorrhage are the temporoparietal region and the cerebellum. Native, nonenhanced CT is the diagnostic modality of choice as an initial diagnostic modality to detect intracranial bleeding.

Blood exhibits different densities on CT or signal intensities on MRI according to the age of the hemorrhage (acute, subacute, or chronic) (◾ Fig. 2.3.1).

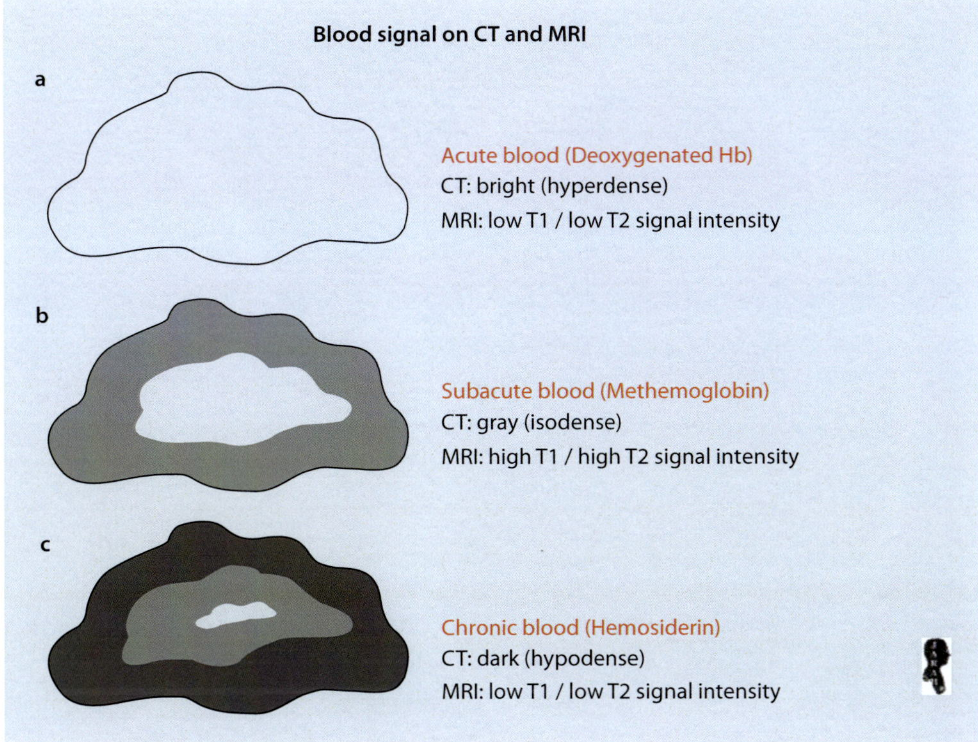


**Fig. 2.3.1** Illustration demonstrates the different hematoma ages and manifestations on CT. (**a**) Acute blood (Deoxygenated Hb). CT: bright (hyperdense). MRI: low T1/ low T2 signal intensity. (**b**) Subacute blood (Methemoglobin). CT: gray (isodense). MRI: high T1/high T2 signal intensity. (**c**) Chronic blood (Hemosiderin). CT: dark (hyperdense). MRI: low T1/low T2 signal intensity

## Epidural Hematoma

Epidural hematoma is a free blood collection located between the inner skull table and the dura matter. It is a life-threatening emergency that usually results from trauma to the middle meningeal artery (85 % of cases).

Patients usually present with nausea, vomiting, and altered consciousness.

### Signs on CT
- The CT typically shows semi-convex-shaped, hyperdense blood collection usually located in the parietotemporal area (Fig. 2.3.2).
- The collected blood does not cross suture lines as the dura matter is firmly attached to the clavaria.
- There is significant mass effect over the ventricles and the brain parenchyma in the acute phase.
- It is almost always acute. However, acute on top of chronic epidural hematoma can occur uncommonly, and it is seen as a semi-convex blood collection with hypodense and hyperdense component (Fig. 2.3.2).

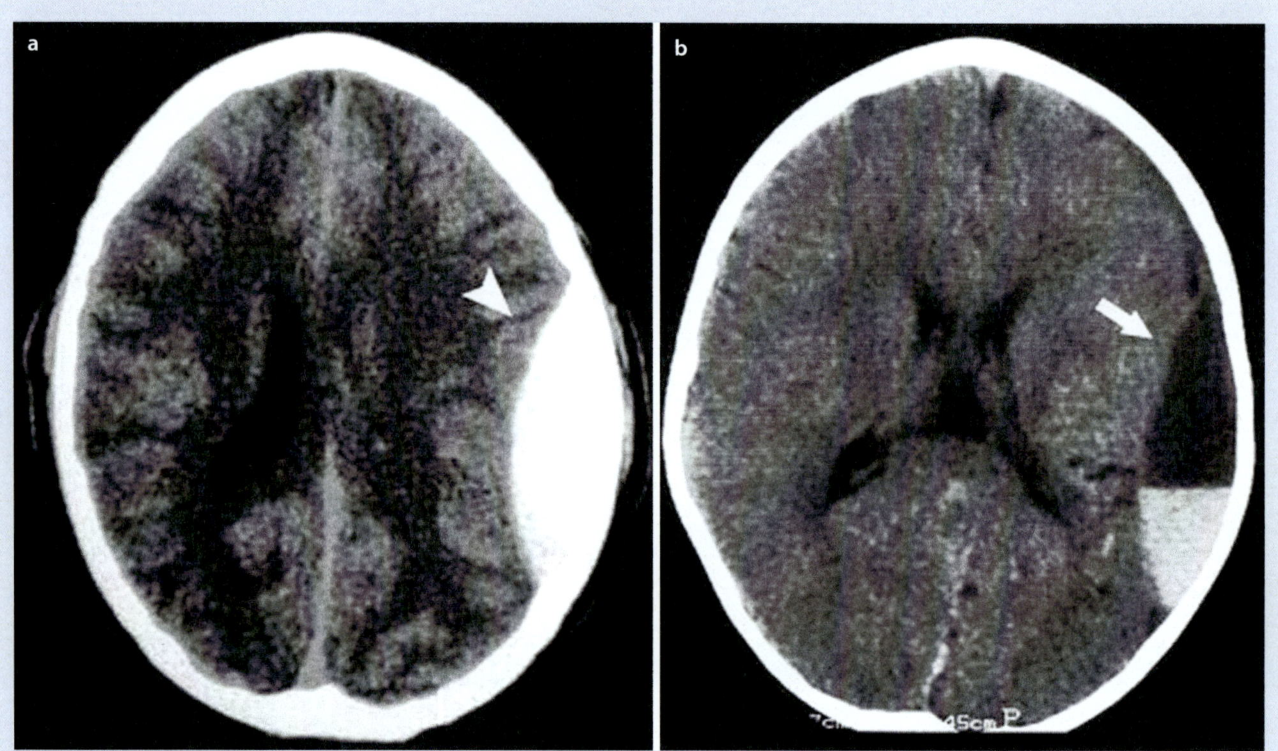

**Fig. 2.3.2** Axial CT images of two different patients show acute epidural hematoma (**a**, *arrowhead*) and acute on top of chronic hematoma (**b**, *arrow*). Notice the mass effect on the left lateral ventricle in (**a**) when the hematoma is acute and lack of the pressure effect on the lateral ventricles in (**b**) when the hematoma is chronic

*Q: When can you find a black (hypodense) hematoma although the bleeding is acute?*

This is a rare condition that is seen when the hemoglobin level in the blood is less than 4 mg/dL, because the hyperdense density that reflects the X-ray photon absorption by the iron in the blood is inadequate.

subdural space to be trapped in little or no absorption. The most common symptom is headache with or without nausea and vomiting; in the acute phase, subdural hygroma behaves like an enlarged intracranial hemorrhage, and in the chronic phase, it behaves like a space-occupying lesion. After traumatic head injury, development of subdural hygroma is noted 6–46 days after the initial trauma.

## Subdural Hematoma

Subdural hematoma is a free blood collection located between the dura matter and the arachnoid. Subdural hematoma usually arises due to emissary vein tear from a minor trauma or due to uncontrolled anticoagulant therapy. Acute subdural hematoma is a clinical emergency, where patients present with signs similar to epidural hematoma. In contrast, chronic subdural hematomas present with less severe symptoms, such as headache, nausea, and vomiting.

### Differential Diagnoses and Related Diseases

*Subdural hygroma* is a collection of cerebrospinal fluid or serum in the subdural space (**Fig. 2.3.4**). It is believed to be caused by chronic subdural hematoma in the elderly or due to intracranial infections in children. Up to 30 % of cases arise after head trauma. The condition is self-limited and is thought to be caused by a tear in the arachnoid that functions as a one-way valve, allowing cerebrospinal fluid to enter the

**Signs on CT**
- Crescent-shaped, hyperdense blood collection usually located in the frontoparietal region (**Fig. 2.3.3**). It can be bilateral in 15 % of cases.
- The bleeding is not bounded by the sutures.
- There is significant mass effect over the ventricles and the cisterns.
- Subdural hematoma can be acute (hyperdense), subacute (isodense), and chronic (hypodense) (**Fig. 2.3.3**). Acute on top of chronic subdural hematoma can occur, and it is seen as crescent-shaped blood collection with hypodense and hyperdense components (sedimentation subacute subdural hematoma).
- Subdural hygroma is seen as a cerebrospinal fluid collection in the subdural space (**Fig. 2.3.4**).

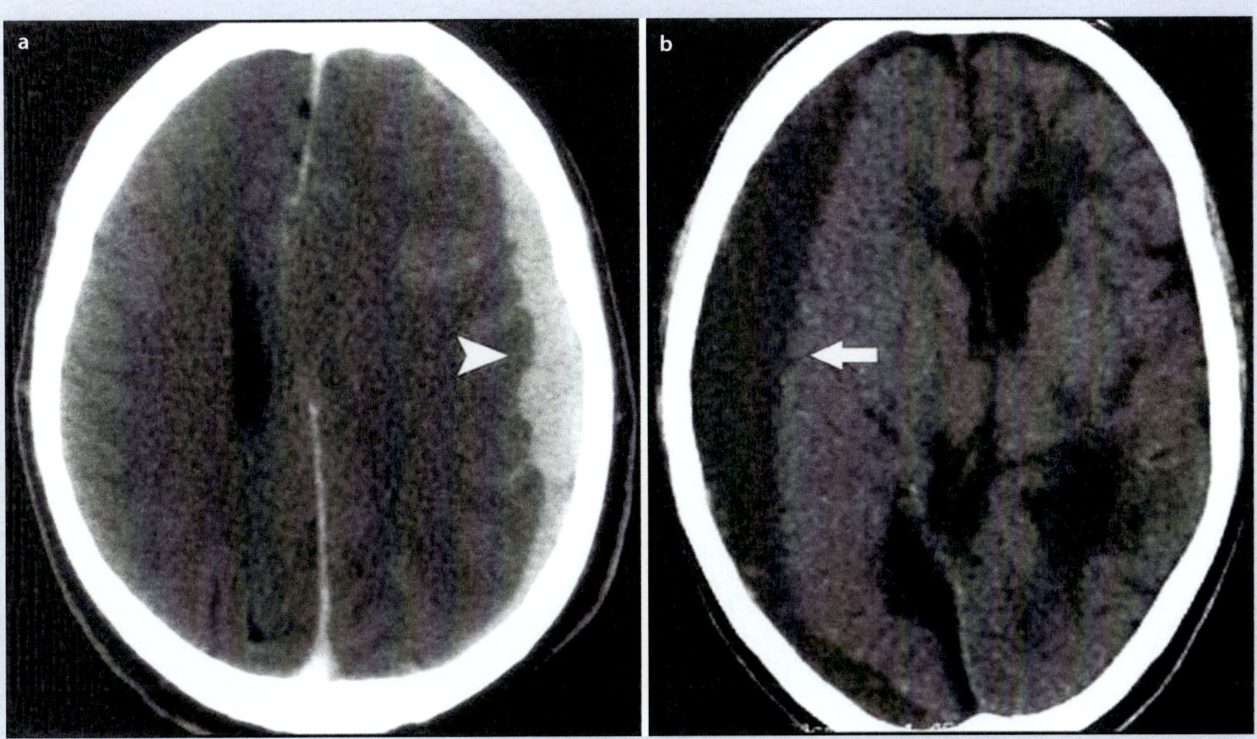

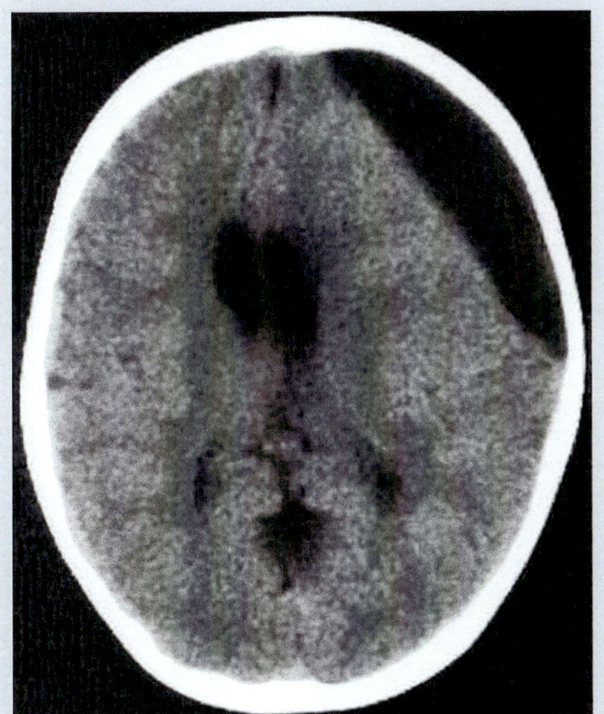

**Fig. 2.3.3** Axial CT images of two different patients show acute subdural hematoma (**a**, *arrowhead*) and chronic subdural hematoma (**b**, *arrow*). Again notice the pressure effect over the lateral ventricles in the acute subdural hematoma (**a**) compared to the chronic subdural hematoma (**b**)

## Subarachnoid Hemorrhage

Subarachnoid hemorrhage is characterized by the presence of free blood within the subarachnoid space and the arachnoid cisterns. It most commonly occurs as a complication of ruptured arterial aneurysms and trauma to the head. Patients typically present with sudden severe headache, nausea, and vomiting with neck stiffness.

**Signs on CT**
- The cerebrospinal fluid spaces and cistern will be seen hyperdense (white) due to blood mixed with cerebrospinal fluid (**Fig. 2.3.5**).
- There is no midline displacement.

**Fig. 2.3.4** Axial brain CT of a patient with a history of posttraumatic brain injury shows large left frontal subdural hygroma

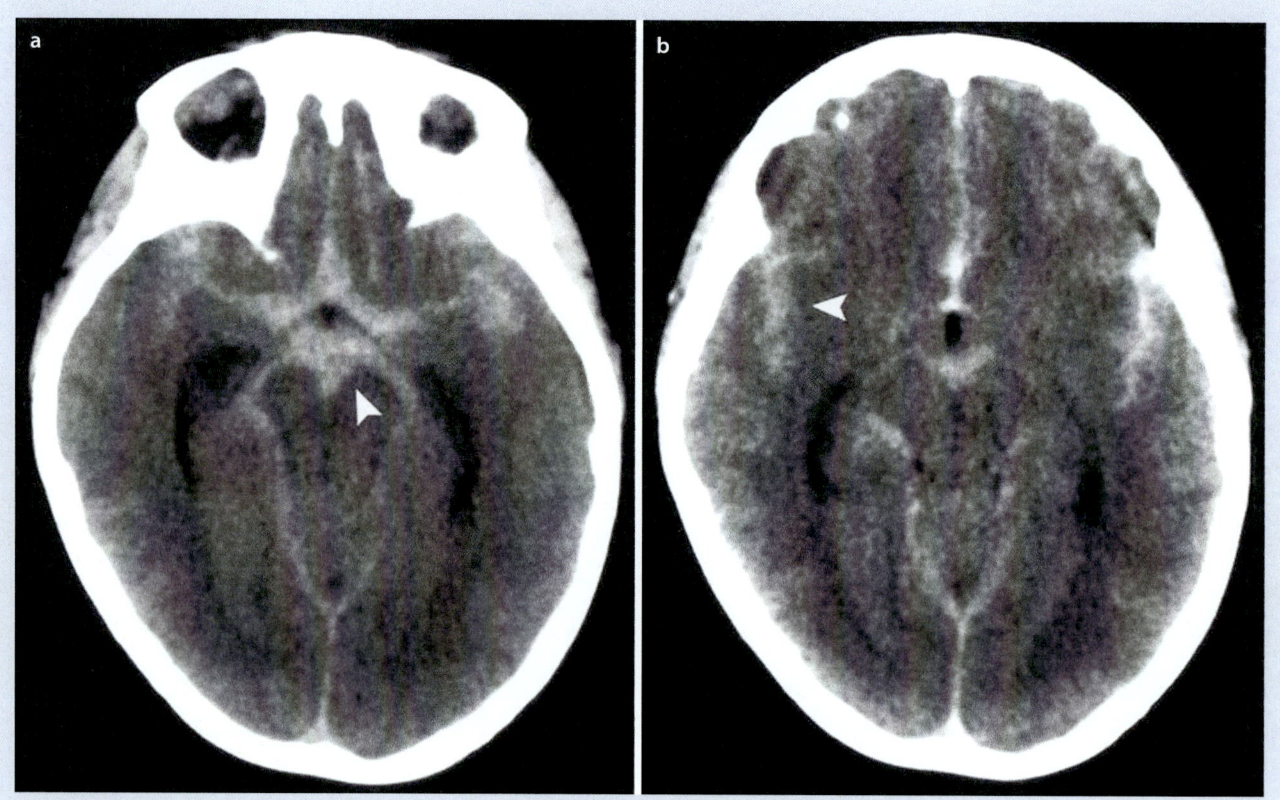

**Fig. 2.3.5** Sequential axial CT images (**a**) & (**b**) of a patient with subarachnoid hemorrhage show hyperdense suprasellar cistern (**a**) and Sylvian fissures (**b**) (*arrowheads*) due to subarachnoid bleeding

## Intracerebral/Intraparenchymal Hemorrhage

Intracerebral hemorrhage is the presence of free blood within the gray or the white brain matter. It commonly arises due to stroke, embolic vascular occlusion, and tumors or after vascular rupture due to head trauma. Hypertension causes bleeding into the basal ganglia in 60 % of cases.

**Signs on CT**
- There is hyperdense blood collection within the brain parenchyma that usually follows a vascular territory (■ Fig. 2.3.6).
- When the bleeding is due to stroke, it is surrounded by a halolike edema (cytotoxic edema), while when it is due to a tumor, a fingerlike edema is seen surrounding the blood collection (vasogenic edema).

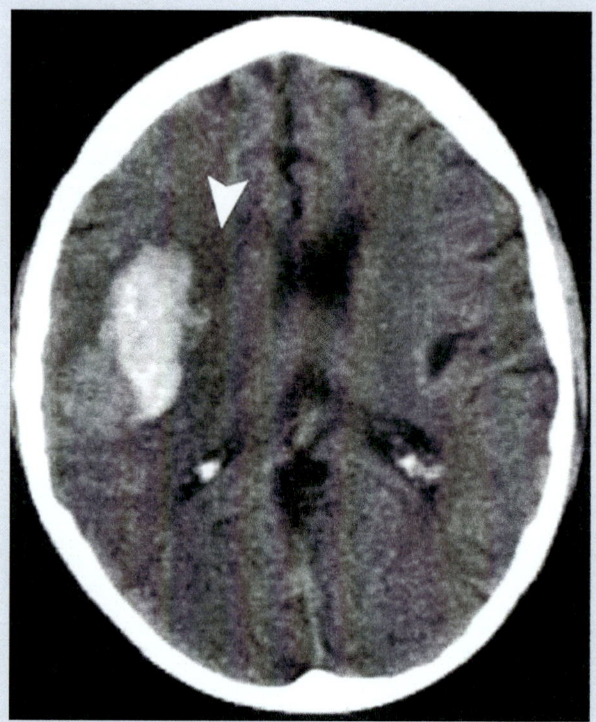

**Fig. 2.3.6** Axial brain CT of a patient with intraparenchymal bleeding in the region of the right middle cerebral artery shows large area of intraparenchymal bleeding surrounded by cytotoxic edema exerting mass effect over the right anterior and posterior horns of the right lateral ventricle (*arrowhead*)

## Intraventricular Hemorrhage

Intraventricular hemorrhage is bleeding into the ventricles. Commonly, it occurs secondary to parenchymal or subarachnoid hemorrhage and associated with diffuse axonal injury of the corpus callosum. Arteriovenous malformation is the most common cause for spontaneous intraventricular hemorrhage in adults. There are two types of intraventricular hemorrhage:

- *Ependymal intraventricular bleeding*: the blood is seen fixed to the ventricular walls.
- *Free intraventricular blood*: the blood is seen located in the posterior horns (gravity dependent).

**Signs on CT**
There is hyperdense blood within the ventricles, either in a free form lying in the posterior horns or encapsulated within the ependymal ventricular wall (◘ Fig. 2.3.7).

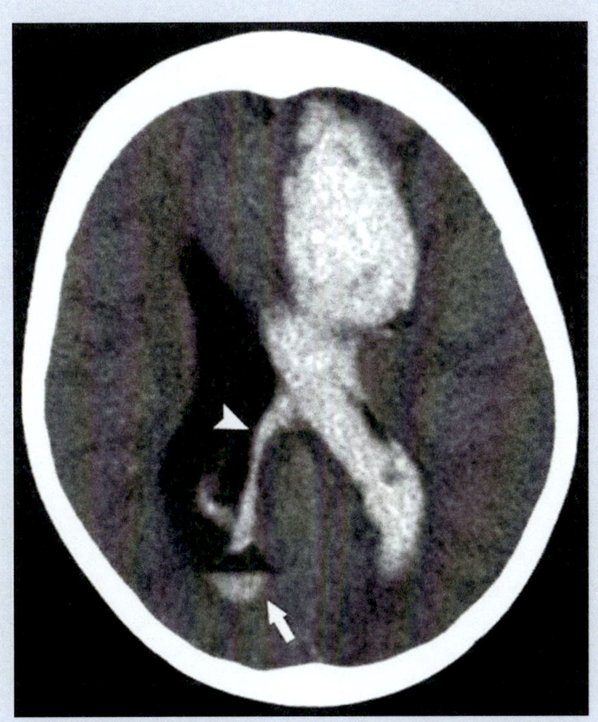

◘ **Fig. 2.3.7** Axial brain CT of a patient with severe intraventricular hemorrhage shows dilated both ventricles due to bleeding, with subependymal (*arrowhead*) and free (*arrow*) intraventricular bleedings also seen

**Signs on MRI**
Chronic bleeding can be detected on T2* images as hypointense intraparenchymal areas (◘ Fig. 2.3.8).

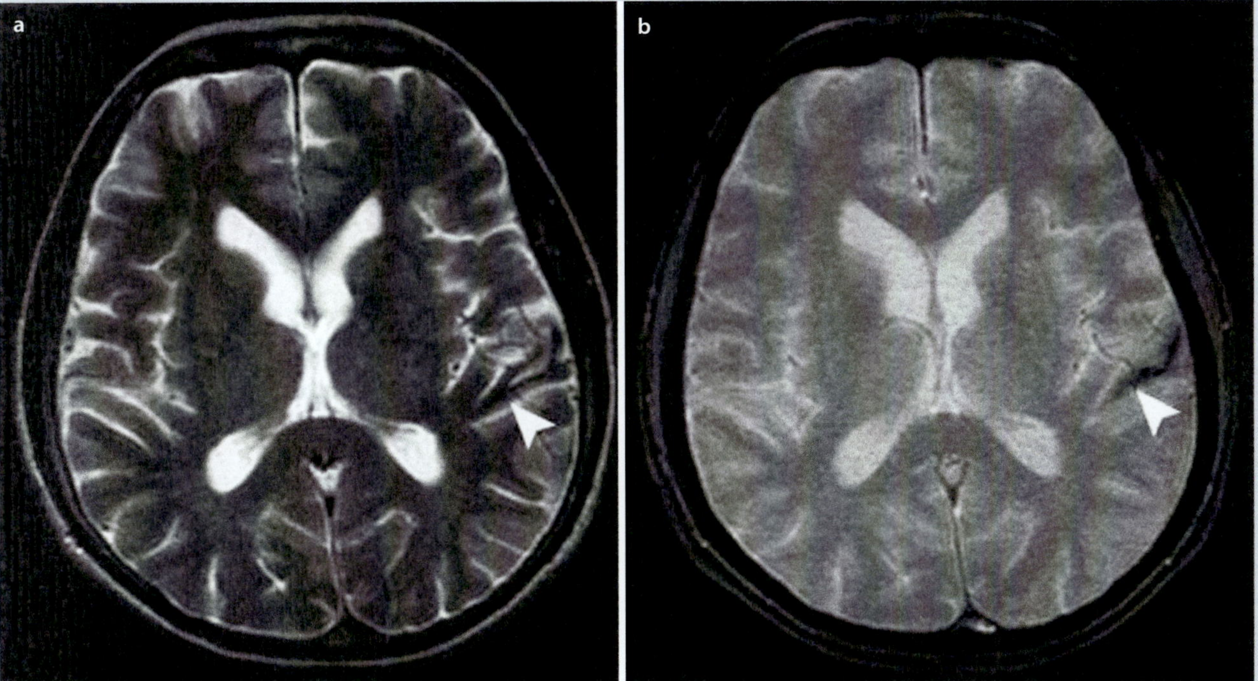

◘ **Fig. 2.3.8** Axial T2W (**a**) and T2* MRI of a patient with previous intraparenchymal bleeding in the left temporal lobe shows area of focal hypointense signal intensity on (**b**) due to hemosiderin. Notice the same area is visible on (**a**) but not as clearly seen as in the T2* image

## Hemorrhage into Malignancy

Hemorrhage into neoplasms accounts for 10% of spontaneous intracranial hemorrhage. It can be seen in 14% of metastases from melanoma and bronchogenic carcinoma and in 5% of cases of gliomas. Bleeding occurs because abnormal tumor vascularity usually occurs in higher-grade malignancies.

**Signs on CT**
- Atypical location for bleeding in a patient with known primary or secondary brain malignancy.
- The signal intensity of the blood is more heterogeneous than that of nonneoplastic hemorrhage. This heterogeneous texture is attributed to the multiple episodes of bleeding with different ages (mixed hypodense and hyperdense pattern).

## Further Reading

Dincsoy MY, et al. Intracranial hemorrhage in hypothalamic low-birth-weight neonates. Child's Nerv Syst. 1990;6: 245–9.

Gross A, et al. Intraventricular hemorrhage originating from choroids plexus angioma in a road accident victim. Z Rechtsmed. 1989;102:409–13.

Heros RC, et al. Cerebral vasospasm after subarachnoid hemorrhage: an update. Ann Neurol. 1983;14:599–608.

Koc RK, et al. Acute subdural hematoma: outcome and outcome prediction. Neurosurg Rev. 1997;20:239–44.

Laguna P, et al. Intracranial hemorrhage in a boy with severe haemophilia A and factor VIII inhibitor. Child's Nerv Syst. 2006;22:432–5.

Masuzawa T, et al. Computed tomographic evolution of post-traumatic subdural hygroma in young adults. Neuroradiology. 1948;26:245–8.

Masuzawa T, et al. Computed tomography evolution of post-traumatic subdural hygroma in young adults. Neuroradiology. 1984;26:245–8.

Moster ML, et al. Chronic subdural hematoma with transient neurological deficits: a review of 15 cases. Ann Neurol. 1983;14:539–42.

Park CK, et al. Spontaneous evolution of post-traumatic subdural hygroma into chronic subdural hematoma. Acta Neurochir (Wien). 1994;127:41–7.

Schellinger PD, et al. Intracranial hemorrhage, the role of magnetic resonance imaging. Neurocrit Care. 2004; 1:31–45.

Schwartz DT. Sensitivity of computed tomography for subarachnoid hemorrhage. Ann Emerg Med. 2009;53(1): 160–1.

Xi G, et al. Intracerebral hemorrhage, pathophysiology and therapy. Neurocrit Care. 2004;1:5–18.

## 2.4    Meningitis

Meningitis is a disease characterized by inflammation of the meninges due to infections or inflammatory disease (e.g., sarcoidosis). Infectious meningitis can be bacterial (e.g., pneumococcus) or viral (e.g., *Haemophilus influenzae*).

Patients with meningitis classically present with fever, neck stiffness, and neurological symptoms. Rarely, meningitis may lead to suprarenal gland suppression, causing patient death due to adrenal gland insufficiency. Infection of the meninges occurs due to hematogenous spread (e.g., bacteremia) or from direct extension from local infectious pathology (e.g., otitis media). Imaging in meningitis is mainly performed to evaluate complications.

**Signs on CT and MRI**
- Meningitis is detected typically as thickened meninges with contrast enhancement. Meningeal enhancement is divided into pachymeningeal and leptomeningeal enhancement. The pachymeninges are the dura matter, with its thick inner meningeal component, and its inner table of the skull (periosteum) component. The leptomeninges are the pia and the arachnoid matters. Pachymeningeal enhancement is seen as enhancement of the inner skull table and meningeal reflections (e.g., falx cerebri) (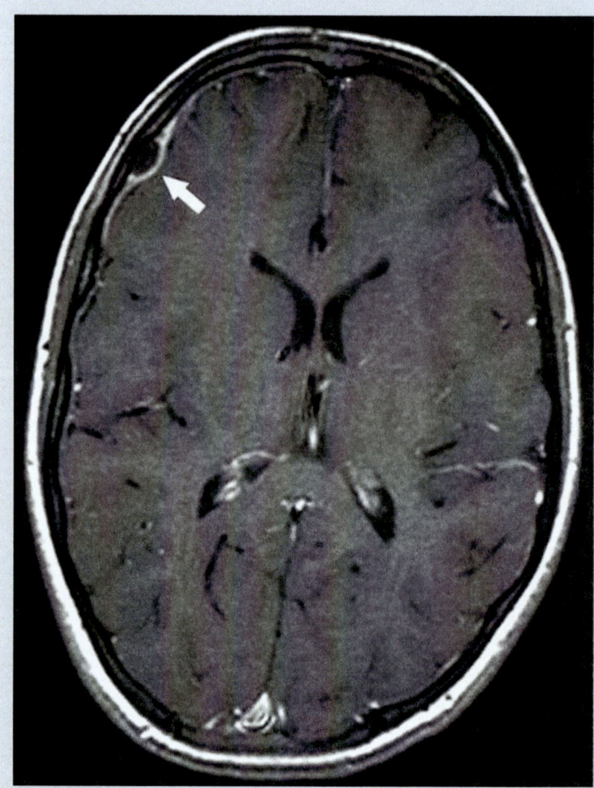 Fig. 2.4.1). In contrast, leptomeningeal

**Fig. 2.4.1**   Axial T1W postcontrast brain MRI shows right frontal pachymeningeal enhancement with epidural abscess formation (*arrow*)

enhancement is seen as thin linear enhancement that follows the pial surfaces, the cortical gyri, and fills the subarachnoid spaces (■ Fig. 2.4.2).

- *Ventriculitis* is seen as an enhancement of the subependymal surface of the ventricles after contrast injection.
- *Subdural pus collection (empyema)* is an extra-axial pus collection that usually results from untreated or chronic meningitis (crescent sign).
- *Abscess* is seen as an area of low density on CT or low T1 and high T2 signal intensities on MRI with uniform rim enhancement after contrast injection (■ Fig. 2.4.3). The abscess is commonly surrounded by vasogenic edema.
- *Subdural hygroma* is a sterile collection of fluid located in the subdural space usually as a sequela of meningitis in children.
- *Hydrocephalus* may arise due to inflammation of the basal meninges blocking the fourth ventricle. It is seen in advanced stages of meningitis. Dilatation of the temporal horns is a definite sign of hydrocephalus.
- *Post meningioencephalic sequela* is a severe advanced stage of meningitis characterized by loss of brain tissue (encephalomalacia) and parenchymal calcification with hydrocephalus (■ Fig. 2.4.4).
- Superior sagittal sinus thrombosis may be seen as a triangular filling defect on axial images (*delta sign*).

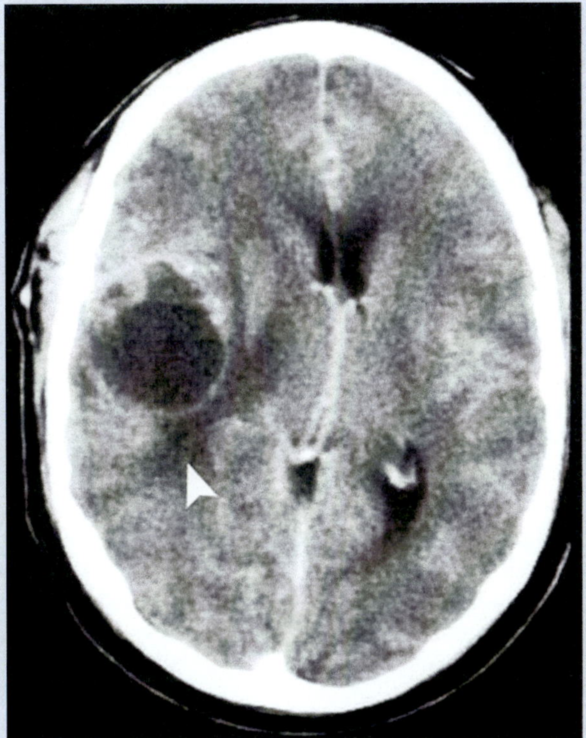

■ **Fig. 2.4.3**  Axial postcontrast brain CT shows right temporal abscess with thin rim enhancement and vasogenic edema (*arrowhead*) that exerts mass effect over the anterior horns of the lateral ventricles

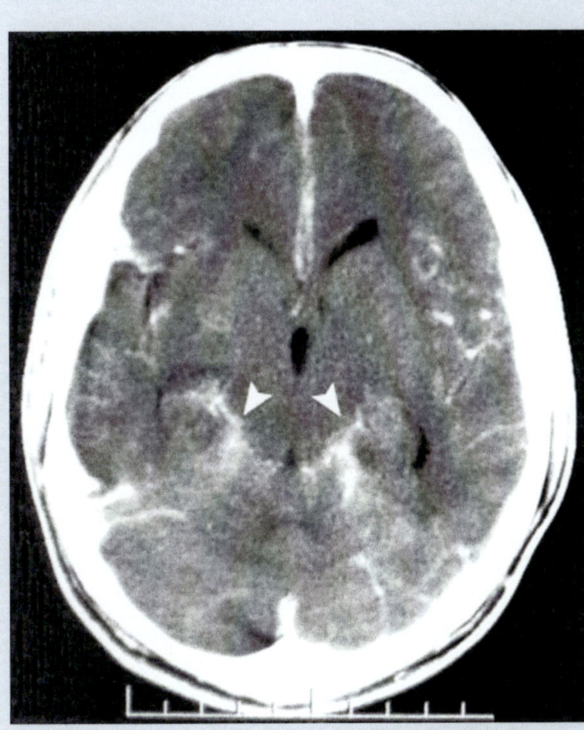

■ **Fig. 2.4.2**  Axial postcontrast brain CT shows enhancement of the leptomeninges around the ambient cisterns (*arrowheads*)

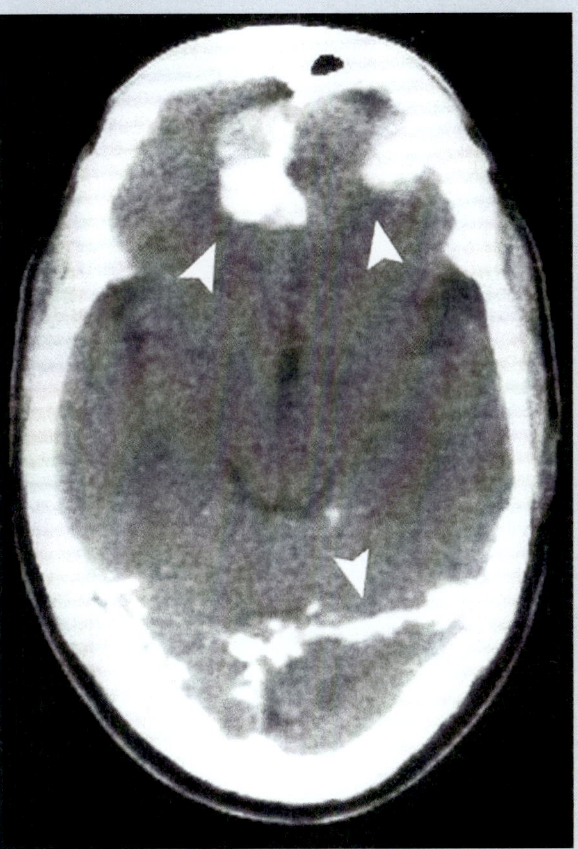

■ **Fig. 2.4.4**  Axial nonenhanced brain CT shows postmeningoencephalic parenchymal and meningeal (falx) calcification (*arrowheads*)

## Differential Diagnoses and Related Diseases

- *Multiloculated hydrocephalus* is a clinicopathological condition characterized by enlarged, loculated ventricles with paraventricular porencephalic cavities. The condition is seen in neonates, commonly as a sequel of ventriculitis complicating neonatal meningitis. Neonates present with hydrocephalus, neurological deterioration, and seizures. Mortality rate is high (>70 %). CT and MRI typically show multiloculated ventricles with irregular borders and internal septae (◨ Fig. 2.4.5).
- *Canalis basilaris medianus* is a congenital anomaly characterized by a well-defined channel seen in the midline of the basiocciput, very close to the anterior rim of the foramen magnum. It is seen on CT or MRI as a linear defect in the midportion of the clivus (◨ Fig. 2.4.6). Although it is an asymptomatic anomaly, it can be the source of recurrent meningitis in children due to transmission of bacteria from the superior nasopharynx into the central nervous system through this basiocciput defect.
- *Vogt–Koyanagi–Harada syndrome* is a rare, sporadic, and systemic disorder mostly seen in adults and characterized by acute panuveitis, meningitis, and cutaneous

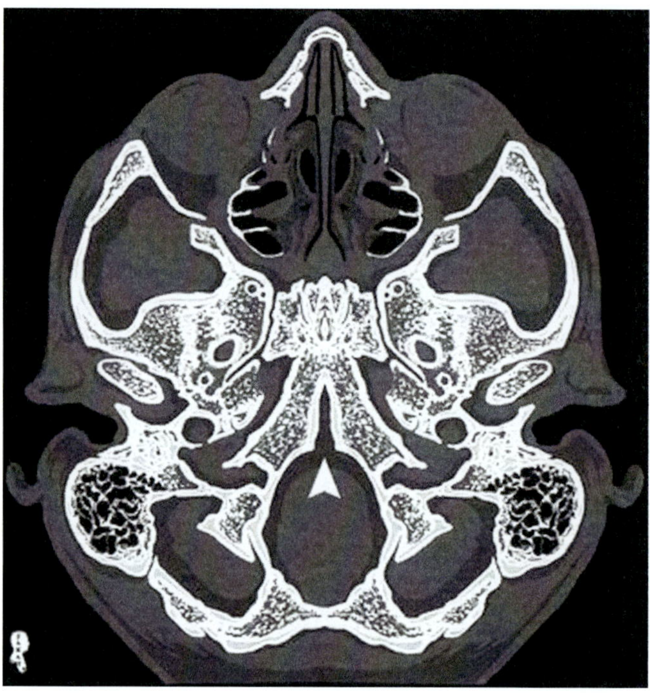

◨ **Fig. 2.4.6**   Axial CT illustration of the base of the skull shows a linear median bony defect of the clivus (canalis basilaris medianus)

manifestations. The disease arises due to a widespread pathology affecting the melanin-forming cells in different organs, typically in dark-skinned people. Uveitis is inflammation of the uvea, which supplies nutrition to the globe and is composed of the iris, ciliary body, and choroid. Any part of the uvea can be involved in the inflammation (e.g., iritis), and patients typically present with a painful eye, with pain in the distribution of the trigeminal nerve (because the ciliary body is supplied by the ophthalmic division of the trigeminal nerve). The disease has three phases: a prodormal phase characterized by fever, severe headache, and tinnitus; an ophthalmic phase characterized by bilateral uveitis and optic disk hyperemia; and a convalescent phase seen weeks after the ophthalmic phase, characterized by premature graying of hair (poliosis), vitiligo, alopecia, painful hearing (dysacousia), tinnitus, and vertigo. Diagnostic criteria include the absence of ocular trauma with the following: (a) bilateral chronic iridocyclitis, (b) posterior uveitis including retinal detachment, (c) neurological signs with signs of meningitis (e.g., neck stiffness), and (d) cutaneous findings of alopecia, vitiligo, or poliosis. Signs on orbital CT or MRI may show choroidal and scleral thickening due to chronic inflammation on postcontrast images or retinal detachment with typical (V-shaped sign) on severe cases (◨ Fig. 2.4.7). Uncommonly, the disease can present with optic neuritis, seen as enhanced optic nerve on postcontrast images on both CT and MRI.

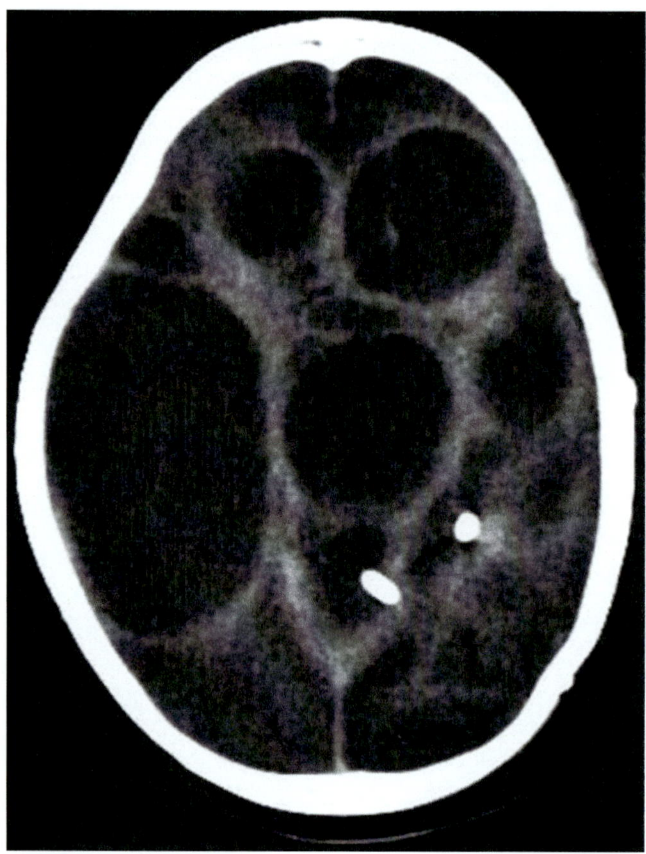

◨ **Fig. 2.4.5**   Axial nonenhanced brain CT of a neonate shows multiloculated hydrocephalus

### Further Reading

Albanese V, et al. Neuroradiological findings in multiloculated hydrocephalus. Acta Neurochir. 1982;60:297–311.

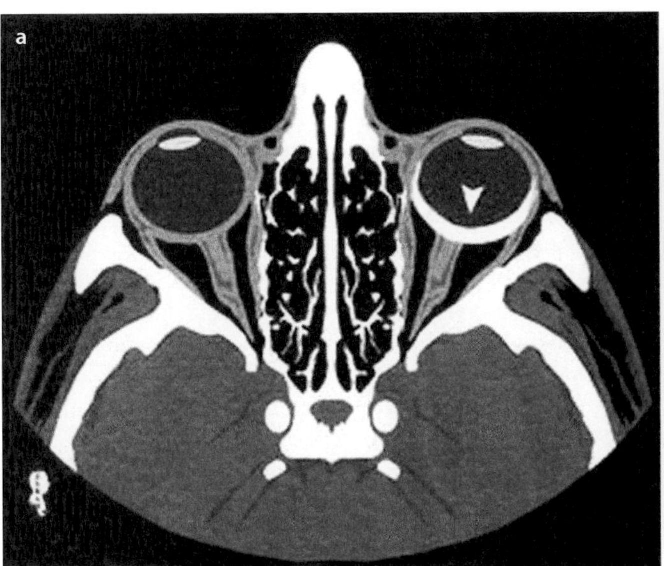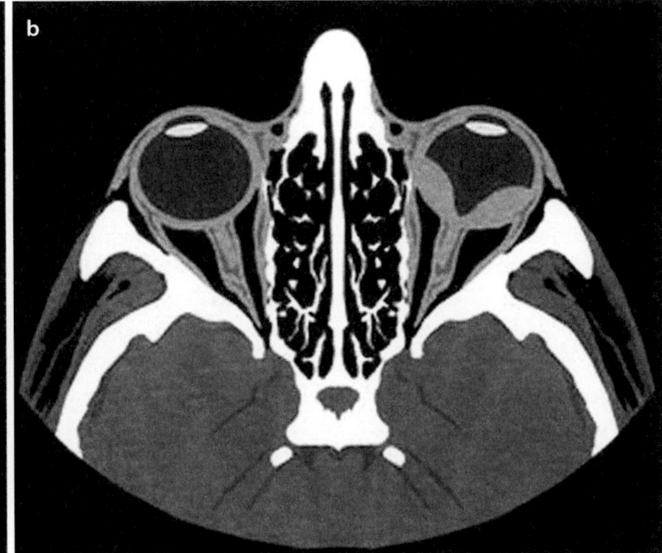

**◘ Fig. 2.4.7** Orbital CT postcontrast (**a**) and nonenhanced (**b**) illustrations of a patient show left eye choroidal/scleral thickening and enhancement due to uveitis in (**a**) (*arrowhead*), with V-shaped sign of retinal detachment in the left eye in (**b**)

Bilaniuk LT, et al. Computed tomography in meningitis. Neuroradiology. 1978;16:13–4.

Gilbert JA, et al. Vogt-Koyanagi-Harada syndrome: case report and review. J Emerg Med. 1994;12:615–9.

Jacquemin C, et al. Canalis basilaris medianus: MRI. Neuroradiology. 2000;42:121–3.

Kamra P, et al. Infectious meningitis: prospective evaluation with magnetization transfer MRI. Br J Radiol. 2004;77: 387–94.

McGehee BE, et al. Bilateral retinal detachment in a patient with Vogt-Koyanagi-Harada syndrome. Emerg Radiol. 2005;11:366–71.

Rao NA, et al. Vogt-Koyanagi-Harada disease diagnostic criteria. Int Ophthalmol. 2007;27:195–9.

Smirniotopoulos JG, et al. Patterns of contrast enhancement in the brain and meninges. RadioGraph. 2007;27: 525–51.

Splendiani A, et al. Contrast-enhanced FLAIR in the early diagnosis of infectious meningitis. Neuroradiology. 2005;47:591–8.

## 2.5 Encephalitis

Encephalitis means inflammation of the brain parenchyma. Brain inflammation can result from different etiologies, most commonly viruses and autoimmune inflammation.

Patients with encephalitis typically present in early stages with headache or flu-like illness, followed by alteration in consciousness, drowsiness, confusion, fever, and seizures. Coma may result in severe cases.

This topic discusses the different kinds of encephalitis with their characteristic radiological features.

## Limbic Encephalitis

The brain can be divided into regions according to functions. The first part is the brain stem, which plays a role in the basic attention, consciousness, arousal, heart and respiration adjustment, temperature control, and sleep–wake cycle control. The second part is the limbic system, which controls the behavior related to food, hormones and sex, jealousy, sadness and love, pleasure, and fight-or-flight responses. The limbic system is composed of the hippocampus, thalamus, hypothalamus, and amygdala. The third part is the rational brain (neocortex), which controls logic, thoughts, speaking, planning, and writing.

Limbic encephalitis (LE) involves inflammation of one structure or more related to the limbic system. LE can be caused by infections (e.g., herpes simplex virus) or autoimmune response.

*Herpes encephalitis* (*HSE*) is caused by herpes simplex virus type 1 or type 2. HSE type 1 is often seen in children and young adults. It starts as an orofacial infection (gingivostomatitis), which lasts for 1–2 weeks, followed by flu-like symptoms. Patients present with fever, headache, and change in mental status. The virus spreads in retrograde fashion along the trigeminal nerve course or the olfactory bulb into the brain. In the brain, the virus has affinity to infect the meninges, temporal lobes, and the inferior frontal lobe. HSE type 1 is the most common cause of encephalitis (95 %). HSV type 2 is a genital form of HSE that affects neonates delivered by mothers, with herpes infection in the birth canal. It is an uncommon type of encephalitis (15 %), and clinical diagnosis is usually confirmed by cerebrospinal fluid (CSF) analysis that reveals high leukocytes and protein content and detection of the herpes virus DNA by serology.

Autoimmune LE has two forms. The first form is called *paraneoplastic limbic encephalitis (PLE)*, which is seen in patients with particular cancers with paraneoplastic manifestations, such as thymus, lung, breast, and testes cancers. PLE is confirmed by detecting paraneoplastic antibodies in the patient blood like immunoglobulin G antibodies, ANNA 1, PCA 1, CV2, MA 2, and ANNA 2 antibodies.

The other form of autoimmune LE is nonPLE, which has the same picture as PLE in the absence of the serum paraneoplastic antibodies. The most common subsyndrome of the nonPLE is *voltage-gated potassium channel (VGKC) antibody-associated encephalitis*. This syndrome is commonly undiagnosed due to the lack of awareness about its existence. The diagnosis of autoimmune LE is important because it responds well to immunosuppressive drugs.

### Signs on CT

- Initially, the scan may be normal or shows hypodense lesions affecting the medial temporal lobes mainly in a bilateral asymmetrical pattern with mass effect and edema (□ Fig. 2.5.1). Areas of necrosis and hemorrhage may be seen on nonenhanced contrast images. Postcontrast images show patchy enhancement. The explanation for the temporal lobe affection lies in the reactivation of the virus from the trigeminal ganglia within Meckel's cave.
- Postencephalitic sequel includes parenchymal calcification and dilatation of ventricles.
- In HSE, the basal ganglia are often spared.

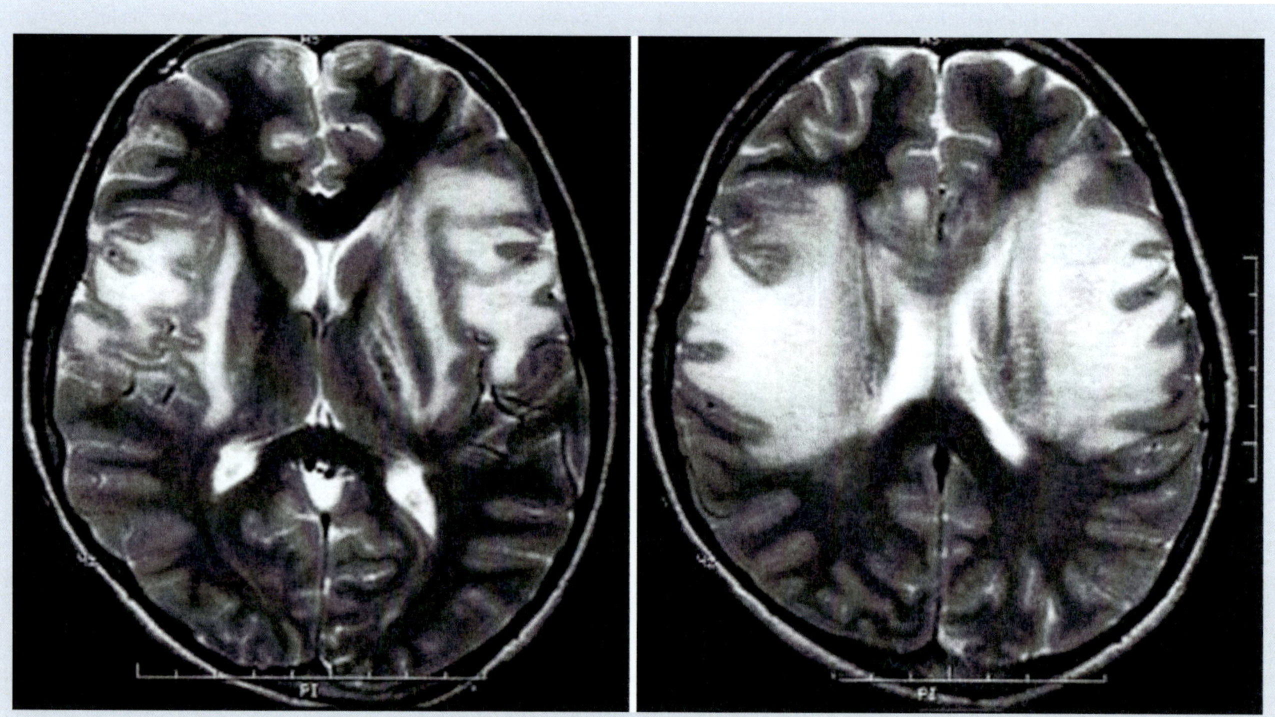

**□ Fig. 2.5.1**   Axial sequential T2W MR images show bilateral symmetrical hyperintense signal intensities affecting the region of the temporal lobes (both white and gray matters) in a patient with herpes encephalitis (HSE)

### Signs on MRI

- In HSE, hyperintense, ill-defined cortical and white matter areas on T2W sequences with edema, mass effect, and gyral enhancement (□ Fig. 2.5.1) are seen. Later in the course of the disease, meningeal enhancement after contrast may be seen due to the spread of the virus to the meninges.

- Autoimmune LE shows the same picture like HSE. Bilateral temporal and hippocampal lesions are typically seen. The main difference is based on the CSF analysis detecting the virus antibodies or the autoimmune antibodies. Also, the history of cancer favors the autoimmune encephalitis.

## Acute Demyelinating Encephalomyelitis (ADEM)

ADEM is an autoimmune demyelinating encephalitis that arises typically as an immune reaction 2 weeks after viral infection with MMR (measles, mumps, rubella), whooping cough infection (pertussis), or after immunization with MMR vaccine.

In ADEM, there is a hypersensitivity reaction affecting myelin and brain vessels (vasculitis). Patients classically present with sudden onset of neurological symptoms reflecting a wide central nervous system disturbance 2 weeks after viral infection or immunization.

ADEM has the same MRI picture as multiple sclerosis (MS). Unlike MS, which has multiple relapsing episodes, ADEM occurs once in life (monophasic course).

*Acute hemorrhagic leukoencephalitis (AHL)* is a severe form of ADEM characterized by intraparenchymal hemorrhage. AHL often arises after an upper respiratory tract infection or allergic reaction. The patient will show features of encephalitis, fever, and impaired consciousness.

**Signs on MRI**

- Large multifocal periventricular lesions with mild mass effect giving high signals in T2 (demyelinating areas) exactly like MS plaques, with asymmetric involvement of cerebral hemispheres ( Fig. 2.5.2). MS plaques are often found bilaterally. The demyelinating plaques show ring enhancement after gadolinium injection in a similar fashion like acute MS plaques.
- Involvement of spinal cord and the cortical gray matter is common.
- Contrast enhancement is not always a feature.
- Typically, ADEM does not involve the corpus callosum.
- Bilateral optic neuritis may occur.
- In AHL, signs of hemorrhagic plaques are found on nongadolinium-enhanced images.

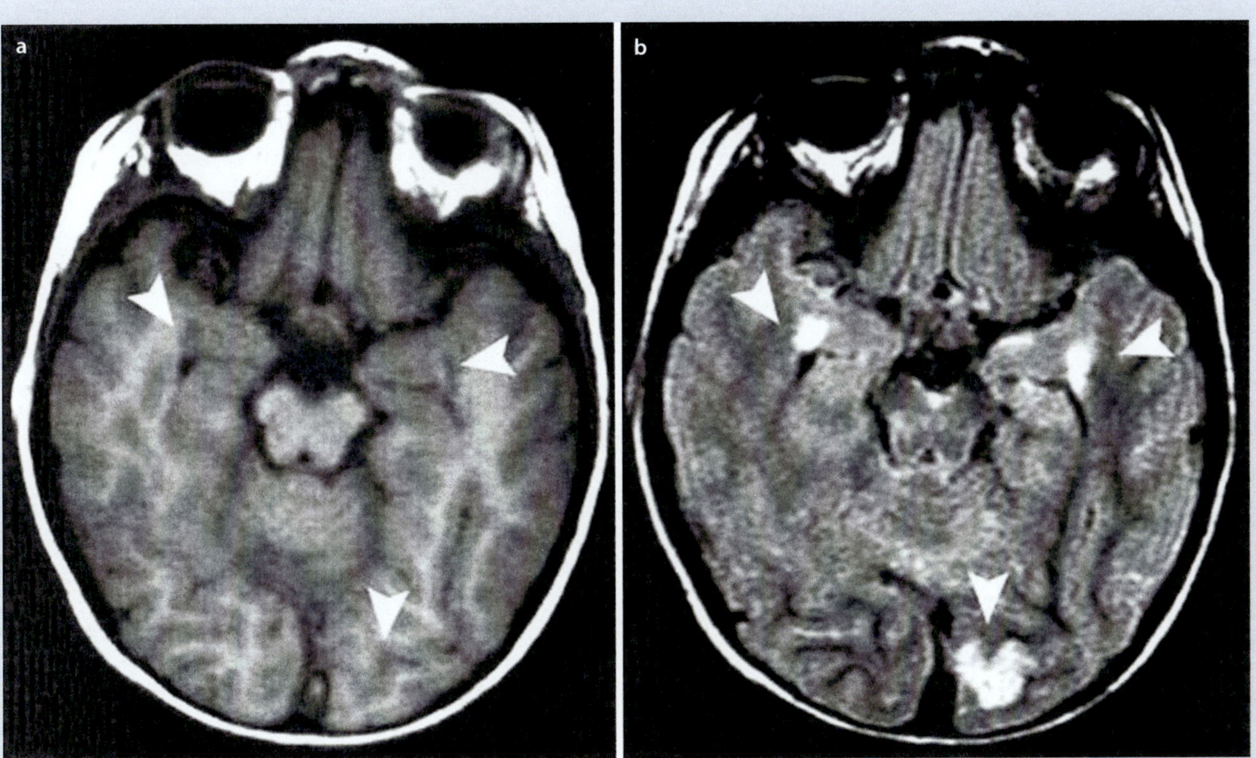

 **Fig. 2.5.2**  Axial T1W (**a**) and FLAIR (**b**) images in a patient with acute demyelinating encephalomyelitis (ADEM) after measles, mumps, and rubella (MMR) vaccination show multifocal hyperintense areas in (**b**) affecting the posterior lobe and the area around the temporal horns of the lateral ventricles (*arrowheads*). The areas are patchy and asymmetrically distributed

*How can you differentiate between MS and ADEM?*
- MS has an acute and chronic phase, while ADEM has only one acute stage.
- MS affects white matter only, while ADEM affects white and gray matters.
- Clinical history of infection or immunization with ADEM.
- Corpus callosum is typically not affected in ADEM, while it is commonly affected in MS.
- ADEM causes bilateral optic neuritis, while MS typically causes unilateral optic neuritis.

## Hashimoto's Encephalitis

Hashimoto's encephalopathy (HE) is defined as a syndrome of persistent or relapsing neurological or neuropsychiatric symptoms, even though the thyroid levels are usually normal.

HE usually affects children in school age, with an incidence of 1.2 % of population. Asymptomatic thyroid goiter can be seen in 85 % of patients.

Patients with HE typically present with different unexplained neurological symptoms like epilepsy, behavioral changes, ataxia, hallucinations, or dementia. Diagnosis needs high level of suspicion. The characteristic feature that confirms HE in a patient with unexplained encephalitis is to find high levels of thyroid antibodies in the serum, which is always abnormally high. In contrast, the thyroid function levels usually are within normal or lower than normal range. The disease responds well to steroid therapy.

**Signs on MRI**
The signs on MRI in HE are nonspecific. The MRI can be normal or show nonspecific features of subcortical white matter changes (not the normal changes seen in a patient with epilepsy) (■ Fig. 2.5.3).

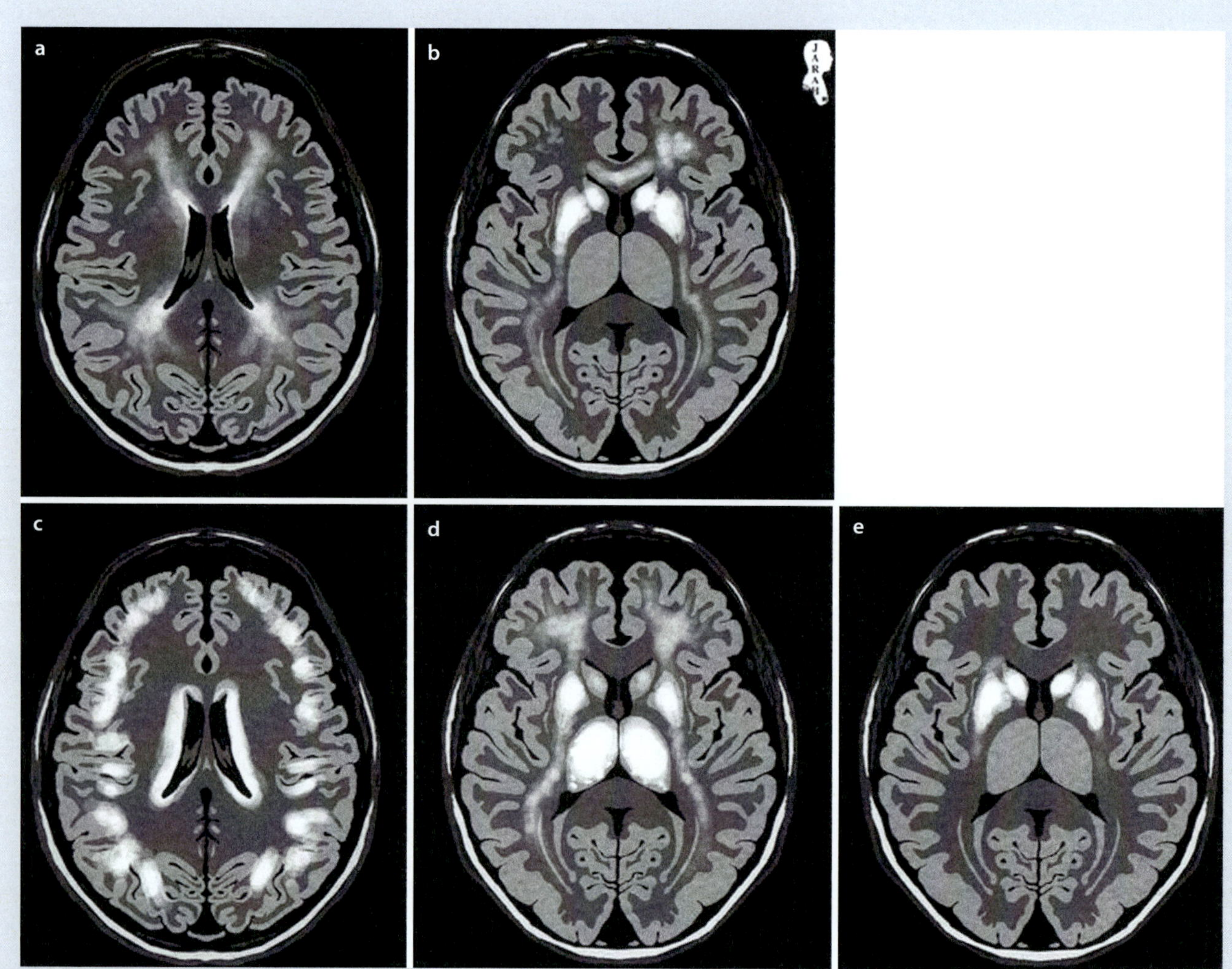

■ **Fig. 2.5.3**    Axial FLAIR MR illustrations demonstrate different brain affection pattern in different types of encephalitis disorders: (**a**) Hashimoto's encephalitis, (**b**) measles encephalitis (ME), (**c**) subacute sclerosing panencephalitis (SSPE), (**d**) Japanese encephalitis (JE), and (**e**) encephalitis lethargica

## Rasmussen Encephalitis (Rasmussen Syndrome)

Rasmussen encephalitis (RE) is a rare, pediatric disease of chronic encephalitis usually effecting one hemisphere. The disease is characterized by partial motor seizures and progressive cognitive deterioration.

RE has an unknown cause, although viral and immunological causes have been suggested. Patients may show high titers of Epstein–Barr virus and cytomegalovirus in the CSF, with high serum GluR3 antibodies supporting the autoimmune and the viral theories.

RE is mostly seen in children (mainly pediatric disease), although few rare adult cases have been reported. RE has three stages, initial, acute, and residual. In the initial stage, the patient suffers from few partial motor seizures. Later in the acute stage, there is increased frequency of the seizures attack. The residual stage is characterized by cortical atrophy and permanent neurological deficits. Histopathology features include gliosis and perivascular cuffing in both white and gray matters.

The key to suspect and diagnose RE is to have a pediatric patient with multiple attacks of epilepsy, increasing in frequency, with serial MRI examinations showing changes and atrophy in one cerebral hemisphere only. Brain biopsy may be needed to confirm the diagnosis in atypical cases. Treatment ranges between antiepileptics, antiviral medications, corticosteroids, and immunosuppressive agents.

### Criteria to Diagnose Rasmussen Encephalitis

- Previously healthy child between 14 months and 14 years.
- Patients present with drug-resistant seizure, usually tonic–clonic or partial seizure.
- There are progressive unilateral neurological deficits that might lead to paresis (bilateral involvement occasionally).

> **Signs on MRI**
> - Hyperintense cortex is seen on T2W or FLAIR images on noncontrast-enhanced images affecting the parieto-frontal or the temporal lobes in acute stages (◘ Fig. 2.5.4). The MRI may be normal initially and then shows signs of unilateral cortical atrophy. Classically, the contralateral hemisphere, basal ganglia, and the posterior fossa are unaffected. However, the head of the caudate nucleus may be affected.
> - In the residual stage, cortical atrophy, ventricular enlargement of the affected side (evacuee dilatation), and caudate nucleus atrophy can be seen with atrophy of the whole cerebral hemisphere. Atrophic changes are predominantly seen in the perisylvian area and the caudate nucleus.

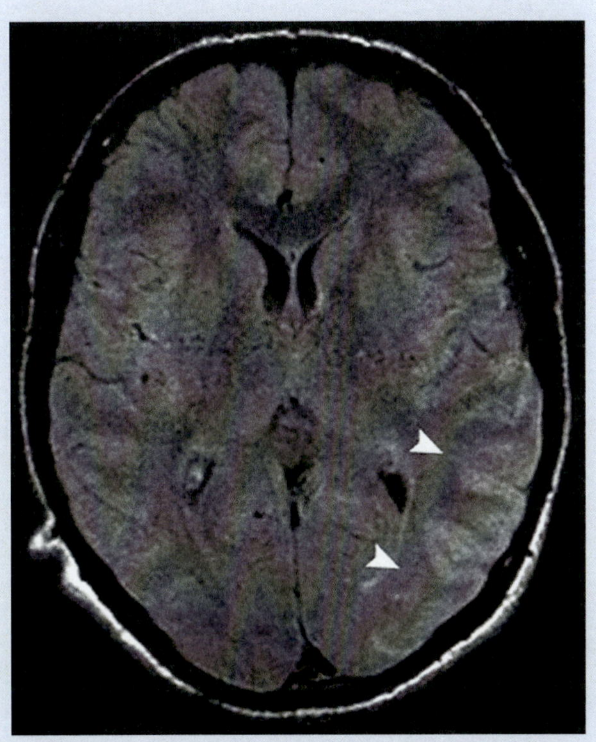

◘ **Fig. 2.5.4** Axial FLAIR image in a child with recurrent epilepsy shows moderate hyperintense cortices in the left temporo-occipital region in a unilateral pattern (*arrowheads*). The patient was diagnosed later as a case of Rasmussen encephalitis (RE)

## Measles Encephalitis

Measles encephalitis (ME) is a brain inflammation due to an acute infection with measles virus. ME is considered rare due to the worldwide spread of MMR vaccine (0.05–0.4 %), yet few sporadic cases are reported in the literature occasionally.

ME starts on the second to sixth day after the development of the rash, but it may precede the rash. Patients present with the usual clinical picture of encephalitis. Diagnosis is made on the basis of identifying high antimeasles antibodies titers in the CSF.

> **Signs on MRI**
> - MRI often shows bilateral T1/T2 hyperintense signal intensities in the basal ganglia and the white matter (◘ Fig. 2.5.3).
> - The frontotemporal areas may be affected in an asymmetric pattern bilaterally.

## Subacute Sclerosing Panencephalitis (SSPE)

SSPE is a well-recognized chronic complication of measles virus, developing 6–12 years after initial measles infection.

SSPE is a rare disease, with an incidence of 1:1,000,000 and a high mortality rate. The majority of patients with SSPE are known to have a previous attack of classical measles years before. Fifty percent of SSPE cases occur after 2 years from the initial measles infection, and patients are between 5 and 15 years of age.

Patients with SSPE often present behavioral changes with jerking movements known as myoclonic seizures. The myoclonic jerking is exacerbated on excitement. Later, develops, with problems in swallowing, speech, and vision. Some patients may develop pyramidal signs with cerebellar signs (e.g., ataxia). Cortical blindness due to occipital lobe involvement or optic nerve edema may occur. The diagnosis of SSPE should be considered in patients with cortical blindness even when other classical findings of SSPE are absent. The duration of the illness can be short (e.g., 6 weeks) or very long (e.g., 10 years).

Diagnosis of SSPE is based on the high serum and CSF antimeasles antibody titer detection. Imaging is helpful in establishing differential diagnosis.

> **Signs on MRI**
> — Commonly, the periventricular and subcortical white matters are affected in SSPE (■ Fig. 2.5.3), with bilateral high T2W and FLAIR signal intensities seen on MRI.
> — The basal ganglia, cerebellum, spinal cord, and corpus callosum are less frequently affected.

## Japanese Encephalitis

Japanese encephalitis (JE) is acute viral encephalitis, caused due to infection with JE virus. JE virus belongs to the *Flaviviridae* family (Flavivirus). The virus is transmitted to humans from its hosts via its carrier, the *Culex tritaeniorhynchus* mosquito. The natural hosts of the JE virus are pigs, birds, dogs, and horses.

Following bite on the human body from an infected mosquito, the virus proliferates in the lymphatic system. From there, it enters the bloodstream and crosses the blood–brain barrier (BBB) to start brain parenchymal inflammation. Patients with JE present with loss of appetite (anorexia), fatigue, headache, and vomiting. The initial stage of the disease is characterized by rapidly progressing fever and nonspecific central nervous system symptoms. The neurological symptoms include rigidity, Parkinson-like symptoms, altered mental status, and seizures. The fever and the systemic symptoms improve gradually after 7–8 days. In 10 % of patients, long-term sequelae may occur, including psychiatric symptoms, motor impairment, and epilepsy.

Diagnosis is confirmed by detection of JE virus antibodies or isolation of the virus from the CSF.

> **Signs on MRI**
> — The classical findings in JE include bilateral symmetrical high signal intensity lesions onT2Wand FLAIR images located in both thalami (■ Fig. 2.5.3). Similar lesions may be found in the basal ganglia, substantia nigra, hippocampus, pons, and cerebral white matter.
> — Hemorrhagic lesions in the thalami may be found occasionally.

## West Nile Encephalitis

West Nile encephalitis (WNE) is encephalitis caused by acute infection with the West Nile virus (WNV). WNW is a positive-strand RNA virus belonging to the *Flaviviridae* family.

WNE is observed in the Middle East and African countries. The virus is transmitted to humans from the *C. tritaeniorhynchus* mosquito from its original hosts; the hosts of the WNV are crows and pigeons. WNV is an "arbovirus." Arboviruses are viruses that are transmitted from one animal host to the next by insects (arthropods). WNV is not transmitted from person to person.

Patients with WNE present with nonspecific febrile illness, lymphadenopathy, skin rash, headache, and body ache. Encephalitis symptoms start when the virus crosses the BBB, resulting in seizures, confusion, paralysis, and behavioral changes that may be mistaken with hysteria.

Diagnosis is based on detecting high titers of WNV antibodies in the CSF.

> **Signs on MRI**
> The scan shows bilateral symmetrical lesions in both thalami, with hemorrhagic tendency. The MRI picture is similar to the JE picture.

## Tick-Borne Encephalitis (Spring–Summer Encephalitis)

Tick-borne encephalitis (TBE) is encephalitis caused by TBE virus, a virus that belongs to the *Flaviviridae* family.

Patients with TBE commonly present with meningitis (49 %), followed by meningoencephalitis (41 %) and meningoencephalomyelitis (10 %). Patients may present with polio-like symptoms with polyradiculitis course. The virus has an affinity to the anterior horn cells in the spinal nerve roots.

Diagnosis is based on confirming the virus antibodies in the CSF.

> **Signs on MRI**
> - The brain MRI shows the same picture like JE and WNE.
> - Polyradiculitis is seen as marked contrast enhancement of the spinal nerve roots on contrast-enhanced images ( Fig. 2.5.5).

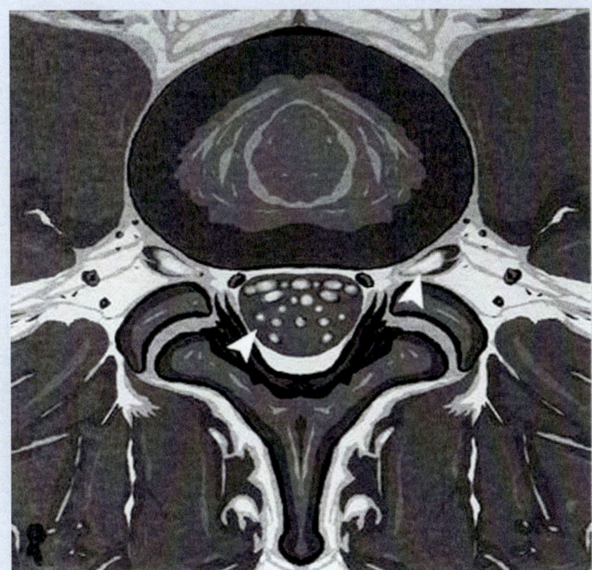

 **Fig. 2.5.5**  Axial postcontrast spinal MR illustration at the level of L3/L4 shows enhanced cauda equina roots and spinal roots representing polyradiculitis (*arrowheads*)

## Murray Valley Encephalitis

Murray Valley encephalitis (MVE) is encephalitis caused by MVE virus, another virus that belongs to the *Flaviviridae* family.

Majority of patients with MV virus are asymptomatic, with only 1:1,000 infected persons developing encephalitis. The symptoms are nonspecific, with neurological residua in 40 % of survivors. Diagnosis is based on detecting the virus antibodies in the CSF.

> **Signs on MRI**
> The brain MRI shows the same picture like JE, TBE, and WNE.

## St. Louis Encephalitis

St. Louis encephalitis is a disease caused by the St. Louis virus, another virus that belongs to the *Flaviviridae* family. The virus was named after it was isolated from the human brain tissue in 1933 during a large epidemic in St. Louis City, USA.

The disease ranges between flu-like illnesses to a life-threatening central nervous system disease. Diagnosis is based on CSF serology.

> **Signs on MRI**
> - The brain MRI shows the same picture like JE, TBE, MVE, and WNE.
> - The substantia nigra is commonly involved in St. Louis encephalitis.

## Encephalitis Lethargica

Encephalitis lethargica (EL) is a rare, mysterious form of encephalitis that was responsible for epidemic disease that killed 500,000 people from about 1917 until 1940. Many investigators link EL with the notorious Spanish flu influenza virus, which is responsible for the influenza epidemic at the end of the First World War. Although the disease is considered historical, few sporadic cases are reported from time to time.

EL typically has three forms: irritable, lethargic, and lethargic with paralysis. The irritable form is characterized by marked restlessness and excitability. The lethargic stage is characterized by a drowsy state and expressionless, masklike face, resembling Parkinson's disease. The third stage is characterized by drowsiness with some form of motor paralysis in the lower extremities and frequent convulsions.

Patients with EL present with characteristic gradual onset of headache, lethargy and asthenia, low-grade fever, cranial nerve palsies, and vomiting, especially in children. Other neuropsychiatric symptoms include Parkinsonian masked face, catatonia, choreiform movements, insomnia, delirium, and profound sweating.

Children with EL present with a wide variety of behaviors that can be regarded as psychopathic. These include personality change, emotional instability, nervousness, restlessness, and destructive and impulsive mood.

EL is one of the causes of juvenile Parkinsonism, mainly the rigid–akinetic form. This can be explained by the fact that the basal ganglia are classically affected in EL.

*Criteria* to diagnose EL include encephalitis with three of the following major criteria, assuming all the known causes of encephalitis have been excluded:
- Neuropsychiatric symptoms
- Sleep disturbance (e.g., insomnia)
- Signs of basal ganglia involvement (e.g., Parkinson-like symptoms)
- Ophthalmic symptoms
- Obsessive–compulsive behavior
- Respiratory irregularity

**Signs on MRI**

MRI of EL patients shows bilateral basal ganglia lesions with high signal intensities on T2W and FLAIR images (▶ Fig. 2.5.3).

## Further Reading


Abe T, et al. Japanese encephalitis. JMRI. 1998;8:755–61.

Alfaresi M, et al. West Nile virus in the blood donors in UAE. Indian J Med Microbiol. 2008;26:92–3.

Arain A, et al. Hashimoto's encephalopathy: documentation of temporal seizure origin by ictal EEG. Seizure. 2001;10:438–41.

Baba Y, et al. Acute measles encephalitis in adults. J Neurol. 2006;253:121–4.

Beleza P, et al. From juvenile Parkinsonism to encephalitis lethargica, a new phenotype of post-streptococcal disorders: case report. Eur J Paediatr Neurol. 2008;12:505–7.

Bender A, et al. Sever tick borne encephalitis with simultaneous brain stem, bithalamic, and spinal cord involvement documented by MRI. J Neurol Neurosurg Psychiatry. 2005;76:135–7.

Benneis C, et al. Encephalitis lethargica following Bartonella henselae infection. J Neurol. 2007;254:546–7.

Bermejo PE, et al. Hemorrhagic acute disseminated encephalomyelitis as first manifestation of systemic lupus erythematosus. J Neurol. 2008;255:1256–8.

Bertoni M, et al. Encephalopathy associated with Hashimoto's thyroiditis: an additional case. Eur J Intern Med. 2003;14:434–47.

Bosanko CM, et al. West Nile virus encephalitis involving the substantia nigra. Neuroimaging and pathologic findings with literature review. Arch Neurol. 2003;60:1448–52.

Collison K, et al. Asymmetric cerebellar ataxia and limbic encephalitis as a presenting feature of primary Sjögren's syndrome. J Neurol. 2007;254:1609–11.

De Tiège X, et al. The spectrum of herpes simplex encephalitis in children. Eur J Paediatr Neurol. 2008;12:72–81.

Deb P, et al. Neuropathological spectrum of Rasmussen encephalitis. Neurol India. 2005;53:156–61.

Feydy A, et al. Brain and spinal cord MR imaging in a case of acute disseminated encephalomyelitis. Eur Radiol. 1997;7:415–7.

Garg RK. Subacute sclerosing panencephalitis. J Neurol. doi:10.1007/s00415-008-9932-6.

Granata T. Rasmussen's syndrome. Neurol Sci. 2003;24:S239–43.

Grubbauer HM, et al. Tick-borne encephalitis in a 3-month-old child. Eur J Pediatr. 1992;151:743–4.

Heo SH, et al. A case of unilateral hemispheric encephalitis. Neurol Sci. 2007;28:185–7.

Kroeger MA, et al. Murray Valley encephalitis virus recombinant subviral particles protect mice from lethal challenge with virulent wild-type virus. Arch Virol. 2002;147:1155–72.

Lacroix C, et al. Acute necrotizing measles encephalitis in a child with AIDS. J Neurol. 1995;242:249–56.

Lury KM, et al. Eastern equine encephalitis: CT and MRI findings in one case. Emerg Radiol. 2004;11:46–8.

Paprocka J, et al. Difficulties in differentiation of Parry-Romberg syndrome, unilateral facial scleroderma, and Rasmussen syndrome. Childs Nerv Syst. 2006;22:409–15.

Parmar RC, et al. Measles encephalitis: a case report of two cases with variable manifestations. Pediatr Int. 2002;44:90–2.

Parquet MC, et al. St. Louis encephalitis virus induced pathology in cultured cells. Arch Virol. 2002;147:1105–19.

Pedersen H, et al. Computed tomographic findings of early subacute sclerosing panencephalitis. Neuroradiology. 1982;23:31–2.

Pfefferkorn T, et al. Tick-borne encephalitis with polyradiculitis documented by MRI. Neuroradiology. 2007;68:1232–3.

Rajesh B, et al. Putaminal involvement in Rasmussen encephalitis. Pediatr Radiol. 2006;36:816–22.

Senol U, et al. Subacute sclerosing panencephalitis: brain stem involvement in a peculiar pattern. Neuroradiology. 2000;42:913–6.

Urbach H, et al. Serial MRI of limbic encephalitis. Neuroradiology. 2006;48:380–6.

van der Meyden CH, et al. Gadolinium ring enhancement and mass effect in acute disseminated encephalomyelitis. Neuroradiology. 1994;36:221–3.

Vasconcellos E, et al. Pediatric manifestations of Hashimoto's encephalopathy. Pediatr Neurol. 1999;20:394–8.

Vilensky JA, et al. Children and encephalitis lethargica: a historical review. Pediatr Neurol. 2007;37:79–84.

Wong SH, et al. Murray Valley encephalitis mimicking herpes simplex encephalitis. J Clin Neurosci. 2005;12:822–4.


## 2.6    Epilepsy

Epilepsy is a chronic neurological disease characterized by recurrent, spontaneous episodes of seizures, which are defined as excessive abnormal neuronal activity of the cortical neurons. Seizures originate either from a localized area within the brain (partial/focal) or arise from both hemispheres simultaneously (generalized).

*Partial seizures* can be associated with loss of consciousness (complex) or occur without loss of consciousness (simple/Jacksonian). Partial seizures can spread from one area to another, ending up in initiating secondary generalized seizure. Patients with partial simple seizures experience mental events like confusion, mild hallucinations, jerking movements, or emotional events (déjà vu phenomenon). In contrast, partial complex seizure patients experience uncontrolled behavior, loss of judgment, and loss of consciousness. Also, patients with partial complex seizures often experience a warning sign such as aura, odd odor, or visual or auditory hallucinations. Partial seizures are resistant to antiepileptic drugs in up to 30 % of cases.

*Generalized seizures* are divided into two types: one type is characterized by episodes of rigidity (tonic), followed by repetitive involuntary movements (clonic), and it is called "grand mal seizure." The other type is characterized by the absence of seizure with sudden, brief (seconds) episode of loss of physical movement, and it is called "petit mal seizure."

*Status epilepticus* is a condition characterized by continuous seizure attack that lasts more for than 5 min and can extend up to 30 min. Status epilepticus can occur as a withdrawal symptom of antiepileptic medications. *Todd's paralysis* is a form of temporary motor weakness experienced by the patient after an episode of seizure.

Epilepsy can be caused by a variety of clinical conditions. Any condition that insults the brain cortex is capable of initiating seizure attacks and epilepsy. Moreover, seizure attacks can be initiated by metabolic abnormalities (e.g., hypercalcemia). The role of brain imaging in epilepsy is to detect anatomical structural abnormalities. It is practical to divide the common causes of epilepsy into five simplified main groups:

- *Mesial hippocampal (temporal) sclerosis* is a disease characterized by atrophy and sclerosis of the hippocampus. Most patients have a history of brain injury before the age of 5 years in the form of febrile convulsion or status epilepticus. Mesial temporal sclerosis is the most common cause of epileptic seizures in adults (40–60 % of cases).
- *Congenital cortical anomalies* constitute up to 50 % of epilepsy cases in children and up to 25 % of adult cases. Anomalies that fall into this group include lissencephaly, pachygyria, polymicrogyria, gray matter heterotopia, and phakomatosis. The frontal lobe is commonly involved in congenital cortical anomalies.
- *Neoplasms* constitute up to 4 % of epilepsy cases, and they are mostly cortical neoplasms like astrocytoma, ganglioglioma, desmoplastic neuroepithelial tumor, and oligodendroglioma. The temporal lobe is commonly involved in cortical neoplasms.
- *Vascular abnormalities* constitute up to 5 % of epilepsy cases and commonly include arteriovenous malformations and cavernous angiomas.
- *Gliosis* is the result of the previous insult to the cortex like postinfarction, postinfection, and posttrauma.

## Differential Diagnoses and Related Diseases

- *Lafora disease* is a very rare, autosomal recessive disease characterized by myoclonic jerks, generalized tonic–clonic seizures, and multisystemic manifestation. *Myoclonus jerks* are brief involuntary contractions of a group of muscles (e.g., hiccups are myoclonus jerks of the diaphragm). The disease is caused by abnormal deposition of polyglucosan in the central nervous system, liver, myocardium, skin, and muscles. Diagnosis is confirmed by skin biopsy that identifies polyglucosan inclusions (*Lafora bodies*) by positive periodic acid Schiff (PAS) stain. Patients present typically before 20 years of age, complaining of multiple

attacks of myoclonic and generalized tonic–clonic seizures, intellectual disturbance, and severe progressive motor and coordination disturbance. Patients often show abnormal liver profile due to liver failure. The disease is frequently seen in countries where consanguineous marriages are common, like the Middle East, India, and Pakistan. Death occurs almost 6–10 years after the first manifestation of the disease.

- *Ulegyria* is a disease characterized by destruction and gliosis of the gray matter in the depth of the sulci with relative preservation of the gyral surfaces, giving the gyri a "mushroom-shaped appearance." Ulegyria commonly arises as a late effect of perinatal and postnatal hypoxia. It tends to occur in a symmetrical fashion in the perisylvian areas.
- *Schinzel–Giedion syndrome* is a rare, autosomal recessive disease characterized by seizures, mental retardation, and spasticity. Other manifestations include characteristic facial features, bitemporal narrowing giving the skull a "figure-of-eight shape," choanal atresia, congenital heart defects, wide occipital synchondrosis, distal phalangeal hypoplasia, and hypospadia.



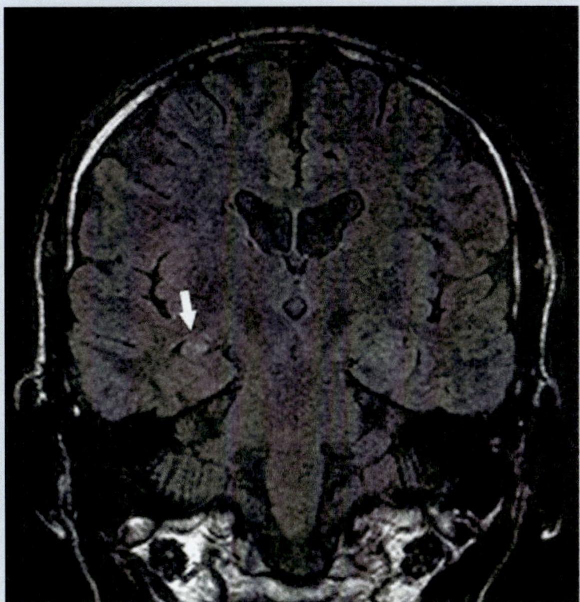

◘ **Fig. 2.6.1**   Coronal T2W brain MRI of a patient with recurrent epilepsy shows mild atrophy of the right hippocampus with higher T2 signal intensity (*arrow*) compared to the left side (mesial temporal sclerosis)

— In *oligodendroglioma*, there is a brain mass with calcifications and minimal brain edema. The lesion is seen predominantly located in the frontal lobe and shows heterogeneous contrast enhancement (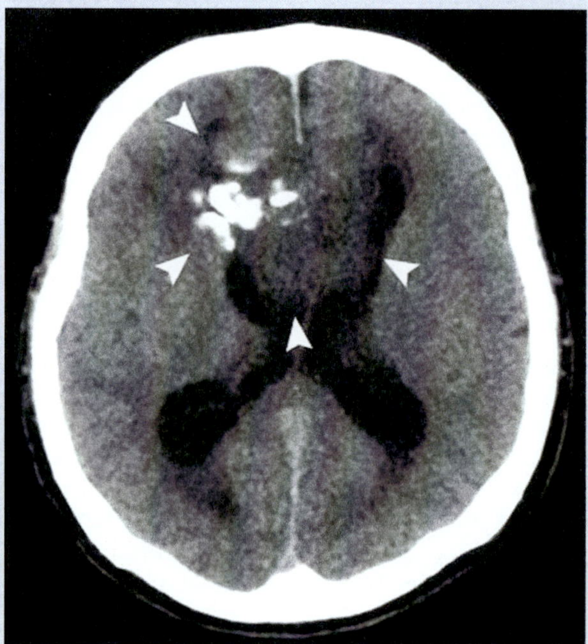 Fig. 2.6.2).
— In *ganglioglioma*, there is a lesion that arises from the frontal or the temporal lobe cortices. Usually, the patient has a history of epilepsy. The lesion can be cystic, solid, or mix. It may show heterogeneous contrast enhancement and rarely shows calcification.
— In desmoplastic neuroepithelial tumor, there is a hypodense lesion located in the temporal lobe cortex on CT, with no specific signal on MRI. Usually, the patient has a history of epilepsy. The tumor shows no contrast enhancement (Fig. 2.6.3).
— In *gliosis*, the cortex shows an area of low signal intensity on T1W and T2W images due to parenchymal fibrosis (Fig. 2.6.4).
— In *cavernous angioma*, there is a honeycomb-like lesion that appears with no edema or mass effect (except in cases of fresh bleeding). The lesion has an isointense signal on T1W and T2W images, with mixed hyperintense (blood) and hypointense (calcium/hemosiderin) signals within it, and surrounded by a hypointense rim of hemosiderin (pathognomonic sign, Fig. 2.6.5). MR angiography shows no vascular malformation, usually because most of the lesion is thrombosed.

**Fig. 2.6.2** Axial nonenhanced brain CT shows a right frontal lobe tumor that abuts the lateral ventricles (*arrowheads*) and shows areas of dense calcifications (oligodendroglioma)

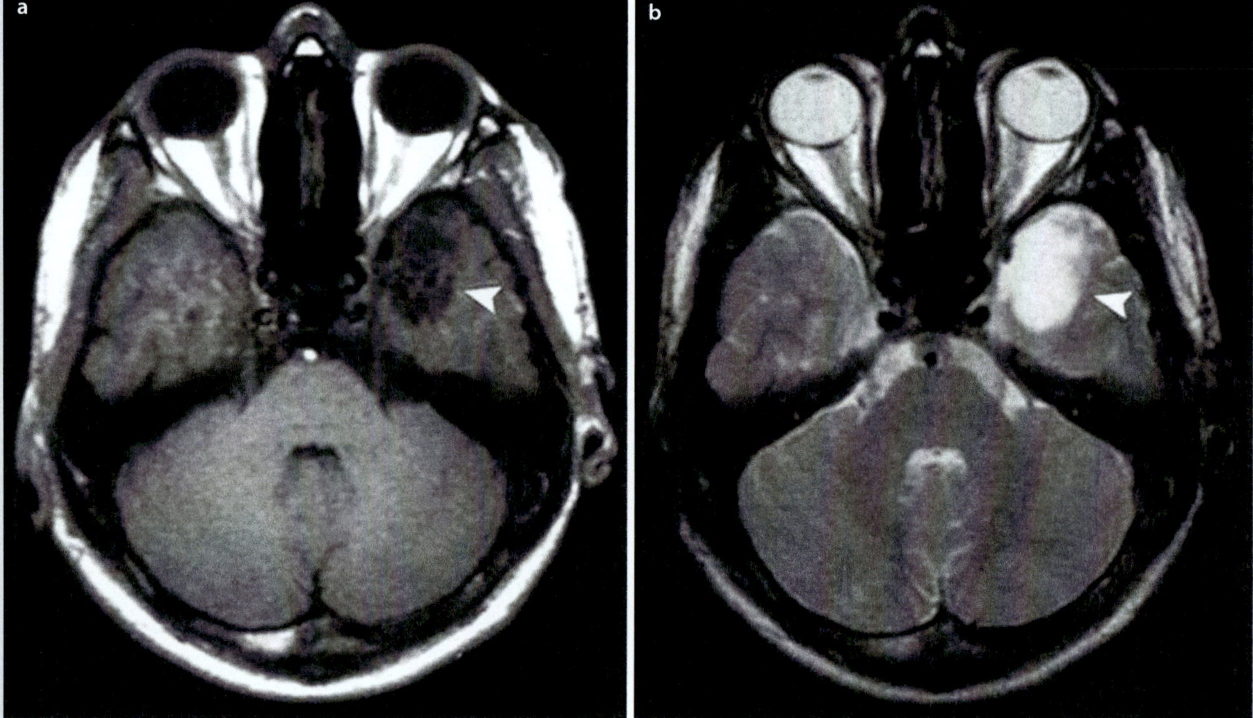

**Fig. 2.6.3** Axial T1W postcontrast (**a**) and T2W (**b**) brain MRI in a patient with epilepsy shows temporal cortical hypointense lesion with high T2 signal intensity and no contrast enhancement (desmoplastic neuroepithelial tumor)

- In *Lafora disease*, brain infarction in the frontal and parietal subcortical white matter areas may be seen after severe seizure attack. On MR

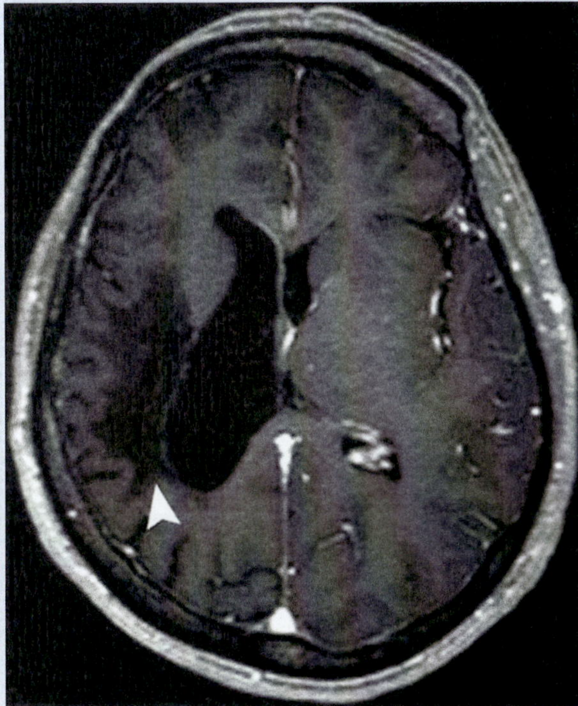

 **Fig. 2.6.4**    Axial T1W postcontrast MRI of a patient with previous brain infarction shows area (*arrowhead*) of hypointensity, with dilatation of the right occipital horn of the lateral ventricle adjacent to it (gliosis)

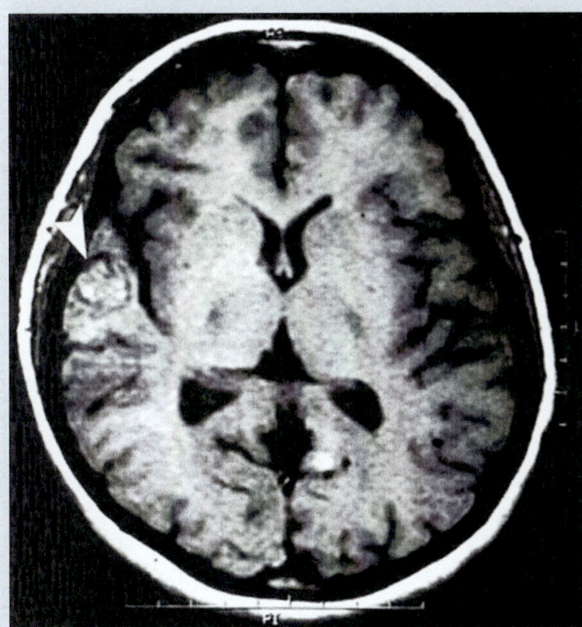

 **Fig. 2.6.5**    Axial T1W brain image shows a hypointense signal intensity ring with multiple areas of different MR intensities (*arrowhead*) located within the right temporal lobe (cavernous angioma)

spectroscopy, there is a characteristic decrease in *N*-acetylaspartate (NAA)/creatine ratio in the frontal lobe and the basal ganglia.

- In *ulegyria*, the MRI scan shows thin gyri in the perisylvian area with abnormal high T2 signal in a bilateral, symmetrical fashion ( Fig. 2.6.6). Unilateral lesions can occur.In *status epilepticus*, the hippocampus shows unilateral or bilateral high signal intensity signal on both T2W and FLAIR images ( Fig. 2.6.7). This sign is usually seen in the acute phase and can extend up to months after the initial attack.

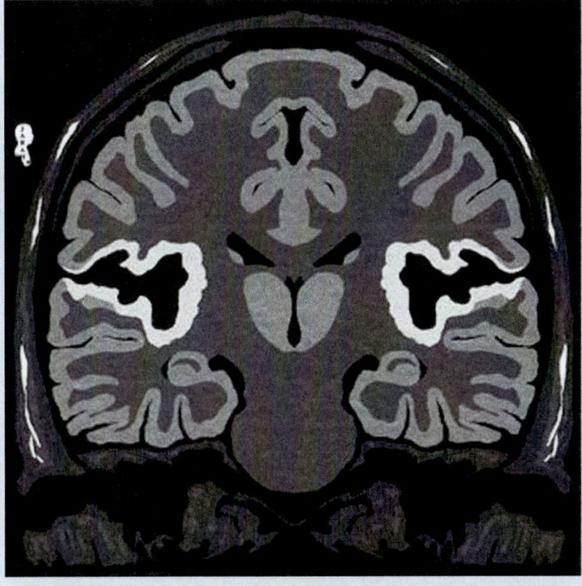

 **Fig. 2.6.6**    Coronal FLAIR brain MR illustration demonstrates the radiological findings in ulegyria

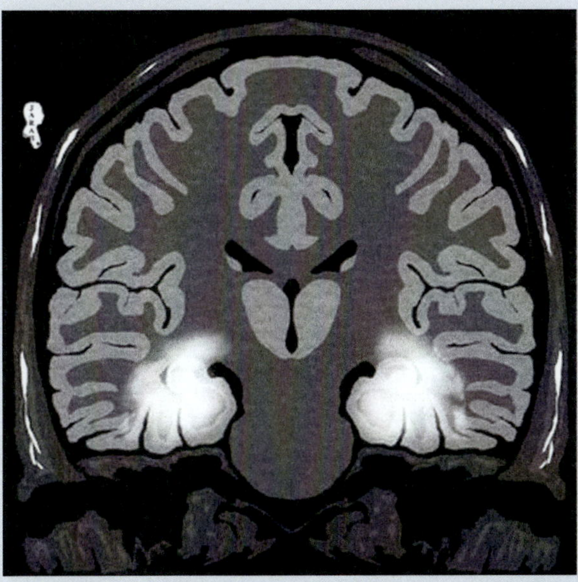

 **Fig. 2.6.7**    Coronal FLAIR brain MR illustration demonstrates the radiological findings in status epilepticus

## Further Reading

Al-Mudaffer M, et al. Clinical and radiological findings in Schinzel-Giedion syndrome. Eur J Pediatr. 2008;167:1399–407.

Deblaere K, et al. Structural magnetic resonance imaging in epilepsy. Eur Radiol. 2008;18:119–29.

Gómez-Garre P, et al. Hepatic disease as the first manifestation of progressive myoclonus epilepsy of Lafora. Neurology. 2007;68:1369–73.

Paesschen WV, et al. Qualitative and quantitative imaging of the hippocampus in mesial temporal lobe epilepsy with hippocampal sclerosis. Neuroimaging Clin N Am. 2004;14:373–400.

Ramos A, et al. Uncommon epileptogenic lesions affecting the temporal lobe. Semin Ultrasound CT MR. 2008;29:47–59.

Sirven JI, et al. MRI changes in status epilepticus. Neurology. 2003;60:1866.

Urbach H. Imaging of epilepsy. Eur Radiol. 2005;15:494–500.

Urbach H, et al. MRI of long-term epilepsy-associated tumors. Semin Ultrasound CT MR. 2008;29:40–6.

Vattipally VR, et al. MR imaging of epilepsy: strategies for successful interpretation. Neuroimaging Clin N Am. 2004;14:349–72.

Vazquez E, et al. Developmental abnormalities of temporal lobe in children. Semin Ultrasound CT MR. 2007;29:15–39.

Villanueva V, et al. MRI volumetry and proton MR spectroscopy of the brain in Lafora disease. Epilepsia. 2006;47:788–92.

## 2.7    Headache

Headache is the most common neurological complaint worldwide. There are over 300 different types and causes of headache, including teeth pain, frontal sinusitis, vision problems (e.g., myopia), hypertension, otitis media, intracranial tumors, and much more. Radiological imaging for headache investigation is often indicated in cases of new-onset headaches, headaches with progressive course, headaches that never alternate sides, and headaches associated with neurological deficits of seizures.

In this topic, some of the common causes of headache with well-defined radiological signs are discussed.

## Migraine

Headache is divided into primary and secondary headaches. Primary headaches include migraine, tension-type headache, cluster headache, and others. Secondary headaches in contrast are attributed to a variety of causes that include vascular, sinusoidal, infectious, and inflammatory causes.

Migraine headache is divided into two main types: migraine with aura and migraine without aura. Migraine aura consists of neurological manifestations that precedes migraine or can occur without it. Typically, the aura develops over 5 min and lasts no more than 60 min. Aura manifestations may include auditory and visual symptoms, numbness, paresthesia, and tingling sensation.

Uncommon manifestations of migraine include cyclical vomiting (2.5 %), which is characterized by unexplained nausea and vomiting. It often occurs in children and lasts for 1–5 h in the absence of gastrointestinal disease. Benign paroxysmal vertigo is characterized by recurrent attacks of vertigo (e.g., five episodes) that last from minutes to hours. Lastly, recurrent attacks of abdominal pain that are accompanied by anorexia, nausea, and some vomiting may be seen in children with migraine, and it is called *abdominal migraine.*

Migrainous infarction can occur when one or more aural symptoms persist beyond 1 h. *Status migrainous* refers to an attack of migraine with headache that lasts >72 h.

### Signs on CT

— In acute migraine, hypodense areas may be seen within the brain parenchyma commonly in the occipitotemporal areas (■ Fig. 2.7.1). These areas enhance after contrast injection. The hypodense areas are thought to represent brain edema and ischemia. Contrast enhancement supports the theory of ischemia. Migraine is thought to be caused by changes in the blood perfusion within the cerebral parenchyma.

— Cerebral vessels angiography is typically normal.

— Infarction is seen as an area of hypodense parenchyma surrounded by cytotoxic edema.

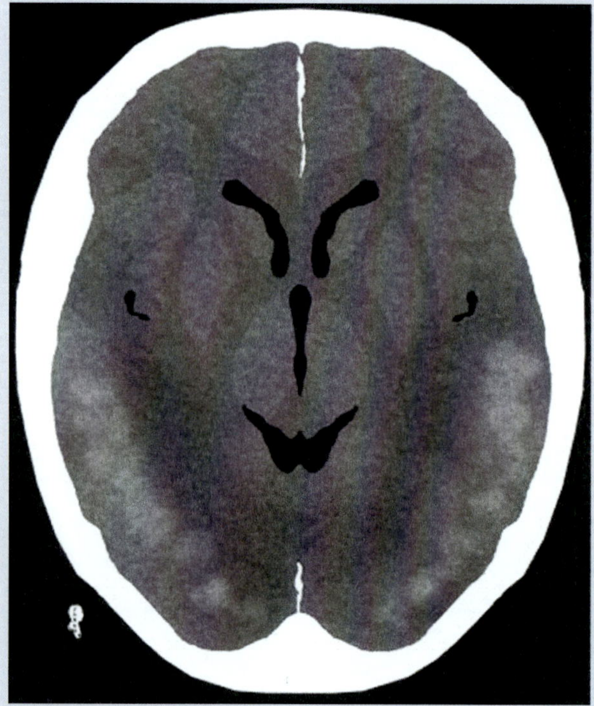

■ **Fig. 2.7.1** Axial brain CT illustration shows bilateral occipital hypodensities, a sign that can be encountered in acute attack of migraine headache due to vasogenic edema

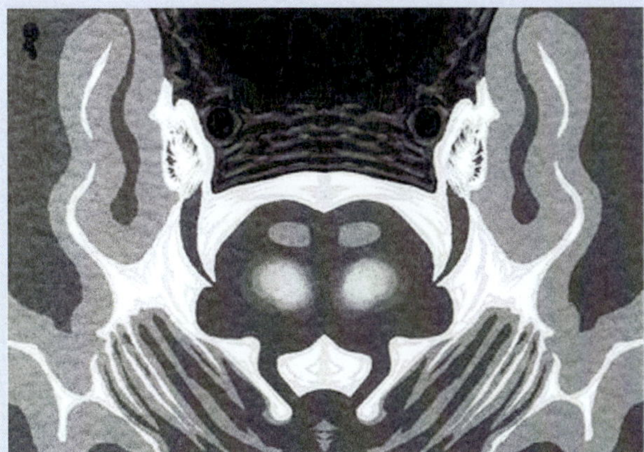

■ **Fig. 2.7.2** Axial brain T2W MR illustration at the level of the pons demonstrates bilateral hyperintense areas, a sign that can be seen in patients with migraine

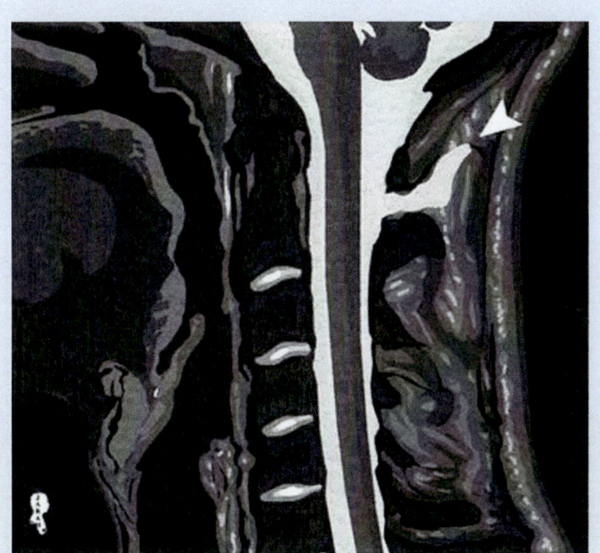

■ **Fig. 2.7.3** Sagittal T2W cervical MR illustration demonstrates cerebrospinal fluid (CSF) leak between the posterior elements of C2 and C3 (*arrowhead*)

## Spontaneous Intracranial Hypotension (Schaltenbrand Syndrome)

Spontaneous intracranial hypotension (SIH) is a disease characterized by a typical headache that is evoked by changing body position from supine to standing position (orthostatic headache). The headache pain lasts for few minutes and improves or disappears after acquiring recumbent or supine position.

Causes of SIH can be due to cervical disk herniation, vigorous activity, sexual activity, minor head trauma, or a violent sneeze or cough.

Other features of SIH include nausea and vomiting, hearing disturbance, and diplopia. SIH headache is either frontal or occipital in location and typically is not relieved by analgesics.



## Idiopathic Intracranial Hypertension (Pseudotumor Cerebri)

Idiopathic intracranial hypertension or pseudotumor cerebri (PTC) is a disease with unknown cause, characterized by papilledema with raised intracranial pressure in the absence of space-occupying lesions, normal CSF composition, and normal neuroimaging findings.

PTC can be seen in patients with particular medical disorders like obesity, hypervitaminosis, venous sinus thrombosis, iron-deficiency anemia, typhoid fever, brucellosis, and oral contraceptive use. In children, the most common cause of PTC is otitis media.

Patients with PTC commonly present with headache, visual disturbance, diplopia, and pulsatile tinnitus or ear noise. The most serious condition in PTC is sudden visual loss. Fundoscopic examination typically reveals optic disk edema (papilledema). PTC can be associated uncommonly with *Parinaud's syndrome* (*dorsal midbrain syndrome*), a disease characterized by upward gaze paralysis, convergence-retraction nystagmus, and light-near dissociation.

sellar floor. Empty sella is one of the radiological signs frequently seen in PTC. The infundibular stalk is seen dipping in the sella beyond the level of the posterior clinoid process (normally, the pituitary gland is connected to the infundibulum at the level of the posterior clinoid process) (◘ Fig. 2.7.4). Most of the sellar space is occupied by CSF.

— Dilated optic nerve sheath due to increased CSF with its perineural subarachnoid space. The optic nerve can be clearly differentiated from the sheath.
— Bilateral, nonsymmetrical intraocular protrusion of the optic nerve, with tortuosity of the orbital optic nerve (due to the increased intracranial CSF pressure) (◘ Fig. 2.7.5).
— Normal size ventricles with no signs of hydrocephalus.

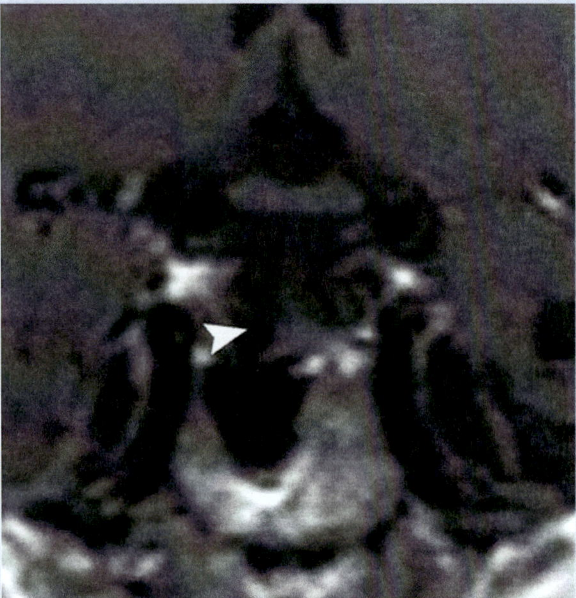

◘ **Fig. 2.7.4**  Coronal nonenhanced MRI of the sella shows marked reduction of the sellar mass (*arrowhead*), with the pituitary stalk seen dipping in the sella beyond the level of the posterior clinoid process (empty sella)

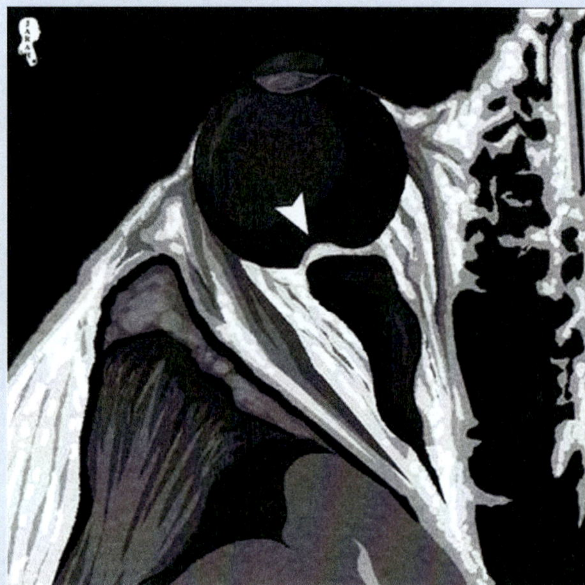

◘ **Fig. 2.7.5**  Axial orbital T1W MR illustration demonstrates bulging of the optic disk due to increased intracranial pressure in a patient with pseudotumor cerebri (PTC) (*arrowhead*)

## Temporal (Giant) Cell Arteritis

Temporal (giant) cell arteritis is a chronic disease of large- and medium-sized vasculitis characterized by granulomatous inflammation of the temporal vessels.

Giant cell arteritis (GCA) is characterized clinically by fever, weakness, anorexia, and headache localized over the area of temporal artery branches. Typically, the area is swollen and the arteries are tender on palpation. The disease is not only confined to the temporal vessels, as the occipital arteries may be affected also. Moreover, vasculitis may affect the central retinal arteries, resulting in partial or complete visual loss (20 % of cases).

Up to 30 % of patients present with mononeuropathies and peripheral polyneuropathies in the arms or legs. Transient ischemic attack or strokes may rarely occur. Aortic or subclavian stenosis with limb claudication may occur in up to 10–15 % of cases. There is unexplained relationship between GCA and polymyalgia rheumatica (PMR). Up to 20 % of patients with PMR develop GCA, while more than 50 % of patients with GCA have PMR.

Laboratory investigations often show high erythrocyte sedimentation rate and C-reactive proteins reflecting active inflammatory process. Moderate to severe anemia is characteristically found due to "toxic" suppression of the bone marrow. Biopsy of the temporal artery classically shows vasculitis characterized by predominance of mononuclear cell infiltrates or granulomatous inflammation, usually with multinucleated giant cells (hence the name).

### Signs on Doppler Sonography
— By placing the ultrasound probe over the dilated temporal vessels, the scan typically shows hypoechoic dark halo surrounding the arterial lumen, reflecting edema of the vessel wall.
— The Doppler signal within the artery may show small systolic peak that indicates arterial occlusion or pseudo-occlusion.
— Reduced or missing vessel wall pulsation.

**Signs on MRI**

Brain MR postgadolinium injection images show characteristic mural enhancement of the temporal arteries with or without the occipital arteries, indicating inflammation ( Fig. 2.7.6). In normal situations, the arterial walls show no or mild mural enhancement.

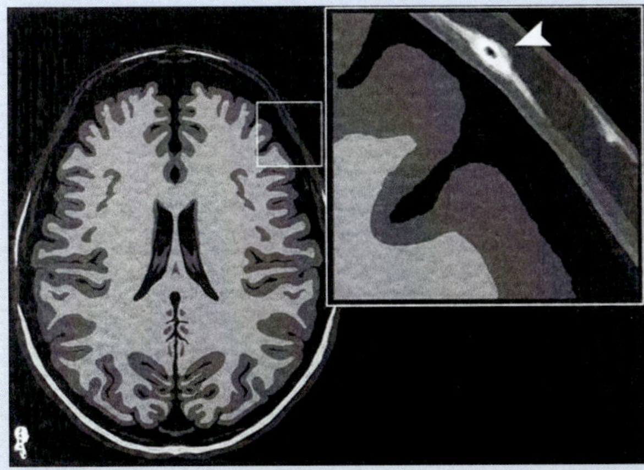

 **Fig. 2.7.6**   Axial brain T1W postcontrast MR illustration demonstrates mural enhancement of the temporal arteries due to inflammation (giant cell arteritis (GCA))

## Further Reading

Alvarez-Cermeno J-C, et al. Cranial computer tomography in pediatric migraine. Pediatr Radiol. 1984;14:195–7.

Atalar MH, et al. Spontaneous intracranial hypotension: clinical and magnetic resonance imaging findings. Eur J Radiol Extra. 2004;51:57–60.

Bley TA, et al. High-resolution MRI in giant cell arteritis: imaging of the wall of the superficial temporal artery. AJR Am J Roentgenol. 2005;184:283–7.

Bousser MG, et al. Ischemic strokes and migraine. Neuroradiology. 1985;27:583–7.

Chansoria M, et al. Pseudotumor cerebri with transient oculomotor palsy. Indian J Pediatr. 2005;72:1047–8.

Chiapparini L, et al. Headache and intracranial hypotension: neurological findings. Neurol Sci. 2004;25:S138–41.

Christoforidis GA, et al. Spontaneous intracranial hypotension: report of four cases and review of the literature. Neuroradiology. 1998;40:636–43.

Firat AK, et al. Spontaneous intracranial hypotension with pituitary adenoma. J Headache Pain. 2006;7:47–50.

Güngör K, et al. Pseudotumor cerebri complicating brucellosis. Ann Ophthalmol. 2002;34:67–9.

Haritanti A, et al. Spontaneous intracranial hypotension. Clinical and neuroimaging findings in six cases with literature review. Eur J Radiol. 2008. doi:10.1016/j.ejrad.2007.10.013.

Kruit MC, et al. Brain stem and cerebellar hyperintense lesions in migraine. Stroke. 2006;37:1109–12.

La Mantia L, et al. Headache and inflammatory disorders of the central nervous system. Neurol Sci. 2004;25:S148–53.

Laldinpuii J, et al. Giant cell arteritis (temporal arteritis): a report of four cases from north east India. Ann Indian Acad Neurol. 2008;11:185–9.

Larner AJ. Late onset migraine with aura: how old is too old. J Headache Pain. 2007;8:251–2.

Lewis DW. Headaches in children and adolescents. Curr Probl Pediatr Adolesc Health Care. 2007;37:207–46.

Lipoton RB, et al. Classification of primary headaches. Neurology. 2004;63:427–35.

Mandelstam S, et al. MRI of optic disc edema in a childhood idiopathic intracranial hypertension. Pediatr Radiol. 2004;34:362.

Mukhopadhyay S, et al. Evaluation of headache in children. Paediatr Child Health. 2008;18:1–6.

Reinhard M, et al. Color-coded sonography in suspected temporal arteritis—experience after 83 cases. Rheumatol Int. 2004;24:340–6.

Salvarani C, et al. Polymyalgia rheumatica and giant-cell arteritis. N Engl J Med. 2002;347:261–70.

Seiden AM, et al. Headache and the frontal sinus. Otolaryngol Clin North Am. 2001;34:227–41.

## 2.8 Multiple Sclerosis and Other Demyelinating Diseases

Demyelinating disorders are a group of diseases characterized by myelin loss. Normally, the white matter before the myelination process is *hydrophilic* (contains a lot of water), which is detected as high T2 signal intensity and low T1 signal intensity on MRI at birth. After axonal myelination, the white matter becomes *hydrophobic* (contains a lot of fat), producing normal MRI signal as high T1 and relatively low T2 signal intensities. In demyelinating diseases, the normal myelin is lost, making the affected parts of the white matter to be hydrophilic again, producing high signal intensity on T2W images (signal of water).

## Multiple Sclerosis

Multiple sclerosis (MS) is a disease of unknown origin characterized by progressive inflammatory demyelinating destruction of the brain and the spinal cord white matter (central nervous system demyelination).

MS is characterized by a remission/regression course, with "dissemination in time and space." The latter sentence means that MS lesions are changing and growing in space as time passes by (in a better or worse clinical course).

MS lesions (plaques) often start around the small venules that penetrate the ependymal layer of the ventricles. These venules are located perpendicular (90°) over the ventricles, making MS plaques classically seen as oval plaques perpendicular to the ventricles because they start around the venules and spread laterally. MS plaques are typically seen in the periventricular white matter, corpus callosum, cerebral peduncles, and spinal cord.

The typical age of incidence is from 10 to 50 years of age. MS usually is not diagnosed before or after this range. Up to 10 % of MS case patients have isolated spinal cord injury. Patients present with neurological symptoms according to the area involved. The classical MS patient triad (of Charcot) is scanning speech, intention tremor, and nystagmus (jerky, back-and-forth movements of the eyes). Internuclear ophthalmoplegia, also known as *medial longitudinal fasciculus syndrome*, is a specific eye disease of MS characterized by medial rectus muscle palsy in attempted lateral gaze and monocular nystagmus in the abducting eye with convergence. Internuclear ophthalmoplegia results from demyelination of the medial longitudinal fasciculus. *Uhthoff's phenomenon* is a term used to describe worsening of MS symptoms after an episode of exercise or increased body temperature (e.g., during hot bath).

*Criteria* for radiological diagnosis of MS (at least three out of the four criteria):

- At least one contrast enhancement plaque or nine hyperintense lesions on T2W or FLAIR images
- At least one infratentorial lesion (including spinal cord)
- At least three periventricular lesions
- At least one subcortical lesion

### Signs on CT

Multiple hypodense periventricular plaques that enhance after contrast administration (in acute phase only)

### Signs on MRI

- Multiple hyperintense T2 signal plaques in the white matter are seen classically at the periventricular area along the lateral ventricles and the occipital horns, the internal capsule, the corpus callosum, the pons, and the middle cerebral peduncles ( Fig. 2.8.1).
- Contrast ring enhancement occurs in acute stage (remission) of the disease only. Contrast study is not recommended after therapy with intravenous steroid administration as active plaques will usually not enhance.
- Minimal surrounding edema.
- *Gliomatous/tumefactive MS* is an MS plaque with a mass effect. The plaque has a mass effect and is enhanced in a ring fashion (ring within a ring), which will be mistaken for a neoplasm or an abscess. Also, the enhanced ring is irregular and the thickness is increased in the side opposite to the ventricle.
- *Dawson's fingers*: they are focal hyperintensities seen on the inferior aspect of the corpus callosum in T2W or FLAIR images ( Fig. 2.8.2).
- *Hyperintense dentate nucleus sign*: this sign describes hyperintense dentate nucleus of the cerebellum, usually in a bilateral fashion on T1W nonenhanced images. This sign is described with

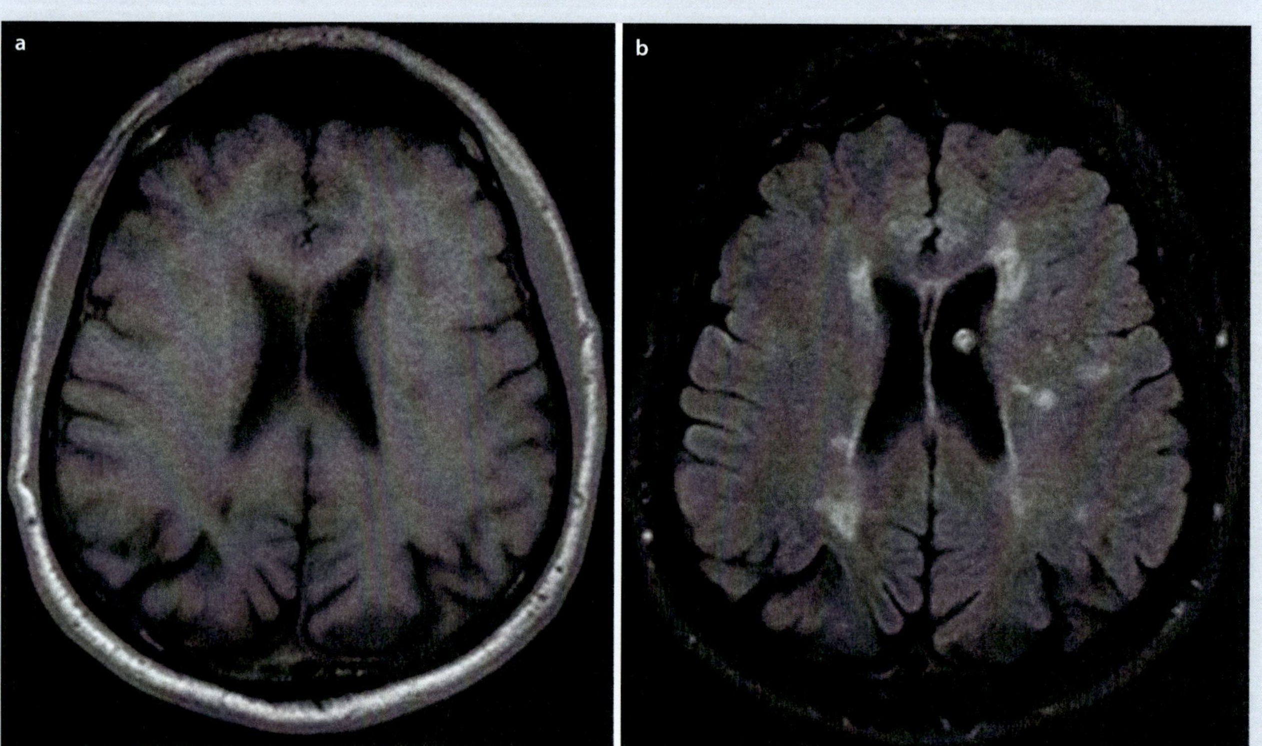

 **Fig. 2.8.1**   Axial T1W (**a**) and FLAIR (**b**) brain MRI in a patient with MS shows classical periventricular white matter lesions (plaques)

secondary progressive MS subtype. *Secondary progressive MS subtype* is a term used to describe an MS patient with gradually progressive worsening clinical course without recovery; it is seen in 10 % of MS patients.

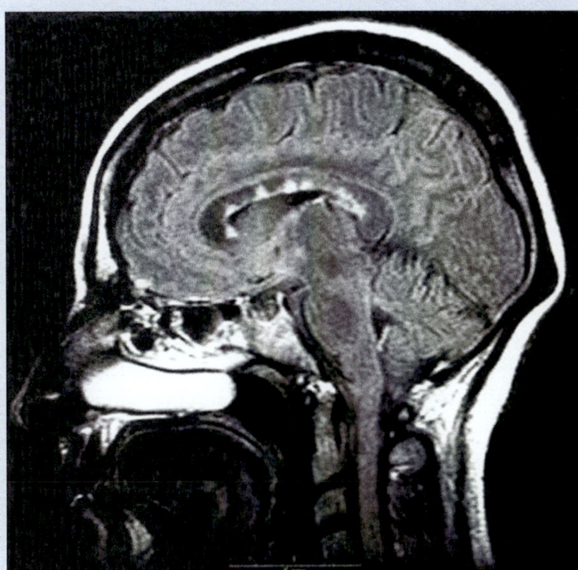



**Fig. 2.8.2** Sagittal FLAIR brain MRI shows that multiple hyperintense lesions within the corpus callosum start from the inferior peripheral surface toward the center (Dawson's fingers)

white matter tracts. DTI results in diffusion-encoded FA map that shows the white matter fibers and tracts. In these maps, bright voxels represent high diffusion anisotropy, whereas dark voxels represent low diffusion anisotropy. A color-coded FA map provides the direction of the white matter fibers. Most MRI machines represent $x$-direction (right to left) in red, $y$-direction (anterior–posterior) in green, and $z$-direction (superior–inferior) in blue.

The white matter fibers can be localized anatomically based on their color-coded FA map. The white matter fibers are classified anatomically into:

- *Commissural fibers*: fibers which connect region of one hemisphere to the other hemisphere (e.g., corpus callosum). These fibers are encoded in red.
- *Association fibers*: fibers which connect different regions of the cerebral cortex in the same hemisphere (e.g., optic radiation). These fibers are encoded in green.
- *Projection fibers*: fibers which connect the cerebral cortex to the subcortical structures (e.g., corticospinal tract). These fibers are encoded in blue.

DTI can be used to localize the affected white matter tracts from the nonaffected white matter tracts in a pathological process, information that is so valuable for the neurosurgeon to plan his surgery, so he can avoid removing healthy functioning tracts in cases of brain tumor resection planning. Also, DTI can be used to monitor the therapy and disease progression in diseases with white matter tract lesions like MS (**Fig. 2.8.3**) and amyotrophic lateral sclerosis, which mainly affects the corticospinal tract.

## The Concept of Diffusion Tensor MR Imaging

Diffusion tensor imaging (DTI), also known as MR tractography, is a highly sophisticated MR method to image white matter tracts and fibers. Diffusion is defined as random translational molecular motion (*Brownian motion*) that results from the thermal energy carried by these molecules. Diffusion can be random (isotropic) or directional (anisotropic) depending on the characteristic of the tissue. The routine diffusion-weighted imaging (DWI) provides a measure of the water molecule displacement in one direction. Since the white matter fibers are multidirectional, multidirectional DWI is needed. This multidirectional diffusion imaging is expressed by a *diffusion tensor*, which expresses the measurement of water diffusion in different directions.

*Diffusivity* is a term used to describe water diffusion per unit time. Pathological conditions alter both the diffusivity and the anisotropic diffusion characteristics of water and metabolites. Tissue anisotropy is measured by fractional anisotropy (FA), which represents the directionality of the

## Neuromyelitis Optica (Devic's Syndrome)

Neuromyelitis optica (NMO) is an unusual acute fulminant variant of MS characterized by unilateral or bilateral optic neuritis with transverse myelitis. The lesions in NMO affect both gray and white matters (unlike typical MS).

Criteria for NMO diagnosis include:

- *Absolute*: optic neuritis, acute myelitis, with no evidence of clinical disease outside the optic nerve or spinal cord
- *Major*: negative brain MRI at onset and spinal cord lesions that extend >3 vertebral segments
- *Minor*: bilateral optic neuritis

Patients may present initially with paroxysmal tonic spasms that typically last 10–30s due to the transverse myelitis. They are characterized by painful spasm and usually mistaken with partial seizures. Prognosis is poor, with more than 50 % of patients developing severe visual loss within 5 years of disease onset.

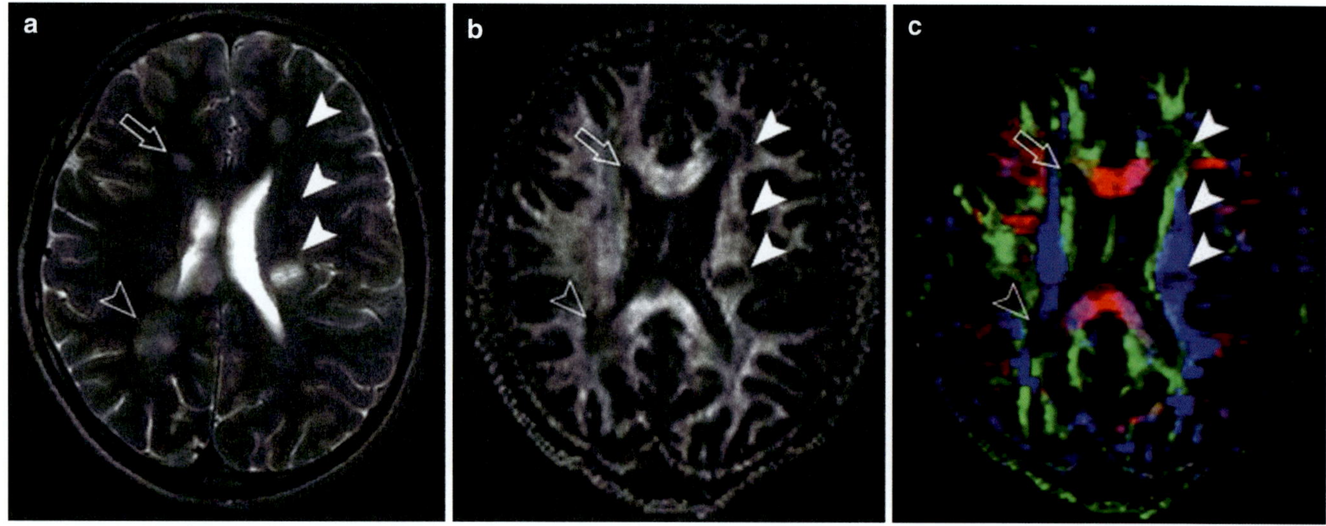

**Fig. 2.8.3** Axial T2W brain MRI (**a**), diffusion-encoded FA map (**b**), and color-coded FA map (**c**) of a 16-year-old patient with MS. By comparing (**a**) with (**b**) and (**c**), the MS plaques can be assessed according to the white matter tract affected: the left superior region of corona radiata (*solid arrowheads*), the right forceps minor of corpus callosum (*hollow arrow*), and the right superior region of corona radiata plus the right forceps major of corpus callosum (*hollow arrowhead*)

### Signs on MRI
- Brain MRI is typically normal.
- Extensive spinal cord lesion with high T2 signal intensity and enhancement postcontrast that extends >3 vertebral segments.
- Unilateral or bilateral optic nerve enhancement after contrast administration reflecting optic neuritis.

## Marburg's Type MS

Marburg's type MS is an acute, malignant, rapidly deteriorating form of MS that can be lethal within 4 weeks of onset if not treated.

Patients with Marburg's MS usually present with hyperacute onset of multifocal neurological deficits and altered consciousness status in different degrees. Death usually occurs when the disease destroys the brain stem.

The disease is characterized by *monophasic* demyelinating encephalopathy (like ADEM), with fulminant progression if not treated. History of infection or recent vaccination may help to differentiate it from acute disseminated encephalomyelitis (ADEM).

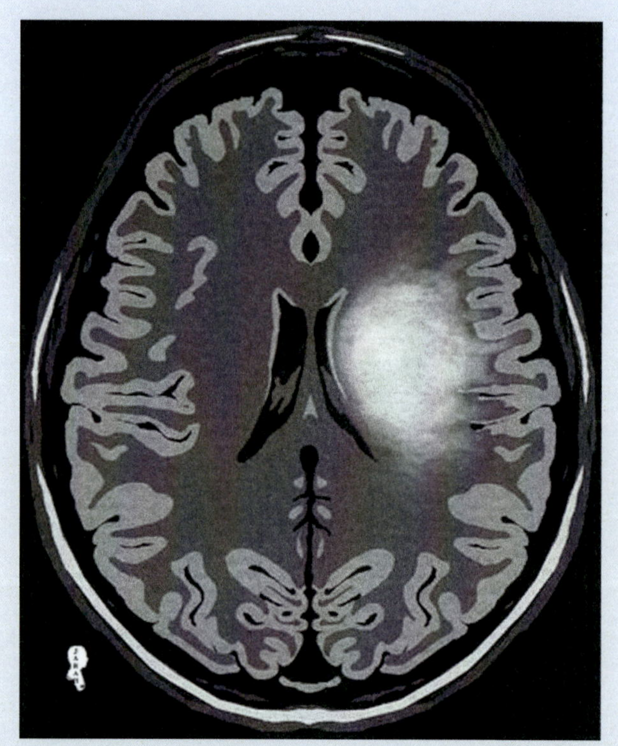

**Fig. 2.8.4** Axial FLAIR brain MR illustration demonstrates large left MS plaque with pressure effect over the lateral ventricle (Marburg's type MS)

### Signs on MRI
Marburg's MS usually is characterized by MS plaques with pressure effect and extensive demyelination (Fig. 2.8.4). Marburg's plaques mimic the tumefactive MS plaques. ADEM plaques in contrast usually are small and located in the periventricular areas.

## Baló Concentric Sclerosis

Baló concentric sclerosis (BCS) is another MS variant characterized by demyelinating plaques like MS, but the main distinctive feature is that these plaques are arranged in concentric layers.

A BCS demyelinating plaque occurs first, and then this plaque is surrounded by a layer of preconditioning proteins at the periphery of the plaque. Later, another demyelinating plaque occurs at the periphery of the protein ring. Another protein ring later might be formed peripherally to the previous demyelinating ring in a desperate attempt to contain the demyelinating process, and so on, producing the ring pattern detected on MRI.

### Signs on MRI
The unique pathology sequence of BCS can be clearly appreciated on MRI as a demyelinating plaque with multiple concentric hyperintense and isointense signal intensities on T2W and FLAIR images (◘ Fig. 2.8.5).

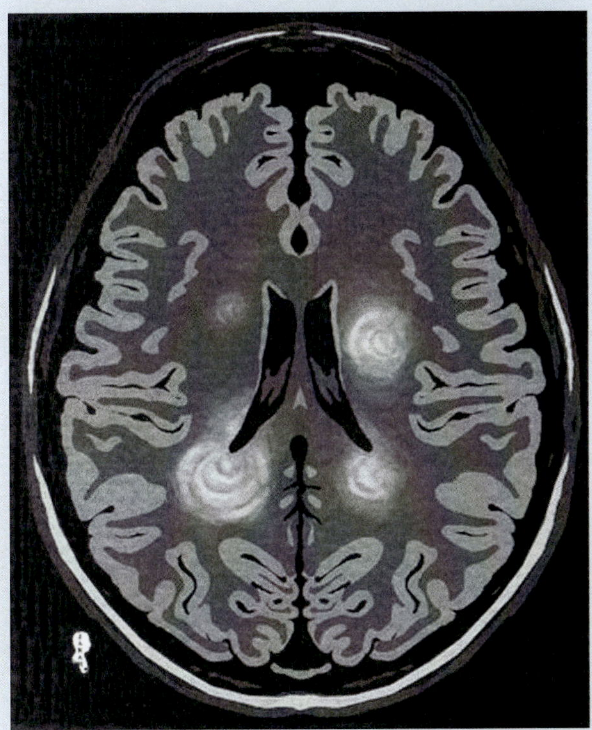

◘ Fig. 2.8.5   Axial FLAIR brain MR illustration demonstrates the concentric MS plaques of Baló concentric sclerosis (BCS)

## Schilder's Disease (Diffuse Myelinoclastic Sclerosis)

Schilder's disease (SD) is a disease presenting in childhood with progressive, diffuse cerebral demyelination similar to MS.

SD diagnosis is very difficult, because it can be mistaken with other leukodystrophies. Diagnosis of SD can be suggested after exclusion of adrenoleukodystrophy. The typical patient is a young female, with MRI picture resembling that of MS. The disease has two types, a self-limiting monophasic type and a progressive relapsing type.

### Signs on MRI
Typically, the lesions of SD are located in the central semiovale, bilaterally, with minimal edema and mass effect (◘ Fig. 2.8.6). After contrast injection, the enhancement is limited to one side of the lesion. The lesions can be solitary or multiple.

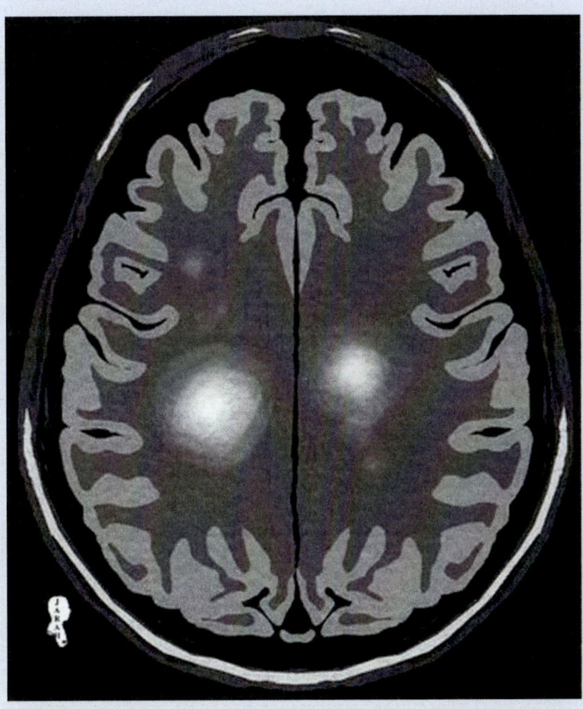

◘ Fig. 2.8.6   Axial FLAIR brain MR illustration demonstrates the MS plaques of Schilder's disease (SD) located in the centrum semiovale bilaterally

## Susac's Syndrome

Susac's syndrome is an uncommon disorder characterized by microvascular angiopathy causing encephalopathy and retinal artery branch occlusion that causes sudden blindness and cochlear hearing loss.

Susac's syndrome is of unknown origin, but autoimmune endotheliopathy theory was suggested to explain its manifestations because it responds to steroid therapy and immunosuppressive therapy. The disease predominantly affects females between 30 and 40 years of age.

Susac's syndrome manifestations usually do not present until advanced stages of the disease. Patients commonly present with the encephalopathy, which include predominantly severe migrainous headache with or without an aura.

The MRI shows multiple lesions that mimic MS and ADEM, leading to it being mistaken for and misdiagnosed with these two common conditions.

**Signs on MRI**
- Multiple lesions affect the gray and white matters seen as high signal intensity lesions on T2W and FLAIR images. The lesions enhance after contrast injection (mimicking MS and ADEM).
- The corpus callosum is affected in its central portion by linear or cystic lesions (characteristic and pathognomonic finding) (Fig. 2.8.7).
- Leptomeningeal enhancement is seen in up to 33 % of cases.

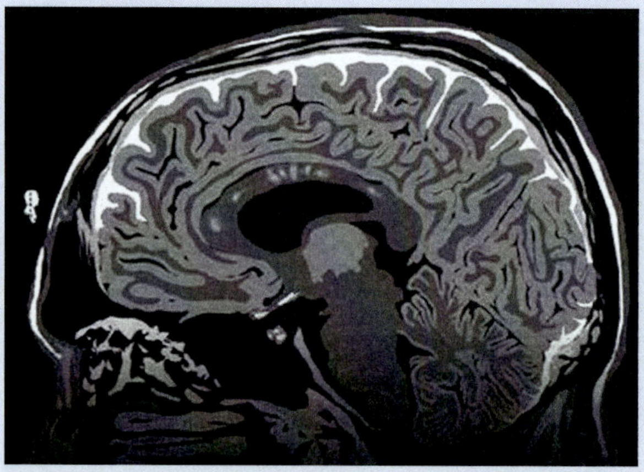

**Fig. 2.8.7** Sagittal FLAIR brain MR illustration demonstrates the characteristic central lesions of the corpus callosum seen in Susac's syndrome

*How to differentiate between Susac's syndrome, MS, and ADEM?*
- Susac's corpus callosum lesions are in the center of the corpus callosum, while the lesions of the corpus callosum in MS (Dawson's fingers) are usually affecting the inferior edges. MS lesions start from the edges toward the center.
- Susac's syndrome affects both gray and white matters, like ADEM, while MS only affects white matter.
- The hearing loss differentiates Susac's syndrome from both ADEM and MS. Both clinical diseases do not present with hearing loss.

## Guillain–Barré Syndrome

Guillain–Barré syndrome (GBS) is a disease characterized by acute inflammatory demyelination of the peripheral nervous system, commonly affecting the nerve roots in the conus medullaris and cauda equina.

Patients with GBS classically present with acute areflexic lower limb flaccid paralysis preceded by respiratory or gastrointestinal infections (e.g., 6 weeks before the onset of symptoms). Infections known to be associated with GBS include *Epstein-Barr virus*, *Mycoplasma pneumoniae*, *Cytomegalovirus*, and *Campylobacter jejuni*, and GBS has been reported after vaccination, surgery, and head trauma. The paralysis is mainly motor, symmetric, and with or without sensory and autonomic disturbances. Up to 50 % of patients experience pain, which is described as severe and occurs with even the slightest of movement.

The disease is caused by autoantibody-mediated reaction against gangliosides and glycosphingolipids. The diagnosis of GBS is determined mainly by the clinical picture and the cerebrospinal fluid (CSF) findings, which classically show high protein counts in 80 % of cases with normal cell count (albuminocytologic dissociation). The role of contrast-enhanced spinal MRI is to exclude other differential diagnosis or to monitor the treatment response.

GBS weakness reaches a nadir at 2–4 weeks after symptom onset. Recovery can be expected within 6–12 months. Some patients have residual paresthesia or persistent minor weakness. Approximately 7–15 % of patients have permanent neurological sequelae. Although GBS is a monophasic disease, about 7–16 % of patients suffer recurrent episodes.

GBS has different variants. An example of GBS variant is *Miller Fisher syndrome*, which is characterized by ophthalmoplegia, areflexia, and cerebellar ataxia. Another example of GBS variants is *polyneuritis cranialis*, which is characterized by acute multiple cranial nerves' demyelination without spinal cord involvement or involvement of the cranial nerves I and II. Diagnosis of polyneuritis cranialis requires exclusion of other causes of multiple cranial nerves palsies (e.g., Garcin's syndrome).

### Differential Diagnoses and Related Diseases

*Garcin's syndrome (hemibase syndrome)* is a very rare syndrome characterized by progressive, unilateral, almost complete paralysis of the cranial nerves due to nasopharyngeal tumor, which invade the skull base and do not affect the brain itself. This disease is seen with cases of tonsillar carcinoma, nasopharyngeal carcinoma, and carcinoma of the base of the skull. Also, it can be caused by invasive infections (e.g., mucormycosis) and paraneoplastic syndromes. MRI typically reveals invasive carcinoma of the skull base or infection that affects the cranial nerves and invades their foramina.

**Signs on Brain and Spinal MRI**
- Classically, GBS shows thickened nerve roots in the conus medullaris and cauda equina with marked enhancement after contrast injection (Fig. 2.8.8). Normally, the nerve root ganglia in the cauda equina and the conus medullaris do not enhance with gadolinium due to the intact blood–brain barrier. Abnormal enhancement of the nerve root ganglia after gadolinium injection is a pathological process that is seen in GBS, arachnoiditis, sarcoidosis, lymphoma, and AIDS-related polyradiculopathy. Due to the previous fact, GBS is essentially diagnosed by the clinical picture and

the CSF analysis. The spinal MRI supports the diagnosis.
- Miller Fisher syndrome classically shows a lesion affecting the brain stem (e.g., glioma).

- Polyneuritis cranialis cerebral MRI shows enhancement of multiple cranial nerves except the cranial nerves I and II.

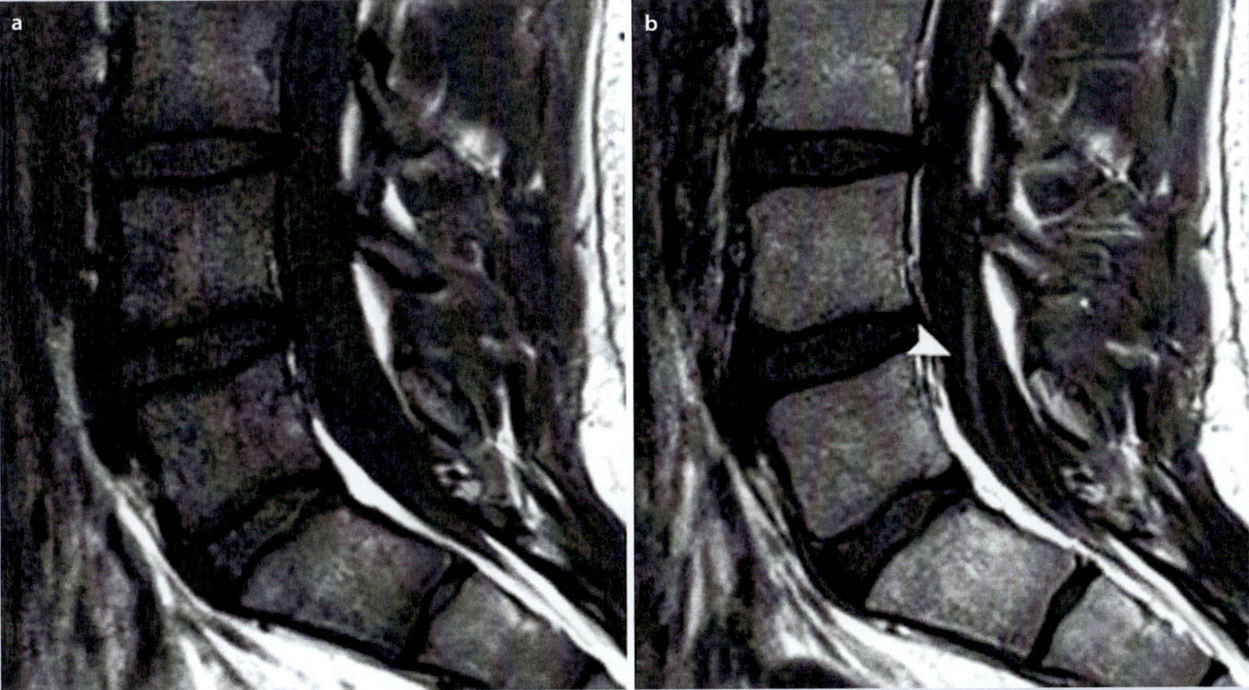


☐ **Fig. 2.8.8** Sagittal T1W (**a**) and T1W postcontrast (**b**) spinal MRI in a 10-year-old boy with flaccid lower limbs and motor deficits shows enhancement of the nerve roots of the cauda equina after contrast injection due to polyneuritis (*arrowhead*)

## Further Reading

Alkan O, et al. Spinal MRI findings of Guillain-Barré syndrome. J Radiol Case Rep. 2009;3:25–8.

Barbareschi M, et al. Schilder disease (1912): report of a case. Ital J Neurol Sci. 1988;9:157–60.

Bielekova B, Kadom N, et al. MRI as a marker for disease heterogeneity in multiple sclerosis. Neurology. 2005;65:1071–6.

Bougias C, et al. Theory of diffusion tensor imaging and fiber tractography analysis. Eur J Radiogr. 2009;1:37–41.

Capello E, et al. Marburg type and Baló concentric sclerosis: rare and acute variants of multiple sclerosis. Neurol Sci. 2004;25:S361–3.

Eluvathingal Muttikkal TJ, et al. Susac syndrome in a young child. Pediatr Radiol. 2007;37:710–3.

Erer S, et al. The first Susac's syndrome case in Turkey. J Neurol Sci. 2006;251:134–7.

Filippi M, et al. Diffusion tensor magnetic resonance imaging in multiple sclerosis. Neurology. 2001;56:304–11.

Fitzgerald MJ, et al. Recurrent myelinoclastic diffuse sclerosis: a case report of a child with Schilder's variant of multiple sclerosis. Pediatr Radiol. 2000;30:861–5.

González Sánchez JJ, et al. A case of malignant monophasic multiple sclerosis (Marburg's disease type) successfully treated with decompressive hemicraniectomy. J Neurol Neurosurg Psychiatry. 2008. doi:10.1136/jnnp.2007.142133.

Gupta SS, et al. Pictorial essay: neurological application and physics of diffusion tensor imaging with 3D fiber tractography. Indian J Radiol Imaging. 2008;18:37–44.

Hahn CD, et al. MRI criteria for multiple sclerosis: evaluation in a pediatric cohort. Neurology. 2004;62:806–8.

Hanemann CO, et al. Baló concentric sclerosis followed by MRI and positron emission tomography. Neuroradiology. 1993;35:578–80.

Houtchens MK, et al. Thalamic atrophy and cognitive in multiple sclerosis. Neurology. 2007;69:1213–23.

Hulcombe JE, et al. Baló concentric sclerosis. J Clin Neurosci. 1999;6:46–8.

Humm AM, et al. Quantification of Uhthoff 's phenomenon in multiple sclerosis: a magnetic stimulation study. Clin Neurophysiol. 2004;115:2493–501.

Iwata E, et al. MR imaging in Guillain-Barré syndrome. Pediatr Radiol. 1997;27:36–8.

Jacob A, et al. Neuromyelitis optica. Ann Indian Acad Neurol. 2007;10:231–9.

Johnson MD, et al. Fulminant monophasic multiple sclerosis, Marburg's type. J Neurol Neurosurg Psychiatry. 1990;53:918–21.

Kastrup O, et al. Balo's concentric sclerosis demonstrated by MRI. Neurology. 2001;57:1610.

Li DKB, et al. MRI T2 lesion burden in multiple sclerosis: a plateauing relationship with clinical disability. Neurology. 2006;66:1384–9.

Maddestra M, et al. Encephalopathy, hearing loss and retinal occlusions (Susac's syndrome): a new case. Ital J Neurol Sci. 1998;19:225–7.

Morosini A, et al. Polyneuritis cranialis with contrast enhancement of cranial nerves on magnetic resonance imaging. J Paediatr Child Health. 2003;39:69–72.

Murata Y, et al. Susac syndrome. Am J Ophthalmol. 2000;129:682–4.

Roccatagliata L, et al. Multiple sclerosis: hyperintense dentate nucleus on unenhanced T1-weighted MR images is associated with the secondary progressive subtype. Radiology. 2009;251:503–10.

Schwarz U, et al. Marburg's encephalitis in a young woman. Eur Neurol. 2002;48:42–4.

Vucic S, et al. Guillain-Barré syndrome: an update. J Clin Neurosci. 2009. doi:10.1016/j.jocn.2008.08.033.

Wingerchuk DM, et al. The clinical course of neuromyelitis optica (Devic's syndrome). Neurology. 1999;53:1107–14.

Wingerchuk DM, et al. Neuromyelitis optica: clinical predictors of a relapsing course and survival. Neurology. 2003;60:848–53.


## 2.9    Parkinsonism

Parkinsonism, previously known as *paralysis agitans*, is a motor disease characterized essentially by resting tremor, rigidity, and poverty of spontaneous movements (bradykinesia).

Parkinsonism essentially arises due to nerve cell degeneration affecting the pigmented cells in the substantia nigra (release dopamine) and the cells within the caudate nucleus and putamen (striatum). Neurofilament eosinophilic inclusions within the neurons in patients with Parkinsonism are called Lewy bodies.

Causes of Parkinsonism can be idiopathic (Parkinson's disease), postencephalitic (e.g., encephalitis lethargica), or drug induced (e.g., metoclopramide). *Pseudoparkinsonism* is a term used to describe Parkinsonism that arises due to arteriosclerosis of the vessels supplying the striatum with perivascular hemorrhages and glial proliferation. It is usually found to affect the older population more than other Parkinsonisms (>60 years). *Hemiparkinsonism* is a term used to describe Parkinsonism features of progressive space-occupying lesion. Other causes of Parkinsonism include brain trauma (e.g., boxers) and Wilson's disease (excess deposition of copper within the liver due to deficiency in its carrier ceruloplasmin).

As previously mentioned, the cardinal clinical manifestations of Parkinsonism include resting tremor, rigidity, and bradykinesia. Resting tremor initially starts unilaterally as a relatively rhythmic alteration contraction of opposing groups of muscles. Tremor initially starts in the distal muscles, affecting the fingers and the hand. *Pill-rolling movement* is a term used to describe characteristic tremor movement, where the thumb repetitively moves on the first two fingers with wrist motion. This tremor characteristically is seen from 2 to 6 s. Other areas that may be affected by tremor include the jaw, tongue, and lips. Parkinsonism tremor is characteristically visualized at rest. It disappears as the patient starts to do a voluntary movement or during sleep.

Rigidity is a term that describes a state of steady muscular tension equal in degree in the opposing muscle groups. This muscular tension is constant whether the limb is moved slowly or rapidly, and this phenomenon is described as *lead pipe resistance*. Sometimes when the rigid limb is moved passively, the examiner can feel a jerky intermittent resistance, and the muscles seem to give way in a series of steps, a phenomenon known as *cogwheel rigidity*.

Bradykinesia can be observed in many aspects along the disease progression. There is loss of the normal swinging of the arms while walking, reduced facial movements (masked face), loss of eye blinking, difficulty in initiating smile, narrow-steps shuffling gait, and cervical and lumbar flexion in the standing position. The writing is shaky and tremulous and characteristically gets smaller as the patient continues to write (micrographia). The speech articulation is disturbed and slurred, with monotone soft voice. Involuntary repetition of words or phrases (palilalia) may be seen. Sensory and deep reflexes are characteristically preserved in Parkinsonism. However, exaggerated orbicularis oris (snout) and orbicularis oculi (glabellar) reflexes are often exaggerated. Tapping on the glabella (forehead) may initiate repetitive eye blinking due to exaggerated reflexes (Myerson's sign).

*Camptocormia* is a rare postural involuntary posture of the trunk characterized by an extreme forward flexion of the thoracolumbar spine induced by walking, standing, or sitting that disappears while the patient is lying supine. Camptocormia can be seen in patients with Parkinsonism, and it is caused by severe paraspinal muscles atrophy.

Mental status changes in Parkinsonism may include depression (30 %), slowness of memory, and global dementia in advanced stages of the disease (20 %).

Postencephalitis Parkinsonism shows the same clinical features as Parkinson's disease (idiopathic form). However, postencephalitis Parkinsonism is characterized by some features that are not usually seen in Parkinson's disease. The cogwheel phenomenon is markedly observed in postencephalitis Parkinsonism. Autonomic nervous system disturbance with drooling of saliva (sialorrhea) and excessive sweating (hyperhidrosis) is commonly associated with postencephalitis Parkinsonism. Hypothalamic disturbance with increased appetite, with development of diabetes mellitus and diabetes insipidus, is more observed with postencephalitis Parkinsonism. Moreover, two important ocular manifestations are observed in postencephalitis Parkinsonism that are not usually seen in Parkinson's disease: oculogyric crises and blepharospasm. *Oculogyric crises* are attacks of involuntary conjugate upward deviation of the eyeballs, whereas *blepharospasm* is a period in which the eyes go nearly or completely shut, causing the patient to be virtually blind during this episode.

## Differential Diagnoses and Related Diseases

*Stiff-man syndrome* is a rare disorder characterized by truncal and proximal limbs rigidity, sporadic spasm, and continuous motor unit activity (CMUA) even at rest. The disease is rare with an incidence of <1 per million in the general population. Stiff-man syndrome diagnostic criteria include stiffness and rigidity in the axial muscles, abnormal axial posture (exaggerated lumbar lordosis), and spasm precipitated by voluntary movement or emotions, CMUA in at least one group of muscles, and the absence of brain stem, pyramidal, extrapyramidal, or lower motor neurons signs. The stiff-man syndrome can be seen in cases of syringomyelia, tetanus, diabetes mellitus type 1, and Hashimoto's thyroiditis. Up to 5 % of cancers may precipitate stiff-man syndrome (e.g., small cell carcinoma of the lung).

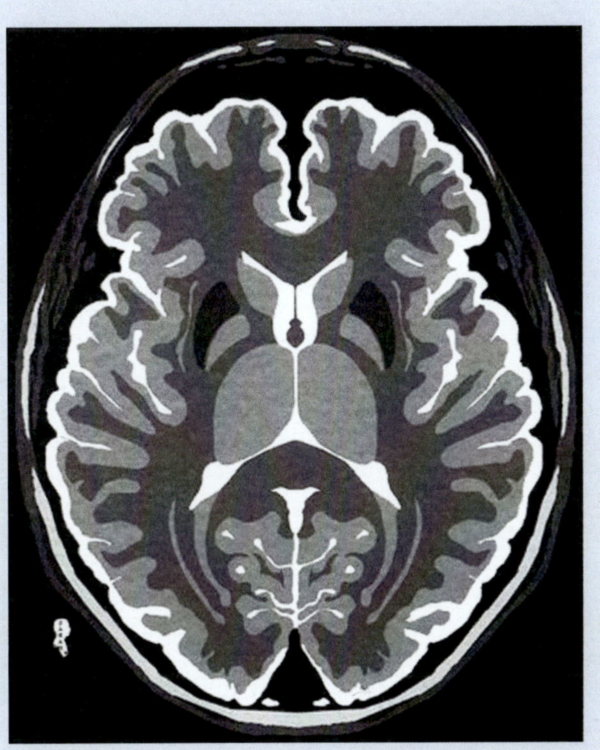

**Fig. 2.9.1** Axial T2W brain MR illustration demonstrates low signal intensity of the putamen bilaterally, a sign of Parkinson's disease

### Signs on MRI
- Generalized brain atrophy with prominent subarachnoid spaces.
- T2W hypointense areas in the putamen and the substantia nigra may be seen due to iron deposition (siderosis) (Fig. 2.9.1).
- Atrophy of the midbrain, cerebellum, and medulla can occur.
- In camptocormia patients, severe paraspinal muscle atrophy with fatty changes in the thoracolumbar region can be seen.

## Further Reading

Agid Y, et al. Biochemistry of Parkinson's disease 28 years later: a critical review. Mov Disord. 1989;4:S126–44.

Andereadou E, et al. Stiff person syndrome: avoiding misdiagnosis. Neurol Sci. 2007;28:35–7.

Benabid AL, et al. Deep brain stimulation of subthalamic nucleus for the treatment of Parkinson's disease. Lancet Neurol. 2009;8:67–81.

Bonneville F, et al. Camptocormia and Parkinson's disease: MR imaging. Eur Radiol. 2008;18:1710–9.

Brown P, et al. The stiff man and stiff man plus syndromes. J Neurol. 1999;246:648–52.

DeJong RN. Parkinsonism. Dis Mon. 1961;7:1–39.

Fowler CJ. Update on the neurology of Parkinson's disease. Neurourol Urodyn. 2007;26:103–9.

Gupta P, et al. Akinetic rigid syndrome: an overview. Ann Indian Acad Neurol. 2007;10:21–30.

## 2.10    Dementia

Dementia is a multifactorial disease characterized by deterioration of the cognitive brain functions. Memory is the most common cognitive brain function lost in dementia. Each brain lobe or region processes different neurological and psychological functions, which can be affected according to the disease causing dementia. The occipital lobe is responsible for the visual activities and processing, the parietal lobe is responsible for spatial navigation, the temporal lobe is responsible for language and memory functions, whereas the frontal lobe is responsible for strategic planning, logic, planning, and social judgment.

The hippocampus is a critical structure for long-term memory storage. Emotions have a powerful influence on learning and memory, and they are controlled by the limbic system.

*The limbic system* is a complex brain network that controls emotions. It was first described by James Papez in 1937 (Papez circuit) and later was completed by Yakovlev in 1948 (Yakovlev circuit). The limbic system is generally composed of five main structures:

- *Limbic cortex* includes the cingulated gyrus and the parahippocampal gyrus. The cingulated gyrus in Latin means "belt bridge."
- *Hippocampal formation* includes the dentate gyrus, the hippocampus, and the subocular complex.
- *Amygdala* is an almond-shaped structure located deep within the temporal lobe beneath the uncus. It controls fear emotions. Amygdala, in conjunction with prefrontal cortex, is involved in retrieval of emotional memories.
- *Septal area* is a gray matter structure that lies immediately above the anterior commissure of the corpus callosum, with extensive reciprocal connections with the hippocampus via the fornix.

- *Hypothalamus* is subdivided into three regions from anterior to posterior: the supraoptic region, the tuberal region (tuber cinereum), and the mammillary bodies.

## Alzheimer's Disease

Alzheimer's disease (AD) is a disease characterized by diffuse cortical brain atrophy with enlargement of the ventricular system.

AD is the most common cause of dementia and is found in up to 10 % of all persons >70 years of age with significant memory loss. The disease is caused by deposition of A amyloid in the neuronal cytoplasm and the cerebral vascular walls. The most important risk factors for AD are old age and a positive family history. *Presenile Alzheimer's disease* is a term used to describe AD that develops in patients <65 years old.

AD starts with memory loss that progress into language and visual–spatial deficits. Memory loss can interfere with the daily activities such as following job instructions or driving. In later stages, loss of judgment and reason often develops. Delusions are common in the later stages of the disease, with 10 % of patients likely to develop Capgras syndrome. *Capgras syndrome* is a form of delusion where the patient believes that a person has been replaced by one or more imposers. The delusion is specific to one person, usually the patient's closest relative.

**Signs on CT and MRI**
- In AD, there is generalized brain atrophy, with bilateral atrophy of the medial temporal lobe and parietal lobe, which are the hallmark signs of AD (◨ Fig. 2.10.1). Usually, there is enlargement of the temporal horns of the lateral ventricles due to parenchymal loss of volume (◨ Fig. 2.10.1).
- In presenile AD, there is striking parietal lobe atrophy with mild medial temporal lobe atrophy. In contrast, in the classical AD, medial temporal lobe atrophy is the hallmark pathology.

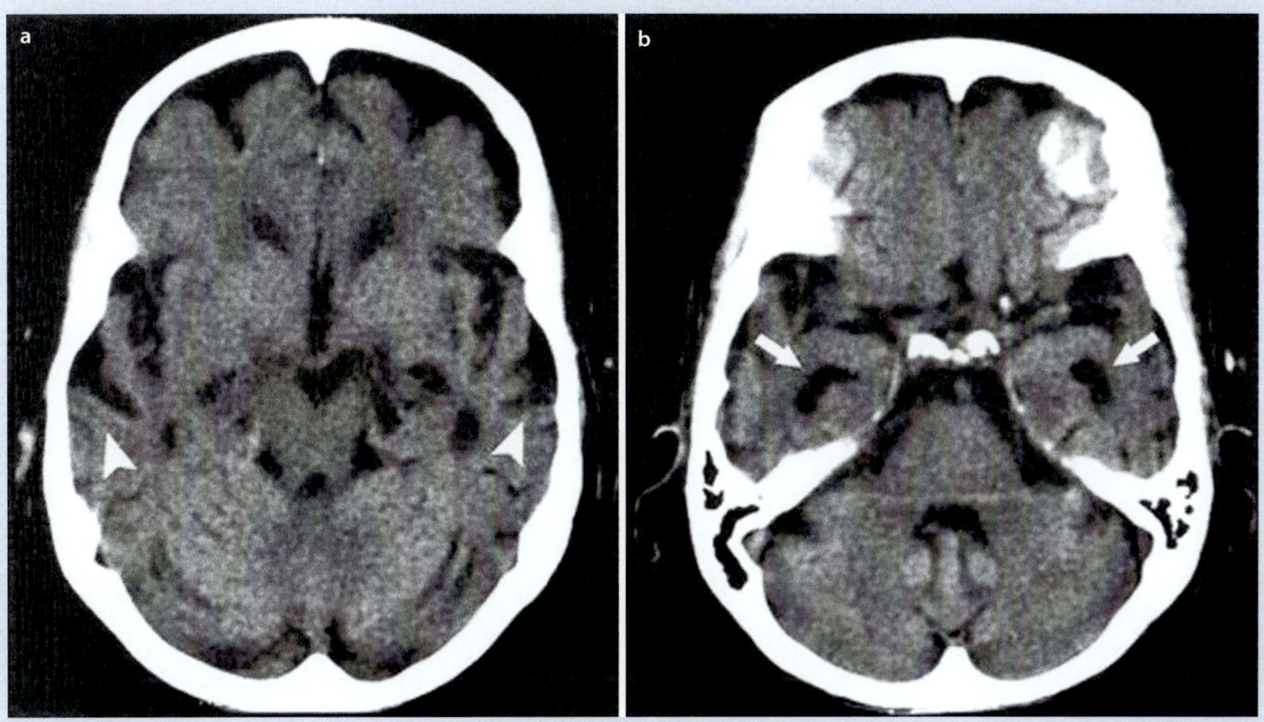

**◘ Fig. 2.10.1** Axial sequential brain CT images of a patient with Alzheimer's disease show generalized brain atrophy, medial temporal lobe atrophy bilaterally in (**a**) (*arrowheads*), bilateral frontal lobe atrophy in (**a**), dilatation of the temporal horns of the lateral ventricles in (**b**) (*arrows*), and dilated prepontine cistern in (**b**)

## Vascular Dementia

Vascular dementia (VaD) is a term used to describe dementia that develops due to vascular lesions involving Papez circuit. *Papez circuit* fibers include the fornix, mammillary bodies, mammillothalamic tracts, cingulated cortex, and anterior thalami. Lesions involving Papez circuit projections result in memory disturbance.

VaD is the second most common cause of dementia after AD and is differentiated from AD by its sudden onset, usually after vascular insult. Stroke is the most common cause of VaD. Two types of strokes are often linked to VaD: watershed infarctions and strategic infarctions.

*Watershed infarctions* occur between two or three vascular territories (◘ Fig. 2.10.2). Anterior watershed infarction is located between the anterior cerebral artery (ACA) and the middle cerebral artery (MCA) territories. Posterior watershed infarction is located between MCA and the posterior cerebral artery (PCA) territories. Internal watershed infarction is located between ACA, MCA, and PCA territories. Watershed infarctions are caused by severe occlusion or stenosis of the internal carotid artery, microemboli, or hypotension. Bilateral watershed infarctions are typically caused by severe brain hypovolemia.

*Strategic infarctions* occur in areas important for normal cognitive function of the brain. Examples of strategic infarctions include:

- Angular gyrus and parietotemporal area (MCA) infarction
- Paramedian thalamic area (PCA) infarction
- Superior frontal or parietal area infarction
- Bilateral thalamic area infarction

## Frontotemporal Lobar Degeneration (Pick's Disease)

Frontotemporal dementia (FTD) is a group of progressive neurodegenerative diseases that include three syndromes: frontal variant FTD, progressive nonfluent aphasia, and semantic dementia.

FTD is the third most common cause of dementia after AD and dementia with Lewy bodies (DLB). It constitutes 5–15 % of all cases of dementia.

Interestingly, studying FTD patients with artistic painting skills revealed development of new visual artistic skills during their illness. In FTD, the posterior parietal and temporal cortices are not frequently affected. These areas mediate the visuospatial and visuoconstructive skills important for drawing, painting, and copying. These new enhanced artistic skills are believed to be attributed to loss of inhibitory activity over the posterior parietotemporal regions involved in visuospatial and visuoconstructive processes.

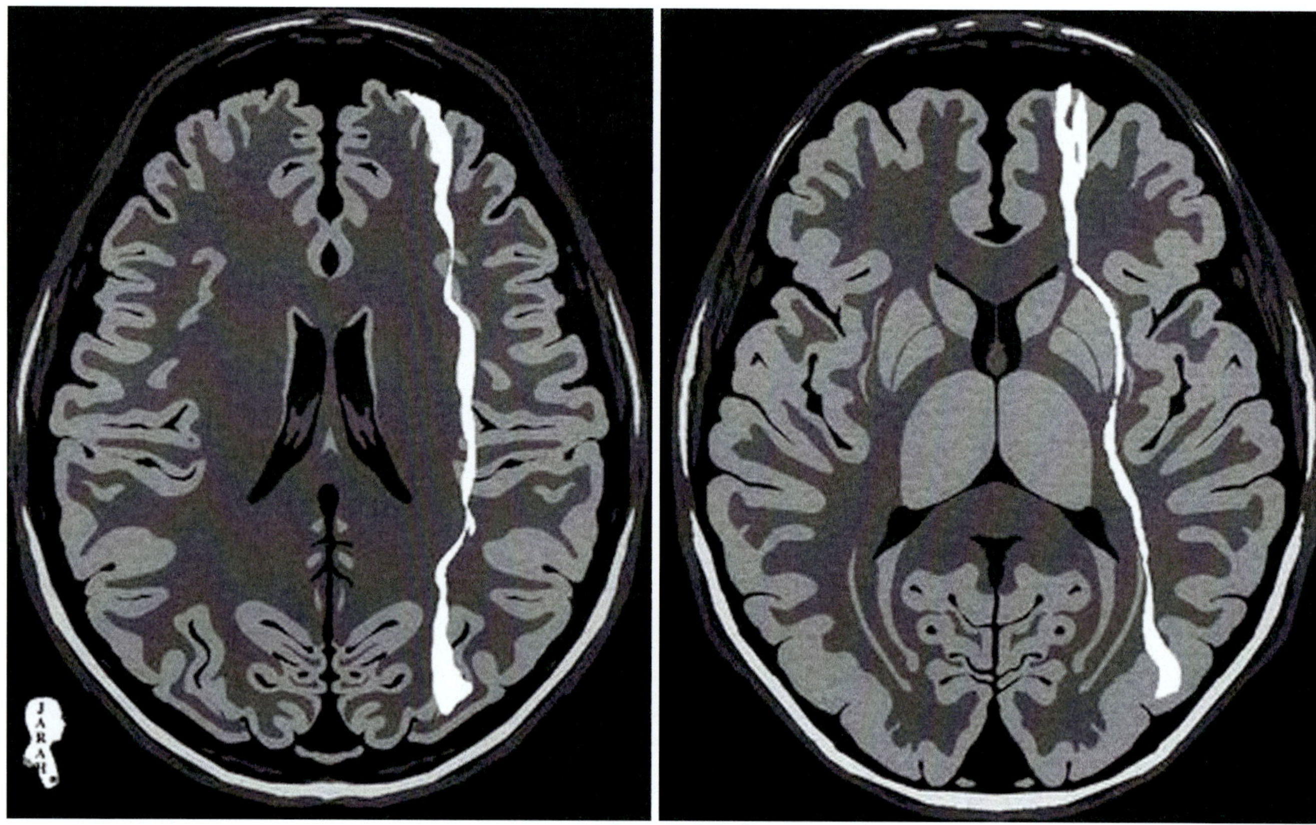

**Fig. 2.10.2**    Axial FLAIR brain MR illustrations demonstrate the watershed zones (*white lines*)

### Signs on MRI
- There is marked atrophy of the frontal and/or the temporal lobes. Frontal lobe atrophy is the hallmark FTD (Fig. 2.10.3).
- Another characteristic finding is asymmetric atrophy of the temporal lobe in one hemisphere, resulting in temporal gyri that appear as sharp as knifes "knife-blade atrophy" (Fig. 2.10.4). Areas of high signal intensity on FLAIR images might be found, presumed to be gliotic changes.

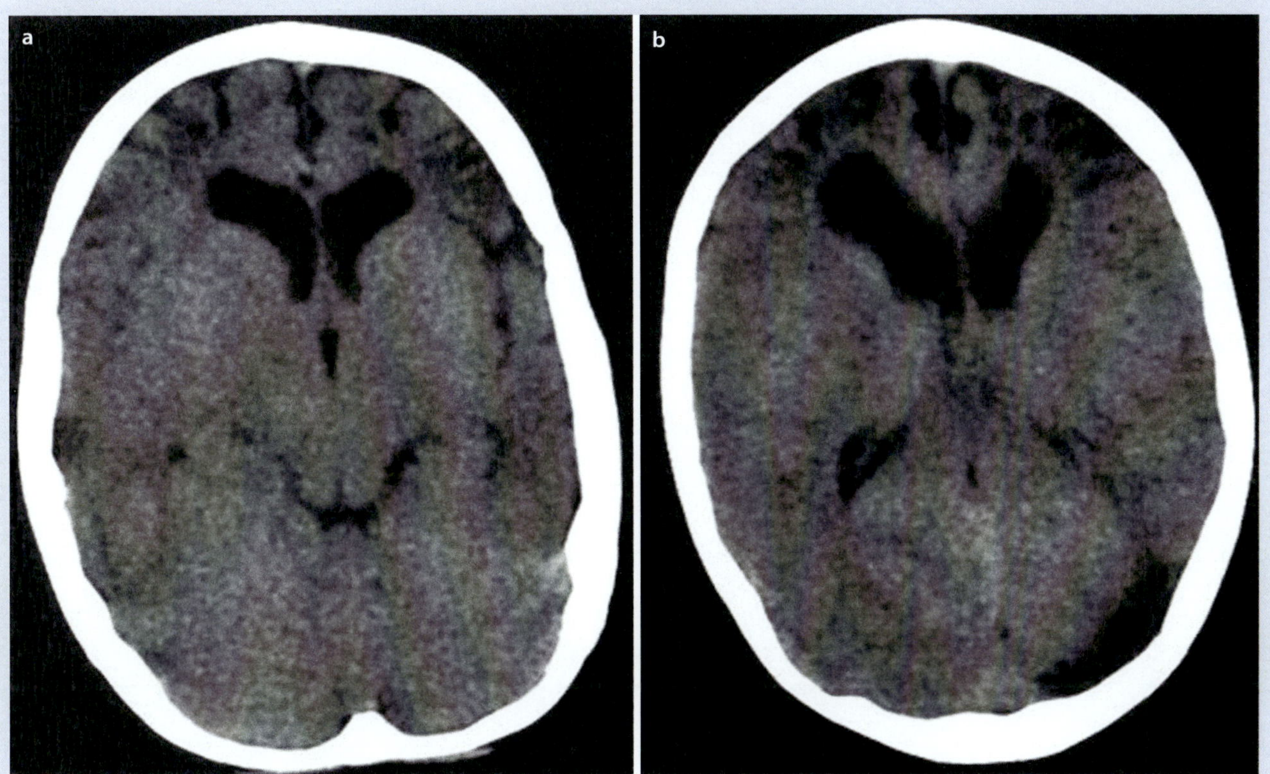

**Fig. 2.10.3** Axial sequential brain CT images of a patient with frontotemporal dementia (FTD) show bilateral frontal lobe atrophy with dilatation of the anterior horns of the lateral ventricles (both **a** & **b**)

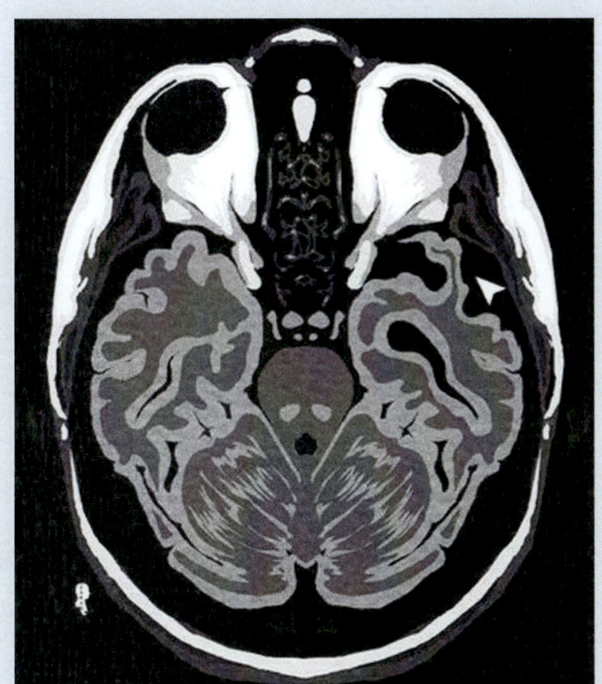

**Fig. 2.10.4** Axial FLAIR brain MR illustrations demonstrate left knife-blade temporal atrophy commonly seen in FTD (*arrowhead*)

## Dementia with Lewy Bodies

DLB is a rare neurodegenerative disorder with features of Parkinsonism (e.g., motor dysfunction) and AD (e.g., dementia).

Current diagnostic criteria of DLB include cognitive impairment with predominant visuospatial dysfunction, recurrent visual hallucinations, and Parkinsonism. Visual hallucinations differentiate DLB from classical Parkinson's disease.

DLB accounts for 25 % of cases of dementia. Pathologically, the disease is characterized by deposition of Lewy bodies in the hippocampus and subcortical nuclei.

## Progressive Supranuclear Palsy (Steele–Richardson–Olszewski Syndrome)

Progressive supranuclear palsy (PSP) is a neurodegenerative, Parkinsonian syndrome characterized by supranuclear vertical gaze palsy, balance disturbance, and limited response to L-dopa.

Early stages of SPS are not usually distinguishable from the classical Parkinson's disease. However, PSP neural deterioration occurs much faster than Parkinson's disease, with many patients dying within 6–7 years from the onset of symptoms. Death is often due to pneumonia, with dysphagia arising in the early stages of PSP. Vertical gaze palsy distinguishes PSP from DLB. Also, DLB is characterized by visual hallucinations, which are not part of the diagnostic criteria of PSP.

In PSP, patients typically present with truncal or neck rigidity, with the absence or with only mild limb involvement and impaired postural reflexes leading to backward falls.

Moreover, limb rigidity and bradykinesia develop in a symmetrical fashion. Resting tremor is uncommon. A patient with the past clinical picture with vertical gaze palsy should assist establishing the PSP diagnosis from Parkinson's disease.

**Signs on MRI**
The MRI shows three characteristic changes: atrophy of the anterior cingulated gyrus, atrophy of the corpus callosum trunk, and atrophy of the midbrain tegmentum, resulting in convexity of its border referred to as "hummingbird sign" (Fig. 2.10.5).

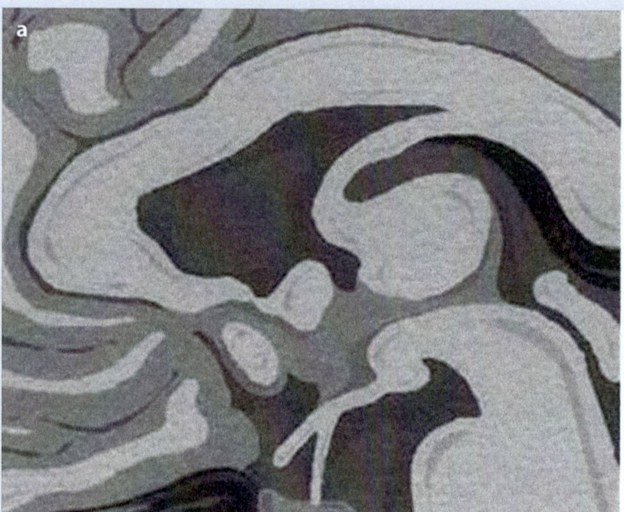

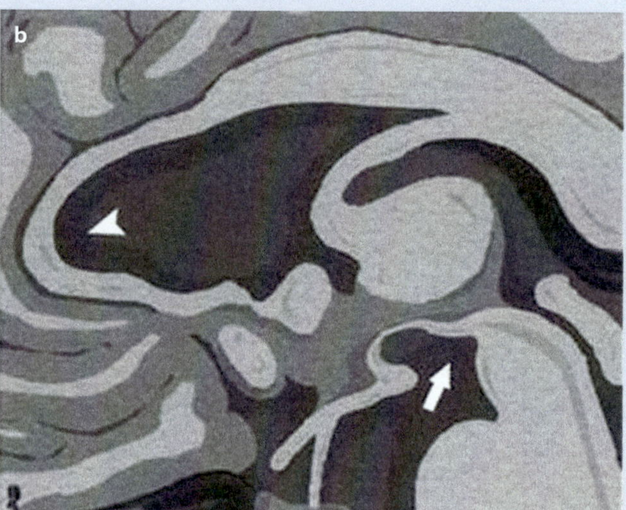

**Fig. 2.10.5**  Sagittal T1W brain MR illustrations demonstrate normal brain stem with corpus callosum (**a**) and atrophied anterior part of the corpus callosum in (**b**) (*arrowhead*) with atrophied brain stem tegmentum in the form of the classical hummingbird sign (*arrow*)

## Multiple System Atrophy (Shy–Drager Syndrome)

Multiple system atrophy (MSA) is a rare disease characterized by Parkinson-like syndrome and degeneration of three systems (autonomic, cerebellar, and extrapyramidal). When atrophy affects the autonomic nervous system mainly, the disease is called *Shy–Drager syndrome*.

MSA arises typically due to olivopontocerebellar atrophy and striatonigral degeneration. Postmortem findings in MSA reveal gliosis and/or neuronal loss in substantia nigra, putamen, caudate nuclei, cerebellar cortex, pontine nuclei, and inferior olive.

Patients with MSA first show signs of Parkinson's disease in their 40s, do not respond to antiparkinsonian medications, and usually succumb to the disease 7–10 years after symptom onset.

**Signs on MRI**
- There is characteristic atrophy of three regions: putamen, pons, and cerebellum (the three systems).
- A characteristic pontine hyperintensity in a cross pattern referred to as *hot cross bun sign* may be seen, and it is a characteristic of this disease (Fig. 2.10.6).
- Abnormal decreased signal in the putamen on T1W and T2W images can be found.

# Subcortical Arteriosclerotic Encephalopathy (Binswanger's Disease)

Subcortical arteriosclerotic encephalopathy (SAE) is a disease characterized by dementia due to arteriosclerosis and occlusion of the deep perforating cerebral arteries and their branches.

SAE is characterized by multiple microinfarctions and focal or diffuse demyelination and gliosis of the periventricular area. Patient usually presents between 40 and 60 years of age with a history of chronic hypertension and multiple stroke episodes. Lack of interest and alteration in mood and personality with loss of appetite for social conducts are among the psychiatric symptoms of the disease. It may be difficult to distinguish Binswanger's disease from AD and other vascular dementias.

> **Signs on MRI**
> — Diffuse periventricular white matter T2 hyperintense signal, ventricular dilatation, and signs of anterior brain atrophy (☐ Fig. 2.10.7). The white matter lesions can be mistaken for multiple sclerosis. However, these lesions characteristically fall in the border between two different vascular supplying systems.

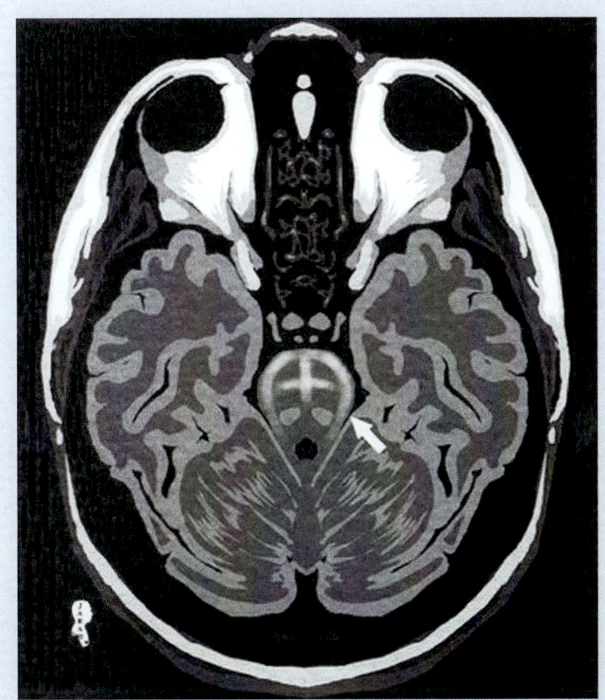

☐ **Fig. 2.10.6** Axial FLAIR brain MR illustrations demonstrate the characteristic "hot cross bun" sign of the multiple system atrophy (MSA) disorder (*arrow*)

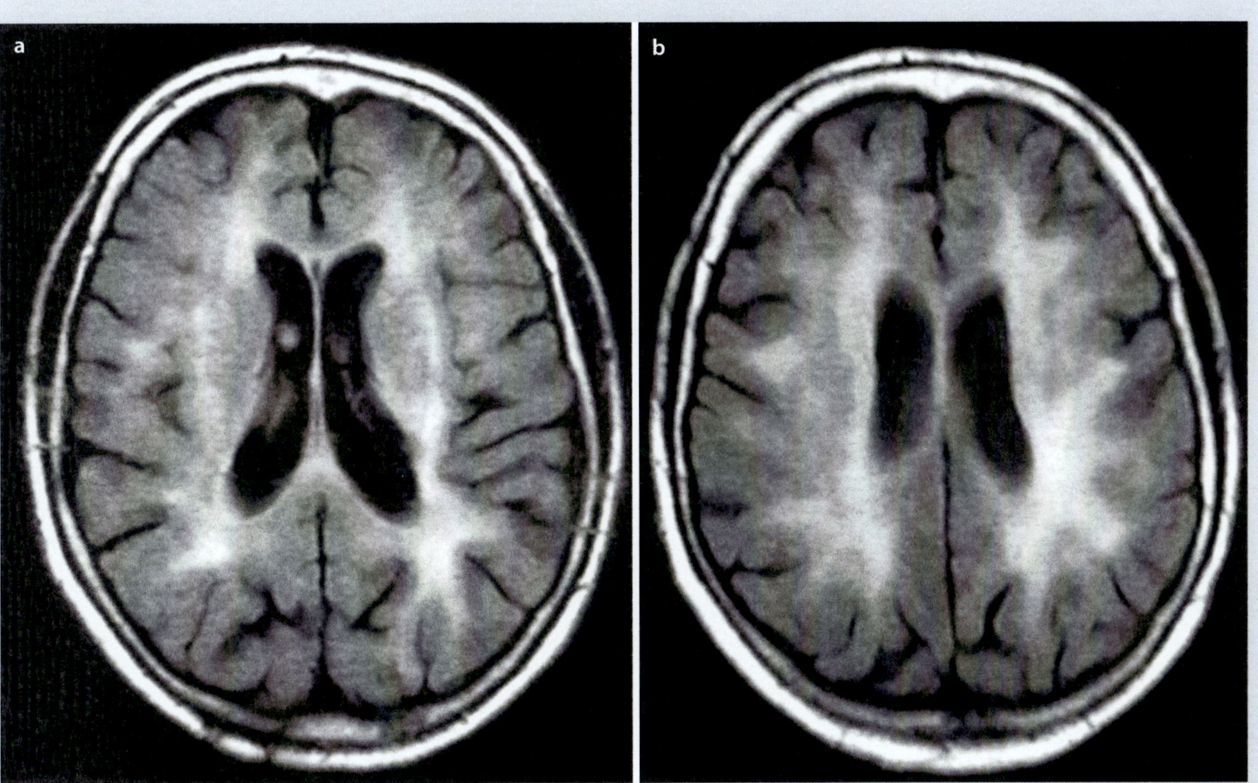

☐ **Fig. 2.10.7** Axial sequential FLAIR brain MRI (**a** & **b**) of a patient with chronic hypertension and dementia shows bilateral symmetrical periventricular white matter diffuse hyperintense signal intensities with mild ventricular dilatation bilaterally without signs of brain atrophy (subcortical arteriosclerotic encephalopathy (SAE)

- There may be T2 hyperintense signal in the basal ganglia, centrum semiovale, and brain stem representing old lacunar (micro)infarctions and Virchow–Robin space dilatation surrounding the perforating arteries (état criblé). *Virchow–Robin (VR) spaces* are perivascular spaces surrounding the walls of vessels as they course from the subarachnoid space through the brain parenchyma. VR spaces surround the walls of arteries, arterioles, and venules. Cerebral veins are not surrounded by VR spaces. VR spaces <2 mm are found normally in all age groups.

As age advances, large VR spaces >2 mm in diameter can be found. VR spaces can be seen as normal variants or part of pathologies (e.g., CADASIL). They are typically seen in the basal ganglia, parallel to the ventricles, and in the midbrain. VR spaces show cerebrospinal fluid signal on MR images (◘ Fig. 2.10.8). Rarely, VR spaces can present with bizarre cystic lesion with pressure over the adjacent structures, which may be mistaken for cystic tumors (e.g., pilocytic astrocytoma).

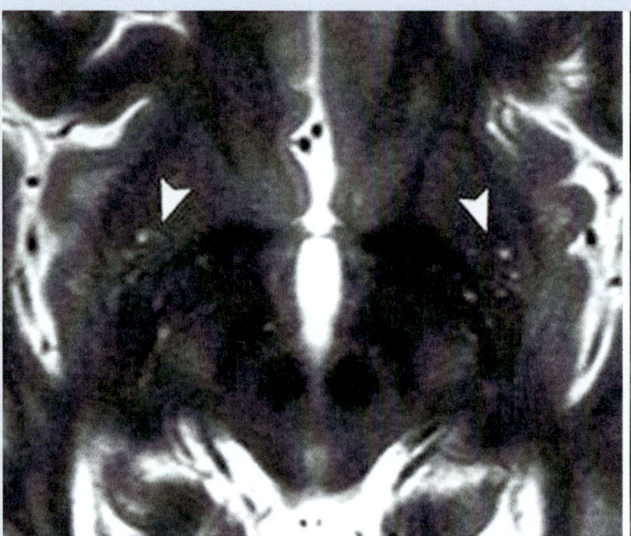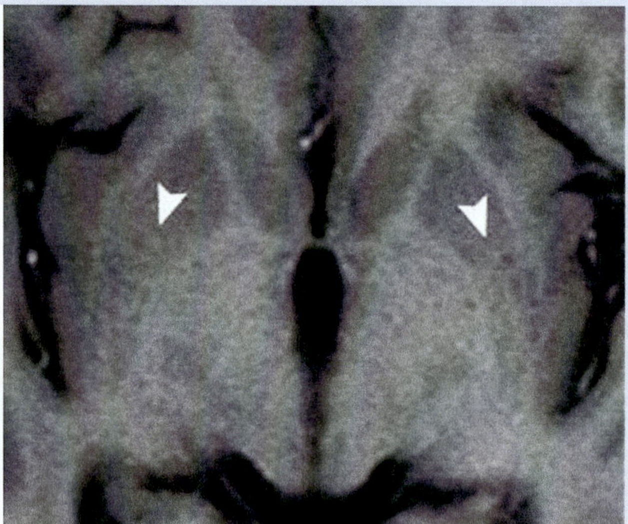

◘ **Fig. 2.10.8**    Coronal T2W (**a**) and T1W (**b**) MRI shows Virchow–Robin space dilatation surrounding the perforating arteries (état criblé) (*arrowheads*)

## Prion Disease

Prion disease, also known as transmissible spongiform encephalopathy, is a group of rare diseases characterized by cognitive dysfunction (dementia), psychiatric symptoms, and variable central nervous system manifestations.

Prion diseases can be found in both animals and human beings. In animals, major prion diseases include chronic wasting disease in deer and elks, scrapie in sheep and goats, and bovine spongiform encephalopathy (BSE) in cattle, notoriously known as "mad cow disease." In human beings, prion diseases include Creutzfeldt–Jakob disease (CJD), Gerstmann–Sträussler–Scheinker disease (GSS), fatal familial insomnia (FFI), and kuru. Human prion diseases are divided into three main categories according to their etiology:

- *Sporadic (most common)*: sCDJ
- *Inherited*: fCDJ, GSS, and FFI
- *Acquired by infections*: vCDJ

*Gerstmann–Sträussler–Scheinker disease* is an autosomal dominant, rare prion disease characterized by progressive spinocerebellar dysfunction, ataxia, spastic paraparesis, and dementia.

FFI is an autosomal dominant prion disease characterized by progressive untreatable insomnia, dysautonomia, and motor signs. MRI in patients with FFI typically shows hypothalamic lesions, which is the hallmark of this disease.

*Kuru* is a disease confined to the Fore linguistic group, a tribe in Papua New Guinea. Kuru is a prion disease linked to ritual tribal cannibalism. The word kuru in Fore language means "to tremble or to shake." The disease is also known as "laughing disease" because the patients present with headache, ataxia, trembling limbs, and laughing or crying episodes without a prior reason.

CJD is a neurodegenerative prion disease with four main forms:

- *Sporadic CJD (sCJD)*: this is the most common form, with an incidence of 1–1.5 per million of population.
- *Familial CJD (fCJD)*: this is a rare form due to mutation in the PrP gene.
- *Iatrogenic CJD (iCJD)*: this form is related to neurosurgeries with cadaveric-derived dura matter or corneal grafts.

— *New variant CJD (vCJD)*: this form is related to consumption of meat infected with BSE. It is generally seen in younger patients than the classical CJD.

sCJD is characterized by rapidly progressing dementia, with 50% chance of death within 5 months of symptom onset. It is typically seen in patients 60–75 years old. Other neurological features include cerebellar ataxia, pyramidal and extrapyramidal signs, and cortical blindness. Death in sCJD patients is most commonly due to pneumonia.

vCJD is linked to consumption of infected cattle meat with BSE. vCJD is seen in younger age than sCJD, and the neurological symptoms are nonspecific, with patients often showing psychiatric and behavioral changes. Incubation period of the disease is approximately 10 years. MRI plays an important role in establishing the diagnosis, since definite diagnosis of prion diseases requires pathological sample examination.

**Signs on MRI**
— In sCJD, the brain shows hyperintense signal changes in the caudate head and the putamen on T2W images (■ Fig. 2.10.9). This sign can be observed in other diseases like carbon monoxide poisoning, hypoglycemia, hemolytic uremic syndrome, and Wilson's disease.
— In vCJD, there are bilateral, almost symmetrical T2 hyperintense lesions found in the pulvinar, the

most posterior thalamic nucleus (*positive pulvinar sign*) (■ Fig. 2.10.10). Normally, the pulvinar is the most hypointense nuclei of the deep gray matter on T2W images. Positive pulvinar sign is a highly sensitive sign of vCJD (■ Fig. 2.10.10).

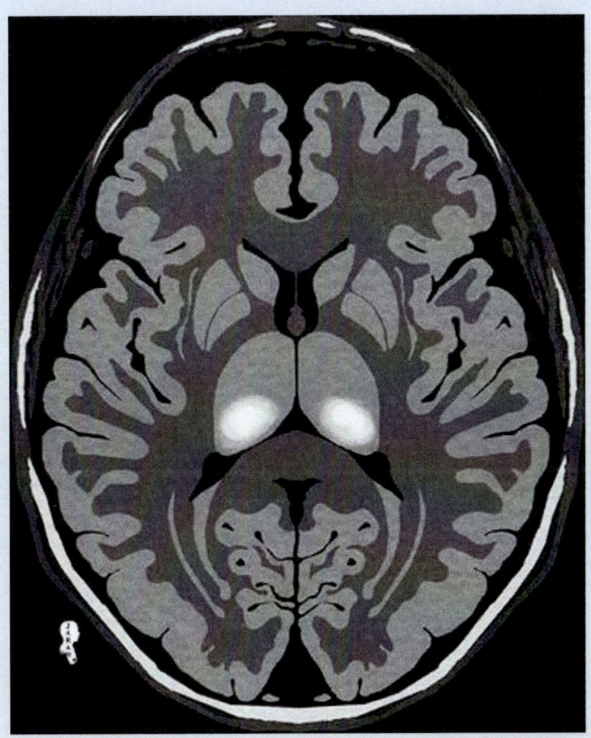

■ **Fig. 2.10.10**   Axial FLAIR brain MR illustration demonstrates the bilateral posterior thalamic (pulvinar) hyperintense lesions in vCJD (positive pulvinar sign)

## Further Reading

Almer G, et al. Fatal familial insomnia: a new Austrian family. Brain. 1999;122:5–16.

Arai K. MRI of progressive supranuclear palsy, corticobasal degeneration and multiple system atrophy. J Neurol. 2006;253 Suppl 3:III/25–9.

Bastos Leite AJ, et al. Thalamic lesions in vascular dementia: low sensitivity of fluid-attenuated inversion recovery (FLAIR) imaging. Stroke. 2004;35:415–9.

Clerici F, et al. Dementia with Lewy bodies with supranuclear gaze palsy: a matter of diagnosis. Neurol Sci. 2005;26: 358–61.

Collie DA, et al. MRI of Creutzfeldt-Jakob disease: imaging features and recommended MRI protocol. Clin Radiol. 2001;56:726–39.

Drago V, et al. What's inside the art? The influence of frontotemporal dementia in art production. Neurology. 2006;67:1285–7.

Guermazi A, et al. Neuroradiological findings in vascular dementia. Neuroradiology. 2007;49:1–22.

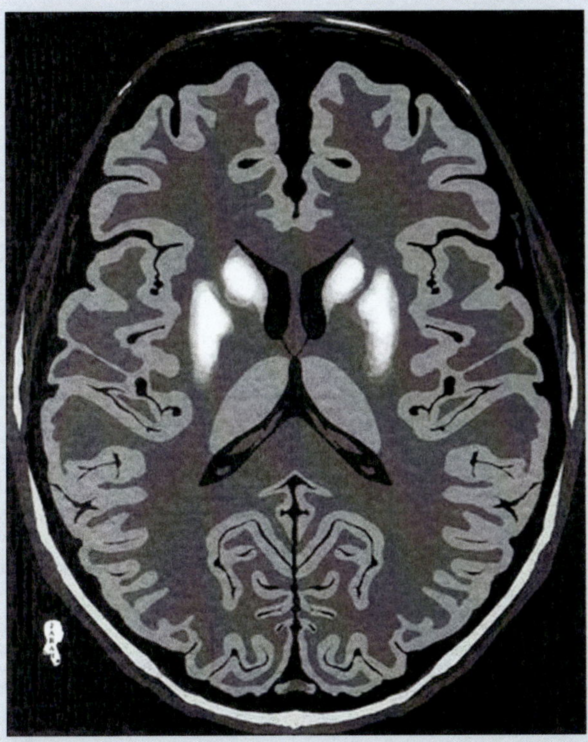

■ **Fig. 2.10.9**   Axial FLAIR brain MR illustration demonstrates the MR signs of sCJD

Kwee RM, et al. Virchow-Robin spaces at MR imaging. RadioGraph. 2007;27:1071–86.

Lucchelli F, et al. The case of lost Wilma: a clinical report of Capgras delusion. Neurol Sci. 2007;28:188–95.

Massano J, et al. Teaching neuroimage: MRI in multiple system atrophy: "hot cross bun" sign and hyperintense rim bordering the putamina. Neurology. 2008;71:e38.

RajMohan V, et al. The limbic system. Indian J Psychiatry. 2007;49:132–9.

Sy M-S, et al. Human prion diseases. Med Clin North Am. 2002;86:551–71.

Uhlenbrock D, et al. The value of T1-weighted images in the differentiation between MS, white matter lesions, and subcortical arteriosclerotic encephalopathy. Neuroradiology. 1989;31:203–12.

Wang Y, et al. Report on the first Chinese family with Gerstmann-Sträussler-Scheinker disease manifesting the codon 102 mutation in the prion protein gene. Neuropathology. 2006;26:429–32.

Wodarz R. Watershed infarctions and computed tomography. A topographical study in cases with stenosis or occlusion of the carotid artery. Neuroradiology. 1980;19:245–8.

## 2.11  Huntington's Disease

Huntington's disease (HD) is a chronic, progressive, autosomal dominant, degenerative disease of the brain characterized by motor, cognitive, and behavioral abnormalities.

Patients with HD initially present between 30 and 50 years of age with chorea. Chorea is an involuntary, jerking, dancing-like movement of the distal limbs (Huntington's chorea). Chorea increases in severity in the first few years of life but eventually fades away again to be replaced by bradykinesia and hypokinesia, which are the real causes of motor disability in HD. In advanced stages, patients develop dysarthria, dysphagia, and impairment of gait and balance.

Psychiatric symptoms can be seen in HD, including depression, personality change, and anxiety. The suicide rate is high, especially in the early stage of the disease.

There is no treatment for HD, and death usually occurs 10–15 years after manifestations of the symptoms.

**Signs on CT and MRI**
- Both scans typically show bilateral symmetrical or asymmetrical caudate nuclei atrophy causing ballooning of the frontal horns (boxcar-shaped frontal horns) (◘ Fig. 2.11.1).
- Brain cortical and white matter atrophy, especially the frontal lobes, can be seen in advanced stages of the disease.

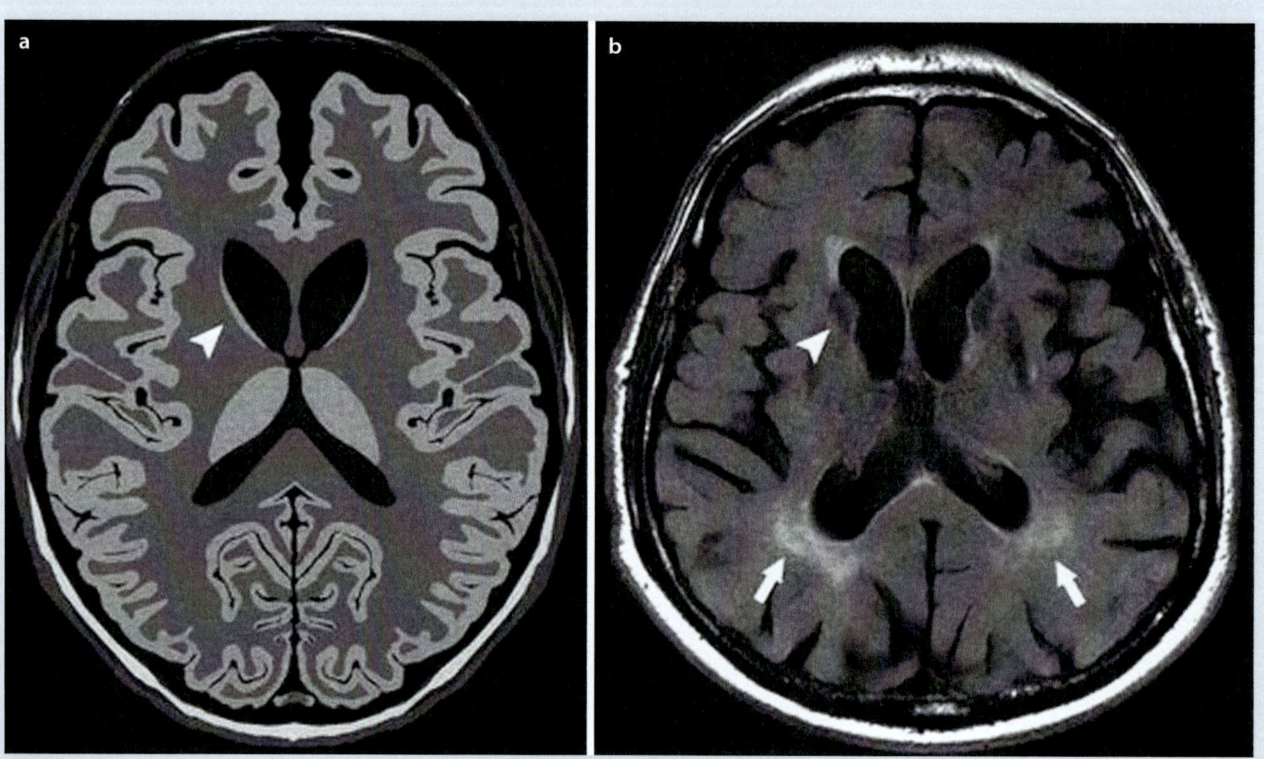

◘ **Fig. 2.11.1**    Axial FLAIR MR illustration (**a**) and FLAIR MRI (**b**) of patients with Huntington's disease (HD) show bilateral caudate nucleus head atrophy and the characteristic boxcar-shaped frontal horns (*arrowheads*)

## Differential Diagnoses and Related Diseases

*Sydenham chorea (rheumatic encephalitis)* is a manifestation of a severe form of rheumatic fever. Sydenham chorea (SyC) is characterized clinically by involuntary and uncoordinated movements, frequent falls, dysarthria, and multiple weaknesses. There is female gender predominance and mean age of 11.7 years at the onset of SyC. The duration of SyC ranges from a week to 2 years with an average duration of 4 months. In rheumatic fever patients, female gender and the presence of carditis can be the risk factors for a longer duration of SyC. Interestingly, patients with previous history of SyC develop psychiatric manifestations later in life, such as obsessive–compulsive disorder, major depressive disorders, or attention deficits. On MRI, basal ganglia hyperintense lesions may be found in patients with SyC.

### Further Reading

Angelini L, et al. Tourettism as clinical presentation of Huntington's disease with onset in childhood. Ital J Neurol Sci. 1998;19:383–5.

Craufurd D. Huntington's disease. Prenat Diagn. 1996;16:1237–45.

Faustino PC, et al. Clinical, laboratory, psychiatric and magnetic resonance findings in patients with Sydenham chorea. Neuroradiology. 2003;45:456–62.

Terrence CF, et al. Computed tomography in Huntington's disease. Neuroradiology. 1977;13:173–5.

## 2.12 Heat Stroke (Pancerebellar Syndrome)

Heat stroke is a medical emergency characterized by a core body temperature >40 °C or more, hot dry skin, and neurological disturbance.

Heat stroke may be environmental due to prolonged exposure to sun heat with hydration, endogenous as in runners during heavy military exercises (exertional heat stroke), or a combination of both. Heat stroke may also develop in other pathological conditions such as infections and neuroleptic malignant syndrome (NMS). NMS is a rare complication of neuroleptic medication therapy (e.g., haloperidol) characterized clinically by hyperpyrexia, muscular rigidity, autonomic dysfunction, altered mental status, and elevation of serum creatine phosphokinase (CK) levels. Patients with NMS typically present with fever and muscle rigidity 24–72 h after the start of treatment with neuroleptic medications; however, NMS may develop weeks to months later. Cerebellar atrophy can be rarely caused by NMS.

The most dramatic effect of heat stroke is observed in the central nervous system, especially the cerebellum. Confusion, delirium, convulsions, myoglobinuria, stupor, and coma are seen in most cases. Downbeat nystagmus, which is defined as a primary position nystagmus with rapid downward phase and slow upward drift, may be seen with heat stroke cerebellar atrophy. Direct thermal insult to the brain may lead to intraparenchymal hemorrhage or stroke.

The most common permanent neurological sequela of heat stroke is *pancerebellar syndrome*, which is characterized by cerebellar atrophy causing dysarthria, irritability, ataxic gait, and poor concentrations. Classically, the patient presents with cerebellar atrophy symptoms weeks to months after the initial heat stroke attack. Cerebellar atrophy is caused by marked degeneration of Purkinje cells with pyknotic nuclei, chemolytic changes, and swollen dendrites. The cerebellar atrophy is indistinguishable from that seen in various degenerative diseases affecting the cerebellum (e.g., alcoholism), so history is very important.

> **Signs on Brain CT and MRI**
> - The initial CT scan may be normal. Follow-up scans after weeks or months may show bilateral cerebellar atrophy with dilatation of the cerebellopontine angle cisterns and the fourth ventricle. No changes in the cerebral hemispheres or the brain stem are noticed classically.
> - Stroke or intraparenchymal hemorrhage may be seen in cases of direct thermal insult.
> - There is an absence of increased intracranial pressure signs.
> - On postcontrast MRI, patchy enhancement of the cerebellum hemispheres may be seen bilaterally.
> - *Neuroleptic malignant syndrome* may show hyperintense T2 white matter lesions affecting the parieto-occipital area. Rarely, cerebellar atrophy may be seen.

### Further Reading

Becker T, et al. MRI white matter hyperintensity in neuroleptic malignant syndrome (NMS) - a clue to pathogenesis? J Neural Transm Gen Sect. 1992;90:151–9.

Deleu D, et al. Downbeat nystagmus following classical heat stroke. Clin Neurol Neurosurg. 2005b;108:102–4.

Manto M, et al. Cerebellar gait ataxia following neuroleptic malignant syndrome. J Neurol. 1996;243:101–6.

McLaughlin CT, et al. MR imaging of heat stroke: external capsule and thalamic T1 shortening and cerebellar injury. AJNR Am J Neuroradiol. 2003;24:1372–5.

Yaqub BA, et al. Pancerebellar syndrome in heat stroke: clinical course and CT scan findings. Neuroradiology. 1987;29:294–6.

## 2.13 Aphasia

Aphasia is a term used to describe the inability to use language. Brodmann has divided the brain into areas according to the cerebral functions. Language is controlled by two main areas: Broca's and Wernicke's areas. *Broca's area (area 45)* occupies the opercular and triangular parts of the inferior frontal gyrus. In contrast, *Wernicke's area (areas 21 and 42)* occupies the posterior part of the superior temporal gyrus.

## Neural Control of Speech

1. *Occipital lobe*: the occipital lobe (Brodmann's areas 17, 18, and 19) receives visual information during reading (*word shapes*) and projects them to different brain regions specialized with language processing.
2. *Angular gyrus*: the dominant angular gyrus (usually the left) receives inputs from the occipital, temporal, and parietal lobes, and it *associates words with the their objects and their meaning*.
3. *Wernicke's area*: Wernicke's area (Brodmann's areas 21 and 42) is the auditory association area responsible for *assembling words into sentences*. Wernicke's area is a region that involves part of the supramarginal gyrus, the angular gyrus, the bases of the middle gyrus, the posterior part of the superior temporal gyrus, and the planum temporale. The *planum temporale* is the superior aspect of the temporal lobe, and it lies in the depth of the Sylvian fissure.
4. *Arcuate fasciculus (Wernicke's arc)*: arcuate fasciculus is an axonal band that transfers information from Wernicke's area (temporal lobe) to Broca's area (frontal lobe). The arcuate fasciculus lies within the *superior longitudinal fasciculus* in the dominant hemisphere (usually the left).
5. *Broca's area*: Broca's area (Brodmann's area 45) occupies the opercular and triangular parts of the left inferior frontal gyrus, and it is the "primary language area" responsible for *words motor articulation planning*.
6. *Motor cortex*: the motor cortex speech (precentral gyrus, Brodmann's area 4) receives inputs from Broca's area regarding spoken sentences to be produced, and it is responsible for *motor articulation of spoken words/ sentences*.
7. *Lips*: the lip is important for the final sound manipulation. The lower lip is much faster and stronger than the upper one.
8. *Tongue*: tongue movement against the hard palate causes the production of the majority of phonemes in English.
9. *Velum/velopharyngeal opening*: for nonnasal speech, the velum closes the gap between it and the nasopharynx (nasopharyngeal opening) during speech by the action of the *levator veli palatini muscle*.
10. *Mandible*: the mandible movement assists in tongue movement. The *mandibular elevators* are temporalis, masseter, and medial pterygoid muscles, and the *mandibular depressors* are *digastric, mylohyoid, geniohyoid*, and *lateral pterygoid muscles*.
11. *Hyoid bone*: the hyoid bone is attached to the larynx, which will cause change in the position of the larynx/ SVT during speaking by the action of attaching muscles, causing different voice resonance. The hyoid moves during mandibular depression.
12. *Supralaryngeal vocal tract (SVT)*: the SVT acts in a manner similar to the tube of a woodwind instrument, filtering the source of acoustic energy emitted from the vocal cords as series of air puffs. The SVT's different cross-sectional areas cause resonance of the sound.
13. *Vocal cords*: the vocal cords vibrate rapidly moving inward and outward during phonation, converting the steady flow of air flowing from the lungs through the trachea into a series of cyclic "puffs" of air that becomes sounds. When vocal cords close, their vibration results in voiced sounds; when they open, this vibration stops, and unvoiced sounds result.
14. *Lung*: speech occurs during expiration, where the outward flow of air from the lungs usually provides the power of speech production.

## Aphasia Pathophysiology and Subtypes

Language production is a very complex mechanism that can be oversimplified by the following models: visual information reaches the *occipital lobe (Brodmann's area 17, 18, and 19)* and processed in various ways, and then the information are projected via the *dominant angular gyrus*, which associates words with the object and its attributes; the words are then transferred to *Wernicke's area*, which assemble them into sentences; Wernicke's area then activates the appropriate motor programs in *Broca's area*, most likely via the *superior longitudinal fasciculus*. Activation of the word's motor program in Broca's area activates the *motor cortex (precentral gyrus, area 4)*. Aphasia can result in disturbance of this neural loop, manifested as:

1. *Broca's aphasia* results in defect in the motor activation of words. The patient tries to produce words, but he is unable to or produces few written or spoken words. However, they may speak or write in a telegraphic way (*only the most meaningful words in a sentence are produced*). Broca's aphasia deprives the motor cortex from the instruction needed to generate language. Broca's aphasia is also known as *expressive aphasia*. On *CT* and *MRI*, Broca's aphasia is detected when the clinical picture shows expressive aphasia with a brain lesion that affects the opercular and triangular parts of the left inferior frontal gyrus (◘ Fig. 2.13.1).
2. *Wernicke's aphasia* results from the inability to assemble sentences. Patients with Wernicke's aphasia are able to produce spoken or written words, but the words or their sequence in a sentence is defective in their linguistic content (*sometimes called cocktail hour speech*). The patient may substitute one letter or a word for another (paraphasia), insert new meaningless words (*neologism*), or string words together in order to convey little or no meaning (*jargon aphasia*). Wernicke's aphasia is also known as *receptive aphasia*. On *CT* and *MRI*, Wernicke's aphasia is detected when the clinical picture shows receptive aphasia with a brain lesion that affects the

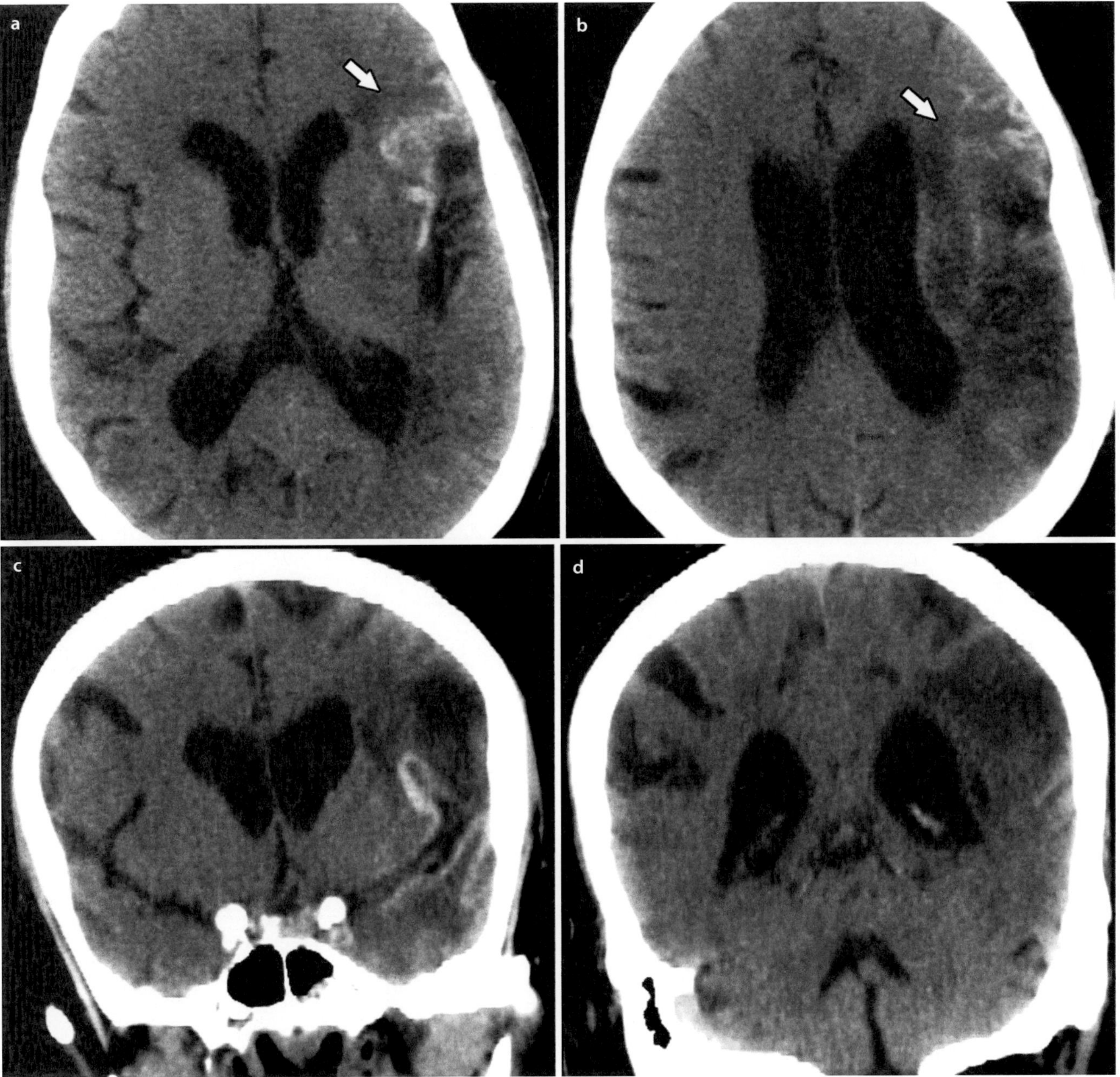

**Fig. 2.13.1** Multiple brain CT postcontrast, axial (**a**, **b**), and coronal (**c**, **d**) images of a patient presented with aphasia; the CT shows left cerebral infarction that affects the frontotemporal area, including the Broca's area (*arrows*). The linear contrast enhancement seen in the images is due to inflammatory hyperemia of acute stroke (luxury perfusion)

left-sided supramarginal gyrus, the angular gyrus, the bases of the middle gyrus, the posterior part of the superior temporal gyrus, and/or the planum temporale (**Fig. 2.13.2**).

3. *Conduction (associative) aphasia*: it is a rare form of aphasia due to damage to the superior arcuate fasciculus, the fibers associating Wernicke's area to Broca's area. The superior arcuate fasciculus lies below the supramarginal gyrus in the temporal lobe. Patients with conduction aphasia are unable to repeat sentences, words, or phrases (hallmark of this condition). Patient's ability to repeat numbers is typically much better than their ability to repeat words. Patients also may have difficulty in finding a word to describe a person or an object. On *MRI*, conduction aphasia can be detected via MR tractography (diffusion tensor imaging), which typically shows lesion affecting the superior longitudinal fasciculus.

4. *Anomic (nominal) aphasia*: it is an inability to name objects, and patients classically know the object or the person's name, but they have difficulty in finding their names. Unlike Wernicke's aphasia, paraphasias are rare. Anomic aphasia usually arises due to destruction of the angular gyrus in the dominant hemisphere (left hemisphere). Speech and comprehension are not

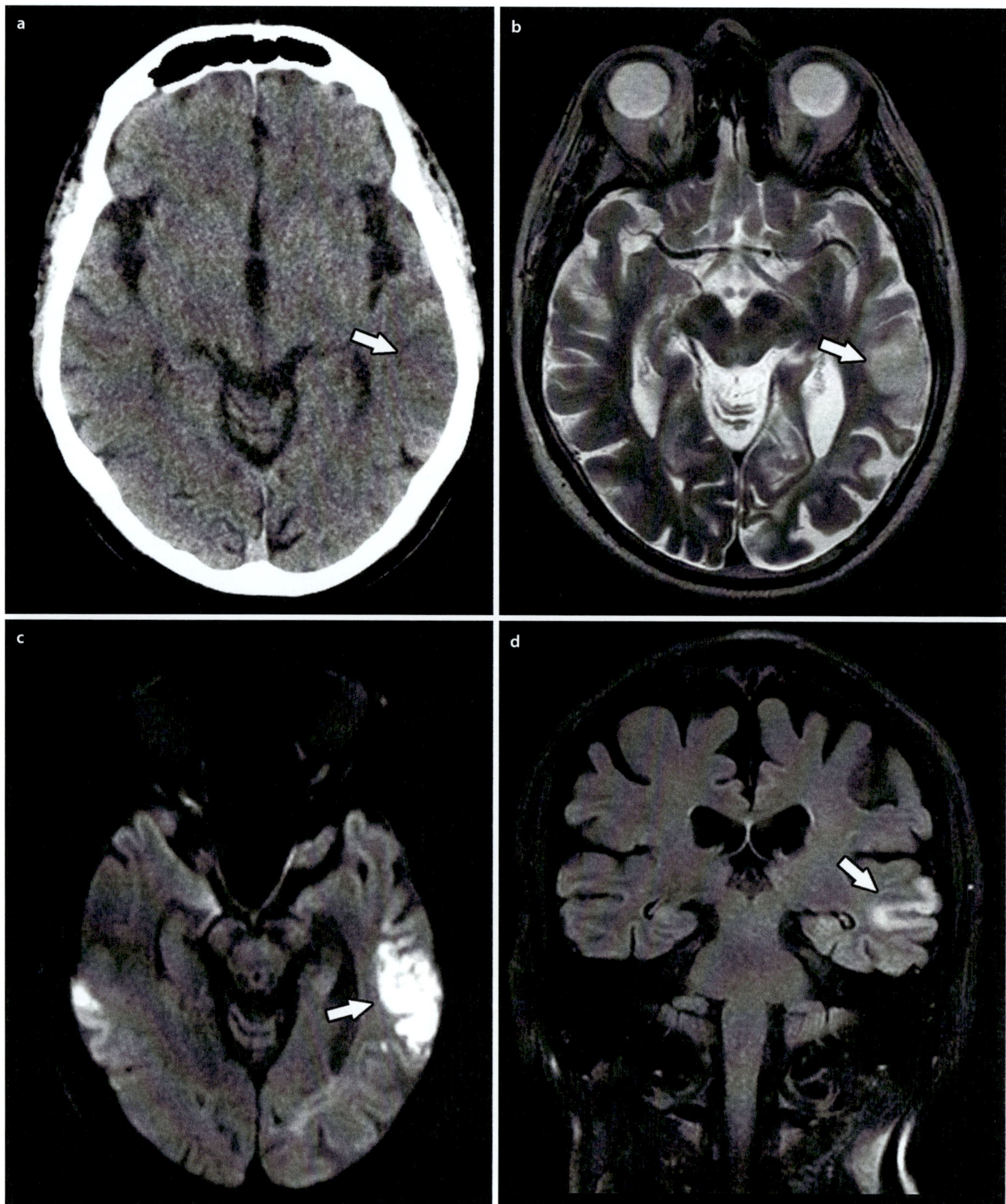



■ **Fig. 2.13.2**   Axial CT (**a**), axial T2W MR image (**b**), axial DW-MR image, (**c**) and coronal FLAIR-T2-MR image (**d**) of a patient with Wernicke's aphasia showing ischemic cerebral insult that involves the left-sided superior and middle temporal gyri (*arrows*)

affected. On *MRI*, a lesion (e.g., infarction) is seen affecting mainly the left angular gyrus.

5. *Global aphasia*: this type of aphasia results from a widespread damage of the language center of the left hemisphere due to anterior and posterior lesions affecting both Broca's and Wernicke's areas together. Typically, global aphasia can arise due to occlusion of the proximal portion of the middle cerebral artery. Patients

suffer from symptoms of both Broca's and Wernicke's aphasias combined. On *CT* and *MRI*, global aphasia imaging typically shows extensive damage to the left (dominant) hemisphere involving both Broca's and Wernicke's regions.

6. *Transcortical sensory aphasia*: it is a very rare form of aphasia that arises when Broca's area, Wernicke's area, and the arcuate fasciculus are undamaged but are cut from the rest of the brain, usually after watershed infarction. The infarcted areas usually are affecting Brodmann's areas 37, 22, and 39. Patients are characterized by well-preserved memory and repetition abilities but are unable to read or write. On *MRI*, transcortical sensory aphasia classically is associated with watershed infarction affecting Brodmann's areas 37, 22, and 39.

7. *Subcortical aphasia*: this aphasia arises due to lesions involving the anterior subcortical area involving the internal capsule and putamen. The lesion affects the language fiber output impairing articulation. On *CT* and *MRI*, a lesion is seen affecting the internal capsule with clinical presentation of aphasia (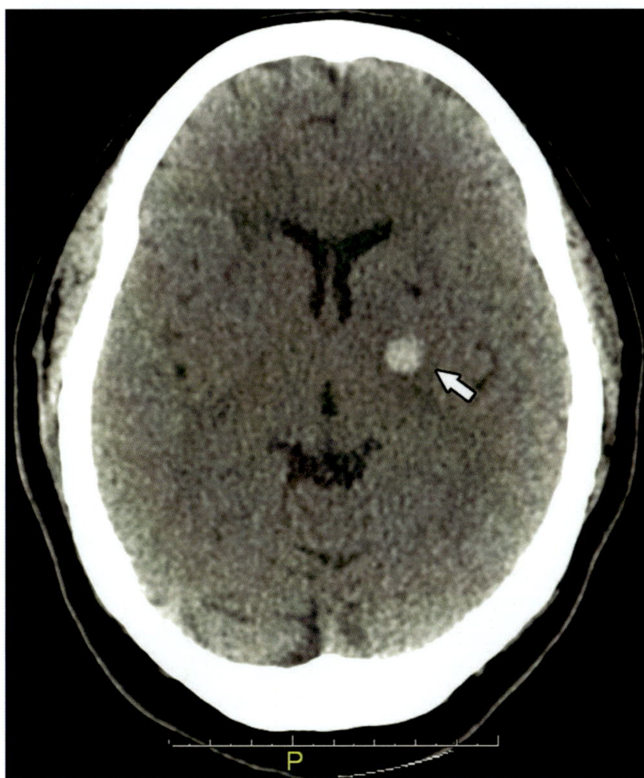 Fig. 2.13.3).

8. *Primary progressive aphasia*: it is a part of frontotemporal degeneration (Pick's disease), which is characterized by deterioration of language for at least 2 years before the onset of cognitive deficits. In its early stages, PPA is often mistaken for Alzheimer's disease, because patients are often presenting with language (naming) impairment. On *MRI*, primary progressive aphasia shows signs of frontotemporal degeneration and asymmetrical left perisylvian region pathology or atrophy.

9. *Akinetic mutism*: it is a rare condition that arises due to acute thalamic lesion, which can be confused with global aphasia. In contrast to global aphasia, akinetic mutism arises due to lesions of the dorsomedial and ventromedial thalamus and usually develops in the acute period of thalamic hemorrhage and tends to show improvement.

## Differential Diagnoses and Related Diseases

*Landau–Kleffner syndrome (acquired epileptic aphasia)* is a rare syndrome characterized by an acquired receptive and expressive aphasia with epileptic seizures in a previously normal child. The disease is diagnosed based on specific clinical and electroencephalography (EEG) criteria. Children with Landau–Kleffner syndrome (LKS) classically present between 3 and 8 years (>50 % of cases) with deafness, behavioral disturbance (>75 % of cases), and loss of auditory verbal understanding (*agnosia*) of speech. EEG classically shows bitemporal, multifocal, or generalized, high-amplitude spikes and wave discharges. The EEG may be normal in the evolutionary stages of the condition and almost always apparent during nonrapid eye movement (REM) sleep. Therefore, children suspected with LKS should have EEG during sleep, especially if the record during awake is normal. The disease cause is unknown; however, cases of LKS have been reported in patients with focal subacute encephalitis, neurocysticercosis, and cerebral arteritis. MRI may show signs of white matter demyelinating lesions affecting the frontal lobe or the centrum semiovale.

## Selected Readings

Barbas H, et al. Frontal-thalamic circuit associated with language. Brain Lang. 2013;126:49–61.

Borovsky A, et al. Lesion correlates of conversational speech production deficits. Neuropsychologia. 2007;45:2525–33.

George A, et al. Primary progressive aphasia: a comparative study of progressive nonfluent aphasia and semantic dementia. Neurol India. 2005;53(2):162–6.

Guenther FH, et al. A neural theory of speech acquisition and production. J Neurolinguistics. 2012;25:408–22.

Honda M. Human speech production mechanisms. NTT Technical Review. 2003;1(2):24–9.

Lee A, et al. The contribution of neuroimaging to the study of language and aphasia. Neuropsychol Rev. 2006;16:171–83.

Lieberman P, et al. The anatomy, physiology, acoustics and perception of speech: essential elements in analysis of the evolution of human speech. J Hum Evol. 1992;23:447–67.

Ozeren A, et al. Global aphasia due to left thalamic hemorrhage. Neurol India. 2006;54(4):415–7.

Perniola T, et al. A case of Landau-Kleffner syndrome secondary to inflammatory demyelinating disease. Epilepsia. 1993;39(2):551–6.

Salamon N, et al. The human cerebral cortex on MRI: value of coronal plane. Surg Radiol Anat. 2005;27:431–43.



**Fig. 2.13.3** Plain brain CT image of a patient presented with aphasia; the CT showed hemorrhagic infarction of the striate arteries that involves the left internal capsule region (*arrowhead*); the CT diagnosis suggests subcortical aphasia, in conjunction with the clinical presentation

## 2.14   Squint (Strabismus)

*Strabismus*, also known as *squint*, is defined as deviation of an eye's visual axis from its normal position (ocular malalignment). The typical clinical manifestation of strabismus is double vision (diplopia). *Diplopia* is a term used to describe double vision, and it occurs when the two eyes are not misaligned in straight ahead gaze or during movement. It can arise due to squint or due to a disease affecting the motor nerves (e.g., *palsies*) or the ocular muscles (e.g., *Grave's disease*).

## Neural Control of Ocular Muscles

1. *Oculomotor nerve (CN 3)*: its nucleus is located in the *midbrain* and supplies all of the extraocular muscles except the *superior oblique muscle* and the *lateral rectus muscle*.
2. *Trochlear nerve (CN 4)*: its nucleus is located in the *midbrain* and supplies the *superior oblique muscle*.
3. *Abducens nerve (CN 6)*: its nucleus is located in the *pons* and supplies the *lateral rectus muscle*.
4. *The medial longitudinal fasciculus (MLF)*: it controls *vertical* eye movement (□ Fig. 2.14.1). Lesions to the MLF cause vertical gaze palsy (*Parinaud's syndrome*).
5. *Paramedian pontine reticular formation (PPRF)*: it controls *horizontal* eye movement.

## Pathophysiology

There are two major types of manifest strabismus:
1. *Concomitant strabismus* (from the Latin *comitare*, accompany): the deviating eye *accompanies* the leading eye in every direction of movement. The angle of deviation *remains the same* in all directions of gaze.

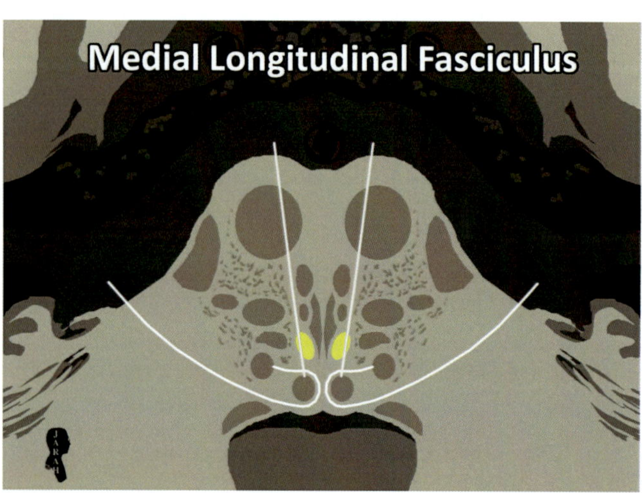


□ **Fig. 2.14.1**   Axial T1W MR illustration demonstrates the normal location of the medial longitudinal fasciculus on MRI (yellow nuclei)

2. *Paralytic strabismus*: it results from paralysis of one or more eye muscles. This form differs from concomitant strabismus in that the angle of deviation *does not remain constant* in every direction of gaze. Concomitant strabismus usually occurs in *children*, whereas paralytic strabismus primarily affects *adults*.

Risk factors for strabismus include family history, low birth weight, maternal cigarette smoking, increasing maternal age, retinopathy of prematurity, and refractive errors. Strabismus is described as:
1. *Esotropia*: the eye is inverted *inward*. Esotropia compromises up to 60 % of all types of strabismus in the West, with up to 90 % of cases occurring before 5 years of age. Esotropia has to be corrected before the age of 7 years since the risk of *amblyopia (the brain shuts down the deviated eye)* is high.
2. *Exotropia*: the eye is inverted *outward*. Exotropia is less commonly seen compared with esotropia, and it is common among Asian population. The disease tends to affect older children than those affected by esotropia, and the risk of amblyopia is lower than esotropia generally.
3. *Hypertropia*: the eye is inverted *upward*. Hypertropia is not common compared to eso- and exotropias, with up to 30 % of cases are associated with the *fourth cranial nerve palsy*. Other causes of hypertropia include Brown's syndrome and primary inferior oblique overaction.
4. *Hypotropia*: the eye is inverted *downward*.

## Related Disorders

1. *Amblyopia*: the brain responds to the childhood strabismus by suppressing the image from the deviating eye to prevent the diplopia, resulting in amblyopia (lazy eye). Amblyopia is not corrected by glasses, and if not treated before the age of 7, the visual loss is irreversible. When strabismus develops in an adult (>7 years of age), it results in double vision (*diplopia*), and it usually arises due to cranial nerve injuries affecting the third, fourth, and sixth cranial nerves, ocular muscle disease (e.g., *Brown's syndrome*), or neuromuscular junction disorder affecting the ocular muscles (e.g., *myasthenia gravis*).
2. *Heavy eye syndrome*: heavy eye phenomenon presents as progressive esotropia and hypotropia in high myopia. It appears to be due to compression of the lateral rectus muscle against the lateral orbital wall by the enlarged myopic globe or due to degeneration of the lateral rectus–superior rectus (LR–SR) band, which joins the lateral and superior rectus muscles. Patients present with acute or subacute strabismus with esotropia that can be misdiagnosed as stroke or mass lesion in the brain.
3. *Congenital fibrosis of the extraocular muscles (CFEOM) syndrome*: it is an autosomal recessive disease present since early infancy characterized by strabismus and congenital nonprogressive restrictive ophthalmoplegia

with or without ptosis. The disease is divided into CFEOM1, CFEOM2, CFEOM3, and Tukel syndrome. CFEOM is caused by mutation of the FEOM1 gene located on chromosome 12p11.2-q12. The main pathological cause of CFEOM is hypoplasia of the superior division of cranial nerve 3 (oculomotor nerve, CN III) branches with maldirection of its fibers.

Congenital fibrosis syndrome may be seen in association with Joubert's syndrome and Marcus Gunn jaw-winking phenomenon. Patients with CFEOM show bilateral severe limitation in vertical gaze with their eyes partially or completely fixed in a strabismic and hypotrophic position due to extraocular muscles fibrosis. The horizontal gaze is normal.

### Signs on MRI

1. The role of MRI in squint is to exclude cerebral lesions (◘ Fig. 2.14.2) and to evaluate the ocular muscles, typically via oculodynamic MRI. *Oculodynamic MRI* is a technique that uses cine MR images to evaluate the eye movement in motion. Typically, T2W images are taken in axial images, and the patient is asked to look to the right and left while the MR is scanning in cine sequence to evaluate the medial and lateral rectus muscles (◘ Fig. 2.14.3). For the superior and inferior rectus muscles, the same technique is used with sagittal images that are taken for each eye.

2. *Heavy eye syndrome*: on MRI (1) the lateral rectus–superior rectus (LR–SR) band is deficient or degenerated causing the lateral rectus muscle to be displaced inferiorly from the globe center. The lateral rectus muscle can be displaced in elderly people between *2* and *4* mm, but in heavy eye syndrome, the lateral rectus is displaced *4.5–6.1* mm from the globe center; (2) the inferior rectus muscle in the affected eye

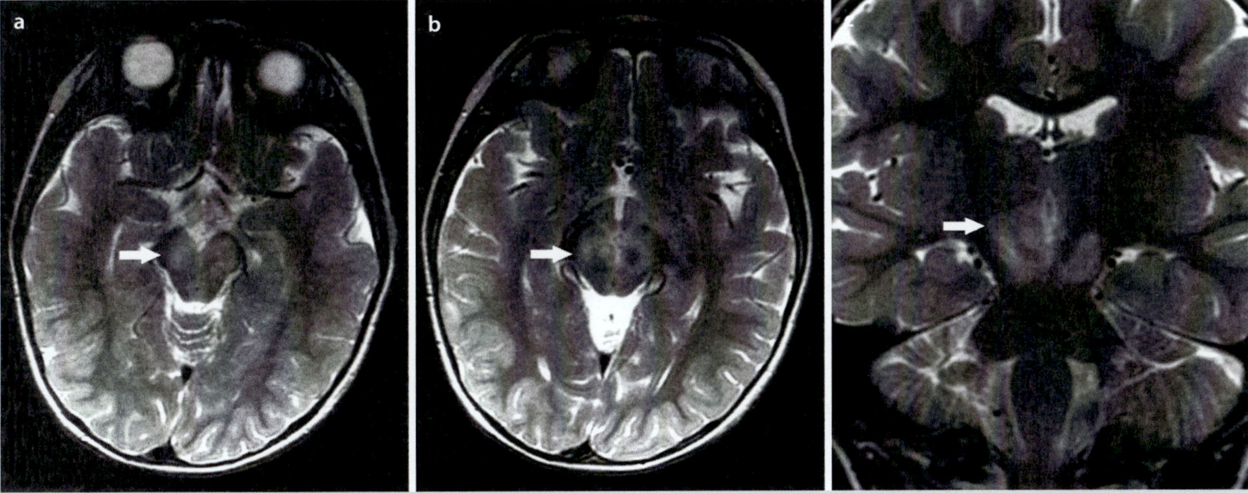

◘ **Fig. 2.14.2**  Axial (**a**, **b**) and coronal (**c**) T2W images of a 2-year-old patient with Coxsackievirus encephalitis presented with strabismus. The inflammatory changes involve the midbrain nucleus bilaterally (*arrowheads*)

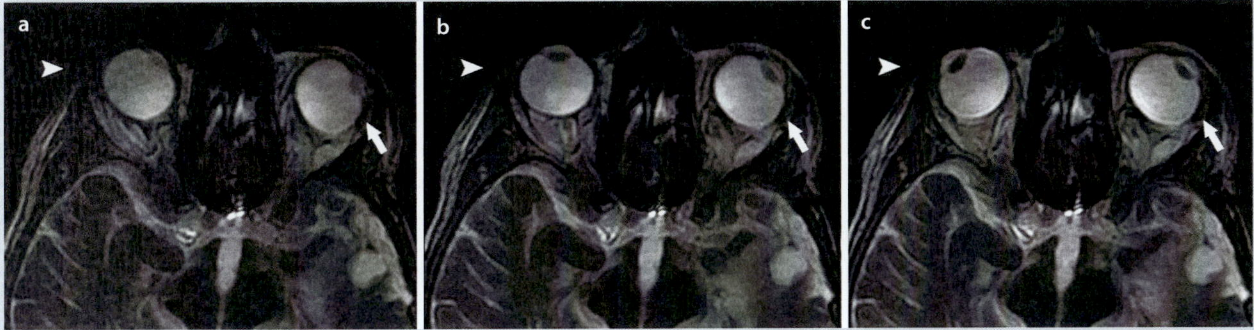

◘ **Fig. 2.14.3**  Sequential, axial, T2W, oculodynamic cine MR images of a 41-year-old patient presented with left-sided third cranial nerve palsy. On the dynamic imaging, the left eye (*arrows*) is seen fixed laterally by the action of an intact lateral rectus and paralyzed medial rectus muscle. The right eye, in contrast, is normally moving when the patient moves the right eye from the left side (**a**) into the right side (**c**) passing through the middle (**b**), when the patient is asked to move his eyes from right to left (*arrowheads*). The left eye remained paralyzed in all images from (**a**) to (**c**)

can show displacement; and (3) the affected eye can show elongation (myopia) with compression over the lateral rectus muscle.

3. *CFEOM*: on MRI, there is agenesis of the corpus callosum, basal ganglia, and cerebellar atrophies, and hypoplasia of the oculomotor nerve may be seen in association with CFEOM syndrome; on T1W coronal orbital images, CFEMO shows high T1 signal intensity on T1W images with small volume ocular muscles. Also, selective involvement and atrophy of the superior rectus–levator muscles are characteristic signs observed in CFEMO.

## References

Demer JL, et al. High-resolution magnetic resonance imaging demonstrate abnormalities of motor nerves and extraocular muscles in patients with neuropathic strabismus. J AAPOS. 2006;10:135–42.

Durnian JM, et al. Treatment of "heavy eye syndrome" using simple loop myopexy. J AAPOS. 2010;14:39–41.

Hickman SJ. Neuro-ophthalmology. Pract Neurol. 2011;11:191–200.

Rutar T, et al. "Heavy Eye" syndrome in the absence of high myopia: a connective tissue degeneration in elderly strabismic patients. J AAPOS. 2009;13:36–44.

Yoshida K, et al. Congenital fibrosis of the extraocular muscles (CFEOM) syndrome associated with progressive cerebellar ataxia. Am J Med Genet A. 2007;134A:1494–501.

## 2.15  Nystagmus

The function of the ocular motor system is to hold images stable on the fovea. Nystagmus is defined as the inability to maintain stable foveal vision, resulting in involuntary oscillation of the eyes (*seeing illusionary movement in the visual field*). It may be congenital or acquired in onset. Congenital nystagmus will present within the first 6 months after birth.

Congenital nystagmus has two main causes of origin: *sensory* and *motor*. *Sensory nystagmus* results from afferent pathway disease of the globes, optic nerves, optic chiasm, or optic tracts in children who lose their vision before 4–6 months of age. A child who sustains bilateral loss of vision after the age of 6 months will not develop sensory nystagmus. *Motor nystagmus*, in contrast to sensory nystagmus, results from an anomaly of the central oculomotor control system. It usually presents within weeks after birth. It is typically binocular and conjugate and is associated with nearly normal visual acuity.

## Neural Control of Eye Movement

1. *Frontal eye field (Brodmann's area 8)*: this is a cerebral cortical region that lies anterior to the premotor cortex (Brodmann's area 5) and is responsible for *voluntary turning both eyes horizontally.*

2. *Higher centers*: higher centers that contribute to the eye movement include the anterior cingulated gyrus and parietotemporal cortex (including the insula and hippocampus).

3. *Thalamus*: a lesion to the posterolateral thalamus can initiate nystagmus.

4. *Midbrain*: apart from holding the oculomotor (CN 3) and trochlear (CN 4) nuclei, the midbrain participates in eye movement via the *interstitial nucleus of Cajal* (⬛ Fig. 2.15.1) and the *rostral interstitial nuclei of the medial longitudinal fasciculus (riMLF)*, both of which are involved in the control of vertical and torsional gaze.

5. *Oculomotor nerve (CN 3 – midbrain)*: it supplies all the ocular muscles except the *lateral rectus muscle* and the *superior oblique muscle*. The oculomotor nucleus receives afferent fibers from the *riMLF* and the *interstitial nucleus of Cajal*.

6. *Trochlear nerve (CN 4 – midbrain)*: it supplies the *superior oblique muscle*, and its nucleus is located on top of the *medial longitudinal fasciculus*.

7. *Abducens nerve (CN 6 – pons)*: it supplies the *lateral rectus muscle*, and it receives inputs from the vestibulocochlear nerve (CN 8) regarding the semicircular canal position in space via the *paramedian pontine reticular formation (PPRF)*. The abducens nucleus sends axons to the *medial rectus muscle* via axons that cross and ascend to the oculomotor nucleus (CN 3) via the *medial longitudinal fasciculus* (⬛ Fig. 2.15.2). The end result is the movement of the medial rectus in the same direction of the lateral rectus muscle during eye movement. Only neurons that innervate the medial rectus muscle in the oculomotor nucleus receive this ascending, crossed input from the abducens nucleus

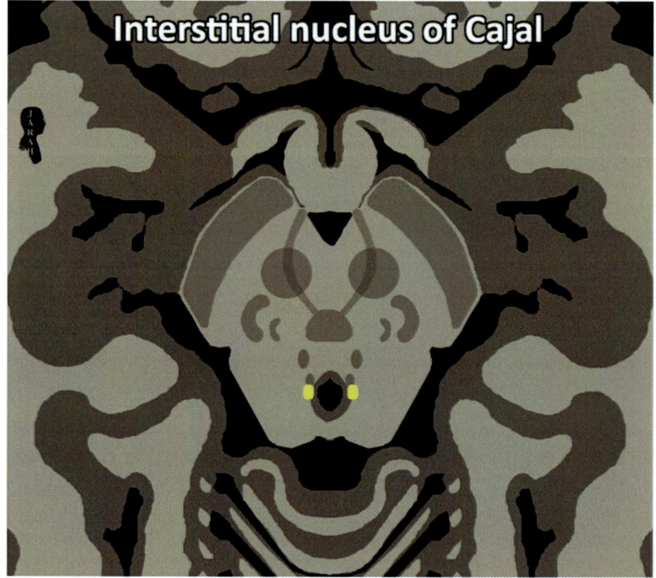


⬛ **Fig. 2.15.1**   Axial T1W MR illustration demonstrates the normal location of the interstitial nucleus of Cajal on MRI (yellow nuclei)

(CN 6). So during head movement, the *right* semicircular canal sends inputs regarding the position of the head in space to the *right* vestibulocochlear nerve. The *right* vestibular nerve sends crossed inputs to the *left* PPRF, which in turn sends neural inputs to the *left* abducens nucleus. The *left* abducens nucleus sends two neural outputs: (1) to the lateral rectus to move via the *left* abducens nerve and (2) to the medial rectus to move to the *right* oculomotor nucleus via the *right* MLF. The past neural pathway is known as the *vestibulo-ocular reflex*,

which is important to stabilize gaze while the head is moving.

8. *Vestibulochochlear nerve (CN 8)*: the vestibular nerve projects its neural input from the semicircular canals to the contralateral abducens nucleus affecting the gaze via the *vestibulo-ocular reflex.*

9. *Semicircular canals*: the semicircular canals send inputs regarding the position of the head in space to the *right* vestibulocochlear nerve, which in turn affect gaze via the *vestibulo-ocular reflex.*

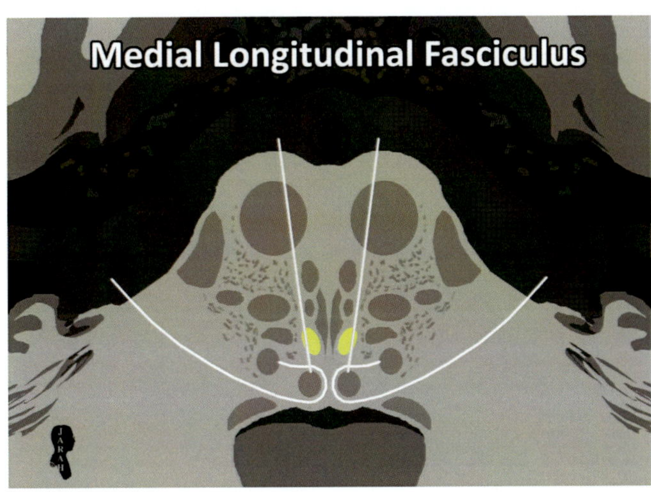


■ **Fig. 2.15.2**   Axial T1W MR illustration demonstrates the normal location of the medial longitudinal fasciculus on MRI (yellow nuclei)

■ **Fig. 2.15.3**   An illustration that demonstrates lesion locations of some nystagmus subtypes

## Nystagmus Subtypes

1. *See-saw nystagmus*: it is an uncommon form of nystagmus characterized by synchronous alternating elevation and intorsion of one eye, with simultaneous depression and extrusion of the other eye, followed by reversal of the vertical and torsional movement in the next half cycle. On *MRI*, sea-saw nystagmus can arise due to (1) suprasellar masses, (2) Chiari malformations, (3) midbrain lesions involving the *interstitial nucleus of Cajal* (■ Figs. 2.15.1 and 2.15.3), (4) lesions involving the *medial and lateral vestibulospinal tracts*, and (5) the absence of the optic nerve decussation (*achiasma*).

2. *Periodic alternating nystagmus*: it is a rare disorder where the patient complains from the acquired periodic alternating nystagmus and often complains of increasing or decreasing oscillopsia for specific time intervals. On

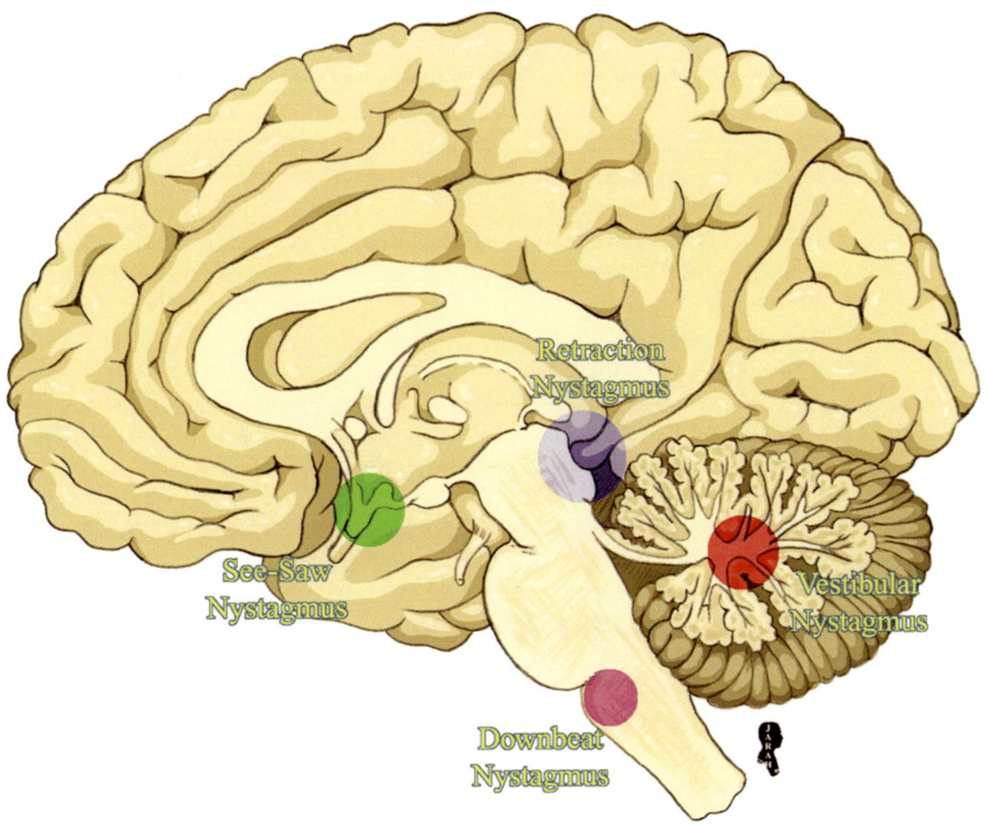

MRI, periodic alternating nystagmus can be caused by vestibular lesions, cerebellar degeneration, brain stem infarctions, and intoxications (e.g., *lithium*).

3. *Horizontal nystagmus*: it is an abnormal eye movement that is restricted to the horizontal axis. On *MRI*, horizontal nystagmus can be caused by vestibular neuritis, otoliths, and superior oblique myokymia. *Superior oblique myokymia* is a rare disorder characterized by recurrent attacks of oscillopsia and double vision with oblique images due to monocular oscillations due to trochlear nerve (CN4) disorder. On *MRI*, SOM is classically caused by vascular compression over CN4 or a lesion in the region CN4.

4. *Torsional nystagmus*: it is a rare condition characterized by torsional eye movement. On *MRI*, torsional nystagmus can be caused by a lesion involving the *riMLF* or the *interstitial nucleus of Cajal* (◻ Fig. 2.15.1).

5. *Downbeat nystagmus syndrome (DNS)*: it is a disease characterized by nystagmus with downward pupil displacement. It can be associated with oculomotor palsy, bilateral ptosis, and hypersomnolence. On *MRI*, there is a lesion involving the *cerebellum* (*involving the bilateral lesion of the flocculus or paraflocculus lobes*) and/or *midbrain* (e.g., *Arnold–Chiari malformation, Basilar invagination, hypomagnesemia, etc.*) (◻ Fig. 2.15.3).

6. *Upward gaze-evoked nystagmus (UGEN)*: it is an uncommon condition reported with organoarsenic compound poisoning characterized by nystagmus when the patient is asked to look upward due to gaze-holding failure, in association with cerebellar ataxia, involuntary movements (*tremors and myoclonus*), attention and memory deficits, and sleep disorders. On *MRI*, there is a lesion in the midbrain involving the *interstitial nucleus of Cajal* (◻ Fig. 2.15.1).

7. *Pendular nystagmus*: it is a rare disorder characterized by monocular or binocular sinusoidal oscillations with a predominant horizontal, vertical, or oblique trajectory. On *MRI*, pendular nystagmus can be caused by optic chiasma lesions, blindness (*<6 months of age*), oculopalatal tremor syndrome (myoclonus), and Pelizaeus–Merzbacher diseases.

8. *Gaze-evoked nystagmus*: it is a rhythmic oscillation of the eyes produced by the attempted maintenance of an extreme eye position probably due to a defective neural integrator. On *MRI*, cerebellar lesion is typically found.

9. *Opsoclonus and ocular flutter (dancing eye syndrome)*: opsoclonus is characterized by repetitive bursts of fast, high-frequency conjugate saccadic oscillations without intersaccadic intervals. The oscillations may have horizontal, vertical, and torsional components and are often triggered by saccades, pursuit, eye closure, and convergence. On *MRI*, dancing eye syndrome can be caused by (1) *cerebellitis (post-viral, e.g., coxsackie B37; post-vaccine)* and (2) *paraneoplastic cerebellar syndrome* (*infants, neuroblastoma; adults, carcinoma of the lung, breast, uterus, or ovary*).

10. *Caloric nystagmus*: it is a term used to describe physiologically induced nystagmus via tilting the head back and irrigating the ear with *warm* water (*causes nystagmus in the same direction of the ear irrigated*) or *cold* water (*causes nystagmus in the opposite direction of the ear irrigated*).

11. *Spasmus nutans*: it is an acquired form of nystagmus that typically presents between *6 and 12 months* of age. The classic triad of spasmus nutans includes (1) *head nodding*, (2) *torticollis*, and (3) *motor nystagmus*. Spasmus nutans typically disappears by age *4 years* and is associated with normal vision.

## References

Sami DA, et al. The achiasmia spectrum: congenitally reduced chiasmal decussation. Br J Ophthalmol. 2005;89:1311–7.

Swash M, et al. Periaqueductal dysfunction (the Sylvian aqueduct syndrome): a sign of hydrocephalus? J Neurol Neurosurg Psychiatry. 1974;37:21–6.

Thompson L, et al. The visually impaired child. Pediatr Clin North Am. 2003;50:225–39.

## 2.16 Erectile Dysfunction

*Erectile dysfunction* is defined as the inability to achieve or maintain an erection of sufficient rigidity to allow vaginal penetration. Impotence can be psychological or physical. Physical impotence can be arterial in origin (e.g., *atherosclerosis*) or venous in origin (e.g., *venous leak*).

## Neural Control Human Sexual Behavior

1. *Frontal lobe*: the frontal lobe sends tonic inhibitory signals to the *periaqueductal gray matter (PAG)*, which causes *social inhibition* of sexual activity.

2. *Temporal lobe*: the temporal lobe mediates *sexual drive/libido*.

3. *Higher centers*: other higher cortical functions that are involved in sexual behavior include the insula and somatosensory region.

4. *Hypothalamus*: it affects human sexual functions via the *medial preoptic area (MPO)* and the *paraventricular nucleus (PVN)*. The PVN contains large neurosecretory cells which secrete vasopressin and oxytocin. The hypothalamus mediates *sexual drive/libido* and *penile erection*.

5. *Amygdala*: it mediates *sexual drive/libido* (*in temporal lobes*).

6. *Midbrain*: it affects human sexual functions via the *periaqueductal gray matter (PAG)* and the *ventral*

*tegmental area (VTA)*. The VTA has an important role in *rewarding behavior*.

7. *Sympathetic nervous system* $(T_{10}–L_2)$: the hypogastric nerve, which arises from the hypogastric plexus at the aortic bifurcation at (L5–S1), supplies the corpora, bladder neck, and prostate. Stimulation of the parasympathetic sacral nerves causes detumescence.

8. *Parasympathetic nervous system* $(S_2–S_4)$: stimulation of the parasympathetic sacral nerves causes erection.

9. *Pudendal nerve*: it originates from the (S2–S4) sacral nerve roots (*Onuf's nucleus*), travels into the ischiorectal fossa (*Alcock's canal*), and transmits autonomic (30 %), sensory (50 %), and motor (20 %) impulses. The pudendal nerve gives sensory and motor fibers to the ischiocavernosus muscle, bulbospongiosus muscle, and penile and perianal skin. In females, it supplies the clitoris.

10. *Neuroendocrine hormones*: gonadal hormones affect the sexual behavior via modifying the cerebral control of lower reflexive mechanisms. The gonadal hormones affect sexual performance rather than sex drives. Multiple gonadal hormone receptors are found within the midbrain, hypothalamus, and amygdala.

## Pathophysiology

Penile erection depends on a complex interaction of *psychological, neural, vascular*, and *endocrine* factors. Erectile dysfunction can arise from abnormalities in one or more of the previous four components:

I. *Arterial erectile dysfunction*: it typically has a gradual onset and is most commonly the result of progressive systemic arteriosclerosis. Arterial erectile dysfunction can arise in patients with hypertension, hypercholesterolemia, and diabetes mellitus and who are smokers.

II. *Venous erectile dysfunction*: venous erectile dysfunction due to venous insufficiency in the presence of adequate arterial inflow is called *veno-occlusive dysfunction* or *venous leakage*. Venous leakage (◘ Fig. 2.16.1) can result from congenital excessively large venous channels through the corpora cavernosa, venous shunts between the cavernosa and the spongiosum, and inadequate compression of the subtunical and emissary veins and may occur with aging or Peyronie's disease.

III. *Neurologic erectile dysfunction*: neurological disease accounts for the second most common cause of erectile dysfunction in older men. It results from disorders of the parasympathetic sacral spinal cord or peripheral efferent autonomic fibers to the penis, which impairs penile smooth muscle relaxation and prevents the vasodilation needed for erection. Common neurological causes of erectile dysfunction in older men include autonomic dysfunction from diabetes mellitus, stroke, Parkinson's disease, cauda equina syndrome (◘ Fig. 2.16.2), and injury to autonomic nerves from radical prostatectomy or proctocolectomy.

IV. *Psychogenic erectile dysfunction*: a classic psychogenic cause in older men is the *Widower's syndrome*, where the older man involved in a new relationship feels guilt and develops erectile dysfunction as a defense against perceived unfaithfulness to his dead spouse.

## Erectile Dysfunction Differential Diagnoses

1. *Neurological causes*: spinal cord lesion (e.g., *cauda equina syndrome*), diabetic neuropathy, and multiple sclerosis

2. *Endocrinological causes*: diabetes mellitus, hypogonadism, and hyperprolactinemia

3. *Vascular causes*: peripheral vascular disease and veno-occlusive disease

4. *Drug-induced causes*: alcohol, cigarette smoking, marijuana, heroin, antidepressants, spironolactone, $H_2$ blockers, statins, amiodarone, opiates, β-blockers, and $Ca^{+2}$ blockers

5. *Local penile causes*: Peyronie's disease, priapism, and penile fracture

6. *Myofascial causes*: can arise due to trigger points affecting the *pyramidalis muscle*

**Fig. 2.16.1** T1W, postcontrast, fat-sat, reconstructed MR image of a 37-year-old male patient erectile dysfunction due to venous leakage investigated by MR cavernosography technique; the left mid- and deep periprostatic venous plexus shows venous leakage (*arrowheads*), 1 min after intracavernous gadolinium injection

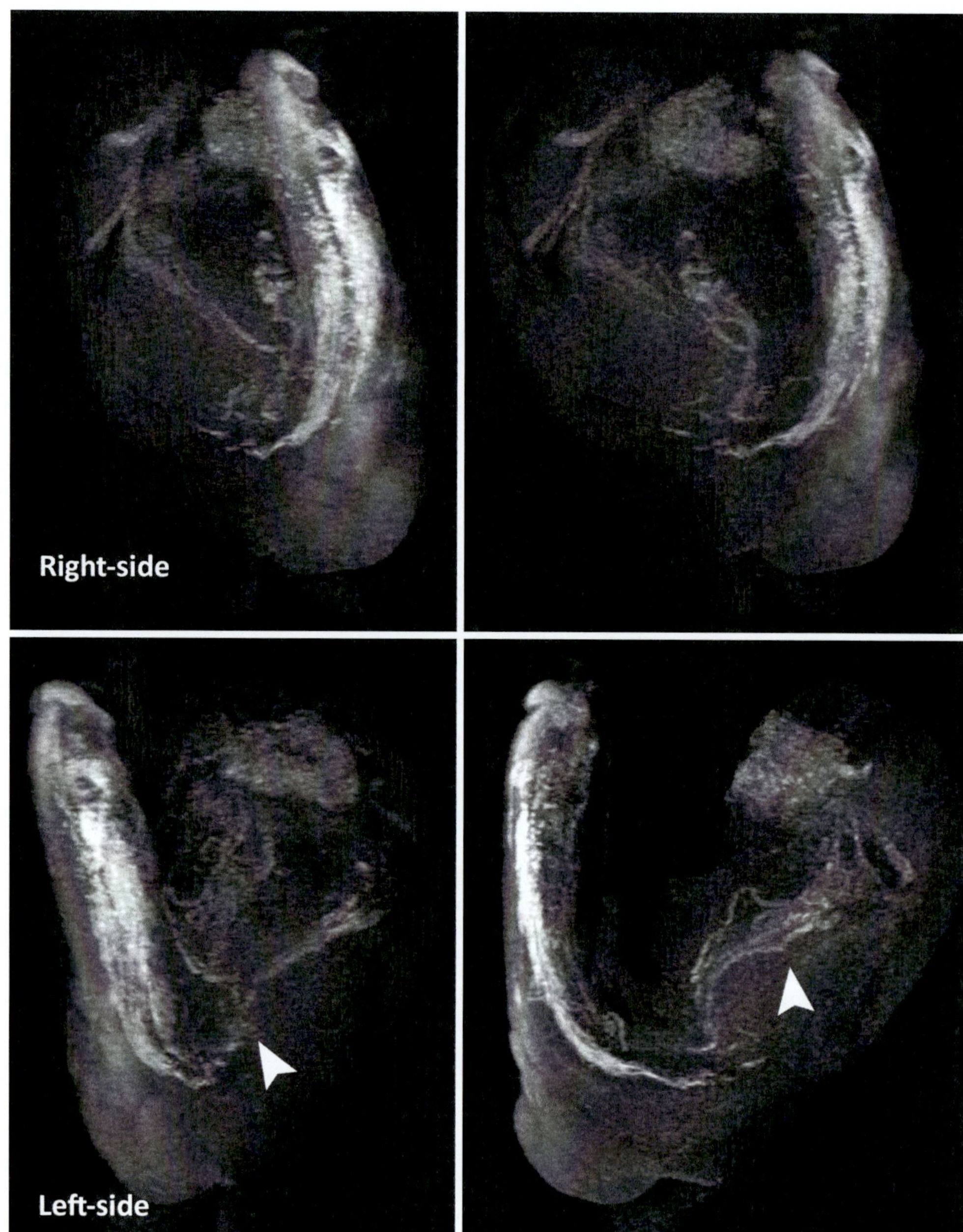

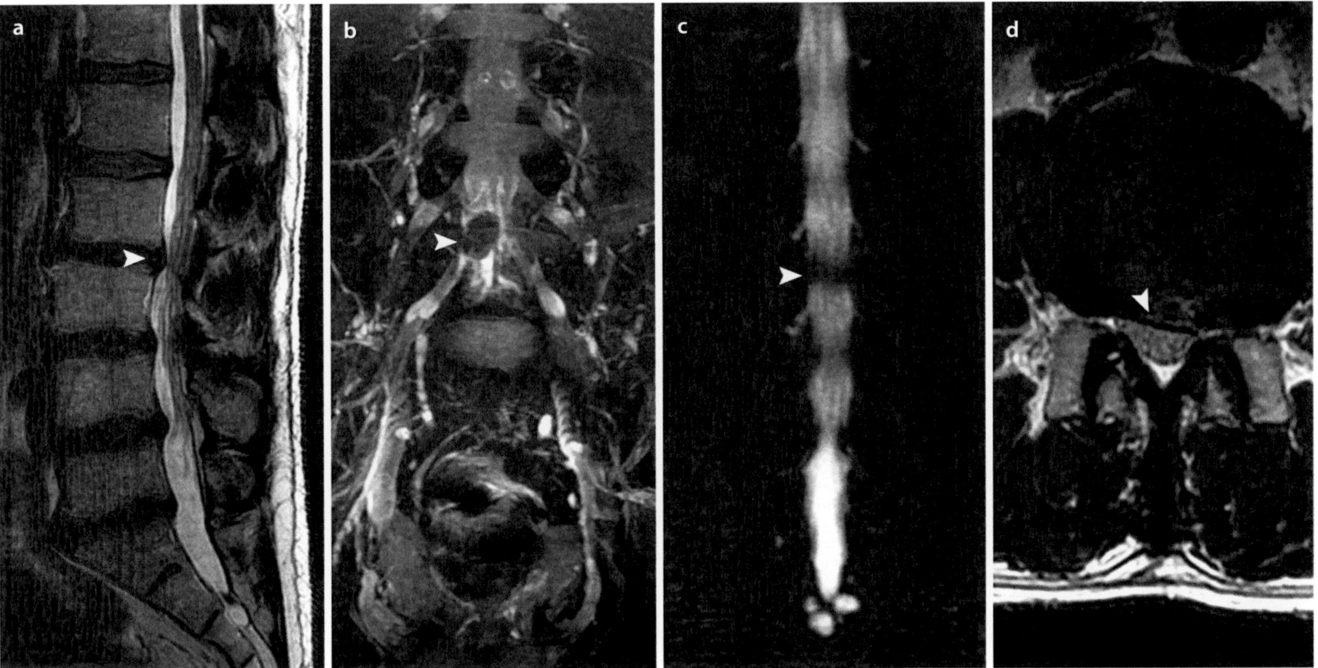

**◻ Fig. 2.16.2** Sagittal T2W (**a**), coronal T2W (**b**), MR myelographic (**c**), and axial T2W (**d**) images of a 53-year-old female patient with cauda equina syndrome seen as intervertebral disk protrusion that impinges over the thecal dural sac causing moderate spinal canal stenosis (*arrowheads*)


## References

Argiolas A. Male erectile dysfunction: chemical pharmacology of penile erection. Drug Discov Today Ther Strateg. 2005;1(2):31–6.

Basson R, et al. Sexual sequelae of general medical disorders. Lancet. 2007;369:409–24.

Bhasin S, et al. Sexual dysfunction in men and women with endocrine disorders. Lancet. 2007;369:597–611.

Carey JC. Pharmacological effects on sexual function. Obstet Gynecol Clin North Am. 2006;33:599–620.

De Silva P. Paraphilias. Psychiatry. 2004;2(1):33–6.

Giuliano F, et al. Neural control of erection. Physiol Behav. 2004;83(2):189–201.

Khan SA, et al. An unusual case of neurogenic sexual dysfunction due to lead exposure. Open Androl J. 2011;3:6–7.

Levin R, et al. The physiology of human sexual function. Psychiatry. 2007;6(3):90–4.

Ramage M. Female sexual dysfunction. Psychiatry. 2007;6(3):105–10.

Rao DS, et al. Vasculogenic arterial and venous surgery. Urol Clin North Am. 2001;28(2):309–19.

Riley A. The physiology of sexual function. Psychiatry. 2004;3(2):3–7.

Shamloul R, et al. Erectile dysfunction. Lancet. 2013;381: 153–65.

Steers WD. Neural pathways and central sites involved in penile erection: neuroanatomy and clinical implications. Neurosci Biobehav Rev. 2000;24:507–16.

Wylie KR. Male sexual dysfunction. Psychiatry. 2007;6(3): 99–104.

# Endocrinology and Metabolism




© Springer International Publishing Switzerland 2017
J.A. Al-Tubaikh, *Internal Medicine*, DOI 10.1007/978-3-319-39747-4_3

## 3.1   Graves' Disease (Hyperthyroidism)

Graves' disease (GD) is an autoimmune disorder characterized by hyperthyroidism, thyroid goiter, and ophthalmopathy. The disease arises due to the production of autoantibodies that auto-stimulates the thyrotropin receptors in the thyroid gland to secrete thyroid hormones.

GD clinical manifestations are mainly due to hyperthyroidism (thyrotoxicosis). Patients are commonly females between the third and fifth decades presenting with thyroid goiter. The thyroid is hypervascular, with venous humming that can be heard by stethoscope in some cases.

Systemic manifestations of hyperthyroidism include rapid weight loss (>10 % of body weight in less than 6 months), profuse sweating and heat intolerance, increased appetite (85 %), anorexia (15 %), increased bowel motion and diarrhea, oligomenorrhea in females, gynecomastia in males due to increased sex hormone-binding proteins, and proximal muscle weakness and muscle wasting due to increased basal metabolic rate. Skin manifestations include skin moisture due to sweating, vitiligo, and pretibial skin thickening due to mucin deposition in the dermis (myxoedema).

Graves' ophthalmopathy is the most characteristic sign of this disease. GD is the most common cause of exophthalmos (abnormal prominent eye) and proptosis (protrusion) of globe in adults. It occurs in 35 % of cases. The proptosis can precede the actual thyroid abnormalities or occur after the disease has been brought under control. Proptoses are commonly bilateral and symmetrical; unilateral proptosis is uncommon.

Proptosis in GD can be explained by:

- Infiltration and deposition of mucopolysaccharidosis (hyaluronic acid) into orbital muscles. The muscles' bellies are characteristically increased in size, while their tendons are spared (fusiform enlargement). The inferior rectus and the medial rectus muscles are the most commonly involved. The lateral rectus is the last muscle to be involved. Hypertrophy of the lateral rectus only can be seen in orbital pseudotumor, and hypertrophy of the superior rectus only can be seen in orbital lymphoma.
- Increased volume of the retrobulbar fat which will push the globe anteriorly.

Clinical signs of Graves' ophthalmopathy include widened palpebral fissure (*Dalrymple's sign*), staring expression with infrequent blinking (*Stellwag's sign*), lid lag on downward gaze (*von Graefe's sign*), and poor convergence (*Möbius's sign*). Up to 5 % of patients with Graves' ophthalmopathy develop optic neuropathy due to compression of the nerve in its canal because of backward herniation of the retro-orbital fat through the optic canal or from hypertrophied ocular muscle belly at the orbital apex.

### Signs on US and Doppler Sonography

- The gland is diffusely hypoechoic and enlarged in size.
- On color Doppler scan, the gland shows bilateral diffuse increase duplex signal due to hypervascularity. This sign is characteristic for GD and is called "thyroid inferno" sign (◘ Fig. 3.1.1).

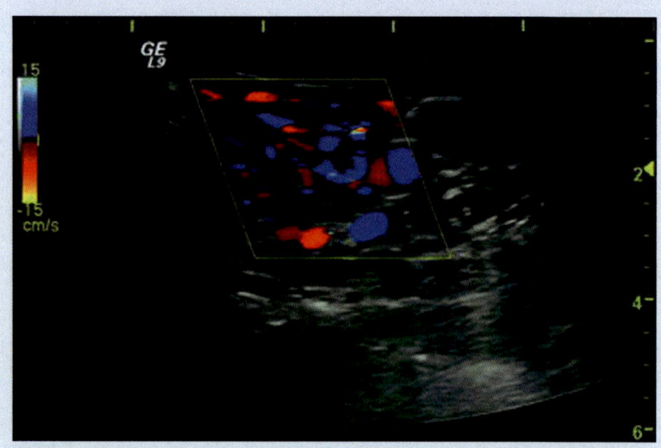

**◘ Fig. 3.1.1**   Color Doppler (Duplex) scan of the thyroid in a patient with Graves' disease shows marked vascular signal due to bruit (thyroid inferno sign)

### Signs of Graves' Ophthalmopathy on CT and MRI

- Bilateral, symmetrical increase in orbital muscles bellies width with spares tendons causing the orbital muscles to have fusiform appearance. The inferior rectus and the medial rectus muscles are characteristically affected (◘ Figs. 3.1.2 and 3.1.3).

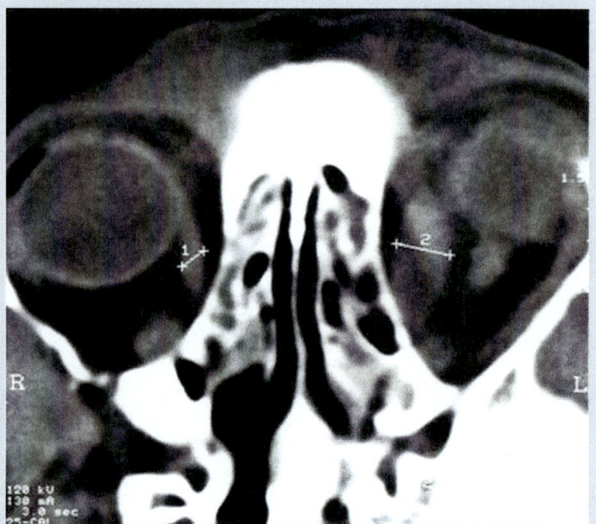

**◘ Fig. 3.1.2**   Axial ophthalmic CT image of a patient with Graves' ophthalmopathy shows marked thickening of the medial rectus muscle of the left eye. Notice the difference in the medial rectus belly thickness (*2*) in comparison with the right eye (*1*)

- Increases in the retrobulbar fat size.
- CT evidence of proptosis is defined as globe protrusion exceeding the interzygomatic line by 21 mm or more on axial images at the level of the lens ( Fig. 3.1.4).
- GD optic neuropathy can be detected if retro-orbital fat is seen extending 4 mm beyond the boundary of the superior orbital fissure or if the optic nerve is seen compressed by a hypertrophied ocular muscle belly at the orbital apex.
- Uncommonly, isolated dilatation of the superior ophthalmic vein may occur in patients with GD, and it can be easily mistaken for carotid–cavernous fistula. CT angiography can confirm the absence of carotid–cavernous fistula.

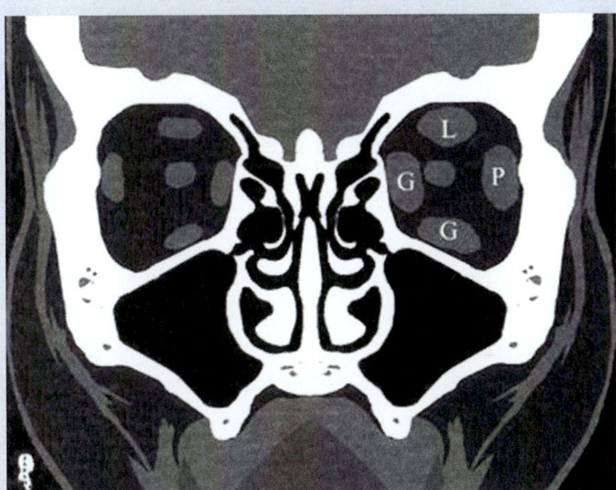


 **Fig. 3.1.3** Coronal sinus and orbital CT illustration shows a differential diagnosis of recti muscles enlargement; the letter *G* stands for Grave's disease, *L* for lymphoma, and *P* for orbital pseudotumor

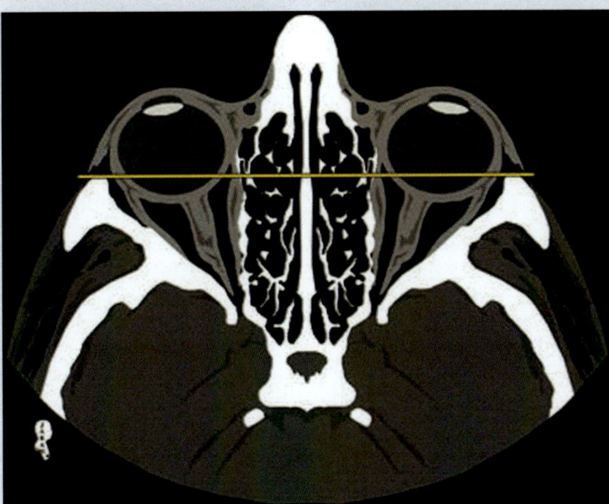

 **Fig. 3.1.4** Axial ophthalmic CT illustration demonstrates the interzygomatic line. A globe that protrudes >21 mm or more across this line is considered proptosis

## Further Reading

Arslan H et al. Power Doppler sonography in the diagnosis of Graves' disease. Eur J Ultrasound. 2000;11:117–22.

Babcock DS. Thyroid disease in pediatric patient: emphasizing imaging with sonography. Pediatr Radiol. 2006;36: 299–308.

Birchall D et al. Graves ophthalmopathy: intracranial fat prolapse on CT images as an indicator of optic nerve compression. Radiology. 1996;200:123–7.

Charkes ND et al. MR imaging in thyroid disorders: correlation of signal intensity with Graves disease activity. Radiology. 1987;164:491–4.

Greer MA et al. Hyperthyroidism. Dis Mon. 1967;13:1–45.

Nugent RA et al. Graves orbitopathy: correlation of CT and clinical findings. Radiology. 1990;177:657–82.

Ralls PW et al. Color-flow Doppler sonography in Graves disease: "thyroid inferno". AJR Am J Roentgenol. 1988;150:781–4.

Rawson RW. Hyperthyroidism. Dis Mon. 1955;1:3–43.

Reed Larsen P. Hyperthyroidism. Dis Mon. 1976;22:1–30.

## 3.2　Hyperparathyroidism

Hyperparathyroidism is a metabolic disease characterized by the metabolic triad of high serum calcium level (hypercalcemia), low serum phosphorus level (hypophosphatemia), and increased calcium and phosphorus renal excretion (hypercalciuria).

Hyperparathyroidism can be caused by increased parathyroid hormone (PTH) release due to parathyroid adenoma or hyperplasia (primary type), chronic renal failure or parathyroid glands insensitivity to elevated serum calcium level (secondary type), or chronic renal failure with autonomous PTH release even after correction of the renal failure (tertiary type). Chronic renal failure causes reduction in serum calcium level, which induces hypersecretion of PTH to elevate serum calcium level. PTH increases serum calcium by increasing osteoclastic activity, promoting vitamin D renal hydroxylation, and promoting tubular renal absorption of calcium.

Hyperparathyroidism generally arises in those endocrine phases of life when endocrine glands are most active or rapidly changing like puberty, during the active phase of sexual life, or after menopause. Thus, hyperparathyroidism is rare before puberty and less commonly starts in later decades.

Symptoms and clinical presentation of hyperparathyroidism are related to its complications. Renal stone formation is one of the most common presentations of hyperparathyroidism. Increased renal excretion and serum calcium level promotes renal calculi formation. Peptic ulcers may occur in association with hyperparathyroidism for unknown reasons. It is speculated that changes in the calcium ion concentration may play a role in parasympathetic nervous system tone, which predisposes to increased secretions of gastric acids by increased vagal activity.

Episodes of acute pancreatitis are commonly associated with hyperparathyroidism for unknown reasons. Thirst and urinary frequency are common symptoms. Muscle fatigue and low back pain are also common complaints, and they are independent of bone changes.

The most common metabolic changes in hyperparathyroidism are observed in the skeletal system. Diffuse osteoporosis and bone resorption are commonly seen in primary hyperparathyroidism. In contrast, diffuse or focal osteosclerosis is observed in secondary hyperparathyroidism. Subperiosteal, subchondral, and subligamentous bone resorptions are the most common findings radiologically.

*Brown tumor* is an eccentrically located, expansile bony lesion uncommonly seen in secondary hyperparathyroidism. In severe hyperparathyroidism, large areas of bone marrow cavity are lost due to bone resorption. This bony resorption leads to microfractures and bleeding in the resorbed areas, which will create a mass-like effect within the trabecular bone. This mass-like structure has a brown pigment in gross section due to hemosiderin content. Gradually, this mass undergoes cystic changes. As the severity of the disease increases, these changes can progress to severe and diffuse type of bone expansion, cystic changes, and bone marrow fibrosis, a condition which is known as *osteitis fibrosa cystica*. Brown tumor mimics giant cell tumor (*osteoclastoma*) radiologically and histologically. Differentiation between the two clinical conditions depends on the presence or absence of hyperparathyroidism manifestations. Osteitis fibrosa cystica is a rare complication of hyperparathyroidism that is seen in advanced stage disease. It is usually seen in young patients <20 years.

*Nephrocalcinosis* is a condition characterized by calcification and calcium deposition within the renal parenchyma, either in the cortex or in the medulla. *Cortical nephrocalcinosis* occurs due to prior insult to the renal cortex like in tuberculosis, ischemia, and glomerulonephritis. Usually it affects one kidney, and the affected kidney is small with global atrophy. *Medullary nephrocalcinosis*, on the other hand, arises due to calcification of the medullary pyramids due to deposition of calcium within the renal tubules. Medullary nephrocalcinosis is the most common type of nephrocalcinosis (95 %) and is caused by systemic hypercalcemic states like in hyperparathyroidism, distal renal tubular acidosis, malignancy, and acute sarcoidosis. Typically, it affects both kidneys in a bilateral and symmetrical fashion, because the cause usually is a systemic disease.

Primary hyperparathyroidism can be a part of *multiple endocrine neoplasia (MEN) syndrome*. MEN syndrome is characterized by the occurrence of tumors involving two or more endocrine glands within a single patient. There are two major types of MEN: MEN type 1 (MEN1, Wermer's syndrome) and MEN type 2 (MEN2, Sipple's syndrome). Both syndromes are inherited as autosomal dominant. MEN1 is characterized by the combined occurrence of parathyroid tumors, pancreatic islet cell tumors (e.g., gastrinoma), and anterior pituitary tumors (e.g., prolactinoma). Associated tumors include adrenal tumors, carcinoid tumors, and lipoma. Although not part of the original description,

meningioma has been reported to occur in patients with hyperparathyroidism due to MEN type 1. MEN type 2, on the other hand, is divided into three subtypes: MEN2a, MEN2b, and MTC only. MEN2a describes the association of medullary thyroid carcinoma (MTC), pheochromocytoma, and parathyroid tumors. MEN2b describes the association of MTC, pheochromocytoma, marfanoid body habitus, mucosal neuromas, and megacolon. Lastly, MTC only is a variant in which MTC is the sole manifestation of this syndrome.

In up to 2 % of normal people, an ectopic parathyroid tissue may be found within the mediastinum. The ectopic parathyroid tissue is commonly located within the anterior mediastinum. An ectopic parathyroid adenoma is rare and should be suspected in a patient with hyperparathyroidism who was operated and the signs and symptoms of hyperparathyroidism persisted (5–10 % of cases). Other areas where ectopic parathyroid tissue may be found include the neck (45 %), upper cervical area (8 %), or along the aortic arch (5 %).

## Differential Diagnoses and Related Diseases

— *Hyperparathyroidism–jaw tumor syndrome* is a rare, autosomal recessive disease characterized by hyperparathyroidism (90 %), ossifying fibroma of the maxilla and/or mandible (30 %), renal cysts and/or tumors (10 %), and uterine tumors. Ossifying fibroma is a benign lesion that arises from cells in the periodontal ligament and is mainly restricted to the tooth-bearing areas of the jaw. The lesion is visualized as a well-demarcated bony lesion composed of fibrocellular tissue and mineralized material. The tumor is typically painless and located at the posterior region of the mandible. Patients are often >35 years old. However, a juvenile form (<20 years) may be seen.

— *Hungry bone syndrome* (HBS) is a rare complication of parathyroidectomy manifested by severe, prolonged, sometimes life-threatening hypocalcemia. The hypercalcemia in hyperparathyroidism is mainly due to increased bone turnover with predominant osteoclastic bone resorption and increased renal tubular absorption of calcium. After parathyroidectomy, the PTH stimulus over the osteoclasts is suddenly removed, stopping the osteoclastic activity, but the osteoblastic activity continues at its high rate, resulting in marked increase in bone uptake of calcium to facilitate bone remodeling. The excessive osteoblastic bony remodeling causes severe hypocalcemia. HBS is seen in 12 % of parathyroidectomy cases, and it is suspected in patients who had parathyroidectomy and presented with persistent hypocalcemia and hypophosphatemia. Predisposing factors for HBS include parathyroid adenoma >5 cm in diameter, high preoperative PTH, calcium, and alkaline phosphatase levels, advanced age, and osteitis fibrosa cystica.

### Signs on Plain Radiographs

- On chest radiograph, tracheal shift due to enlarged parathyroid adenoma may be the first sign detected in an asymptomatic patient.
- On abdominal radiographs, urinary tract calcium calculi are seen as radio-opaque lesions in the renal area or the urethral course.
- Cortical nephrocalcinosis is often detected as a unilateral renal "eggshell calcification," while medullary nephrocalcinosis is detected as multiple, punctuated calcification seen within the kidney shadows in a bilateral symmetrical fashion (◘ Fig. 3.2.1).

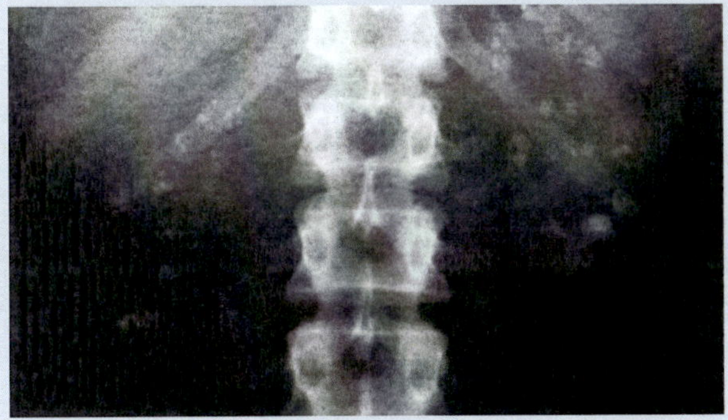

◘ **Fig. 3.2.1**  A plain radiograph of the kidneys in a patient with medullary nephrocalcinosis shows bilateral, almost symmetrical, punctuated calcification within the renal shadow

### Signs on Skeletal Radiographs

- Diffuse osteoporosis and lytic bony lesions are commonly found in primary hyperparathyroidism.
- Widening of sacroiliac joints due to subchondral bone resorption can be seen.
- *Salt and pepper skull appearance*: this occurs due to resorption of the trabecular bone in the skull and replacement of the resorbed bone by a newly formed connective tissue causing loss of integrity in the shape of the skull bones (◘ Fig. 3.2.2).
- The vertebral bodies in secondary hyperparathyroidism show sclerosis of the end plates (Rugger–Jersey spines) (◘ Fig. 3.2.3).
- *Subperiosteal cortical resorption* typically occurs in the hand, especially at the radial aspect of the middle phalanx, which is a specific sign seen in both primary and secondary hyperparathyroidism (◘ Fig. 3.2.4).
- *Brown tumor* is seen as a well-circumscribed cystic bony lesion which can cause bone expansion.

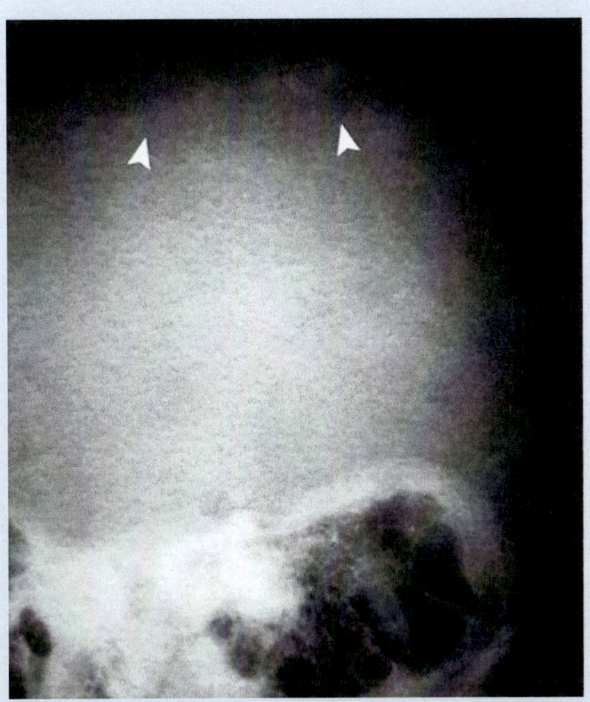

◘ **Fig. 3.2.2**  A lateral plain radiograph of the skull shows mild salt and pepper skull lesions in a patient with primary hyperparathyroidism

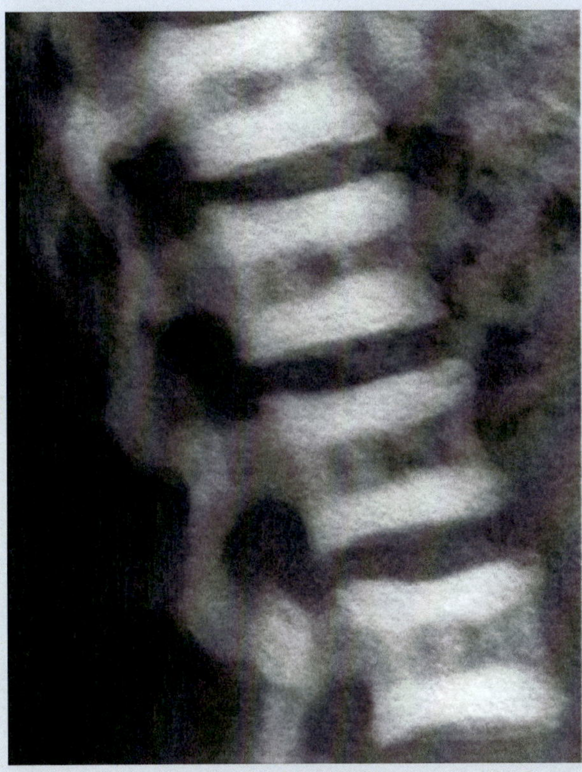

◘ **Fig. 3.2.3**  A lateral spine radiograph of a patient with secondary hyperparathyroidism shows diffuse vertebral end plate sclerosis (Rugger–Jersey spines)

There are often multiple lytic lesions found together. When the hyperparathyroidism is treated, the brown tumor undertows ossification and will transform into a bone island (sclerotic lesion). The most common areas for brown tumors are the pelvis, rib, long bone diaphysis, clavicle, and mandible (◘ Fig. 3.2.5).

— *Subligamentous bone resorption* at the sites of ligament insertion into bone can be seen. It is commonly observed at the elbows over the olecranon, plantar aspect of the calcaneus, and the superior pole of the dorsal aspect of the patella.

— *Chondrocalcinosis* occurs due to deposition of calcium pyrophosphate dehydrate into the cartilage of the joints (metastatic calcification). It is found in up to 40 % of hyperparathyroidism cases.

— *Osteitis fibrosa cystica* presents as a lytic expansile bony lesion that mimics metastatic bone disease (◘ Fig. 3.2.6).

— Diffuse osteosclerosis is commonly seen in patients with secondary hyperparathyroidism (◘ Fig. 3.2.7).

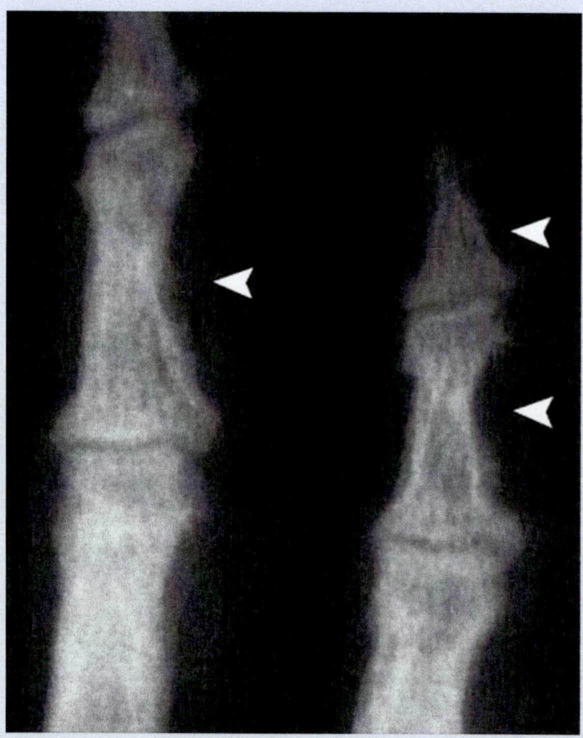

◘ **Fig. 3.2.4**    A plain radiograph of the fingers shows radial side subperiosteal resorption of the middle and distal phalanges (*arrowheads*), a specific sign of prolonged hyperparathyroidism

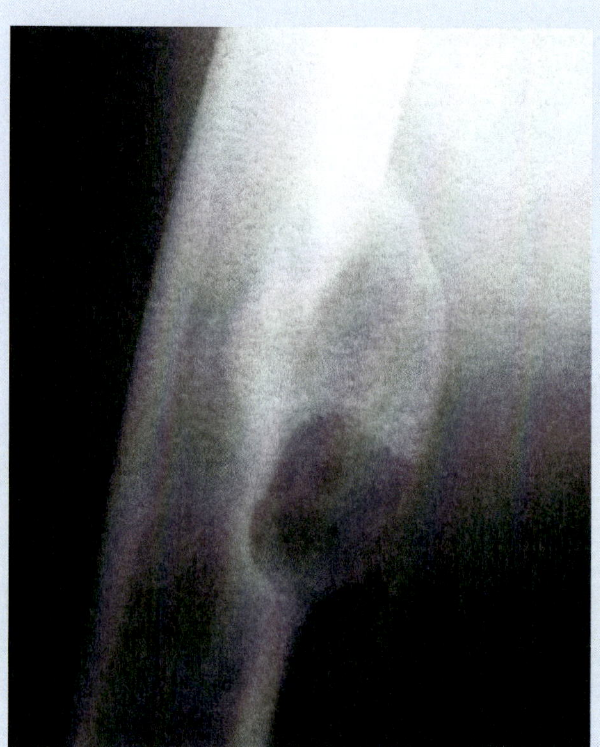

◘ **Fig. 3.2.5**    A femoral diaphyseal lytic, expansile bony lesion in a patient with prolonged hyperparathyroidism. Pathological biopsy proved to be brown tumor

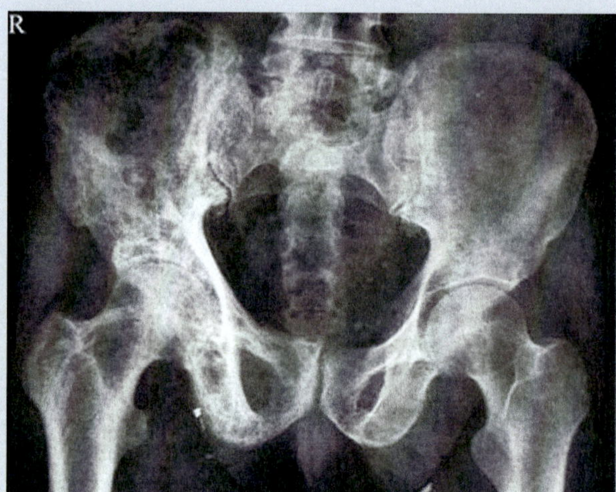

◘ **Fig. 3.2.6**    A plain hip radiograph of a patient with prolonged undiagnosed hyperparathyroidism. The right side of the hip shows numerous bony lytic and sclerotic lesions with a semi-moth-eating appearance that was initially thought to be Paget's disease. Bone biopsy proved to be osteitis fibrosa cystica

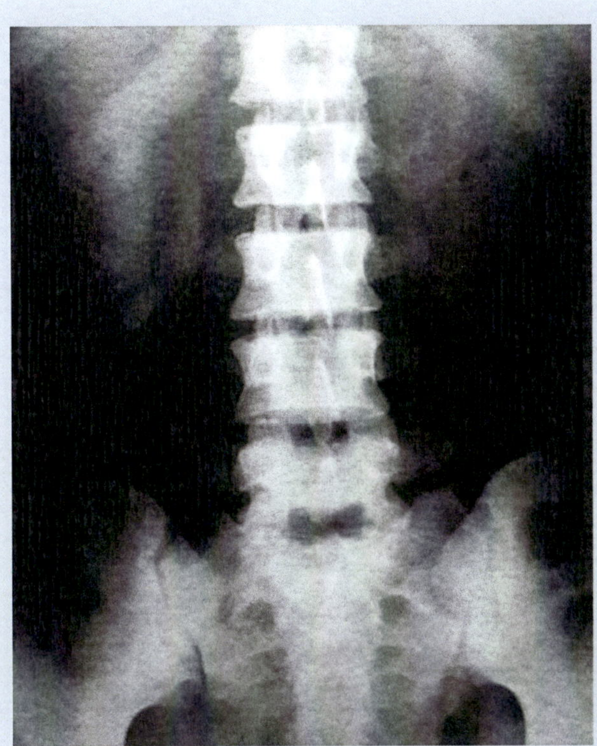



■ **Fig. 3.2.7** A plain abdominal radiograph of a patient with secondary hyperparathyroidism shows diffuse osteosclerosis

### Signs on US
- Thyroid ultrasound often shows oval or round hypoechoic mass in the posterior inferior poles of the thyroid (usually <3 cm in diameter) representing parathyroid adenomas. The mass has a well-defined echogenic line separating the adenoma from the thyroid gland representing the capsule. The mass shows internal cystic changes, mixed echogenicity, or calcification as the size exceeds 3 cm in diameter.
- Renal calculi are seen as hyperechoic lesions with posterior shadowing.
- Medullary nephrocalcinosis is detected as hyperechogenic renal pyramids.

### Signs on Doppler Sonography and PD
The parathyroid adenoma typically shows high blood flow signal and perfusion, especially at the peripheral portion of the adenoma.

### Signs on CT and MRI
- On CT, parathyroid adenoma is detected as a well-defined mass located in the posterior/inferior pole of the thyroid with intense enhancement after contrast administration. On MRI, the mass shows intermediate T1 and high T2 signal intensities with intense enhancement after contrast injection.
- Ectopic parathyroid adenoma is identified as an anterior mediastinal mass with high contrast enhancement (similar to the usual parathyroid adenomas). The ectopic parathyroid mediastinal adenoma is classically <2 cm in diameter.
- Brown tumors have characteristically low T2 signal intensity due to hemosiderin content. It shows early intense enhancement after contrast injection due to marked vascularity. Fluid–fluid levels may be observed within the tumors in some cases due to intramural bleeding.
- *Ossifying fibroma* is seen on CT as a well-demarcated lytic lesion with mixed mineralized material (up to 50 % are purely lytic lesions). The lytic lesion typically is expansile and may mimic fibrous dysplasia with its ground-glass appearance if the matrix is extensively calcified (■ Fig. 3.2.8). On MRI, ossifying fibroma typically shows low to intermediate signal intensity on both T1W and T2W images with homogeneous contrast enhancement after contrast injection.
- The salt and pepper skull appearance seen in plain radiograph can be seen on MRI as bone resorption (■ Fig. 3.2.9).

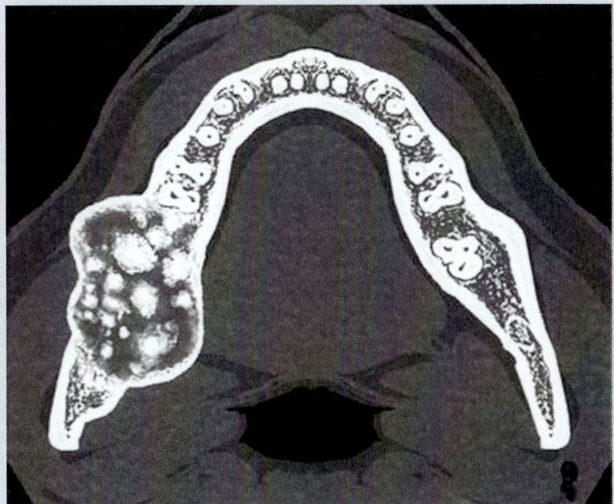

■ **Fig. 3.2.8** A CBCT dental illustration shows ossifying fibroma as lytic expansile bony lesion with mixed calcified matrix

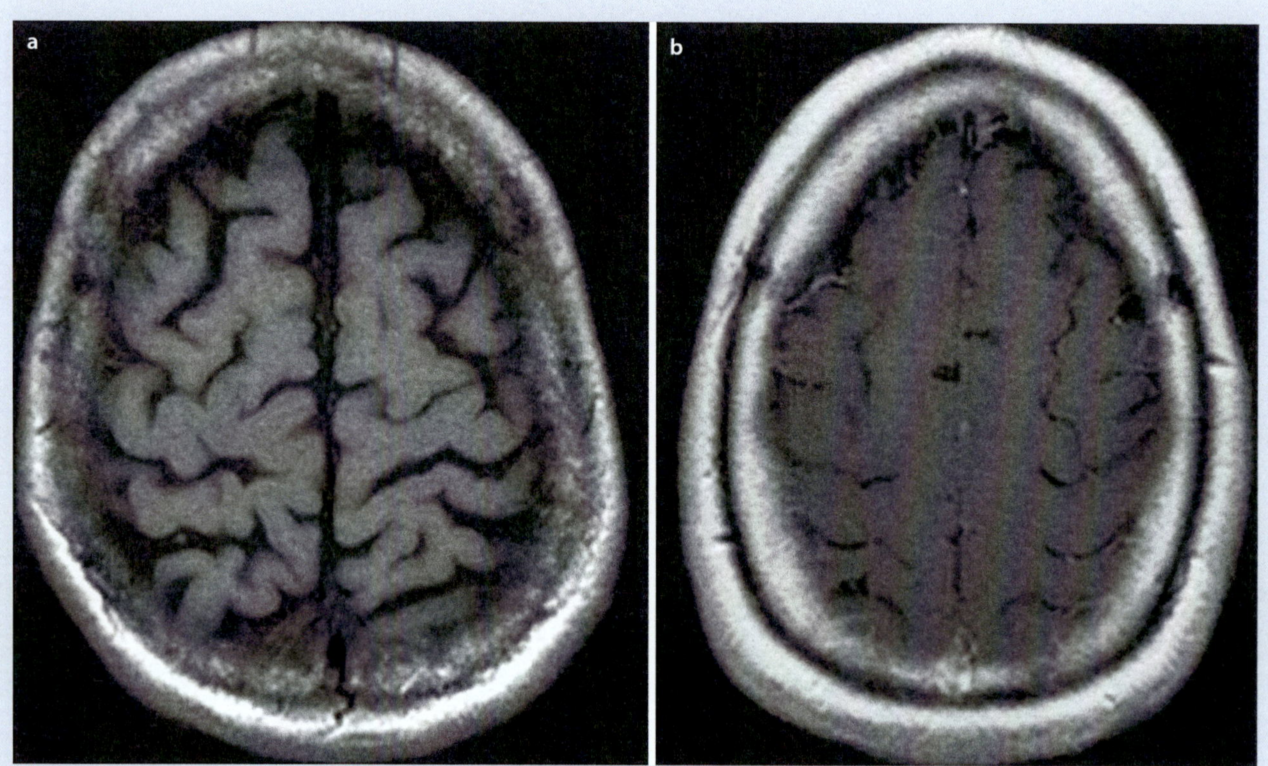

**Fig. 3.2.9** Two different patients with T1W image MRI of the brain. In image (**a**), there is marked bone resorption of the inner surface of the skull in a patient with prolonged primary hyperparathyroidism (salt and pepper skull appearance). Compare the skull bones with the normal skull in image (**b**)

## Further Reading


Ahuja AT et al. Imaging of primary hyperparathyroidism – what beginners should know. Clin Radiol. 2004;59: 967–76.

Bertolini F et al. Multiple ossifying fibromas of the jaw: a case report. J Oral Maxillofac Surg. 2002;60:225–9.

Eggert P et al. Nephrocalcinosis in three siblings with idiopathic hypercalciuria. Pediatr Nephrol. 1998;12:144–6.

Falchetti A et al. Multiple endocrine neoplasia type I variants and phenotypes: more than nosological issue. J Clin Endocrinol Metab. 2009;94:1518–20.

Ghanaat F et al. Hungry bone syndrome: a case report and review of the literature. Nutr Res. 2004;24:633–8.

Hsieh M-C et al. Pathologic fracture of the distal femur in osteitis fibrosa cystica simulating metastatic disease. Arch Orthop Trauma Surg. 2004;124:489–501.

Kabala JE. Computed tomography and magnetic resonance imaging in diseases of the thyroid and the parathyroid. Eur J Radiol. 2008;66:480–92.

Krudy AG et al. The detection of mediastinal parathyroid glands by computed tomography, selective arteriography, and venous sampling. Radiology. 1981;140:739–44.

McDonald DK et al. Primary hyperparathyroidism due to parathyroid adenoma. Radiographics. 2005;25:829–34.

Reuter K et al. Unsuspected medullary nephrocalcinosis from furosemide administration: sonographic evaluation. J Clin Ultrasound. 1985;13:357–9.

Rypins EL. Osteitis fibrosa cystica at unusual age. J Bone Joint Surg Am. 1933;15:509–12.

Schmidt BP et al. Hyperparathyroidism-jaw tumor syndrome: a case report. J Oral Maxillofac Surg. 2009;67: 423–7.

Smith D et al. Hungry bones without hypocalcemia following parathyroidectomy. J Bone Miner Metab. 2005;23:514–5.

Takeshita T et al. Brown tumor with fluid-fluid levels in a patient with primary hyperparathyroidism: radiological findings. Radiat Med. 2006;24:631–4.

Wang Q et al. Power Doppler imaging findings in multilocular giant parathyroid adenoma which caused hypercalcaemic crisis. J Laryngol Otol. 1998;112:769–99.


## 3.3    Growth Hormone Diseases

The human growth hormone (GH) is a polypeptide consisting of 188 amino acids and having a molecular weight of 21,500. GH from other species shares partial sequences of amino acids in common with human GH (e.g., bovine GH).

These partial sequences consist of active cores, which are pharmacologically active. Thus, it may be not necessary to synthesize the entire bovine GH molecule to yield an actively working substance in humans.

GH disorders result from either excess or reduction of its secretion within the body. The normal GH is secreted in two cyclic rhythms: one in the morning and the other in the evening.

## Growth Hormone Insufficiency (Hypopituitarism)

GH insufficiency (hypopituitarism) can be idiopathic (primary) or due to pituitary gland tumor (secondary). Idiopathic GH insufficiency children exhibit growth retardation, delayed puberty, and hypothyroidism without elevated thyroid-stimulating hormone (TSH) level. Growth retardation is assumed if the child falls more than three standard deviations below the mean for his/her age and also if the child's growth rate is <50 % of the anticipated growth rate over a period of 1 year.

*Pituitary stalk interruption syndrome (PSIS)* is a form of GH insufficiency due to abnormal pituitary stalk. Children with PSIS have pronounced GH insufficiency, with or without other anterior pituitary hormonal deficiencies.

**Signs on Skeletal Radiographs**
- Plain skeletal radiographs can be used to accurately assess bone age according to the bone maturation. Each bone in the body starts to ossify at a certain age. By imaging certain bones within the body, assessing their ossification maturation, and comparing it to a standard reference of bone maturation of the patient's current age, the radiologist can easily assess the patient bone maturation rate. This method is a valuable tool that can detect GH abnormalities in a relatively short time with much accuracy.
- Both hands and elbows are often X-rayed, and the shapes of all epiphyses of the radius, ulna, carpals, metacarpals, and all the phalanges are assessed in comparison with a standard reference. Delayed bone maturation can be seen in GH insufficiency and hypothyroidism.
- The normal appearance of primary ossification centers of the wrist: capitate (2–3 months), hamate (3 months), triquetral (2–3 years), lunate (3 years), trapezium (3–4 years), trapezoid (4 years), scaphoid (4–5 years), pisiform (8–9 years), ulnar epiphysis (6–7 years), and radial epiphysis (1 year).

- The normal appearance of primary ossification centers of the elbow (CRITOE): capitulum (6 months), radial head (5 years), internal (ulnar) epicondyle (6–7 years), trochlea (9 years), olecranon (9–10 years), and external (radial) epicondyle (10–11 years).
- By applying the previous primary ossification centers age to a skeletal radiograph of a child, radiologists can estimate roughly the age of that child. However, precise age estimation should be assessed using a standard reference (■ Fig. 3.3.1).

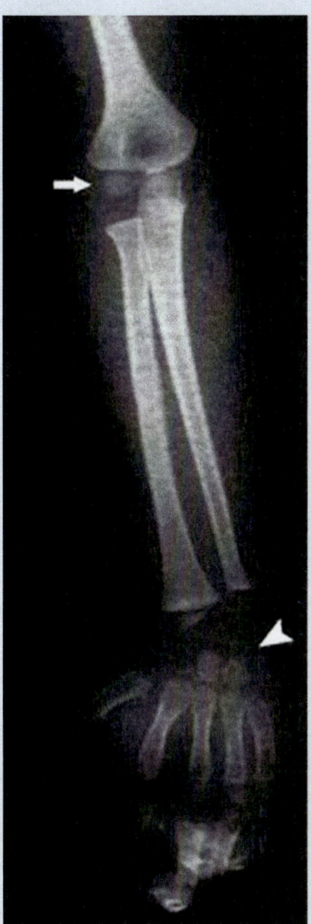

■ **Fig. 3.3.1** A plain radiograph of the hand, wrist, and forearm in a 4-year-old boy with growth retardation shows skeletal maturation retardation. Although the child's age is 4 years, only the capitate and hamate bones are ossified (*arrowhead*), which commonly start ossification at 2–3 months. At 4 years of age, we expect the scaphoid, lunate, and trapezium to be seen too. Moreover, the elbow shows only the ossification center of the capitulum (*arrow*), which starts to ossify at 6 months of age. It seems as if the patient's age has been stunted at 6–12 months old

### Signs on MRI

The pituitary on MRI in patients with GH insufficiency shows absence or marked thinning of the pituitary stalk, reduced size of the anterior pituitary, lack of the normal posterior pituitary high signal, and presence of a high signal nodule in the region of the infundibular recess of the third ventricle representing ectopic posterior pituitary (◘ Fig. 3.3.2).

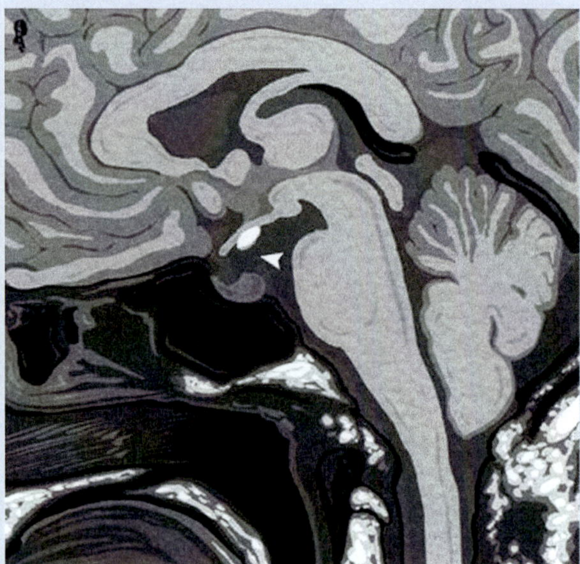

◘ **Fig. 3.3.2**    Sagittal T1W sella MR illustration demonstrates interruption of the pituitary stalk with ectopic high T2 signal intensity characteristic of ectopic neurohypophysis and pituitary stalk interruption syndrome (PSIS) (*arrowhead*)

## Acromegaly and Gigantism

Excess GH pituitary release or GH abuse in body builders results in two disorders named acromegaly and gigantism. The term acromegaly was used for the first time by "Pierre Marie" in France in 1886 describing patients with characteristic hands and feet (acro) hypertrophy (megaly). Acromegaly literally means hypertrophy of the extremities. The disease has been described in historical writings, especially in people whose body development is considerably greater than normal and who are looked upon as giants. It is even described in the Jewish Talmud by the Biblical name *sarua* that refers to abnormal growth of a single limb, which rendered a priest unfit to serve in the temple.

Acromegaly is an adult disease characterized by increased production of the GH resulting in characteristic body changes. When the excess GH release starts in adolescence with open epiphyses, the condition is called "gigantism." The common etiology in both cases is a pituitary adenoma that

increases GH production. GH causes retention of nitrogen with an overall anabolic effect. It also increases the transport of amino acids in the tissues and their release into proteins and mobilizes lipids from adipose tissue increasing their oxidation as a source of energy, thus sparing muscle glycogen. Due to previous GH effects, an athlete who abuses GH may realize an improvement in performance and strength with the use of GH supplements. Amino acid supplements of arginine, ornithine, and lysine, in combination or alone, can stimulate the production of endogenous GH. GH release can be also stimulated by some medications like L-dopa, clonidine, and propranolol. Athletes with GH abuse may develop acromegaly or acromegalic-like state with complications similar to acromegaly.

Patients with acromegaly are characterized by overgrowth of the terminal parts of the skeleton (e.g., hands) and the soft-tissue parts of the viscera. The earliest complaints include headache, visual defects in 30 % of patients (bitemporal), fatigability, asthenia, and sweating. Later, the size of the head, hands, and feet starts to grow progressively.

Patients with acromegaly develop characteristic appearance. The facial features become coarse and thickened, with enlargement of the nose. Protrusion of the mandible (prognathism), tongue enlargement, widening of the teeth, vertebral kyphosis, skin thickening, and protrusion of the supraorbital ridges are also characteristic features. The heart, spleen, liver, and kidneys may be enlarged. Patients with acromegaly show higher tendency toward gastrointestinal cancers (e.g., colon cancer).

Women with acromegaly show high incidence of intrauterine bleeding or amenorrhea. In both males and females, there is gradual loss of libido, and testicular or ovarian atrophy may develop later in life.

Other hormonal abnormalities may be found in patients with acromegaly. Thyroid enlargement usually occurs due to hypertrophy with increased thyroid function rate. Inappropriate lactation due to hyperprolactinemia may be found in some patients. Increased serum phosphorus level is a characteristic feature of acromegaly due to increased tubular reabsorption. Adrenal gland hypertrophy without signs of cortical hyperfunction may occur. Lastly, large patients with acromegaly develop diabetes mellitus due to the diabetogenic effect of GH which increases the serum blood glucose level. Most of the hormones in the body increase the serum glucose blood level like glucagons, cortisol, and GH. Only insulin is capable of reducing the serum glucose blood level.

Patients with gigantism exhibit the same clinical and radiological features as acromegaly. The characteristic feature in gigantism is the tall height of the patients. Increased GH production delays the closure of the epiphyses, so patients will start to grow in height beyond the normal age of epiphyseal closure. This may result in patients reaching a height of up to 2.4 m according to the historical medical literature.

### Differential Diagnoses and Related Diseases

*Van Buchem disease* is a rare hereditary disorder characterized by endosteal hyperostosis of the skull and the mandible due to excessive lamellar bone deposition with narrow Haversian canals. The disease has both autosomal dominant and recessive forms. Clinically, van Buchem disease may resemble acromegaly but not radiologically. Patients with van Buchem disease present with thickening of the bridge of the nose, deafness due to petrous bone thickening, eye abnormalities due to stenosis of the optic canal, and cranial nerve palsies due to hyperostosis at the base of the skull (◘ Fig. 3.3.3).

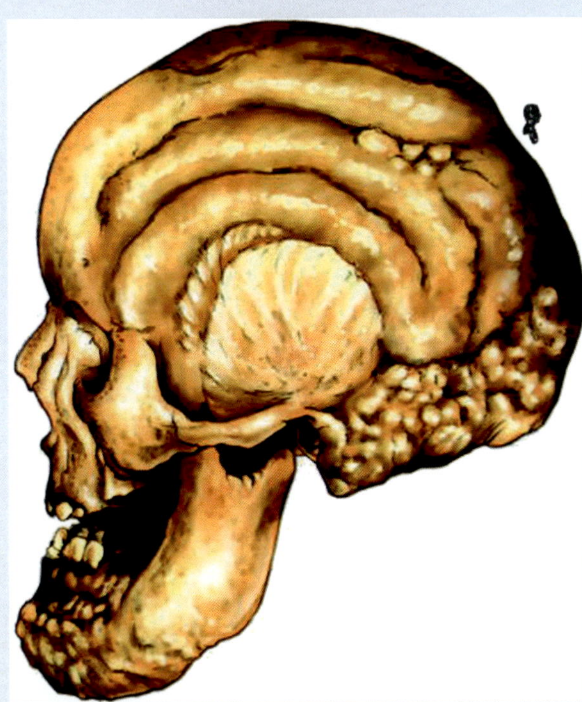

◘ **Fig. 3.3.3** An illustration of the skull in a lateral view shows the gross pathological changes seen in van Buchem disease. Notice the enlargement and thickening of the mandible, with sclerosis of the skull base and calvarium

### Signs on Skeletal Radiographs

- Increased thickness of the flat bones of the skull (◘ Fig. 3.3.4).
- Enlargement of the sinuses and mastoid air cells (◘ Fig. 3.3.4).
- Enlargement of the external occipital protuberance (◘ Fig. 3.3.4).
- Enlargement of the sella turcica (due to adenoma). The posterior clinoid processes may show signs of erosions.

- Enlargement of the vertebrae, especially in their transverse diameter.
- Increased size and widening of the distal phalangeal tufts (spade-like appearance) (◘ Fig. 3.3.5).
- Increased soft-tissue thickening of the heel pad (normal up to 23 mm in men and 21 mm in women).
- Hypertrophic osteoarthritis of the joints.
- *Locking of the metacarpals* is a relatively rare condition that can be seen in patients with acromegaly. The condition is characterized by a hooklike osteophytes formation in the heads of the metacarpal bones. As the patient makes a fist or grasps something, the volar distal part of the proximal phalanx will be locked against the osteophyte in the metacarpal head, locking the finger in the grasping position.
- *Hyperostosis frontalis interna* is a condition where thickening of the inner surface of the frontal bone may be seen in some cases with acromegaly.
- In van Buchem disease, there is generalized skull hyperostosis, mandibular hyperostosis and enlargement, ribs and clavicular thickening, and diaphyseal endosteal sclerosis that spares the bone ends, especially in the phalanges. Unlike acromegaly, there is no dental widening or mandibular prognathism.

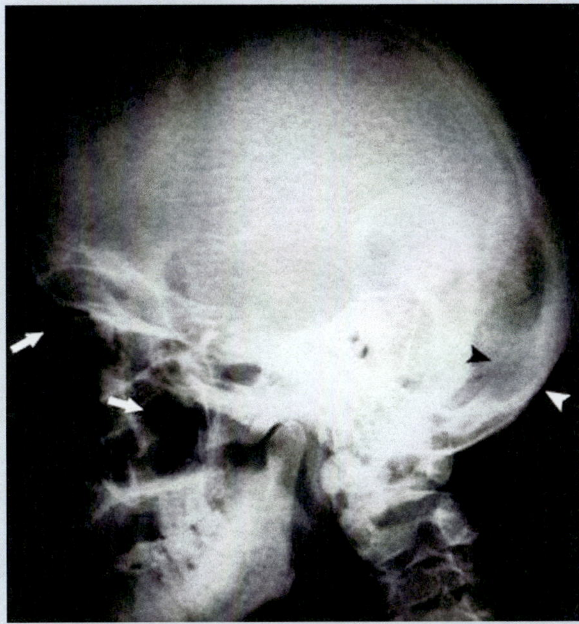

◘ **Fig. 3.3.4** A lateral skull radiograph of a patient with acromegaly shows thickened occipital bone (*arrowheads*) and enlargement of the frontal and maxillary sinuses (*arrows*)

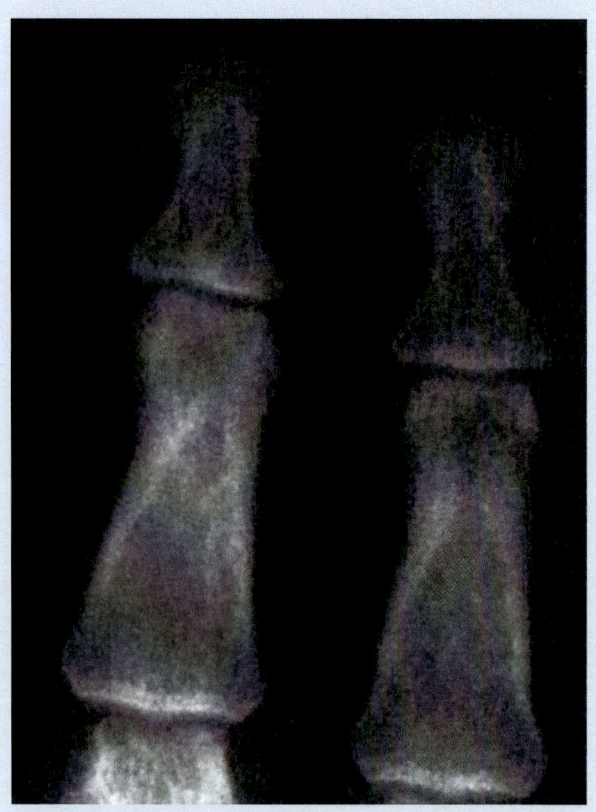

**Fig. 3.3.5** Anteroposterior plain radiograph of the third and fourth fingers of a patient with acromegaly shows widening of the distal phalangeal tufts (spade-like appearance)

**Signs on Brain MRI**
- Pituitary adenoma is seen as a bulging lesion in the superior or inferior aspect of the pituitary gland with low T1/high T2 signal. The adenoma is hypointense compared to the normal pituitary tissue on postcontrast images (■ Fig. 3.3.6).
- Indirect signs of pituitary adenoma include convex upper border of the gland with shifted pituitary stalk. When the cavernous internal carotid artery is completely surrounded by the tumor, then the cavernous sinus is mostly invaded by the tumor.

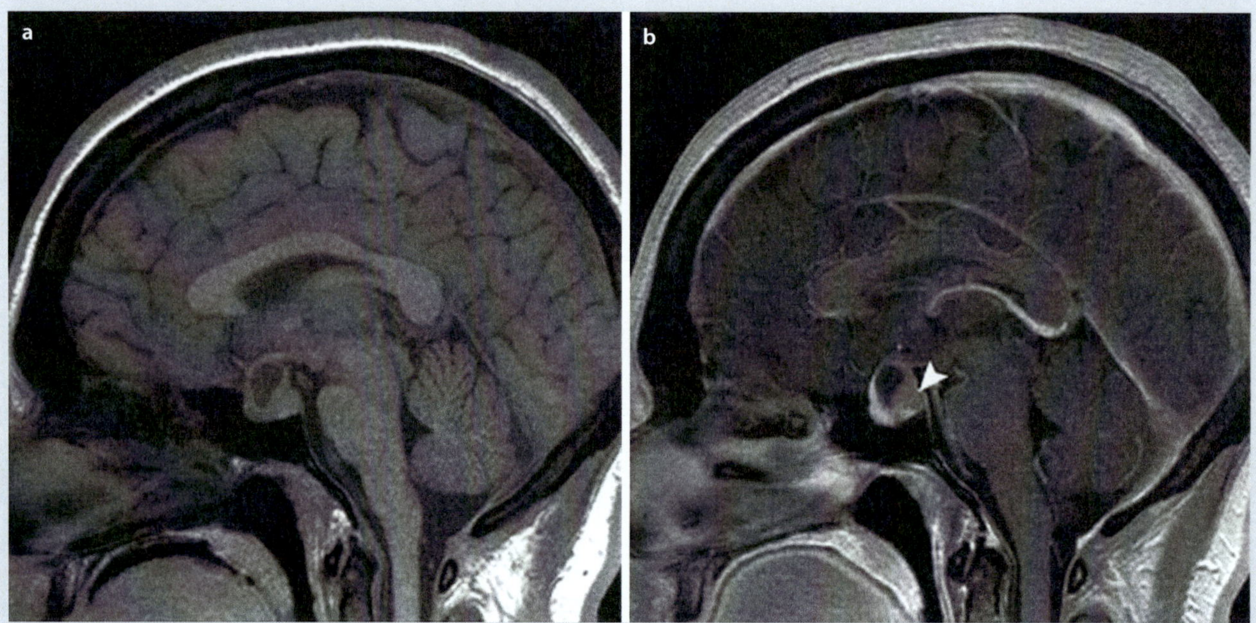

**Fig. 3.3.6** Sagittal T1W (**a**) and T1Wpostcontrast (**b**) sella MRI in a patient presented with features of acromegaly. The MR examination showed macroadenoma with cystic changes. The adenoma is detected as a mass with low contrast enhancement (*arrowhead*) compared with the highly enhanced normal pituitary tissue due to its rich blood supply

## Growth Hormone Insensitivity (Laron Syndrome)

Laron syndrome (LS) is a rare, autosomal recessive, congenital disease characterized by GH receptors gene defects, resulting in lack of body tissue response to GH.

Patients with LS present with dwarfism, severe growth retardation, and characteristic facial features. Most cases are reported from patients with Oriental Jewish origin or patients originating in the Mediterranean area like Arab, Turkish, Iranian, and Pakistani origin.

Patients with LS typically have small chin (micrognathia), underdeveloped facial bones, smaller head circumference according to age, protruding forehead, and saddle nose deformity due to nasal bone underdevelopment. The teeth are defective and crowded due to micrognathia. The hair is silky and shows frontal and temporal thinning. Alopecia is often seen in males ( Fig. 3.3.7).

Patients are usually obese due to underdevelopment of bones and muscles. The children and even adults have very high-pitched voices due to narrow oropharynx. Hands and feet are small (acromicria). The genitalia and gonads are small since birth, and males show delayed puberty more than females. LS patients do not have real pubertal growth spurt.

Laboratory investigations show severe hypoglycemia in neonates that improves with age, low serum alkaline phosphatase and creatinine, low serum cholesterol, and low-density lipoproteins.

Hormonal investigations show increased serum GH levels with very low serum levels of insulin-like growth factor-I (IGF-I). IGF-I is the anabolic effector hormone of GH. Prolactin levels may be elevated due to a drift phenomenon to the GH secretion. Serum insulin level is usually high with hypoglycemia.

> **Signs on Radiographs**
> - Generalized bone maturation delay and osteoporosis.
> - Epiphyseal closure occurs after age 16–18 in girls and 20–22 in boys.
> - Underdeveloped facial bones, with thin diploe of the skull.
> - Atlantoaxial joint degeneration and spinal stenosis is often observed.
> - Os odontoideum may be seen. Os odontoideum is a situation where the axial den (odontoid process) is hypoplastic, absent, or separated from the axis body as a congenital variant (not due to previous trauma). It is due to failure of the three dens ossification centers to fuse together with the axis body. It is seen as a round ossicle with smooth edges over the axis body in open mouth view (best view to evaluate the dens). It may be impossible to differentiate os odontoideum from a previous old dens fracture without history.

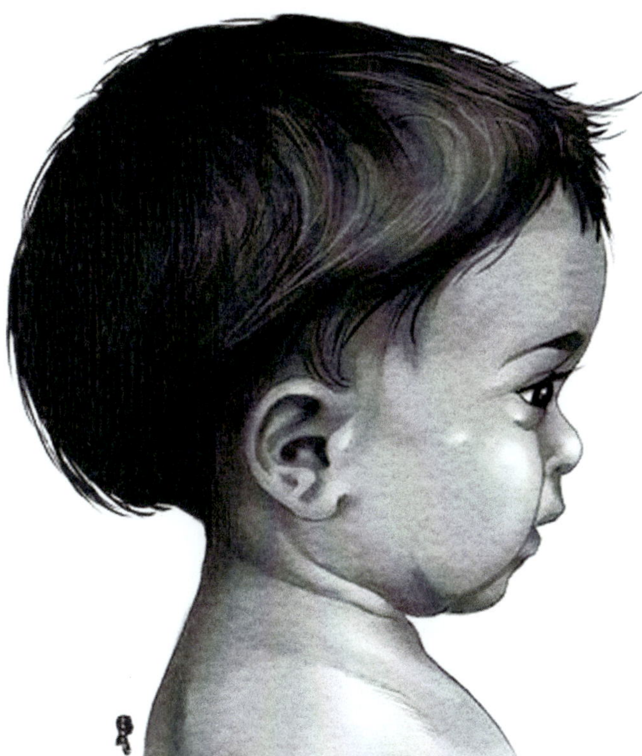

 **Fig. 3.3.7** An illustration of a child demonstrates the characteristic features of Laron syndrome (LS) like micrognathia, silky hair with temporal thinning, saddle nose deformity, and mildly protruding forehead

## Carney's Complex

Carney's complex (CNC) is a rare disease characterized by the formation of multiple endocrine and nonendocrine tumors, spotty skin pigmentation, myxomas, and endocrine overactivity. The disease is also known as *NAME syndrome* (nevi, atrial myxoma, myxoid neurofibromata, and freckles) and *LAMB syndrome* (lentigines, atrial myxoma, mucocutaneous myxomas, and blue nevi).

CNC condition has an autosomal dominant mode of inheritance. *Carney's syndrome* is a different clinical condition characterized by a triad of several neoplasms including gastric epithelioid leiomyosarcoma, pulmonary chondroma, and extra-adrenal paraganglioma. Patients with CNC are diagnosed by fulfilling two or more of the CNC diagnostic criteria.

### Carney's Complex Major Diagnostic Criteria

- *Lentiginosis and blue nevi*: Lentigo is a brownish-black flat macule that is typically found in the lips, around the inner canthus of the eye, axilla, or genitals (Fig. 3.3.8). When the macules are found diffusely in the body, the condition is called "lentiginosis." The other characteristic skin lesion found in CNC is blue skin nevi.
- *Cutaneous myxomas*: These are seen on the trunk as small red papules.
- *Cardiac myxoma*: It is the most common component of CNC. Cardiac myxoma is a gelatinous tumor, and it is the most common primary cardiac neoplasm in adults (50 % of cardiac neoplasms). Ninety percent of cases are seen in adult women between 30 and 60 years of age. Most cases are sporadic. Patients usually present with CNS symptoms, fatigue, arthralgia, fever, anemia, and weight loss. Twenty percent of myxomas are asymptomatic. Patients with CNC cardiac myxoma are younger than patients with sporadic myxoma (an average age of 24 years).

- *Acromegaly*: CNC patients can develop acromegaly due to GH-releasing pituitary micro-/macroadenoma.
- *Primary pigmented nodular adrenocortical disease (PPNAD)*: It is a rare disease of children and young adults below 20 years of age. It can be the first manifestation of CNC. Pathologically, the adrenal shows small black, brown, red, or yellow nodules separated by atrophic adrenal cortex. Diagnosis is essentially based on histological findings. PPNAD is one of the common causes of ACTH-independent Cushing's syndrome.
- *Large-cell calcifying Sertoli cell tumor (LCCSCT)*: Bilateral germ cell tumors of the testes are the initial presentation of CNC in 20 % of cases. Diagnosis is strengthened by the detection of high serum levels of estrogen or androgen.
- One or more of the following cancers: breast fibromyxomas (25 % of cases), osteochondromyxoma, follicular thyroid carcinoma, and psammomatous melanotic schwannoma.

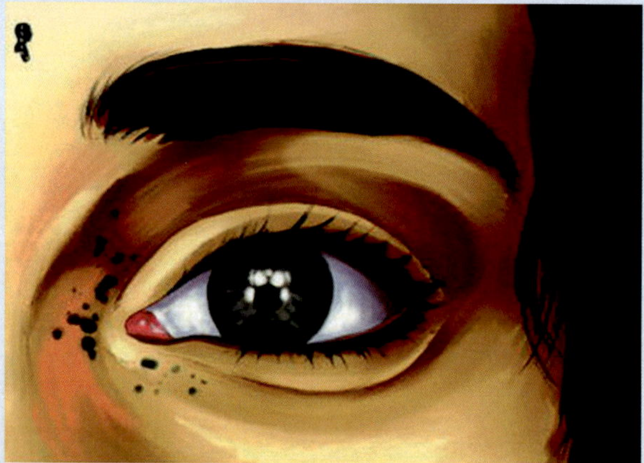

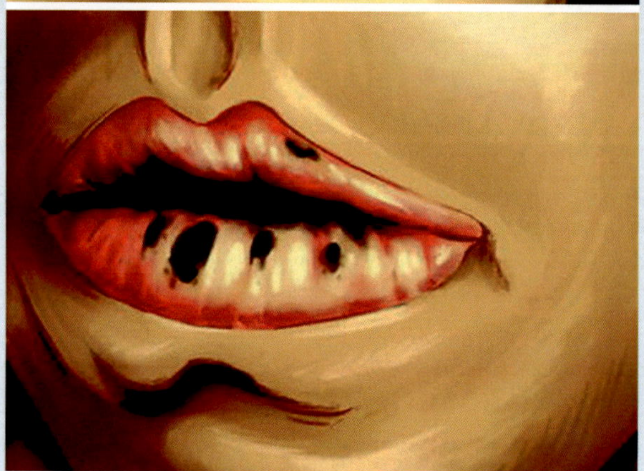

**Fig. 3.3.8**   An eye and lip illustration demonstrates the lentigo pigmented lesions found in the inner canthus and the lips in a patient with Carney's complex (CNS)

### Signs on US

In LCCSCT, the testes show multiple, round, well-defined, large (5–10 mm) echogenic calcification with acoustic shadowing representing the stromal tumors.

### Signs on MRI

- *Cardiac myxoma*: myxoma typically appears as a heterogeneous mass on T2W images with a narrow-based attachment located in the interatrial septum at the area of fossa ovalis (90 % of cases). Eighty percent of myxomas arise in the left atrium and 10 % in the right atrium. Calcification is frequently seen, and the mass shows heterogeneous contrast enhancement. The location of the tumors is very characteristic.
- *LCCSCT* are detected as multiple high T2 intratesticular masses with hypointense areas representing calcifications (Fig. 3.3.9).
- Sella MRI may show pituitary adenoma especially in patients with signs of acromegaly.
- *PPNAD*: the adrenal glands may be normal or show limbs macronodularity (>5 mm in size).

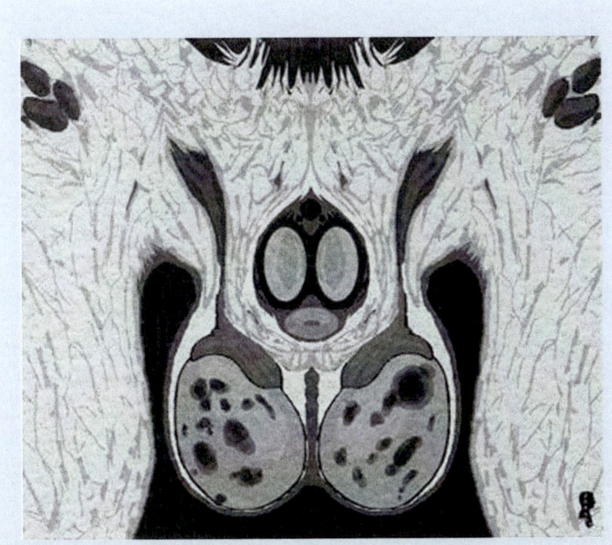



## Further Reading

Boikos SA et al. Pituitary pathology in patients with carney complex: growth-hormone producing hyperplasia or tumors and their association with other abnormalities. Pituitary. 2006;9:203–9.

Cazabat L et al. PRKAR1A mutations in primary pigmented nodular adrenocortical disease. Pituitary. 2006;9:211–9.

Chakraborty PP et al. Laron's syndrome in two siblings. Indian J Pediatr. 2007;74:870–1.

Daughaday WH et al. The pituitary in disorders of growth. Dis Mon. 1962;8:1–47.

Doppman JL et al. Cushing syndrome due to primary pigmented nodular adrenocortical disease: findings at CT and MR imaging. Radiology. 1989;172:415–20.

Elster AD. Imaging of the sella: anatomy and pathology. Semin Ultrasound CT MR. 1993;14:182–94.

Fisher MS. An unusual bone change in acromegaly. Skeletal Radiol. 1978;3:177–8.

Frohman LA. Diseases of hypothalamic releasing factors. Dis Mon. 1976;22:1–37.

Haupt HA. Anabolic steroids and growth hormones. Am J Sports Med. 1993;21:468.

Jacobs P. Van Buchem disease. Postgrad Med J. 1977;53:497–506.

Kaplan SA. Human growth hormone. Dis Mon. 1968;14:1–33.

Kornerich L et al. Laron syndrome abnormalities: spinal stenosis, Os odontoideum, degenerative changes of the atlanto-odontoid joint, and small oropharynx. AJNR Am J Neuroradiol. 2002;23:625–31.

Laron Z. Growth hormone insensitivity (Laron syndrome). Rev Endocr Metab Disord. 2002;3:347–55.

Laron Z. Laron syndrome (primary growth hormone resistance or insensitivity): the personal experience 1958–2003. J Clin Endocrinol Metab. 2004;89:1031–44.

Mateus C et al. Heterogeneity of skin manifestations in patients with Carney syndrome. J Am Acad Dermatol. 2008;59:801–10.

Ron E et al. Acromegaly and gastrointestinal cancer. Cancer. 1991;68:1673–7.

Tani Y et al. Locking of the metacarpophalangeal joints in a patient with acromegaly. Skeletal Radiol. 1999;28:655–7.

Vandersteen A et al. Cutaneous signs are important in the diagnosis of rare neoplasia syndrome Carney complex. Eur J Pediatr. 2009;168:1401–4.

Wyszynski DF. Dysmorphology in the Bible and the Talmud. Teratology. 2001;64:221–5.

## 3.4 Osteoporosis

Osteoporosis is a group of disorders characterized by reduced bone mass or density in the absence of defect in bone mineralization. Osteoporosis can arise due to unknown reasons (primary) or due to pathological conditions (secondary).

Bones reach their peak density in the third decade of life and then decrease gradually at the rate of 0.25–1 % per year. This percentage is higher in women at the menopause, which may reach up to 8 % per year. Osteoporosis affects the axial skeleton more than the perpendicular skeleton, while osteomalacia (excess un-mineralized bone matrix) affects the perpendicular skeleton more than the axial skeleton. Osteoporosis starts to show itself on radiographs when 30–60 % of bone mass is lost.

## Primary Osteoporosis

Primary osteoporosis is a term used to describe reduction in bone density in the absence of a specific clinical condition that explains this bone density reduction. It is divided into juvenile, idiopathic, and postmenopausal types.

*Idiopathic juvenile osteoporosis* is osteoporosis that affects children and young adults and is typically seen before puberty. Patients present with difficulties and gait abnormalities and multiple fractures that typically involve the metaphyses of distal tibias and the vertebral bodies. Pain in the heels and the lower back is a common complaint. Diagnosis of this condition is established after exclusion of all cases that may present with similar manifestations (e.g., osteogenesis imperfecta and homocysteinuria).

*Idiopathic osteoporosis* is a term used to define osteoporosis seen in patients between 20 and 45 years of age with the same clinical features as the juvenile form. *Postmenopausal osteoporosis* is seen in women who have undergone natural menopause or after oophorectomy. Primary osteoporosis affects mainly the hip more than any other area in the skeleton.

*Vacuum phenomenon*, also known as "intervertebral cleft sign," is a term used to describe a condition characterized by accumulation of gas, mostly nitrogen (95 %), within the vertebral bodies, intervertebral disks, and synovial joints. The gas is produced from the surrounding soft tissues, and its accumulation mechanism is poorly understood. The main hypothesis of vacuum phenomenon suggests ischemic origin. Osteonecrosis of the vertebral end plates with negative pressure between the bone fragments is mandatory to release gas from the surrounding tissue, a situation that can be classically seen in osteoporotic vertebral fractures and collapse. Vacuum phenomenon is also seen in osteonecrosis due to long-term corticosteroid therapy, diabetes mellitus, arteriosclerosis, multiple myeloma, and alcoholism.

The main differential diagnosis of the intravertebral vacuum phenomenon is gas produced by osteomyelitis and malignancies. In infectious gaseous production, the gas has high pressure and tends to accumulate in small collections, plus extends into the adjacent soft tissues, which is not seen in vacuum phenomenon where gas is limited to the bony or intradiskal areas.

*Kümmel's disease* is a term used to describe vacuum phenomenon within a vertebra that arises from vertebral end plates osteonecrosis and vertebral collapse. Kümmel's disease represents healing failure of an osteoporotic vertebral fracture with the formation of pseudoarthrosis (false joint).

### Signs on Plain Radiograph and CT

- Thinning of the cortex (compact bone) is the main radiographic feature of osteoporosis (Fig. 3.4.1). It is best seen in the second metacarpal bone diaphysis. Normally, the cortex in the mid-shaft of the second metacarpal should be almost one third the thickness of the metacarpal width. This sign is seen in up to 50 % of cases.
- *Dowager's hump* is an osteoporotic multiple thoracic vertebrae causing wedge deformities (Fig. 3.4.2).
- *Pathologic fractures* mostly occur at the neck of the femur, distal radius, and humeral neck.
- *Intracortical tunneling* is a sign of rapid bone loss. It is typically seen as long lucent lines parallel to the long axis of the bone (Fig. 3.4.3). When the tunneling is severe, a double cortical line is seen.
- *Diffuse bone resorption* occurs in 50 % of cases and is characterized by loss of the trabecular bone.
- *Linear translucent bands* of 4–8 mm thickness are seen within the bone in radiograph. They are commonly seen with disuse osteoporosis and leukemic patients.
- *Patchy bone resorption*: seen as multiple lucent patches usually in the carpal or tarsal bones. It can be mistaken with lytic lesions of Ewing's sarcoma and multiple myeloma (Fig. 3.4.4).

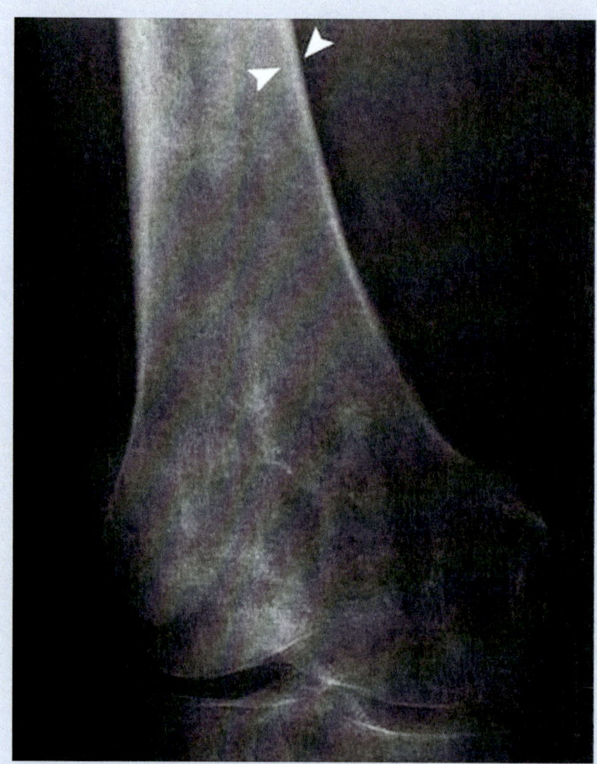

**Fig. 3.4.1**   A plain radiograph of the knee shows diminished bone mineral density (BMD) with thinning of the cortex (*arrowheads*)

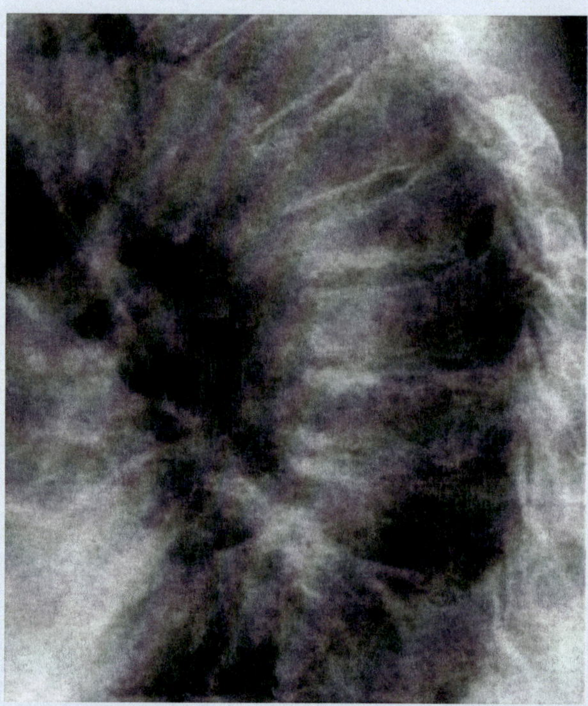

**Fig. 3.4.2**   A lateral thoracic vertebrae radiograph shows kyphosis of the thoracic vertebrae due to osteoporosis (dowager's hump)

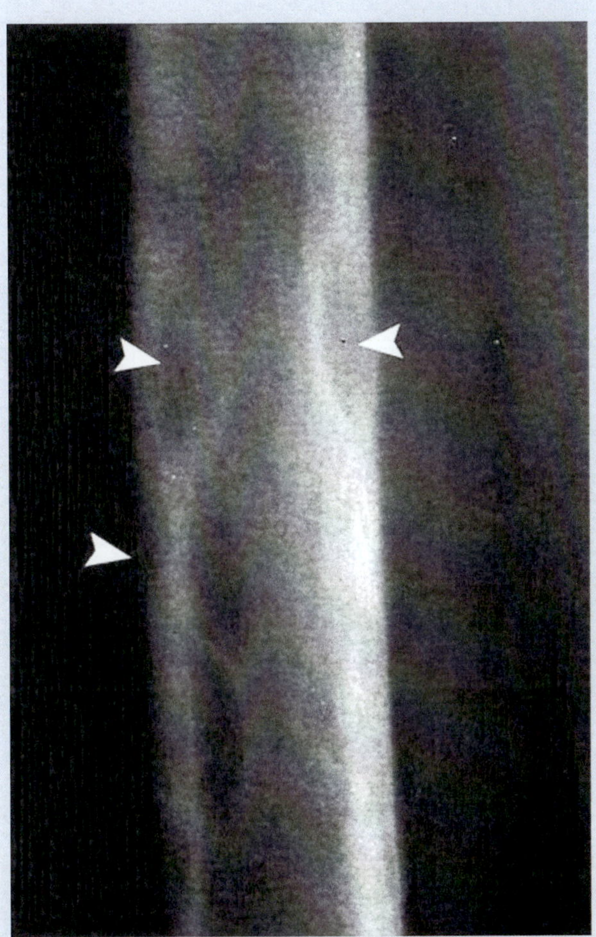

**Fig. 3.4.3** A plain radiograph of osteoporosis of the femoral shaft demonstrates clearly the intracortical tunneling sign (*arrowheads*)

- Vacuum phenomenon is seen as a gas collection in a collapsed vertebra or in intervertebral disk space (Fig. 3.4.5).
- *Singh index* is a simple method to estimate the level bone mineral density (BMD) on radiograph by analyzing the changes in the trabecular pattern of the proximal femur. A scale of six grades is classically described, with the first grade showing only basic trabecular structures (low BMD, severe osteoporosis), and the sixth grade showing trabecular structures in all areas of the proximal femur (high BMD, normal bone).

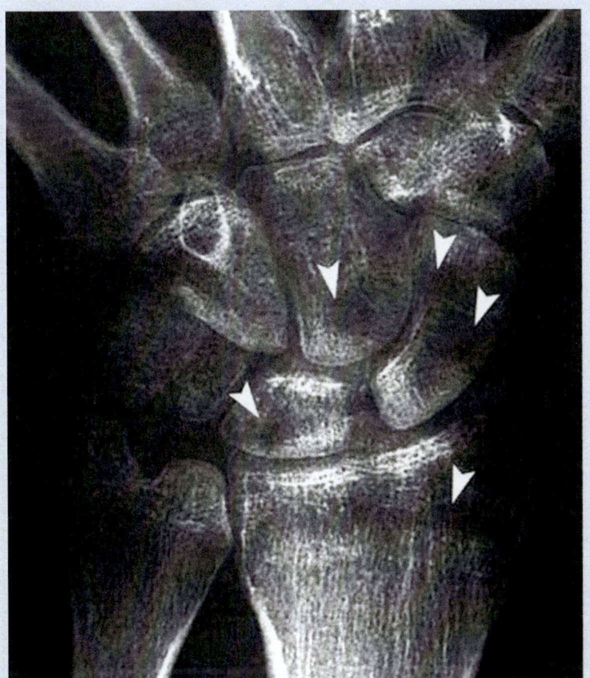

**Fig. 3.4.4** Anteroposterior plain wrist radiograph in a patient with osteoporosis shows patchy areas of radiolucent opacities representing patchy osteoporosis (*arrowheads*)

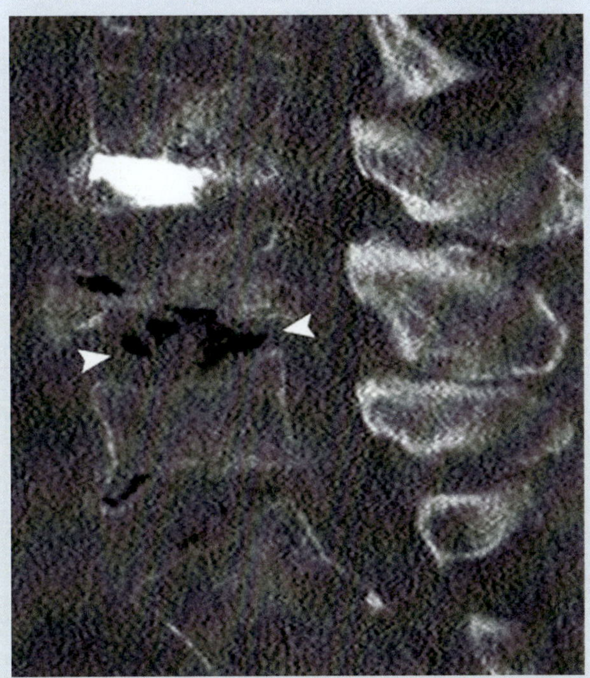

**Fig. 3.4.5** Sagittal lumbar CT image in a patient with osteoporosis shows severe osteopenia, collapse of L4 vertebra (vertebra plana), and vertebroplasty of L3, with gas formation located in the intervertebral disk space between L4 and L5 (*arrowheads*)

### Signs on MRI

- The area of vacuum phenomenon may appear as an area of fluid signal intensity on T2W images. This finding is explained by the fact that fluid replacement tends to fill the area of vacuum gas on long supine position. This T2 flow signal depends on the time of scanning. In the first 10 min of the scan, the vacuum area is seen as a hypointense area on T2W images. The signal turns into T2 hyperintense signal between 20 and 40 min after positioning.
- In *Kümmel's disease*, the vertebral end plates are seen compressing over the fractured area in flexion. In extension, the gap between the fractured end plates open. Intervertebral air can be seen on CT and MRI, with no signs of inflammation on T2W images.

### Dual Energy X-Ray Absorptiometry (DEXA) Scan

- DEXA scan is a quantitative method for measuring bone mass by using low-energy X-ray beam. The bone mass is measured in units of gram per cubic centimeter of bone. The World Health Organization (WHO) defines the *T*-scores as follows: between +1 and −1 indicates normal bone; between −1 and −2.5 indicates osteopenia; and osteoporosis is diagnosed when the *T*-score is less than −2.5.

*Pitfall*: sclerosis and osteophytes in the vertebral column can increase the values of the DEXA scan giving a false impression of a good bone density. For this reason, DEXA report should always be written after comparison of the results with plain frontal and lateral radiographs of the vertebral column to avoid misinterpretation.

## Secondary Osteoporosis

Secondary osteoporosis is seen in association with other clinical conditions such as endocrine diseases (e.g., Cushing's syndrome), nutritional diseases (e.g., scurvy), drug induced (e.g., heparin), neoplasms (e.g., multiple myeloma), metabolic diseases (e.g., diabetes mellitus), and chronic inflammatory conditions (e.g., rheumatoid arthritis). Radiological manifestations are same as primary osteoporosis.

## Regional Migratory Osteoporosis of the Hip (Bone Marrow Edema Syndrome)

Regional migratory osteoporosis (RMO) is a rare condition characterized by migrating arthralgia of weight-bearing joints in the lower limbs (hips, knees, and ankles).

RMO typically affects males between 50 and 60 years of age presenting with pain confined to a single joint. Patients experience progressive pain in one joint that can last from weeks to months. Peak intensity of the pain is experienced usually in the second and third months after the initial presentation. There is no history of trauma or signs suggesting joint infection (e.g., septic arthritis). The symptoms resolve spontaneously often between 4 and 11 months after presentation.

### Signs on Radiographs

Typically, there is osteopenia of the affected joint compared to the other joint which normally shows no osteopenia (unless the patient is generally osteoporotic). Unfortunately, this sign is seen after 3–6 weeks from the start of symptoms. Remineralization of the affected area may take up to 2 years to complete after the symptoms are resolved.

### Signs on MRI (Four Morphological Criteria at T1W Images Are Needed to Indicate RMO of the Hip)

- The bone marrow edema must involve the femoral head and often spares the subchondral bone resulting in a thin rim of unaffected subchondral marrow. The edema may extend to the femoral neck.
- The bone marrow lacks the definite margins or transitional zone between the lesion and the adjacent marrow.
- The signal is homogeneous with areas of high- or low-intensity foci.
- The signal intensity of the marrow is moderately reduced. All the above four criteria must be evaluated on T1W images.
- Joint effusion is seen in 75 % of patients.
- *RMO of the knee* has the same diagnostic criteria as the RMO of the hip and typically involves the lateral femoral condyle, although it can affect any part of the knee (◘ Fig. 3.4.6).

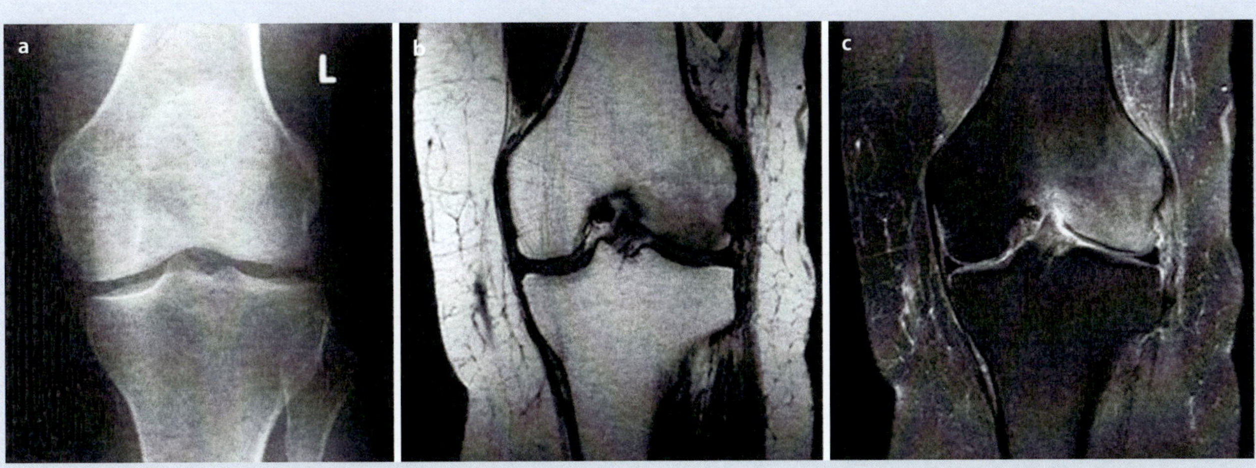

**⬛ Fig. 3.4.6**  Anteroposterior plain radiograph of the left knee (**a**), with coronal T1W image (**b**) and coronal PD image (**c**) of a 57-year-old lady who presented with nonspecific knee pain for 3 weeks' duration. The plain radiograph shows no signs of obvious pathology or diminished bone density. On the MR images, the lateral femoral condyle showed bone marrow edema signal with no sign of a fracture of cortical destruction. The knee showed no signs of abnormalities that explain the knee pain. The diagnosis was regional migratory osteoporosis (RMO) of the knee and the patient was advised a 3-month MRI follow-up examination

### RMO Differential Diagnoses

- *Avascular necrosis*: usually with history of trauma, steroid use, chemotherapy, or renal disease. No such history is associated with RMO. Risk factors for RMO include low dietary calcium and tobacco smoking.
- *Reflex sympathetic dystrophy*: there are atrophic skin changes and history of neurological disease, which are not seen in RMO.
- *Chronic recurrent multifocal osteomyelitis*: has the same picture as RMO on MRI, but plain radiographs show both lytic and sclerotic lesions, which is not characteristic of RMO.

## Further Reading

Akpinar E et al. The intravertebral vacuum phenomenon. Eur J Radiol Extra. 2008;66:e55–7.

Aloia JF et al. Risk for osteoporosis in black women. Calcif Tissue Int. 1996;59:415–23.

Cahir JG et al. Regional migratory osteoporosis. Eur J Radiol. 2008;67:2–10.

Freedman BA et al. Kummel disease: a not-so-rare complication of osteoporotic vertebral compression fracture. J Am Board Fam Med. 2009;22:75–8.

Goldring SR et al. Metabolic bone disease: osteoporosis and osteomalacia. Dis Mon. 1981;27:1–103.

Hauschild O et al. Evaluation of Singh index for assessment of osteoporosis using digital radiography. Eur J Radiol. 2009;71:152–8.

Karantanas AH. Acute bone marrow edema of the hip: role of MR imaging. Eur Radiol. 2007;17:2225–36.

Kumpan W et al. The intravertebral vacuum phenomenon. Skeletal Radiol. 1986;15:444–7.

Libicher M et al. The intravertebral vacuum phenomenon as a specific sign of osteonecrosis in vertebral compression fractures: results from a radiological and histological study. Eur Radiol. 2007;17:2248–52.

Lorenc RS. Idiopathic juvenile osteoporosis. Calcif Tissue Int. 2002;70:395–7.

Lutwak L et al. Osteoporosis. Dis Mon. 1963;9:1–39.

Sarli M et al. The vacuum cleft sign: an uncommon radiological sign. Osteoporos Int. 2005;16:1210–4.

Vande Berg BC et al. Bone marrow edema of the femoral head and transient osteoporosis of the hip. Eur J Radiol. 2008;67:68–77.

Williamson MR et al. Osteoporosis: diagnosis by plain chest film versus dual photon bone densitometry. Skeletal Radiol. 1990;19:27–30.

## 3.5    Rickets and Osteomalacia

Rickets is a group of conditions characterized by accumulation of nonmineralized bony matrix (osteoid) within the skeleton in children, while osteomalacia is an accumulation of nonmineralized bony matrix in the mature skeleton of adults (the bone quantity is normal, but the bone quality is abnormal).

Understanding bone physiology and metabolism is crucial for understanding the pathology of rickets and osteomalacia. Bones are made up of bony cells surrounded by extracellular matrix. The extracellular matrix has organic and inorganic components. The *organic* component, also called "osteoid," is made of type I collagen fibers embedded in a ground substance composed of proteoglycans and other components. The osteoid is secreted by the osteoblasts, and it accounts for 35 % of the bone mass. In contrast, the *inorganic* component is composed of osteoid plus calcium and pyrophosphate (mineral salts). The inorganic materials are what give bone its density and account for 65 % of the bone mass. Rickets and osteomalacia are diseases of matrix mineralization, while osteoporosis is a disease of bony matrix.

After osteoid mineralization, the mineralized collagens are arranged in either woven or lamellar pattern. *Woven bone* is immature bone with its fibers not arranged in any direction. Normally it presents in life as a transitional stage and then is replaced by lamellar bone. Woven bone is not found in mature skeleton normally; however, it is produced during healing of fractures or remodeling (callus formation). Its presence indicates abnormality when found in mature skeleton. *Lamellar bone*, on the other hand, is mature bone with its fibers arranged in a certain pattern to withstand mechanical pressure. The mature skeleton is made only of lamellar bone, and the fibers are arranged in vertical form in the cortical bone and arranged in transverse form in the trabecular bone. Some sheets of lamellar bone are circumferentially arranged around a bundle of blood vessels and lymphatics, forming what are known as "Haversian canals or osteons." These Haversian canals are found in the cortical bone and arranged along the long axis of the bone, and they communicate with each other through channels of interstitial lamellae.

The *physis* is the cartilaginous growth plate in immature skeleton which is responsible for adding length to bone. The growth plate functions as a one-way barrier to blood vessels, allowing the blood from epiphyseal capillaries to supply the metaphysis but not vice versa.

Hormones that affect bone metabolism and hemostasis include the parathyroid hormone (PTH) and the active form of vitamin D, 1,25-dihydroxyvitamin D (1,25(HO)$_2$D). PTH is secreted in response to low plasma calcium concentration. PTH promotes bone formation on the physiological level, but it causes bone resorption at high concentrations. Vitamin D undergoes two hydroxylation steps in the liver and the kidney before it becomes metabolically active, promoting calcium absorption from the intestines. Calcitonin is a hormone that opposes the action of both PTH and vitamin D.

From the latter explanation of the bone metabolism, any condition that can result in hormonal imbalance or matrix mineralization defects can result in the development of rickets or osteomalacia. Causes of rickets include:

- Acquired rickets due to vitamin D deficiency (most common form).
- Congenital rickets due to vitamin D enzyme hydroxylation deficiency.
- Congenital rickets due to vitamin D resistance and receptors mutation.

- Congenital rickets due hypophosphatemia (low phosphates). It can be X-linked, autosomal dominant, or autosomal recessive.
- Acquired rickets due to hypocalcemia.
- Acquired rickets due to renal failure. Reasons for developing rickets or osteomalacia are loss of the hydroxylation step of vitamin D and raised PTH levels.

Patients with rickets often present with bowing of the legs, swollen joints, bone pain, and muscle weakness. Patients with rickets due to vitamin D resistance may present with alopecia.

## Differential Diagnoses and Related Diseases

*Dent's disease* is a rare disease characterized by X-linked recessive hypophosphatemic rickets, idiopathic low molecular weight proteinuria, and X-linked recessive nephrolithiasis. Patients with this disorder commonly present with hypercalciuria, nephrocalcinosis, and renal failure at advanced stage of the disease. Radiological investigations in these patients include plain radiographs of the bone to show signs of rickets and renal ultrasound to detect urinary stones and medullary calcinosis.

**Signs of Rickets on Plain Radiograph**
- Flaring of the epiphysis.
- Bending of the diaphysis of long bones, commonly the tibia (◨ Fig. 3.5.1).
- Cupping deformity of the metaphysis due to herniation of the hypertrophied physis into the metaphysis (◨ Fig. 3.5.2). The metaphyses may also show fine bony speculation (◨ Fig. 3.5.3).
- *Looser's zone fracture (pseudofractures)* is a very distinctive feature of osteomalacia, which is characterized by a fracture through a large osteoid area within the bone. This type of fracture is rare and tends to occur in the scapula or the pelvis.
- *Rachitic rosary* is swelling of the costochondral junction of the middle ribs.
- Osteomalacia presents with signs of osteopenia on radiographs. It cannot be differentiated from osteoporosis with radiographs alone. History of chronic renal failure is a helpful clue.
- Rickets due to hypophosphatemia are usually associated with craniosynostosis (e.g., scaphocephaly).
- Skull radiographs in patients with rickets show soft skull bones (craniotabes), flattening of the skull, hot-cross-bun skull (caput quadratum), and delayed closure of the fontanels.
- Hypocalcemic rickets characteristically show hypoplasia of the dental enamel, whereas abscesses of the teeth occur more often in rickets due to hypophosphatemia.

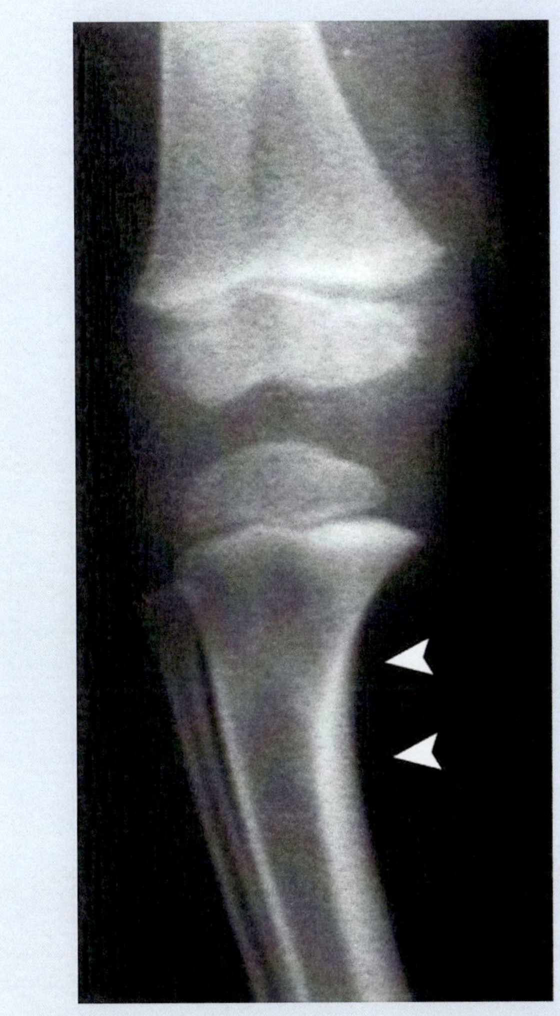

**Fig. 3.5.1** Anteroposterior plain radiograph of the right knee in a child with rickets shows mild bowing of the proximal tibial metaphysis (*arrowheads*)

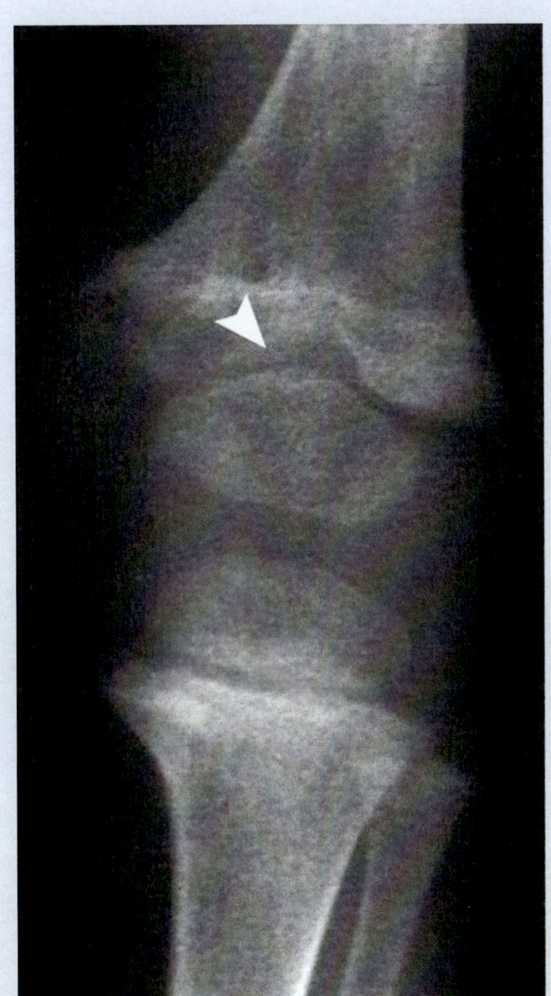

**Fig. 3.5.2** Anteroposterior plain radiograph of the left knee in a child with rickets shows focal cupping of the distal femoral metaphysis (*arrowhead*)

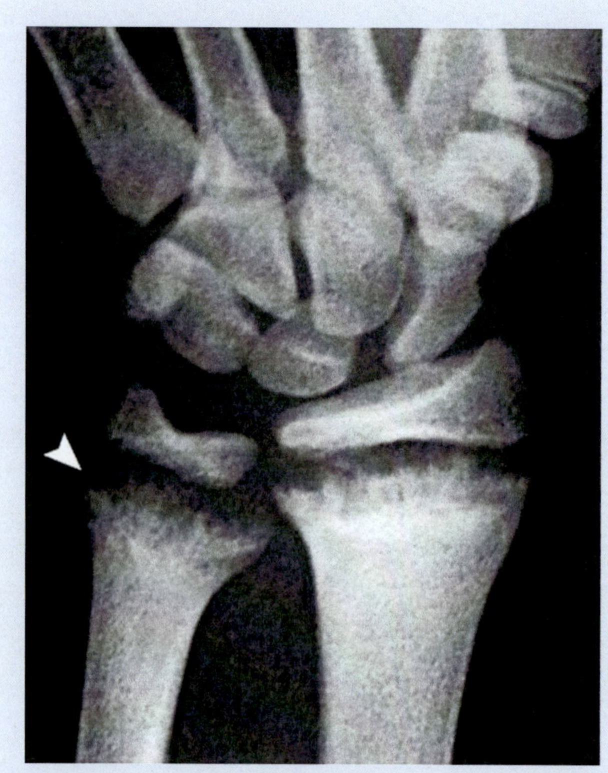

**Fig. 3.5.3** A plain wrist radiograph of a patient with rickets shows metaphyseal bony speculations (*arrowhead*)

## Further Reading

Brickley M et al. Evaluation and rickets interpretation of residual rickets deformities in adults. Int J Osteoarchiol. 2008. doi:10.1002/oa.1007.

Cheong HI et al. Phenotype and genotype of Dent's disease in three Korean boys. Pediatr Nephrol. 2005;20:455–9.

Currarino G. Sagittal synostosis in X-linked hypophosphatemic rickets and related diseases. Pediatr Radiol. 2007;37:805–12.

DeJong AR et al. Pseudotumor cerebri and nutritional rickets. Eur J Pediatr. 1985;143:219–20.

Mays S et al. Skeletal manifestations of rickets in infants and young children in a historic population from England. Am J Phys Anthropol. 2006;129:362–74.

McBride A et al. Vitamin D-resistance rickets (X-linked hypophosphatemic rickets). Curr Orthop. 2007;21:369–99.

Ramavat LG. Vitamin D, deficiency rickets at birth in Kuwait. Indian J Pediatr. 1999;66:37–43.

Tosetto E et al. Dent's disease and prevalence of renal stones in dialysis patients in Northeastern Italy. J Hum Genet. 2006;51:25–30.

## 3.6    Scurvy

Scurvy is disease that arises due to vitamin C deficiency. Most cases of scurvy arise due to severe malnutrition, alcoholism, and drug abuse.

Vitamin C (ascorbic acid) functions as a cofactor, enzyme complement, co-substrate, or a strong antioxidant in a variety of metabolic activities. It provides electrons needed to reduce molecular oxygen. It also works as a cofactor for collagen synthesis and norepinephrine synthesis. Vitamin C is present in marine fish, vegetables, and citrus fruits (in high concentrations).

Vitamin C absorption occurs in the small intestine and is excreted by the kidneys. The maximum concentration of vitamin C is found in the pituitary gland, leukocytes, the brain, adrenals, and the eye.

Patients with scurvy usually present with irritability, limb pain, and tenderness with pseudoparalysis. Unusual manifestations of scurvy include subdural and subarachnoid hemorrhage, hematuria, melena, pleural hemorrhage, and retro-orbital hemorrhage causing proptosis. Patients improve within 2 days to 1 week from starting vitamin C therapy. Scurvy is often found in children, and radiographic abnormalities are rare before 6 months of age.

### Signs on Plain Radiograph

- *Subperiosteal hemorrhage* is seen as elevated periosteum from the bone ( Fig. 3.6.1).
- *Wimberger's sign*: sclerotic rim surrounding the epiphysis in children.
- *White line of Frankel*: dense sclerotic metaphyseal line over the metaphysis ( Fig. 3.6.2).
- *Pelkin's fracture*: metaphyseal avulsion fracture.
- Scurvy is a frequent cause of osteoporosis in children ( Fig. 3.6.2), and it can predispose to slipped distal femoral epiphysis due to epiphysiolysis.

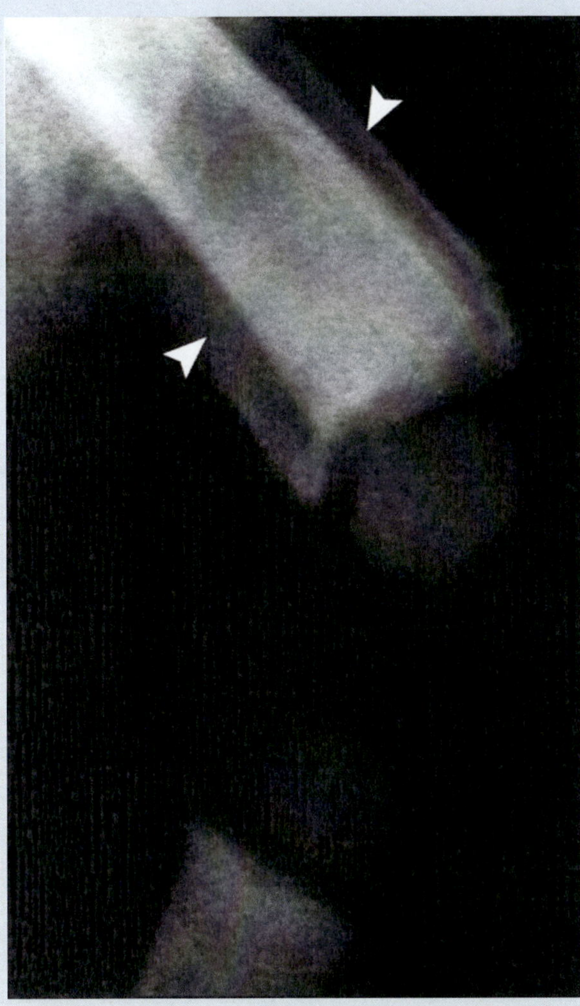

 **Fig. 3.6.1**  Anteroposterior left femoral radiograph shows periosteal hemorrhage in a baby with scurvy seen as radiolucent shadow that surrounds the distal femur shaft (*arrowheads*)

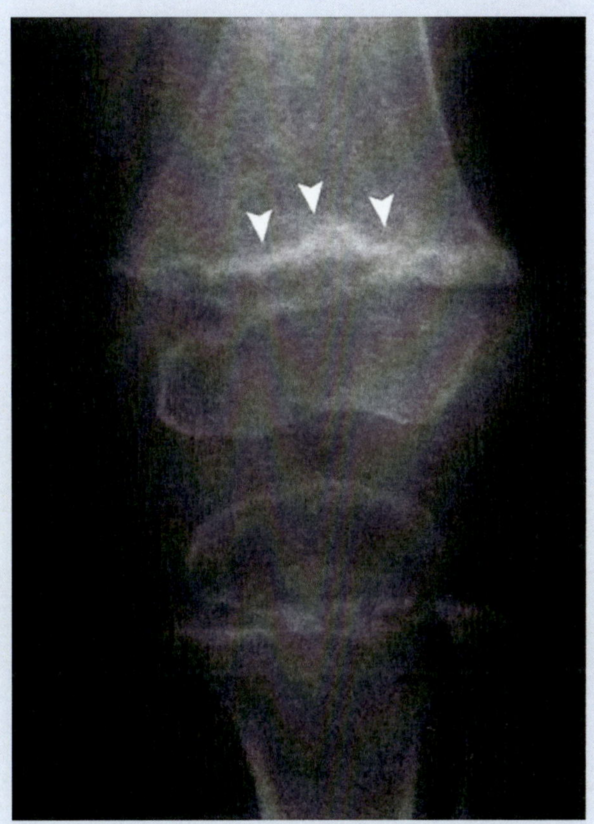

 **Fig. 3.6.2**  Anteroposterior plain knee radiograph in another child with scurvy shows dense sclerotic metaphyseal line (*white line of Frankel*). Notice the diffuse osteoporosis affecting the entire knee joint

### Further Reading

Akikusa JD et al. Scurvy: forgotten but not gone. J Paediatr Child Health. 2003;39:75–7.

Brickley M et al. Skeletal manifestations of infantile scurvy. Am J Phys Anthropol. 2006;129:163–72.

Firth N et al. Oral lesions in scurvy. Aust Dent J. 2001;46:298–300.

Ratageri VH et al. Scurvy in infantile tremor syndrome. Indian J Pediatr. 2005;72:883–4.

Suvarna J et al. Hemorrhagic pleural effusion: can it be scurvy? Indian J Pediatr. 2007;74:1050–1.

Verma S et al. Unilateral proptosis and extradural hematoma in a child with scurvy. Pediatr Radiol. 2007;37:937–9.

## 3.7    Fluorosis

Fluorosis is a clinical condition characterized by excessive ingestion of fluoride, which causes toxicity and systemic manifestations that can be disabling.

Fluoride is an element that is found in water, soil, and air. It results from the combination of the "fluorine" gas with different natural elements. Fluoride can be found in food, seawater, and tea. Each cup of tea may supply 0.3–0.5 mg of fluoride. The safe daily intake of fluoride for an adult is <4 mg/day. Skeletal fluorosis results from ingesting fluoride >10 mg/day for at least 10 years.

Fluorosis classically results from ingestion of water or food with high fluoride content in endemic areas. Fluorosis toxicity may also develop from chronic intake of sodium fluoride as a long-standing therapy for osteoporosis, using Teflon-coated pots, chewing tobacco, and the overuse of niflumic acid (nonsteroidal anti-inflammatory drug).

Fluoride absorption in the body can be reduced by taking calcium or magnesium salts. In contrast, phosphate, sulfates, and molybdenum increase gastrointestinal absorption of fluoride and lead to fluoride toxicity.

Up to 99 % of the absorbed fluoride combines with the mineralized bones, mostly in the teeth, pelvis, and vertebrae. Dental fluorosis deposits mainly in the enamels and causes brown or black dental pigmentation (◘ Fig. 3.7.1). Pitting, chipping, and mottling of the teeth may also occur.

Patients with fluorosis often complain from pain in the joints and back, which is often mistaken with rheumatic disorders like rheumatoid arthritis and ankylosing spondylitis. Back stiffness, limb paresthesia, and restricted spine movement are early signs of fluorosis. In severe form of back fluorosis, the vertebral column becomes one continuous column of bones due to calcification of the paravertebral ligaments, a condition known as *poker back* (◘ Figs. 3.7.2 and 3.7.5). Development of genu varum, genu valgum, and kyphosis may occur. Involvement of the ribs by fluorosis results in a barrel-shaped chest with restricted respiratory breathing. Abdominal breathing becomes the main breathing mechanism in severe cases.

Neurological manifestations of fluorosis usually are related to the spinal cord compression due to vertebral canal stenosis. Patients experience radiculopathy and difficulty in walking due to muscle weakness. Cranial nerve compression may occur when fluorosis affects the skull base foramina.

Some patients develop hyperparathyroidism for unknown reasons. It is thought that the resistance of the osteoclastic activity by the sclerotic bones causes parathyroid hormone overactivity.

Diagnosis is confirmed by detecting high level of fluoride in the urine (main path of fluoride excretion), serum, and bone. A 24 h sampling of urine is the most reliable method for confirming fluorosis. The serum alkaline phosphatase level is usually high.

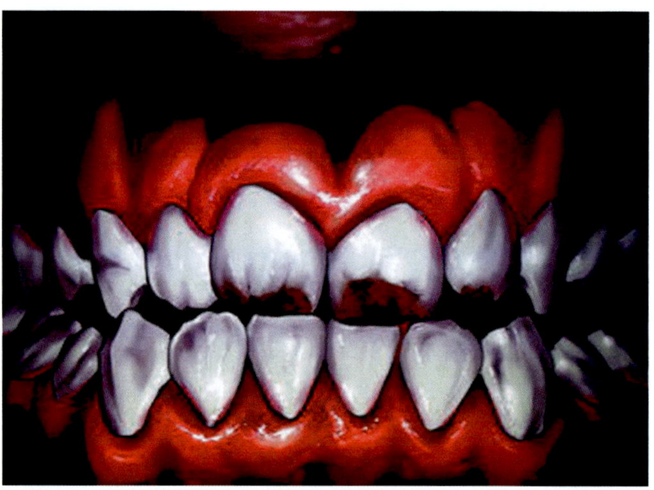

◘ **Fig. 3.7.1**    An illustration demonstrates the clinical appearance of dental fluorosis

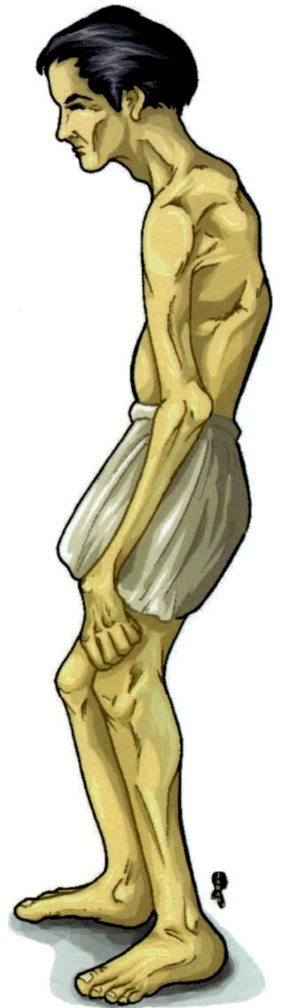

◘ **Fig. 3.7.2**    An illustration demonstrates a patient with poker back due to fluorosis

## Signs on Radiographs

- The axial skeleton is mainly affected in the form of sclerosis of the trabecular bone and thinning of the cortical bone, mostly affecting the vertebrae and the iliac wings (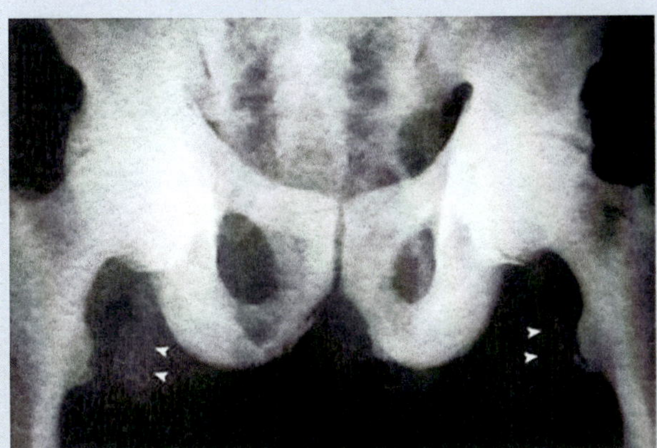 Fig. 3.7.3). Although the pelvis shows sclerosis, the long bones may show osteopenia. A theory to explain this finding states that bones which accumulate fluoride are resistant to the osteoclastic activity of bone remodeling. The hyperparathyroidism resulting from fluorosis causes high resorption of the long bones which do not contain fluorosis, but not of the sclerotic axial bones. This may explain the mixed sclerotic–osteoporotic radiological picture seen in fluorosis.
- Subperiosteal new bone formation causes the long bones to become uneven ( Fig. 3.7.4).
- Ligament calcification is a very characteristic sign of fluorosis, affecting commonly the sacrotuberous and the petroclinoid ligaments. Paravertebral ligament calcification causes vertebral column restriction ( Fig. 3.7.5).
- Prominence of the occipital protuberance with formation of exostosis occasionally is another minor manifestation.

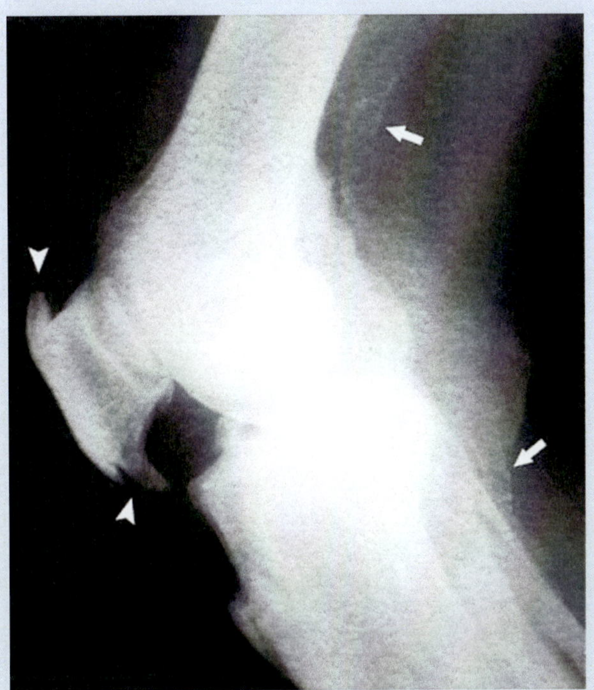

**Fig. 3.7.4** Lateral knee radiograph of the same patient shows diffuse sclerosis with sclerosis and osteophytes formation of the quadriceps and patellar tendons insertion at the superior and the inferior poles of the patella (*arrowheads*). Sclerosis of the popliteal vessels can be observed too (*arrows*)

**Fig. 3.7.3** Anteroposterior pelvis radiograph shows severe systemic fluorosis with diffuse skeletal sclerosis. Calcification can be seen affecting even the femoral vessels (*arrowheads*)

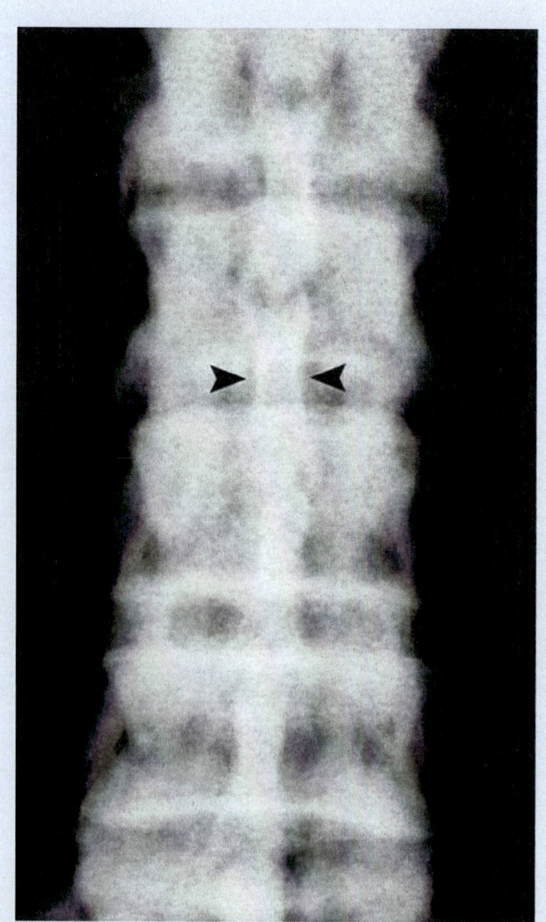

**Fig. 3.7.5** Anteroposterior plain radiograph of the thoracic spines of the same patient shows severe vertebral and paravertebral ligaments sclerosis (poker back). Calcification of the supraspinous ligament results in the classical "dagger sign" that is usually seen in ankylosing spondylitis (*arrowheads*)

## Further Reading

Boillat MA et al. Radiological criteria of industrial fluorosis. Skeletal Radiol. 1980;5:161–5.

Gupta RK et al. Compressive myelopathy in fluorosis: MRI. Neuroradiology. 1996;38:338–42.

Lian Z-C et al. Osteoporosis – an early radiographic sign of endemic fluorosis. Skeletal Radiol. 1986;15:350–3.

Mithal A et al. Radiological spectrum of endemic fluorosis: relationship with calcium intake. Skeletal Radiol. 1993;22:257–61.

Tamer MN et al. Osteosclerosis due to endemic fluorosis. Sci Total Environ. 2007;373:43–8.

Whyte MP et al. Skeletal fluorosis and instant tea. Am J Med. 2005;118:78–82.

## 3.8   Lead Poisoning (Plumbism)

Lead poisoning is a clinical condition which arises either due to direct ingestion of the lead metal compounds (e.g., in water) or by inhalation of lead oxide fumes. Ingestion of lead compounds is often seen in children, whereas in adults it is often due to occupational lead inhalation. In children, lead toxicity can be also due to pica (e.g., dirt eating), inhalation of toxic fumes, or ingestion of lead-based paints.

The effect of lead poisoning is mainly noticed in the growing bone. When lead is ingested or inhaled, its ions deposit on the hydroxyapatite crystal preferentially in the zone of provisional calcification in the growth plate (physis). Lead mainly inhibits osteoclastic remodeling without affecting the osteoblasts, resulting in an increase in the thickness and the trabeculae at the metaphyses. This is seen on plain radiographs as a dense band of bones at the metaphyses of long bones (dense metaphyseal band sign).

Dense metaphyseal band sign may be seen as a normal variant in healthy children following prolonged exposure to sunlight. The cause of this phenomenon is unknown, but it may involve overproduction of endogenous vitamin D. Other causes of dense metaphyseal band sign include vitamin D toxicity, congenital hypothyroidism, and recovery from scurvy.

### Signs on Radiograph
- Dense metaphyseal bands are seen as thick radio-opaque bone at the metaphysis of long bones, especially at the wrists and knees. All of the other bone structures are normal (**Fig. 3.8.1**).
- The presence of a dense metaphyseal band at the proximal fibula is a strong indication of lead toxicity.

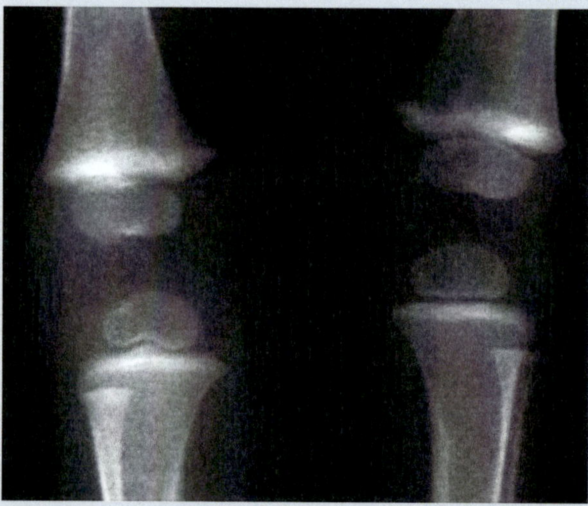

**Fig. 3.8.1** Anteroposterior plain radiograph of both knees in a child with lead poisoning shows dense metaphyseal band sign in the distal femur and the proximal tibia of both knees. The right proximal fibular metaphysis shows also the dense metaphyseal band as a strong indication of lead poisoning

## Further Reading

Blickman JG et al. The radiologic "lead band" revisited. AJR Am J Roentgenol. 1986;146:245–7.
Nagaraj BR et al. A rare case of lead poisoning – a case report. Indian J Radiol Imaging. 2005;15:67–8.
Raber SA. The dense metaphyseal band sign. Radiology. 1999;211:773–4.
Wiwanitkit V et al. Lead intoxication: a summary of the clinical presentation among Thai patients. Biometals. 2006;19:345–8.

## 3.9    Adrenal Glands Abnormalities

The adrenal glands are a pair of retroperitoneal endocrinal glands located above the kidneys. Each gland is composed of a cortex derived from the mesoderm and a medulla derived from the neural crest.

The cortex is composed of three layers: *zona fasciculate* that secretes cortisol, *zona glomerulosa* that secretes aldosterone, and *zona reticularis* that secretes androgens. The medulla secretes epinephrine and norepinephrine. Adrenal masses are divided into functioning and nonfunctioning tumors depending on whether they secrete hormones or not.

*Cortical bodies* are islands of ectopic chromaffin tissues (adrenal cortical tissues) found in the broad ligament of the uterus, spermatic cord, or epididymis. A tumor of the ectopic adrenal tissues is called *paraganglioma*. Paragangliomas can be found in the paraspinal region, in the pineal gland, and in the urinary bladder.

On MRI and CT, the thickness of the adrenal limbs can be compared with the thickness of the adjacent diaphragmatic crus. The normal glands width should not exceed that of the adjacent diaphragmatic crus (normally <5 mm). Both adrenals are found at the level of T12. The right gland is located posterior to the IVC, while the left gland is adherent to the left diaphragmatic crus.

## Cushing's Syndrome

Cushing's syndrome (CS) is a disease characterized by multiple systemic manifestations due to chronic exposure to excess glucocorticoids, often due to adrenal hyperplasia. *Cushing's disease* is a pathological condition with similar clinical manifestations as CS, but it arises due to increase glucocorticoid production secondary to an adrenocorticotropic hormone (ACTH)-secreting pituitary adenoma. *Pseudo-Cushing's syndrome* is a term used to describe any condition that results in distortion of the hypothalamic–pituitary–adrenal axis.

The clinical manifestations of CS are attributed to the chronic exposure to glucocorticoids; however, none of these symptoms or signs is pathognomonic of the syndrome. Progressive central obesity is the most common sign of CS. Fat accumulation in the cheeks results in a "moon" face appearance. Enlarged fat pads that fill the supraclavicular fossae and obscure the clavicles making the neck appear

shortened are characteristic signs of CS. Up to 5 % of patients have increased retro-orbital fat content that may cause exophthalmos.

Hypertension, menstrual abnormalities, oligomenorrhea, insomnia, and impaired short-term memory are well-known manifestations of CS. In obese persons and patients with CS, renal pelvis lipomatosis may develop. *Renal pelvis lipomatosis* is a condition characterized by excess proliferation of the encapsulated fat cells in the renal pelvis. The proliferated fat causes mass effect on the intrarenal collecting system but rarely leads to symptoms. *Replacement lipomatosis of the kidney* is an uncommon extreme form of renal pelvis lipomatosis where the lipomatosis is accompanied by atrophied or destructed kidney.

Skin manifestations include skin atrophy, easy bruisability, and purple cutaneous striae due to skin stretching. Hyperpigmentation can be seen in CS due to increased ACTH release, which induces melanocytes pigment overproduction. When CS is associated with excess androgens secretion, oily skin, acne, increased libido, female virilization, and temporal balding may be seen.

### Differential Diagnoses and Related Diseases

*Nelson's syndrome* is a rare disease characterized by skin hyperpigmentation after bilateral CS adrenalectomy. The main mechanism of development of this condition can be explained by hyperactive pituitary function. The loss of the partial cortisol inhibition on the pituitary ACTH secretion after adrenalectomy causes the pituitary to secrete a very large amount of ACTH that may promote growth of an anterior pituitary adenoma. Serum ACTH levels are excessively high in patients with Nelson's syndrome. The prevalence of Nelson's syndrome after bilateral adrenalectomy ranges from 8 to 29 %, with a time interval between the adrenalectomy and the development of the disease ranging from 6 months to 24 years.

### Signs on Skeletal Radiographs

Osteoporosis and pathological bone fractures are commonly seen in chronic cases of CS due to the osteolytic effect of glucocorticoids on the bones.

### Signs on CT and MRI

- Adrenal hyperplasia is checked by detecting bilateral increased thickness of the adrenal limbs (>5 mm). The adrenal limbs appear thicker than the adjacent diaphragmatic crus, with the preservation of the gland's general shape (◘ Fig. 3.9.1).

- In Cushing's disease and Nelson's syndrome, anterior pituitary adenoma is often found (◘ Fig. 3.9.2).
- Renal pelvis lipomatosis shows proliferation of hypodense fat at the renal pelvis. Replacement lipomatosis of the kidney is seen as a fatty mass at the renal pelvis with markedly atrophied renal parenchyma (◘ Fig. 3.9.3).

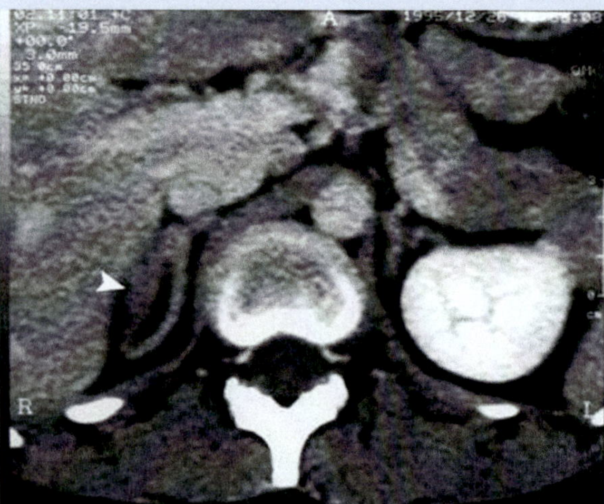

◘ **Fig. 3.9.1**  Axial postcontrast CT image of a patient with adrenal hyperplasia shows enlargement of the lateral limb of the right adrenal gland (*arrowhead*)

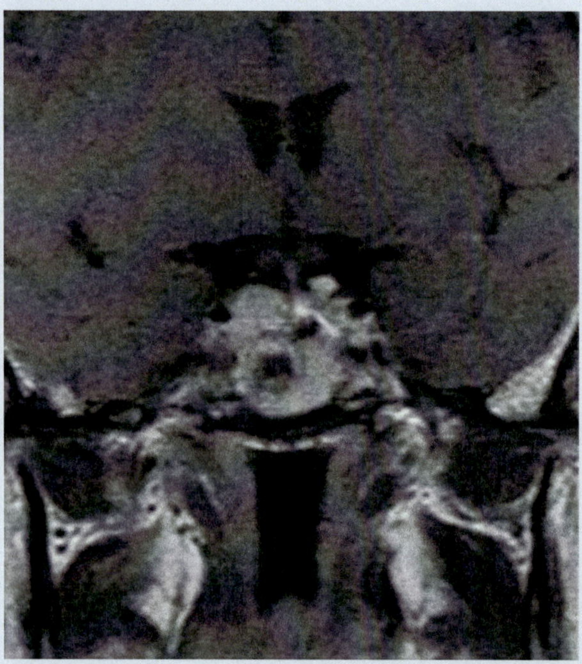

◘ **Fig. 3.9.2**  Coronal T1W postcontrast MRI of the sellas shows large pituitary adenoma with inner cystic changes and infiltration of the left cavernous sinus in a patient with Nelson's syndrome. The patient had bilateral adrenalectomy in 1994, and he developed pituitary adenoma in 2006

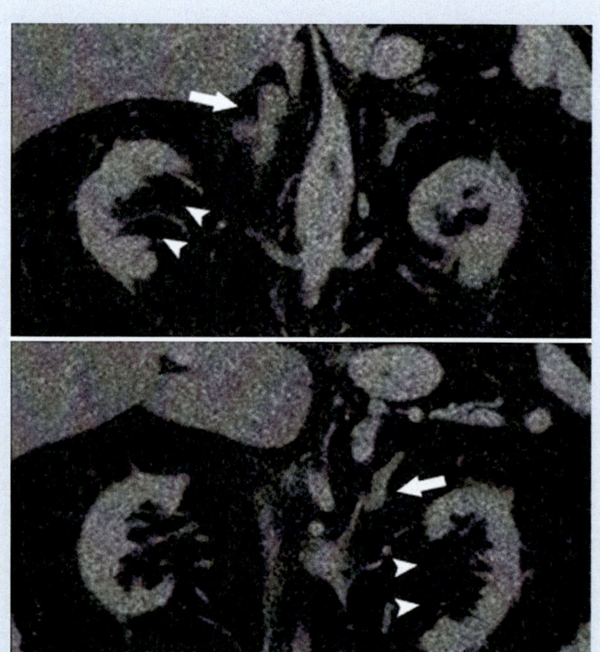

◘ **Fig. 3.9.3**  Coronal sequential nonenhanced CT images of another patient with Cushing's syndrome (CS) show bilateral renal pelvis lipomatosis (*arrowheads*) and bilateral adrenal hyperplasia (*arrows*). Notice how the right adrenal gland is markedly thickened

## Conn's Syndrome (Hyperaldosteronism)

Conn's syndrome is a clinical pathological condition characterized by hypertension and hypokalemia due to excess secretion of aldosterone. Conn's syndrome commonly arises due to adrenal adenoma (80 %) or adrenal hyperplasia (20 %).

Aldosterone secretion is mainly stimulated by plasma sodium depletion. Acute hemorrhage is a potent stimulus for aldosterone secretion. Aldosterone facilitates sodium absorption and facilitates potassium excretion in the kidney. Increased aldosterone secretion can occur in some conditions that are not related to a true pathology such as anxiety, adaptation to hot weather, high potassium intake, low sodium intake, and pregnancy (second and third trimesters).

### Differential Diagnoses and Related Diseases
- *Liddle syndrome* is a rare autosomal dominant pediatric disorder characterized by failure to thrive, hypertension, metabolic alkalosis, hypokalemia, and an abnormally decreased rate of aldosterone and renin secretion. In this disease, the nephron acts as if it were exposed to a large amount of aldosterone even when the aldosterone is absent. Children with Liddle syndrome present classically with a triad of hypertension, hypokalemia, and metabolic alkalosis.

- *Gordon syndrome* is a rare autosomal dominant disease characterized by hypertension, hyperkalemia, hyperchloremia, and normal renal glomerular function. Inconstant features include short stature and muscle weakness. The basic abnormality is related to excessive renal sodium retention, causing suppression of renin and aldosterone.
- *Bartter syndrome* is a disease characterized by hyperplasia of the juxtaglomerular apparatus and hyperreninism leading to secondary hyperaldosteronism, metabolic alkalosis, severe hypokalemia, and normal blood pressure. Up to 80 % of patients have peculiar facies, distinguished by triangular face, large eyes, and protruded ears. A milder form of Bartter syndrome associated with hypocalciuria and hypomagnesemia is called *Gitelman syndrome*.

**Signs on CT**
- Adrenal hyperplasia: like CS.
- Adrenal carcinoma shows focal nodular enlargement of one or more adrenal limbs (>5 mm), with contrast enhancement after contrast injection. Regional lymphadenopathy may be found.

## Addison's Disease

Addison's disease (AD) is a clinical condition that arises due to decreased or absent glucocorticoids.

AD typically results from adrenal hypofunction, usually when >90 % of the gland cortex is destroyed. Patients with AD often present with hypotension, salt-craving, and hyperpigmentation due to increase ACTH secretion from the pituitary. The most common causes of AD are tuberculosis and autoimmune diseases. The disease is diagnosed by clinical picture and biochemistry, not by imaging. Imaging is often used to confirm the bilateral adrenal atrophy.

**Differential Diagnoses and Related Diseases**
- *Wolman's disease* is a rare neonatal, autosomal recessive, lysosomal storage disorder that manifests within the first week of life as striking hepatosplenomegaly, poor feeding, abdominal distension, and loose stool and vomiting. Liver cirrhosis and pulmonary failure may occur later in life due to lipid storage disease. Death usually occurs within the first year of life.
- *Allgrove syndrome* (*triple A syndrome*) is a rare disease characterized by *a*drenal hypoplasia and insufficiency, *a*chalasia, and *a*lacrima (lacks of teardrops). The disease has an autosomal recessive mode of inheritance, and it is one of the ACTH insensitivity inherited diseases. Patients usually develop adrenal insufficiency (AD) in the first two decades of life. In contrast, symptoms of achalasia start from the early 6 months of age or early childhood.
- *Triple H syndrome* is a disease characterized by dysfunctional triad of the hypothalamic–pituitary axis (e.g., isolated ACTH deficiency), the hippocampus (e.g., impairment of anterograde memory), and hair follicles (e.g., alopecia universalis).

**Signs on CT**
- Whether the cause is tuberculosis or autoimmunity, both glands typically appear shrunken with calcifications due to chronic destruction and atrophy (Fig. 3.9.4).
- In *Wolman's disease*, CT of the abdomen examination shows hepatosplenomegaly with bilateral adrenal calcifications. The clinical picture plus the CT findings are usually sufficient to confirm the diagnosis of Wolman's disease.
- In *Allgrove syndrome*, CT usually shows bilateral adrenal hypoplasia like AD but often in a child patient.

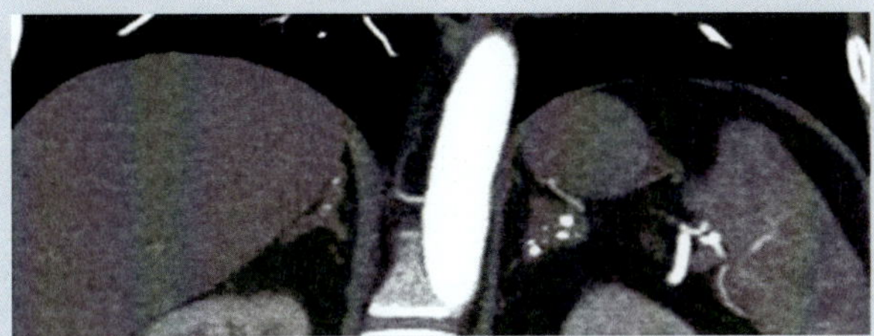

**Fig. 3.9.4** Coronal postcontrast CT image of a patient with Addison's disease (AD) shows bilateral adrenal calcification (classical finding)

## Pheochromocytoma

Pheochromocytoma is an adrenal medullary tumor that arises from chromaffin cells of the sympathetic system with increase secretion of catecholamine.

Pheochromocytoma is one of the most common causes of malignant hypertension. It is usually suspected in a young patient (<30 years) with history of hypertension. Classic pheochromocytoma symptoms are summarized by 5 Ps: high blood pressure, *pain* (abdomen or heart), *perspiration, palpitation,* and *panic* attacks.

Pheochromocytoma has a classical "rule of 10 %": 10 % bilateral, 10 % inherited as autosomal dominant, 10 % extra-adrenal (paragangliomas), and 10 % occurring with von Hippel–Lindau syndrome.

Extra-adrenal intra-abdominal pheochromocytoma is usually detected in the para-aortic area at the level of the celiac axis and the renal hilum, paracaval area at the level of the renal hilum, and the retrocaval area.

Rarely, paraganglioma may be found in the bladder wall. Patients present with signs of pheochromocytoma during micturition due to catecholamine release during *micturition attack*, and it is seen in 50 % of cases. Although most cases of bladder paragangliomas are sporadic, they can be associated with phakomatosis (e.g., von Hippel–Lindau syndrome).

— Bladder paraganglioma is detected usually as a single mass with well-defined or lobulated border that may show cystic necrosis and circumferential ring calcification (highly suggestive).

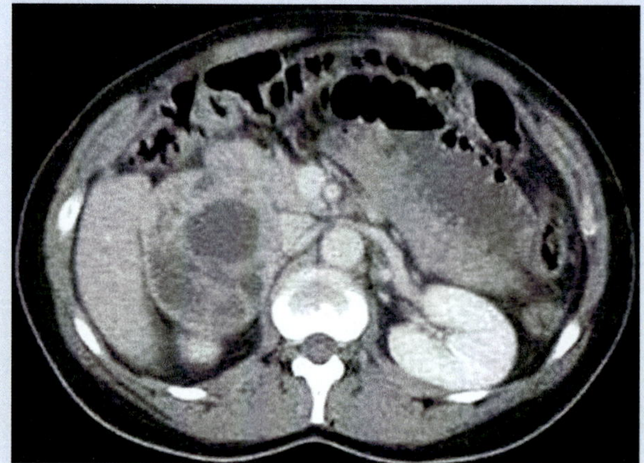

**Fig. 3.9.5**  Axial, delayed postcontrast CT image of a patient with pheochromocytoma shows large mass in the area of the adrenal gland with multiple cystic changes inside the mass

### Signs on CT

— Pheochromocytoma is detected as round, homogeneous adrenal mass with intense contrast enhancement due to hypervascularity. The mass can show internal calcifications or cystic changes (**Fig. 3.9.5**). Rarely, pheochromocytoma can present like a cystic mass that mimics hydrated cyst (cystic pheochromocytoma).

### Signs on MRI

Pheochromocytoma shows typically low T1 signal intensity and intense high T2 signal intensity and marked contrast enhancement after contrast injection (**Fig. 3.9.6**). The fact that pheochromocytoma has intense T2 signal intensity is useful to detect ectopic paragangliomas, which shows the same MR signal characteristics.

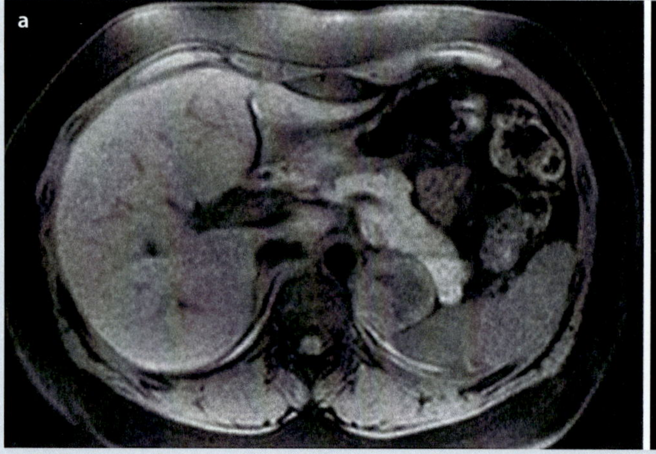
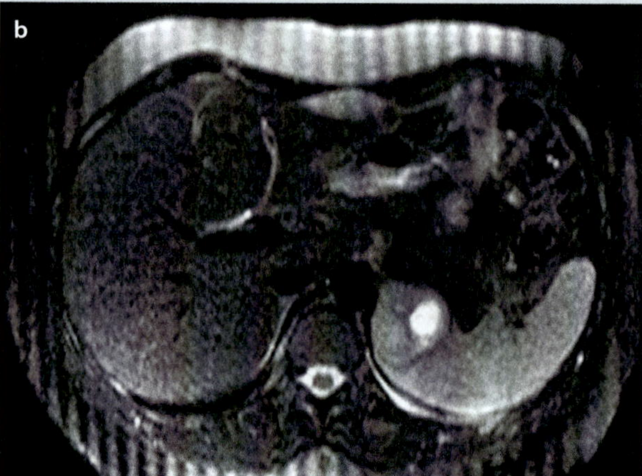

**Fig. 3.9.6**  Axial T1W (**a**) and T2W (**b**) nonenhanced MRI of a patient with left adrenal pheochromocytoma shows low signal intensity tumor in (**a**) and the intense T2 signal intensity of the tumor in (**b**)

## Neuroblastoma

Neuroblastoma is a pediatric malignant tumor that arises from immature neuroblasts from the adrenal medulla or the sympathetic chain. When the tumor histopathologically contains mature ganglion cells, it is called *ganglioneuroblastoma*. Both tumors are usually diagnosed <10 years of age.

Neuroblastoma constitutes for up to 15 % of childhood cancer fatalities, and it is the second most common retroperitoneal mass in children after Wilms' tumor (nephroblastoma). The most common complaint is pain or abdominal fullness. Other uncommon symptoms include Horner's syndrome, limping, or irritability due to metastasis (Hutchinson's syndrome).

> **Differential Diagnoses and Related Diseases**
> - *Hutchinson's syndrome* is characterized by neuroblastoma, extensive skeletal metastasis (especially skull), bone pain, and proptosis due to orbital metastasis.
> - *Pepper syndrome* is characterized by neuroblastoma and hepatomegaly due to extensive metastases.

> **Signs on CT and MRI**
> Neuroblastoma is detected as a large posterior mediastinal, pelvic, or retroperitoneal mass with calcification, cystic changes, or hemorrhage. A fluid–fluid level within the cystic changes indicates hemorrhage within the tumor. Rib or pedicular erosions can be seen in cases of mediastinal neuroblastoma. A full metastasis workup by scintigraphy, PET/CT, or whole-body MRI should be performed.

## X-Linked Adrenoleukodystrophy

X-linked adrenoleukodystrophy (ALD) is X-linked recessive, peroxisomal disease characterized by accumulation of very long chain of fatty acids (called birefringent striations) within the brain, the adrenal cortex, and the testicular interstitial glands. Adrenal insufficiency (AD) occurs in 10 % of cases.

ALD is both demyelinating and dysmyelinating disease. Demyelinating diseases are characterized by the formation of normal myelin, and then the myelin is destroyed. In contrast, dysmyelinating diseases are characterized by the formation of abnormal nonfunctioning myelin.

Pathologically, ALD is characterized by "three zone of demyelination": the outer zone is made of external actively demyelinating white matter; the middle zone is made of inflammatory demyelinating process in varying stages with inflammatory cell infiltration (sudanophilic macrophages); and the central inner zone is made up of burned-out axons with gliotic scar. Initially, ALD affects the parieto-occipital area. As the disease progresses, the temporal and frontal areas are affected too.

Male children with ALD often present between 4 and 8 years of age with progressive disturbance of gait, disturbance in vision and hearing, gradual deterioration in school work, behavioral changes, and dementia.

> **Signs on CT**
> - Low-density white matter affecting mainly the occipital lobes and corpus callosum (almost always).
> - Frontal and temporal lobes might be affected in advanced stages of the disease.

> **Signs on MRI**
> - Variable high T2 signal intensities affecting the occipitoparietal lobes bilaterally and symmetrically representing the three zones of demyelination (almost pathognomonic appearance) (◘ Fig. 3.9.7).
> - Contrast enhancement occurs in the early acute phases along the outer margin of the demyelinating area (outer zones), while the center does not enhance (gliotic inner zone).
> - MR spectroscopy shows low *N*-acetylcysteine concentration and high choline, glutamate, and glutamine concentrations.

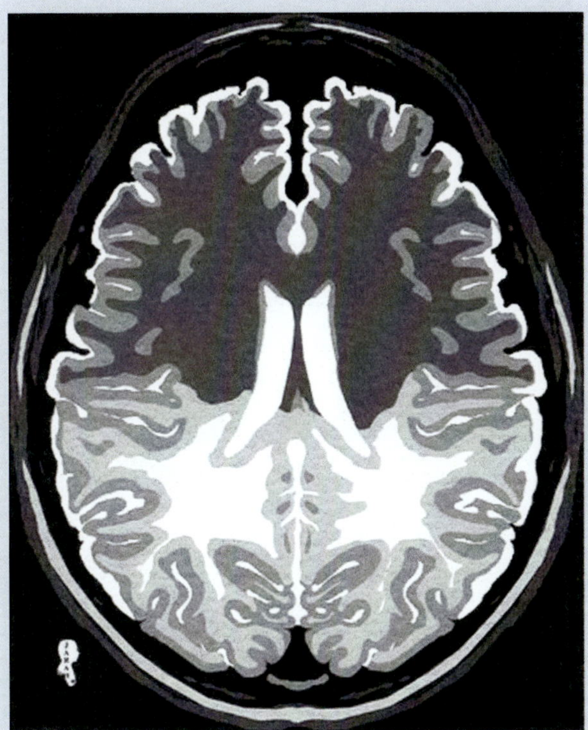

◘ **Fig. 3.9.7** Axial brain T2W MR illustration shows the three areas of demyelination in bilateral parieto-occipital area typically seen in X-linked adrenoleukodystrophy (ALD)

## Testicular Adrenal Rest Tumors

During embryogenesis, development of the primitive adrenal cortex occurs close to the gonads. Testicular adrenal rest tumors (TARTs) are tumors that arise from aberrant adrenal cortical tissues located in the testes from the primitive adrenal cortex residuals.

TARTs are usually felt as palpable testicular mass. The aberrant testicular adrenal rests may proliferate and grow in conditions with high ACTH levels like congenital adrenal hyperplasia, AD, Nelson's syndrome, and CS. In congenital adrenal hyperplasia, neonates present with bilateral testicular masses with or without salt wasting. TARTs can lead to precocious puberty and male infertility in patients with congenital adrenal hyperplasia.

### Signs on US
TARTs are seen as multifocal, possibly bilateral hypoechoic masses within the testes. The masses may be mistaken for tumors or infarctions.

### Signs on MRI
TARTS are detected as bilateral low T1 and T2 signal intensity lesions with marked contrast enhancement after contrast injection ( Fig. 3.9.8).

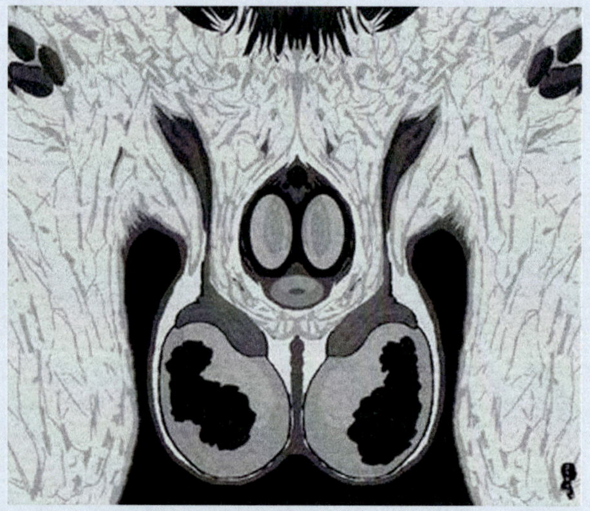

 **Fig. 3.9.8**   Coronal T2W MR illustration shows bilateral low T2 signal intensity lesions demonstrating testicular adrenal rest tumors

### Further Reading

A. J et al. Luetscher. Aldosteronism. Dis Mon 1964;10(5): 1–46.

Assadi FK et al. Liddle syndrome in a newborn infant. Pediatr Nephrol. 2002;17:609–11.

Assie G et al. The Nelson's syndrome…revisited. Pituitary. 2004;7:209–15.

Dogra V et al. Sonographic appearance of testicular adrenal rest tissue in congenital adrenal hyperplasia. J Ultrasound Med. 2004;23:979–81.

Elsayes KM et al. Adrenal masses: MR imaging features with pathologic correlation. Radiographics. 2004;24:S73–6.

Garel L et al. Nephrocalcinosis in Bartter's syndrome. Pediatr Nephrol. 1988;2:315–7.

Juan YH et al. Adrenal nodular hyperplasia with so called testicular tumor of adrenogenital syndrome (adrenal rests of both testes): a case report and review of the literature. Chin J Radiol. 2008;33:41–6.

Kannan CR. Diseases of the adrenal cortex. Dis Mon. 1988;34:601.

Kasar PA et al. Allgrove syndrome. Indian J Pediatr. 2007;74:959–61.

Lockhart ME et al. Imaging of adrenal masses. Eur J Radiol. 2002;41:95–112.

Low G et al. Characteristic imaging findings in Wolman's disease. Clin Radiol Extra. 2004;59:106–8.

Ma ES et al. Tuberculous Addison's disease: morphological and quantitative evaluation with multidetector-row CT. Eur J Radiol. 2007;62:352–8.

Madrigal G et al. Bartter syndrome in Costa Rica: a description of 20 cases. Pediatr Nephrol. 1997;11:296–301.

Martinez-Aguayo A et al. Testicular adrenal rest tumors and Leydig and Sertoli cell function in boys with classical congenital adrenal hyperplasia. J Clin Endocrinol Metab. 2007;92:4583–9.

Mayo-Smith WW et al. From the RSNA refresher courses, state-of-the-art adrenal imaging. Radiographics. 2001;21:995–1012.

Otal P et al. Imaging features of uncommon adrenal masses with histopathologic correlation. Radiographics. 1999;19:569–81.

Puura A et al. Gordon syndrome and succinylcholine. J Inherit Metab Dis. 2005;28:1157–8.

Renken NS et al. Magnetic resonance imaging of the adrenal glands. Semin Ultrasound CT MR. 2005;26:162–71.

Rha SS et al. The renal sinus: pathologic spectrum and multimodality imaging approach. Radiographics. 2004;24: S117–31.

Shoaib SA et al. Primary hyperaldosteronism (Conne syndrome): MR imaging findings. Radiology. 2000;214:527–31.

Stikkelbroeck NMML et al. Testicular adrenal rest tumors. Eur Radiol. 2003;13:1597–603.

Waragi M et al. MRI of adrenoleukodystrophy involving predominantly the cerebellum and brain stem. Neuroradiology. 1996;38:788–91.

## 3.10   Sex Hormone Abnormalities

There are multiple pathological conditions that result in abnormalities in the estrogen–androgen levels in both males and females. Androgen is a term that refers to a compound, natural or synthetic, that controls or maintains the male masculine characteristics.

Radiology can help establish the diagnosis of many endocrinal pathological conditions that are related to abnormal levels of estrogen and androgen when combined with the clinical history, clinical examination, and laboratory investigations.

## Polycystic Ovary Disease (Stein–Leventhal Syndrome)

Polycystic ovary disease (PCOD) results from inability of the mature follicular cyst to release its ova, resulting in formation of a follicular cyst.

Women with PCOD commonly present with amenorrhea, anovulation, infertility, and hirsutism; the latter symptom is due to increased levels of androgen. Criteria to diagnose PCO require two of the following features with exclusion of other causes:

- Presence of polycystic ovaries confirmed by ultrasound or MRI.
- Elevated levels of estrogen and androgen, with low levels of follicle-stimulating hormone (FSH) and luteinizing hormone (LH).
- Oligomenorrhea or amenorrhea. Up to 80 % of women with oligomenorrhea have PCOD.

> **Signs on MRI**
> The typical feature of PCOD includes bilateral slightly enlarged ovaries with low-intensity central stroma accompanied by multiple, small (<1 cm) follicular cysts arranged at the peripheries (◘ Fig. 3.10.1). Enlargement of the central stroma is an important sign differentiating this condition from other conditions with follicular cysts (e.g., ovarian hyperstimulating syndrome).

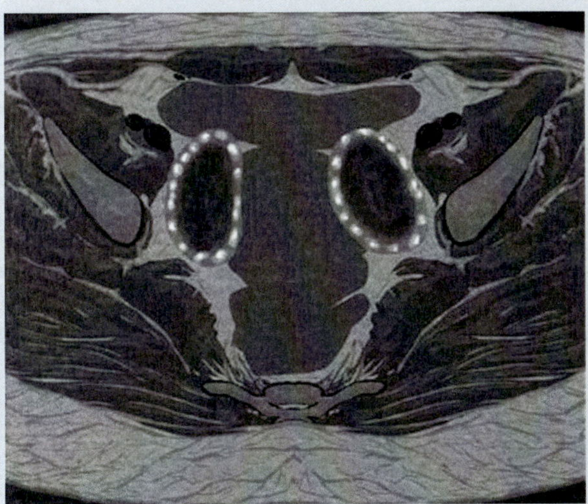

◘ **Fig. 3.10.1** Axial T2W fat-sat MR illustration demonstrates polycystic ovary disease (PCOD) seen as bilateral ovarian central hypointense stroma surrounded by peripheral multiple small cysts

## Precocious Puberty

Precocious puberty is a condition characterized by premature development of secondary sexual characteristics before 8.5 years in girls and 9.5 years in boys. Delayed female puberty is defined as a girl who shows no signs of secondary sexual characteristics by the age of 13 or absence of menstruation after age of 15. In contrast, delayed male puberty is defined as a male who shows no signs of secondary sexual characteristics by the age of 14.

Puberty is initiated by increasing the release of hypothalamic secretion of gonadotropin-releasing hormone (GnRH), which stimulates the release of anterior pituitary gonadotropins (LH and FSH). The gonadotropic hormones stimulate Leydig cells in males to release testosterone and ovarian follicles in females to release estrogen.

Precocious puberty is divided into isosexual and heterosexual from a clinical standpoint. *Isosexual precocious puberty* refers to physical sexual development that is appropriate to the individual (e.g., female with early feminine characteristics). In contrast, *heterosexual precocious puberty* refers to physical changes that are consistent with those of the opposite sex (e.g., female with early male characteristics).

Isosexual precocious puberty is further divided into two types: central or true (gonadotropin dependent) and peripheral or incomplete (gonadotropin independent). Central precocious puberty (CPP) arises due to an increase in the release of gonadotropin and sex steroids due to premature activation of the hypothalamic–pituitary axis. In contrast, peripheral precocious puberty (PPP) arises due to excess release of gonadal sex steroids due to a peripheral cause (e.g., adrenal tumor).

CPP is characterized by true isosexual physical characteristics and gonads maturation. The girl exhibits all features of true puberty. In contrast, PPP is characterized by early secondary sexual characteristics without gonads maturation (incomplete). Maturation is incomplete with usually only one type of sexual characteristic developing early. In girls, if ovarian estrogen secretion predominates, breast development is the major manifestation of precocious puberty (premature thelarche). In contrast, if adrenal steroid secretion and early and rogenization predominate, pubic hair development in the absence of virilization is the major manifestation of precocious puberty (premature adrenarche). In summary, PPP indicates that the sexual development is not mediated by the pituitary gland.

In CPP, a disease, often a tumor, results in the early activation of the hypothalamic–pituitary axis. This early activation releases GnRH from the hypothalamus, which facilitates the release of FSH and LH from the adenohypophysis. The most common central lesion causing CPP is hypothalamic and tuber cinereum hamartomas. Hamartoma is defined as a group of normal cells in an abnormal configuration.

Radiological evaluation of a child with precocious puberty should include bone age assessment, ultrasound for the testes or the ovaries to exclude tumors, and MRI of the sella.

### Differential Diagnoses and Related Diseases

*McCune–Albright syndrome* is a rare disease which affects young females characterized by polyostotic fibrous dysplasia, precocious puberty, and skin hyperpigmentation (café au lait spots).

### Signs on Plain Radiographs

Bone age determination is an important step in evaluating a precocious puberty patient. Children with premature adrenarche or thelarche often show normal or slightly advanced bone age.

### Signs on US

- In true precocious puberty, both testes are enlarged in males, and both ovaries are enlarged in females. In PPP, a tumor may be found in the testes or the ovaries.
- Patients with McCune–Albright syndrome show large asymmetric ovaries bilaterally. The ovarian volume is the largest among all types of causes of precocious puberty (e.g., >4 cm³). This large volume is often due to single or multiple cystic lesions with autonomous hormonal secretion.

### Signs on MRI

Tuber cinereum hamartoma is seen as an isointense lesion, up to 2 cm in diameter, and is located at the region of the tuber cinereum, which lies between the pituitary stalk and the mammillary bodies. The lesion has low T1 and high T2 signal intensities and does not enhance after contrast administration (because they are normal cells but disorganized) (◘ Fig. 3.10.2).

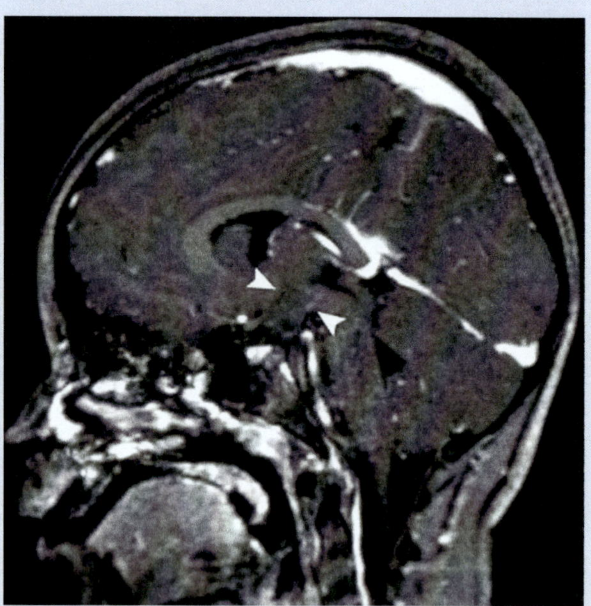

◘ **Fig. 3.10.2**   Sagittal T1W postcontrast image of a patient with tuber cinereum hamartoma shows a lesion (*arrowheads*) located at the area of the tuber cinereum of the hypothalamus with no contrast enhancement

## Van Wyk and Grumbach Syndrome

Van Wyk and Grumbach syndrome (VWGS) is a disease of young girls characterized by precocious puberty due to overproduction of FSH and LH and delayed bone maturation due to juvenile hypothyroidism.

The patient typically is a female child presenting with breast enlargement, enlarged labia minora, and estrogenic changes in vaginal smear, with absence of pubic hair. Irregular vaginal bleeding and spontaneous ovarian hyperstimulation syndrome (*hyperraction luteinaris*) may be seen. Hyperraction luteinaris is a condition characterized by high serum levels of human chorionic gonadotropins (hCG) due to an intrinsic cause like normal pregnancy or gestational trophoblastic disease (e.g., hydatidiform mole). The same condition is often produced in females receiving exogenous hCG to induce ovulation.

Patients with VWGS suffer from juvenile hypothyroidism with delayed bone maturation in the first place. The lower level of thyroid hormone may provoke the hypothalamus to secrete thyroid-stimulating hormone (TSH). The excessive response by elevated TSH can cause pituitary hypertrophy, which in turn secretes higher levels of adenohypophyseal hormones. The excess levels of adenohypophyseal hormones are responsible for the precocious puberty and the other features of the disease.

Laboratory investigations in VWGS characteristically show low thyroxin ($T_4$ and $T_3$) levels, high TSH level, and high FSH and LH levels.

### Signs on Plain Radiograph

Patients with VWGS typically show signs of osseous bone mineralization delay with bone age below their current age when radiographic bone age assessment is carried out. VWGS is the only form of precocious puberty in which the bone age is delayed.

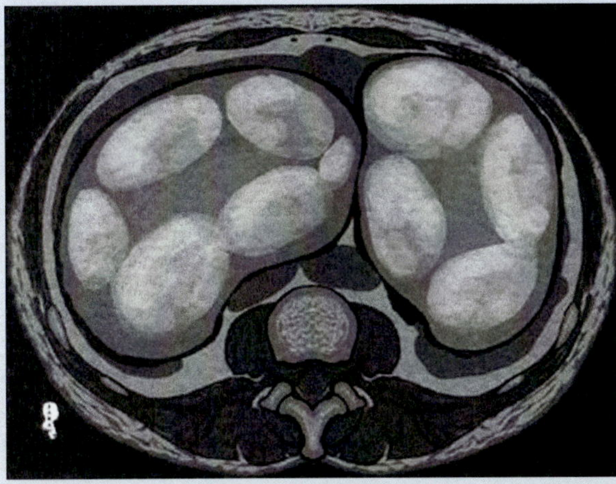

◘ **Fig. 3.10.3** Axial T2W MR illustration demonstrates bilateral enlarged ovaries with large cysts of almost uniform size within (hyperraction luteinaris)

## Gynecomastia

Gynecomastia is defined as benign breast enlargement in males due to proliferation of the glandular breast tissue. In contrast, pseudo-gynecomastia is defined as increase in the breast size in males due to increased breast fatty content (e.g., like in obesity).

Physiological gynecomastia in males is seen in three age peaks. The first is in neonates due to transplacental passage of estrogen. The second is seen in mid-adolescent boys (10–14 years) due to imbalance between serum estrogen and androgen levels. The third is seen in patients aged 50–80 years old.

Pathological gynecomastia is related to increased serum level of estrogen in males or reduced serum androgen level. Causes of pathological gynecomastia can be idiopathic (25 %), drug related in 15 % of cases (e.g., cimetidine), Klinefelter's syndrome, and testicular tumors of the germ cell.

Testicular tumors are rare and classically are divided into germ cell tumors and stromal tumors. Stromal tumors make up approximately 5 % of testicular tumors and may arise from Leydig, Sertoli, theca, granulosa, or lutein cells. When stromal elements coexist with germ cell elements, the tumor is called "gonadoblastoma." Leydig cells are cells that secrete testosterone and are found within the testicular interstitium in males, while Sertoli cells are supporting cells and phago-cytes. They form a junction with one another forming a blood–testis barrier. Sertoli cells are located within the seminiferous tubules in males.

Leydig cell tumors constitute approximately 2 % of testicular tumors and commonly seen in male children between 3 and 6 years old, as well as adults between 30 and 50 years of age. Patients present with painless scrotal swelling, and the tumors are hormonally active in up to 30 % of cases. Serum androgen or estrogen levels are high causing precocious puberty, gynecomastia, or impotence.

Testicular Sertoli cell tumors are rare, and they lead to feminization and gynecomastia in males. A distinct subtype of Sertoli cell tumors is called "large-cell calcifying Sertoli cell tumor," which is found in genetic syndromes like Peutz–Jeghers syndrome and tuberous sclerosis. Sertoli cell tumors may develop metastases in 10–15 % of cases. In women, ovarian Sertoli–Leydig cell tumors are a common cause of virilization in young women.

Primary testicular germ cell tumors may regress spontaneously with formation of distant metastases, a phenomenon known as "burned-out germ cell tumor." The phenomenon is poorly understood and is believed to be caused by high tumor metabolic rate that makes the tumor outgrow its blood supply. Patients present with normal size testes and widespread germ cell tumor metastases, making physicians look for the primary germ cell tumor in extragonadal regions like in the thoracic mediastinum, retroperitoneum, or the pineal gland, which all return negative in the end.

The role of imaging in gynecomastia is reserved to search for tumors that may cause gynecomastia, assuming no other cause is found by history and clinical examination.

### Signs on Plain Radiographs
Gynecomastia is detected as unilateral or bilateral breast shadow enlargement (◘ Fig. 3.10.4).

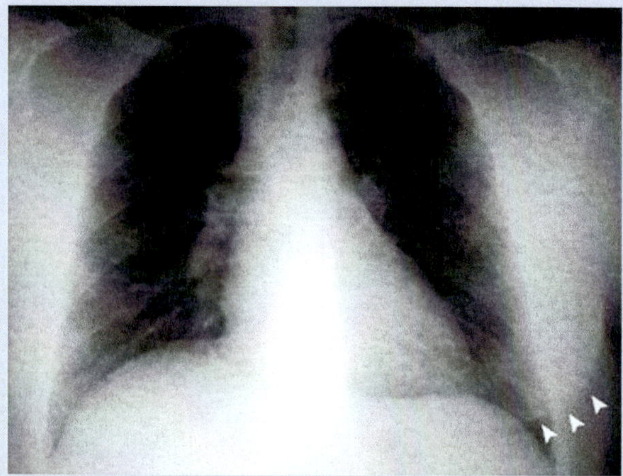

◘ **Fig. 3.10.4**    A plain chest radiograph of a patient with gynecomastia demonstrates unilateral enlarged breast shadow

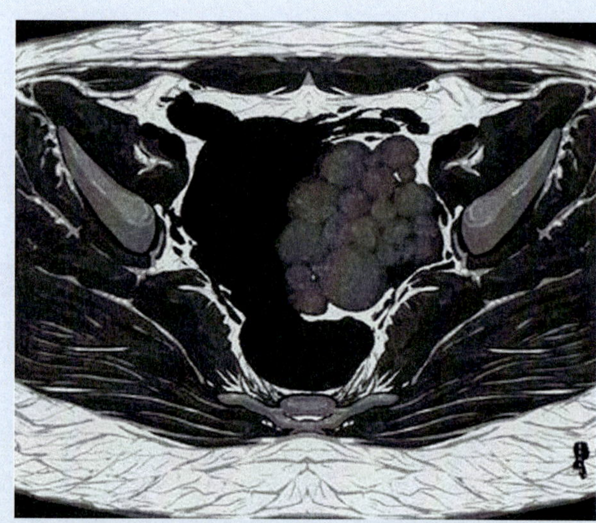

◘ **Fig. 3.10.5**    Axial T1W nonenhanced MR illustration demonstrates left-sided multilobulated ovarian mass with internal small cystic lesions representing ovarian Sertoli cell tumor

### Signs on US
- *Leydig cell tumors* are seen as hypoechoic lesions within the testes with peripheral vascularity on color Doppler sonography. Larger tumors show cystic changes and mixed echo-texture. Large-cell calcifying Leydig cell tumors are detected as multiple areas of high echogenicity with acoustic shadowing representing calcification.
- *Testicular Sertoli cell tumors* are seen usually as bilateral hypoechoic lesions with areas of dense echogenic foci due to calcified scars (burned-out appearance) or as multicystic lesion arranged in a "spoke wheel" configuration.

### Signs on MRI
- *Testicular Sertoli cell tumors* show low T1 and high T2 signal intensity with marked contrast enhancement after contrast injection. History and elevated androgen or estrogen serum levels are important supportive tools for diagnosis.
- *Ovarian Sertoli cell tumor* is detected as unilateral, multilobulated mass with or without internal cysts. The mass can show low T2 signal depending on the extents of fibrous stroma. After contrast injection, the cells show intense heterogeneous contrast enhancement (◘ Fig. 3.10.5).

## Intersex Disorders

Intersex disorders are a group of diseases characterized by ambiguous genitalia and abnormalities in sexual differentiation. *Ambiguous genitalia* are defined as external genitalia that do not have a typical male or female anatomic appearance. A person's phenotypic sex results from the differentiation of the Müllerian ducts and external genitalia under the influence of hormones and transcription factors.

There are four main categories of intersex disorders: female pseudohermaphroditism, gonadal dysgenesis, true hermaphroditism, and male pseudohermaphroditism. Imaging plays a role in detecting abnormalities in the internal pelvic sex organs and early detection of malignant masses formed within these organs. There is an increased prevalence of stromal and gonadal tumors in patients with intersex disorders. Image analysis included evaluation of the presence or absence of the uterus, ovaries, testes, penis, and clitoris.

### Female Pseudohermaphroditism
Female pseudohermaphroditism is a female genetically (46, XX) with two ovaries for gonads, but their external genitalia show a variable degree of virilization due to exposure to excess androgens in utero. *Virilization* refers to male sexual characteristics due to androgen exposure.

Female pseudohermaphroditism most commonly arises due to *congenital adrenal hyperplasia (CAH)*. In CAH, there are enzymatic defects in cortisol production pathway at certain key positions. These enzymatic defects cause excessive accumulation of the intermediate steroid compounds that are produced before the metabolic block. Some of these intermediate steroids are converted into androgenically active substances. This excess androgen exposure causes virilization of the external genitalia, which is manifested commonly as enlarged clitoris (clitoromegaly).

### Signs on US

CAH is seen as enlarged adrenals located above the kidneys with a "cerebriform pattern" (the adrenal glands have multiple coils that look like cerebral gyri). The adrenal gland limbs are commonly over 20 mm long, 4 mm wide, and with normal corticomedullary differentiation.

### Signs on MRI

— MRI demonstrates masculinized external genitalia with normal ovaries, fallopian tubes, uterus, and vagina. The clitoris mimics a small penis due to prominent corpora cavernosa and corpus spongiosum ( Fig. 3.10.6).
— The vagina and the uterus may be filled with urine due to urogenital sinus formation.

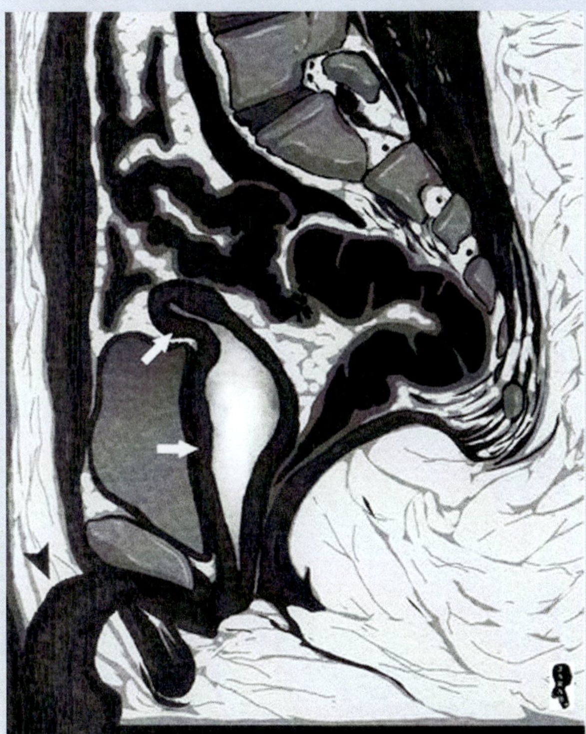

 **Fig. 3.10.6** Sagittal T1W pelvic MR illustration demonstrates enlarged clitoris with prominent corpora cavernosa and corpus spongiosum (*black arrowhead*) with normal vagina and uterus (*white arrows*) in a patient with female pseudohermaphroditism

### Male Pseudohermaphroditism

In male pseudohermaphroditism, patients are genetically male (46, XY) with two testes for gonads, but their external genitalia show a variable degree of feminization due to a defect in the testes or testosterone metabolism.

The phenotype of the male pseudohermaphroditism ranges from completely female external genitalia to a mild male phenotype with hypospadia or cryptorchidism. *Cryptorchidism* is a condition characterized by both abnormal testicular development and failure of the intra-abdominal testes to descend into the scrotum. The testes may be located at any point along the normal descent route. This condition can be seen in up to 30 % in premature infants and up to 8.8 % in full-term infants.

Male pseudohermaphroditism can be classified into eight groups according to the etiology:
— *Leydig cell failure*: Leydig cells are testicular cells that secrete testosterone in males. Failure of testosterone secretion results in male pseudohermaphroditism.
— *Testosterone synthesis defects*: any cause of testosterone synthesis results in male pseudohermaphroditism.
— *Androgen insensitivity syndrome* (AIS) (*Morris syndrome*): this syndrome, also known as *testicular feminization syndrome*, arises due to insensitivity of the body cells to testosterone due to mutation of the steroid-binging receptors. Children with AIS exhibit a female external genitalia, although the karyotype is (46, XY), and testes are located internally. Most patients with AIS are not diagnosed until puberty, when they are investigated for amenorrhea.
— *5α-Reductase deficiency* is an autosomal recessive condition characterized by a defect in conversion of testosterone to the active form dihydrotestosterone through the enzyme 5α-reductase.
— *Persistent Müllerian duct syndrome* (*PMDS*): as mentioned before, Sertoli cells are supporting cells and phagocytes. In the embryo, Sertoli cells secrete anti-Müllerian inhibitory substances that cause apoptosis and regression of the Müllerian ducts, facilitating the male phenotype development. Failure of Sertoli cells to secrete the Müllerian inhibitory substances results in male pseudohermaphroditism.
— *Testicular dysgenesis*: abnormal formation of the testes can result in male pseudohermaphroditism.
— *Congenital anorchia* (*vanishing testes syndrome*) is a disease where the testes are absent. Loss of the testes before 8 weeks' gestation results in a male (46, XY) with female external and internal genitalia. A loss of testes function after the critical male differentiation period at 12–14 weeks' gestation results in a normal male phenotype externally with anorchia internally.
— *Exogenous source*: due to insult to the male development mechanism in utero, often due to maternal ingestion of progesterone or estrogen or various environmental hazards.

## Differential Diagnoses and Related Diseases

- *PAGOD (Mecham) syndrome* is an extremely rare disease characterized by pulmonary artery hypoplasia, agonadism, omphalocele/diaphragm defect, and dextrocardia. Most infants die shortly after birth due to cardiopulmonary problems.
- *Denys–Drash syndrome (DDS)* is a disease characterized by male pseudohermaphroditism, progressive glomerulopathy, and urinary tract tumors (e.g., Wilms' tumor). Nephropathy starts in infancy as a diffuse mesangial sclerosis and rapidly progresses to end-stage renal failure by the age of 3 years. DDS have overlap manifestations with Mecham syndrome, which is characterized by congenital diaphragmatic hernia, double vagina, sex reversal, and cardiac malformations. Unlike DDS, those with Mecham syndrome do not develop Wilms' tumor.
- *Fraser syndrome* is a disease characterized by male pseudohermaphroditism, progressive glomerulopathy, and urinary tract tumors (e.g., Wilms' tumor). Unlike DDS, nephropathy is a steroid-resistant focal segmental sclerosis, and it starts in childhood and progresses to end-stage renal failure by the second or third decade of life. Both Fraser and DDS may present with congenital diaphragmatic hernias.
- *Aarskog (facial–digital–genital) syndrome* is a disease characterized by characteristic short status and facial features (e.g., hypertelorism), digital abnormalities (e.g., short fingers), and genital abnormalities (e.g., cryptorchidism). Radiographic findings of Aarskog syndrome show maxillary hypoplasia, hypoplasia of terminal phalanges of fingers, spina bifida occulta, and hypoplastic middle phalanges of the toes. Children with Aarskog syndrome may show features of growth hormone deficiency.
- *LEOPARD syndrome* is a disease characterized by lentigines (pathognomonic), electrocardiographic (ECG) conduction defects, ocular hypertelorism, pulmonary stenosis, abnormal genitalia, retardation of growth, and sensorineural deafness. To establish LEOPARD syndrome diagnosis, lentigines and two of the other characteristic features need to be fulfilled. The disease has an autosomal dominant mode of inheritance.

### Signs on US

Cryptorchidism can be detected by US as an isoechoic or hypoechoic mass relative to the normal testes located in the inguinal canal (70 % of cases) or the prescrotal region just beyond the external inguinal ring (20 %).

### Signs on CT and MRI

- Both testes are present either in the scrotum or in the inguinal canal (undescended testes). The external genitalia are incompletely masculinized or frankly ambiguous. Prostatic tissue appears to be present.
- *AIS*: patients with AIS may show cystic lesions within the pelvis representing residual parts of the Müllerian system. It is important to screen patients with male pseudohermaphroditism radiologically because of the high risk of malignant transformation of the nonfunctioning Müllerian system residuals. Bilateral gonadectomy is recommended in patients with AIS because of the high incidence of seminomas.
- *PMDS*: patients with PMDS are males with uterus and fallopian tubes inside their pelvis. Two forms are present, the male and the female forms. The male form, also called *hernia uteri inguinale*, is characterized by a male with one testis descended in the scrotum and the other testis located at the contralateral ovary position in the pelvis. In the female form, the phenotype is of a female with a hypoplastic, blind-ended uterus located behind the bladder. The testes are bilaterally located in the "ovarian" position (not within the scrotum) (◘ Fig. 3.10.7).

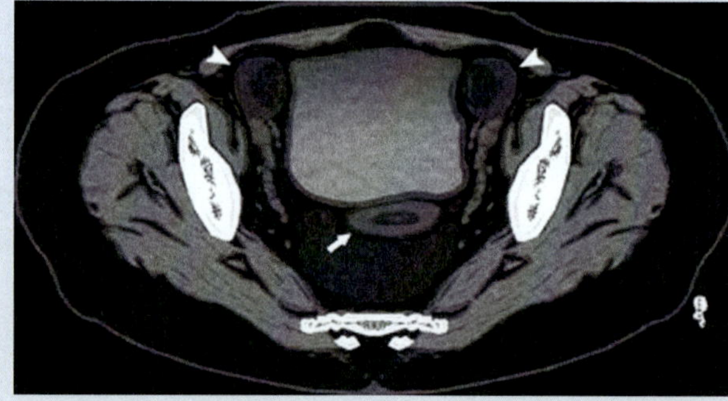

◘ **Fig. 3.10.7**  Axial pelvic CT illustration demonstrates the female form of persistent Müllerian duct syndrome (PMDS). The uterus is detected behind the bladder (*arrow*), and the testes are located at the position of the ovaries bilaterally (*arrowheads*)

### True Hermaphroditism

In true hermaphroditism, patients have both ovaries and testes for gonads, often due to chromosome mosaicism (*chimerism*).

There are three types of true hermaphroditism:

- *Lateral true hermaphroditism*: patients have a testis on one side and an ovary on the other side in the pelvis.

- *Unilateral true hermaphroditism*: patients have both a testis and an ovary on one side and a testis or an ovary on the other side of the pelvis.
- *Bilateral true hermaphroditism*: patients have both a testis and an ovary on both sides of the pelvis.

Patients with true hermaphroditism also show ambiguous genitalia, with hypospadia, cryptorchidism, and incomplete fusion of the labioscrotal folds.

### Signs on MRI
- The external genitalia are ambiguous.
- There are both testes and ovaries found in the pelvis according to the type (lateral, unilateral, or bilateral).
- Hypoplastic uterus is found in almost all cases.

### Gonadal Dysgenesis
Patients with gonadal dysgenesis are male pseudohermaphroditism with Müllerian duct structures. Gonadal dysgenesis disorders are a spectrum of anomalies that include pure gonadal dysgenesis, partial gonadal dysgenesis, and mixed gonadal dysgenesis. In pure gonadal dysgenesis, patients have bilateral streak gonads (dysfunctional gonads without germ cells). In mixed and partial gonadal dysgenesis, there is one testis on one side and a streak gonad on the other side.

Gonadal dysgenesis is characterized by defect in the sex determination region on chromosome Y (SRY). The infant initially starts as a male karyotype (46, XY), but due to the failure in the SRY, the testes are not developed and the female development takes place (sex reversal), despite the presence of the Y chromosome. The patient is a female with XY karyotype and Müllerian derivatives including uterus, fallopian tubes, and cervix. Turner syndrome (45, XO) is an example of gonadal dysgenesis disorder.

*Swyer syndrome* is an uncommon form of pure gonadal dysgenesis. The male child with Swyer syndrome looks female externally, but the karyotype is (46, XY) with a non-functioning Y chromosome. Patients with Swyer syndrome may have *multiple pterygium syndrome*, which is characterized by multiple body contractures since birth with webbing of the neck, elbows, knees, and intracrural areas.

Streak gonads should be removed surgically because the risk of malignant transformation within the first two decades of life can reach up to 30 % of cases.

### Signs on MRI
The patient shows both testes and Müllerian duct derivatives (e.g., uterus) (◘ Fig. 3.10.8).

Streak gonads are difficult to detect and usually seen as low signal intensity stripes on T2W images. High signal intensity of streak gonads on T2W images could represent a sign of malignant transformation.

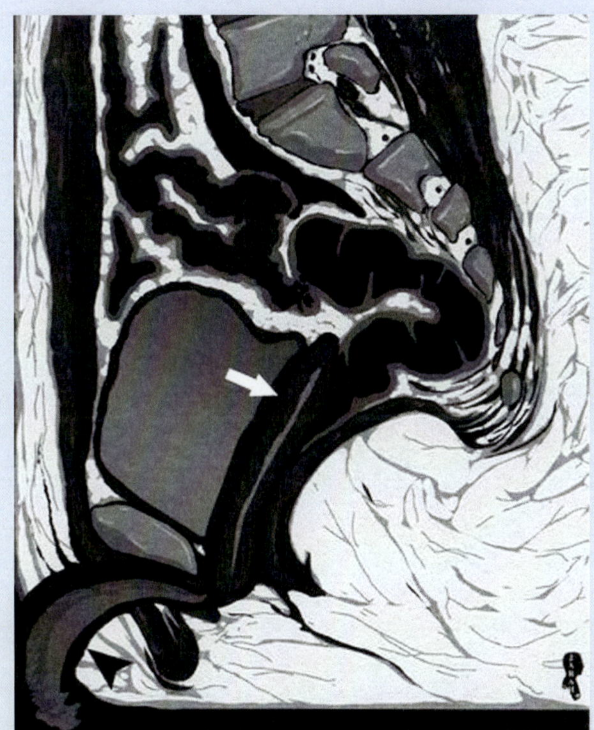

◘ **Fig. 3.10.8** Sagittal T1W pelvic MR illustration demonstrates findings in a patient with gonadal dysgenesis. There is vagina with absent uterus representing Müllerian duct derivatives (*white arrow*), in the presence of the penis (*black arrowhead*)

## Further Reading

Angle B et al. XY gonadal dysgenesis associated with a multiple pterygium syndrome phenotype. Am J Med Genet. 1997;68:7–11.

Aso C et al. Gray-scale and color Doppler sonography of scrotal disorders in children: an update. Radiographics. 2005;25:1197–214.

Browne LP et al. Van Wyk and Grumbach syndrome revisited: imaging and clinical findings in pre- and postpubertal girls. Pediatr Radiol. 2008;38:538–42.

Chavhan GB et al. Imaging of ambiguous genitalia: classification and diagnostic approach. Radiographics. 2008;28:1891–904.

Chen H-Y et al. Pure XY gonadal dysgenesis and agenesis in monozygotic twins. Fertil Steril. 2006;85:1059.e9–11.

Cho HY et al. Hydrothorax in a patient with Denys-Drash syndrome associated with diaphragmatic defect. Pediatr Nephrol. 2006;21:1909–12.

Choi HK et al. MR imaging of intersexuality. Radiographics. 1998;18:83–96.

Christensen JD et al. The undescended testis. Semin Ultrasound CT MR. 2007;28:307–16.

Elon Gale M. Hermaphroditism demonstrated by computed tomography. AJR Am J Roentgenol. 1983;141:99–100.

Erdem CZ et al. Polycystic ovary syndrome: dynamic contrast-enhanced ovary MR imaging. Eur J Radiol. 2004;51:48–53.

Franceschi R et al. Prevalence of polycystic ovary syndrome in young women who had idiopathic central precocious puberty. Fertil Steril. 2009. doi:10.1016/j.fertnstert.2008.11.016.

Hedlund GL et al. Disorders of puberty: a practical imaging approach. Semin Ultrasound CT MR. 1994;15:49–77.

Hernanz-Schulman M et al. Sonographic findings in infants with congenital adrenal hyperplasia. Pediatr Radiol. 2002;32:130–7.

Hyun G et al. A practical approach to intersex in the newborn period. Urol Clin North Am. 2004;31:435–43.

Jagadhish LCTK. Van Wyk and Grumbach syndrome (a syndrome of incomplete isosexual precocity and juvenile hypothyroidism). Armed Forces Med J India. 2002;58:343–5.

Johnsen DE et al. MR imaging of the sellar and juxtasellar regions. Radiographics. 1991;11:727–58.

Jung SE et al. CT and MRI findings of sex-cord stromal tumor of the ovary. AJR Am J Roentgenol. 2005;185:207–15.

Karabulut N et al. Stromal tumor of the sex cord in a woman with testicular feminization syndrome: imaging features. AJR Am J Roentgenol. 2002;178:1496–8.

Kim JB et al. A case of PAGOD syndrome with hypoplastic left heart syndrome. Int J Cardiol. 2007;114:270–1.

Kodama M et al. Aarskog syndrome with isolated growth hormone deficiency. Eur J Pediatr. 1981;135:273–6.

Narlawar RS et al. Persistent mullerian duct syndrome with teratoma in an ectopic testis: imaging features. Eur Radiol. 2001;11:955–8.

Sharafuddin MJA et al. MR imaging diagnosis of central precocious puberty: importance of changes in the shape and size of the pituitary gland. AJR Am J Roentgenol. 1994;162:1167–73.

Wang Y-C et al. Maternal and female fetal virilization caused by pregnancy luteoma. Fertil Steril. 2005;84:509.e15–7.

Woodward PJ et al. Tumors and tumorlike lesions of the testes: radiologic-pathologic correlation. Radiographics. 2002;22:189–216.

Wu H-C et al. Persistent Müllerian duct syndrome with seminoma: CT findings. AJR Am J Roentgenol. 2000;174:102–4.

Yagubyan M et al. LEOPARD syndrome: a new polyaneurysm association and an update on the molecular genetics of the disease. J Vasc Surg. 2004;39:897–900.

Yanai Y et al. Androgen insensitivity syndrome with serous gonadal cyst. Fertil Steril. 2008;90:2018.e9–11.

## 3.11  Sheehan Syndrome (Postpartum Hypopituitarism)

Sheehan's syndrome (SS), previously known as *Simmonds' disease* (*pituitary cachexia*), is a rare condition characterized by infarction and necrosis of the anterior pituitary gland (adenohypophysis) due to postdelivery hemorrhage.

The normal pituitary gland shows physiological changes in size according to age: infants and children 6 mm in diameter, men and postmenopausal women 8 mm in diameter, and childbearing women 10 mm in diameter, and women in late pregnancy and puerperium may reach up to 12 mm in diameter. SS is attributed to an increased size of the pituitary gland during pregnancy, which may compress over the superior hypophyseal artery and thereby cause a mild ischemia. If sudden change in the arterial pressure occurs during or after delivery due to severe hemorrhage or hypotension, arterial spasm in the small vessels and pituitary infarction (apoplexy) may occur. However, SS may rarely occur without postpartum bleeding.

Patients with SS are characterized by postpartum delivery hemorrhage, hypovolemia, and disseminated intravascular coagulation (DIC), usually due to retained placenta products. A relatively small sella size was suggested as a risk factor for the development of SS.

SS patients often present after a period of 6 months to 24 years after a hemorrhagic delivery with different clinical manifestation according to the progression of the condition. Acute manifestations of SS include pituitary apoplexy. Patients present with sudden headache (95 %) due to stretching and irritation of the dura matter in the wall of the sella, because it is supplied by the meningeal branches of the trigeminal nerve. Other features include ocular paresis due to abducens and oculomotor nerve compression within the cavernous sinus and vomiting (69 %) due to increased intracranial pressure or meningeal irritation.

Chronic or delayed manifestations of SS are all related to adenohypophysis dysfunction with a wide spectrum of symptoms. The most common manifestation is postpartum lactation failure (agalactia). Growth hormone is one of the earliest hormones lost in SS, and it may result in constitutional symptoms like weakness, malaise, and fatigue. Amenorrhea and postpartum menstruation failure are other common complaints in SS. Residual pituitary function may be sufficient to conceive in some patients, which means that the presence of pregnancy is not against SS in patients who suffered from pituitary apoplexy in the past. Secondary hypothyroidism and adrenocortical insufficiency may occur. Interestingly, women with SS may show premature pale aging face with fine wrinkling around the mouth and the eyes due to long-term growth hormone and estrogen deficiency that result in skin aging.

Apart from the hormonal abnormalities, laboratory findings in SS include normocytic normochromic anemia, hyponatremia, and hypoglycemia.

## Signs on CT

In pituitary apoplexy, CT will show an enlarged pituitary gland with hyperdense areas as a sign of hemorrhage and hypodense areas as a sign of necrosis (Fig. 3.11.1). Contrast injection shows hyperdense rim enhancement with hypodense center due to infarction.

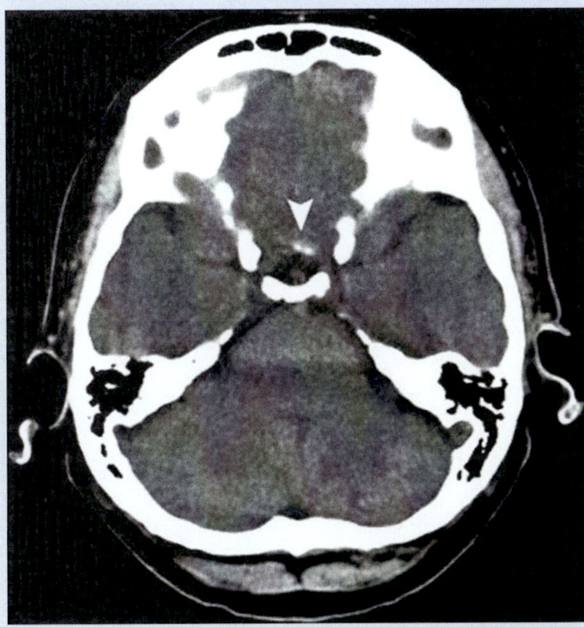

Fig. 3.11.1 Axial unenhanced brain CT shows hyperdense area in the region of the sella as an area of hemorrhagic infarction in a patient with Sheehan's syndrome (SS) (*arrowhead*)

## Signs on MRI

- The normal postpartum pituitary is hyperintense on T1W images and can measure up to 12 mm in diameter. In the acute stage of SS, the pituitary is enlarged (>12 mm) and bulging under the optic chiasma. Areas of hypointensity on T1W and hyperintensity on T2W images representing infarction may be seen. After gadolinium injection, the gland shows thick homogeneous peripheral ring enhancement with hypointense center due to infarction and hyperemia (Fig. 3.11.2).
- In the chronic stage of SS, the MR scan usually shows empty sella.

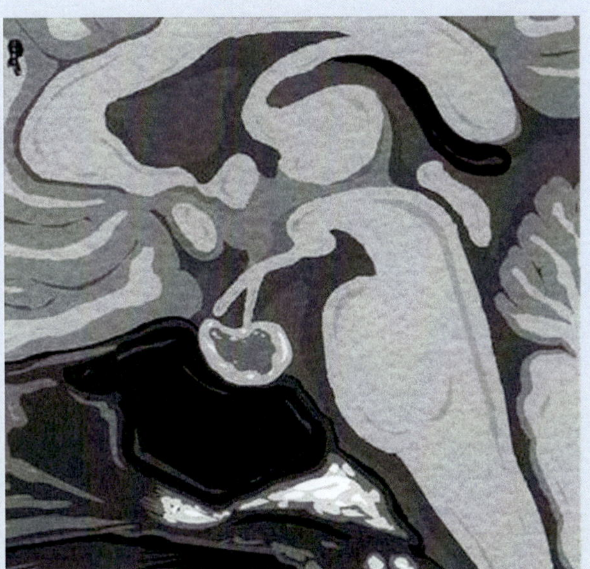

Fig. 3.11.2 Sagittal T1W postcontrast MR illustration of the sella demonstrates a thick rim enhancement in a patient with SS due to pituitary apoplexy

## Further Reading

Dejager S et al. Sheehan's syndrome: differential diagnosis in the acute stage. J Intern Med. 1998;244:261–6.

Gokalp D et al. Sheehan's syndrome as a rare cause of anaemia secondary to hypopituitarism. Ann Hematol. 2009;88:405–10.

Keleştimur F. Sheehan's syndrome. Pituitary. 2003;6:181–8.

Vaphiades MS et al. Sheehan syndrome: a splinter of the mind. Surv Ophthalmol. 2003;48:230–3.

Weiner HA. Simmond's disease. Yale J Biol Med. 1937;10: 31–9.

# Nephrology




© Springer International Publishing Switzerland 2017
J.A. Al-Tubaikh, *Internal Medicine*, DOI 10.1007/978-3-319-39747-4_4

## 4.1   Hypertension

Hypertension is a disease characterized by an increase in systolic blood pressure >140 mmHg and in diastolic blood pressure >100 mmHg. Hypertension is 90 % primary (without a cause) and 10 % secondary to an organic cause. Radiological modalities are mainly used to detect secondary causes of hypertension.

Secondary causes of hypertension include the following:

- *Renovascular diseases*: atherosclerosis (adults), fibromuscular dysplasia (children), vasculitis (polyarteritis nodosa (PAN) and Takayasu arteritis (TA)), and renal artery aneurysm.
- *Adrenal causes*: pheochromocytoma, primary hyperaldosteronism, and Cushing's syndrome.
- *Renal parenchymal diseases*: chronic glomerulonephritis, diabetic nephropathy, lupus nephritis, polycystic kidney disease, and page kidney.
- *Aortic diseases*: coarctation of the aorta and midaortic syndrome.
- *Other causes*: brain tumors, congenital AVM, carcinoid tumors, acromegaly, and hypercalcemia.

## Renal Artery Stenosis

Renal artery stenosis (RAS) constitutes 1–5 % of patients with hypertension. Atherosclerosis is the commonest cause of renovascular hypertension in adults, while renal artery fibromuscular dysplasia is the most common cause of renovascular hypertension in children. Atherosclerosis RAS often affects the proximal part of the artery, while fibromuscular dysplasia often involves the middle and the distal part in a form of small stenotic and aneurysmal dilatation, giving the so-called beaded appearance on angiography.

RAS is suspected as a cause of hypertension in the following situations:

- Hypertension in a patient <30 years of age or a patient >50 years
- Hypertension that is resistant to three antihypertensive regimens
- Sudden renal functions worsening in a hypertensive patient
- Sudden development or worsening of hypertension in any age
- Unilateral small kidney
- Renal impairment after treatment with angiotensin-converting enzymes (ACE) inhibitors

RAS is commonly diagnosed by color-coded duplex scanning by two methods: direct and indirect. The direct method involves measuring the blood velocity directly within the renal artery (■ Fig. 4.1.1). In contrast, the indirect method involves measuring the blood velocity within the segmental and interlobar intrarenal vessels (■ Fig. 4.1.2). The indirect method is insensitive for less than 60 % RAS.

The resistance index (RI) is the maximal systolic velocity minus the end-diastolic velocity divided by the maximal velocity. Increase in renal artery RI is seen in RAS, transplant rejection, acute tubular necrosis, graft infections, and obstructive hydronephrosis. The RI tends to be high in patients with chronic renal disease.

*Goldblatt kidney* is a condition where the kidney starts to release rennin to overcome RAS, leading to renovascular hypertension. *Page kidney*, on the other hand, is a condition where the kidney is compressed from an adjacent pathology that causes cortical ischemia. The kidney releases rennin to overcome the ischemia, leading to renovascular hypertension.

### The Normal Renal Artery Waveform Parameters

- The normal renal artery waveform shows low resistance, continuous profile through the cardiac cycle, with an RI <0.7. Also, the normal main renal artery waveform has an early systolic peak (ESP) (■ Fig. 4.1.3).
- *The renal-aortic ration (RAR)* is defined as the maximum peak systolic velocity (PSV) of the renal artery divided by the maximum PSV of the aorta at the level of the superior mesenteric artery (SMA). A high false RAR can be seen in cases of abdominal aortic aneurysm, and aortic PSV <40 cm/s, or aortic PSV >125 cm/s. Also, RAR should not be used in the assessment of renal artery aneurysm for young patients or patients with renal artery stents.
- The normal interlobar and segmental arteries display an ESP at the beginning of the systole. The ESP is absent when the arterial stenosis is >60 %. The Doppler angle should be <30°; otherwise, the peak will not be demonstrated.
- *The systolic acceleration time (SAT)* is defined as the time measured from the start of the systolic upstroke to the first ESP. Normally it is <0.07.

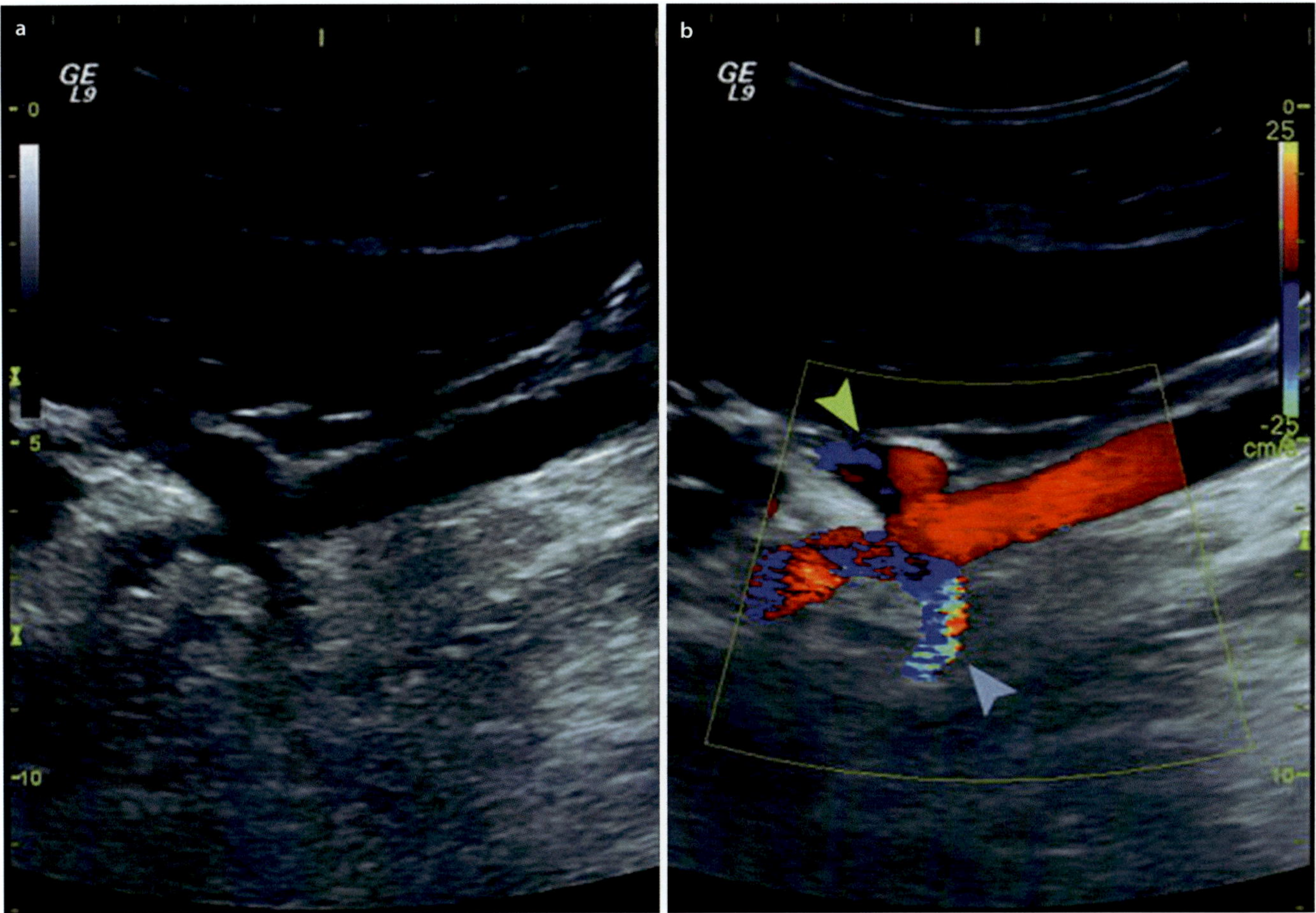

**◘ Fig. 4.1.1** Color Doppler sonogram of the aorta shows a normal anatomy of the renal arteries (banana peel view) in gray mode in (**a**) and Duplex-colored mode in (**b**) taken while the patient is in the lateral decubitus position. The right renal artery is clearly detected in (**b**) (*yellow arrowhead*), and the left renal artery is also detected well in this position (*blue arrowhead*)

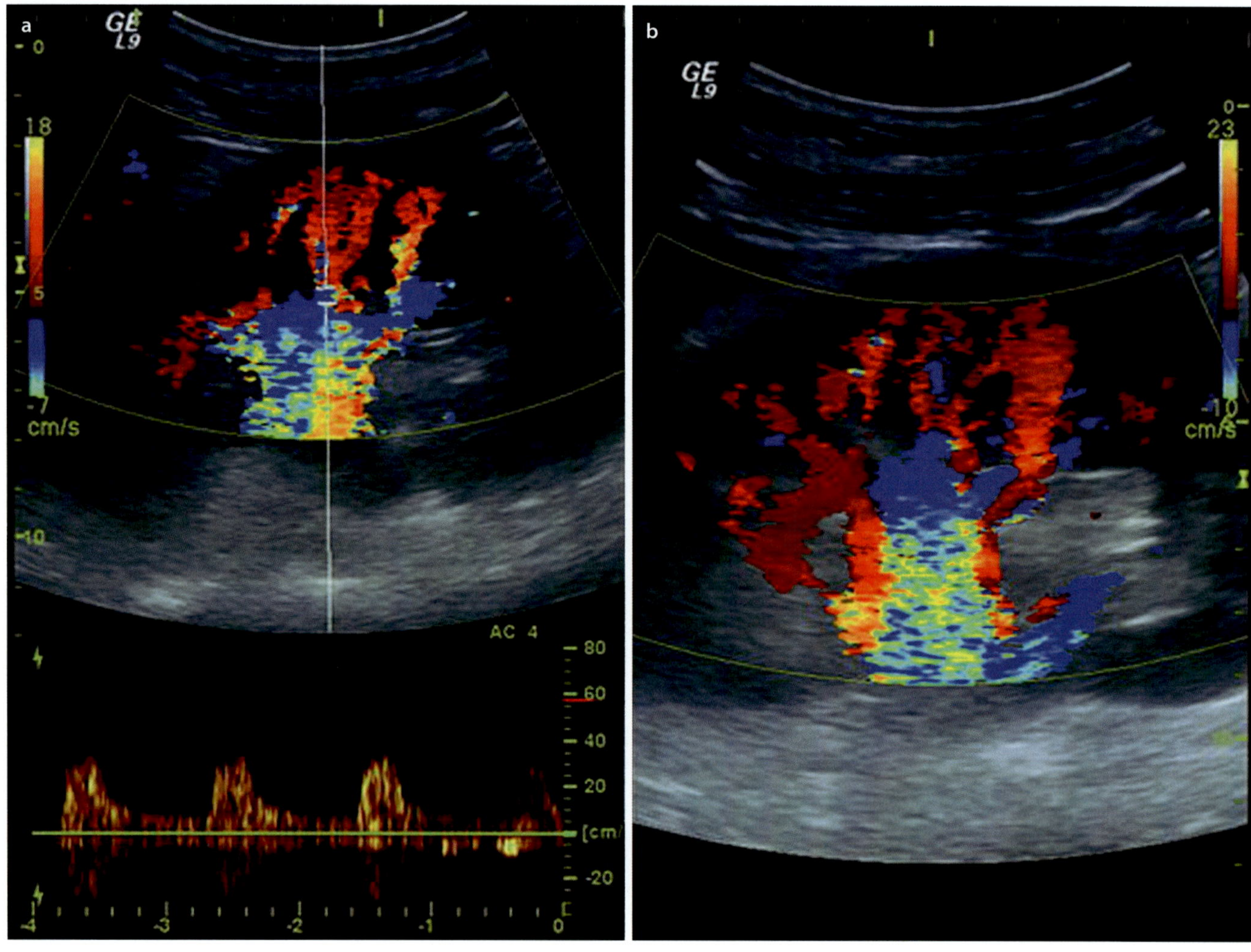



**Fig. 4.1.2** Color Doppler sonogram of the left kidney demonstrates its vascular anatomy in (**b**) and arterial waveform detection in (**a**) to assess the arterial vascular supply as an indirect method for detecting RAS

**Signs of Direct RAS on Doppler Sonography**
- High renal parenchymal echogenicity that may reach or exceed the liver echogenicity (signs of renal parenchymal damage). A kidney disease can cause renal artery-resistant waveform, which may be mistaken with RAS.
- Normal RAR (<3.5) and the normal renal PSV (<180 cm/s). Sixty percent RAS shows RAR <3.5, with PSV between 180 and 200 cm/s. There is no poststenotic turbulence (mosaic pattern/aliasing artifact) with RAS <60%. A 60–99% RAS shows RAR >3.5, PSV >200 cm/s, and poststenotic turbulence.

**Signs on Indirect RAS on Doppler Sonography**
- Absence of the ESP.
- An accelerated time peak >100 ms is consistent with >60% stenosis.
- *Tardus parvus waveform* consists of slow, damped systolic acceleration (tardus) and rounding and flattening of the systolic peak (parvus).
- More than (−5) difference between the two kidneys RI.
- Kidney size <9 cm or the difference in size between the two kidneys >2 cm in diameter (normal kidney size = 9–12 cm in diameter).

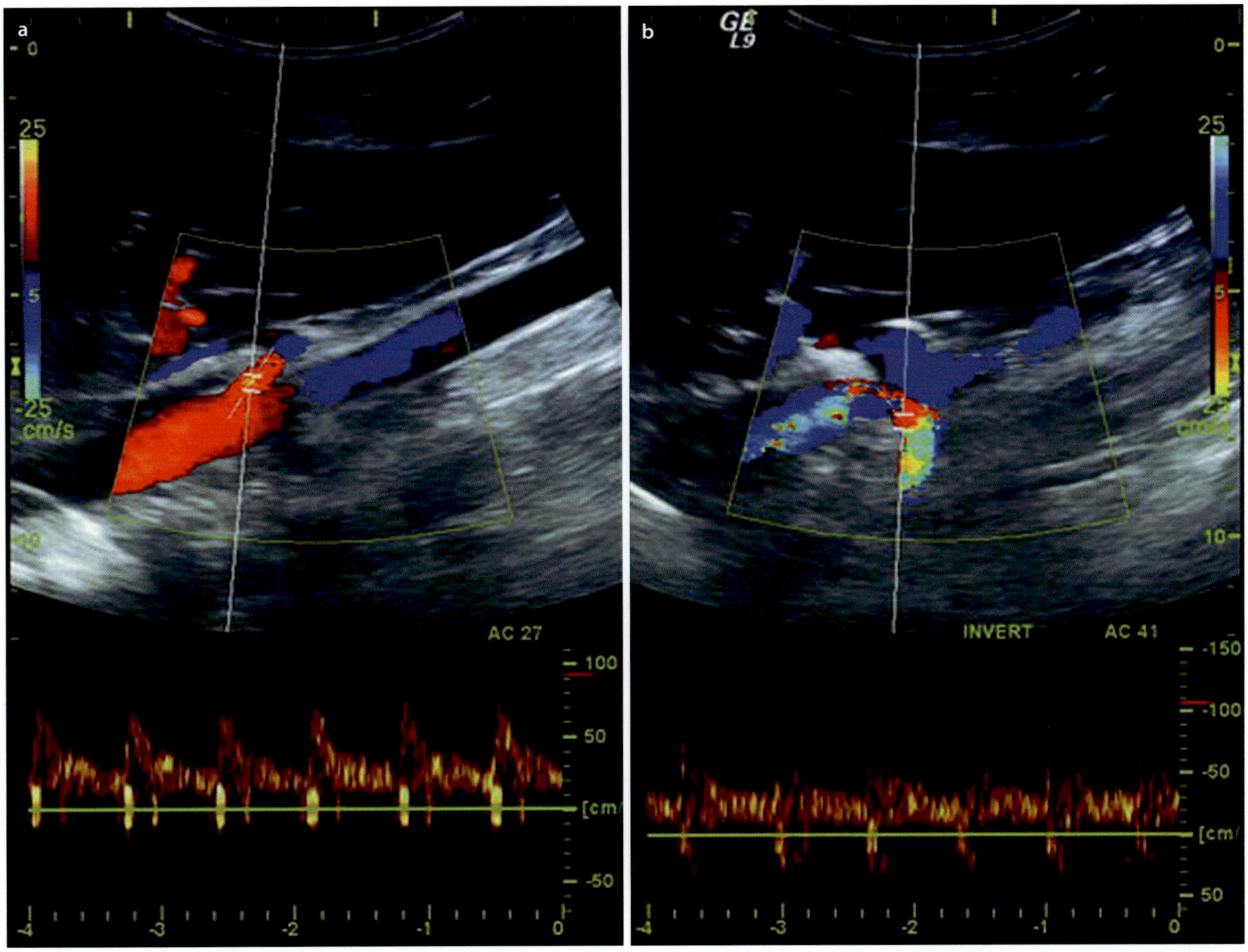

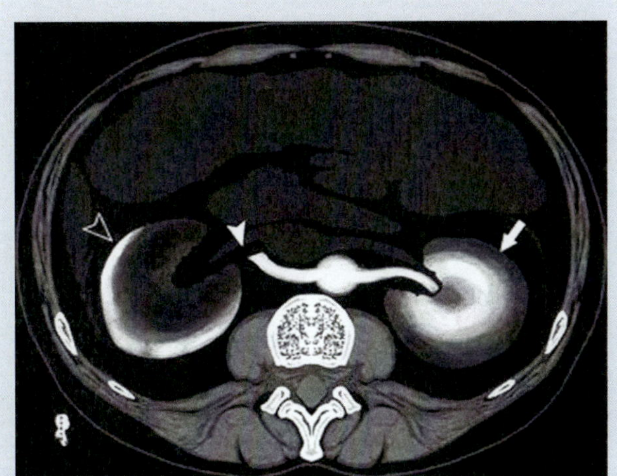

**Fig. 4.1.3** Color Doppler sonogram of the renal arteries demonstrates normal arterial waveform of the right renal artery (**a**) and the left renal artery (**b**)

### Signs on CT

— *Arterial cut-off sign*: the course of the renal artery is seen interrupted on contrast-enhanced images. It is a sign of renal artery obstruction (**Fig. 4.1.4**).

— *Rim sign of vascular compromise*: the kidney fails to enhance on contrast-enhanced images, with a thin rim of subcapsular enhancement seen paralleling the renal margin (**Fig. 4.1.4**). This sign is caused by renal medullary arterial perfusion interruption in cases of renal artery obstruction, with preserved perfusion of the renal cortex by the capsular perforating vessels. This sign can be seen in cases of renal vein thrombosis, renal arterial occlusion, and acute tubular necrosis.

— *Reverse rim sign*: this sign is seen as hypodense renal cortex against a contrast-enhanced background of intact medullary arterial perfusion (**Fig. 4.1.4**). This sign is seen in cases of compromised renal arterial perfusion in cases of cortical necrosis.

**Fig. 4.1.4** Axial postcontrast-enhanced CT illustration shows the arterial cut-off sign (*solid arrowhead*), rim sign of vascular compromise (*open arrowhead*), and reverse rim sign (*arrow*)

### Signs on MRA

- Magnetic resonance angiography (MRA) demonstrates the aortic vessels clearly, and it is mostly used after detection of RAS on Doppler sonography for surgical planning (◘ Fig. 4.1.5).

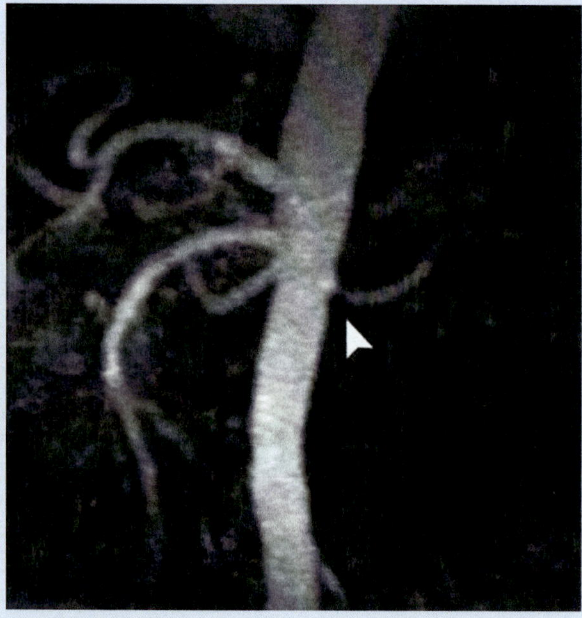

◘ **Fig. 4.1.5**  MRA image shows >50 % stenosis of the left renal artery (*arrowhead*) in a patient with peripheral vascular disease

## Coarctation of the Aorta

Coarctation of the aorta is a condition characterized by aortic lumen narrowing, most commonly located below the origin of the left subclavian artery (the aortic isthmus near the ligamentum arteriosum), causing hypertension below the level of the narrowing.

Patients with aortic coarctation often present with severe hypertension that does not respond to antihypertensive medication and chest pain that radiates to the back. Patients with aortic coarctation carry the risk of aortic dissection, which is characterized by aortic wall intimal tear and leaking of the blood in between the aortic wall layers.

When it is chronic, aortic coarctation causes dilatation of the internal mammary and intercostals arteries. Chronic high-pressure pulsation of the intercostals arteries over the inferior aspect of the ribs may result in rib notching. Coarctation of the aorta can be seen in up to 30 % in patients with bicuspid aortic valve.

*Pseudocoarctation of the aorta* is a relatively rare condition characterized by kinking of the aorta at its isthmus near the ligamentum arteriosum without lumen narrowing. Pseudocoarctation resembles true coarctation; differentiation is possible by looking for changes of the collateral circulation, where there will be no enlarged peripheral vessels, signs of pressure gradients, or rib notching. The condition is symptomless and can be associated with congenital bicuspid aortic valve.

### Signs on Chest Radiograph

- In chronic cases of aortic coarctation, the ribs show irregular lower border representing rib notching (◘ Fig. 4.1.6). This condition can be also seen in other conditions affecting the intercostals neurovascular bundle like superior vena cava obstruction syndrome and neurofibromatosis of the intercostals nerves.
- The aortic arch is often bulging with dilatation of the aortic knuckle (◘ Fig. 4.1.7).
- Pseudocoarctation of the aorta is seen as elongated aortic knuckle appearing like a posterior mediastinal mass.

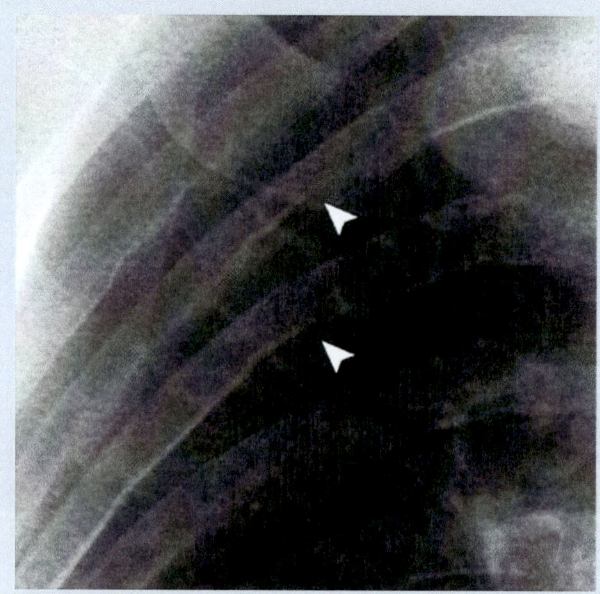

◘ **Fig. 4.1.6**  Plain chest radiograph shows rib notching in a patient with severe aortic coarctation since 12 years (*arrowheads*)

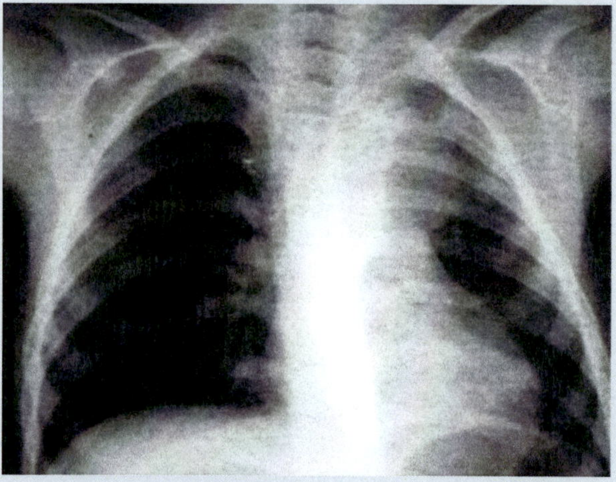

◘ **Fig. 4.1.7**  Posteroanterior plain chest radiograph in a patient with coarctation of the aorta shows bulging of the aortic knuckle

### Signs on CT and MRI

- Aortic coarctation classically is seen in sagittal reformatted images as a narrowing of the aortic lumen located at the area of the aortic isthmus, giving the classic "inverted shape of 3" (Fig. 4.1.8).
- Aortic dissection is seen as hypodense layer found within the aortic lumen on postcontrast-enhanced images representing the false lumen (Fig. 4.1.9). *Stanford type A* dissection involves dissection of the ascending aorta and the arch up to the origin of the left subclavian artery. *Stanford type B* dissection involves dissection of the descending aorta below the origin of the subclavian artery. Type A is managed surgically, while type B is managed medically, providing evidence of end-organ ischemia not being present.
- Aortic pseudocoarctation is seen on axial CT images as higher than normal located arch, with a well-defined enhancing vascular mass located near the aortic arch, representing the kinked portion of the arch.

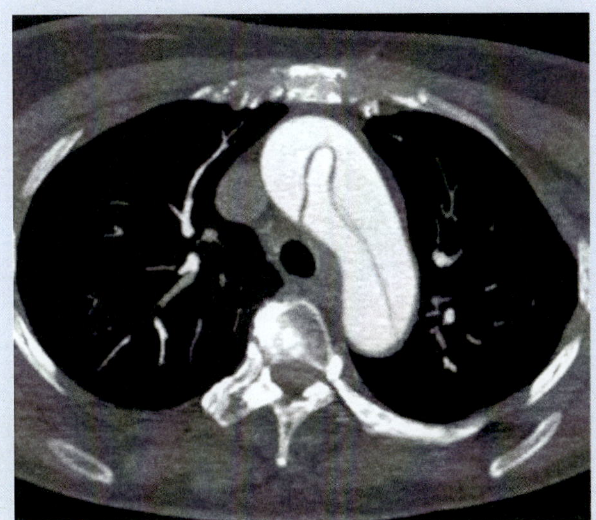

**Fig. 4.1.9**   Axial CT angiography shows the classical intimal flap in a patient with aortic dissection Stanford type A

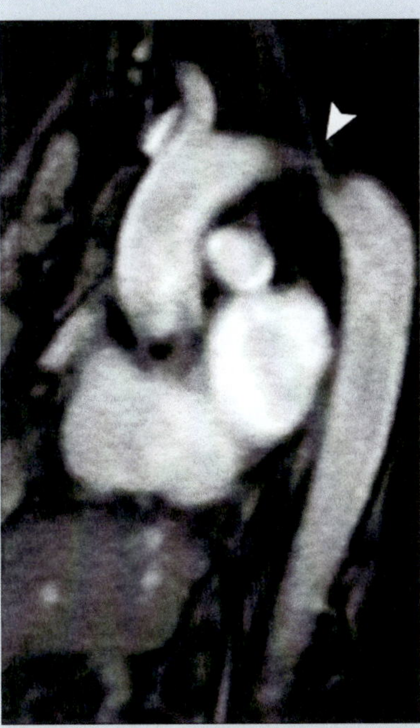

**Fig. 4.1.8**   Sagittal MRA of a patient with coarctation of the aorta shows the inverted shape of 3, which is a characteristic of this condition (*arrowhead*)

## Polyarteritis Nodosa

Polyarteritis nodosa is a rare disease characterized by aneurysmal, nodular lesions that affect the medium-sized and small-sized arteries due to fibrinoid necrotizing vasculitis.

Vasculitides are a diverse group of diseases characterized by inflammation and necrosis of all three coats of the vessels (intima, media, and adventitia). They are divided into large-sized vessel vasculitis (e.g., Takayasu and giant cell arteritis), medium-sized vessel vasculitis (e.g., polyarteritis nodosa and Kawasaki disease), and small-sized vessel vasculitis (e.g., Wegener's granulomatosis and Henoch–Schönlein purpura).

Polyarteritis nodosa commonly causes multiple arterial aneurismal wall formation, plus fragmentation and degeneration of the adventitia layer. Necrosis starts in the media layer and spreads to involve the entire width of the vascular wall. This inflammation and necrosis are associated with eosinophilic infiltration, fibrin deposition, and destruction of the elastic tissue and the intima layer. Vascular thrombosis or an aneurysm, mainly at the vessels bifurcation or the hilar region of viscera, may occur. Later, a granuloma is formed at the area of previous inflammation with fibroblast proliferation. A healed stage is characterized by vascular recanalization and formation of a nonvascularized fibrous mass that completely replaces a section of the vessel wall. The disease rapidly progresses once started, and death may result from strokes or myocardial infarctions within 2–3 months after onset.

Any organ can be affected by PAN, including the central and peripheral nervous system. The kidney is the most commonly involved (80–90 %), followed by the gastrointestinal (GI) tract (50–70 %). Clinically, patients present with vague signs and symptoms like fever, myalgia, headache, and malaise. Renal artery involvement, especially at the renal hilum, often results in rapidly progressing hypertension. Involvement of the GI tract may present with lower GI bleeding, abdominal pain, and vomiting (6 % of cases). Peripheral nervous system involvement compromises the nervous tissue blood supply causing polyneuropathy. Other lesions involve pericarditis, myocardial infarction, and purpuric skin rash. Up to 30 % of patients test positive to hepatitis B surface antigens, and up to 50 % of patients have arthralgias.

Laboratory investigations usually show leukocytosis with eosinophilia (4 %), anemia, uremia, and high erythrocyte sedimentation rate.

### Signs on Angiography or MRA

Polyarteritis nodosa is suggested by detection of multiple aneurysms up to 1 cm in diameter within the renal, mesenteric, hepatic, or central venous vasculature. This finding is not pathognomonic since it can be seen in patients with necrotizing angiitis associated with drug abuse. The history and the high suspicion of PAV with this angiographic picture help to differentiate the two entities.

### Signs on CT

- The bowel walls are thickened and show white-attenuated target sign after contrast injection.
- CT angiography shows multiple aortic aneurysms in the branches of the SMA or the celiac trunk.
- In *spotted nephrogram*, small vessel occlusion in cases of PAN may cause patchy perfusion of the kidney on IVU or contrast-enhanced CT due to multiple infarctions (◘ Fig. 4.1.10). This sign can be also seen in scleroderma and hypertensive nephrocalcinosis.

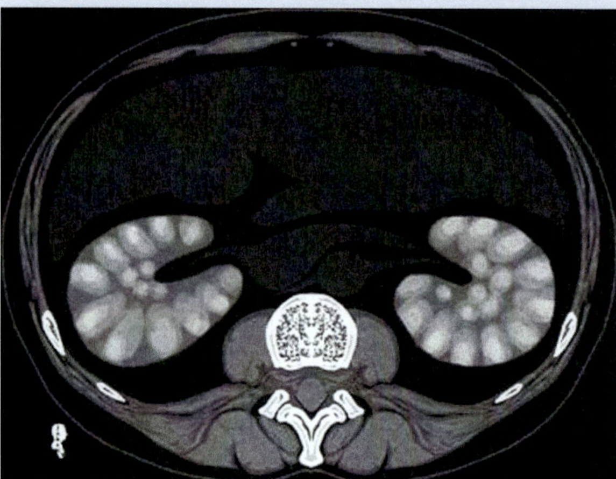

◘ **Fig. 4.1.10**   Axial CT illustration demonstrates the spotted nephrogram that may be seen in patients with polyarteritis nodosa

## Takayasu Arteritis

Takayasu arteritis is a rare, granulomatous disease characterized by inflammation of the large vessel walls, leading to progressive stenosis, aneurysms, or limb ischemia. The disease affects mainly the aorta and its major branches.

TA affects mainly young females between 20 and 30 years of age, who present with nonspecific systemic inflammatory symptoms like fever, night sweat, weight loss, myalgia, and arthralgia. TA has two main phases with different clinical presentations, an early and a late phase. The early phase is characterized by nonspecific inflammation in the blood vessels walls affecting the media and the adventitia layers. These nonspecific inflammatory changes are responsible for the nonspecific, systemic inflammatory symptoms. In contrast, the late phase is characterized by arterial symptoms with no systemic symptoms. The absence of the systemic symptoms in the late phase is attributed to the development of systemic collaterals; however, this is not seen in all patients. In the late phase, the coronary arteries might be affected. Hypertension, arterial stenosis, aneurysms, and dissection all can be seen in late phase of TA.

### Criteria for TA Diagnosis (TA Diagnosis Requires at Least Three Criteria)

- Age of presentation <40 years.
- Limbs claudication.
- Decrease one or both brachial arteries pulse.
- Blood pressure difference of the extremities >10 mmHg.
- Bruit heard over the aorta or the subclavian arteries.
- Angiographic abnormalities include arterial occlusion, stenosis, or aneurysms of the aorta or its main branches. Commonly, these abnormalities are observed bilaterally.

### Signs on CT and CT Angiography

- In the acute phase, there is thickening of the great vessel wall without signs of calcification due to inflammation and intramural hematomas (especially the aorta) (◘ Fig. 4.1.11).
- The thickened vascular wall may show enhancement in early contrast phase due to inflammatory hyperemia.
- Aneurysmal dilatation of the aortic root or its major branches is mainly observed in late chronic phase of the disease.
- Signs of dissection, stenosis, or occlusion of the major vessels may be seen (◘ Fig. 4.1.12).

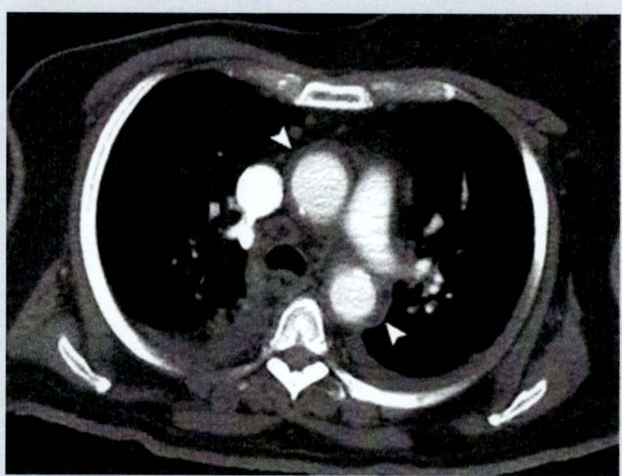

◘ **Fig. 4.1.11**   Axial CT angiography in a 50-year-old female patient presented with nonspecific systemic inflammatory symptoms with absent right arm pulsation and limb claudication. Patient was suspected to have Takayasu arteritis by the attending physician. CTA confirmed the acute thickening of the aortic wall (*arrowheads*), with occlusion of the right subclavian artery and multiple aneurysms affecting the carotid arteries (not shown)

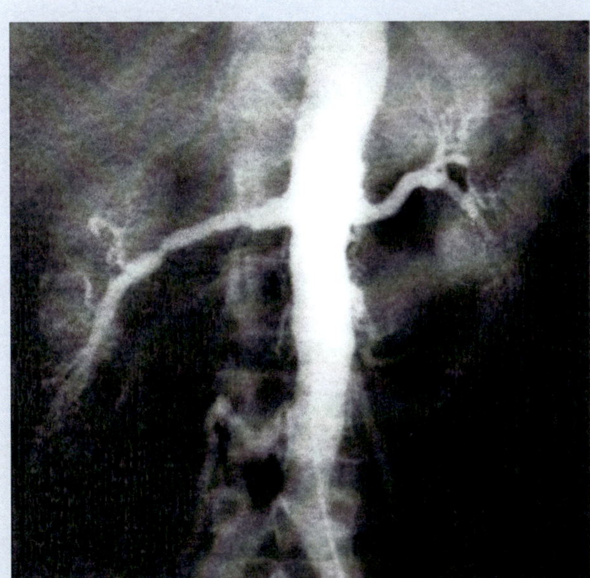

**Fig. 4.1.12** Aortic-renal angiography in a patient with chronic Takayasu arteritis shows multiple small stenoses and dilatations affecting the right renal artery and the abdominal aorta in a milder degree

## Midaortic Syndrome

Midaortic syndrome (MAS) is a nonspecific arteritis that affects the midportion of the abdominal aorta and its main branches.

MAS classically starts from the infrarenal part of the aorta and progresses proximally to involve the renal arteries (80 %), SMA, and the celiac artery (25 %). MAS mainly affects children and young adults who typically present with renovascular hypertension due to bilateral RAS. If untreated, the disease is fatal by the age of 30, with many patients experiencing intracranial bleeding due to malignant hypertension. The inferior mesenteric artery (IMA) and the common iliac arteries are almost never involved.

- **How Can You Differentiate Between MAS and TA?**
- Takayasu arteritis often presents with systemic symptoms of fever, malaise, and weight loss. These features are not part of MAS.
- MAS affects mainly children and young adults, while Takayasu arteritis mainly affects females between 20 and 30 years of age.
- MAS exclusively affects the mid-abdominal aorta, while Takayasu arteritis involves any vessels and can even affect the pulmonary artery, causing pulmonary hypertension.

**Signs on Doppler Sonographs**
- Stenosis of the mid-abdominal aorta.
- Renal artery stenosis is often seen unilaterally or bilaterally.

**Signs on CT Angiography**
- The aorta shows stenosis typically from the infrarenal portion and extends proximally to involve the renal arteries, IMA, or the celiac.
- The IMA and the common iliac vessels are spared.

## Preeclampsia

Preeclampsia is a pregnancy-related condition characterized by hypertension, lower leg edema, and proteinuria. In contrast, eclampsia is a life-threatening condition characterized by the same symptoms as preeclampsia plus tonic–clonic seizures.

Hypertensive disorders occur in about 3–10 % of all pregnancies, and the incidence of preeclampsia ranges between 10 and 15 % in primigravida (first birth) and 5.7–7.3 % in multiparas (multiple pregnancies). Hypertension in preeclampsia is diagnosed after 20 weeks of gestation by a diastolic blood pressure >90 mmHg stable over 4 h or one measurement of diastolic blood pressure >110 mmHg. Proteinuria is defined as a concentration of protein of 0.1 g/L or more in at least two random urine samples collected 4 h or more apart or as 0.3 g/L in a 24 h urine collection in the absence of urinary tract infection.

Patients with preeclampsia usually present with hypertension (hallmark of the disease), lower leg edema, proteinuria, headache, visual symptoms, and epigastric pain. The absence of hypertension in the presence of edema and proteinuria does not exclude the diagnosis of preeclampsia. The liver is uncommonly affected by preeclampsia (10 % of cases). When liver dysfunction occurs, mild elevation of serum enzymes is common.

*HELLP syndrome* is a disease characterized by hemolytic anemia (Hb <11 g/dL), elevated liver enzymes, low platelet count that predisposes to thrombocytopenia (<100,000/μL), and subcapsular liver hematoma. The incidence of HELLP syndrome is 2–12 % of preeclampsia cases. Patients often present with epigastric pain (65 %), nausea and vomiting (50 %), and nonspecific symptoms. Severe hypertension is not a constant or a frequent finding in HELLP syndrome.

**Signs on CT or MRI**
- In patients with HELLP syndrome, the imaging findings include subcapsular hematoma, hepatomegaly with bulging of the left lobe, fatty liver, free abdominal ascites, bilateral pleural effusions, or bilateral basal lobes atelectasis (**Fig. 4.1.13**).

**4**

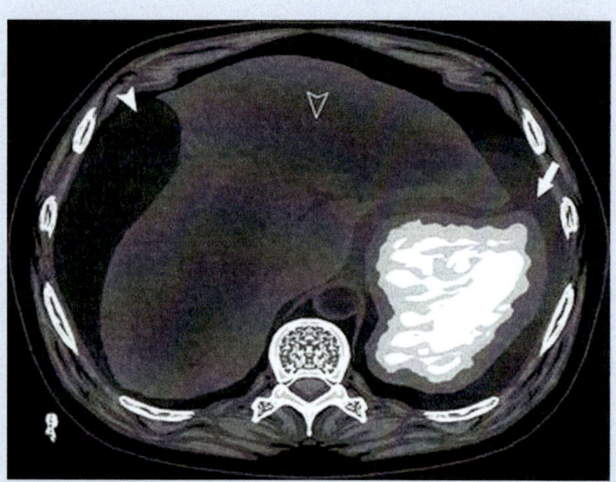

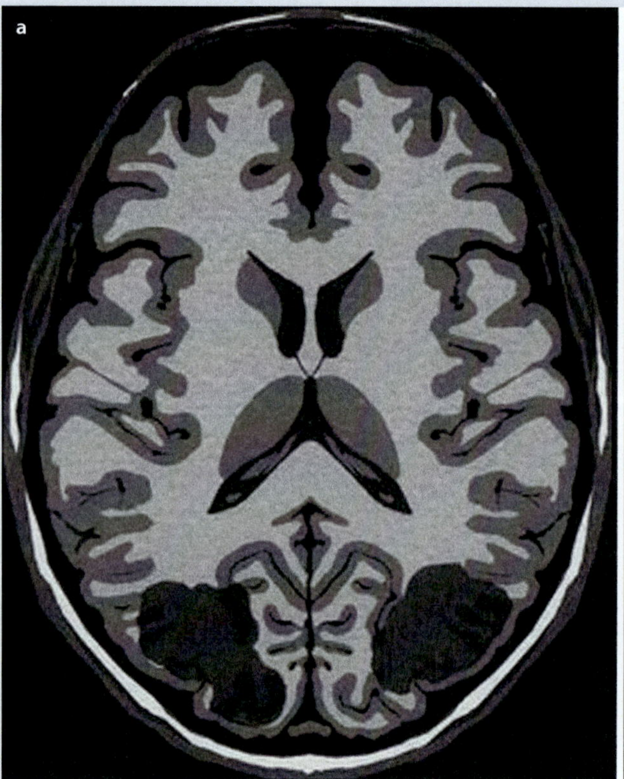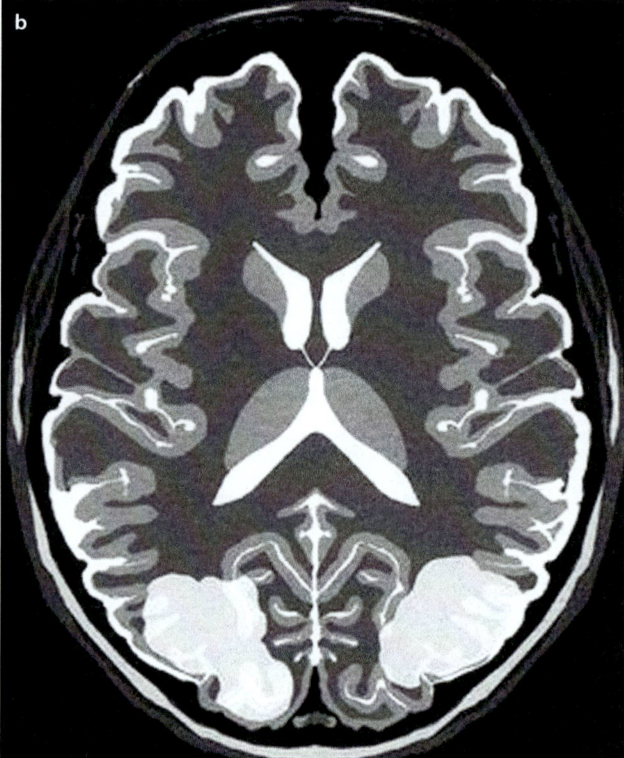

**Fig. 4.1.13** Axial abdominal postcontrast CT illustration demonstrates signs of HELLP syndrome. There is hepatic subcapsular hematoma (*solid arrowhead*), fatty liver changes (*open arrowhead*), and ascites (*arrow*)

## Reversible Posterior Leukoencephalopathy Syndrome (Hypertensive Encephalopathy)

Reversible posterior leukoencephalopathy syndrome (RPLES) is a disease with unknown cause characterized by cerebral demyelination in the posterior white matter areas of the brain (occipital lobes). PRLES is thought to be caused by increased permeability of the blood–brain barrier in the posterior circulation.

PRLES is typically seen in patients with hypertension and eclampsia and patients on immunosuppressive and cytotoxic drugs like cephalosporin and methotrexate. PRLES is a reversible condition once the cause is removed (e.g., control hypertension). If the cause persists, it will lead to cerebral infarction. Patients will present with headache, vertigo, vomiting, seizures, and altered mental status.

### Signs on CT and MRI
— On CT, there are symmetrical, noncontrast-enhancing hypodensities located in the posterior region of the occipital and the parietal lobes.
— On MRI, symmetric low T1 signal intensity with high T2 and FLAIR signal intensities in the region of the occipital and the parietal lobes (**Fig. 4.1.14**).
— There is cytotoxic edema and restricted water diffusion (high DWI signal intensity) in cases of infarction.

**Fig. 4.1.14** Axial T1W (**a**) and T2W (**b**) MR illustrations demonstrate bilateral almost symmetrical low T1 and high T2 signal intensity lesions located in the posterior lobes. This sign with a history of hypertension is diagnostic of RPLES

## Nephroptosis (Floating Kidney)

Nephroptosis, also known as floating or wandering kidney, is a condition characterized by renal descent of 5 cm or more (or two vertebral bodies) when the patient moves from supine to an upright position.

Nephroptosis occurs more commonly in slim women (ten times more common than in males) and affects the right kidney more than the left (20 % of cases). Causes of nephroptosis include multiple pregnancies, rapid loss of retroperitoneal fat, variation in the shape of the spinal cord, shallow Gerota's fossa, and direct renal trauma.

Patients with nephroptosis are rarely symptomatic. Symptomatic patients typically present with history of flank pain in the upright position that reduces or is relieved by lying down. The pain is attributed to intermittent functional excretory obstruction, forceful traction of the renal artery causing renal ischemia, or traction of the perirenal nerves. The most severe manifestation of nephroptosis is *Dietl's crisis*. Dietl's crisis is a condition characterized by violent paroxysmal colicky flank pain, tachycardia, nausea, chills, oliguria, hypertension, and transient hematuria or proteinuria. The condition is caused by acute hydronephrosis due to kinking or vascular obstruction of the ureters.

On physical examination, the lower pole of the kidney can be palpated on deep inspiration. The examiner's finger should reach over the upper pole of the kidney and push it down to the navel. On Dietl's crisis, the kidney is tender on palpation and may be enlarged.

Historically, nephroptosis is used to be corrected by *nephropexy*, a surgical procedure characterized by suturing part of the renal capsule to the surrounding abdominal wall and vertebral column.





## Riley–Day Syndrome (Familial Dysautonomia)

Riley–Day syndrome (RDS) is a rare inherited disorder characterized by infantile hypertension, postural hypotension, and recurrent attacks of unexplained fever due to autonomic nervous system dysfunction.

As a rule, RDS manifests in infancy, which is important to assume the diagnosis. The major features are often seen in an infant or a child with recurrent attacks of unexplained fever, hypertension, and vomiting. Infants commonly have excessive drooling with swallowing difficulties, making them prone to recurrent aspiration pneumonia. Aspiration pneumonia is the main cause of death in patients with RDS.

Hypertension of RDS is characteristically associated with excitement. Intermittent attacks of hypertension with vomiting may cause RDS to be confused with infantile pheochromocytoma. Postural hypotension can be demonstrated in most patients beyond 2 years of age, and it can be so marked as to give rise to "blackout spells" when the patient stands.

## Stafne's Bone Defect of the Mandible

Stafne's bone defect of the mandible is a rare cyst-like bony defect with cortical bone thickening with continuity from the base of the mandible around the gonial angle of the mandible, under the mandibular canal on panoramic radiography or cone-beam CT. Most cases are seen in hypertensive patients from 40 to 60 years old. The bony defect is symptomless.

Stafne's mandibular bony defect is considered as a complication of long-standing hypertension and thought to be caused by high-pressure exertion by the facial artery over the mandible (■ Fig. 4.1.15).

## Hypertensive Heart Disease

Patients with long-standing hypertension develop left ventricle hypertrophy due to raised left ventricular wall tension, which may lead to coronary microangiopathy of the mid-wall portion of the left ventricle wall. *Hypertensive heart disease* is a term used to describe a hypertensive patient with cardiac failure due to diastolic heart dysfunction with normal systolic heart function (normal ejection fraction).

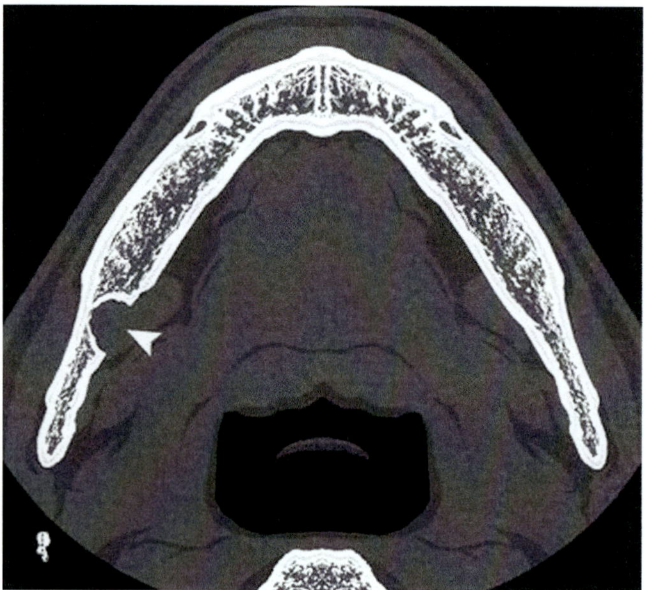



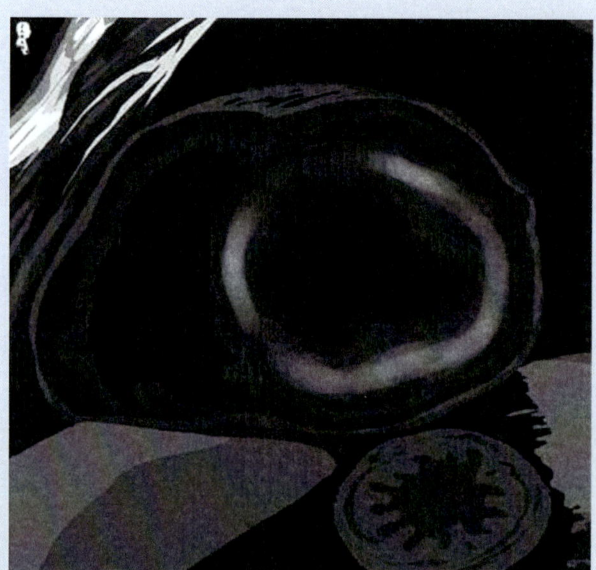

■ **Fig. 4.1.16**   Short-axis dark-blood postcontrast cardiac MR illustration demonstrates left ventricular concentric hypertrophy with intramural enhancement representing MR findings in hypertensive heart disease

Left ventricular hypertrophy can be generalized, reducing the internal cavity (concentric hypertrophy), or localized to the interventricular septum (eccentric hypertrophy). Left ventricular hypertrophy in hypertensive patients is usually concentric and typically found in moderate to severe hypertension in middle-aged and elderly patients. Left ventricular hypertrophy can cause atrial fibrillation and arrhythmias. Also, left ventricular hypertrophy in hypertensive patients is associated with three- to fourfold increase in the risk of stroke, a two- to threefold increase in coronary heart disease, and a threefold increase in peripheral arterial disease.

### Signs on Cardiac MRI
— Patients with left ventricular hypertrophy due to hypertensive heart disease can show intramural, mid-wall, or subendocardial delayed contrast enhancement (e.g., >15 min), mostly due to myocardial ischemia, necrosis, or fibrosis (■ Fig. 4.1.16). Patients with delayed contrast enhancement on cardiac MRI may show ST-segment depression or T-wave inversion on electrocardiogram.

## Further Reading

Akpunonu BE, et al. Secondary hypertension: evaluation and treatment. Dis Mon. 1996;42(10):609.

Andersen K, et al. Myocardial delayed contrast enhancement in patients with arterial hypertension: initial results of cardiac MRI. Eur J Radiol. 2009;71:75–81.

Ando H, et al. Abnormal collateral arterial system in Takayasu's arteritis and Lariche's syndrome evaluated by whole body acquisition using multislice computed tomography. Int J Cardiol. 2007;121:306–8.

Applegate KE, et al. Spontaneous colonic ischemia in a patient with Riley-Day syndrome. Pediatr Radiol. 1995;25:312–3.

Barber NJ, et al. Nephroptosis and nephropexy - hang up on the past? Eur Urol. 2004;46:428–33.

Bulum J, et al. Takayasu's arteritis and chronic autoimmune thyroiditis in a patient with type 1 diabetes mellitus. Clin Rheumatol. 2005;24:169–71.

Canyigit M, et al. Imaging characteristics of Takayasu arteritis. Cardiovasc Intervent Radiol. 2007;30:711–8.

Chen P, et al. Color and power Doppler imaging of the kidneys. World J Urol. 1998;16:41–5.

Das BB, et al. Midaortic syndrome presenting as neonatal hypertension. Pediatr Cardiol. 2008;29:1000–1.

Dineen R, et al. Imaging of acute neurological conditions in pregnancy and the puerperium. Clin Radiol. 2005;60:1156–70.

Dyer RB, et al. Classic signs in uroradiology. Radiographics. 2004;24:S247–80.

Ferrazzani S. Hypertension in pregnancy. Saudi J Kidney Dis Transpl. 1999;10(3):298–312.

Fujita T, et al. Takayasu arteritis evaluated by multi-slice computed tomography in old man. Int J Cardiol. 2008;125:286–7.

Ha HK, et al. Radiologic features of vasculitis involving the gastrointestinal tract. Radiographics. 2000;20:779–94.

Hartman RP, et al. Evaluation of renal causes of hypertension. Radiol Clin North Am. 2003;41:909–29.

Hoenig DM, et al. Nephroptosis: a "disparaged" condition revisited. Urology. 1999;54:590–6.

Lewis III VD, et al. The midaortic syndrome: diagnosis and treatment. Radiology. 1988;167:111–3.

Lip GYH, et al. Hypertensive heart disease. A complex syndrome or a hypertensive 'cardiomyopathy'? Eur Heart J. 2000;21:1653–65.

Moss SW. Floating kidneys: a century of nephroptosis and nephropexy. J Urol. 1997;158:699–702.

Olivier H, et al. Renovascular disease: Doppler ultrasound. Semin Ultrasound CT MRI. 1997;18(2):136–46.

Rooholamini SA, et al. Imaging of pregnancy-related complications. Radiographics. 1993;13:753–70.

Shimizu M, et al. CT analysis of the Stafne's bone defects of the mandible. Dentomaxillofac Radiol. 2006;35:95–102.

Son JS, et al. Pseudocoarctation of the aorta associated with the anomalous origin of the left vertebral artery: a case report. Korean J Radiol. 2008;9:283–5.

Soulez G, et al. Imaging of renovascular hypertension: respective values of renal Doppler US, and MR angiography. Radiographics. 2000;20:1355–68.

Stadlmaier E, et al. Midaortic syndrome and celiac disease: a case of local vasculitis. Clin Rheumatol. 2005;24:301–4.

Strohmeyer DM, et al. Changes of renal blood flow in nephroptosis: assessment by color Doppler imaging, isotope renography and correlation with clinical outcome after laparoscopic nephropexy. Eur Urol. 2004;45:790–3.

Taneja K, et al. Pseudocoarctation of the aorta: complementary findings on plain film radiography, CT, DSA, and MRA. Cardiovasc Intervent Radiol. 1998;21:439–41.

Van Hoe L, et al. Liver involvement in HELLP syndrome: CT and MRI findings in two patients. Eur Radiol. 1995;5:331–4.

## 4.2  Polycystic Kidney Disease

Polycystic kidney disease (PKD) is a disease characterized by the development of multiple cysts within the kidneys in bilateral fashion. A cyst is defined as a fluid-filled sac lined with a single layer of tubular epithelium. A cystic kidney is defined as a kidney that contains three or more cysts.

Simple renal cyst is the most common renal anomaly. Up to 22 % of symptomless patients over 70 years old or older have at least one renal cyst. There are three types of PKD: autosomal dominant (adult) PKD, autosomal recessive (infantile) PKD, and acquired PKD.

### Autosomal Dominant Polycystic Kidney Disease

Autosomal dominant polycystic kidney disease (ADPKD) is the fourth cause of chronic renal failure throughout the world. The disease has an autosomal dominant mode of inheritance as its name states, with a positive family history of ADPKD elicited in 60 % of patients.

ADPKD is typically seen in adults, with both kidneys affected in a bilateral, almost symmetrical, fashion. The kidneys are enlarged in size as the disease progresses. In a patient <30 years old with a positive family history of ADPKD, the presence of two cysts, either unilateral or bilateral, is sufficient to make the diagnosis. In patients >30 years old with a positive family history of ADPKD, at least two cysts in each kidney are sufficient to make the diagnosis.

Patients with ADPKD present with bilateral renal cysts with enlarged kidneys (100 %), renal pain (60 %), hematuria (42 %), hypertension (75 %), colonic diverticuli (80 %), and hepatic cysts (57 %). Potential causes of hematuria in ADPKD include renal stones formation (20 %) and glomerulonephritis.

Hypertension arises in 75 % of ADPKD with normal renal functions. Cyst expansion is believed to alter blood flow by glomerular compression, which results in the release of rennin, leading to the formation of angiotensin II.

Hepatic cysts occur in 57 %of patients with ADPKD, and they are rare before puberty. Hepatic cysts are believed to originate from cystic dilatation of the bile ducts. Patients may present with right upper quadrant pain due to liver capsule stretching and hepatomegaly.

Colonic diverticuli are seen in up to 80 % of patients with ADPKD, usually with end-stage renal disease. Patients with ADPKD are at risk of cerebral aneurysm rupture, which has a prevalence of <5 %. ADPKD patients with positive family history of cerebral arteries aneurysm have an increased incidence of developing cerebral aneurysm (22 %) than ADPKD patients with no family history of cerebral aneurysm (5 %). ADPKD patients with aneurismal rupture present with signs of intracranial bleeding or subarachnoid hemorrhage such as severe headache, neck stiffness, and altered consciousness, with nausea and vomiting.

Rare manifestations of ADPKD include coronary arteries or abdominal aorta aneury sm, mitral valve prolapse, aortic regurgitation, pancreatic cysts (10 %), splenic cysts (5 %), and inguinal hernias. Patients with ADPKD may develop seminal vesicle cysts, which present clinically as painful ejaculation, prostatitis, urinary tract obstruction, or epididymitis.

**Signs on US**
- The kidneys show multiple echo-free parenchymal cysts with typical posterior shadowing.
- Liver, pancreatic, or splenic cysts may be seen (Fig. 4.2.1).

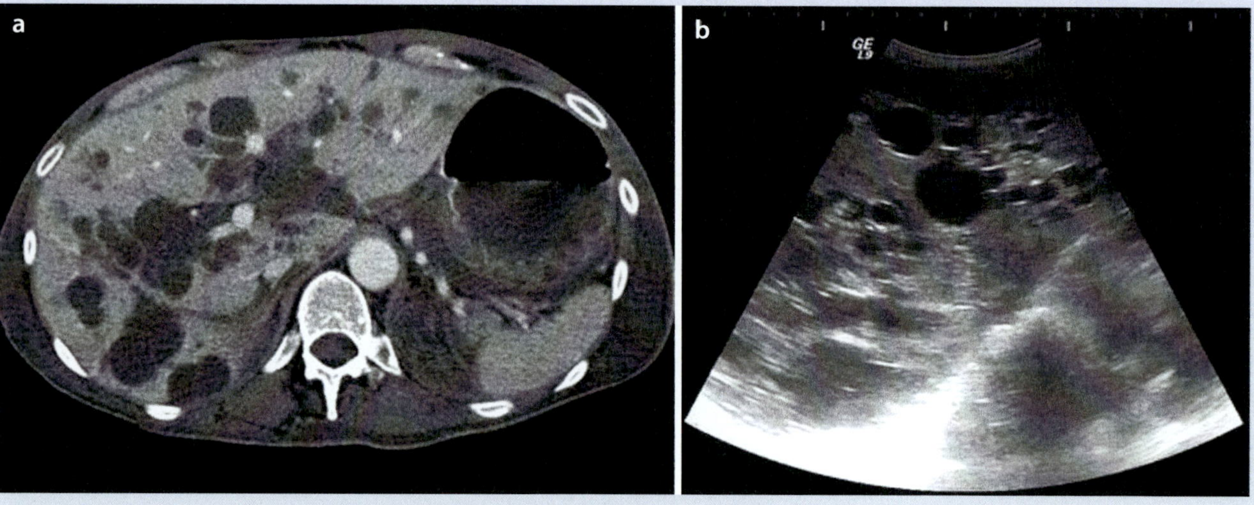

**Fig. 4.2.1** Axial CT postcontrast (**a**) with liver ultrasound (**b**) images show multiple liver cysts in a patient with ADPKD

**Signs on CT**
- Typically, both kidneys are enlarged with multiple cysts of variable sizes (Fig. 4.2.2).
- Hyperdense calculi may be seen within the renal pelvis or the ureters.
- Hepatic, pancreatic, or splenic cysts may be seen (Fig. 4.2.1). Intrahepatic cystic bile duct dilatation (Caroli's disease) can be associated with PKD in up to 70 % of cases.

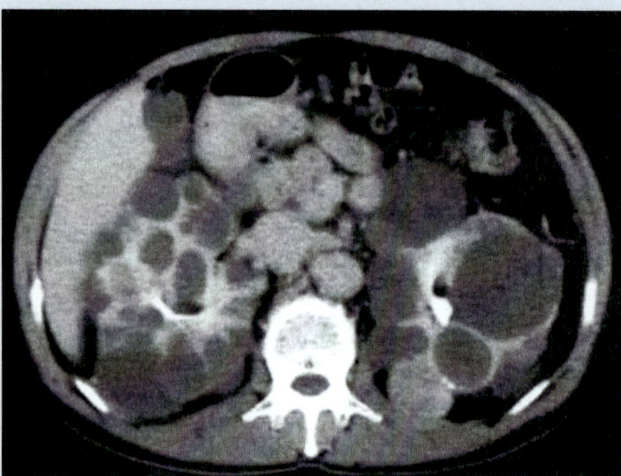

**Fig. 4.2.2** Axial CT urography image in a patient with ADPKD shows bilateral mildly enlarged kidneys with multiple cysts

**Signs on MRI**
- Cerebral MR angiography should be performed for ADPKD patients with positive family history of cerebral aneurysms as a screening examination. These aneurysms are classically saccular aneurysms that occur at the bifurcation of cerebral vessels and resemble a berry in size and shape (*berry aneurysm*). Up to 80 % of berry aneurysms arise from the circle of Willis, and 20 % arise from the posterior fossa.
- Seminal vesicle cyst is detected as unilocular cyst with fluid signal located at the posterolateral aspect of the urinary bladder. The cyst may be associated with ipsilateral ejaculatory duct dilatation that may protrude into the urinary bladder mimicking ectopic ureterocele.

## Autosomal Recessive Polycystic Kidney Disease

Autosomal recessive polycystic kidney disease (ARPKD) is a rare genetic disease with prevalence of 1:20,000 live births. ARPKD typically starts in neonates and infants as early renal failure. Infant's death usually occurs within the first year of life, unless renal transplantation is considered.

The kidneys are massively enlarged with numerous cysts. Hepatic fibrosis is very common in ARPKD (60 %). Hypertension occurs in almost all cases. Pregnant women with an infant with ARPKD typically display oligohydramnios.

### Signs on CT

- Both kidneys are massively enlarged while maintaining a reniform shape (Fig. 4.2.3).

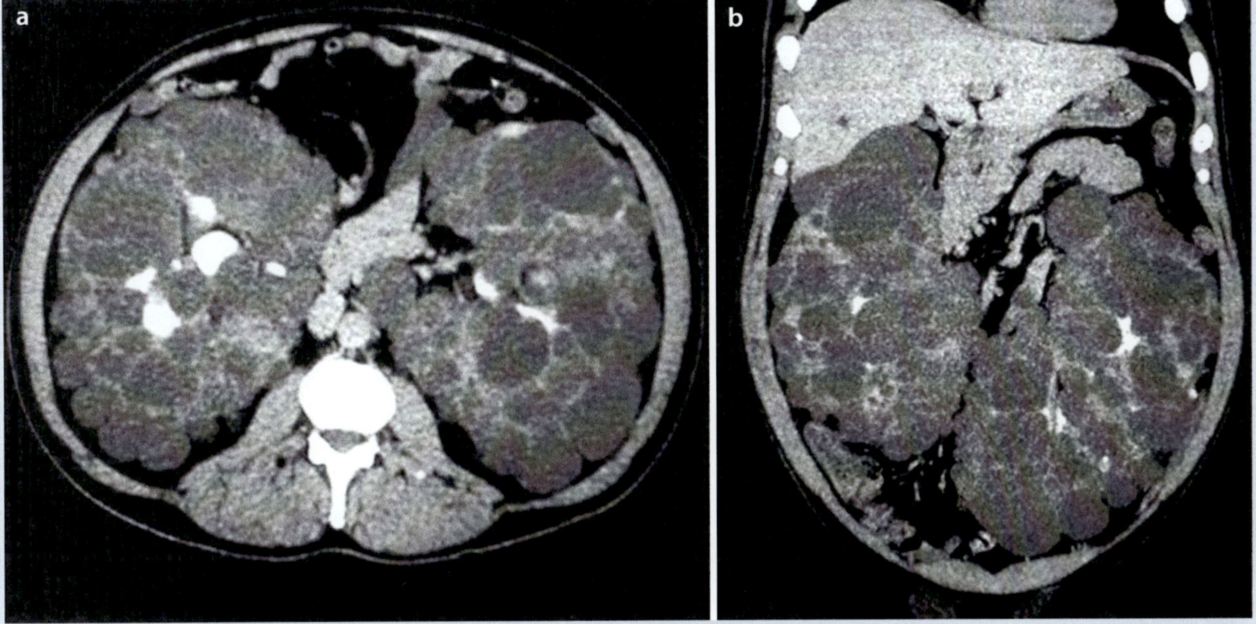

**Fig. 4.2.3** Axial (**a**) and coronal (**b**) CT urography images in a child with ARPKD show massively enlarged kidneys with numerous small cysts bilaterally

## Acquired Polycystic Kidney Disease

Acquired polycystic kidney disease (APKD) is typically seen in chronic renal failure and dialysis. Chronic potassium depletion in humans has been associated with the development of renal cysts (e.g., primary hyperaldosteronism). Some investigators use the term "multiple cystic kidney disease" for this condition to differentiate it from the true congenital polycystic kidney disease.

In contrast to ADPKD and ARPKD, the kidney size is usually normal or smaller than normal. Also, the acquired polycystic kidney has a tendency for malignant transformation.

### Signs on CT

- Bilateral normal size or shrunken kidneys with multiple cysts (Fig. 4.2.4).
- Signs of other complication of end-stage disease or adrenal hyperplasia (hyperaldosteronism) may be seen.

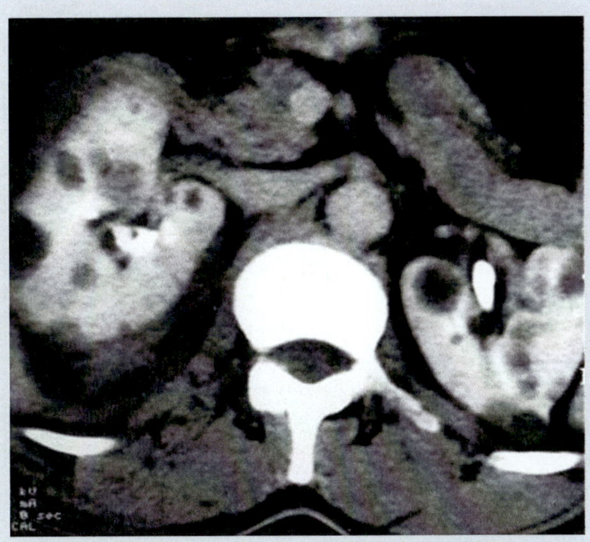

**Fig. 4.2.4** Axial CT urography in a patient with acquired polycystic kidney disease shows bilateral normal-sized kidneys with small cysts

## Differential Diagnoses and Related Diseases

*Nephronophthisis* is an uncommon autosomal dominant disorder characterized by a triad of anemia, salt-wasting, and abnormal levels of nitrogen-containing compounds like urea and creatinine (azotemia) due to tubulointerstitial nephritis. Patients are usually young adults or children presenting with end-stage renal failure. Due to its nonspecific symptoms, definite diagnosis is usually established by kidney biopsy, which classically shows tubular basement membrane disintegration, tubular cyst formation, and tubulointerstitial fibrosis. The disease has three forms: infantile, juvenile, and adolescent. Nephronophthisis can be associated with retinitis pigmentosa (Senior–Løken syndrome), cerebellar ataxia and cerebellar vermis hypoplasia (Joubert syndrome), oculomotor apraxia (Cogan's syndrome), hepatic fibrosis and biliary duct proliferation (Boichis syndrome), phalangeal cone-shaped epiphysis (Saldino-Mainzer disease/conorenal syndrome), hypopituitarism (RHYNS syndrome), ectodermal dysplasia (Sensenbrenner syndrome), and Leber's amaurosis (Arima-Dekaban syndrome). Brain MRI shows the characteristic "molar tooth sign" due to superior cerebellar vermis hypoplasia of Joubert syndrome. On ultrasound, kidneys show multiple cysts up to 2 cm in size, characteristically located at the renal medulla, with hyperechoic cortex and loss of the corticomedullary differentiation. Many researches consider the clinical presentation of nephronophthisis with ultrasound picture of medullary renal cysts as being characteristic and sufficient to establish the diagnosis without the need for renal biopsy. However, renal medullary cysts may be absent in 30% of cases, so the absence of medullary renal cysts does not rule out the diagnosis.

### Further Reading

Blowey DL, et al. Ultrasound findings in juvenile nephronophthisis. Pediatr Nephrol. 1996;10:22–4.

Capisonda R, et al. Autosomal recessive polycystic kidney disease: outcomes from a single-center experience. Pediatr Nephrol. 2003;18:119–26.

Grossman H, et al. Sonographic diagnosis of renal cystic diseases. AJR. 1963;140:81–5.

Martinez JR, et al. Polycystic kidney disease: etiology, pathogenesis and treatment. Dis Mon. 1995;41(11):693–765.

Roche CJ, et al. Selections from the buffet of food signs in radiology. Radiographics. 2002;22:1369–84.

Salomon R, et al. Nephronophthisis. Pediatr Nephrol. 2009;24:2333–44.

Vauthey JN, et al. Adult polycystic disease of the liver. Br J Surg. 1991;78:524–7.

## 4.3    Renal Failure

A renal parenchymal disorder (RPD) is a term used to describe a disease that involves one or more compartments o the renal parenchyma. When this parenchymal injury causes impairment of renal functions, the term "renal failure" is applied to the disease as a progression of parenchymal injury.

The human body contains around one million nephrons in each kidney. The "nephron" is the functional unit of the kidney, and it is composed of glomerulus and a tubule. The normal renal parenchyma is divided into:

1. *Glomeruli (cortex)*: it is the functional unit of the kidney, and it is responsible for plasma ultrafiltration. Another part of the cortex is the *juxtaglomerular apparatus* and the *cortical proximal and distal tubules*, which are responsible for processing the primary urine, thereby maintaining body homeostasis.

   The glomerulus is a tuft of capillaries lined by epithelial cells. The endothelial cell and epithelial cell sandwich the basement membrane, and these structures together constitute a sieve which results in a glomerular ultrafiltrate passing into Bowman's space at the start of the tubule.

   The average adult glomerular filtration rate (GFR) is 125 ml/min/1.73 m$^2$. Therefore, the glomeruli of a healthy adult filter 180 L of plasma each day (around 120 times the normal daily adult urine production).

2. *Renal tubules (cortex and medulla)*: the renal tubules include the proximal tubule (*lies in the cortex*), the loop of Henle (*lies in the medulla*), the distal tubule (*lies in the cortex*), and the collecting duct (*lies in the medulla*).

   Each renal tubule is responsible for reabsorption or secretion of different metabolites. The reabsorption may be across the tubular cells (transcellular) or passively across the tight junctions in between tubular cells (paracellular).

3. *Interstitium*: it refers to the "connective tissue" of both compartments (cortex and medulla) including the lymphatic tissue.

4. *Renal vessels*: these include the intrarenal and the arcuate arteries.

## Examples of Renal Parenchymal Disorders According to Their Anatomical Involvement

A. *Glomerulonephritis (acute nephritis syndrome)*: presents mainly with hematuria and hypertension. Other signs include proteinuria and impaired renal function (e.g., *oliguria*). Oliguria defined as a urine volume < 400 ml/24 h/1.73 m$^2$ body surface area (BSA). Serum complements is an important test to be done in a patient suspected with glomerulonephritis.

B. *Renal tubular disorder*: presents mainly with polyuria/polydipsia and electrolytes imbalance (e.g., *metabolic acidosis, metabolic alkalosis, hyponatremia, hypokalemia,* etc.). Chronic renal tubular disease results in failure to thrive, nephrolithiasis, nephrocalcinosis (mainly medullary type), refractory rickets and osteomalacia, and hypertension.

C. *Renal interstitial disorder*: typically present with chronic renal failure due to renal parenchymal fibrosis and atrophy. Examples of renal interstitial disorders include analgesic nephropathy (e.g., *NSAIDs, Chinese herbs*), toxic materials (e.g., *lithium, lead, cadmium*), interstitial nephritis (e.g., *Lupus nephritis, Sjögren's syndrome*), infections *(CMV, nephropathia epidemica)*, and granulomas (e.g., *sarcoidosis, TB*).

D. *Renal vascular disorders*: typically present with hypertension (e.g., *vasculitis, nutcracker syndrome, hemolytic uremic syndrome, etc.*)

Acute renal failure (ARF) is a disease characterized by decrease/impaired renal functions. ARF can be subdivided into three main subtypes based on the etiology:

1. *Prerenal ARF*: the main cause is hypoperfusion of the kidney that can be due to hemorrhage, shock, hepatorenal syndrome, renal artery stenosis (RAS), and congestive heart failure. Prerenal ARF can occur in patients with RAS who are treated with ACE inhibitors or angiotensin II blockers (*which are normally highly secreted by the kidney to overcome RAS*). A patient who develops ARF with ACE inhibitors or angiotensin II blockers should be investigated for RAS. In children, the most common causes of prerenal ARF include sepsis, hyperviscosity, dehydration, and heart disease (*patent ductus arteriosus and coarctation of the aorta*).

2. *Renal ARF*: it is caused by a disease that affects the renal parenchyma itself (*glomerular, tubular, interstitial, or vascular*).

3. *Postrenal ARF*: it is caused by obstruction of the urine outflow at different levels:
   (a) *Ureter*: stones, strictures, and retrocaval course
   (b) *Bladder*: neurogenic bladder, bladder carcinoma, and stones (rare)
   (c) *Prostate*: benign prostatic hyperplasia and prostate cancers

Signs of ARF include oliguria, increased serum blood-urea nitrogen (BUN) and creatinine levels, increased uric acid levels, metabolic acidosis, hyponatremia, hyperkalemia (*if not corrected pharmacologically consider dialysis*), hyperphosphatemia, hypocalcemia, anemia (*due to decreased erythropoiesis*), leukopenia, and platelet dysfunctions. Urinalysis shows low urea and creatinine levels, proteinuria, and low concentrations of chloride, sodium, and potassium. Other signs of ARF include nausea and vomiting, brown tongue, gastrointestinal bleeding, left heart failure, and maybe pericarditis. Neurological manifestations include fatigability, muscle twitching, and maybe excessive sleeping (hypersomnolence).

In a busy radiology department, many of the ultrasound referrals are from the nephrology and/or the urology department. Renal ultrasound is an essential integral part of the investigation of many renal disorders because of its easy accessibility, its high accuracy, lack of radiation exposure, and lack or radiological contrast exposure. It is the intention of this theme to concentrate on the sonographic signs of different renal disorders that will help the radiologist to characterize the renal status for the referring clinician.

### Signs on Ultrasound

1. *Normal kidney* is ovoid shape with a diameter of 9–12 cm, width 4–6 cm, and normal thickness of the parenchyma 15–25 mm; the pyramids are more echo-poor than the cortex (*good contrast in children, less in elderly persons*); and the cortex is hypoechoic compared to the liver.

2. For *renal size*, the mean right renal length is $10.74 \pm 1.35$ cm and mean left renal length is $11.10 \pm 1.15$ cm, measured as the longest diameter obtained on a posterior oblique image. Asymmetry in renal size can be suggestive of ischemic renal disease (2 cm difference between the two kidneys is a significant measurement of ischemic lesion).

3. *Renal volume* is measured via the following equation: volume (V) = craniocaudal diameter × anteroposterior diameter × transverse diameter × 0.5233. To adjust it to the patient's body size, the volume is then divided by the patient's body mass index (V/BMI × 25). The normal renal volume after adjustment to the body mass index is 231–281. Increased renal volume > 281 means nephromegaly.

4. *Parenchymal echogenicity* is a nonspecific sign that reflects nephropathy, which is classified as the following: *grade 0*, echogenicity poorer than that of the liver parenchyma (normal finding); *grade I*, echogenicity identical to that of the liver parenchyma (normal finding); *grade II*, echogenicity more intense than that of the liver parenchyma (pathological finding); and *grade III*, echogenicity identical to that of the renal sinus (pathological finding). Parenchymal echogenicity varies also with the patient's age (*it is increased in newborn babies up to 6 months of age due to elevated cellularity and in elderly patients due to fibrosis*).

5. *On normal Doppler sonography*, the renal artery shows diameter of 5–8 mm, maximum velocity ($V_{max}$) of 60–180 cm/s, intrarenal RI = 0.6–0.7, and < 10 % difference between right and left kidney. The intrarenal RI is measured from the arcuate arteries (at the corticomedullary junction) or interlobar arteries (adjacent to medullary pyramids). Three to five reproducible waveforms from each kidney are obtained, and RIs from these waveforms are averaged to arrive at mean RI values for each kidney (**□** Fig. 4.3.1).

   In children, it is common for the mean RI to exceed 0.70 through the first year of life, and a mean RI greater than 0.70 can be seen through at least the first 4 years of life. In elderly patients without renal insufficiency, the normal RI can also exceed 0.70. An RI difference greater than 0.10 between the kidneys is seen only with true obstructive renal disease.

6. In *acute renal failure*, morphological abnormalities in B-mode are only seen in 11 % of patients. However,

almost 70 % of patients show intrarenal elevated RI (>0.7) and normal or low RI in prerenal causes (<0.7) on Doppler sonography.

7. In *chronic renal failure*, renal size < 8 cm is a sign of chronic renal failure. Reduced renal volume is a negative prognostic sign and correlates histopathologically with the degree of atrophy, necrosis, and fibrosis. It can be seen in chronic glomerulonephritis, papillary necrosis, hereditary nephropathy, widespread nephrosclerosis, and end-stage chronic renal failure. In patients with chronic renal failure, RI > 0.80 on Doppler sonography predicts progression of nephropathy more accurately than creatinine clearance and proteinuria, showing sensitivity (64 %) and specificity (98 %).

8. *Nephromegaly* is detected when the renal length size is > 13 cm in length or renal volume > 281. In newly diagnosed diabetics, the kidney size is normal or enlarged (>13 cm in diameter) due to glomerular hyperfiltration.

   *Nephromegaly with high renal volume* can be seen in renal hyperfiltration due to insulin therapy, acute tubular necrosis (ATN), acute interstitial nephritis, accumulating diseases (*amyloid, glycogen, lipids*), and liver cirrhosis. Particularly ATN leads to a substantial increase in the anteroposterior diameter of both kidneys, while the length is generally normal.

9. In *nephrocalcinosis*, the hypoechoic medulla appears echogenic with or without shadow reflection in *medullary nephrocalcinosis*, and the cortex appears echogenic with or without shadow reflection in *cortical nephrocalcinosis*. Cortical nephrocalcinosis usually arises due to ischemic injury.

10. *Hyperechoic medullae* can be seen in medullary fibrosis or nephrocalcinosis due to gout, medullary sponge kidney, primary hyperaldosteronism, hyperparathyroidism, glycogenosis, and Wilson's disease.

11. For *hyperechoic corticomedullary junction*, this sign is not specific to a disease but can be seen in diabetes, pseudoxanthoma elasticum, and arterial hypertension.

12. *Diffusely hypoechoic kidney* is an uncommon sign that can be seen in acute pyelonephritis, lymphoma, and nephroblastomatosis.

13. *Glomerular diseases* show normal kidneys in US examination until later stages of the disease. In later stages of the disease, the kidney shrinks (size < 8 cm), and the cortex starts to show increased echogenicity due to inflammation with or without fibrosis (◘ Fig. 4.3.2). In contrast to tubulointerstitial diseases, the RI on Doppler sonography is usually normal in glomerular diseases (mean = 0.58).

14. In *tubulointerstitial nephritis*, the hallmark of tubulointerstitial nephritis is increased *medullary* echogenicity, which correlates with the degree of glomerular sclerosis and interstitial fibrosis. The RI on Doppler sonography is almost always high (>0.75) in interstitial parenchymal pathologies.

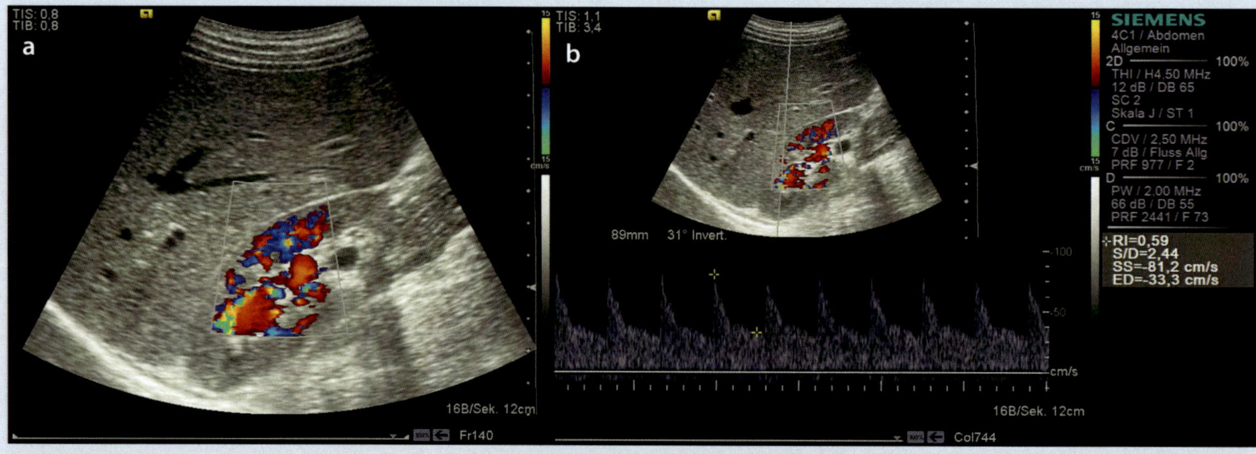


◘ **Fig. 4.3.1** Ultrasound image B-mode (**a**) and Doppler mode (**b**) of a normal kidney

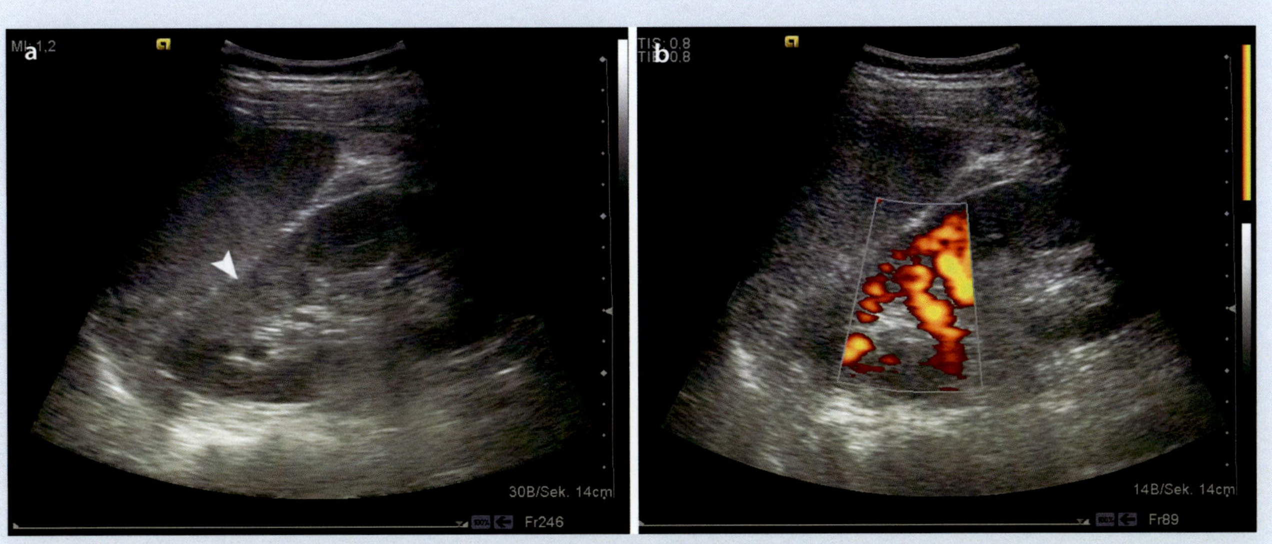

**Fig. 4.3.2** Ultrasound image B-mode (**a**) and power Doppler mode (**b**) of a left kidney with glomerulonephritis due to Streptococcal infection. A localized area of hyperechoic cortex is detected (*arrowhead*) with subsequent hyperemia on power Doppler mode (**b**)

## References

Abernethy LJ, et al. Fibromuscular dysplasia of the renal artery in a child: detection by Doppler ultrasound and correction by percutaneous transluminal angioplasty. Pediatr Radiol. 1989;19:539–40.

Arnerlöv C, et al. Dynamic sonography with provocation of pain for diagnosis of symptomatic mobile kidneys. Eur J Surg. 2001;167:218–21.

Bagga A, et al. Approach to renal tubular disorders. Indian J Pediatr. 2005;72(9):771–6.

Beland MD, et al. Renal cortical thickness measured at ultrasound: is it better than renal length as an indicator of renal function in chronic kidney disease? AJR. 2010;195:W146–9.

Buturovic-Ponikvar J, et al. Ultrasonography in chronic renal failure. Eur J Radiol. 2003;46:115–22.

Christian MT. Renal tubular disorders. Paediatr Child Health. 2010;20(6):266–73.

Fiorini F, et al. The role of ultrasonography in the study of medical nephropathy. J Ultrasound. 2007;10:161–7.

Fredericks BJ, et al. Glomerulocystic renal disease: ultrasound appearances. Pediatr Radiol. 1989;19:184–6.

Meola M, et al. Color Doppler sonography in the study of chronic ischemic nephropathy. J Ultrasound. 2008;11:55–73.

Mercado-Deane MG, et al. US of renal insufficiency in neonates. Radiographics. 2002;22:1429–38.

Riccabona M. Renal failure in neonates, infants, and children: the role of ultrasound. Ultrasound Clin. 2006;1:457–69.

Ries M, et al. Parapelvic kidney cysts: a distinguishing feature with high prevalence in Fabry disease. Kidney Int. 2004;66:978–82.

Tublin ME, et al. The resistive index in renal Doppler sonography: where do we stand? AJR. 2003;180:885–92.

Vester U, et al. The diagnostic value of ultrasound in cystic kidney diseases. Pediatr Nephrol. 2010;25:231–40.

# Cardiology




© Springer International Publishing Switzerland 2017
J.A. Al-Tubaikh, *Internal Medicine*, DOI 10.1007/978-3-319-39747-4_5

## 5.1    Acute Chest Pain

Acute chest pain is one of the most common complaints encountered in medical emergency departments. Chest pain is divided into cardiac and noncardiac chest pain. Causes of cardiac chest pain include angina pectoris (stable and unstable), myocardial infarction (MI) (ST-segment elevation and non-ST-segment elevation), myocarditis, etc. Noncardiac chest pain includes diseases of the great vessels, esophagitis, pneumonia, etc.

This topic discusses the use of radiology in detecting acute chest pain and how the radiologist can contribute in assessing causes of acute chest pain in emergency departments.

## Acute Coronary Syndrome

Acute coronary syndrome (CAS) is a term used to describe symptoms and manifestations of myocardial ischemia induced by coronary artery disease.

The most important components of CAS are angina pectoris and its severe complication MI. *Angina pectoris* is a term used to describe transient myocardial ischemia in the absence of myocardial cell death. In contrast, *MI* is a term used to describe myocardial cell death and necrosis due to ischemia.

Patients with angina pectoris classically present with retrosternal chest pain, which radiates to the neck and the left shoulder, accompanied by a sensation of numbness in the fingers. Associated symptoms include tachycardia, dyspnea, and possibly arrhythmia. The chest pain in angina pectoris typically lasts <10 min in duration. Patients with MI classically present with the symptoms of angina pectoris in a severe fashion. The retrosternal chest pain is severe and associated with autonomic nervous system hyperactivity, causing profound sweating and at times loss of consciousness. The chest pain typically may last up to 30 min in duration.

MI can be transmural involving the whole thickness of the myocardial wall due to complete occlusion of the coronary artery. MI can also be subendocardial, which is classically seen in coronary arterial spasm and hypertension due to hypoperfusion. The vascular supply of the endocardium is the part of the heart wall that is most sensitive to hypoperfusion.

Cardiac CT is used in patients with acute chest pain to rule out three main conditions (triple rule out): acute MI, pulmonary embolism (PE), and aortic dissection. Cardiac CT can also be used to detect calcium plaques within the coronary arteries in a technique known as "calcium scoring."

*Calcium scoring* is a method that quantifies the atherosclerotic plaques within the coronary vessels. The calcium score is used to assess the risk of heart events, not to detect coronary stenosis. The basic idea of calcium scoring is to perform a noncontrast CT of the heart to detect calcified plaques (◘ Fig. 5.1.1). Once a calcified plaque is identified in the coronary arteries, the examiner encircles the plaque by a cursor, and a special program will measure the plaque attenuation and express it as a number in Hounsfield units as a

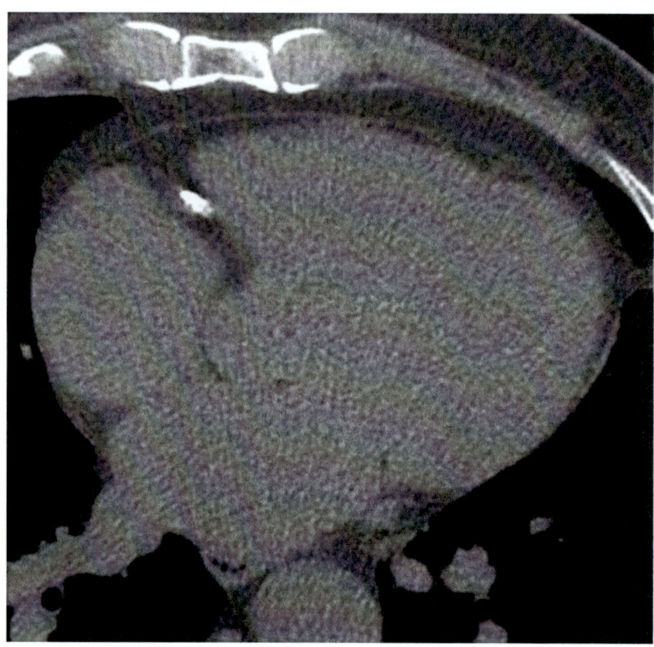

◘ **Fig. 5.1.1**    Axial nonenhanced cardiac CT examination for calcium scoring shows calcified plaque in the right coronary artery

score (Agatston score). Each coronary branch is measured separately and then the numbers added to give a total calcium burden score. The score predicts the probability of heart attacks in the next 5–10 years on the current status of the patient without treatment modifications.

Uncalcified atherosclerotic plaques take up to 15 years before they are calcified and visualized in a calcium scoring study or noncontrast CT study. The uncalcified (vulnerable) plaque appears inhomogeneous or with low density on CT scan ($25 \pm 15$ HU). Uncalcified and partially calcified plaques are more associated with ACS than are calcified plaques, because they are unstable and can be dislodged, initiating a coronary embolic attack.

Cardiac MRI in CAS patients is mainly used to study myocardial wall motion (*myocardial function study*), perfusion (same as the *thallium perfusion study*), viability, and ejection fraction measurement like cardiac Doppler study (*phase-contrast flow quantification*). The role of cardiac MRI postinfarction is to identify viable (salvageable) myocardium, which is mainly detected by the (*myocardial viability study*).

The basic concept of the myocardial viability study is to detect how much viable (alive and contractile) myocardium is left after MI. The technique depends upon the fact that gadolinium diffuses into the myocardial interstitial spaces after its injection into the body. As long as the myocardial membrane (sarcolemma) is intact, the gadolinium is pumped out of the intracellular compartment and concentrated in the extracellular compartment until it is washed out 10 min after its injection. This scenario occurs with normal and viable myocardium. If the myocardium is diseased or infarcted, the gadolinium will diffuse inside the extra- and intracellular compartments, which makes its clearance take longer time than 10 min. Myocardial contrast enhancement that exceeds 10 min from gadolinium injection is called "late gadolinium enhancement," which is considered pathological, and the test is considered positive for nonviable myocardium.

Loss of cardiac wall motion, which is assessed in the myocardial function study, is another important sign of nonviable myocardium. However, there are two situations where the myocardium is viable but is not contracting: myocardial stunning and hibernating myocardium. *Myocardial stunning* is a situation where the cardiac muscles are viable, but they do not contract as a transient phenomenon after MI (like penumbra after stroke). *Hibernating myocardium* is a situation where the cardiac muscles are viable, but are not contracting after reestablishing coronary perfusion due to a long period of chronic perfusion abnormalities. This situation is typically seen in patients with long-standing, compromised coronary perfusion who have undergone coronary artery bypass surgery (CABG). Although the perfusion is normally established after a long period of hypoperfusion, the muscles are not contracting due to a long period of cardiac muscle ischemia and hypofunction.

### Signs on Chest Radiographs
- Indirect signs of CAS include aortic calcification of aorta or coronary arteries calcification.
- If the MI is complicated by heart failure, signs of pulmonary edema may be detected such as upper lobe vessel cephalization and enlarged cardiac silhouette (◘ Fig. 5.1.2).

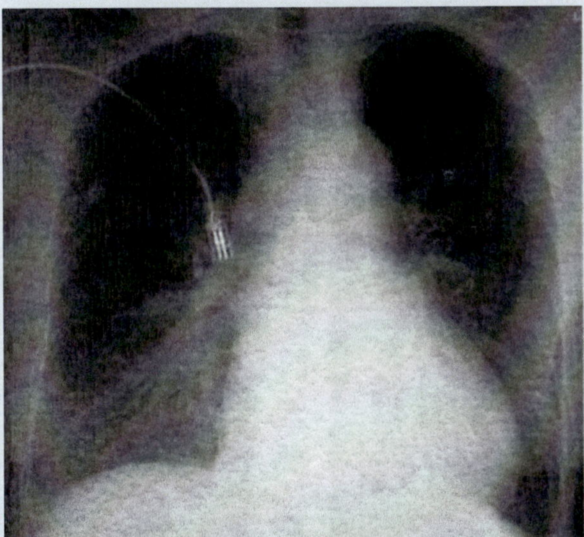

◘ Fig. 5.1.2   Anteroposterior chest radiograph of a bedridden patient with myocardial infarction (MI) shows congested hilar vessels and beginning of pulmonary edema

### Signs on Cardiac CT
- In a patient with acute chest pain, detection of calcified plaques on the nonenhanced coronary vessels with absence of signs of aortic dissection or embolism confirms the diagnosis of CAS. However, absence of the coronary calcified plaques does not rule out CAS because uncalcified plaques can be present. Up to 50 % of patients with sudden cardiac arrests show calcified lesions in their coronary arteries (◘ Fig. 5.1.1).
- MI may be seen as a subendocardial ventricular hypodense area depending upon the blocked coronary artery and its vascular territory.
- Post-myocardial infarction calcification and ventricular dilatation may occur (◘ Fig. 5.1.3).

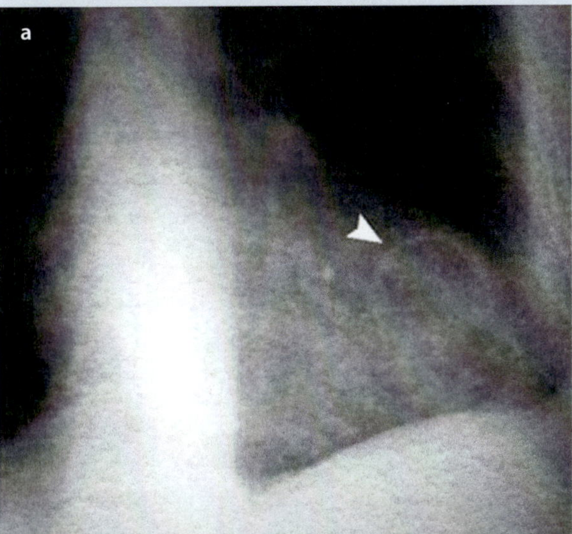

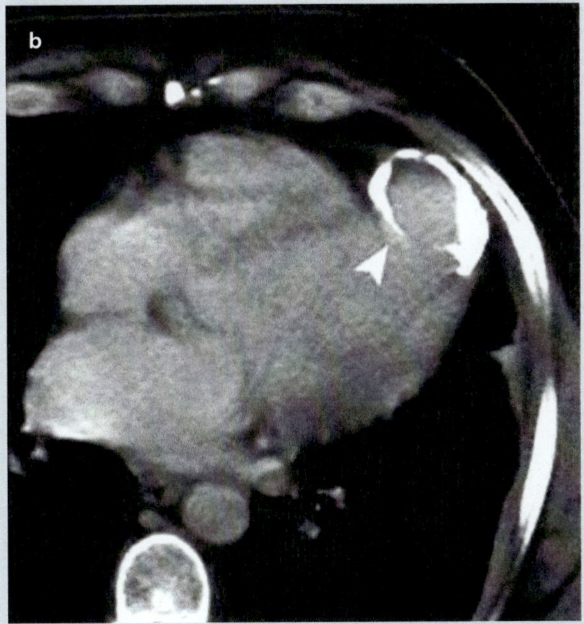

◘ Fig. 5.1.3   Posteroanterior chest radiograph (**a**) and thorax CT (**b**) shows focal apical left ventricular dilatation with calcified rim due to old MI of this region (*arrowheads*)

### Signs of MI on MRI

— Wall motion abnormalities (akinesia or hypokinesia) on cine MRI.
— Contrast enhancement on delayed images (>10 min). There are four patterns of late contrast enhancement of MI: *First pattern* is subendocardial enhancement with sparing of the subepicardial region (■ Fig. 5.1.4a). *Second pattern* is full-thickness myocardial wall enhancement (■ Fig. 5.1.4b). *Third pattern* is full-thickness myocardial wall enhancement, with subendocardial hypointense area, representing a severe edema compressing the intramural vessels (■ Fig. 5.1.4c). *Fourth pattern* is seen as a dark hypointense area that represents the infracted area surrounded by a rim enhancement (■ Fig. 5.1.4d). The fourth pattern is seen in extensive MI with less viable myocardium.
— Stunned and hibernating myocardium is visualized as wall motion abnormalities (akinesia or hypokinesia) in cine MRI with no contrast enhancement on delayed images (>10 min).

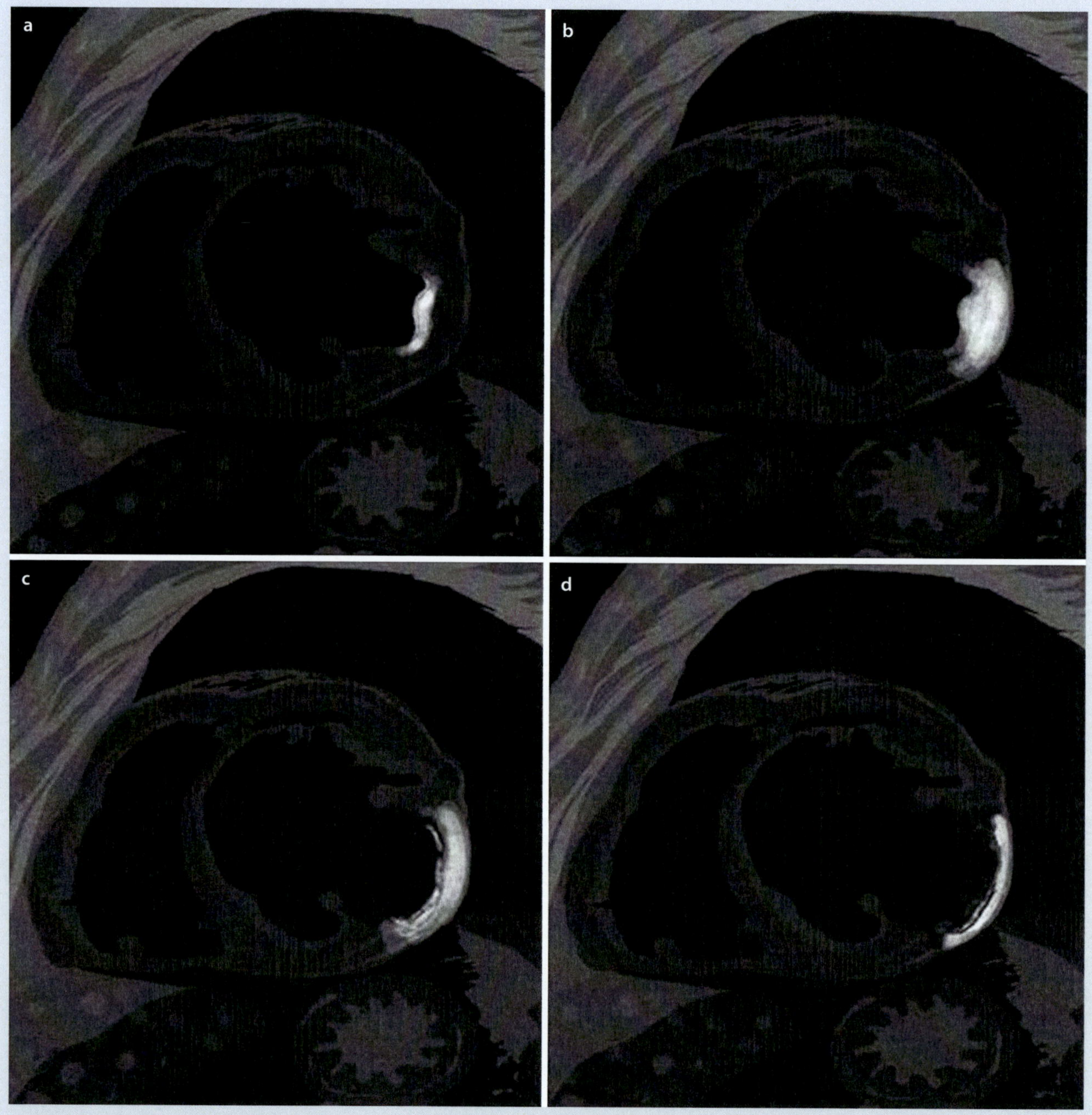

■ **Fig. 5.1.4**  Short-axis dark-blood T1W postcontrast cardiac MR illustrations show different pattern of myocardial enhancement after MI: (**a**) subendocardial enhancement with sparing of the subepicardial region; (**b**) full-thickness myocardial wall enhancement; (**c**) full-thickness myocardial wall enhancement, with subendocardial hypointense area; and (**d**) dark hypointense area represents the infarction surrounded by a rim enhancement

*Why does atherosclerosis not develop in the veins and is only seen in the arteries, although the cholesterol circulates in the blood in both veins and arteries?*

This occurs because the arterial pulsation assists in the deposition of the cholesterol molecules within the intima. Normally, the pulmonary arteries do not pulsate, but when pulmonary hypertension develops, the high pressure blood within the arteries evokes the arterial wall to pulsate, resulting in developing atherosclerosis within the pulmonary arteries.

## Acute Pulmonary Embolism

Acute pulmonary embolism (PE) is an emergency situation characterized by closure of a pulmonary artery by an embolus causing pulmonary ventilation–perfusion mismatch or, in a worse scenario, pulmonary infarction.

The bronchial circulation only supplies nutrients and does not participate in gas exchange in normal situations. However, in PE, the bronchial circulation responds with enlargement and hypertrophy and participates in blood oxygenation due to decreased pulmonary flow and ischemia.

PE is categorized according to severity into two main types: acute sub-massive and acute massive PE. Acute sub-massive PE is characterized by <50 % occlusion of the pulmonary vascular bed, whereas acute massive PE is characterized by >50 % occlusion of the pulmonary vascular bed.

Patients with acute PE often describe acute sudden chest "gunshot-like" pain with progressive dyspnea, tachycardia, and cyanosis. Many patients have a history of deep venous thrombosis (DVT), varicose veins, immobilization, or recent pelvic surgery. A dislodged part of the initial thrombus, mostly from the lower limbs, travels through the venous circulation until it blocks an arterial pulmonary vessel in the chest as an embolus, causing pulmonary vascular congestion. If this congestion persists, pulmonary infarction occurs.

In small percentage of patients, the unresolved thrombus after treatment can be incorporated into the vessel wall and covered by a layer of epithelium. This thrombus organization causes intravascular stenosis of the affected lumen, resulting in the development of pulmonary hypertension and cor pulmonale.

Acute PE is best diagnosed by V/Q scan (ventilation–perfusion nuclear scan study) in circulatory stabilized patient. The scan typically shows pulmonary ventilation–perfusion mismatch. In unstable acute PE patients, CT pulmonary angiography is the initial examination of choice.

### Signs on Chest Radiograph
- Radiographs are normal in 12 % of cases.
- Pulmonary infarction can appear as a patchy radio-opaque shadow on chest radiograph, which cannot be differentiated from patchy pneumonia or pulmonary contusions. Therefore, the radiographic signs have to be correlated with the history and the clinical data.
- *Hampton's hump*: is a wedge-shaped radio-opaque patch that is round shaped, located at the lung periphery, and directed from peripheral toward the hilum (◘ Fig. 5.1.5). This patch represents wedge-shaped infarction of the peripheral lung parenchyma.
- PE can be accompanied by Hemorrhagic pleural effusion.

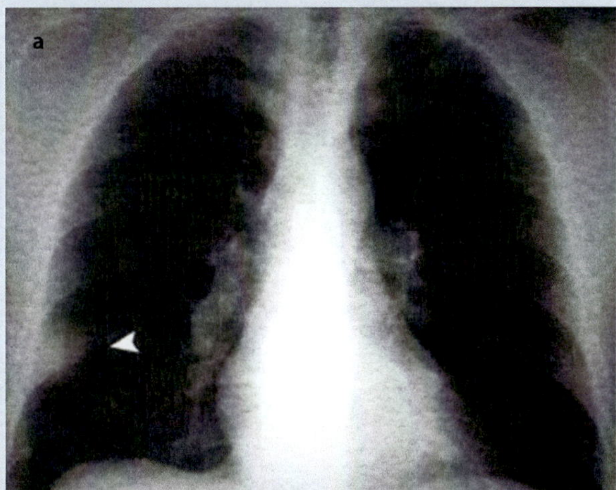
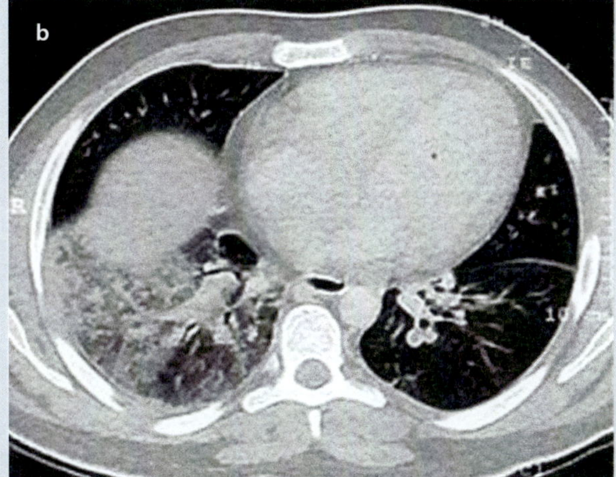

◘ **Fig. 5.1.5** Posteroanterior chest radiograph (**a**) and chest HRCT in two different patients with pulmonary infarction show Hampton's hump in (**a**) (*arrowhead*) and basal area of pulmonary parenchymal consolidation due to infarction in (**b**)

### Signs on Doppler Sonography

- Doppler sonography should be performed for patients with PE or patients with high risk of DVT who show signs of respiratory distress (e.g., bedridden patients).
- DVT is diagnosed on Doppler sonography when an intravenous echogenic material is detected (e.g., thrombus), the vein is distended and noncompressible (most specific and diagnostic sign), and there is loss of color duplex signal within the vein. The thrombus should be followed by the probe to detect its free edge, and an observation of labile, freely moving edge on real-time sonography should be reported. A labile, free edge thrombus has a high risk of embolization (□ Fig. 5.1.6).

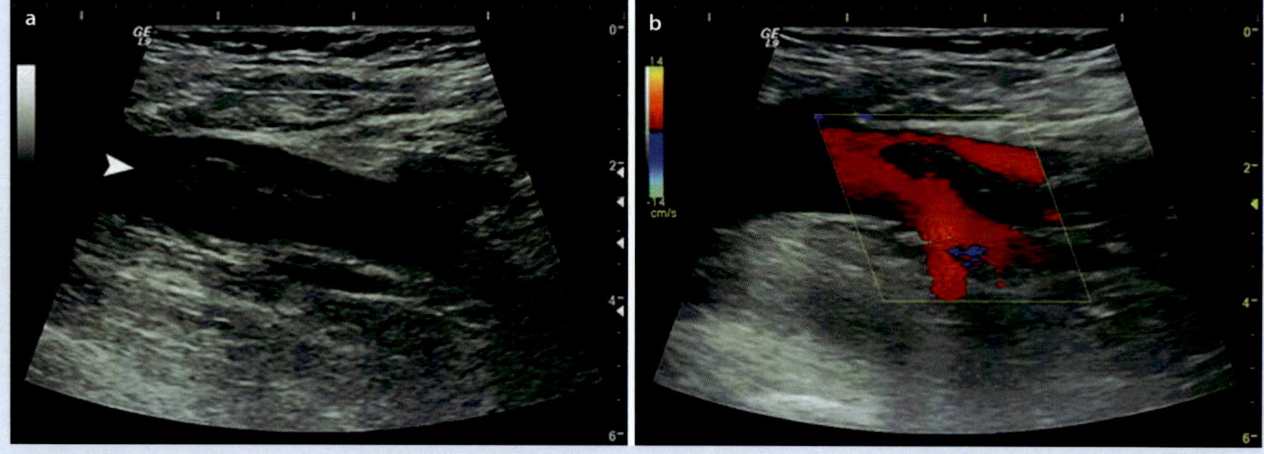

□ **Fig. 5.1.6**  Sagittal, Doppler sonography (**a**) and Duplex (**b**) images of a patient with DVT show hypoechoic material within the external iliac vein with free labile edge

### Signs on CTA

- PE is detected as complete filling defect with failure to enhance the entire lumen (complete thrombosis). The thrombosed vessel may be enlarged, and the thrombus may appear hyperdense on non contrast-enhanced images.
- Partial filling defect of a pulmonary vessel surrounded by areas of contrast material enhancement (□ Fig. 5.1.7) may be seen.
- Pulmonary infarction is visualized as a wedge-shaped area of lung parenchyma with high density located in the periphery of the lung, with the base lying along the pleura (□ Fig. 5.1.5).
- Areas of lobar atelectasis in PE may show contrast enhancement.
- Chronic PE is visualized as a peripheral intra-arterial wall filling defect. Calcification of the organized thrombus may be seen.
- *Saddle thrombus* is a term used to describe a big thrombus that abuts over the bifurcation of the main pulmonary arteries (□ Fig. 5.1.7).
- Signs of right ventricular enlargement might be seen in CT with displacement of the ventricular septum toward the left ventricle, as a sign pulmonary hypertension.
- Areas of mosaic lung parenchyma pattern with pruning of the pulmonary vessels may be seen (□ Fig. 5.1.8).

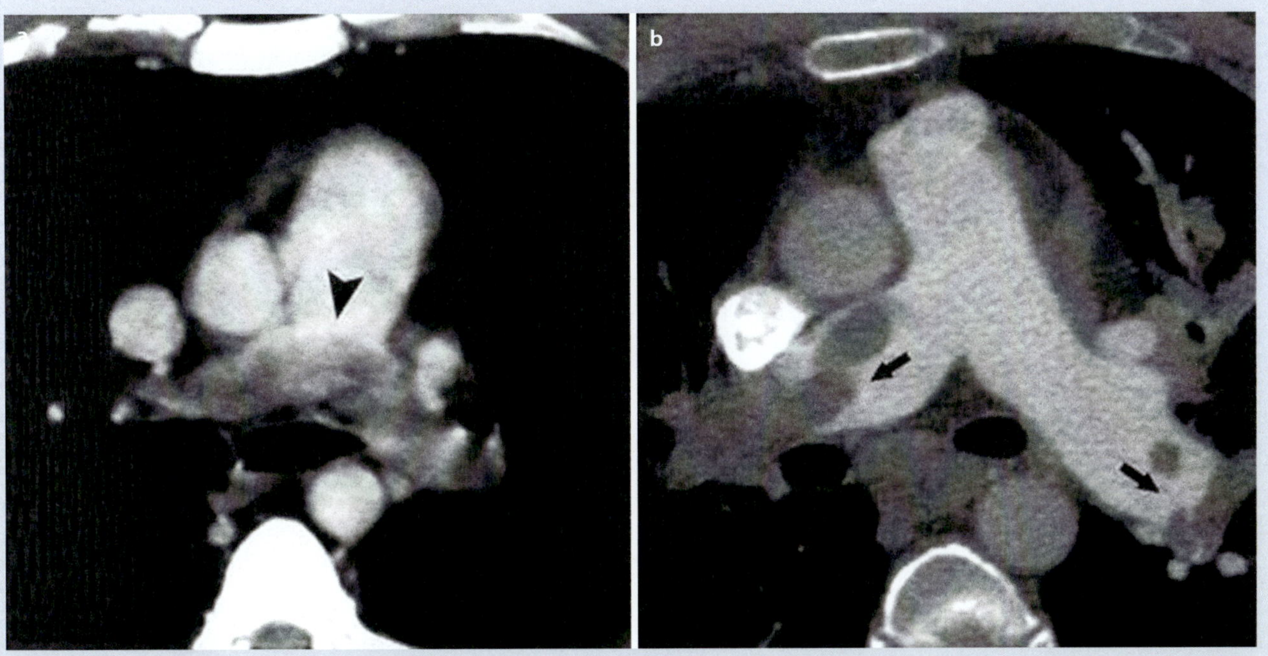

**Fig. 5.1.7** Axial pulmonary CTA of two different patients (**a** and **b**) with pulmonary embolism (PE) shows saddle thrombus in (**a**) (*arrowhead*) and distal complete thrombosis of the right pulmonary artery with partial thrombosis of the distal part of the left pulmonary artery (*arrow* in **b**)

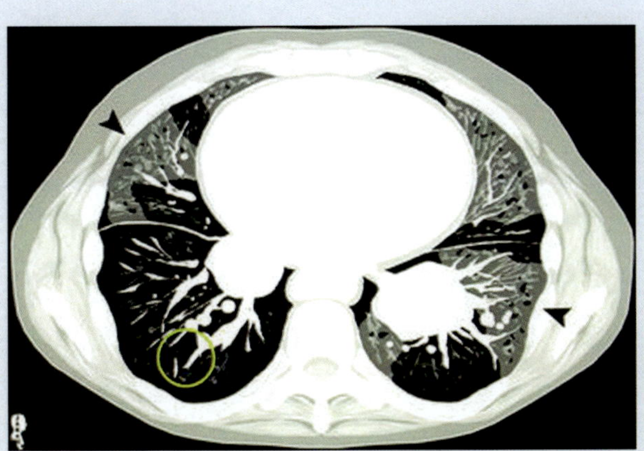

**Fig. 5.1.8** Axial chest HRCT lung window illustration shows mosaic pulmonary parenchymal pattern (*arrowheads*) and pruning of the pulmonary arteries (*yellow circle*)

## Aortic Dissection

The term *acute aortic syndrome* is applied to multiple acute chest pain presentations that are caused by thoracic aortic diseases, including aortic dissection, aortic intramural hematoma (IMH), and penetrating atherosclerotic ulcer.

*Aortic dissection* is a condition characterized by separation of the aortic intima with presence of blood in a false lumen between the intima and the medial layers of the aortic wall.

The intima is the innermost layer of the aortic wall. Aortic wall intimal tear starts typically at sites of highest intramural pressure and wall tension. After intimal tear, the blood flow inside the tear dissects its way between the intima and the media layer, creating a false lumen. The structure between the true and the false lumen is called "intimal flap," which is the key diagnosis of aortic dissection on radiological examinations.

The most common predisposing factors of aortic dissection are systemic hypertension, bicuspid aortic valve, aortic coarctation, and Marfan's syndrome. Patients typically present with sudden acute chest pain that is described as "tearing" sensation and classically radiation to the back.

## Aortic Dissection Is Classified According to the Stanford and Debakey Classifications

### Stanford Classification

*Type A*: this type involves the ascending aorta, and it is managed surgically. This type carries the risk of spontaneous rupture into the pericardium resulting in pericardial tamponade, or it can continue dissection to involve the coronary arteries (right coronary more than the left). Patients with this type can also develop aortic regurgitation (50 % of cases).

*Type B*: this type involves the descending aorta only. The site of dissection is typically just distal to the subclavian artery, near the insertion of the ligamentum arteriosum. When the dissection involves both the descending and the ascending aorta, it is classified as type A. This type is managed medically; however, in the current era, even type B is managed with endovascular stent across the origin of the dissection.

### Debakey Classification

*Type I* involves ascending aorta only.
*Type II* involves the ascending and the descending aorta.
*Type III* involves the descending aorta only.

## Differential Diagnoses and Related Diseases

*Vascular Ehlers–Danlos syndrome* is a disease characterized by joint hypermobility, skin abnormalities (e.g., easy bruising), fragility of intestinal and genitourinary organs, and vascular fragility leading to dissection or rupture of medium to large muscular arteries. The disease has an autosomal dominant mode of inheritance and caused by mutation in collagen type 3 gene (COL3A1). The dissection arises in vascular Ehlers–Danlos syndrome that occurs typically without preceding aneurysm.

### Signs on Radiographs

There is mediastinal widening with obliteration of the aortic knuckle on plain radiographs.

### Signs on CTA

- The key diagnostic finding in aortic dissection is identification of the intimal flap, which appears as a thin "line" of soft tissue within the aortic lumen separating the false lumen from the true lumen (◧ Fig. 5.1.9).
- The true lumen shows higher enhancement than the false lumen, because filling of the false lumen is slower than the true lumen. Moreover, the false lumen may show signs of intravascular thrombosis.
- In the ascending aorta, the false lumen is typically the more anterior lumen, while in the descending aorta, it is typically the more posterior lumen.

- Coronary artery dissection can be suspected when the intimal flap is detected at or near the site of a coronary ostium. When this sign is identified, coronary CTA should be performed to detect the extension of the dissection.
- Pericardial hemorrhagic effusion may be detected as highly attenuated fluid within the pericardial space (40–50 HU).

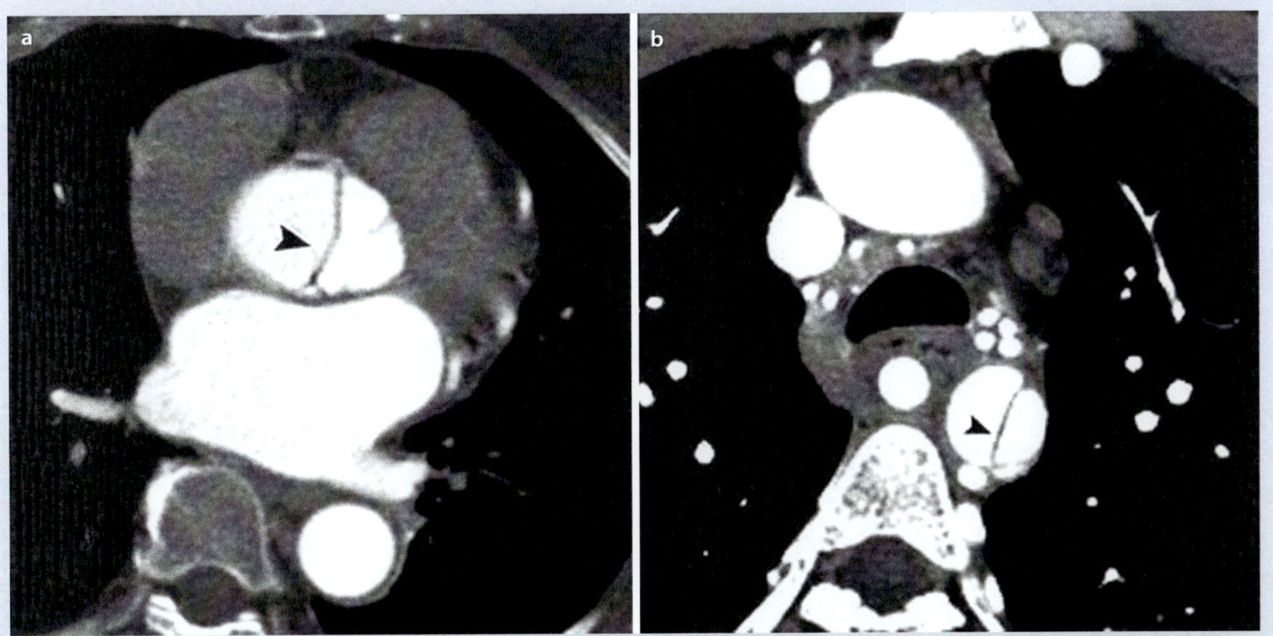



**Fig. 5.1.9** Axial cardiac CTA of two different patients with aortic dissection Stanford type A (**a**) and Stanford type B (**b**) shows the classic intimal flap (*arrowheads*) separating the true from the false lumen

## Aortic Intramural Hematoma

*IMH* is a condition characterized by rupture of the vasa vasorum, the network of vessels that supply the aorta itself, resulting in bleeding within the aortic wall, mostly within the media layer.

IMH is clinically indistinguishable from aortic dissection. Patients present with signs of acute aortic syndrome consisting of sudden chest pain that is radiating to the back or chest depending on which part of the aorta is affected. IMH accounts for 10–30 % of cases of acute aortic syndrome, and it may be caused by hypertension, blunt trauma, or penetrating atherosclerotic ulcer. In contrast to aortic dissection, no intimal tear flap is identified in this condition. However, the hematoma can progress into a true dissection if the aortic wall continues to enlarge in thickness by the hematoma >5 cm.

### Signs on CTA
On contrast-enhanced scan, the aortic wall show a crescentic area of wall thickening that may show high attenuation if the bleeding is fresh. There is no intimal flap (**Fig. 5.1.10**).

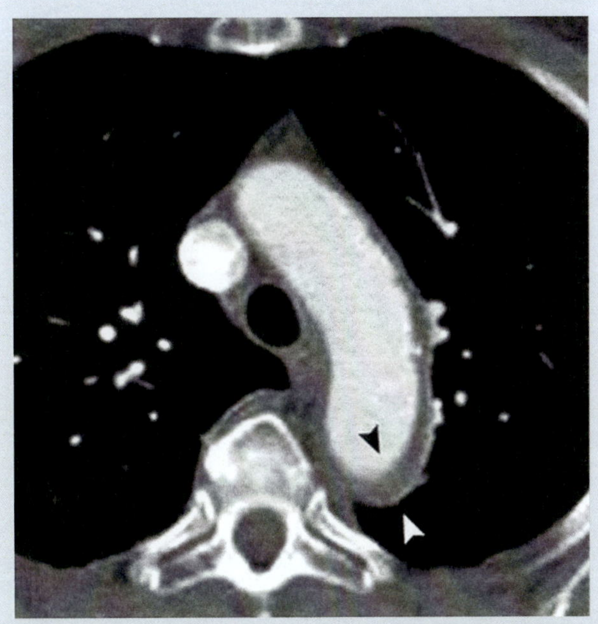

**Fig. 5.1.10** Axial cardiac CTA shows posterior aortic arch focal area of aortic wall thickening due to intramural hematoma (*arrowheads*)

## Penetrating Atherosclerotic Ulcer

*Penetrating atherosclerotic ulcer* is a condition that results from ulceration and break of an aortic atherosclerotic plaque resulting in an intimal defect. This defect causes bleeding within the aortic wall surrounding the ulcer, which will result in IMH formation or pseudo-aortic aneurysm formation.

> **Signs on CTA**
> The scan will show an area of intimal defect within the aorta with the formation of saccular pseudoaneurysm, IMH, or periaortic mediastinal hematoma (□ Fig. 5.1.11).

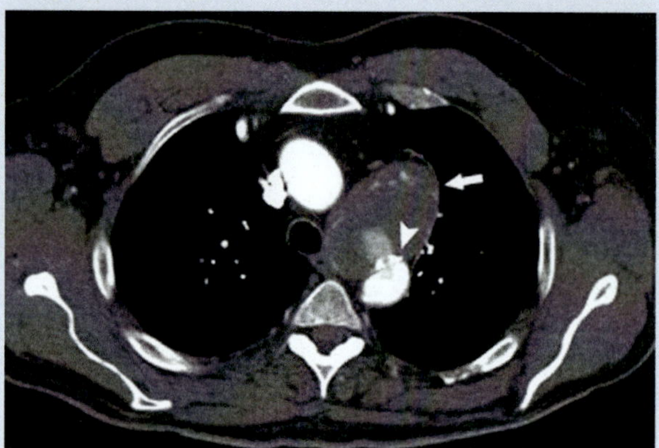

□ **Fig. 5.1.11**  Axial cardiac CTA shows an area of aortic wall ulceration of the descending thoracic aorta (*arrowhead*) with a jet of bleeding into the aortic wall creating a periaortic mediastinal hematoma (*arrowhead*)

### Further Reading

Birchard KR. Acute aortic syndrome and acute traumatic aortic injury. Semin Roentgenol. 2009. doi:10.1053/j.ro.2008.10.002.

Castañer E, et al. Congenital and acquired pulmonary anomalies in the adult: radiologic overview. RadioGraphics. 2006;26:349–71.

Choe YH, et al. Comparison of MDCT and MRI in the detection and sizing of acute and chronic myocardial infarcts. Eur J Radiol. 2008;66:292–9.

De Becker J, et al. Marfan and Marfan-like syndromes. Artery Res. 2009;3:9–16.

Hoffmann U, et al. Cardiac CT in emergency department patients with acute chest pain. RadioGraphics. 2006;26:963–80.

Jeudy J, et al. Nontraumatic thoracic injuries. Radiol Clin N Am. 2006;44:273–93.

Oliver TB, et al. Spiral CT in acute non-cardiac chest pain. Clin Radiol. 1999;54:38–45.

Winter-Muram HT, et al. Suspected acute pulmonary embolism: evaluation with multi-detector row CT versus digital subtraction pulmonary arteriography. Radiology. 2004;233:806–15.

## 5.2    Diseases of the Great Vessels

The great vessels include the aorta, the superior and inferior vena cava, the pulmonary artery, and the pulmonary veins. There are multiple medical conditions affecting the great vessels that require imaging to assess their complications, establish their diagnosis, or monitor their therapy response. This topic discusses some of the common medical conditions where radiology plays an important role in their diagnosis and assessment.

### Thoracic Aortic Aneurysm

Thoracic aortic aneurysm (TAA) is a disease characterized by dilatation of the wall of the aorta affecting its three layers (intima, media, and adventitia). In contrast, pseudo-aortic aneurysm is a condition characterized by saccular dilatation of the outer most layers of the aortic wall (media and/or adventitia) with an intact inner wall layer (intima).

The most common cause of TAA is atherosclerosis, while the most common cause of pseudo-aortic aneurysm is aortic trauma violating the wall integrity. TAA originates in the ascending aorta (50 %), descending aorta (40 %), and the aortic arch (10 %). In contrast, pseudo-aortic aneurysm usually arises at three basic levels: the aortic root, the aortic isthmus, and the aortic diaphragm.

Patients with TAA are typically in their 50s and 70s and usually are asymptomatic. Up to 30 % of patients present with complications due to TAA rupture. Pain or dysphagia due to mass effect over the adjacent mediastinal structure may be seen uncommonly.

TAA expands at a rate of 0.5 cm per year, with an increased risk of rupture when it is >5 cm in diameter. Patients with TAA >6 mm may present with spontaneous bleeding resulting in hemomediastinum or periaortic hematoma formation.

### Differential Diagnoses and Related Diseases

- *Marfan's syndrome* is a disease characterized by ocular, musculoskeletal, central nervous system, and cardiovascular complications. Marfan's syndrome patients are known to suffer from aortic root dilatation in up to 80 % of cases. Patients may suffer also from mitral valve prolapse, or dissection of the aorta.
- *Loeys–Dietz syndrome* is a disease characterized by aortic aneurysm and dissection, with widespread arterial tortuosity/aneurysms (seen in the thoracic aorta and neck vessels mainly). The disease has an autosomal dominant mode of inheritance. The disease is divided into two types: type I Loeys–Dietz syndrome is characterized by craniosynostosis, hypertelorism, bifid uvula, cleft palate, and/or arterial aneurysms and tortuosity; type II lacks the hypertelorism, craniosynostosis, and cleft palate.
- Aortoduodenal syndrome is a very rare disease characterized by obstruction of the duodenum by aneurysmal dilatation of the abdominal aorta. Patients classically present with abdominal pain, bilious vomiting, and pulsatile abdominal mass.

### Signs on Radiographs

- Aortic aneurysm is detected as a marked dilatation of the aortic knuckle and mediastinal widening (◘ Fig. 5.2.1).
- Bronchial compression or erosion of the thoracic vertebrae due to mass effect and chronic pressure causing anterior scalloping may be seen on lateral views.
- Aortic wall calcification may be seen.

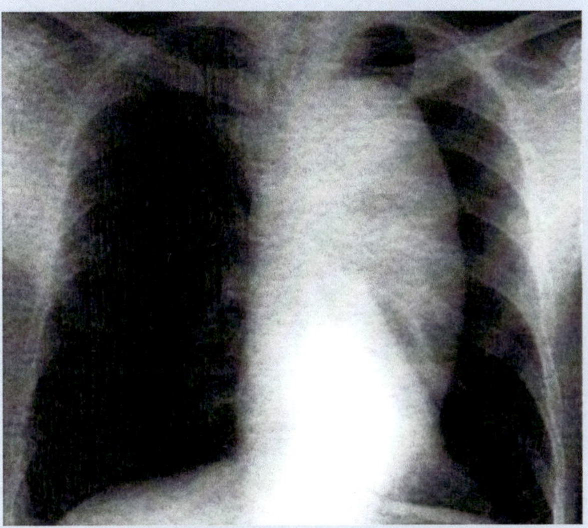

◘ **Fig. 5.2.1** Posteroanterior chest radiograph of a patient with thoracic aortic aneurysm (TAA) shows marked dilatation of the aortic knuckle and the descending thoracic aorta

### Signs on CTA

- The thoracic aorta is considered dilated when its diameter is >4 cm (◘ Fig. 5.2.2).
- Periaortic hematoma is detected as a hypodense mass located in the mediastinum surrounding the aorta. If the bleeding is fresh, the hematoma may show high density (◘ Fig. 5.2.3).
- Aortic wall calcification may be seen.

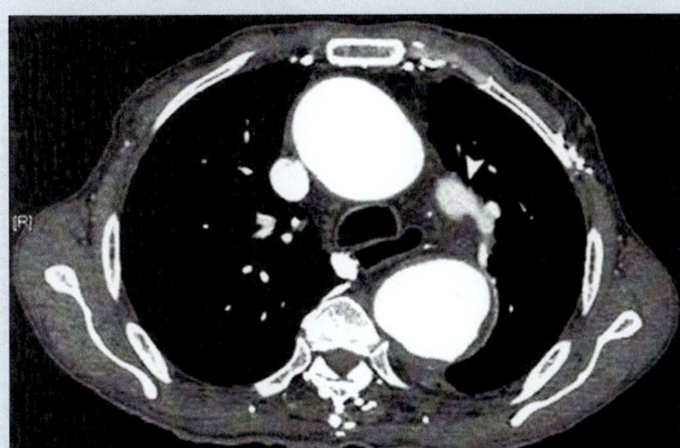

◘ **Fig. 5.2.2** Axial thoracic CTA demonstrates TAA with fresh blood leak into the mediastinum (*arrowhead*)

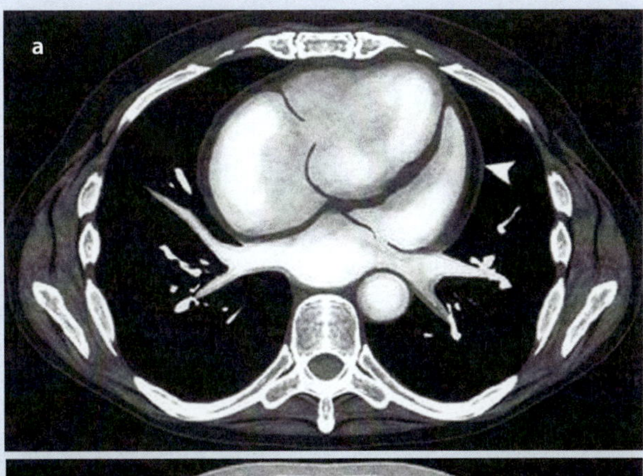

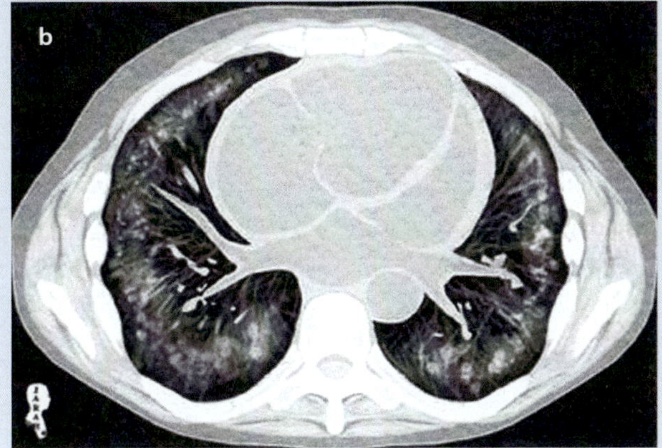

◘ **Fig. 5.2.3** Axial mediastinal window (**a**) and lung window (**b**) HRCT illustrations of a patient with pulmonary veno-occlusive disease (PVOD) show right-sided heart chambers dilatation with normal left heart chambers size. In (**b**), the lung parenchyma shows bilateral diffuse linear interstitial lung pattern. Notice also the small pericardial effusion in (**a**) (*arrowhead*)

## Pulmonary Hypertension

Pulmonary hypertension (PHT) is a disease characterized hemodynamically by a mean pulmonary artery pressure >25 mmHg at rest (normal level, 10 mmHg) or >30 mmHg during exercise (normal level, 15 mmHg) with increased pulmonary vascular resistance.

Causes of PHT can be divided into two main groups: a group with pathology is confined to the arterial side of the pulmonary circulation (*precapillary PHT*) and a second group with pathology confined to the venous circulation, between the capillary bed and the left atrium (*postcapillary PHT*). When the cause of the PHT is unknown, it is called "idiopathic or primary" PHT, and when the cause of the PHT is known, it called "secondary" PHT.

### Causes of PHT

- *Precapillary PHT*: primary PHT, congenital heart defects with left-to-right shunt, pulmonary embolism, parasites (e.g., schistosomiasis), and talcosis (lung disease due to talc crystals inhalation).
- *Postcapillary PHT*: primary veno-occlusive disease, mitral stenosis, and mediastinal fibrosis.

*Primary PHT* is an idiopathic condition characterized by precapillary PHT in the absence of an identifiable cause. Patients typically present with dyspnea (60 %), fatigue, angina, cor pulmonale, and Raynaud's phenomenon. Typically, the patient is a young or middle-aged female. Risk factors associated with primary PHT include portal hypertension, collagen vascular disease, pregnancy, and women who use contraceptive pills.

Congenital heart defects associated with left-to-right shunts predispose to PHT. Common defects with PHT include atrial septal defects, ventricular septal defects, and truncus arteriosus. *Eisenmenger syndrome* is an advanced stage of PHT associated with congenital heart defects. The disease is characterized by dyspnea, cyanosis, generalized fatigue, and syncope. Patients with Eisenmenger syndrome may die at a young age due to cardiac arrhythmias, which are common features of this disease. Patients may also develop paradoxical embolus passing from the right side of the heart to the left through a heart defect.

*Pulmonary veno-occlusive disease* (PVOD) is a rare idiopathic disease characterized by postcapillary PHT, in the presence of normal left atrial and left ventricular pressures. PVOD is characterized by PHT, congestive heart failure, and interstitial pulmonary edema with a normal wedge pressure on cardiac catheterization. The pathological findings in PVOD show extensive and diffuse occlusion of pulmonary veins by fibrous tissue, which may be loose edematous or dense and sclerotic. Patients present with dyspnea, flu-like symptoms, and hemoptysis. It commonly affects children (30 % of cases), transplant patients, and pregnant women. The disease may be misdiagnosed initially as interstitial lung disease (◘ Fig. 5.2.3).

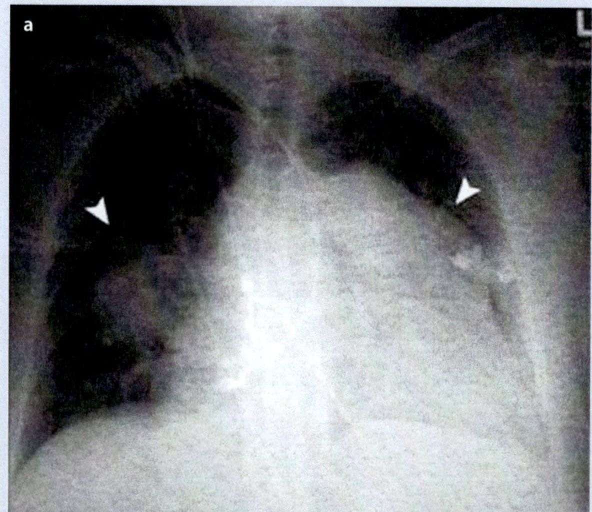
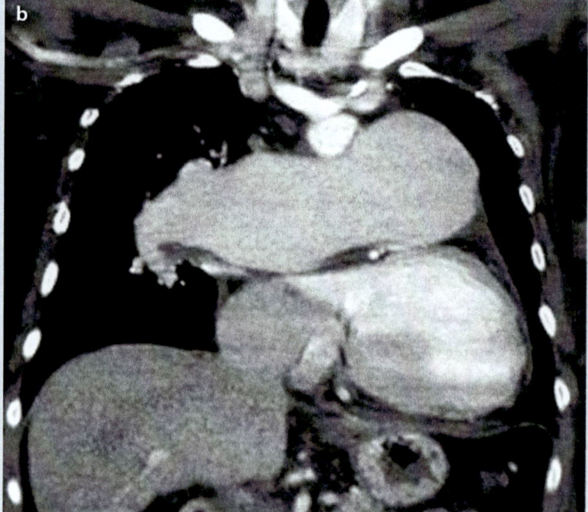

◘ **Fig. 5.2.4** Anteroposterior chest radiograph (**a**) and coronal CTA (**b**) of a patient with primary pulmonary hypertension (PHT) shows massively dilated pulmonary arteries (*arrowheads*)

### Signs on Chest Radiograph
- The pulmonary vasculature diminishes in caliber as it extends from the center toward the periphery (pruning), with a mean width of the right descending pulmonary artery >24 mm (normal <17 mm in width).
- Dilatation of the right and left main pulmonary arteries (◘ Fig. 5.2.4).
- Signs of right ventricular enlargement, right atrial enlargement, or left atrial enlargement (mitral stenosis).
- POVD is suggested radiographically when the radiograph shows signs of pulmonary PHT associated with pulmonary interstitial edema and normal-sized left atrium. The interstitial edema is visualized as a diffuse linear interstitial pattern. Mediastinal hilar lymphadenopathy may be present.

### Signs on HRCT and CTA
- PHT is diagnosed when the mean diameter of the pulmonary artery is >29 mm, with a segmental artery-to-bronchus ration >1:1 in three or four pulmonary lobes (◘ Fig. 5.2.4).
- The lung parenchyma shows mosaic pattern of lung attenuation due to variation in parenchymal perfusion.
- Arteriography shows symmetric enlargement of the central arteries with tapering subsegmental vessels toward the peripheries (pruning).
- The right ventricle is considered dilated when the ratio of its diameter to the diameter of the left ventricle is greater than 1:1, with bowing of the interventricular septum toward the left ventricle.

- Right ventricular hypertrophy is confirmed when the myocardial wall thickness is >5 mm (normally <4 mm).
- Signs of pericardial thickness with small pericardial effusion can be seen in a percentage of patients with PHT without an obvious reason.
- In *PVOD*, classical CT finding shows the combination of diffuse linear interstitial lung pattern with or without mosaic ground glass opacities, dilated pulmonary arteries, right-sided heart chambers dilatation, mediastinal lymphadenopathy, and pericardial or pleural effusion, with normal-sized left atrium and pulmonary veins (Fig. 5.2.3).

## Coral Reef Aorta

Coral reef aorta is a rare condition characterized by excessive calcification of the suprarenal and juxtarenal aorta resembling the growth of hyperplastic bone, in the absence of abnormalities in serum calcium levels.

Coral reef aorta can cause malignant hypertension due to significant abdominal aortic lumen stenosis or renal artery stenosis when it involves the renal arteries. Other complications include blue toe syndrome due to dislodged ulcerated atherosclerotic plaques.

### Signs on CT
On nonenhanced images, the aorta shows hard, irregular, and gritty intra-aortic mass of calcification. In contrast to the typical appearance of atherosclerosis of the great vessels, which follows the curve of the vessel wall, the calcification in coral reef aorta is irregular and protrudes into the lumen (Fig. 5.2.5).

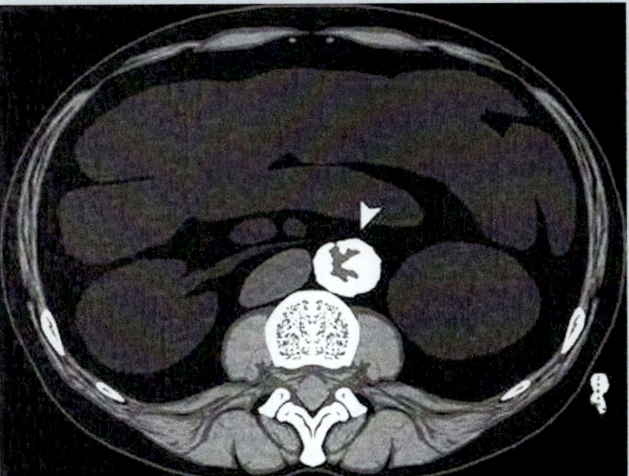

**Fig. 5.2.5** Axial abdominal CT illustration demonstrates coral reef aorta seen as diffusely calcified arterial wall with projection of the calcified plaques into the aortic lumen (*arrowhead*)

## Superior Vena Cava Syndrome

Superior vena cava syndrome (SVCS) is a disease characterized by a triad of edema of the upper torso, venous distension of the neck, and chylothorax. SVCS arises due to extrinsic or intrinsic SVC obstruction, causing disturbance of the venous backflow from the head and neck region and formation of venous collaterals.

Extrinsic causes of SVCS include bronchogenic carcinoma or lymphoma compressing the SVC (80 % of cases). Intrinsic causes of SVCS are mostly due to thrombosis, most commonly due to intravenous catheter use. Other causes of intrinsic SVCS include thrombus propagation from the subclavian veins to the SVC due to thoracic outlet syndrome.

Patients with SVCS typically present with marked cyanosis and swelling involving the head and neck region and the upper extremities, with development of superficial collateral circulation. Complications include pulmonary embolism (5–35 % of cases), thrombophlebitis, sepsis, and thrombus propagation into intracranial sinuses or veins. In some patients, blood may be "sucked" into the thorax during inspiration, but because of the limited ventricular filling, the neck veins may become further distended (Kussmaul's sign).

In infants, SVCS has been linked with the formation of hydrocephalus, called *extraventricular obstructive hydrocephalus* (EVOH). The mechanism of hydrocephalus is believed to be caused by decrease in cerebrospinal fluid absorption at the level of the arachnoid granulation secondary to the elevated venous pressure. EVOH can be seen in up to 91 % in infants with SVCS. Complications of EVOH include hemorrhagic infarction and seizures.

### Signs on Chest Radiographs
- Pleura effusion (chylothorax).
- The chest may show the cause of SVCS if the reason was obstruction from a mediastinal tumor.
- Rib notching may present with long-standing SVC obstruction.

### Signs on Superior Vena Cavography
There is partial or complete SVC filling defect with formation of numerous venous collaterals (Fig. 5.2.6).

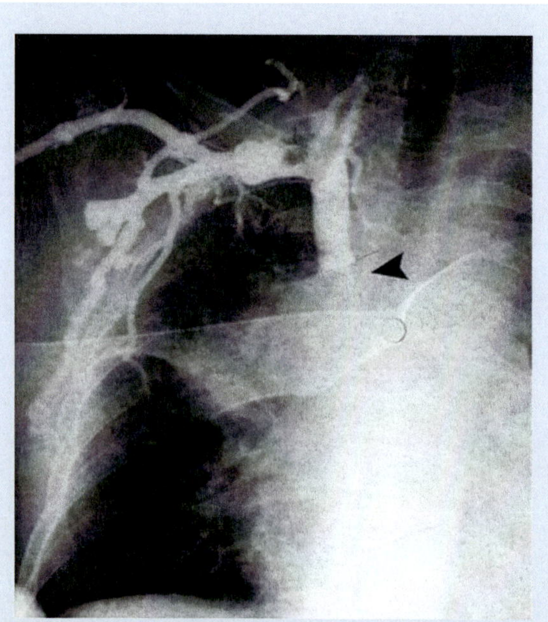

**Fig. 5.2.6** Superior vena cava venography shows occlusion of the superior vena cava (SVC) due to thrombosis (*arrowhead*)

### Signs on Chest CT
- Mediastinal masses (e.g., bronchogenic carcinoma) can be found in cases of extrinsic SVC obstruction.
- After contrast injection, partial or complete filling defects representing SVC thrombosis can be seen in cases of intrinsic SVC obstruction.

### Signs on Brain CT
In infants with EVOH, brain CT may be normal in early stages or show signs of ventricular dilatation due to hydrocephalus.

### Further Reading


Akpinar E, et al. PVOD suggested by MDCT and clinical findings in a pregnant woman. Emerg Radiol. 2008; 15:193–5.

Beghetti M, et al. Eisenmenger syndrome. A clinical perspective in a new therapeutic era of pulmonary arterial hypertension. JACC. 2009;53:733–40.

Deitch JS, et al. Abdominal aortic aneurysm causing duodenal obstruction: two case reports and review of the literature. J Vasc Surg. 2004;40:543–7.

Frazier AA, et al. Pulmonary vasculature: hypertension and infarction. RadioGraphics. 2000;20:491–524.

Gotway MB, et al. Thoracic aorta imaging with multislice CT. Radiol Clin N Am. 2003;41:521–43.

Johnson PT, et al. Loeyz-Dietz syndrome: MDCT angiography findings. AJR. 2007;189:W29–35.

Karmazyn N, et al. Neuroimaging findings in neonates and infants from superior vena cava obstruction after cardiac operation. Pediatr Radiol. 2002;32:806–10.

Rosenberg GD, et al. Blue toe syndrome from a "coral reef" aorta. Ann Vasc Surg. 1995;9:561–4.

Rosenberger A, et al. Superior vena cava syndrome: a new radiologic approach to diagnosis. Cardiovasc Intervent Radiol. 1980;3:127–30.

Schulte K-M, et al. Coral reef aorta: a long-term study of 21 patients. Ann Vasc Surg. 2000;14:626–33.

Takagi H, et al. Aortoduodenal syndrome. J Vasc Surg. 2006;43:851.


## 5.3    Myocardial Diseases (Cardiomyopathies)

Cardiomyopathies are a group of diseases with different etiologies, all characterized by cardiac muscle dysfunction. Cardiomyopathies are an important cause of arrhythmias and sudden cardiac death in young patients. Three types of cardiomyopathies have been described by the World Health Organization (WHO):
- *Hypertrophic cardiomyopathy* (*HCM*) is characterized by inappropriate left ventricular hypertrophy, with preservation of the myocardium contractility.
- *Dilated cardiomyopathy* (*DCM*) is characterized by ventricular dilatation with contractility dysfunction. Most secondary causes of cardiomyopathies are related to this type.
- *Restrictive cardiomyopathy* (*RCM*) is characterized by diastolic dysfunction and restricted contractility.

Other uncommon forms of cardiomyopathies include athlete's heart, arrhythmogenic right ventricular dysplasia (ARVD), noncompaction cardiomyopathy (NCCM), and peripartum cardiomyopathy. Each of the classic three forms and the uncommon forms of cardiomyopathies are discussed below.

### Hypertrophic Cardiomyopathy

Primary HCM is a disease characterized by inappropriate myocardial hypertrophy in the absence of a cause (e.g., hypertension). In contrast, secondary HCM can be seen due to diseases of protein deposition (e.g., amyloidosis).

Cardiac muscle hypertrophy in HCM is described as "concentric" or "eccentric." *Concentric heart hypertrophy* means increased heart muscle bulk and wall thickness, and it is best assessed on cardiac MRI by looking at the heart thickness in the short-axis view. *Eccentric heart hypertrophy* means general increase in the heart muscles with preservation of the normal cardiac wall thickness (isometric).

Patients with HCM often present with symptoms that include ischemic cardiac pain and arrhythmias, although most patients may be asymptomatic. HCM is the most common cause of sudden cardiac death in athletes. Up to 25 % of HCM patients have left ventricle outflow tract (LVOT) obstruction due to the thickened interventricular septum. *Venturi effect* is a term used to describe LVOT obstruction by hypertrophic interventricular septum during systole, which causes retrograde jet flow toward the mitral valve, causing anterior mitral valve leaflet regurgitation.

*Athlete's heart* is a physiological cardiac hypertrophy. Sports are divided into endurance sports (e.g., weight lifting) and dynamic sports (e.g., running). Endurance sports cause concentric cardiac hypertrophy (<12 mm) thickness, while dynamic sports cause eccentric cardiac hypertrophy that may reach (13 mm) in thickness.

Differentiation between athlete's heart and HCM can be difficult by imaging alone. However, evidences of bizarre electrocardiogram (ECG) patterns, female sex, abnormal left ventricular filling, and marked left ventricular enlargement all favor HCM. Moreover, athlete's heart shows reduction in the heart muscle wall thickness from 2 to 5 mm after a 3-month period of athletic abstaining, a feature that is not seen in true HCM.

## Differential Diagnoses and Related Diseases

- *Yamaguchi syndrome*, also known as *apical HCM*, is a disease characterized by HCM that is confined to, or located primarily in, the left ventricle (LV) apical region. Up to 40 % of patients are asymptomatic. ECG leads show characteristic deeply inverted T wave, which might be mistaken for coronary ischemic disease.
- *Barth syndrome* is an X-linked recessive disorder characterized by HCM, neutropenia, skeletal myopathy, growth delay, hypocholesterolemia, and urinary excretion of 3-methylglutarate, 3-methylglutaconate, and 2-ethyldracrylate.
- *Romano–Ward syndrome* is an autosomal dominant disease characterized by long ECG QT interval, cardiac arrhythmia, and occasional incidence of HCM.
- *Jervell and Lange-Nielsen syndrome* is an autosomal recessive disease characterized by long ECG QT interval, cardiac arrhythmia, sensorineural hearing loss, syncopal attacks evoked by emotional stress, and occasional HCM.





- Abnormal, late (>10 min) patchy contrast enhancement of the hypertrophic muscles is found in 79 % of patients of HCM, probably due to small-vessel disease and ischemia.
- Venturi effect is seen as an area of signal void and mitral valve regurgitation with LVOT obstruction on cine images during systole.
- *Yamaguchi syndrome* shows hypertrophic left ventricular apex, causing the left ventricular cavity to exhibit characteristic "spade-like" configuration.
- *Athlete's heart* is visualized as mild increase in the left ventricular myocardial wall thickness that does not exceed 13 mm in thickness on short-axis views. There is no abnormal wall enhancement after contrast injection.

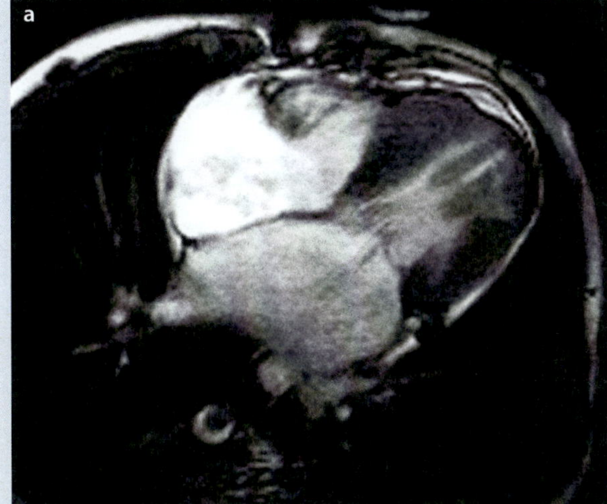


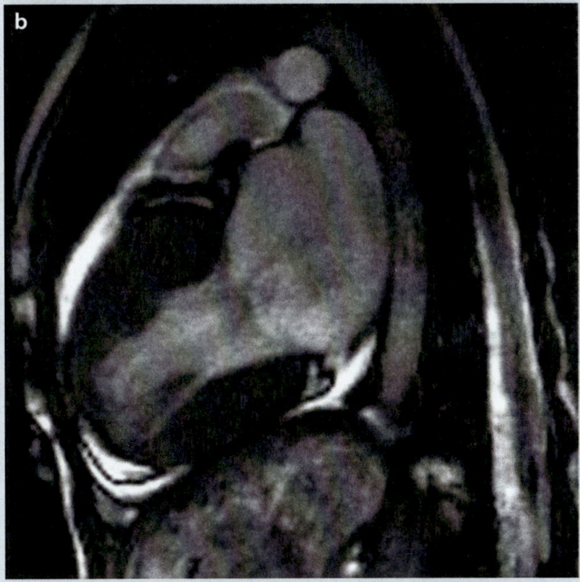


◘ **Fig. 5.3.1**  Four-chamber white blood cardiac MRI (**a**) and two-chamber view (**b**) show concentric hypertrophic cardiomyopathy (HCM). Notice the thickened chordae tendineae in (**a**)

## Dilated Cardiomyopathy

DCM is characterized by left ventricular or biventricular dilatation with impaired systolic function.

The most common presentation of DCM is left-sided heart failure. Causes can be due to alcoholism (50 % of cases), cocaine abuse, and hyper- and hypothyroidism. Contrast-enhanced MRI for DCM study is mainly indicated to differentiate primary DCM (e.g., without a cause) from secondary (e.g., postmyocardial infarction) DCM.

### Signs on Chest Radiographs

The cardiac heart is markedly enlarged with increased cardiothoracic ratio due to cardiac muscles dilatation (◘ Fig. 5.3.2).

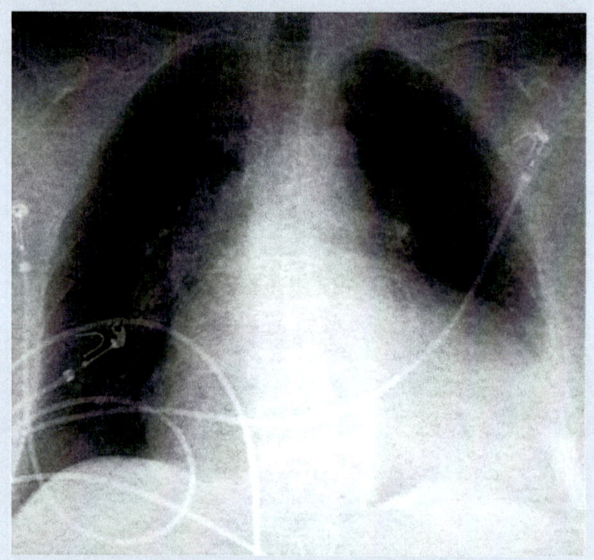

◘ **Fig. 5.3.2**   Anteroposterior chest radiograph of a bedridden patient shows massively dilated heart due to dilated cardiomyopathy (DCM)

### Signs on MRI

- There is marked dilatation of the heart ventricles, often with global wall motion abnormalities on cine MR images. Focal wall motion abnormalities are more commonly seen in DCM due to ischemic heart disease (e.g., postmyocardial infarction) (◘ Fig. 5.3.3).
- Secondary DCM usually shows late contrast enhancement, depending on its primary cause (e.g., myocardial infarction): the contrast uptake reflecting areas of degeneration, necrosis, and fibrosis. In contrast, primary DCM shows no late contrast enhancement. The contrast enhancement can be subendocardial or transmural.
- Intraventricular thrombus may be found.

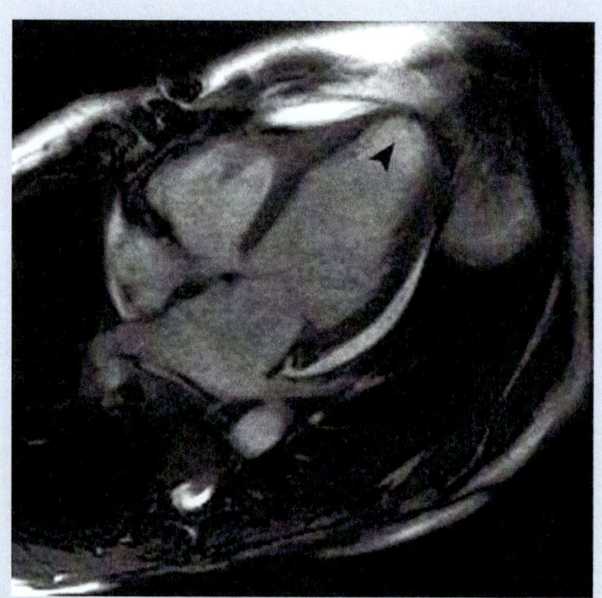

◘ **Fig. 5.3.3**   Four-chamber white blood cardiac MRI shows left ventricular apical dilatation due to previous myocardial infarction (*arrowhead*)

## Restrictive Cardiomyopathy

RCM is a disease characterized by ventricular filling defect. RCM can be caused by diseases that disturb the myocardial integrity such as amyloidosis, sarcoidosis, metastasis, and glycogen storage diseases.

Patients may present with signs of congestive heart failure because of ventricular contractility restriction in a similar fashion to constrictive pericarditis. Cardiac MRI in RCM is used to differentiate restrictive pericarditis from RCM.

### Signs on Chest Radiographs

The heart size is generally enlarged due to atrial dilatation or due to the development of congestive heart failure.

### Signs on MRI

The ventricular chamber dimensions and thickness are within normal range, with both atria enlarged as a direct sign of right ventricular and left ventricular filling resistance.

## Arrhythmogenic Right Ventricular Dysplasia

*ARVD* is a rare, progressive disease characterized by infiltration and replacement of the right ventricle free wall myocardium with fibro-fatty tissue, which causes contractility dysfunction and right ventricular dilatation.

ARVD is one of the causes of arrhythmias and sudden cardiac deaths because this fibro-fatty tissue causes electrical instability of the right ventricular wall. ARVD is familial in up to 50 % of cases, with an autosomal dominant mode of inheritance. The disease has a male predominance. Patient is typically a young male (30 years) complaining from arrhythmias initiated by exercise.

> **Signs on MRI**
> — There is right ventricular bulging and dilatation, thinning of the right ventricle free wall (2–6 mm in thickness), and high signal intensity seen within the myocardium on T1W images representing fat infiltration within the myocardium (diagnostic key) (❑ Fig. 5.3.4). If fatty infiltration cannot be

> demonstrated, right ventricular trabeculation also fulfills the criteria of ARVD, presuming the clinical picture also suggests it.
> — Abnormal wall motion is demonstrated on cine images.

## Noncompaction Cardiomyopathy (Spongy Myocardium)

NCCM is a rare, distinct cardiomyopathy characterized by arrest of the left ventricular muscle compaction during embryonal development, causing left ventricular myocardial trabeculation with deep intertrabecular recesses that makes the left ventricular myocardium looks like sponge.

NCCM commonly affects the LV; however, the right ventricle can be involved occasionally. The disease has an incidence of 0.05 % in the general population and can occur as an isolated case or associated with other cardiac anomalies. The clinical picture is variable. Patients may show no symptoms, while others may show signs of severe heart failure and arrhythmias.

> **Signs on MRI**
> The left ventricular walls look thickened with prominent ventricular trabeculations within them (diagnostic feature) (❑ Fig. 5.3.5).

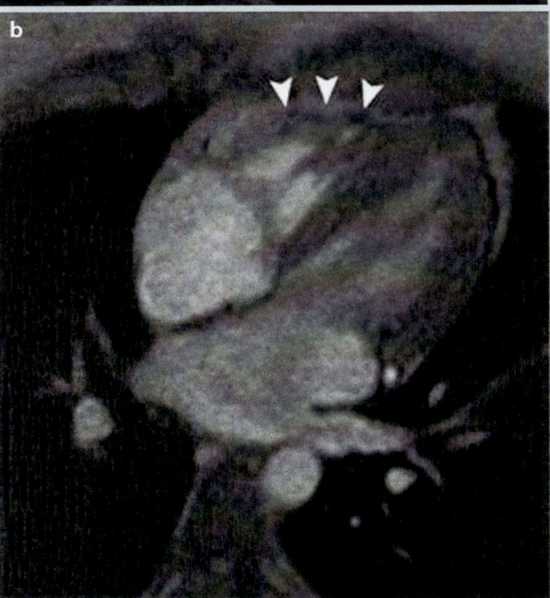

❑ **Fig. 5.3.4** Four-chamber white blood cardiac MRI during diastole (**a**) and systole (**b**) of a patient with arrhythmogenic right ventricular dysplasia (ARVD) show thinning of the left ventricle (LV) wall with hyperintense signal within the wall representing fibro-fatty changes (*arrows*)

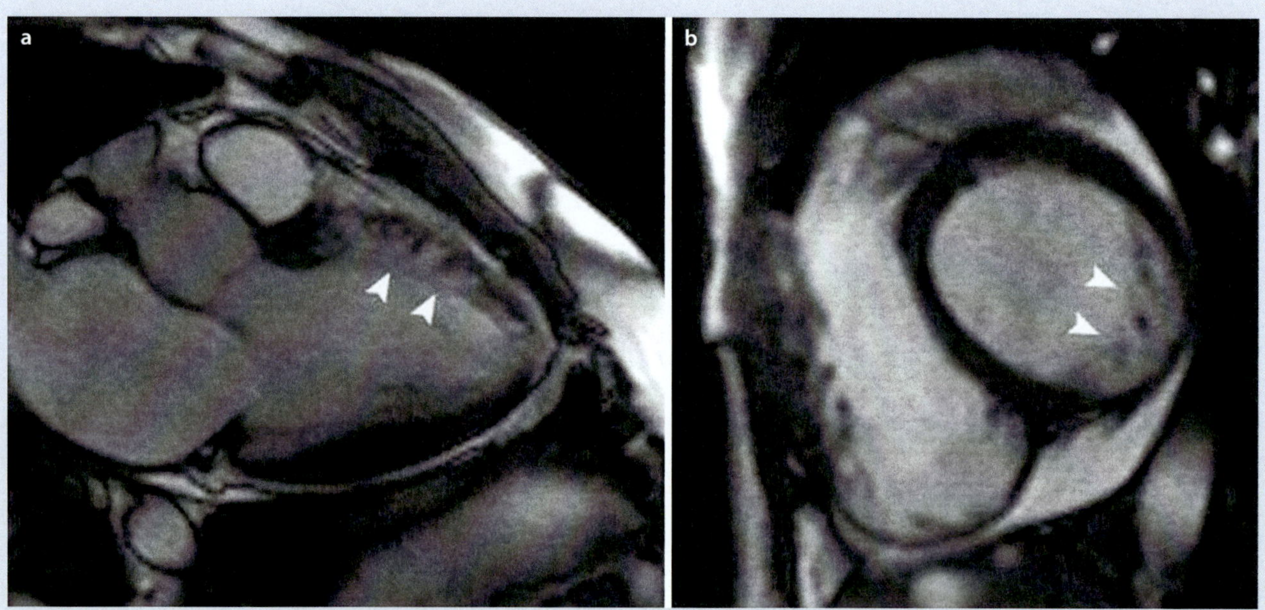



**Fig. 5.3.5**    Three-chamber white blood cardiac MRI (**a**) and short-axis view (**b**) show LV trabeculation in a patient with noncompaction cardiomyopathy (NCCM) (*arrowheads*)

## Peripartum Cardiomyopathy (Cardiomyopathy of Pregnancy)

Peripartum cardiomyopathy is defined as heart failure that occurs during the last 4 weeks of a term pregnancy or the first 5 months after delivery.

Peripartum cardiomyopathy is a rare condition with an incidence of 1:15,000 postpartum women. Exclusion of previous heart disease is essential before making the diagnosis of peripartum cardiomyopathy. There is a 50 % risk of thromboembolic complications associated with peripartum cardiomyopathy.

### Further Reading

Alhabshan F, et al. Extent of myocardial noncompaction: comparison between MRI and echocardiographic evaluation. Pediatr Radiol. 2005;35:1147–51.

Bachou T, et al. A novel mutation in the G4.5 in a Greek patient with Barth syndrome. Blood Cells Mol Dis. 2009;42:262–4.

Burch GE, et al. Heart muscle disease. Dis Mon. 1968;14:1–68.

Duygu H, et al. Apical hypertrophic cardiomyopathy might lead to misdiagnosis of ischemic heart disease. Int J Cardiovasc Imaging. 2008;24:675–81.

Hamamichi Y, et al. Isolated noncompaction of the ventricular myocardium: Ultrafast computed tomography and magnetic resonance imaging. Int J Cardiothorac Imaging. 2001;17:305–14.

Hedrich O, et al. Sudden cardiac death in athletes. Curr Cardiol Rep. 2006;8:316–22.

Isbell DC, et al. The evolving role of cardiovascular magnetic resonance imaging in nonischemic cardiomyopathy. Semin Ultrasound CT MRI. 2006;27:20–31.

Leon MB, et al. Hypertrophic cardiomyopathy. Dis Mon. 1981;28:1–87.

Malouf J, et al. Apical hypertrophic cardiomyopathy in a father and a daughter. Am J Med Genet. 1985;22:75–80.

Oduncu V, et al. Images in cardio-thoracic surgery. Biventricular noncompaction presenting with stroke. Eur J Cardiothorac Surg. 2008;33:737.

Reardon W, et al. Consanguinity, cardiac arrest, hearing impairment, and ECG abnormalities: counselling pitfalls in the Romano-Ward syndrome. J Med Genet. 1993;30:325–7.

Rochitte CE, et al. The emerging role of MRI in the diagnosis and management of cardiomyopathies. Curr Cardiol Rep. 2006;8:44–52.

Schwartz PJ, et al. The Jervell and Lange-Nielsen syndrome: natural history, molecular basis, and clinical outcome. Circulation. 2006;113:783–90.

Sparrow P, et al. Cardiac MRI and CT features of inheritable and congenital conditions associated with sudden cardiac death. Eur Radiol. 2008. doi:10.1007/s00330-008-1169-5.

Zandrino F, et al. Magnetic resonance imaging of athlete's heart: myocardial mass, left ventricular function, and cross-sectional area of the coronary arteries. Eur Radiol. 2000;10:319–25.

Zenovich AG, et al. Hypertrophic cardiomyopathy with apical aneurysm. Circulation. 2004;110:e450.

## 5.4    Endocarditis

Endocarditis is a term used to describe acute or chronic inflammation of the cardiac chamber's interior. Although the most common cause of endocarditis is infectious agents, other rare causes of endocarditis can be encountered uncommonly.

# Infective Endocarditis

Infective endocarditis (IE) is a disease that results from bacterial colonization of the platelet fibrin vegetation on the surface of the heart endothelium by circulating microorganisms.

IE can be acute or subacute. Acute IE is caused by highly virulent bacteria infecting even a healthy valve, whereas subacute IE occurs in a patient with prosthetic or defective heart valve with low virulent bacteria. The bacteria in the acute IE are present in the blood as septicemia, while in the subacute IE, a bacteremia is sufficient to initiate the disease.

The acute IE embolus initiates abscess and pyemia in the tissue in which it is deposited because of the high virulent bacteria within it. In contrast, subacute emboli cause localized effect within the vessels or the organs such as mycotic aneurysms and infarction due to vascular occlusion.

Classically, patients with IE are patients with known previous injury to their heart valves (e.g., patients with past history of rheumatic fever) who present with signs of fever and night sweat, typically weeks after dental or surgical procedures. Nowadays, intravenous drug abusers (IVDAs) are the most common population at risk of developing IE.

The most common infectious organisms causing IE include *staphylococci, streptococci, Candida albicans, Coxiella burnetii* (Q fever), and the HACEK organisms (*Haemophilus parainfluenzae, Haemophilus aphrophilus, Actinobacillus [Haemophilus] actinomycetemcomitans, Cardiobacterium hominis, Eikenella* species, and *Kingella* species).

Patients with IE typically present with fever, anorexia, weight loss, malaise, night sweat, bacteremia, evidence of active vasculitis, septic emboli, and immunologic vascular phenomenon. However, the previous typical stigmata are not always present, and the symptoms may be nonspecific, especially among IVDA patients.

*The modified Duke criteria for IE diagnosis*: Diagnosis of IE must fulfill two major criteria, 1 major plus 3 minor, or 5 minor criteria.

## Major Criteria

- Positive blood culture
- Two separated blood cultures consistent with IE organisms (e.g., *Staphylococcus aureus*) in the absence of the primary focus
- Evidence of endocardial involvement
- Positive echocardiogram for heart valves vegetations
- New partial dehiscence of prosthetic valve
- New valvular regurgitation

## Minor Criteria

- Predisposing heart condition (e.g., congenital heart disease)
- Fever
- Vascular phenomenon (septic arterial emboli, intracranial or conjunctival hemorrhage, Janeway's lesions)
- Immunologic phenomenon (glomerulonephritis, Osler's nodes, Roth's spots, or rheumatoid factor)
- Positive blood culture that does not meet major criteria or serological evidence of infection

The cardiac complications of IE include valvular heart defect, mostly affecting the mitral valve followed by the aortic valve. The valvular disease in the subacute form is due to stenosis and long-term fibrosis, whereas in the acute form, the valvular disease or insufficiency arises due to acute valvular destruction. The most common valves involved are the left-sided heart valves, except in IVDAs, where infection in the right-sided valves is as common as in the left side. Left-sided heart failure is the end product of mitral or aortic valves insufficiency when the tricuspid or the pulmonary valves are also involved. Extra-cardiac manifestations of IE are mostly related to septic vascular emboli, vascular phenomenon, and immunological phenomenon. The organs most commonly affected are the central nervous system, the thorax, the vascular system, the spleen, the kidneys, and the skin.

Neurological manifestations of IE are the most common complications, and they involve embolic strokes (15–20 % of cases). The septic embolic stroke may precede the diagnosis of IE in up to 75 % of IE complicated by strokes. Septic embolic strokes rate increases in patients with IE when the vegetation is >10 mm in diameter. Rarely, the septic emboli may result in the formation of brain abscess or meningitis. *S. aureus* is the most common organism causing embolic strokes. Mycotic arterial aneurysm involving the cerebral vessels with intracranial hemorrhage is seen in 2–10 % of IE cases. Mycotic aneurysm is formed secondary to septic emboli injuring the vascular endothelium intima of the vasa vasorum and implanting infectious focus or due to vasculitis. Patients with mycotic aneurysms may present with headaches and neurological deficits. Mortality can reach up to 80 % if the mycotic aneurysm is ruptured. Streptococci are the most common organisms causing mycotic aneurysms.

Thoracic IE complications are seen when IE affects the right side of the heart. Complications include septic emboli (65–75 % of cases) and pulmonary infarction, pneumonia, empyema, abscess formation, and mycotic aneurysm of the pulmonary arteries. IVDA patients are affected by pulmonary septic emboli in up to 75 % of cases.

Splenic abscesses are the most common abdominal extra-cardiac manifestations of IE (55 % of cases) and occur due to septic emboli dissemination. The abscess formation can be single or multiple. Renal involvement may occur in up to 66 % of patients in the form of glomerulonephritis or renal infarction due to septic emboli.

Musculoskeletal complications of IE include spondylodiscitis (1.8–5 % of cases), sacroiliitis, septic arthritis, and osteomyelitis, all which are explained by septic emboli dissemination. However, aseptic, self-limiting arthralgia with low back pain may occur in up to 44 % of cases.

Skin manifestations of IE are explained by vasculitis that results from deposition of circulating immune complexes on various endothelial locations. The most common skin lesions in IE are Osler's nodes and Janeway's lesions. *Osler's node is a* tender, erythematous, nonhemorrhagic lesion with white center located at the fingers pads (□ Fig. 5.4.1), whereas

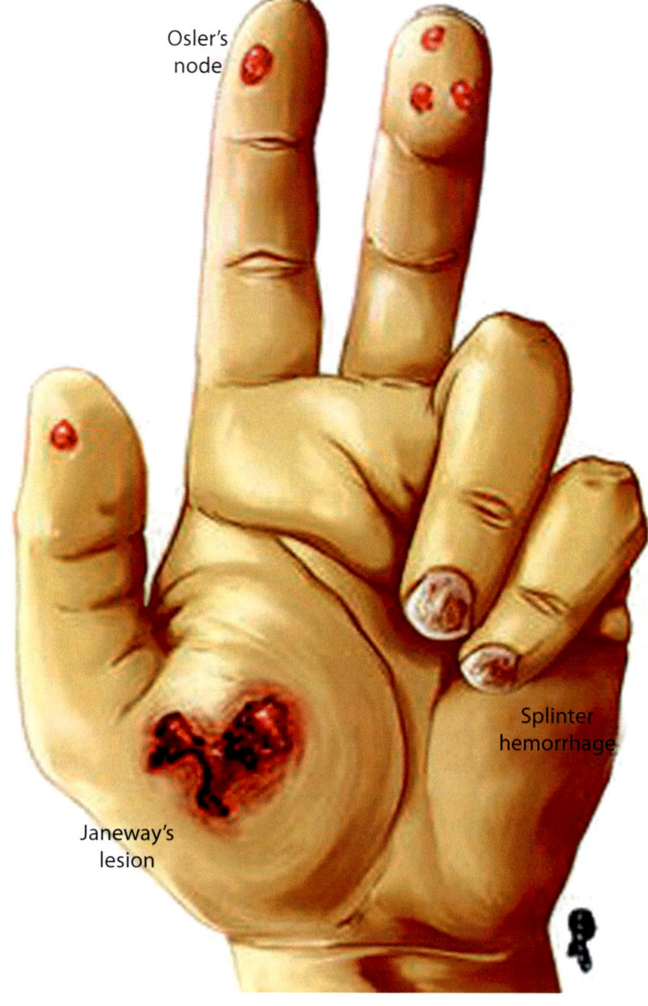




**Fig. 5.4.1**   A hand illustration of a patient with IE shows Osler's nodes, Janeway's lesion, and splinter hemorrhage

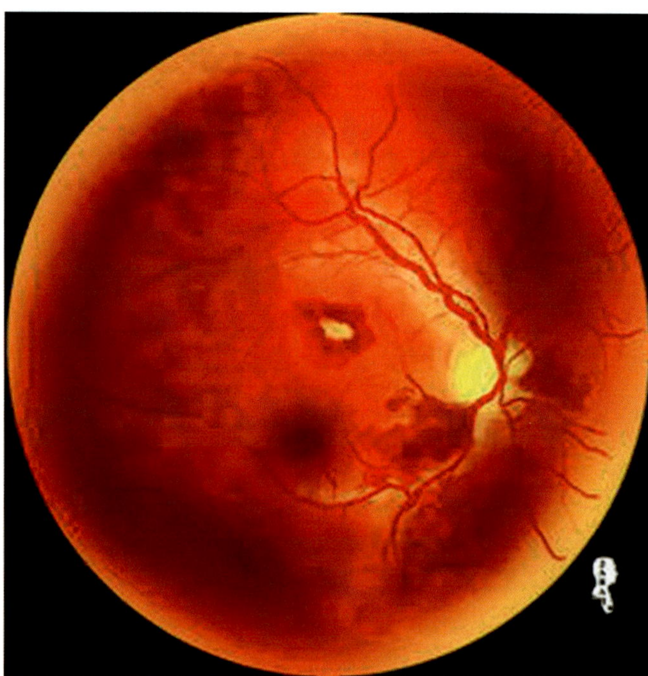

**Fig. 5.4.2**   A fundoscopic illustration demonstrating Roth's spots as multiple hemorrhages within the vitreous humor

*Janeway's lesions* are non-tender, small hemorrhagic, and slightly nodular lesions located at the palms and soles (**Fig. 5.4.1**). *Splinter hemorrhage* is another lesion found in IE, which is characterized by extravasation of blood from the longitudinally located vessels of the nail bed (**Fig. 5.4.1**). Splinter hemorrhage is seen as small areas of bleeding under the nails, commonly affecting the fingernails more than the toes. *Roth's spots* are areas of retinal bleeding within the globe, which is seen on fundoscopy (**Fig. 5.4.2**). Clubbing of fingers occurs due to chronic toxemia in the subacute form.

### Signs on CT and CTA

- On cardiac CT, vegetations are seen as round lesions located at the heart valves (**Fig. 5.4.3**). Lesions >10 mm in diameter have a high risk of embolization.
- In the brain, embolic strokes are often multiple and typically are located at the corticomedullary junction extending to the gray matter. Up to 90 % of septic embolic strokes are in the middle cerebral artery (MCA) vascular territory.
- Cerebral mycotic aneurysms are most commonly seen at the distal branches of the MCA and multiple in 29 % of cases.
- Single or multiple splenic abscesses are seen as hypodense lesions within the spleen on nonenhanced scan. The lesions typically show rim enhancement after contrast injection.
- Renal infarction is detected as a peripheral wedge-shaped area that fails to enhance after contrast injection. The "cortical rim sign" can be seen in 50 % of cases.

### Signs on Chest Radiographs

- Signs of heart failure with enlarged cardiothoracic ratio (>55 %), and pulmonary edema is seen in up to 65 % of cases in patients with clinical signs of heart failure.
- Empyema is detected as a pleural effusion with thick irregular meniscus sign that is immobile on decubitus views.

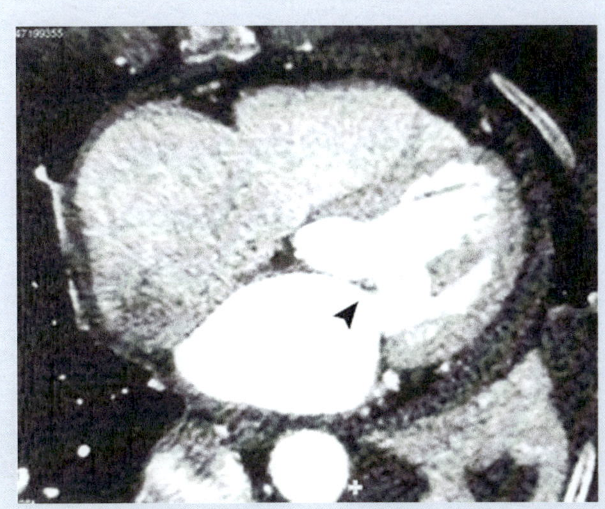

**Fig. 5.4.3** Axial cardiac CTA of a patient with IE shows mitral valve vegetation (*arrowhead*)

## Löffler's Endocarditis (Eosinophilic Endomyocardial Disease)

Löffler's endocarditis (LE) is a rare disease characterized by eosinophilic vasculitis, inflammation, and fibrosis of the myocardium associated with peripheral systemic eosinophilia. It can be primary (idiopathic hypereosinophilia) or secondary to some types of malignancies (e.g., leukemia).

Infiltration of the myocardium by eosinophils causes myocarditis, which is transformed later into myocardial fibrosis and can be superimposed by thrombus formation within the myocardium (mural thrombus). The myocardial fibrosis later on results in restrictive myocardial normal movement similar to the mechanism of restriction encounter in restrictive cardiomyopathy, which results in heart failure. When the fibrosis extends to the papillary muscles and chordae tendineae, disruption of the atrioventricular valves occurs (mitral or tricuspid valves insufficiency).

LE has poor prognosis with high mortality due to heart failure, sudden death, or thromboembolism. Systemic eosinophilic vasculitis can cause multiple infarctions in the brain, kidney, and lungs.

The most characteristic finding in LE which should be indicative is the presence of high eosinophilia in the routine white blood count (CBC), associated with fever and signs of cardiac failure.

The eosinophilia can be absent in chronic cases of LE, where the clinical picture shows the picture of restrictive endocarditis instead of the acute picture of the disease, which is characterized by eosinophilia and cardiac enlargement due to inflammation.



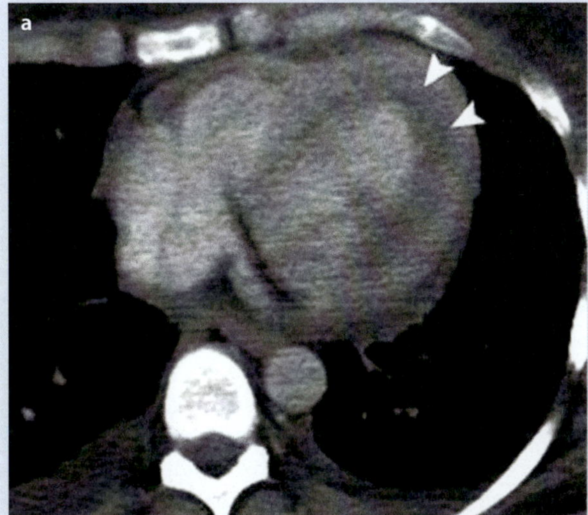
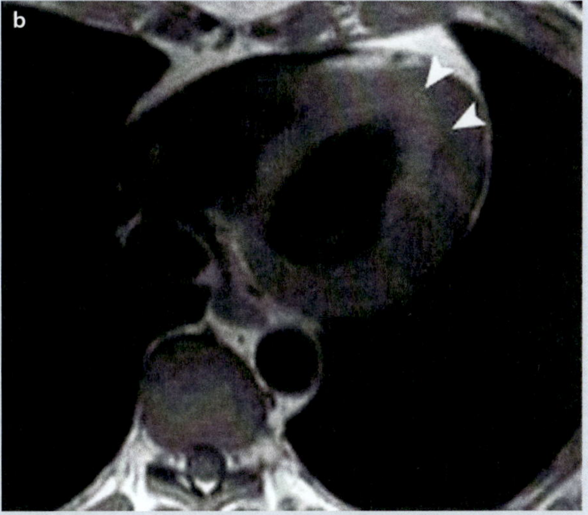

**Fig. 5.4.4** Axial cardiac CT (**a**) and dark-blood MRI (**b**) of a patient with Löffler's endocarditis (LE) showing hypertrophic left ventricle myocardium with subendocardial hypodensities in (**a**) (*arrowheads*) and hypertrophic left ventricle myocardium with subendocardial hyperintensities in (**b**) due to myocardial inflammation and edema

## Marantic Endocarditis (Nonbacterial Thrombotic Endocarditis)

Nonbacterial thrombotic endocarditis (NBTE) is a condition characterized by nonbacterial heart valves vegetation composed of sterile masses of platelets and fibrin fibers. The term is partly a misnomer, because myocardial inflammation is absent.

NBTE is most commonly associated with end-stage malignancies like those of the breast, lung, and colon. Also, NBTE can be seen uncommonly with autoimmune diseases like systemic lupus erythematosus (SLE) (*Libman–Sacks endocarditis*).

Libman–Sacks vegetations are noninfective verrucous vegetations that develop mainly on the mitral valves and maybe the aortic valve. Libman–Sacks vegetations are found in approximately 1 of 10 patients with SLE. Libman–Sacks endocarditis may be differentiated from IE by measuring the white blood count (high in IE and expected to be low during lupus flare), the C-reactive protein (high in IE and possibly suppressed in SLE), and the antiphospholipid antibody level (moderate to high levels in SLE and unlikely to be high in IE).

The vegetation is believed to be caused by the state of hypercoagulability secondary to malignancies or autoimmune diseases. The vegetations are usually <3 mm in diameter and can present with multiple systemic embolic attacks involving the cerebral nervous system or the vascular system (e.g., blue toe syndrome). The vegetations rarely alter valve function or produce murmurs. *Blue toe syndrome* is a condition characterized by sudden onset of acute pain and cyanosis in one or more toes due to embolic event (☐ Fig. 5.4.5).

A blood culture is considered negative after three or more sets of blood cultures incubated for a week fail to demonstrate growth. The most common causes of culture negative endocarditis are antibiotic therapy prior to the blood cultures and infection due to fastidious organisms. NBTE should be considered when a patient with suspected IE fails to demonstrate positive blood culture and fails to respond to antibiotic therapy or in a patient with multiple cerebral strokes due to unknown cause. Early recognition of NBTE will lead to early detection of occult malignancy or autoimmune disease.

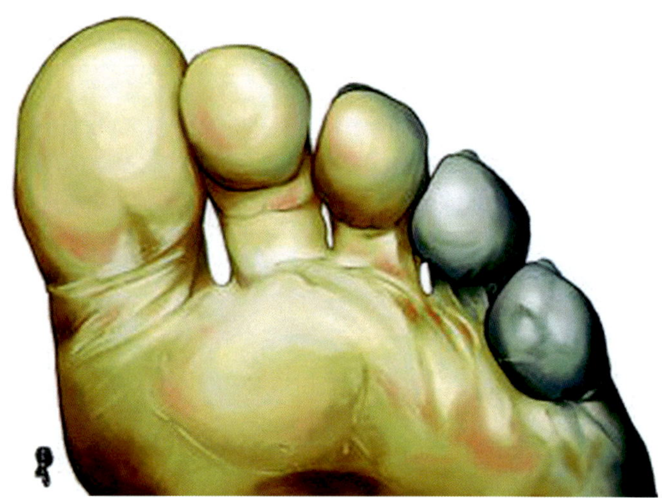

☐ **Fig. 5.4.5**   An illustration demonstrating the gross appearance of blue toe syndrome

## Further Reading


Bayer AS, et al. Diagnosis and management of infective endocarditis and its complications. Circulation. 1998;98:2936–48.

Colen TW, et al. Radiologic manifestations of extra-cardiac complications of infective endocarditis. Eur Radiol. 2008;18:2433–45.

Fanale MA, et al. Some unusual complications of malignancies. Case 2. Marantic endocarditis in advanced cancer. J Clin Oncol. 2002;20:4108–14.

Farrior JB, et al. A consideration of the difference between a Janeway's lesion and an Osler's node in infectious endocarditis. Chest. 1976;70:239–43.

Fellah L, et al. Combined assessment of tricuspid valve endocarditis and pulmonary septic embolism with ECG-gated 40-MDCT of the whole chest. AJR. 2007;189:W228–30.

Files MD, et al. A child with eosinophilia, Loeffler endocarditis, and acute lymphoblastic leukemia. Pediatr Cardiol. 2009;30:530–2.

Freedman LR. Endocarditis updated. Dis Mon. 1979;26:1–51.

Friday BB, et al. Systemic complications of infective endocarditis. Circulation. 2005;112:e324.

Hirschmann JV, et al. Blue (or purple) toe syndrome. J Am Acad Dermatol. 2009;60:1–20.

Joshi SB, et al. Marantic endocarditis presenting as recurrent arterial embolization. Int J Cardiol. 2009;132:e14–6.

Kleinfeldt T, et al. Hypereosinophilic syndrome: a rare case of Loeffler's endocarditis documented in cardiac MRI. Int J Cardiol. 2009. doi:10.1016/j.ijxard.2009.03.059.

Lofiego C, et al. Ventricular remodeling in Loeffler endocarditis: implications for therapeutic decision making. Eur J Heart Fail. 2005;7:1023–6.

Mahlab K, et al. Diagnosis of Candida endocarditis by computed tomography scanning. IMAJ. 2006;8:442–4.

Moyssakis I, et al. Libman-Sacks endocarditis in systemic lupus erythematosus: prevalence, associations, and evolution. Am J Med. 2007;120:636–42.

Saladi RN, et al. Idiopathic splinter hemorrhages. J Am Acad Dermatol. 2004;50:289–92.

Singh V, et al. Marantic endocarditis (NBTE) with systemic emboli and paraneoplastic cerebellar degeneration: uncommon presentation of ovarian cancer. J Neurooncol. 2007;83:81–3.

Yalonetsky S, et al. Mitral valve destruction by Hodgkin's lymphoma-associated Loeffler endocarditis. Pediatr Cardiol. 2008. doi:10.1007/s00246-007-9135-6.

## 5.5  Pericardial Diseases

The pericardium is a double-walled sac that encloses the heart. The outer sac is called the "fibrous pericardium," and the inner sac is called the "serous pericardium." The serous pericardium is composed of an outer (parietal) layer and an inner (visceral) layer separated by potential space (pericardial cavity). Both the fibrous and the serous layers are continuous with the adventitia of the great vessels.

The anterior aspect of the fibrous pericardium is attached to the left half of the sternum and to the fourth, fifth, and sixth left costal cartilages. Inferiorly, it is attached to the central tendon of the diaphragm. Only the fibrous pericardium below the fifth or sixth intercostal space is sensitive to pain, while the remaining fibrous and entire serous pericardium is insensitive. When this pain-sensitive area is stimulated by a disease, pericardial pain is perceived as pain in the neck and trapezius muscle via the phrenic nerve, which enters the spinal cord at the fourth and fifth cervical segments.

The pericardial cavity contains normally 20–50 mL of serous fluid, although the sac has a potential space of 80–100 mL. The pericardial fluid is absorbed by the lymphatics found near the base of the heart. The blood supply of the pericardium comes from the internal thoracic artery via the pericardiophrenic artery.

*Pericardial effusion* is a disease characterized by excess fluid within the pericardial cavity that exceeds 50 mL. Like pleural effusion, this fluid can be classified into transudative or exudative based on the protein content. The pericardial fluid can be edematous (e.g., in uremia) and hemorrhagic (e.g., in trauma), contain pus (e.g., infective endocarditis), or contain lymph (e.g., due to rupture of the thoracic duct). When the pericardial fluid is severe enough to compromise the heart contractility, the condition is called *pericardial tamponade*, and it is a medical emergency. Between 150 and 250 mL of fluid must be present within the pericardial cavity to cause a cardiac tamponade.

*Pericarditis* is a condition characterized by inflammation of the pericardium, which can be acute or chronic. Pericarditis can arise due to infections, autoimmune diseases, and granulomatous diseases. Patients with pericarditis often present with symptoms due to inflammation, pericardial effusion or tamponade, or constriction and/or restriction due to fibrosis.

Symptoms of pericarditis include acute sudden neck or upper arm pain that is exaggerated by body movements, respiration, swallowing, and rarely by heart beat. The pain may be relieved by leaning forward, which will stabilize the pericardial sac and reduce the movement of the pain-sensitive area. When the peripheral diaphragmatic pleura are inflamed, epigastric pain is felt, which can be seen in up to 50 % of patients with acute idiopathic pericarditis. Moreover, dull abdominal pain in the right upper quadrant may be felt due to congestion of the abdominal viscera in cases of tamponade and pericardial constriction. Other symptoms include fever, dyspnea, and paroxysmal nocturnal dyspnea in complicated cases. *Paradoxical pulse* is a normal pulse variation representing the fact that the systolic pressure is less during inspiration than during expiration in a normal person. An accentuation of this normal respiratory variation may be found in patients with pericarditis with tamponade. Also, in patients with tamponade, an alternation of a weak pulse and a strong pulse in the presence of a regular rhythm may be found (*pulsus alternans*).

A pleural effusion may accompany pericarditis in all stages of the disease (>50 % of cases). In patients with large pericardial effusion, an area of dullness of variable size can be found in the region of the inferior angle of the scapula where there is normally bronchial breathing (Ewart's sign). This sign is explained by the fact that large pericardial effusion forces the heart and the great vessels backward, thereby compressing the lung and the bronchi.

Chronic pericarditis, like any chronic inflammation, is characterized by calcification and fibrosis. Pericardial fibrosis due to chronic inflammation with pericardial space limitation is called *constrictive pericarditis*. Constrictive pericarditis can occur due to tuberculosis, radiation, and previous pericardiotomy, and up to 49 % are idiopathic. Patients with constrictive pericarditis often present with signs of right-sided heart failure and atrial fibrillation in up to 40 % of cases. Clinical signs of liver enlargement, ascites, and peripheral edema may be seen in patients with constrictive pericarditis due to congestive heart failure. On auscultation, patients with acute and constrictive pericarditis have pericardial friction rub, in which a sound is heard during heart beat cycle due to friction of the fibrous pericardium layers. Pericardial rub is a diagnostic clinical sign of pericarditis.

*Pneumopericardium* is a rare condition characterized by the presence of air within the pericardial cavity. Pneumopericardium can occur as a complication of pneumomediastinum, pneumothorax, or pericardial fluid aspiration.

## Differential Diagnoses and Related Diseases

- *Dressler's syndrome*, also known as "*postmyocardial infarction syndrome*," is a disease seen as early as 10 days and as late as 2 years following myocardial infarction characterized by fever, pericarditis or pleuritis with hemorrhagic effusion, and pneumonia with gross hemoptysis. The disease has a tendency for recurrence.
- *CACP syndrome* is an uncommon disease characterized by camptodactyly, noninflammatory arthropathy, coxa vara, and pericarditis. The disease is related to a group of

diseases known as *familial arthropathy diseases*. The disease arises due to hypertrophies synovium in the absence of synovitis (in contrast to rheumatoid arthritis or its juvenile form), which is typically detected by synovial biopsy. Patients affected present with arthropathy usually since childhood. Camptodactyly is a congenital or acquired nontraumatic flexion deformity of the proximal interphalangeal (PIP) joint of one or several fingers, which is usually bilateral in CACP syndrome. Noninflammatory arthropathy involves large joints such as the elbows, knees, and ankles. Coxa vara is a horizontally oriented femoral neck. Mild noninflammatory pericarditis with pericardial effusion occurs in 30 % of cases. The condition may be mild or self-limited. MRI studies classically show hypertrophied synovium with rim-like enhancement of the fluid-filled bursae, a feature that distinguishes CACP syndrome from rheumatoid arthritis, which shows synovial hypertrophy, signs of soft tissue hyperemia, and diffuse contrast enhancement.

### Signs on Chest Radiographs

- Pericardial effusion is detected as increased heart enlargement on serial radiographs. The pericardial effusion starts to show radiographic abnormalities when the pericardial fluid exceeds 250 mL in adults (◘ Fig. 5.5.1).
- Constrictive pericarditis can be detected when calcification of the pericardium occurs (◘ Fig. 5.5.2). Calcified pericardium is visualized as a wide area of calcification that follows the heart silhouette.
- Pneumopericardium is visualized as an air surrounding the heart contour (◘ Fig. 5.5.3).

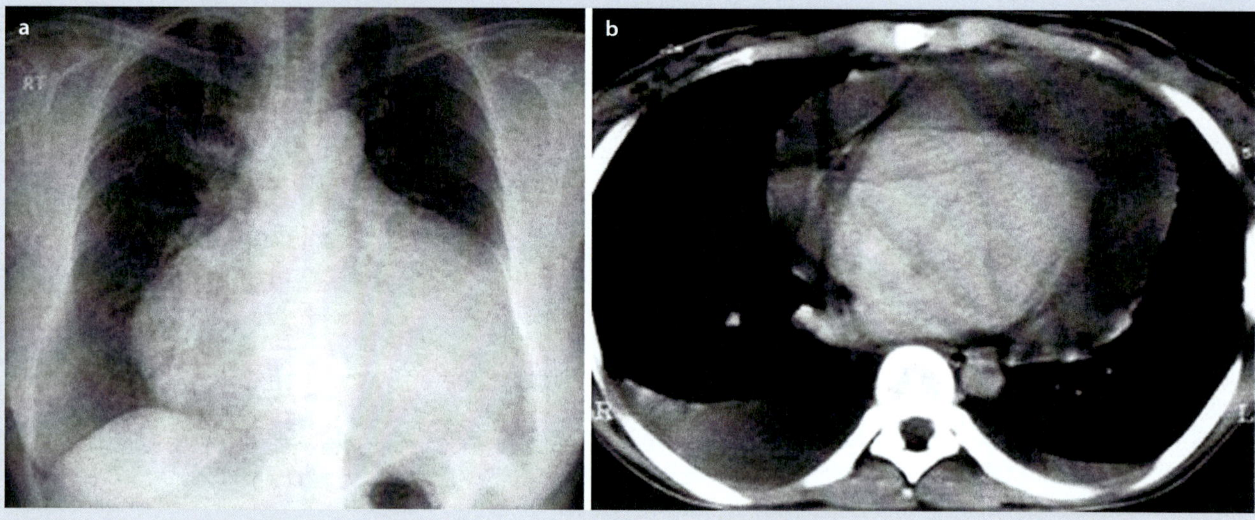

◘ **Fig. 5.5.1**   Posteroanterior chest radiograph (**a**) and axial chest CT of two different patients with pericardial tamponade show massive heart enlargement in (**a**) due to pericardial effusion, and hypodense material is seen surrounding the heart due to marked pericardial effusion in (**b**). Also, bilateral pleural effusion can be seen in (**b**)

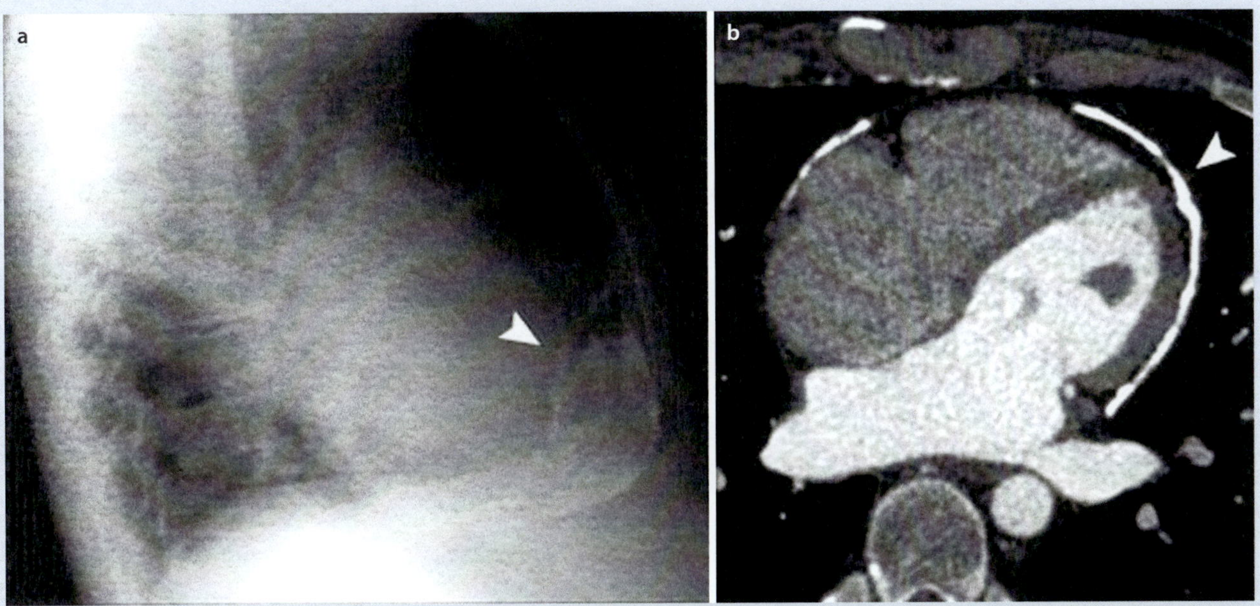

 **Fig. 5.5.2** Lateral chest radiograph (**a**) and axial chest CT of two different patients with constrictive pericarditis show calcified pericardium (*arrowheads*)

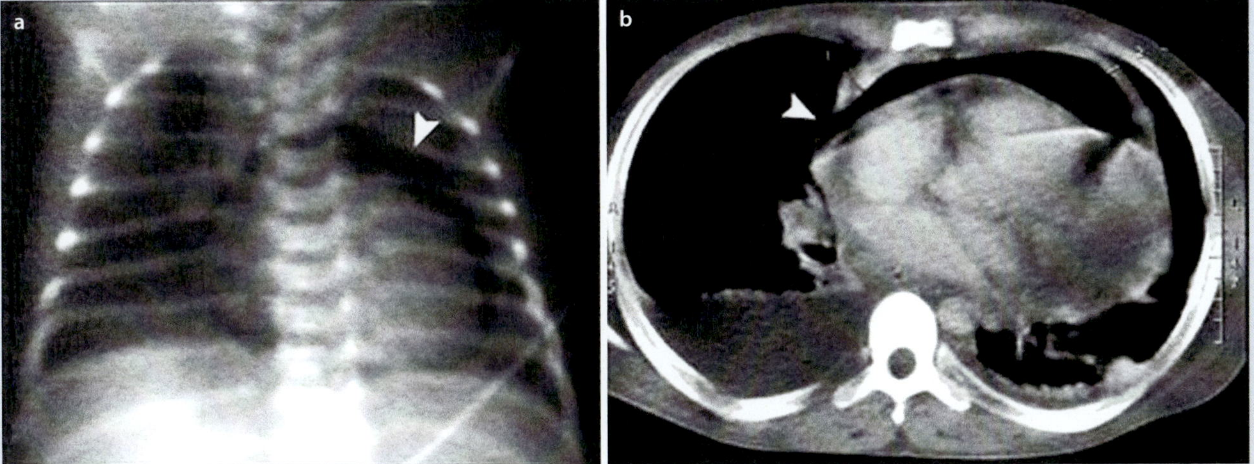

 **Fig. 5.5.3** Posteroanterior chest radiograph (**a**) and axial chest CT of two different patients with pneumopericardium show air surrounding the heart in (**a**) and (**b**) (*arrowheads*)

### Signs on CT and MRI
- Pericardial effusion and tamponade are seen as fluid signal intensity material located within the pericardial space ( Fig. 5.5.1). The normal pericardial space should not exceed 4 mm in width. On CT, the fluid can have high density if it is hemorrhagic (e.g., >80 HU). On MRI, the signal intensity of the fluid is variable according to the content of the fluid (e.g., high T1 and T2 signal intensities if it is hemorrhagic).
- The normal pericardium is visualized on MRI as a thin hypointense line surrounding the heart outlined by the high-intensity pericardial fat, which normally should not exceed 3 mm in thickness. Acute pericarditis on CT and MRI is diagnosed when the pericardium is >3 mm in thickness and enhances after contrast injection ( Fig. 5.5.4).
- Constrictive pericarditis shows diffuse thickening and irregularities of the pericardium with or without calcification. Pericardial calcification is a diagnostic sign of constrictive pericarditis ( Fig. 5.5.2). Normal or near normal thickening of the pericardium does not rule out constrictive pericarditis.
- Pneumopericardium is seen as an air that surrounds the heart within the pericardial space ( Fig. 5.5.3).

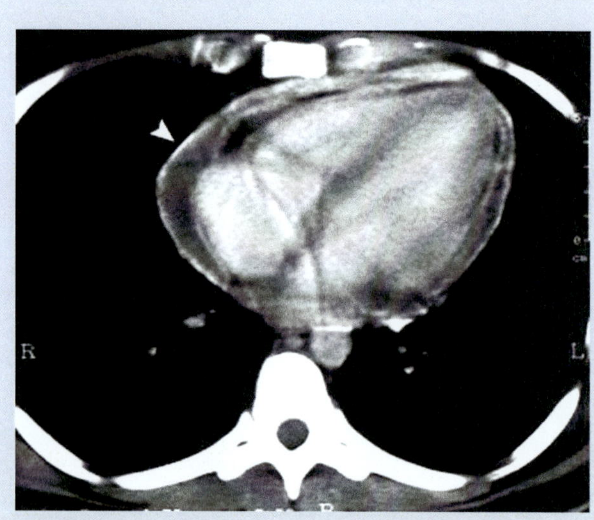

**Fig. 5.5.4** Axial postcontrast cardiac CT with contrast shows pericardial enhancement (*arrowhead*) with moderate pericardial effusion in a patient with acute pericarditis

Glockner JF. Imaging of pericardial diseases. Magn Reson Imaging Clin N Am. 2003;11:149–62.

McIntosh HD. Pericarditis. Dis Mon. 1964;10:1–39.

Oberholzer K, et al. Pneumomediastinum and pneumopericardium due to malignant subcarinal lymphadenopathy: CT demonstration. Eur Radiol. 1997;7:583–5.

Spiegel R, et al. Eosinophilic pericarditis: a rare complication of idiopathic hypereosinophilic syndrome. Pediatr Cardiol. 2004;25:690–2.

Talreja DR, et al. Constrictive pericarditis in 26 patients with histologically normal pericardial thickness. Circulation. 2003;108:1852–7.

Weiser NJ, et al. The postmyocardial infarction syndrome: the nonspecificity of the pulmonary manifestations. Circulation. 1962;25:643–50.

Yousefzadeh DK, et al. The triad of pneumonitis, pleuritis, and pericarditis in juvenile rheumatoid arthritis. Pediatr Radiol. 1979;8:147–50.

## Further Reading

Al-Mayouf SM. Familial arthropathy in Saudi Arabian children: demographic, clinical, and biochemical features. Semin Arthritis Rheum. 2007;36:256–61.

Choi B-R, et al. Camptodactyly, arthropathy, coax vara, pericarditis (CACP) syndrome: a case report. J Korean Med Sci. 2004;19:907–10.

# Rheumatology



© Springer International Publishing Switzerland 2017
J.A. Al-Tubaikh, *Internal Medicine*, DOI 10.1007/978-3-319-39747-4_6

## 6.1    Rheumatoid Arthritis

Rheumatoid arthritis (RA) is a chronic, multisystemic, nonspecific inflammatory disease with unknown etiology that primarily affects the joints and the skeletal muscles.

RA is diagnosed by qualifying certain criteria. Four of the following criteria should be present for more than 6 months to fulfill the diagnosis of RA:

- Morning stiffness that lasts at least an hour before maximal improvement
- Soft-tissue swelling and arthritis in a bilateral symmetrical fashion of at least three joints (polyarthritis)
- Swelling of the metacarpophalangeal, proximal phalangeal, or wrist joints
- Subcutaneous rheumatoid nodules
- A positive test for rheumatoid factor
- Radiographic signs of RA

In joints, the main pathology of RA is related to synovial inflammation and proliferation. The normal synovium is attached to the inner joint capsule in synovial joints. The articulating surface of the joint is covered with cartilage except for a small region at the insertion of the joint capsule. This area is covered only by synovium, and it is called the "bare area." Synovial inflammation and bone erosions start from this area in RA. The granulation tissue (pannus) that results from the chronic synovial inflammation adheres and extends to the articular cartilage and the subchondral surface. This extension causes bone resorption and articular adhesions that may ossify and leads to bony fusion. Intraarticular loose bodies may develop as a consequence of the inflammatory process. The loose intra-articular bodies are composed of destroyed cartilage or hypertrophied synovium.

RA affects mainly women between 30 and 40 years of age. Any joint in the body can be affected by RA, but the disease often affects the small joints of the hands excluding the terminal phalanges. Wrists, knees, and feet are also commonly affected by RA. Patients often present with morning stiffness, small joints swelling due to tenosynovitis, muscular pain, and stiffness commonly after a period of immobilization. Extra-articular manifestations of RA make the disease mixed in its early stage with systemic lupus erythematosus (SLE). SLE, however, may be seen in patients with chronic RA.

Nervous system manifestations in RA can be categorized into four groups: central nervous system rheumatoid nodules, cerebral vasculitis, cervical myelopathy due to atlanto-axial subluxation, and peripheral neuropathy. The atlantoaxial subluxation may lead to the development of *double crush syndrome*. The double crush hypothesis refers to the concept that a single lesion in the course of a nerve predisposes that nerve to a second lesion further along its course. This phenomenon is often observed in patients with thoracic outlet syndrome, where compression of the brachial plexus can result in the development of carpal tunnel syndrome. Median nerve neuritis (carpal tunnel syndrome), Raynaud's phenomenon, and hyperemia of the palms (liver palms) may be seen in cases of rheumatoid peripheral neuropathy and sympathetic nervous system hyperactivity. Moreover, the cervical manifestations of RA can be seen as rheumatoid discitis and myelopathy due to thickening of the dura. Rheumatoid discitis arises due to annulus fibrosis and replacement of the normal intravertebral disk by rheumatoid pannus.

*Rheumatoid nodules* (10–20 %) are seen in juxta-articular surfaces or on the extensor surfaces of the arm and elbows, especially the olecranon surface. Rheumatoid nodules consist histologically of three zones: a central zone of necrotic tissue, a middle zone of histiocytes and monocytes, and an outer zone of chronic inflammatory granulation tissue. They can affect any part of the body including the heart, larynx, eye, Achilles' tendon, and lungs. The presence of rheumatoid nodules is indicative of severe disease. An uncommon complication of rheumatoid nodule includes breakdown of the overlying skin and discharge of the content (*fistulous rheumatism*). Rarely, rheumatoid nodules may present as linear, elongated, cord-like subcutaneous bands.

Moderate hypochromic normocytic anemia can be found in chronic RA due to anemia of chronic disease. Diseases that can be associated with RA are psoriasis (8 %), ulcerative colitis, amyloidosis, and asthma. Lymphadenopathy can be seen in cases of RA.

*Rheumatoid nodulosis* (RN) is a rare, benign RA variant characterized by the presence of subcutaneous rheumatoid nodules with absence of synovitis, absence of systemic manifestations in benign course, and mild radiological findings. Classically, the presence of rheumatoid nodule is a sign of advanced RA with poor prognosis. As a rule, the benign course of the disease and the mild radiological findings are what differentiate RA from RN. RN is found in up to 25 % of classical RA cases and presents between ages 30 and 50 years. RN has a male predominance (81 %), whereas RA has a female predominance. The subcutaneous rheumatoid nodules in RN appear at the onset of clinical symptoms and are usually observed over bony surfaces like the back of the hands and the olecranon (❐ Fig. 6.1.1).

*CNS manifestations of RA* include vasculitis, pachymeningitis, leptomeningitis, rheumatoid nodules formation, stroke, seizures, and encephalopathy. The diagnosis of cerebral manifestation of RA must be supported by high titers of RF and anticyclic citrullinated peptide (anti-CCP), clinical symptoms of RA, and good response to immunosuppressive therapy. Classically, CNS manifestations of RA are associated with subcutaneous rheumatic nodules, cutaneous vasculitis, and peripheral neuropathy (advanced stage of the disease).

## Differential Diagnoses and Related Diseases

- *Juvenile rheumatoid arthritis (JRA)* is a form of RA that emerges before 16 years of age. It has similar manifestations like adult RA.
- *Still's disease* is a rare disease of unknown origin characterized by episodes of spiking fever, skin rash, hepatosplenomegaly, and JRA. It affects 20 % of patients with

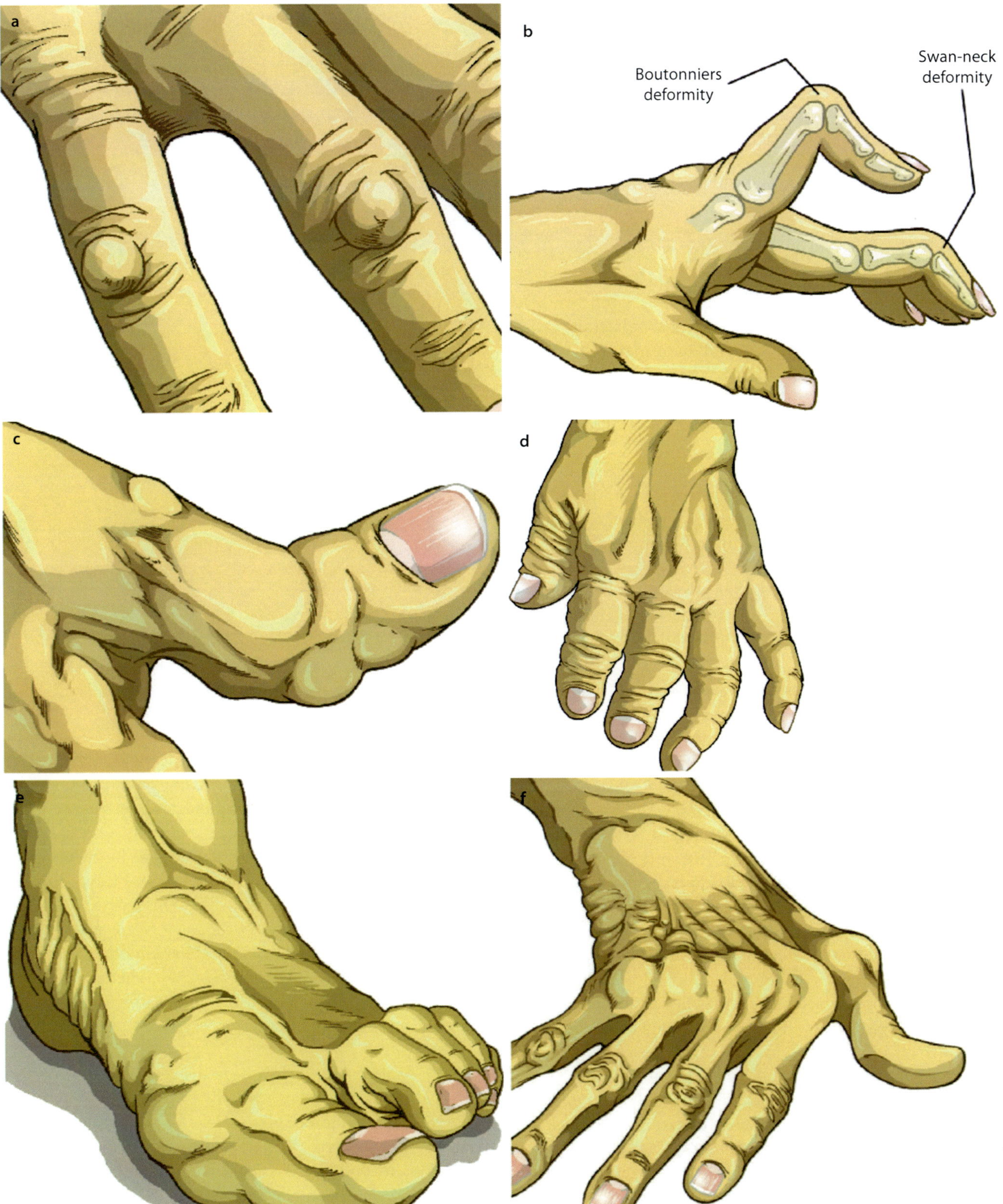



**Fig. 6.1.1** An illustration demonstrates different manifestations of rheumatoid arthritis (RA) in the hand: (**a**) rheumatoid nodulosis, (**b**) Boutonnière and swan-neck deformities, (**c**) hitchhiker thumb deformity, (**d**) opera-glass hand, (**e**) hammertoe deformity, and (**f**) ulnar deviation

JRA, and RF and antinuclear antibodies are negative. It is usually a disease of exclusion.

- *Caplan's syndrome* is a disease characterized by the association of RA with coal worker's lung (pneumoconiosis). On radiographs, the disease is characterized by multiple, well-defined, round opacities 0.5–5 cm in size that mimic pulmonary metastases, representing of necrobiotic rheumatoid lung nodules. Calcification of these opacities is common.
- *Felty's syndrome* is a disease characterized by the triad of RA, splenomegaly, and leucopenia. It is a rare extra-articular manifestation of RA and affects less than 1 % of patients. Felty's syndrome patients are often women between 55 and 65 years of age, with long-standing RA (10–15 years). Hepatomegaly and abnormal liver profile are seen in up to 65 % of cases, with hepatic nodular hyperplasia being the most common hepatic lesion found in these patients. Leg ulceration with hyperpigmentation occurs in 25 % of cases.
- *Pseudo-Felty's syndrome* (*large granular lymphocyte syndrome*) is a disease characterized by RA and proliferation of large granular lymphocytes (LGL). LGLs are a distinct subset of peripheral blood mononuclear cells, with a natural killer activity. Patients present clinically with RA, splenomegaly, and leucopenia similar to classic Felt's syndrome. The only distinction is the laboratory detection of abnormal high levels of LGLs in the blood.
- *Progressive pseudorheumatoid dysplasia* (*PPsRD*) is a rare, autosomal recessive disease characterized by polyarthralgia, multiple joint contractures, prominent interphalangeal joints, and short stature. The disease starts to manifest between 3 and 4 years as progressive cartilage destruction in the absence of synovitis. Rheumatoid factor is typically negative, and genetic testing shows positive WISP3 gene. The disease can be mistaken for JRA and Scheuermann's disease. In contrast to JRA, PPsRD lacks the lymphadenopathy and fever that can be seen in Still's disease. The disease is diagnosed clinically by identifying enlarged carpometacarpal joint bilaterally (■ Figs. 6.1.1 and 6.1.2). The disease is essentially diagnosed radiologically due to its typical radiological features, with genetic and rheumatoid factor laboratory testing as supporting tests for final confirmation.
- *Lupus polyarthritis* is one of the major manifestations of SLE arthritis in SLE and is characterized by mild arthralgia, tenosynovitis, almost absent erosive changes on radiographs, and joint deformities without bone destruction. Concurrence of RA and SLE is termed *rhupus*.
- *Remitting seronegative symmetrical synovitis with pitting edema* (*RS₃PE syndrome*) is a disease characterized by sudden onset of symmetrical synovitis with pitting edema of the extremities. Although the etiology is unknown, RS₃PE syndrome is known to co-occur with diseases like RA, polymyalgia rheumatica, paraneoplastic syndromes, chronic gout, lymphoma, and *Mycoplasma* pneumonia.

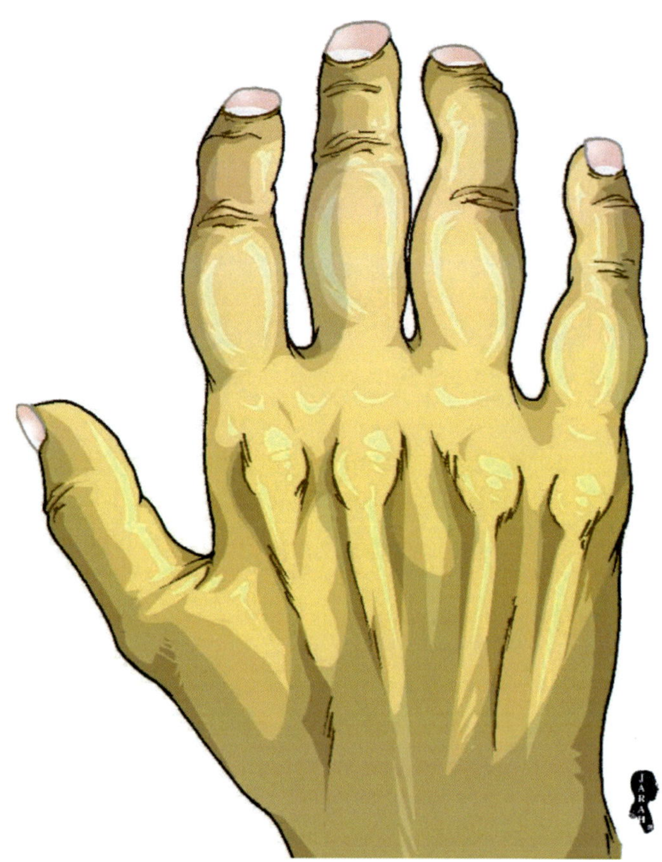

■ **Fig. 6.1.2**  An illustration demonstrates the enlarged carpometacarpal and proximal metacarpophalangeal joints in progressive pseudorheumatoid dysplasia (PPsRD)

Constitutional symptoms like fever, fatigue, and weight loss are reported. Patients classically present with symmetrical polyarthritis of both hands and feet particularly affecting the MCP and PIP joints, with pitting edema that can be mistaken with RA. Other joints can be affected like the wrists, shoulder, knees, and ankles. RS₃PE syndrome is characteristically associated with high serum CRP and ESR levels, with seronegative RF and ANA levels. Characteristically, the serum level of vascular endothelial growth factor (VGEF) is higher than any other rheumatic disorder, and it helps to establish the diagnosis with the radiological findings. The condition responds well to steroid therapy.

- *Jaccoud's arthropathy* is a nonerosive, chronic, progressive, almost painless arthropathy characterized by severe deformities and joint subluxations of the hands and feet with well-preserved functions. In the hands, Jaccoud's arthropathy presents classically with painless ulnar deviation and swan-neck and boutonnière deformities of the fingers and thumb, making the disease easily mistaken for RA. Jaccoud's arthropathy is classically seen in cases of long-standing rheumatic fever, SLE, scleroderma, sarcoidosis, dermatomyositis, and rarely psoriasis. However, the disease can present in the absence of other diseases (idiopathic Jaccoud's arthropathy).

### Signs on Plain Radiographs

- Osteoporosis that can be generalized or focal (juxta-articular), due to hyperemia and disuse (◗ Figs. 6.1.3 and 6.1.4).
- Joint space narrowing due to destruction of the articular surface (◗ Figs. 6.1.3 and 6.1.4). Typically, the distal interphalangeal joint (DIP) is spared in RA.
- Marginal erosions and subchondral cysts formation (geodes) (◗ Fig. 6.1.3). Up to 47 % of patients develop erosions within 1 year after onset of RA.
- *Boutonnière deformity* is flexion at the proximal interphalangeal joint (PIP) and hyperextension at the DIP (◗ Figs. 6.1.1 and 6.1.5).
- *Swan-neck deformity* is hyperextension at the PIP and flexion at the DIP (◗ Fig. 6.1.1).
- *Mallet finger* is a rare finding that is characterized by laxity at the insertion of the extensor tendon on the distal phalanx, thus causing the distal phalanx to drop.
- *Hitchhiker thumb deformity* is flexion at the proximal metacarpophalangeal joint of the thumb and hyperextension at the DIP joint (◗ Figs. 6.1.1 and 6.1.6).
- *Mutlans deformity* (*opera-glass hand*) is a severe hand deformity seen in rapidly progressing RA characterized by severe osteoporosis and phalangeal resorption that causes shortening of the fingers. The carpal and metacarpal bones are commonly resorbed and crumbled due to intercarpal/metacarpal ligaments disruption (◗ Figs. 6.1.1 and 6.1.7). Grossly, the fingers are shortened and the skin is wrinkled, giving the impression that the phalanges were retraced one into another like opera glass (◗ Fig. 6.1.1).
- In *Hammertoe deformity*, the toe is bent at the middle joint, so that it resembles a hammer (Fig. 6.1.1). It is commonly seen affecting the second, third, or fourth toes.
- Due to muscular atrophy, shifting deformities can arise in hands (ulnar deviation), or feet (fibular deviation) (◗ Fig. 6.1.1).
- In the humerus, RA can cause *high-riding shoulder* due to rotator cuff tear.
- In the hip joint, RA causes migration of the femoral head in an axial fashion in the hip joint. In contrast, osteoarthritis causes migration of the femoral head in a superior fashion. Involvement of the foot may occur in up to 90 % of cases. The first and the fifth metatarsophalangeal joints are affected in up to 50 % of cases (◗ Fig. 6.1.4).
- *Atlantoaxial subluxation* is present when the distance between the posterior aspect of the anterior arch of the atlas and the odontoid process is >3 mm in adults or >5 mm in children on flexion

◗ **Fig. 6.1.3**　Plain radiograph of the hand of a patient with RA shows diffuse osteoporosis and reduced space narrowing between the carpal bones and between the carpal bones and the distal radioulnar joint with formation of geodes (*arrowheads*)

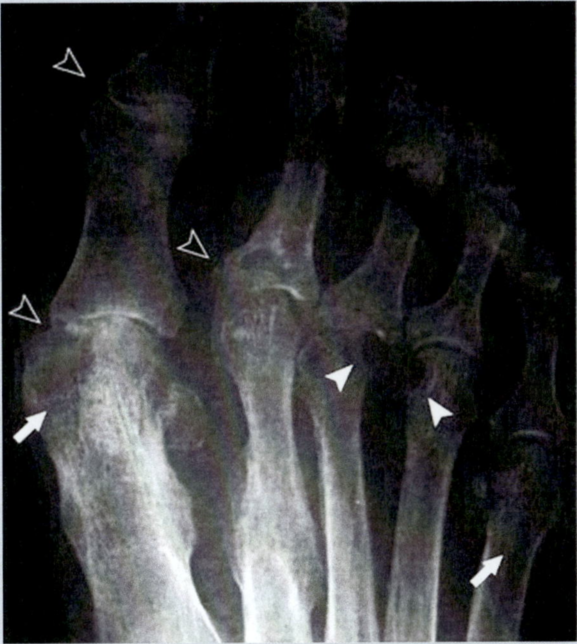

◗ **Fig. 6.1.4**　A plain radiograph of a patient foot with RA shows marginal erosions of the metatarsals (*solid arrowheads*), joint space narrowing of the metatarsophalangeal and interphalangeal joints (*hollow arrowheads*), and patchy osteoporosis (*arrows*) There is old mid-diaphyseal fracture with callus formation of the second metatarsal bone

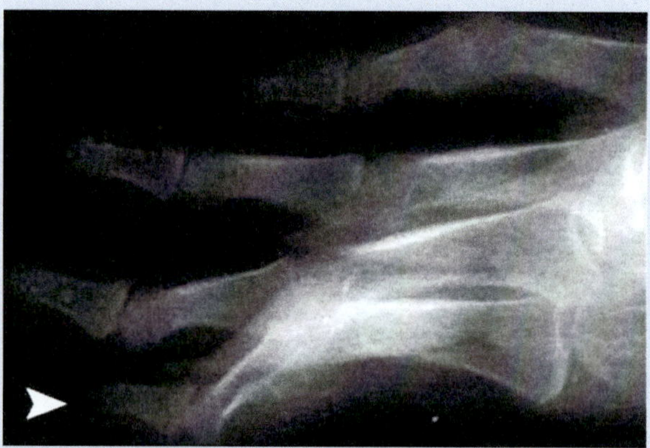

**Fig. 6.1.5** Lateral plain radiograph of the fingers of a patient with RA shows Boutonnière deformity (*arrowhead*)

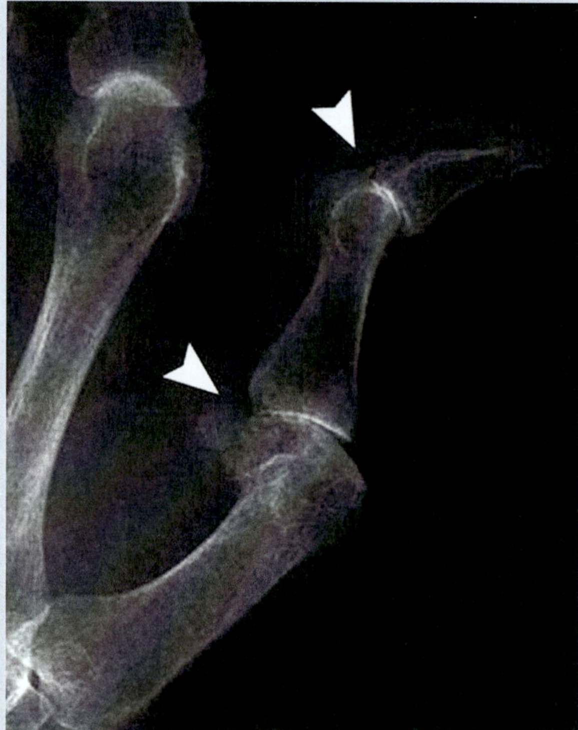

**Fig. 6.1.6** Plain radiograph of the thumb shows flexion at the proximal metacarpophalangeal joint of the thumb and hyperextension at the DIP joint (*arrowheads*) (Hitchhiker thumb deformity)

radiographs. Atlantoaxial subluxation arises in RA with an incidence of 16–36 % of cases, presumably secondary to synovitis causing laxity or tearing of the transverse atlantoaxial ligament (**Fig. 6.1.8**). The atlantoaxial subluxation can progress into atlantoaxial dissociation.

— *Atlantoaxial impaction* occurs when both the facets of the atlas and axis collapse due to erosions. The atlas will articulate with the body of the axis instead of the odontoid process. On lateral

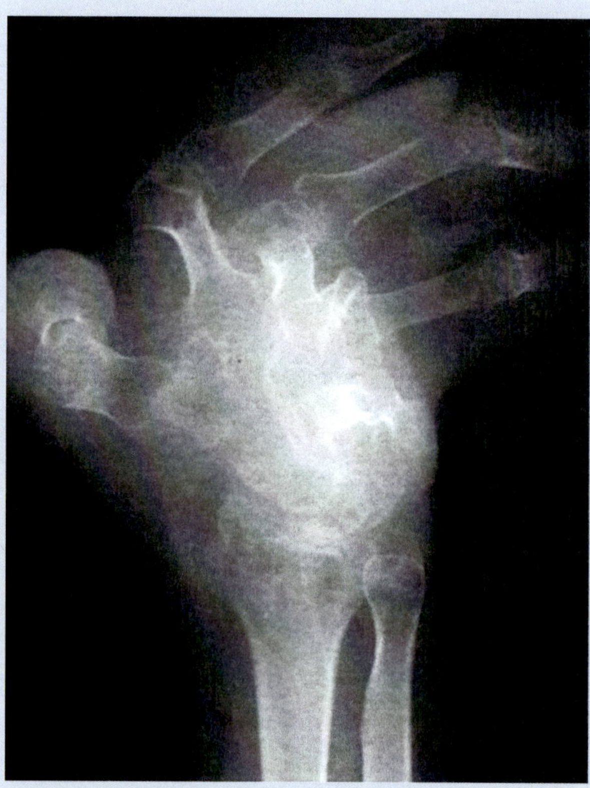

**Fig. 6.1.7** Plain radiograph of the hand of a patient with RA shows crumbling of the carpal bones with severe deformity of the hand plus osteoporosis (Mutlans deformity)

radiographs, the odontoid process will be seen inside the foramen magnum.

— *In juvenile rheumatoid arthritis*, there is fusion between the carpometacarpal joint of the index and middle fingers and enlargement of the epiphysis and the metaphysis end of long bones.

— In *Still's disease*, radiographic features in the hands are a mix between RA and psoriasis arthropathy with affection of the DIP joints in a similar fashion to psoriasis arthropathy erosions.

— Lung fibrosis can be seen in long-standing RA (**Fig. 6.1.9**).

— In *PPsRD*, patients are classically young presenting with widening of the metaphyses of long bones involving the proximal femur and the distal knee, epimetaphyseal enlargement of the metacarpal heads and the phalanges, mega os trigonum, and flattened vertebrae (platyspondyly) with narrowed disk spaces and irregular endplates mimicking Scheuermann's disease. The flattened vertebrae and irregular endplates are seen mainly in the thoracic region in Scheuermann's disease, whereas in PPsRD, the flattened vertebrae with irregular endplates involve the whole spine almost equally (key diagnostic feature).

- In *RS₃PE syndrome*, in contrast to RA, plain radiographs show absent joint erosions.
- In Jaccoud's arthropathy, in contrast to RA, plain radiographs of the hands typically show joint deformities in the absence of bone erosions or cartilage destruction.

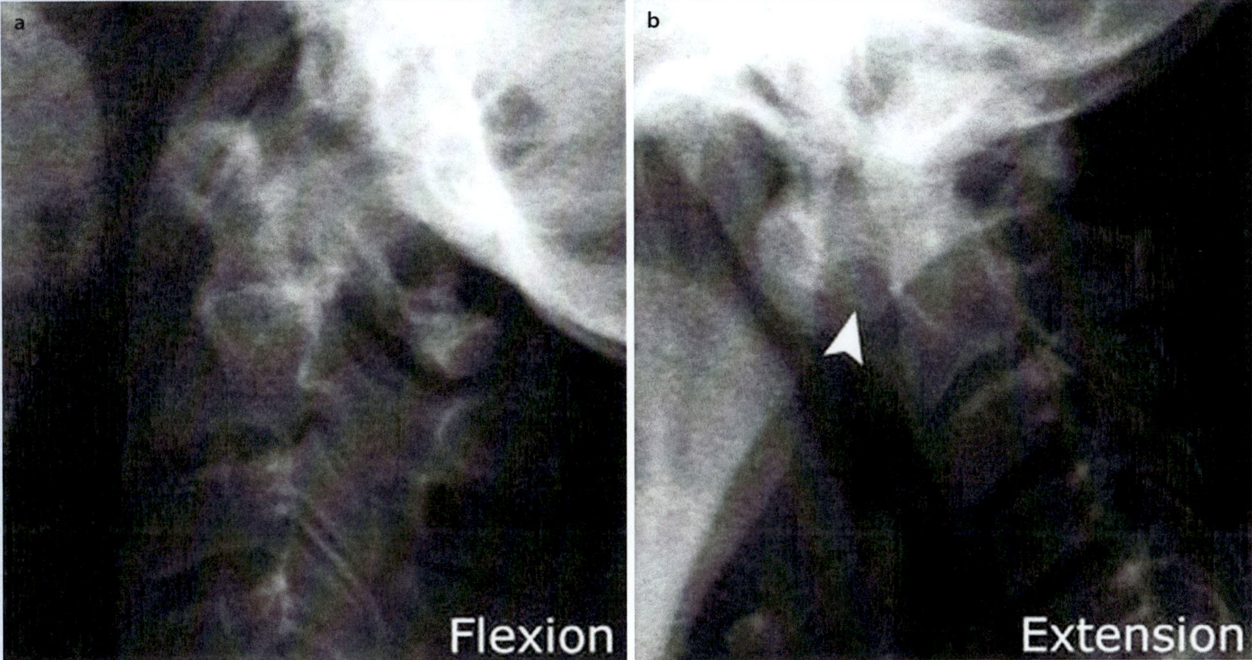


**Fig. 6.1.8** Lateral plain radiograph of the atlantoaxial joint of a patient with atlantoaxial subluxation due to RA shows a significant gap between the anterior arch of the atlas (**a**) and the odontoid process (*arrowhead*) on extension radiograph (**b**)

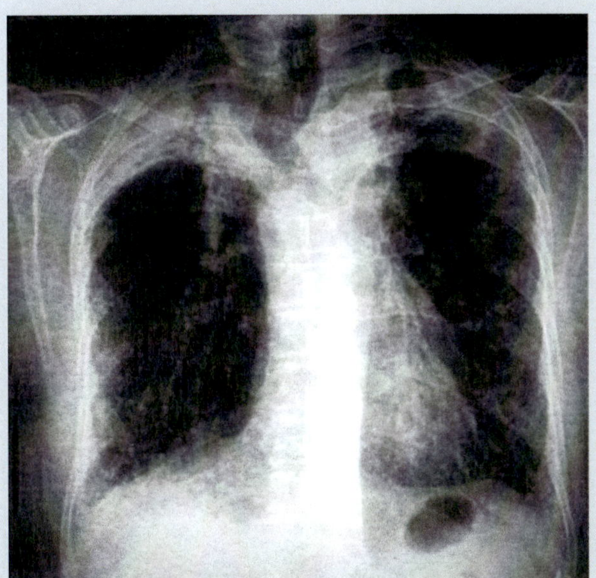

**Fig. 6.1.9** Posteroanterior chest radiograph of a patient with RA shows diffuse reticulonodular interstitial pattern reflecting lung fibrosis

### Signs on MRI

- Different manifestations of inflammation can be seen involving high signal intensity on T2W images of the muscles, bone marrow, tendons, and the articular surface due to effusion. After contrast injection, enhancement of the thickened synovium (pannus) can be seen, and it is a typical sign of RA.
- Extensor carpi ulnaris tendinitis is a typical finding in early RA. On T2W images, fluid signal is observed around the tendon sheath with change in the tendon signal intensity.
- *Popliteal* (*Baker*) *cyst* is a synovial juxta-articular cyst filled with fluid collection that is lined by synovial cells that may, or may not, communicate with the joint. Baker's cyst is a synovial cyst that is located in the posteromedial aspect of the knee and represents a fluid extension through a slit-like communication between knee joint and the gastrocnemius–semimembranosus bursa. The cyst is typically seen as a fluid collection that passes between the gastrocnemius tendon and the

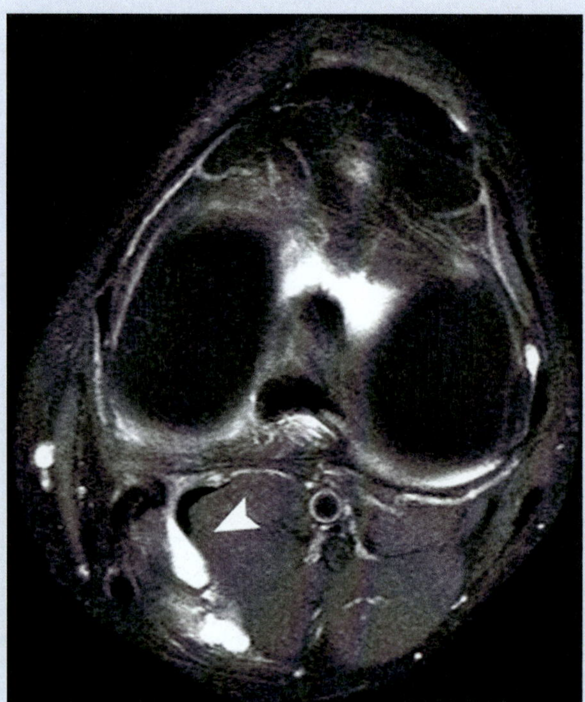



**Fig. 6.1.10** Axial PD knee MRI shows popliteal (Baker) cyst seen as a fluid collection that passes between the gastrocnemius tendon and the semimembranosus tendon (*arrowhead*)

semimembranosus tendon (Fig. 6.1.10). The cyst may show rim enhancement after contrast injection that mimics neoplasm. Rupture of the cyst may present with severe sudden pain that mimics thrombophlebitis or deep venous thrombosis. If the cyst is large enough to compress the popliteal artery, calf claudication arises rarely.

— *Rice bodies* are small, rice-like hypointense bodies seen inside large joints like the knee and hip joints due to cartilage destruction or synovial proliferation (Fig. 6.1.11). Rice bodies are an uncommon feature and very characteristic of RA.

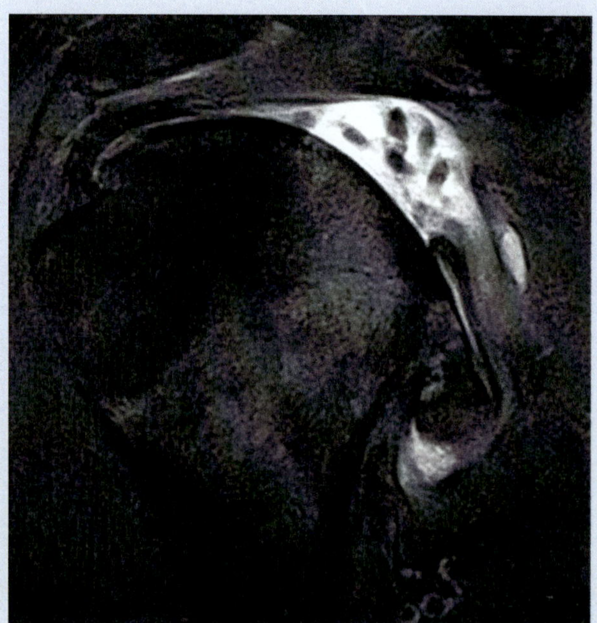

**Fig. 6.1.11** Coronal STIR shoulder MRI shows right shoulder joint effusion with multiple intra-articular hypointense lesions (rice bodies). Differential diagnosis of such sign is synovial chondromatosis, which classically shows intra-articular calcification best demonstrated on plain shoulder radiograph

— *Cerebral rheumatic nodules* are seen as focal parenchymal lesions with high signal intensities on T2W and FLAIR images, associated with adjacent leptomeningeal enhancement (Fig. 6.1.12). Rheumatoid pachymeningitis may occur rarely.
— In *PPsRD*, the whole vertebral column shows flattened vertebrae with irregular endplates and multiple intervertebral disk herniations along almost the whole spine. Remember that the MRI picture is seen in a child or a young man, not in a geriatric person with diffuse degenerative changes.
— In $RS_3PE$ *syndrome*, MRI typically shows signs of tenosynovitis with synovium thickening and enhancement postcontrast injection.

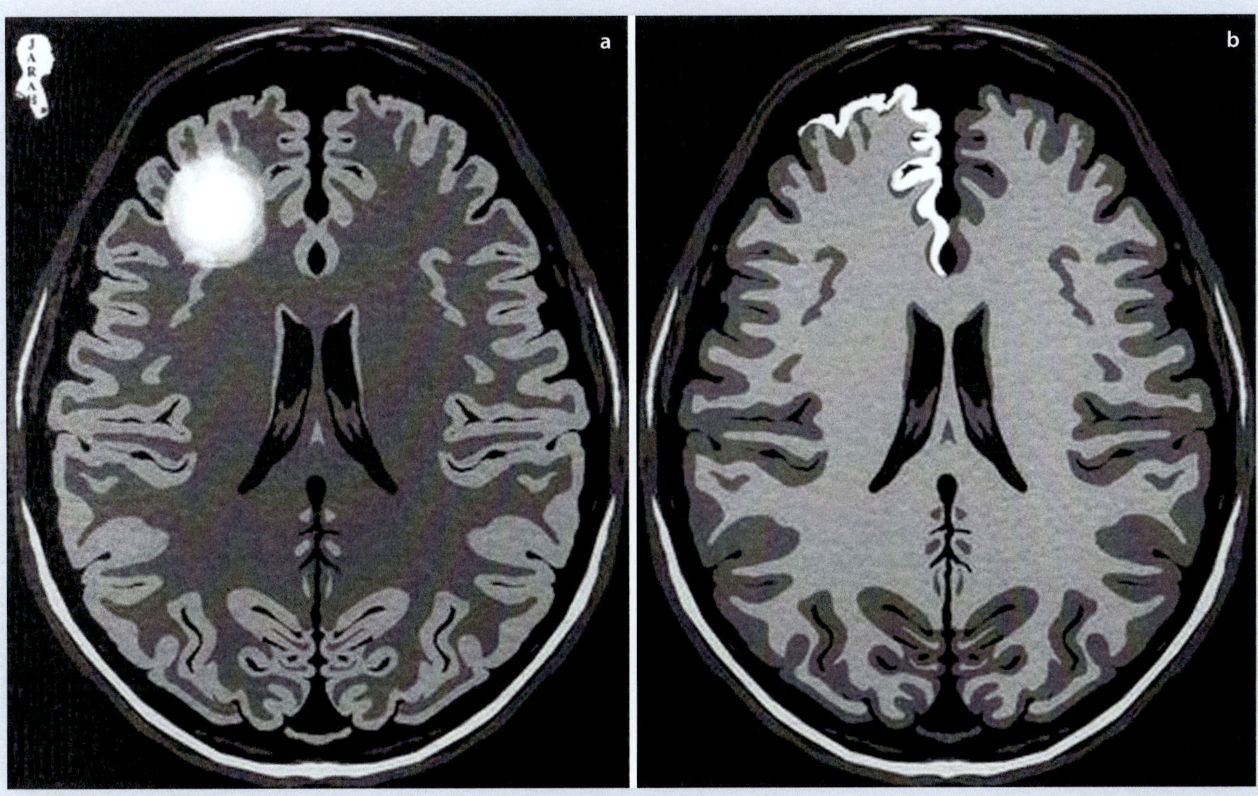

**Fig. 6.1.12**    Axial brain FLAIR (**a**) and T1W postcontrast (**b**) MR illustrations demonstrate the classical findings of cerebral rheumatoid nodule. There is T2 hyperintense lesion on (**a**) associated with leptomeningeal enhancement of the adjacent meninges (**b**)

## Further Reading


Bancroft LW, et al. Cysts, geodes, and erosions. Radiol Clin North Am. 2004;42:73–87.

Beaman FD, et al. MR imaging of cysts, ganglia, and bursae about the knee. Radiol Clin North Am. 2007a;45:969–82.

Bednařik J, et al. Median nerve mononeuropathy in spondylotic cervical myelopathy: double crush syndrome? J Neurol. 1999;246:544–51.

Bordel Gómez MT, et al. Rheumatoid nodulosis: report of two cases. JEADV. 2003;17:695–8.

Calatayud J, et al. Nodular pulmonary amyloidosis in a patient with rheumatoid arthritis. Clin Rheumatol. 2007;26:1797–8.

Cellerini M, et al. MRI of cerebral rheumatoid pachymeningitis: report of two cases with follow-up. Neuroradiology. 2001;43:147–50.

Ehl S, et al. Clinical, radiographic, and genetic diagnosis of progressive pseudorheumatoid dysplasia in a patient with sever polyarthropathy. Rheumatol Int. 2004;24:53–6.

Galvão V, et al. Profile of autoantibodies in Jaccoud's arthropathy. Joint Bone Spine. 2009;76:356–60.

Goñi MA, et al. Rheumatoid nodulosis: a puzzling variant of rheumatoid arthritis. Clin Rheumatol. 1992;11:396–401.

Hurd ER. Extraarticular manifestations of rheumatoid arthritis. Semin Arthritis Rheum. 1979;8:151–76.

Kaya A, et al. Clinical and radiological diagnosis of progressive pseudorheumatoid dysplasia in two sisters with sever polyarthropathy. Clin Rheumatol. 2005;24:560–4.

Mampaey S, et al. Progressive pseudorheumatoid dysplasia. Eur Radiol. 2000;10:1832–5.

Manganelli P, et al. Remitting seronegative symmetrical synovitis with pitting edema in a patient with myelodys-plastic syndrome and relapsing polychondritis. Clin Rheumatol. 2001;20:132–5.

Marik I, et al. Dominantly inherited progressive pseudorheumatoid dysplasia with hypoplastic toes. Skeletal Radiol. 2004;33:157–64.

Paci R, et al. Neuroradiological picture of cerebral vasculitis in rheumatoid arthritis. Neuroradiology. 1983;25:343–5.

Ragan C, et al. Rheumatoid arthritis. Dis Mon. 1955;1:2–51.

Rosenstein ED, et al. Felty's and pseudo-Felty's syndromes. Semin Arthritis Rheum. 1991;21:129–42.

Sivas F, et al. Idiopathic Jaccoud's arthropathy. APLAR J Rheumatol. 2005;8:60–2.

Solomon WM, et al. Chronic absorptive arthritis or opera-glass hand: report of eight cases. Ann Rheum Dis. 1950;9:209–20.

Sommer OJ, et al. Rheumatoid arthritis: a practical guide to the state-of-the-art imaging, image interpretation, and clinical implications. RadioGraphics. 2005;25:381–98.

Sugisaki K, et al. Remitting seronegative symmetrical synovitis with pitting edema (RS3PE) syndrome following spontaneous rupture of a gouty tophus. Mod Rheumatol. 2008;18:630–3.

Tada Y, et al. Flexor tenosynovitis of the ahnd as an initial manifestation of systemic lupus erythematosus. Mod Rheumatol. 2000;10:173–5.

Tehranzadeh J, et al. Advanced imaging of early rheumatoid arthritis. Radiol Clin North Am. 2004;42:89–107.

Unlu Z, et al. Magnetic resonance imaging findings in a case of remitting seronegative symmetrical synovitis with pitting edema. Clin Rheumatol. 2005;24:648–51.

Weissman BNW, et al. Prognostic features of atlantoaxial subluxation in rheumatoid arthritis patients. Radiology. 1982;144:745–51.

Wu Y, et al. Jaccoud's arthropathy and psoriatic arthritis, a rare association. Rheumatol Int. doi:10.1007/s00296-009-1017-1.

Zolcinski M, et al. Central nervous system involvement as a major manifestation of rheumatoid arthritis. Rheumatol Int. 2008;28:281–3.


## 6.2    Ankylosing Spondylitis (Marie–Strümpell Disease)

Ankylosing spondylitis (AS) is a chronic, progressive inflammatory disease of unknown origin that affects the axial skeleton (vertebral column plus the pelvis) and is characterized by bilateral sacroiliitis, stiffness of the axial joints (ankylosis), and syndesmophytes formation.

AS is a rheumatoid factor seronegative arthritis that is positively associated with HLA-B27. HLA stands for human leukocyte antigen (HLA) system. In the body, there are two classes of HLA antigens. Class I HLA is expressed by the human cells for histocompatibility, so the body knows that these cells are its own cells. Class I HLA antigens have an important role in transplant rejection. Class II HLA antigens are expressed by the immunocompetent cells including macrophages, Langerhans cells, B cells, and some T cells. HLA-B27 antigen is associated with AS in 90 % of cases. However, only 5 % of patients with positive HLA-B27 develop AS.

Patients with AS often present with back stiffness, low back ache, and discomfort in the thighs and buttocks. Extraskeletal manifestations include anterior uveitis, ascending aortitis, and bronchiolitis obliterans with organizing pneumonia (cryptogenic organizing pneumonia).

*Cauda equina syndrome* is an uncommon complication of AS. Patients classically present with symptoms related to compression of the cauda equina such as low back and lower extremities pain, impotence, overflow incontinence, cutaneous sensory defects (paresthesia), and motor dysfunction. Up to 30 % of patients describe severe burning or shooting pain in the lower limbs.

### Signs on Radiograph

- *Sacroiliitis* involvement is almost always in a bilateral and symmetrical fashion in AS (90 % of cases). However, unilateral involvement may occur in 10 % of cases. Radiological findings include multiple small erosions (rat bite erosions) along the iliac side of the joint. In the advanced stage of the disease, the erosions increase in size and widen the sacroiliac joint. Later, sclerosis of the sacroiliac joint occurs (◘ Fig. 6.2.1).
- *Vertebral bodies squaring* is an early manifestation of AS that arises due to inflammation of the peripheral fibers of the annulus fibrosis at their attachment to the upper and lower corners of the vertebral bodies (enthesitis). Enthesitis means inflammation of the entheses, the location where a tendon or a ligament is inserted into a bone. Erosions of the vertebral body at these areas make the vertebral body look square in shape (◘ Fig. 6.2.2).
- *Syndesmophytes* are paravertebral ossifications that resemble osteophytes, except that they arise vertically from one vertebra to the other (◘ Fig. 6.2.3), while osteophytes run in a horizontal fashion along the vertebral bodies. When the syndesmophytes are diffusely affecting the vertebral column, the vertebral column is said to have a "bamboo spines appearance" (◘ Fig. 6.2.4). Syndesmophytes are ossifications of the annulus fibrosus–longitudinal ligament complex as a healing process after enthesitis.

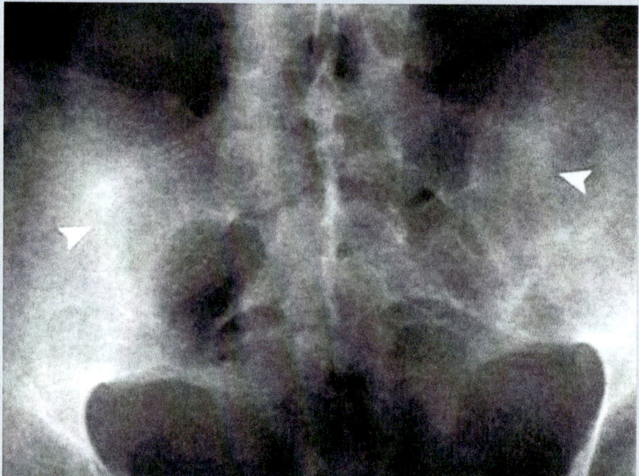

◘ **Fig. 6.2.1**    Anteroposterior plain radiograph of the hip of a patient with advanced ankylosing spondylitis (AS) shows complete sclerosis of the sacroiliac joints bilaterally (*arrowheads*)

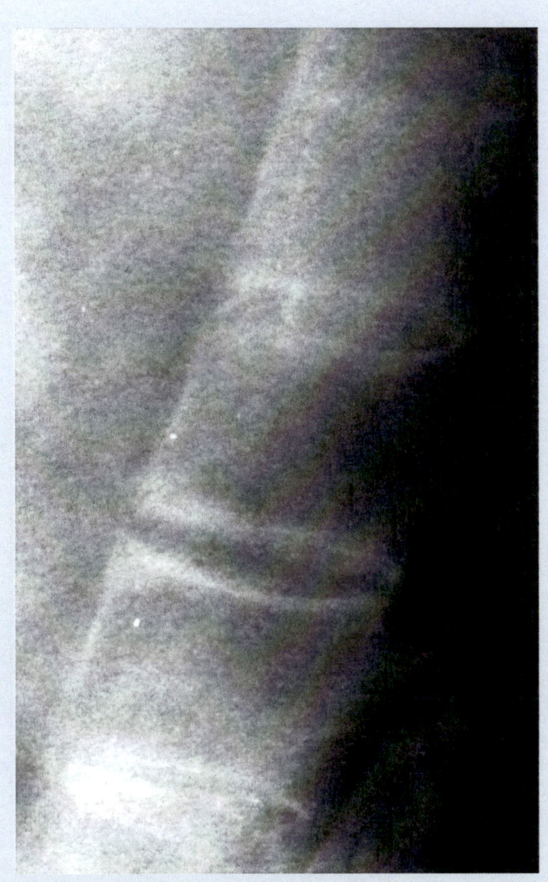



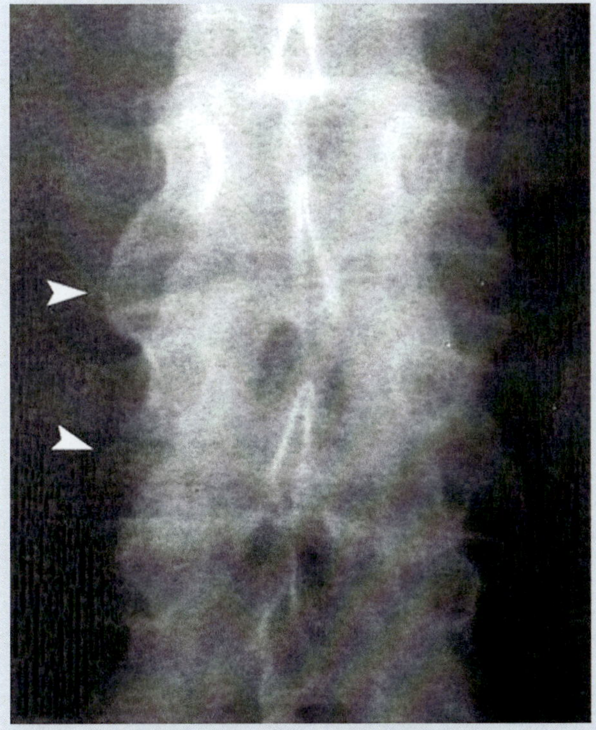



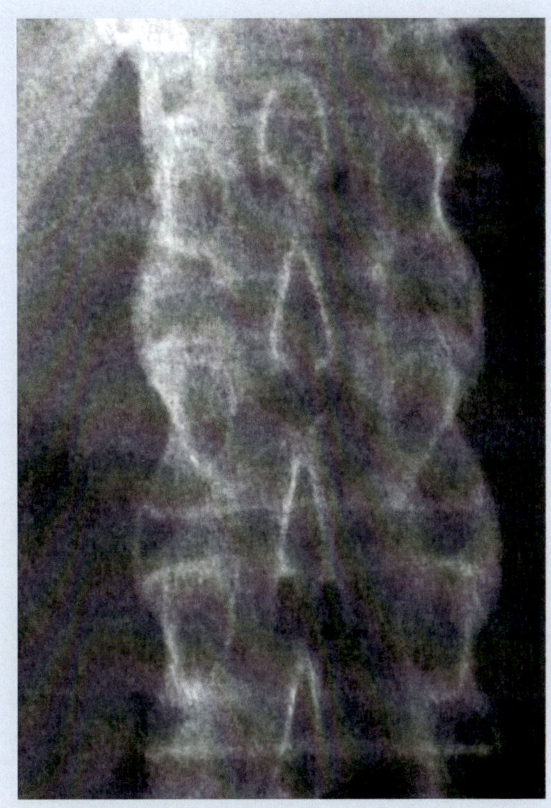

**Fig. 6.2.4**   Anteroposterior plain radiograph of the thoracic vertebrae shows the classic appearance of bamboo spines

- *Dagger sign* is longitudinal radio-opaque line seen along the vertebral column representing calcification of the supraspinous ligament (Fig. 6.2.5).
- *Trolley track signs* are three dense radio-opaque lines seen along the vertebral column representing calcification of the supraspinous and ankylosis of the facets joints.

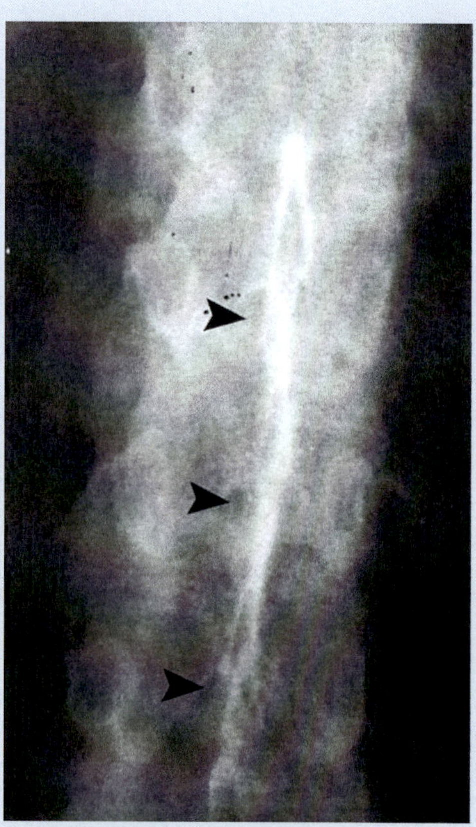



## Signs on MRI

- *Cauda equina syndrome* typically presents as enlargement of the thecal sac, multiple dorsal diverticula, with asymmetric scalloped erosions of the bony canal.
- *Romanus lesion* is enthesitis at the insertion of the annulus fibrosus–longitudinal ligament complex. There is low T1 signal intensity, high T2 signal intensity, and marked contrast enhancement within the annulus fibrosus at the discovertebral junction, indicating active enthesitis (◘ Fig. 6.2.6). When the active enthesitis starts to heal, it forms syndesmophytes.
- *Anderson lesion* is a focal erosive change in the vertebral endplate that resembles bacterial discitis (◘ Fig. 6.2.7). Typical features of Anderson lesion include disk space narrowing, focal bone destruction at the vertebral endplate adjacent to the disk, surrounding sclerosis, and local kyphosis. Differentiation between bacterial discitis and Anderson disease can be difficult in patients with AS. However, the vertebral disk is typically involved in bacterial discitis, while in Anderson lesion, the disk signal is generally preserved or shows degeneration. Moreover, perivertebral effusion and intradiscal effusion are commonly found with bacterial discitis, whereas they are rare with Anderson lesion. After

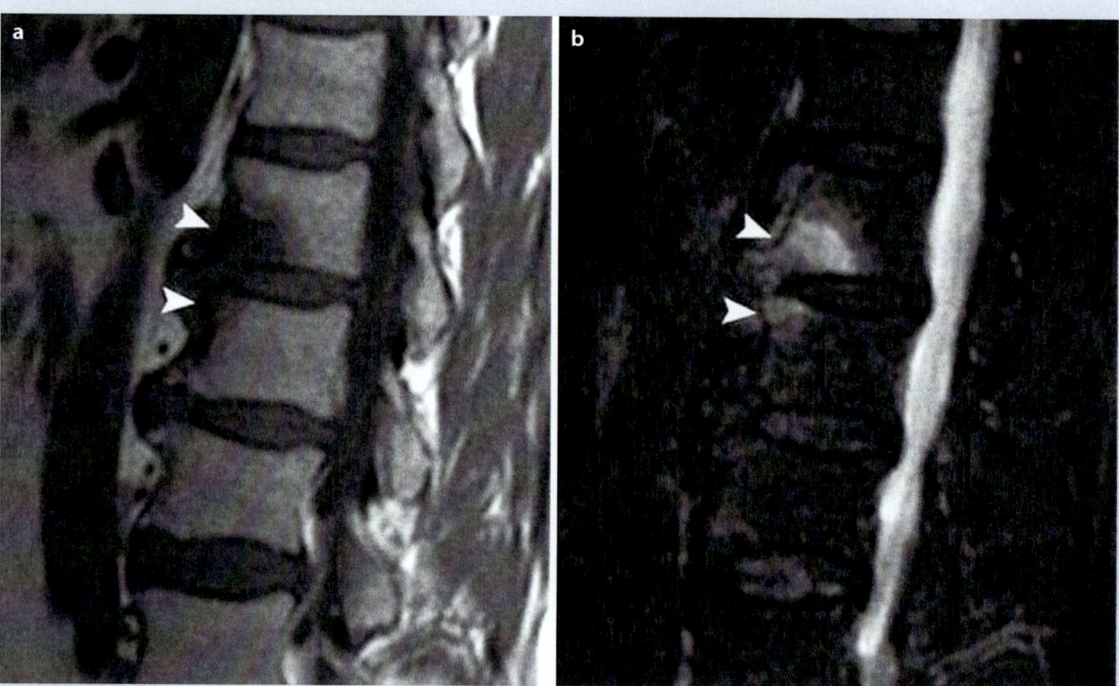

◘ **Fig. 6.2.6**    Sagittal thoracic T1W (**a**) and STIR (**b**) MRI show enthesitis at the anterior superior and anterior inferior vertebral endplates of two adjacent vertebrae (Romanus lesion) (*arrowheads*)

contrast injection, both Anderson lesion and bacterial discitis show contrast enhancement. Bacterial discitis high T2 signal intensity is due to hyperemia and edema, while enhancement in Anderson lesion is due to granulation tissue formation.

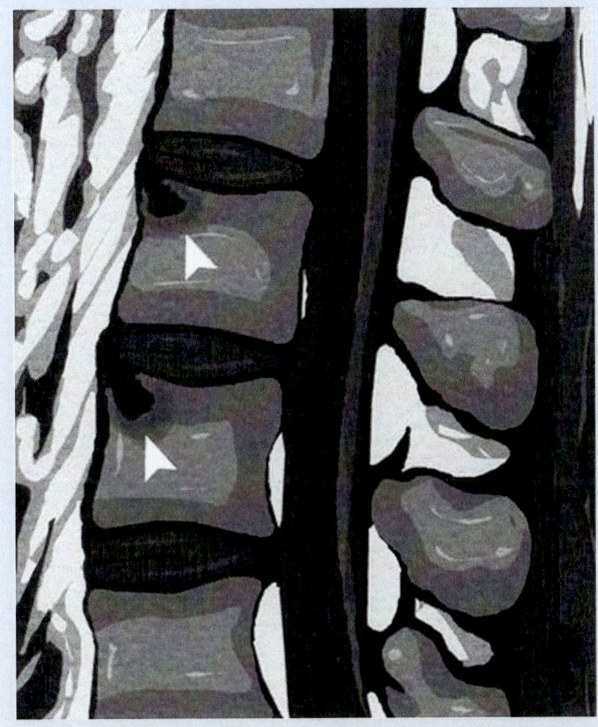



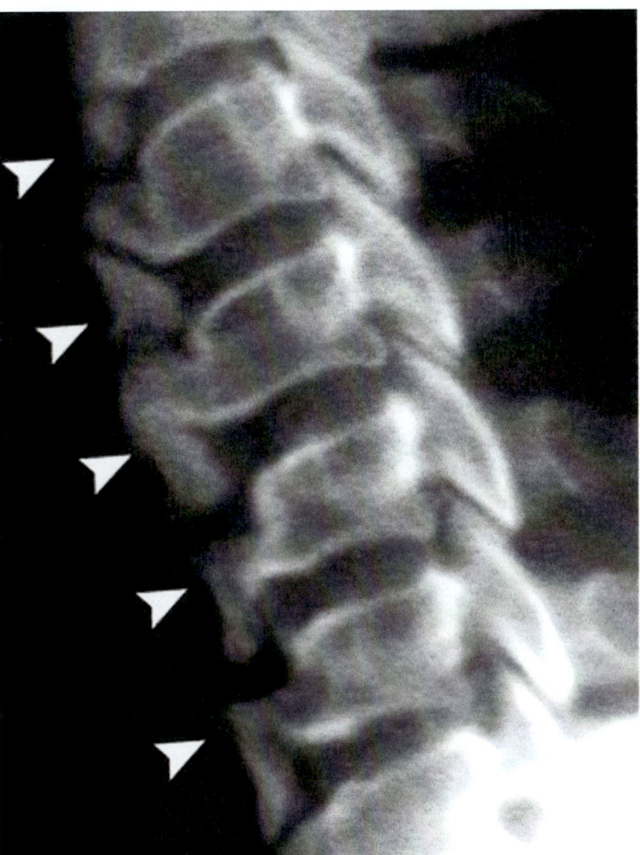



## Differential Diagnoses and Related Diseases

– *SAPHO syndrome* is a rare musculoskeletal disease of unknown origin characterized by *Synovitis, Acne, Pustu-losis* of the palmar and plantar skin surfaces, *Hyperostosis* of the bones, and *Osteitis*. Patients with the adult form of SAPHO syndrome usually present with unilateral sacroiliitis and syndesmophytosis that may mimic the radiographic picture of AS.

– *Diffuse idiopathic skeletal hyperostosis (DISH)* is a disease characterized by multisegmental vertebral fusion due to ligamentous calcification and ossification. The disease is commonly seen in the cervical and the thoracic vertebrae. Patients are usually above 70 years of age presenting with neck pain and stiffness. DISH can be mistaken with AS. Characteristic radiological signs of DISH include flowing vertebral ossification of at least four contiguous vertebral bodies, broad band of ossification along the anterolateral aspect of each vertebra (▶ Fig. 6.2.8), absence of degenerative disk disease, and absence of sacroiliac joints disease.

## Further Reading

Jevtic V, et al. Marginal erosive discovertebral "Romanus" lesions in ankylosing spondylitis demonstrated by contrast enhanced Gd-DTPA magnetic resonance imaging. Skeletal Radiol. 2000;29:27–33.

Jordana X, et al. The coexistence of ankylosing spondylitis and diffuse idiopathic skeletal hyperostosis-a postmortem diagnosis. Clin Rheumatol. 2009;28:353–6.

Lee Bennett D, et al. Spondyloarthropathies: ankylosing spondulitis and psoriatic arthritis. Radiol Clin North Am. 2004a;42:121–34.

Pham T. Pathophysiology of ankylosing spondylitis: what's new ? Joint Bone Spine. 2008;75:656–60.

Quagliano PV, et al. Vertebral pseudoarthrosis with diffuse idiopathic skeletal hyperostosis. Skeletal Radiol. 1994;23:353–5.

Sant SM, et al. Cauda equina syndrome in ankylosing spondylitis: a case report and review of the literature. Clinical Rheumatol. 1995;14:224–6.

Soeur M, et al. Cauda equina syndrome in ankylosing spondylitis. Anatomical, diagnostic, and therapeutic considerations. Acta Neurochir. 1981;55:303–15.

Tsuchiya K, et al. Discovertebral lesion in ankylosing spondylitis: differential diagnosis with discitis by magnetic resonance imaging. Mod Rheumatol. 2002;12:113–7.

Uppal SS, et al. Ankylosing spondylitis and undifferentiated spondyloarthropathies in Kuwait: a comparison between Arabs and South Asians. Clin Rheumatol. 2006;25:219–24.

## 6.3   Gout Arthritis

Gout is a clinical condition characterized by increased serum uric acid levels (hyperuricemia) with deposition of uric acid monocrystals in the synovial fluid, initiating acute inflammatory reaction that leads to arthritis. Gout is the most common cause of inflammatory arthritis in men >40 years of age.

Hyperuricemia is defined as urate levels >7 mg/dL in men and menopausal women or urate levels >6 mg/dL in premenopausal women. Plasma urate level >7 mg/dL exceeds the saturation for urate solubility at normal body temperature and blood PH.

Not every patient with hyperuricemia develops symptoms of gout. Gout can result from impaired uric acid clearance by the kidney (primary gout), or due to increased production of uric acid for a variety of causes, increased turnover of nucleic acids, or from decreased clearance of uric acid (secondary gout). Up to 80 % of cardiac transplant patients develop hyperuricemia, and 10 % develop gout after a mean of 1.5 years posttransplantation.

Uric acid monocrystals are needle-shaped negatively birefringent crystals, and they are the main product of purine catabolism. They deposit within the synovium or the renal parenchyma forming chalky-white deposits that initiate painful arthritis and renal disease. High uric acid precipitation within the renal tubules can result in uric acid renal stones formation.

In gout arthritis (GA), deposition of the urate crystals (tophi) within the synovial fluid and the synovial membrane causes inflammation. With time, a soft-tissue pannus forms within the joint which will start to erode the intra-articular cartilage and the subchondral bone. The monosodium urate crystals may also deposit in the tendon, ligaments, bursae, and other organs like the ear, nose, and skin.

Rarely, gout can involve the spines resulting in sclerotic bony lesions, cervical pain, or paraplegia if the spinal cord is affected.

It takes 4–6 years for gout to cause detectable radiographic signs, and the patients are usually treated before the radiological signs start to appear. Because of this, GA radiographic features are not commonly seen, although they have characteristic patterns.

**Signs on Plain Radiographs and MRI**
- There are typically cortical bony erosions with well-defined sclerotic margin in the absence of osteoporosis (■ Figs. 6.3.1 and 6.3.2). Disuse osteopenia may occur in late stages of the disease.

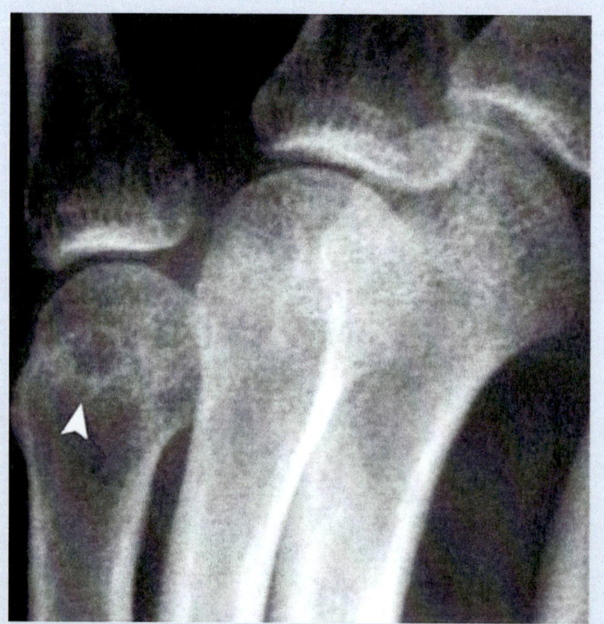

■ **Fig. 6.3.1**   Plain radiograph of the metacarpal heads shows bony erosion with sclerotic margin in the absence of osteoporosis (*arrowhead*), a typical finding of gout arthritis (GA)

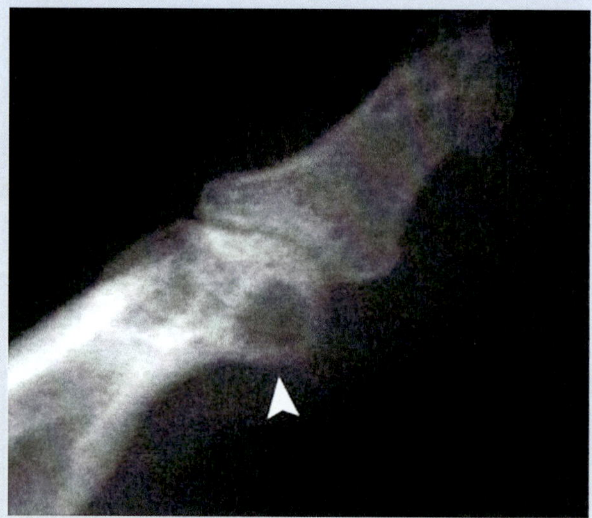

■ **Fig. 6.3.2**   Plain radiograph of a finger shows bony erosion with sclerotic rim in the middle phalanges (*arrowhead*)

- *Podagra* is a term used to describe gout tophi affecting the metatarsophalangeal joint of the great toe; it is seen as erosion of the first metatarsal bone often associated with para-articular soft-tissue swelling (■ Fig. 6.3.3). Podagra shows signs of inflammation when the process of tophus formation is active (■ Fig. 6.3.4).
- Cartilage calcification (chondrocalcinosis) can be seen in up to 40 % of patients.
- Vertebral gout may present as an osteolytic vertebral lesion with sclerotic margin.

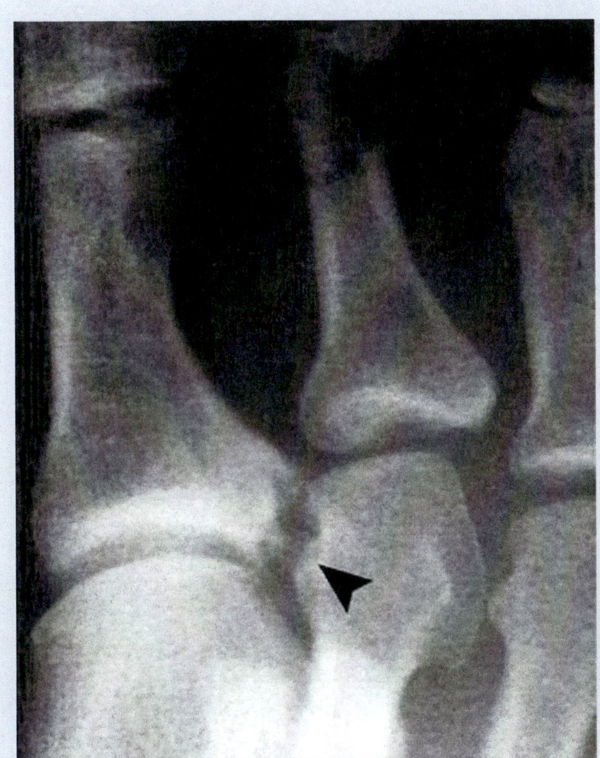



Fig. 6.3.3 Plain radiograph of the foot of a patient with chronic gout shows marginal erosion of the proximal phalanges (*arrowhead*)

## Differential Diagnoses and Related Diseases

*Lesch–Nyhan syndrome (LNS)* is an X-linked recessive metabolic disease characterized by defective purine metabolism that results in uric acid overproduction. The disease arises due to genetic absence or near absence of the enzyme hypoxanthine-guanine phosphoribosyltransferase (HGPRT). Patients with LNS present with involuntary movements in a combination of chorea and athetosis (choreoathetosis), spasticity, and psychiatric abnormalities in the form of compulsive self-mutilation. Recurrent formation of renal uric acid stones is commonly encountered in LNS due to hyperuricemia. Laboratory findings show increased levels of uric acid in the urine, cerebrospinal fluid, and serum. Plain radiographs can show GA. Renal ultrasound can be used to screen for renal stones in these patients. Brain MRI may show caudate nuclei head atrophy with widening of the anterior lateral horns of the lateral ventricles (  Fig. 6.3.5). Furthermore, very prominent prepontine cisterns with mild to moderate midbrain atrophy have been reported in some patients.

### Further Reading

Agarwal K, et al. Fine needle aspiration cytology of gouty tophi with review of the literature. J Cytol. 2007;24:142–5.

Cabot J, et al. Tophaceous gout in the cervical spine. Skeletal Radiol. 2005;34:803–6.

Chang PC, et al. Tophaceous gout of the first costochondral junction in a heart transplant patient. Skeletal Radiol. 2006;35:684–6.

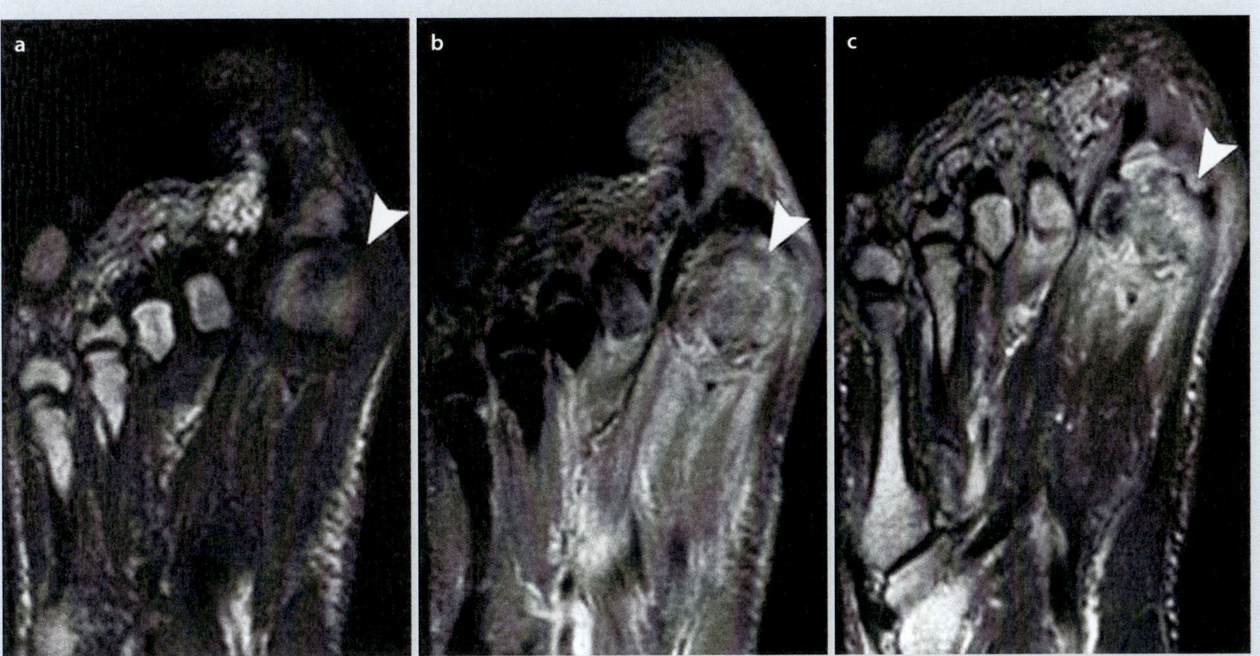



Fig. 6.3.4 Coronal T1W (**a**), STIR (**b**), and T1W postcontrast foot MRI of a patient investigated for gout with foot pain localized to the big toe show hypointense signal intensity due to edema of the first metatarsal head in (**a**), hyperintense T2 signal intensity in (**b**), and marked contrast enhancement (**c**) of the first metatarsal head and the surrounding soft tissues due to active inflammatory process (*arrowheads*)

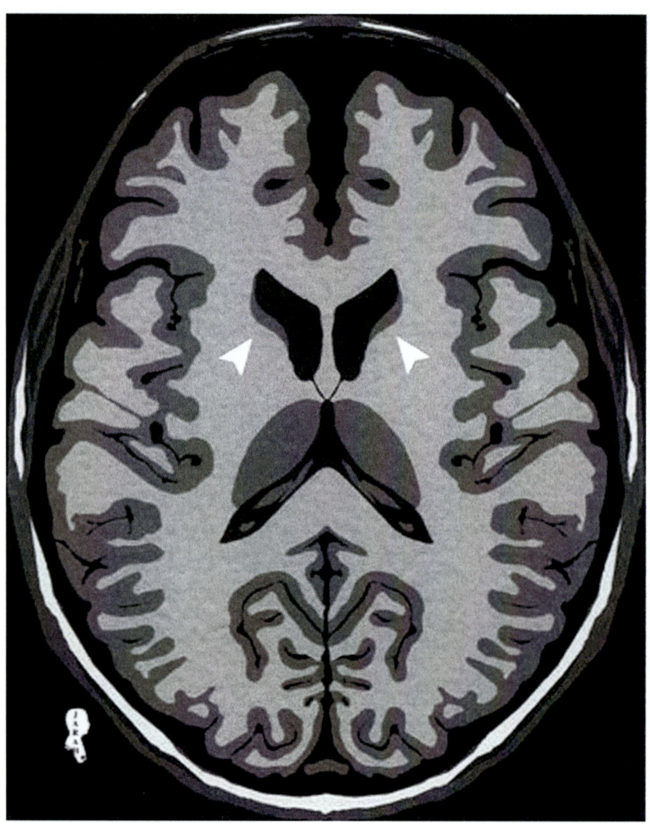



**Fig. 6.3.5** Axial T1W brain MR illustration demonstrates bilateral caudate nucleus atrophy (*arrowheads*) in a patient with Lesch–Nyhan syndrome (LNS)

Harris JC, et al. Craniocerebral magnetic resonance imaging measurments and findings in Lesch-Nyhan syndrome. Arch Neurol. 1998;55:547–53.

Jacobson JA, et al. Radiographic evaluation of arthritis: inflammatory conditions. Radiology. 2008a;248:378–89.

Jajić I, et al. Gout in the spine and sacro-iliac joints: radiological manifestations. Skeletal Radiol. 1982;8:209–12.

Monu JUV, et al. Gout: a clinical and radiological review. Radiol Clin North Am. 2004;42:169–84.

Rosenfeld DL, et al. Serial renal songraphic evaluation in patient with Lesch-Nyhan syndrome. Pediatr Radiol. 1994;24:509–12.

## 6.4    CPPD and HADD

Calcium pyrophosphate dihydrate crystal deposition disease (CPPD) and hydroxyapatite crystal deposition disease (HADD) are diseases characterized by deposition of insoluble crystals within the joints and periarticular soft tissues, initiating inflammatory destructive reaction. Other clinically important calcium-containing crystal deposition diseases include tricalcium phosphate (TCP) and octacalcium phosphate (OCP) diseases.

## Calcium Pyrophosphate Dihydrate Crystal Deposition Disease

CPPD, also known as *pseudo-gout* and *chondrocalcinosis*, is a disease characterized by calcium pyrophosphate crystal deposition within the *articulating cartilage*, leading to cartilage inflammation and later to joint destruction in a similar fashion to gout arthritis.

CPPD is classified based on its etiology into hereditary, idiopathic, or secondary to metabolic disorders (e.g., vitamin D intoxication). The disease is age related, with an incidence of 5% in patients >70 years and nearly 50% in patients >90 years. Many patients present with gout-like arthritic episodes characterized by joint synovitis, malaise, and fever that last from 1 day to 4 weeks. Up to 50% of patients develop progressive degeneration of multiple joints. The most frequently involved joints are the knees, wrists, metacarpophalangeal joints, and the hips.

Pyrophosphate deposition involves both hyaline cartilage and fibrocartilage joints like symphysis pubis, annulus of the spine, triangular fibrocartilagenous complex (TFCC) of the wrist, and menisci. CPPD can occur in high incidence with other diseases like gout, hyperparathyroidism, and hemochromatosis.

CPPD diagnosis is established by identifying the pyrophosphate crystals within the synovial fluid after aspiration. Plasma and uric acid levels of pyrophosphate are typically not elevated (differential point from gout).

### Signs on Plain Radiograph

- *Chondrocalcinosis*: cartilage calcification is the hallmark of CPPD. Chondrocalcinosis is usually observed in medial and lateral compartments of the knee, wrist TFCC, and the symphysis pubis (Fig. 6.4.1).
- *Pseudo-Charcot's joint*: severe joint destruction that mimics Charcot's joint may be observed occasionally.
- Normal bone density with occasional subchondral cysts.
- *SLAC wrist deformity*: Scapholunate Advanced Collapse is a pathological situation characterized by loss of the cartilage between the scaphoid bone and the radius, causing the scaphoid to indent the radius and the capitate to collapse, thus disturbing the scapholunate joint articulation (Fig. 6.4.2).
- *Generalized chondrocalcinosis*: a pathological condition characterized by involvement of more than one group of joints with cartilage calcification (e.g., knees, wrists, plus vertebral disks).

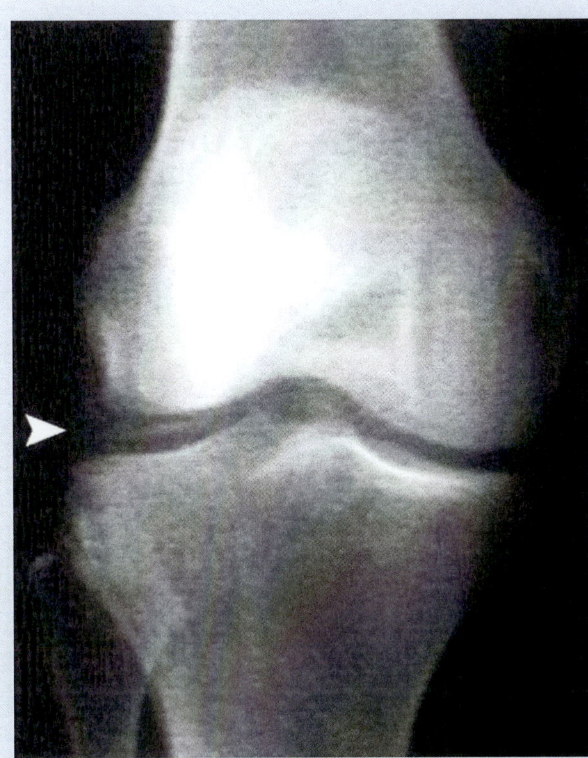

**Fig. 6.4.1** Anteroposterior knee radiograph shows calcification of the lateral meniscus due to CPPD chondrocalcinosis (*arrowhead*)

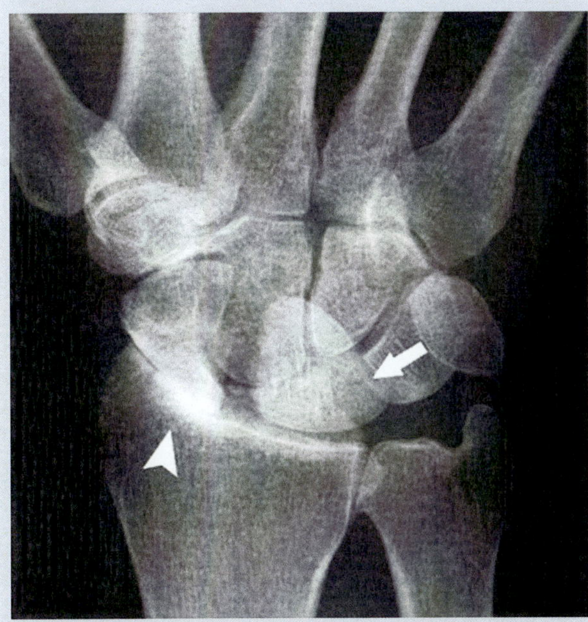

**Fig. 6.4.2** Plain hand radiograph shows scaphoid indenting the distal radius with sclerosis (*arrowhead*) and collapse of the capitate from its normal position (*arrow*) (SLAC wrist deformity)

## Hydroxyapatite Crystal Deposition Disease

HADD, also known as *calcific periarthritis* and *peritendinitis calcarea*, is characterized by hydroxyapatite crystal deposition in the soft tissues, especially the tendons.

The most characteristic feature of this disease is *tendon calcification* within the body, especially around the shoulder. Moreover, crystal deposition and calcification tend to occur characteristically around the joints (periarticular). HADD can be sporadic, or associated with long-term hemodialysis for renal insufficiency.

Patients with HADD can be asymptomatic or present with recurrent attacks of arthritis in the area of crystal deposition. Shoulder pain is the commonest complaint since supraspinatus tendon calcification is common in HADD.

HADD is characterized by three pathological phases: silent, mechanical, and adhesive. The silent phase is characterized by crystal deposition that is completely within the tendon. The mechanical phase is characterized by enlargement of the deposits with starting of impingement-like symptoms (e.g., bursitis). The adhesive phase is characterized by generalized disability and limitation of motion. When the adhesive phase occurs in the shoulder, the condition is called *adhesive capsulitis* or *frozen shoulder*. Hydroxyapatite crystals are commonly deposited in damaged tissues (dystrophic calcification).

HADD calcification is often monoarticular, although it can be polyarticular. Involvement of the joints of the feet and toes is rare (<1 %). There are two syndromes associated with HADD due to crystal deposition around the joints: calcific periarthritis with bone resorption (acute HADD arthritis) and rapid destructive arthritis of the shoulder (Milwaukee shoulder syndrome).

*Calcific periarthritis with bone resorption* is characterized by inflammation of the calcified focus with resorption of the bone beneath it. The condition mimics bone sarcoma, especially if periostitis develops. Biopsy can be avoided if the location of the osteolytic lesion is characteristic of HADD (near a tendon insertion), and other manifestations of HADD exist in the body.

*Milwaukee shoulder syndrome* is a disease characterized by destructive shoulder arthropathy, bloodstained joint effusion (80 %), and chronic tears of the rotator cuff tendon. Patients are typically elderly women with a mean age of 72 years. Symptoms range from none to severe shoulder pain with joint effusion. Most patients have symptoms dating from several years back. Bilateral shoulder involvement is common, and knees arthropathy is found in 50 % of patients.

### Differential Diagnoses and Related Diseases

*Crowned dens syndrome* (CDS) is a rare clinical condition characterized by deposition of pyrophosphate or calcium hydroxyapatite crystals around the odontoid process of the axis vertebra and its ligaments, especially ligamentum flavum. Inflammatory signs and high erythrocyte sedimentation rate (ESR) are present in up to 30 % of cases.

The patients often present with acute attack of neck pain, neck rigidity, and fever, mimicking acute meningitis or spondylodiscitis. CDS affects mostly females, with up to 45 % of cases found in patients above 85 years of age.

### Signs on Radiographs

- Calcification of the supraspinatus and infraspinatus tendons is a very characteristic feature of HADD (◘ Figs. 6.4.3 and 6.4.4). The calcification typically starts in the site of tendon insertion or the critical zone. The *critical zone* is the part of the supraspinatus tendon 1 cm proximal to its insertion into the greater tubercle of the humerus.
- Areas of calcifications are noticed in the periarticular soft tissues.
- Calcification within the carpal bones, ligaments, and wrist tendons is commonly seen.
- Always suspect HADD in a calcification that is observed near a joint, at tendon insertion, near muscular attachment, or after trauma (dystrophic).
- In *Milwaukee shoulder syndrome*, there is glenohumeral joint destruction, narrowing, and sclerosis. Upward subluxation of the humeral head can be seen, indicating long-standing rotator cuff tendon disruption. Periarticular calcification is noticed in 40 % of cases. Pseudoarthrosis between the humeral head, coracoid, and acromion is common. Knees involvement is similar to that of CPPD arthropathy.
- In *crown dens syndrome*, radio-opaque calcifications with different sizes and shapes are seen around and above the superior part of the odontoid process, giving the shape of a "crown on a head" appearance. CDS can be mistaken with cervical block vertebra (Klipple–Feil anomaly type 1).

### Further Reading

Baysal T, et al. The crown dens syndrome: a rare form of calcium pyrophosphate dihydrate crystal deposition disease. Eur Radiol. 2000;10:1003–5.
Curtis W, et al. Calcium hydroxyapatite deposition disease. RadioGraphics. 1999;10:1031–48.

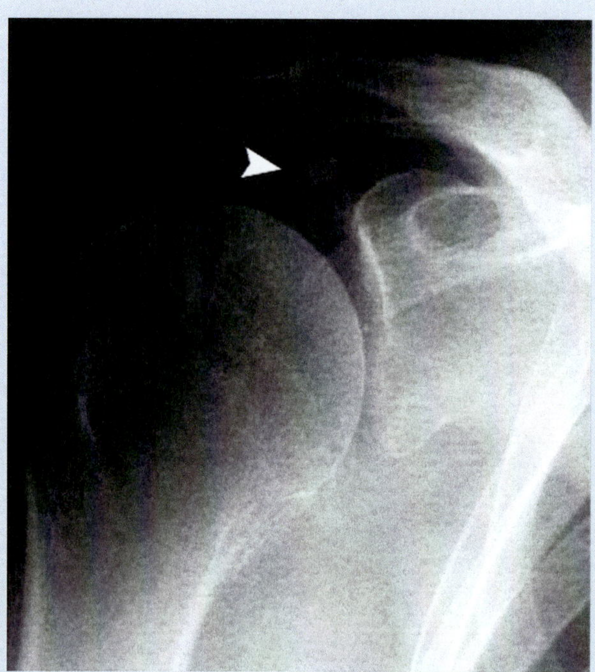


◘ **Fig. 6.4.3**  Plain radiograph of the shoulder shows calcification in the area of the supraspinatus tendon due to HADD (*arrowhead*)

Fam AG, et al. Hydroxyapatite pseudopodagra. A syndrome of young women. Arthritis Rheum. 1989;32:741–7.
Hayashi M, et al. Idiopathic widespread calcium pyrophosphate dihydrate crystal deposition disease in young patient. Skeletal Radiol. 2002;31:246–50.
Nguyen VD. Rapid destructive arthritis of the shoulder. Skeletal Radiol. 1996;25:107–12.
Steinbach LS. Calcium pyrophosphate dihydrate and calcium hydroxyapatite crystal deposition disease: imaging perspectives. Radiol Clin North Am. 2004;42:185–205.Talbott JH. Gout. Dis Mon. 1957;3:1–39.
Till G, et al. Calcium pyrophosphate dihydrate crystal deposition disease: a report of a case. JCCA. 1988;32:23–7.
Vargas A, et al. Calcium pyrophosphate dihydrate crystal deposition disease presenting as a pseudotumor of the temporomandibular joint. Eur Radiol. 1997;7:1452–3.

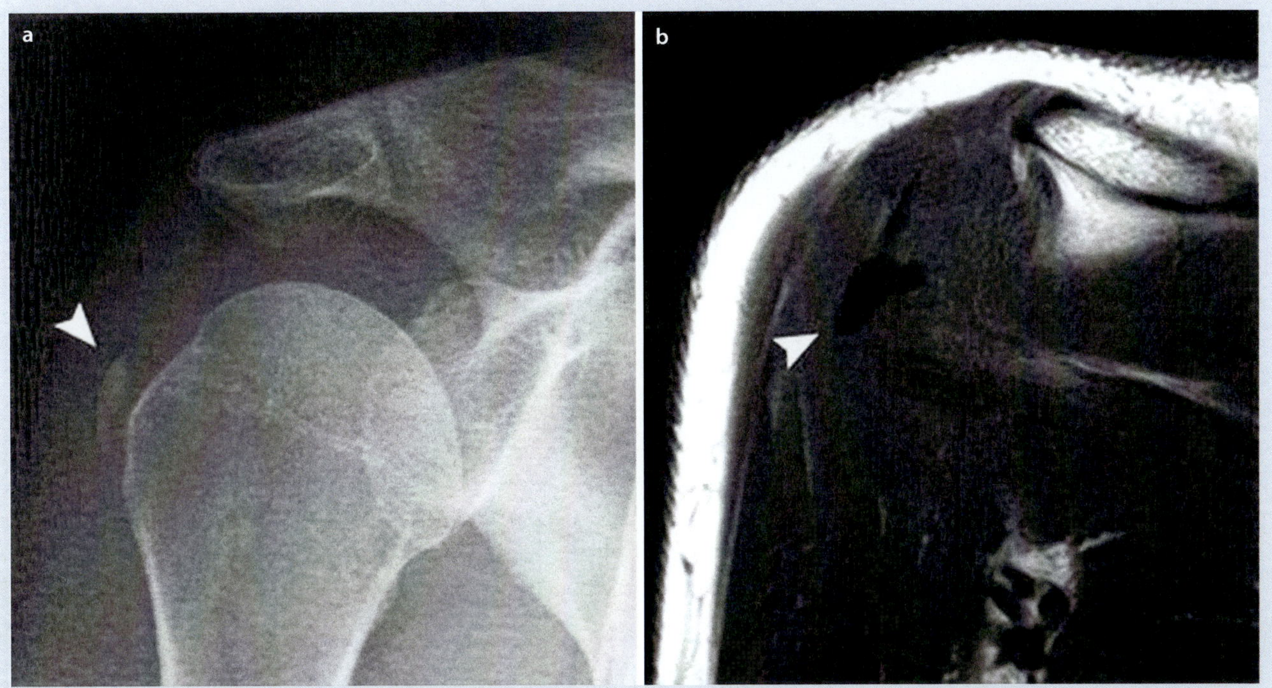

**Fig. 6.4.4** Plain radiograph of the shoulder (**a**) and T1W shoulder MRI (**b**) show calcification area within the infraspinatus tendon due to HADD (*arrowheads*)

## 6.5 Osteoarthritis

Osteoarthritis (OA) is a clinical condition that arises primarily from cartilaginous defect in the joint, which leads to cartilage degeneration and bone-to-bone friction resulting in joint destruction and osteophytes formation.

The hallmarks of OA are:

- *Joint space narrowing*: due to loss of the cartilaginous surface of the joint.
- *Osteophytes formation*: osteophytes are small extra bony growths commonly seen at the margins of the affected joint. Osteophytes formation is the body's palliative attempt to increase the articular surface area. They are formed in the areas of low stress, classically at the margins of the joint, because vascularization of the subchondral bone is high.
- *Subchondral sclerosis*: new bone (callus) formation at the areas of articular cartilage loss due to bone-to-bone friction and trabecular bone microfractures.
- *Subchondral cysts (geodes)*: cystic lesions formed in the subchondral bone due to trabecular bone microfractures with deposition of hemorrhagic, myxoid, and adipose material within these fractured trabeculae. Later, a cyst forms in these fractured trabeculae instead of bone healing.

*Primary OA* is a term used when OA develops with no predisposing factor (e.g., trauma), and it can be classified into three subtypes: genetically determined OA (type 1), estrogen-hormone-dependent OA (type 2), and aging-related OA (type 3). Genetically determined OA is commonly seen in middle-aged women and occurs almost exclusively in the hands. It affects the distal and proximal interphalangeal (DIP and PIP) joints and the base of the thumb in bilateral symmetrical fashion. Primary OA must be bilaterally symmetrical to be diagnosed. Estrogen-dependent OA is seen in females after menopause or patients with hysterectomy due to loss of the effect of estrogen on the cartilage, bone, synovium, ligaments, and muscles. It affects mostly the knees and is seen perimenopausally or within 5 years of natural menopause or hysterectomy.

*Secondary OA* is the most common form, which develops after a pathological event that violates the articular cartilage integrity. Joint trauma, metabolic abnormalities (e.g., ochronosis), and bleeding into joints (hemarthrosis) are common causes of secondary OA. The incidence of OA increases with age, but it is not a natural outcome of it (not every old person develops OA).

*Erosive OA* is a severe form of primary OA that presents clinically with an acute inflammatory process of swelling, erythema of the joint, and limitation in function. Erosive OA is predominantly seen in the hands of postmenopausal women, and it can be confused with rheumatoid arthritis. It has the same distribution as primary OA (bilateral and symmetrical), but is associated with severe osteoporosis and erosions in the hands (it occurs only in hands). Erosions of erosive OA affect the central portion of the articular surface, unlike rheumatoid arthritis which affects margins of the articular surface.

*Rapid destructive osteoarthritis (Postel's osteoarthritis)* is an uncommon type of hip OA where destruction of the bone and cartilage occurs within a matter of weeks to months. The cause of this disorder is unknown. Cases might be seen with disorders like ochronosis, hemochromatosis, and drug-induced arthropathy (especially indomethacin). Patients are usually women presenting with severe progressive pain classically in a single hip joint.

### Signs on Plain Radiographs and MRI

- The radiological hallmarks for OA are its four main signs: narrowing of joint space, bone sclerosis, subchondral cysts, and osteophytes formation ( Fig. 6.5.1).
- *Normal bone density* (no osteoporosis) differentiates OA from rheumatoid arthritis which is characteristically associated with osteoporosis of the affected joint due to hyperemia and synovial inflammation.
- *Subchondral cysts* (*geodes*) are seen as cystic lesions located below the articular cartilage. On MRI, the cysts show fluid signal intensity on T2W images (high signal) ( Fig. 6.5.2).
- *Heberden's nodes* are osteophytes that are seen at the DIP joints. They are commonly seen in primary OA, mainly in the index and the middle fingers ( Fig. 6.5.3).
- *Bouchard's nodes* are osteophytes that are seen at the PIP joints ( Fig. 6.5.3).
- *Ganglion cyst formation* is a myxoid, tumorlike, cystic lesion that is surrounded by dense connective tissue and filled with gelatinous material. It is typically located in the epiphysis of long bones. Ganglion cysts are typically round or tubular, unilocular or multilocular lesions with often sharply defined internal septa ( Fig. 6.5.4). They may show rim enhancement following contrast injection. Ganglion cysts can be found juxta-articular, intraosseus, and periosteal in location. Sometimes they are difficult to differentiate from synovial cysts based on imaging alone.
- *Gullwing sign* describes wavy contours of the base of the distal phalanx resembling the wings of a seagull due to small osteophytes formation on both sides of the articular surface.

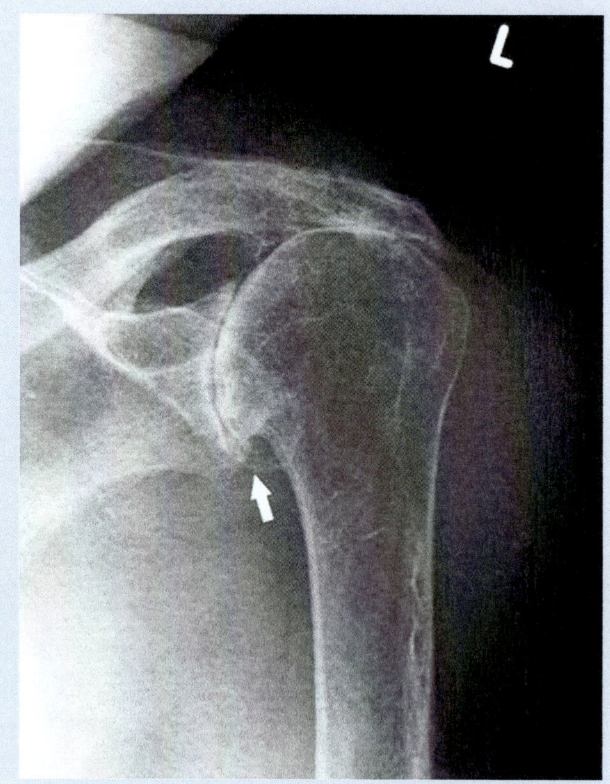


 **Fig. 6.5.1**    Plain shoulder radiograph shows the classical signs of OA: narrowing of the joint space, sclerosis of the humeral head and the glenoid fossa, and osteophyte formation at the base of the humeral head (*arrow*)

- *Thumb-base osteoarthritis* (*rhizarthrosis*) is OA that occurs at the trapeziometacarpal joint and the trapeziometacarpal joint of the thumb ( Fig. 6.5.5).
- *Central erosions* of the interphalangeal joints (characteristic of erosive arthritis).
- *Hallux rigidus* is a term used to describe OA of the first metatarsophalangeal joint (the big toe). The appearance of accentuated transverse skin crease overlying the big toe at the DIP joint is commonly associated with hallux rigidus ( Fig. 6.5.6).
- In *rapid destructive osteoarthritis*, the radiographic features may mimic osteonecrosis of the hip joint. Septic arthritis must be excluded by synovial fluid aspiration before diagnosing rapid erosive OA.
- In OA of the hip joint, superior migration of the femoral head may occur ( Fig. 6.5.7).

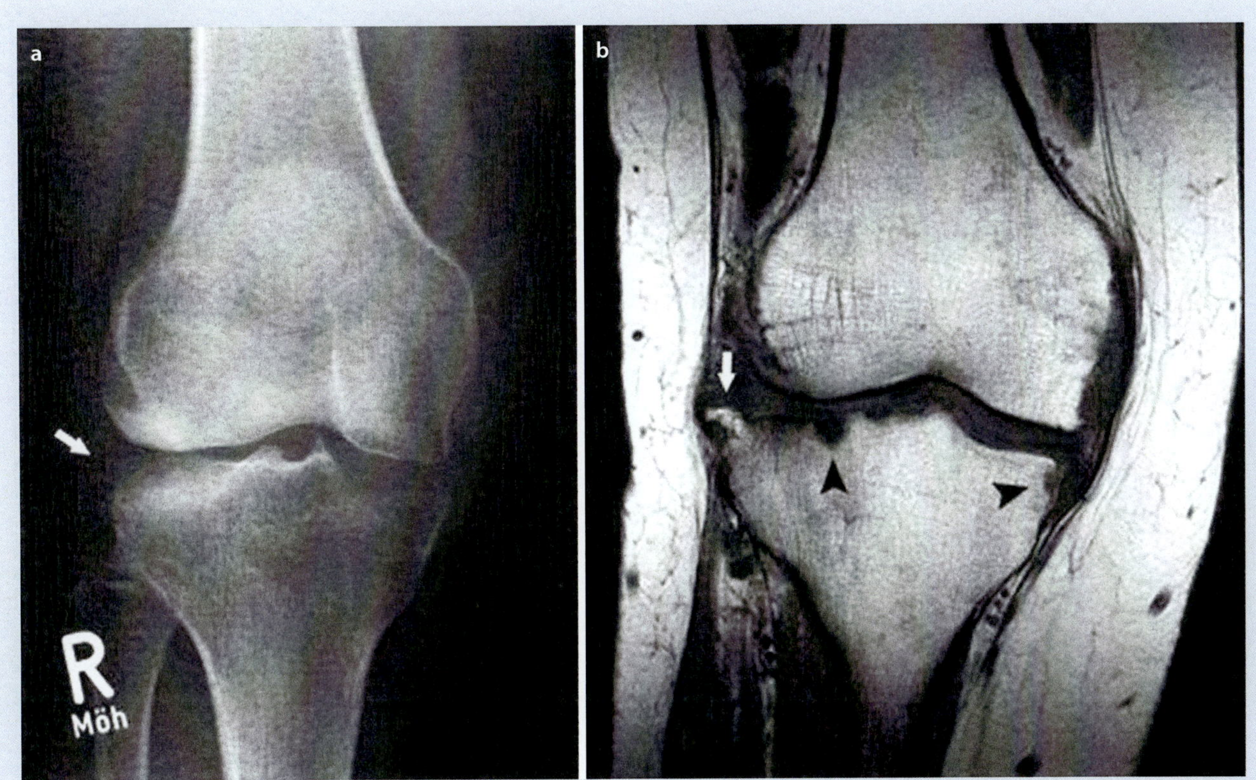

**Fig. 6.5.2** Plain knee radiograph (**a**) and coronal T1W knee MRI of the same patient shows subchondral cysts (*black arrowheads*) and marginal osteophyte (**b**) in the lateral tibial plateau (*white arrows*)

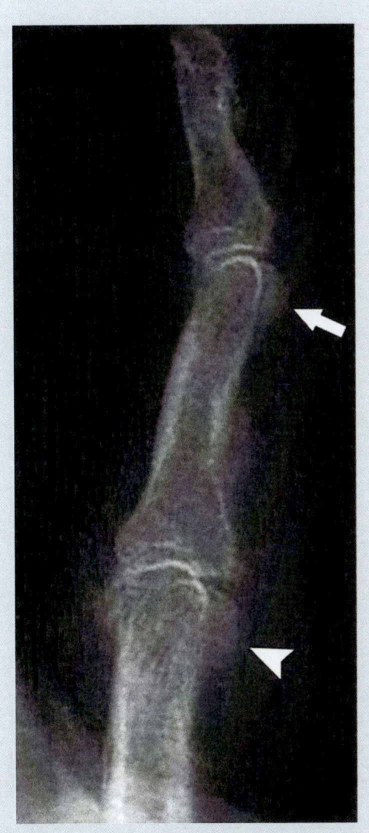

**Fig. 6.5.3** Plain radiograph of the finger shows both Heberden's node (*arrow*) and Bouchard's node (*arrowhead*)

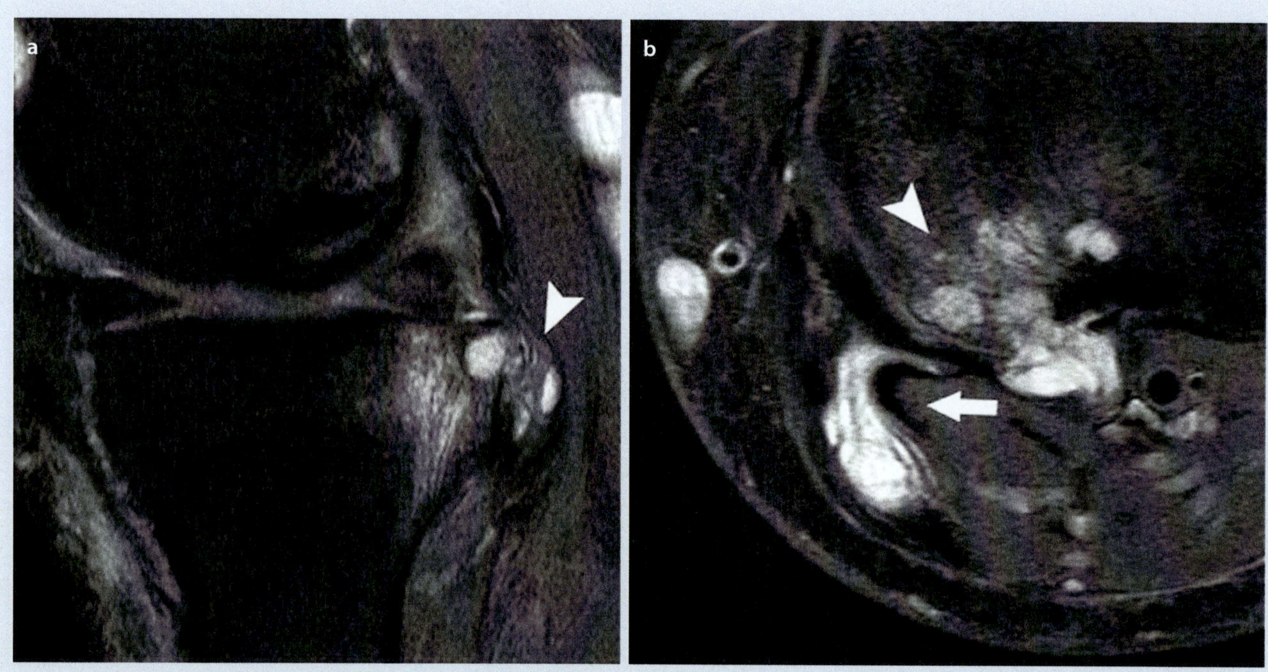

**Fig. 6.5.4** Sagittal (**a**) and axial (**b**) PD knee MRI shows juxta-articular intraosseous ganglion cysts formation in the posterior part of the tibia with bone marrow edema due to knee OA (*arrowheads*). A small Baker cyst can be seen as a secondary finding (*arrow*)

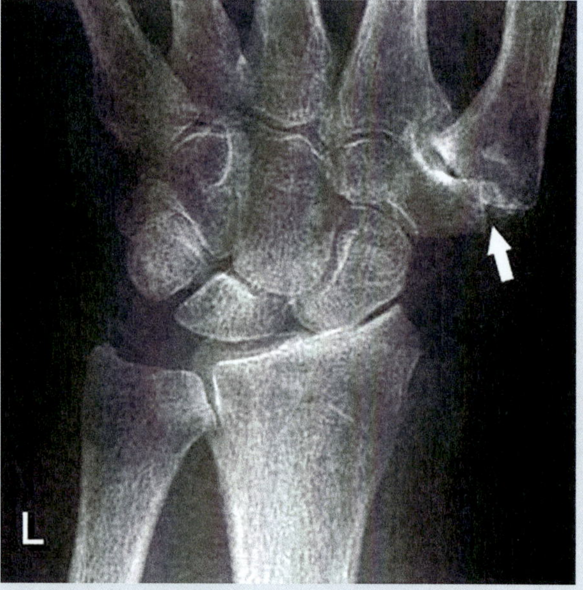

**Fig. 6.5.5** Plain radiograph of the hand shows OA of the base of the thumb (*arrow*)

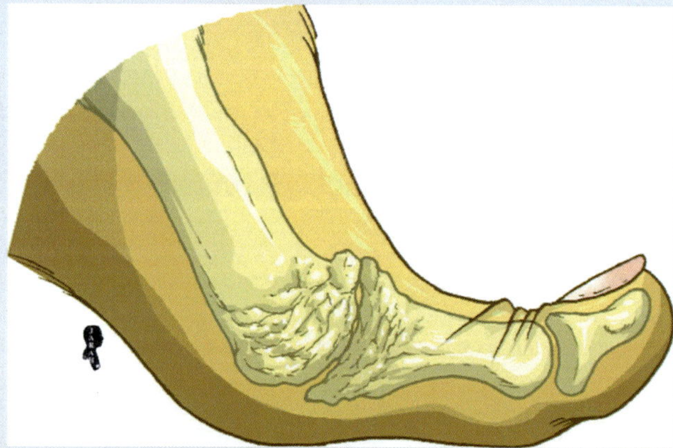

**Fig. 6.5.6** An illustration demonstrates hallux rigidus with its accentuated transverse skin crease

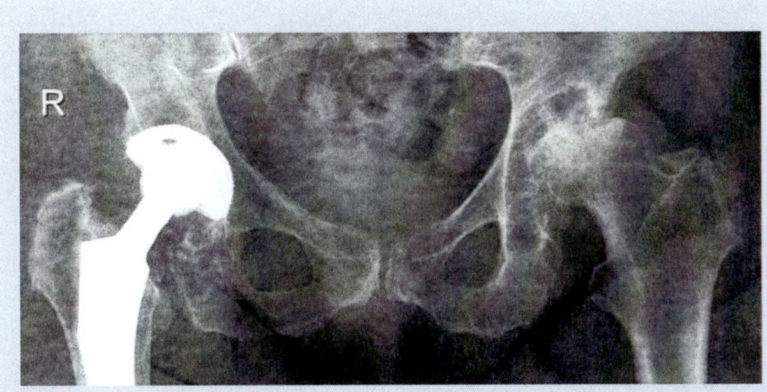



**Fig. 6.5.7** Anteroposterior plain radiograph of the pelvis shows severe OA of the left hip joint with superior displacement of the femoral head. Notice the total right hip joint replacement due to previous OA of the right hip joint

## Further Reading

Beaman FD, et al. MR imaging of cysts, ganglia, and bursae about the knee. Radiol Clin North Am. 2007b;45:969–82.

Corrà T, et al. Ochronotic arthropathy: rapid destructive hip osteoarthritis associated with metabolic disease. Clin Rheumatol. 1995;14:474–7.

Gupta KB, et al. Radiographic evaluation of osteoarthritis. Radiol Clin North Am. 2004;42:11–41.

Kijowski R, et al. Correlation between radiographic findings of osteoarthritis and arthroscopic findings of articular cartilage degeneration within the patellofemoral joint. Skeletal Radiol. 2006;35:895–902.

Theiler R, et al. Reduced vitamin A tolerance in a hyperlipidemia patient with rapid destructive and hyperostotic osteoarthritis of the hip. Clin Rheumatol. 1994;13:293–8.

Weiss E, et al. Osteoarthritis revisited: a contemporary review of aetiology. Int J Osteoarchaeol. 2007;17:437–50.

## 6.6    Psoriasis and Psoriatic Arthritis

Psoriasis is an idiopathic genetic, multifactorial disease characterized by the formation of large, sharply defined, sliver-white scaly cutaneous plaques on the extensor surfaces of the knees and elbows, genitalia, scalp, and lumbosacral area. Psoriasis comes from the Greek word "spora," which means itch.

Psoriasis can present as erythematous plaques (psoriasis vulgaris) or pustules (psoriasis pustulosa). The psoriatic skin lesions are characterized by hyperproliferation of the epidermal keratinocytes, and inflammatory cell cutaneous infiltration in which neutrophils and lymphocytes predominate. The earliest psoriatic lesion is an erythematous papule surmounted by a fine scale and is characteristically sharply demarcated from surrounding normal skin. If the scale of psoriasis is lifted, multiple, minute areas of bleeding will form (*Auspitz sign*).

Predisposing factors of psoriasis include emotional trauma, infections (e.g., β-hemolytic streptococci), sunlight, hormonal changes (e.g., pregnancy), medications (e.g., antimalaria drugs), and cigarette smoking. Many patients experience worsening symptoms in winter. *Köbner's phenomenon* is a term used to describe the formation of psoriatic lesions in an area of previous trauma. *Inverse psoriasis* is a term used to describe a condition in which the psoriasis involves the flexor surfaces rather than the extensor surfaces.

*Psoriatic arthritis* (*PsA*) is an inflammatory, rheumatoid factor-negative arthritis that is associated with psoriasis. PsA is found in 5–7 % of patients with psoriasis. PsA can occur in up to 40 % of severe psoriasis cases. Up to 60 % of PsA patients are HLA-B27 positive, and they are young adults aged 35–55 years.

Skin psoriasis precedes PsA in 70 % of cases and occurs concomitantly with PsA in 15 % of cases. However, PsA may precede psoriasis skin lesions in 10–30 % of cases.

PsA is characterized by bone erosions with new bone formation, which is the most distinguishing character of PsA differentiating it from other seronegative spondyloarthritis disorders. PsA is characterized by the formation of periostitis, enthesitis, and distal joint distribution in the extremities. Moreover, PsA arthritis can be symmetrical mimicking rheumatoid arthritis and asymmetrical, affecting the axial skeleton, mimicking ankylosing spondylitis. Because of these reasons, the history of psoriasis plus the absence of serological tests for rheumatoid factor are essential criteria to establish the diagnosis of PsA.

Hyperuricemia may be found in association with PsA as a result of increased purine metabolism due to high cell turnover. However, gout arthropathy is rarely developed in association with PsA.

Enthesitis is the inflammation at the site of attachment of a tendon or a ligament to the joint capsule (e.g., plantal fasciitis). The concept of an "enthesis organ" states that the enthesis together with the adjacent fibrocartilage, periosteum, synovial, and bursal membrane should be viewed as a unique "organ." PsA is considered as a disease affecting the enthesis organ, unlike rheumatoid arthritis which is a disease essentially affecting the synovium. Entheses may be fibrous (located at the metaphyses or diaphyses of long bones) or fibrocartilaginous (located at the apophyses and epiphyses of long bones). Both types are found in the spine.

*Sinus tarsi syndrome* may occur in patients with PsA. The sinus tarsi is a bony compartment bounded by the talus, the calcaneus, the talonavicular, and posterior subtalar joints and is continuous with the tarsal canal medially. The sinus tarsi contain fat, nerve endings, vessels, and ligaments (cervical and interosseous ligaments). Sinus tarsi syndrome is a clinical condition characterized by pain and paresthesia in the lateral side of the ankle. The causes of sinus tarsi syndrome include hemorrhage or inflammation of the synovial recesses of the sinus tarsi. Other causes include ganglion cyst formation within the sinus tarsi.

### Differential Diagnoses and Related Diseases

*SAPHO syndrome* is a disease characterized by Synovitis, Acne, Pustulosis of the palmar and plantar skin surface (psoriasis vulgaris), Hyperostosis of bones (e.g., sternoclavicular joint), and Ostitis. SAPHO syndrome can occur with PsA in 2 % of cases.

### Signs on Radiographs (In General, the Radiographic Features Are Either Erosive or Proliferative Changes)

- Osteoporosis is mild or absent in spite of severe bone erosions. Erosions typically start at the margins and then progress toward the center.
- Bone erosions start from the periphery of the joint and extend to the articular surface. The distal interphalangeal joints (DIPJs) of the hands and feet are commonly affected.
- The sacroiliac joint is affected in a unilateral or bilateral pattern (sacroiliitis occurs in up to 40 %).
- Periosteal reaction is seen at the affected bones as fuzzy appearance, which is characteristic for the bony proliferation associated with psoriatic arthritis (◘ Fig. 6.6.1).
- *Sausage fingers or toes* are soft-tissue swelling of the affected fingers or toes due to tenosynovitis. It is seen in 40 % of psoriatic patients (◘ Fig. 6.6.2).
- *Ivory phalanx* is a characteristic lesion of PsA that most often occurs in the distal phalanx of the great toe. It is seen as a dense appearance of the distal interphalangeal joint due to sclerosis plus periosteal and endosteal new bone formation.
- *Pencil and cup deformity* is seen in a severe form of marginal erosion, with one end of the joint forming the cup and the other a pencil that projects into this cup. It is mostly seen in the DIP joints of the fingers. The pencil tip is represented by the distal end of the metatarsal or metacarpal bone with the cup represented by the eroded articular surface of the opposing phalanx.
- *Non-marginal bridging* is seen in the axial skeleton as excess bone formation that usually begins toward the vertebral bodies and curves upward. In contrast, syndesmophytes in ankylosing spondylitis begin at the corner of the vertebral body and extend vertically.

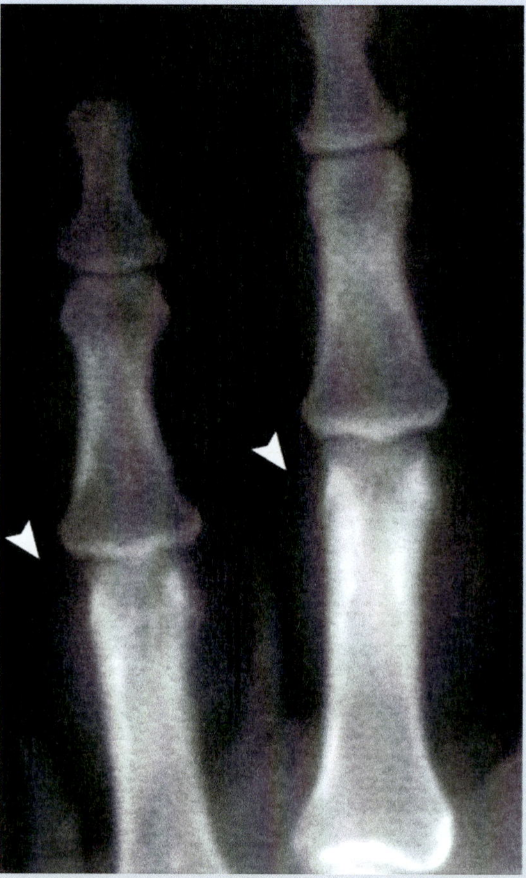

◘ Fig. 6.6.2   Plain radiograph of the fingers in a patient with psoriasis shows soft-tissue swelling (*arrowheads*) of the PIP joints (sausage fingers)

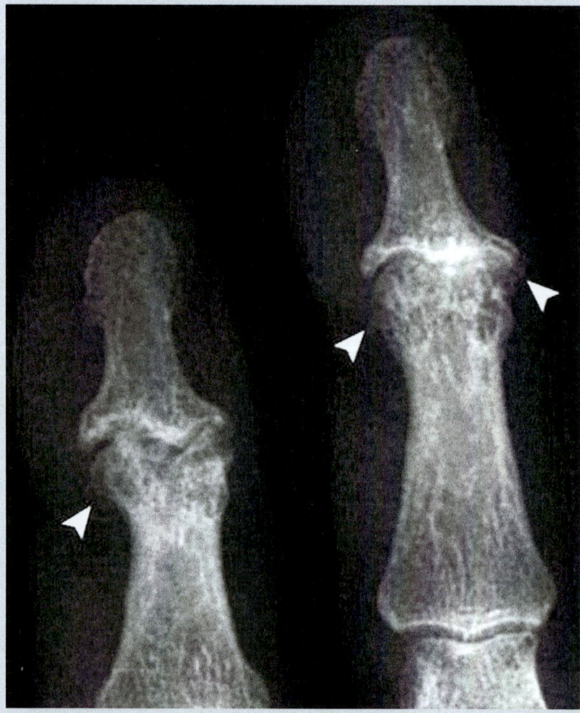

◘ Fig. 6.6.1   Plain radiograph of the distal fingers in a patient with psoriasis shows narrowing of the DIP joints and marginal new bone formation (*arrowheads*)

### Signs on MRI

- Tenosynovitis is defined as high T2 signal intensity surrounding a low T2 intensity tendon (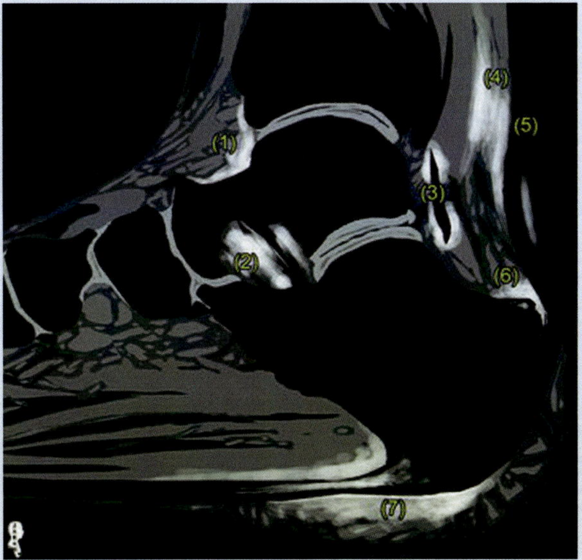 Fig. 6.6.3).
- In the foot, PsA can develop Achilles tendinitis, which is seen as thickened Achilles' tendon with high signal intensity within the tendon (Fig. 6.6.3).
- Plantal fasciitis is seen as a T2 high signal intensity at the site where the plantar fascia is inserted into the calcaneus (enthesitis) (Fig. 6.6.3).
- In sinus tarsi syndrome, there are low T1 and high T2 signal intensities within the sinus tarsi, with or without loss of the cervical or the interosseous ligaments (Figs. 6.6.3 and 6.6.4).



**Fig. 6.6.3** Sagittal STIR ankle MR illustration demonstrates types of foot pathologies seen in psoriatic arthritis: (*1*) synovitis, (*2*) sinus tarsi syndrome, (*3*) tenosynovitis, (*4*) Achilles peritendinitis, (*5*) Achilles tendonitis, (*6*) retrocalcaneal bursitis, and (*7*) plantar fasciitis

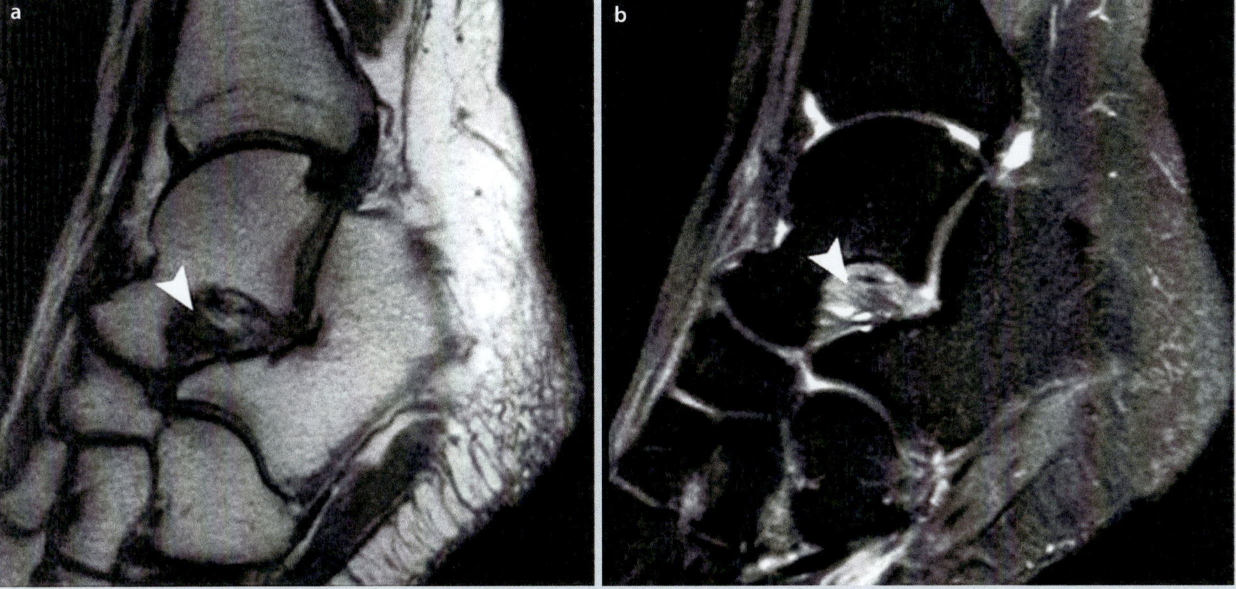



**Fig. 6.6.4** Sagittal T1W (**a**) and STIR (**b**) ankle MRI of a patient with chronic sinus tarsi syndrome show mild hyperintense signal within the sinus tarsi with disruption of the interosseous ligament (*arrowhead*)

## Further Reading

Baden HP, et al. Psoriasis. Dis Mon. 1973;19:1–45.

Bellet JS, et al. Intertriginous pustular psoriasis. J Am Acad Dermatol. 2009;60:679–83.

Benjamin M, et al. Magnetic resonance imaging of entheses. Part 1. Clin Radiol. 2008;63:691–703.

Herbst RA, et al. Guttate psoriasis triggered by perianal streptococcal dermatitis in a four-year-old boy. J Am Acad Dermatol. 2000;42:885–7.

Jacobson JA, et al. Radiographic evaluation of arthritis: inflammatory conditions. Radiology. 2008b;248:378–89.

Jiaravuthisan MM, et al. Psoriasis of the nail: anatomy, pathology, clinical presentation, and a review of the literature on therapy. J Am Acad Dermatol. 2007;57:1–27.

Lee Bennett D, et al. Spondyloarthropathies: ankylosing spondulitis and psoriatic arthritis. Radiol Clin North Am. 2004b;42:121–34.

Leung YY, et al. Psoriatic arthritis as a distinct disease entity. J Postgrad Med. 2007;53:63–71.

Prasad PVS, et al. A clinical study of psoriatic arthropathy. Indian J Dermatol Venerol Leprol. 2007;73:166–70.

Tan AL. Imaging of seronegative spondyloarthritis. Best Pract Res Clin Rheumatol. 2008;22:1045–59.

Vun YY, et al. Generalized pustular psoriasis of pregnancy treated with narrowband UVB and topical steroids. J Am Acad Dermatol. 2006;54:S28–30.

Zelickson BD, et al. Generalized pustular psoriasis in childhood. Report of thirteen cases. J Am Acad Dermatol. 1991;24:186–94.

Zuhal Erdem C, et al. MR imaging features of foot involvement in patients with psoriasis. Eur J Radiol. 2008;67:521–5.

## 6.7    Baastrup's Disease (Spinout Process Impingement Syndrome)

Baastrup's disease (BD) is a pathological condition characterized by close approximation and contact of adjacent spinout processes, an appearance known as "kissing spines," leading to reactive bone and cartilage formation in the spinous processes, causing sclerosis, enlargement, and flattening of the involved spines, with calcification of the interspinous and supraspinous ligaments (◘ Fig. 6.7.1).

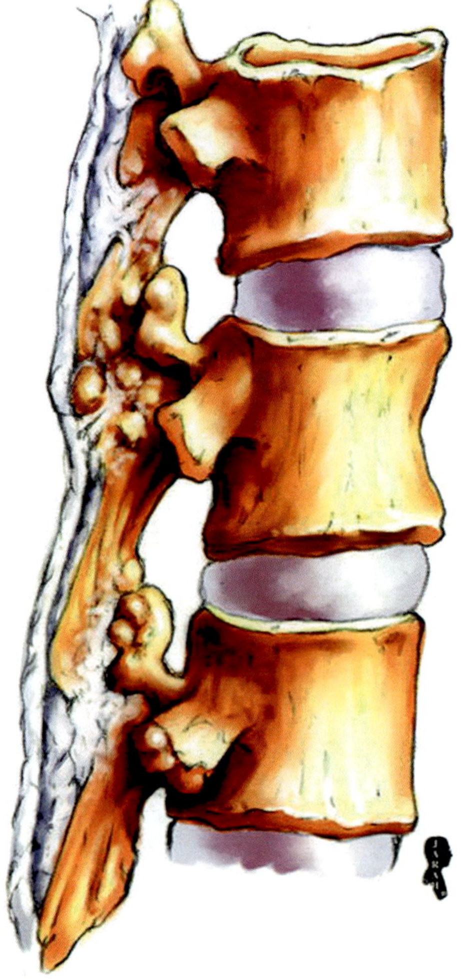

◘ **Fig. 6.7.1**    An illustration of the thoracic vertebrae demonstrates the gross appearance of the kissing spines and the calcification of the interspinous and supraspinous ligaments in Baastrup's disease

BD most commonly occurs in the lumbar spines. Cervical spines can be affected rarely. Patients typically present with back pain exacerbated on spine extension, which is relieved by flexion. The pain arises due to irritation of the periosteum or adventitial bursae between abutting spinous processes.

## Signs on Plain Radiograph

There is close approximation of the spinous processes with sclerosis, osteophytes formation, and hyperlordosis (Fig. 6.7.2).

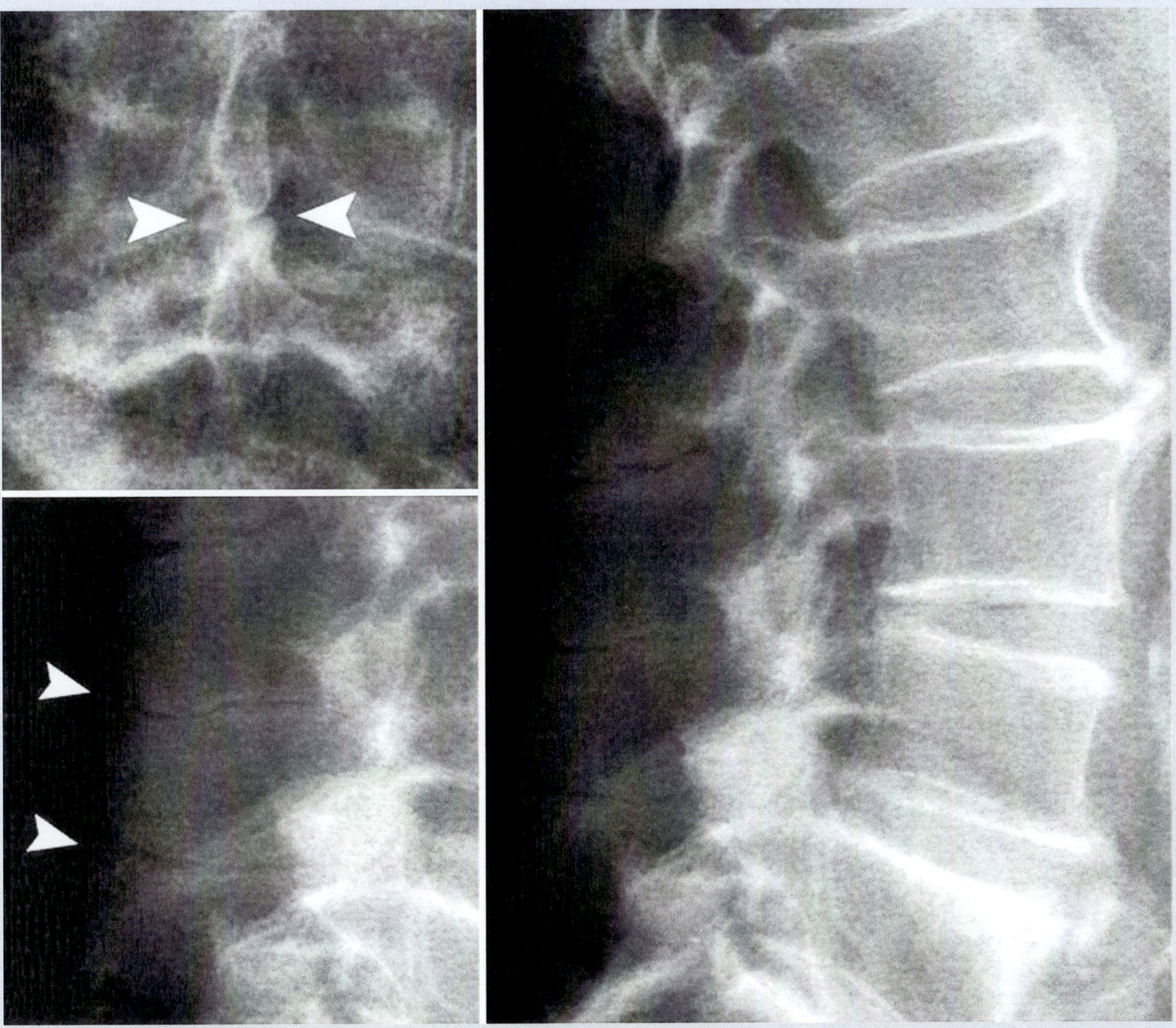

**Fig. 6.7.2**  Lateral and anteroposterior plain radiograph of the vertebral column in the thoracolumbar region shows flattened spinous processes of the lumbar vertebrae with sclerosis and close approximation (*arrowheads*), typical findings in Baastrup's disease of the spines

## Signs on MRI

There is approximation of the spinous processes, usually in the lumbar spines. Bone marrow edema is often seen in active disease, typically located in the spinous processes.

## Further Reading

Hui C, et al. Two unusual presentations of Baastrup's disease. Clin Radiol. 2007;62:495–7.

Lin E. Baastrup's disease (kissing spine) demonstrated by FDG/PET CT. Skeletal Radiol. 2008;37:173–5.

Pinto PS, et al. Spinous process fracture associated with Baastrup disease. J Clin Imaging. 2004;28:219–22.

## 6.8    Scheuermann's Disease (Juvenile Kyphosis Dorsalis)

Scheuermann's disease (SD) is a disease characterized by juvenile thoracic kyphosis with minimal deformity and few clinical symptoms (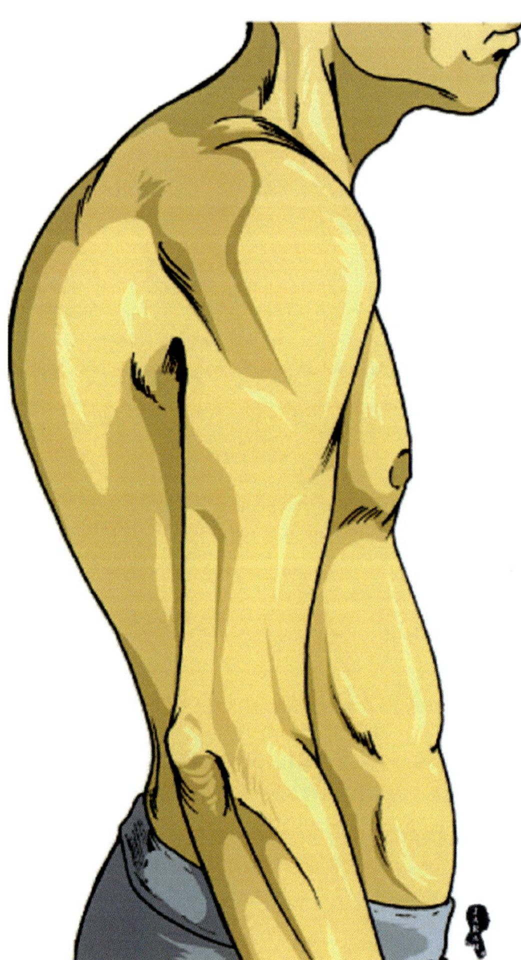 Fig. 6.8.1). The disease has an autosomal dominant pattern of inheritance, with an incidence of 1 % of population.

The normal disk space is composed of two end plates, central nucleus pulposus, and an outer annulus fibrous tissue (annulus fibrosus) surrounding the nucleus pulposus. Due to age process or repetitive trauma, the nucleus pulposus loses its watery content, and the annulus fibrosus develops cracks and fissures. When this occurs, the nucleus pulposus extrudes through the annulus fibrosus fissures. Extrusion of the nucleus pulposus into the vertebral end plates results in Schmorl's node and limbus vertebra, while extrusion through the annulus fibrosus results in disk degenerative disease (disk hernia). *Schmorl's node* is nucleus pulposus extrusion into the end plates and then into the vertebral body. In contrast, *limbus vertebra* is extrusion of the nucleus pulposus below the ring apophysis, separating it from the body of the vertebra. SD is characterized by the presence of Schmorl's node and multiple end plate irregularities due to nucleus pulposus extrusion.

Although the etiology of SD is unknown, Scheuermann proposed that the kyphosis resulted from avascular necrosis of the vertebral body's apophysis ring, but it is now generally believed to be a form of disk degeneration. *Kyphosis* is a term used to describe posterior convex curvature of the spine. Normal vertebral kyphosis is located in the cervicolumbar areas and does not exceed 25–45°. Any kyphosis exceeding this range is considered pathologic. Kyphosis is classified into:

- *Arcuate kyphosis*: kyphosis with long arc. This type is seen in SD, osteoporosis, and ankylosing spondylitis.
- *Angular kyphosis*: kyphosis with short arc. This type is seen in vertebral pathologic or compressive fractures, and spondylitis.

SD can be associated with scoliosis in 15 % of cases. *Scoliosis* is defined as an abnormal lateral curvature of the vertebral column. It can be classified into:

- *Rotoscoliosis*: scoliosis with rotation of the vertebra in the axial plane (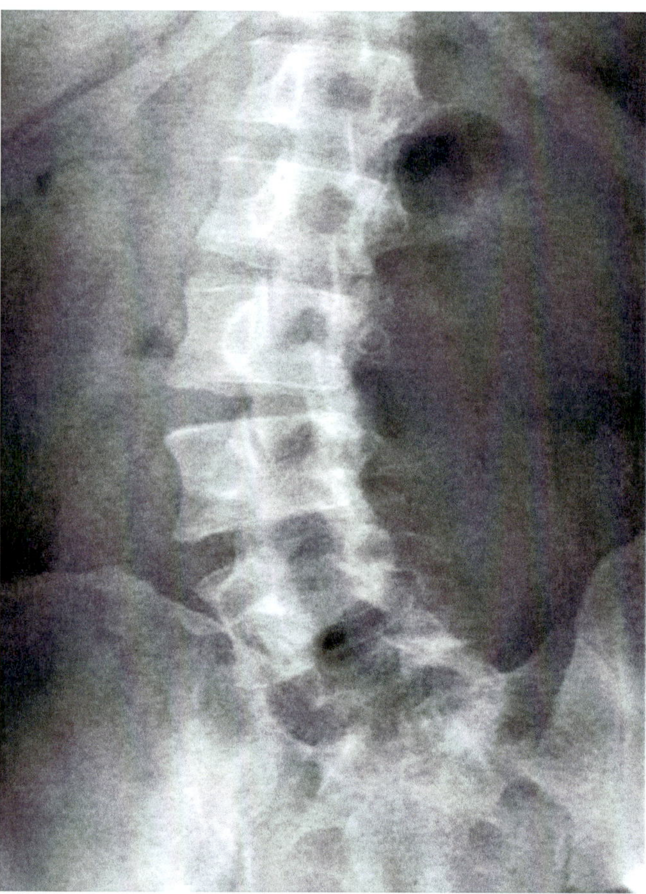 Fig. 6.8.2)
- *Kyphoscoliosis*: scoliosis plus kyphosis
- *S-shaped scoliosis*: double lateral deviation of the vertebral column (Fig. 6.8.3)

**Fig. 6.8.1**    An illustration demonstrates thoracic kyphosis in a young patient with Scheuermann's disease (SD)

**Fig. 6.8.2**    A plain abdominal radiograph of a patient shows right rotoscoliosis

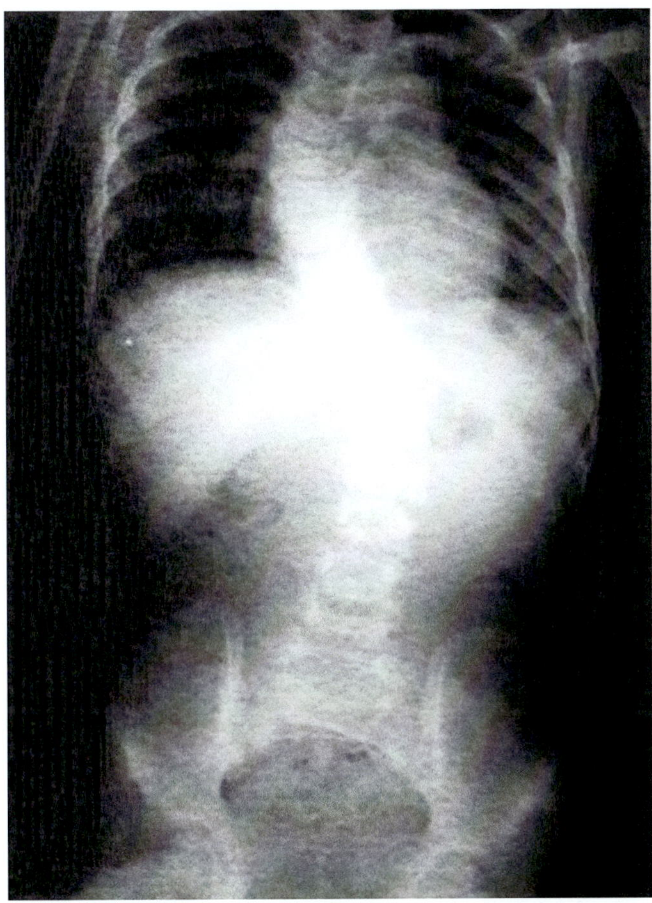

**Fig. 6.8.3** A plain abdominal radiograph of a patient with Marfan's syndrome shows right S-shaped scoliosis

– *C-shaped scoliosis*: single lateral curve of the vertebral column

Neurological symptoms of SD are rare in general and usually arise due to spinal cord compression. There are three types of neural compression reported in SD:
– Extradural spinal cyst
– Compression of the cord at the apex of the kyphos
– Disk hernia at the apex of the kyphos

## Criteria for Scheuermann's Disease Diagnosis

– More than 5° of wedging of at least three adjacent vertebrae at the apex of the kyphosis
– End plate irregularities
– A thoracic kyphosis of more than 45°

### Signs on Radiographs, CT, and MRI
– Increased thoracic kyphosis with compensatory lumbar hyperlordosis (■ Fig. 6.8.4).
– Wedging of at least three consecutive vertebrae (>5°) with end plate irregularities (■ Fig. 6.8.4).
– End plate irregularities, loss of disk space height, and Schmorl nodes. Schmorl node is defined as localized depression of the superior or inferior end plates >3 mm in diameter (■ Fig. 6.8.5).
– Limbus vertebra is visualized as separation of the ring apophysis from the vertebral body (■ Fig. 6.8.6).
– Scoliosis in 15 % of cases.

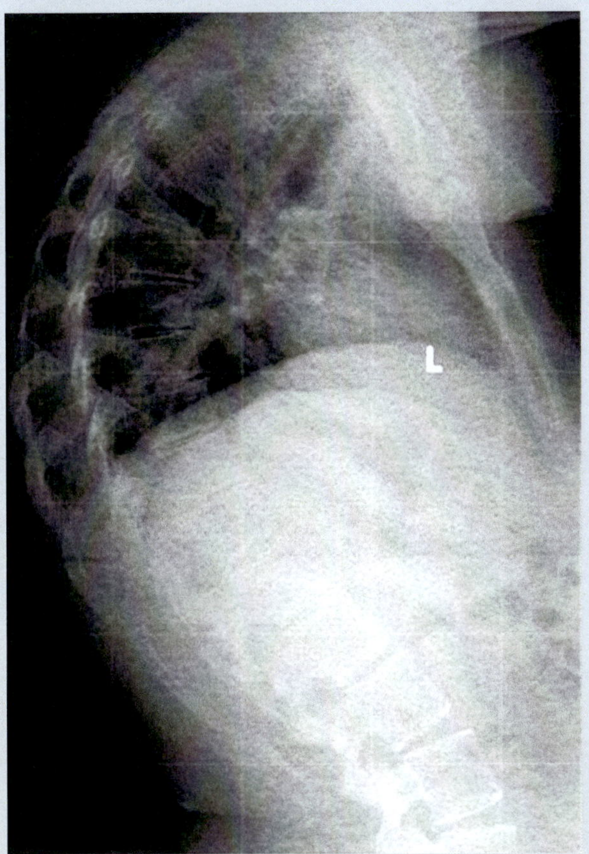


**Fig. 6.8.4** Lateral plain radiograph of the thoracic spine of an 18-year-old girl with SD shows marked thoracic kyphosis with wedging of more than three adjacent vertebrae

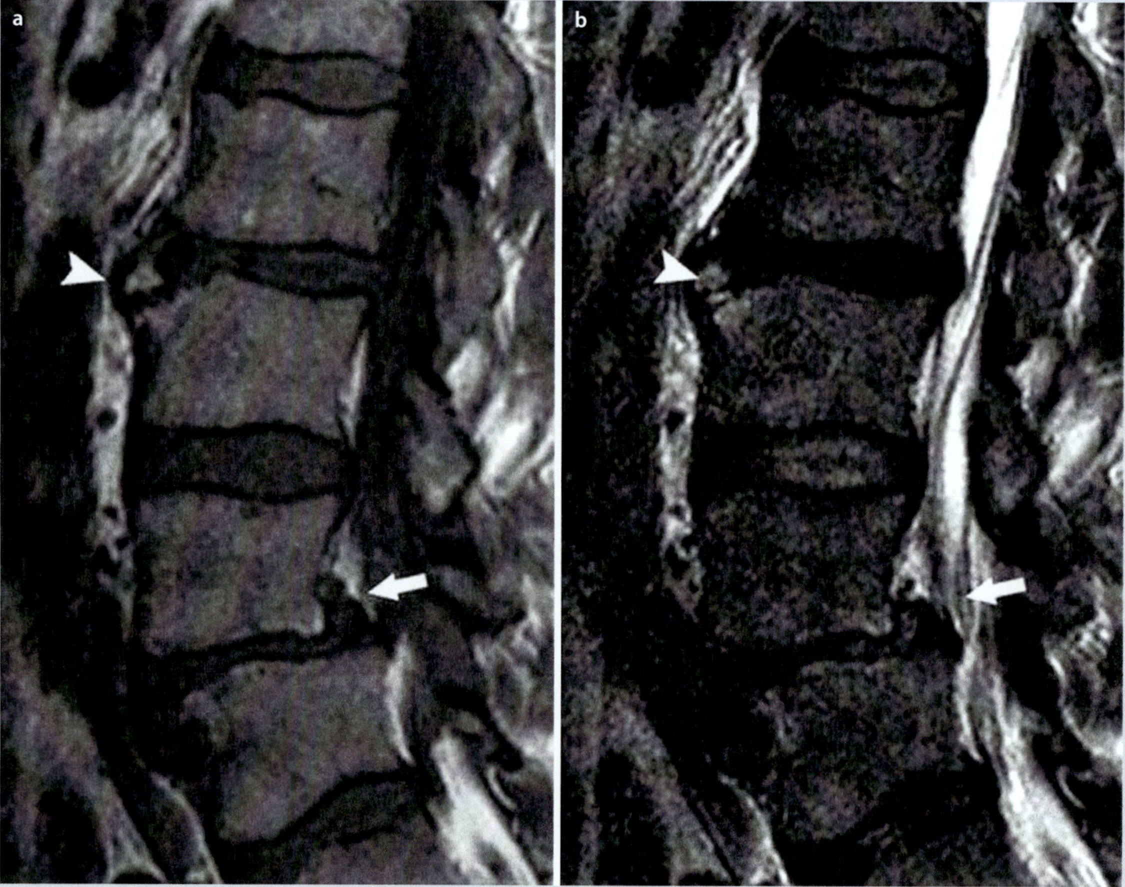

**Fig. 6.8.5** Sagittal (**a**) and axial (**b**) T2W image MRI of a patient with SD shows Schmorl's node seen as localized depression of the superior end plates >3 mm in diameter due to extrusion of the nucleus pulposus into the end plates (*arrowheads*)

**Fig. 6.8.6** Sagittal T1W (**a**) and T2W (**b**) MRI of a patient with vertebral column osteochondrosis shows L2 limbus vertebra (*arrowheads*) and L4/L5 grade 1 (<25 %) spondylolisthesis (*arrows*). Notice the active bone marrow edema around the bone fragment of the anterior superior end plate of L2 in (**b**)

## Further Reading

Alexander CJ. Scheuermann's disease. Skeletal Ardiol. 1977;1:209–21.

Arlet V, et al. Scheuermann's kyphosis: surgical management. Eur Spine J. 2005;14:817–27.

Kapetanos GA, et al. Thoracic cord compression caused by disk herniation in Scheuermann's disease. A case report and review of the literature. Eur Spine J. 2006;15 suppl 5:S553–8.

Paajanen H, et al. Disc degeneration in Scheuermann disease. Skeletal Radiol. 1989;18:523–6.

Swischunk LE, et al. Disk degeneration in childhood: Scheuermann's disease, Schmorl's nodes, and the limbus vertebra: MRI findings in 12 patients. Pediatr Radiol. 1998;28:334–8.

## 6.9 Sjögren Syndrome (Myoepithelial Sialadenitis)

Sjögren syndrome (SS) is a chronic, systemic autoimmune disease characterized by infiltration of the acinar cells of the salivary and lacrimal glands by lymphocytes, causing dry eye (*xeropthalmia*), dry mouth (*xerostomia*), and inflammation of the cornea and the conjunctiva (*keratoconjunctivitis*).

SS is classified as secondary (*Sicca syndrome*) when it is associated with other connective tissue disorders (e.g., rheumatoid arthritis) and primary when it occurs without any manifestation of other connective tissue disorders.

## Criteria to Diagnose SS Include

– Symptoms and signs of ocular dryness (e.g., positive Schrimer's test)
– Symptoms and signs of mouth dryness
– Evidence of autoimmune disease (e.g., positive rheumatoid factor)
– Exclusion of lymphoma, sarcoidosis, and acquired immunodeficiency syndrome

SS causes salivary glands inflammation (*sialadenitis*) that leads to parenchymal destruction and salivary gland dilatation (*sialectasia*).

Patients with SS are commonly perimenopausal women who often develop multiple systemic manifestations that include mouth dryness, which affects eating, speaking, and may lead to teeth decay; extreme fatigue occurs in 50 % of patients, which is more troublesome than the exocrine symptoms; intermittent polyarthritis affecting the small joints in asymmetrical fashion; dry skin (50 %), esophageal dysmotility (up to 90 %), vaginal atrophy and dyspareunia; and interstitial nephritis. Patients with SS have risk for developing lymphoma, and they should be closely monitored.

Patients with SS may also develop neuropsychiatric manifestations. Brain manifestations include aseptic meningoencephalitis and multiple sclerosis-like symptoms (25 % of cases). Psychiatric manifestations include Alzheimer-type dementia, poor attention and concentration, and memory deficits. Rarely, neuromyelitis optica may coexist in patients with SS. In children, although it is rare, SS is characterized by bilateral parotid enlargement. Very rarely, SS may be associated with amyloidosis.

Laboratory investigation reveals high titer of SS-A antibodies and SS-B antibodies plus rheumatoid factor in 50 % of cases.

### Signs on Sialography

On both conventional and MR-sialography, the affected salivary gland shows mottled appearance with cystic changes due to destruction of the gland parenchyma (sialectasia). Four stages of sialectasia are classically described:

- *Stage 1* (*punctuate*): multiple dots <1 mm in size (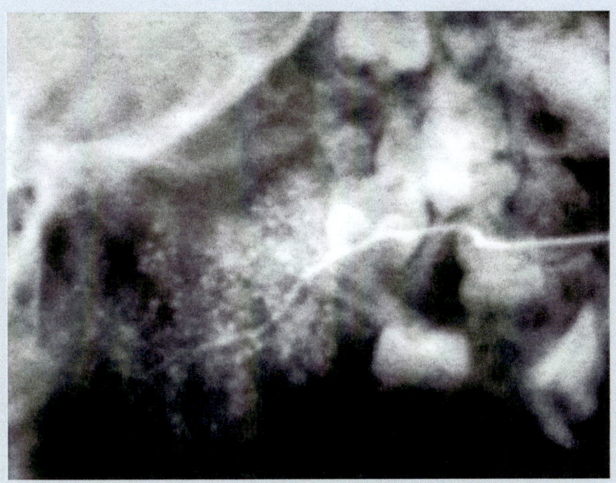 Fig. 6.9.1)
- *Stage 2* (*globular*): multiple dots 1–2 mm in size
- *Stage 3* (*cavitary*): multiple dots >2 mm in size
- *Stage 4* (*destructive*): multiple irregular and widened ducts due to gland inflammation (*sialodochitis*)

**Fig. 6.9.1** Lateral conventional sialography radiograph in a patient with submandibular sialectasis grade 1–2 seen as diffuse multiple punctuated dots between 1 and 2 mm in diameter

### Signs on CT

- In the acute phase, the affected glands are bilaterally enlarged with parenchymal nodules of variable size and formation of cysts, giving a honeycomb appearance (Fig. 6.9.2).

— The salivary glands often show signs of fibrosis and size shrinkage in advanced stages of the disease.

— The lacrimal glands might be bilaterally and symmetrically enlarged (■ Fig. 6.9.3).

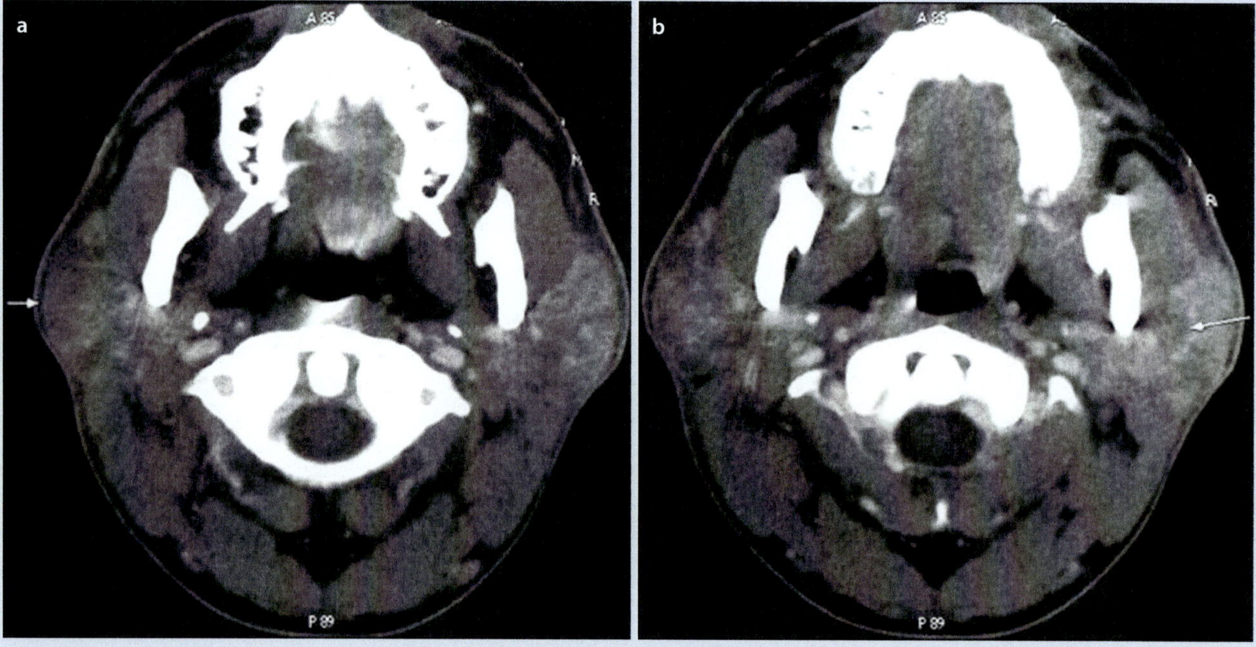

■ **Fig. 6.9.2** Sequential postcontrast head CT images (**a**) and (**b**) of a patient with Sjögren syndrome (SS) show bilateral parotid gland bulging and enlargement (*arrows*)

### Signs on Brain MRI

Brain MRI shows multifocal T2 hyperintensities located in the subcortical and periventricular white matter (■ Fig. 6.9.4), enlargement of the sulci, and ventricular dilatation. These manifestations are often seen in 50 % of patients with focal neurological deficits or psychiatric manifestations.

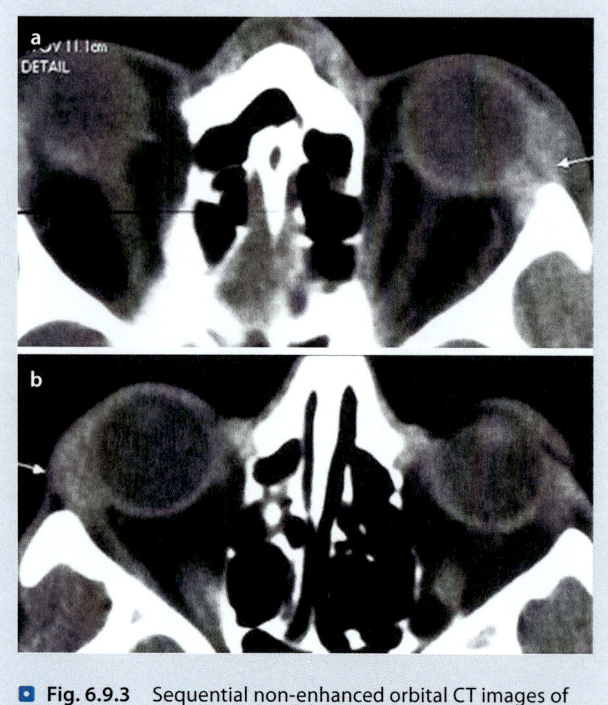

■ **Fig. 6.9.3** Sequential non-enhanced orbital CT images of the same patient with Sjögren syndrome (SS) show bilateral lacrimal glands enlargement (*arrows* in **a** and **b**)

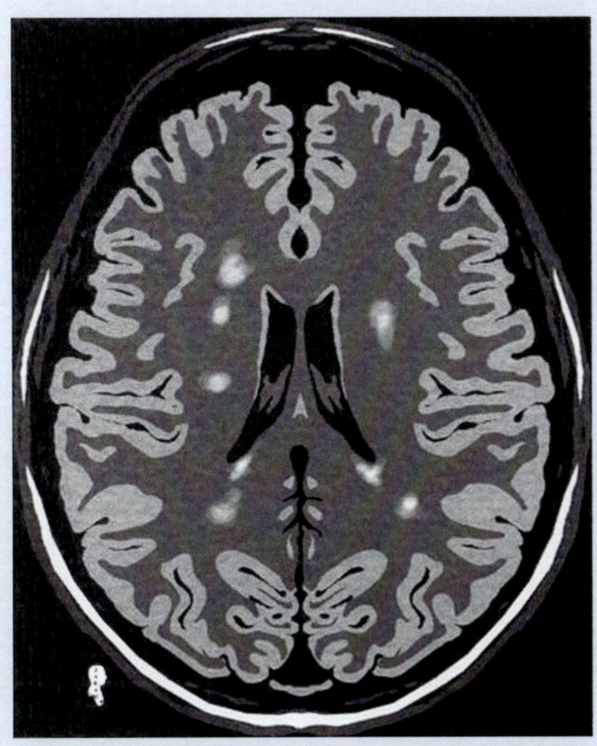

**Fig. 6.9.4** Axial FLAIR brain MR illustration demonstrates patchy areas of high T2 signal intensity lesions within the white matter as presentation of neuro-Sjögren syndrome (SS)

### Signs on Parotid MRI
- Bilateral, almost symmetrical enlargement of the parotid glands (**Fig. 6.9.5**).
- Low T1/high T2 multiple cysts are seen within the parotid and lack of enhancement ("salt and pepper" appearance) (**Fig. 6.9.5**).
- Chronic disease can lead to gland shrinkage, microcysts formation, and calcifications.

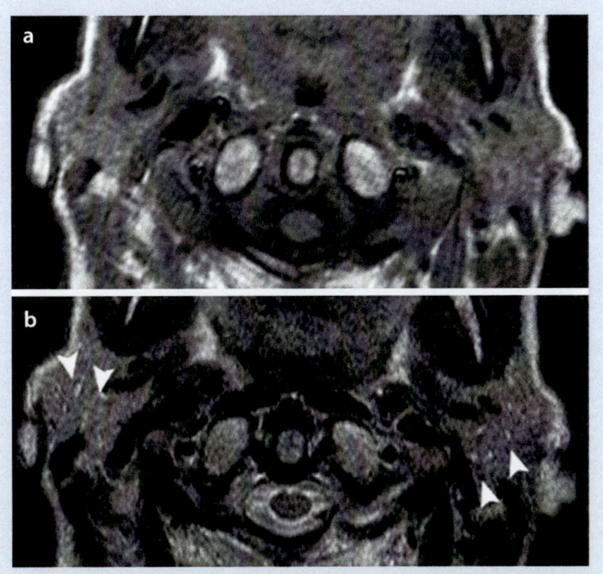


**Fig. 6.9.5** Axial T1W (**a**) and T2W (**b**) images of a patient with Sjögren syndrome (SS) show bilateral moderate parotid glands enlargement with fine, small cysts formation within the gland (*arrowheads*)

## Further Reading

Adžić TN, et al. Multinodular pulmonary amyloidosis in primary Sjögren's syndrome. Eur J Int Med. 2008;19:e97–8.

Kalk WWI, et al. Parotid sialography for diagnosing Sjögren syndrome. Oral Surg Oral Med Oral Pathol Oral Radiol Endod. 2002;94:131–7.

Kassan SS, et al. Clinical manifestations and early diagnosis of Sjögren's syndrome. Arch Intern Med. 2004;164:1275–84.

Kobayashi I, et al. Complications of childhood Sjögren syndrome. Eur J Pediatr. 1996;155:890–4.

Madani G, et al. Inflammatory conditions of the salivary glands. Semin Ultrasound CT MRI. 2006;27:440–51.

Mataró M, et al. Magnetic resonance abnormalities associated with cognitive dysfunction in primary Sjögren syndrome. J Neurol. 2003;250:1070–6.

Mizuno Y, et al. Recurrent parotid gland enlargement as an initial manifestation of Sjögren syndrome in children. Eur J Pediatr. 1989;148:414–6.

Ohbayashi N, et al. Sjögren syndrome: comparison of assessments with MR sialography and conventional sialography. Radiology. 1998;209:683–8.

Tristano AG, et al. A case of Sjögren's syndrome with acute transverse myelitis and polyneuropathy in a patient free of sicca symptoms. Clin Rheumatol. 2005;25:113–4.

Varghese JC, et al. A prospective comparative study of MR Sialography and conventional sialography of salivary duct disease. AJR. 1999;173:1497–503.

Yoon YH, et al. Sialectasis of Stensen's duct: an unusual case of recurrent check swelling. Eur Arch Otorhinolaryngol. doi:10.1007/s00405–008–0702–0.

## 6.10  Behçet Disease

Behçet disease (BD) is a relatively rare rheumatological disease characterized by the triad of aphthous oral ulcers, genital ulcers, and ocular inflammation (uveitis). The disease is named after its first describer, the Turkish dermatologist Hulusi Behçet, in 1937.

## Clinical Criteria to Diagnose BD Require a Combination of Three or More of the Following Findings

- Recurrent aphthous stomatitis (79 %). The lesions are punched out with rolled edges.
- Recurrent genital ulcers, mainly seen on the scrotum or labial majora, which heal by scar formation.
- Anterior or posterior uveitis, presenting with pain, blurry vision, and redness.
- Vasculitis of cutaneous or large vessels.
- Mono- or oligoarthritis affecting the knees in particular.
- Meningoencephalitis.
- Cutaneous hyperactivity to minor trauma.

BD lesions are characterized by chronic inflammation of the soft tissues with neutrophilic infiltration, which is characteristic of BD lesions regardless of the disease stage.

BD is a multisystemic disease with many manifestations. Documented complications of BD are those that affect the gastrointestinal tract (GI), large vessels (vasculitis and thrombophlebitis), musculoskeletal system (myonecrosis and arthritis), renal system (proteinuria and hematuria), and the nervous system (neuro-BD).

Myonecrosis should be considered in patients with known BD presenting with acute onset of muscle pain and edema in the absence of signs and symptoms of infection. Renal BD is mainly caused by secondary amyloidosis (AA-type) and glomerulonephritis.

Neuro-BD has three patterns of presentation: the first pattern is seen as brain parenchymal lesions presenting in stroke-like lesions and brain stem syndrome; the second pattern is migraine headache (64 %), papilledema, and increased intracranial hypertension; and the third pattern presents in the form of meningitis-like disease.

The esophagus is involved in 50 % of patients usually in its midportion. Patients with esophageal involvement often present with substernal pain, dysphagia, and occasional hematemesis. Esophageal varices may develop when the superior vena cava is obstructed due to thrombophlebitis (*superior vena cava syndrome*). Thrombophlebitis may involve the hepatic veins resulting in *Budd–Chiari syndrome* (liver congestion and cirrhosis due to hepatic veins outflow obstruction).

GI manifestations of BD may mimic the manifestations of Crohn's disease (CD) radiologically and even pathologically. However, involvement of the rectum and anus is rare in BD; perforation is more common in BD than CD, no cobblestoning in BD, and the GI disease is usually milder in BD than in CD.

Diagnosis is essentially clinical, and atypical presentation can be misleading and delay the diagnosis.

### Signs on Enteroclysis

Distal ileum inflammation and aphthous ulceration are seen in up to 80 % of patients with GI manifestations of BD. Pseudopolyp formation is seen in 35 % of cases.

### Signs on MRI

- In the muscles, myonecrosis presents with soft-tissue inflammation in the form of soft-tissue mass with high signal intensity on T2W images and rim contrast enhancement on postgadolinium injection images.
- In the brain, multiple, round, small (>5 mm) white matter high T2 signal intensity lesions on FLAIR and T2W images, usually in the juxtacortical region (◘ Fig. 6.10.1). Brain stem lesions and atrophy can be seen.

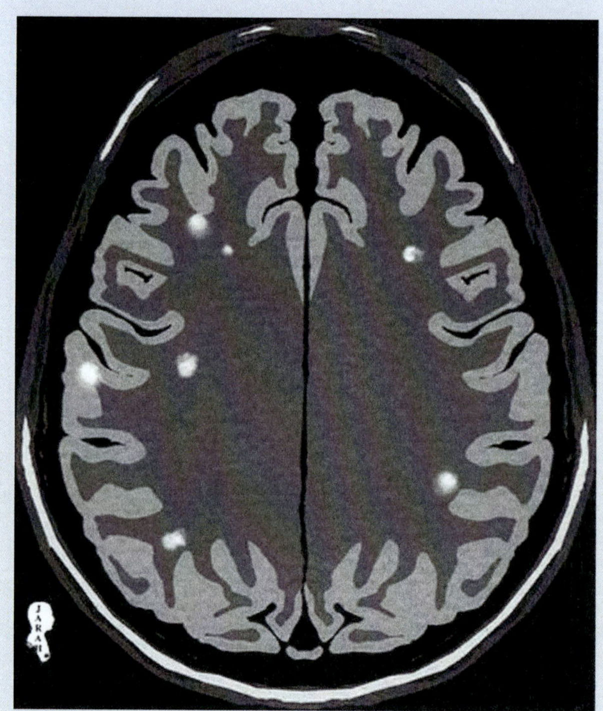

◘ **Fig. 6.10.1**    Axial FLAIR brain MR illustration demonstrates the neurological findings in neuro-Behçet disease

## Further Reading

Akpolat T, et al. Renal Behçet's disease: an update. Semin Arthritis Rheum. 2008;38:241–8.

Bank I, et al. Dural sinus thrombosis in Behçet's disease. Arthritis Rheum. 1984;27:816–8.

Benjilali L, et al. Chylothorax and chylopericardium in a young man with Behçet disease. Joint Bone Spine. 2008;75:740–52.

Ebert EC et al. Gastrointestinal manifestations of Behçet's disease. Dig Dis Sci. doi:10.1007/s10620–008–0337–4.

Hwang I, et al. Necrotizing villitis and decidual vasculitis in placentas of mothers with Behçet disease. Human Pathol. 2009;40:135–8.

Jäger HR, et al. MRI in neuro-Behcet's syndrome: comparison of conventional spin-echo and FLAIR pulse sequences. Neuroradiology. 1990;41:750–8.

Korman U, et al. Enteroclysis findings of intestinal Behcet disease: a comparative study with crohn disease. Abdom Imaging. 2003;28:308–12.

La Mantia L, et al. Headache and inflammatory disorders of the central nervous system. Neurol Sci. 2004;25:S148–53.

Oktay Kaçmaz R, et al. Ocular inflammation in Behçet disease: incidence of ocular complications and loss of visual acuity. Am J Opthalmol. 2008;146:828–36.

Stubbs AY, et al. Myonecrosis in Behcet's disease. Skeletal Radiol. 2008;37:357–60.

## 6.11 Sharp Syndrome (Mixed Connective Tissue Disease)

Mixed connective tissue disorder (MCTD) is a rare disease characterized by a combination of clinical features similar to systemic lupus erythematosus (SLE), scleroderma, and polymyositis and unusually high titers of antibody to RNase-sensitive ribonucleoprotein complex (RNP).

MCTD patients have mixed features of rheumatological symptoms that do not match a certain rheumatological category. For example, polyarthritis, myositis, and hypergammaglobulinemia are more common in MCTD than in scleroderma. Also, polyarthritis and hypergammaglobulinemia are more frequently found in MCTD than in polymyositis. Esophageal hypermotility, pulmonary hypertension, and absence of renal disease are typical features of MCTD. Moreover, the detection of serological antibodies to RNP is very specific for MCTD and very rarely found in other rheumatic or connective tissue disorders.

Patients with MCTD may show neurological signs like seizures, psychosis, headache, gait disturbance, and polyneuritis. Trigeminal neuralgia has been reported in patients with MCTD and seen frequently when the patient has more symptoms toward scleroderma. In contrast, MCTD with more symptoms toward SLE shows neurological symptoms like gait ataxia, transverse myelitis, and optic neuropathy. MCTD is one of the rare causes of "treatable dementia."

MCTD should be considered in a patient when his/her symptoms and signs cannot be confined to a sole rheumatological disease.

### Signs on Radiograph and CT

Chest radiograph or CT may show signs of pulmonary hypertension (e.g., prominent pulmonary trunk) (◘ Fig. 6.11.1).

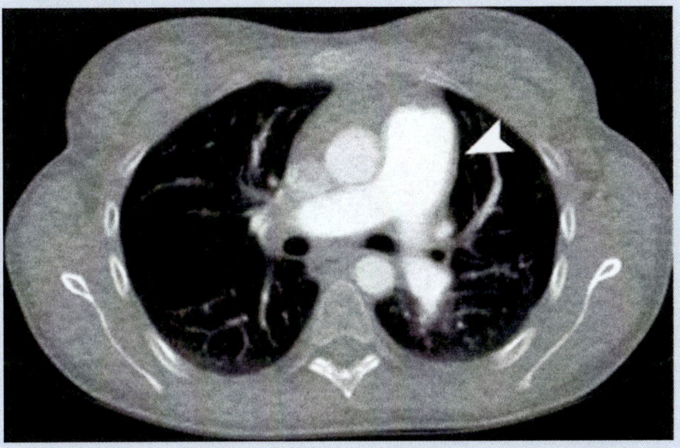

◘ **Fig. 6.11.1**    Axial postcontrast CT angiography of the pulmonary vessels in 32-year-old woman with Sharp's syndrome shows mildly dilated pulmonary trunk (28 mm) due to newly developed pulmonary hypertension (*arrowhead*)

### Signs on Brain MRI

- Optic or trigeminal neuritis is seen as contrast enhancement of the nerve after gadolinium injection due to the hyperemia and inflammation (the normal nerve does not enhance after contrast injection).
- Transverse myelitis shows enlargement of the cord with diffuse hyperintense signal of the spinal cord on T2W images in the affected segment (◘ Fig. 6.11.2). The affected segment enhances in an inhomogeneous pattern after contrast administration. Cord atrophy occurs in chronic cases. On axial segments, the high signal on T2W images occurs on both sides of the cord, giving a "snake-eye appearance."

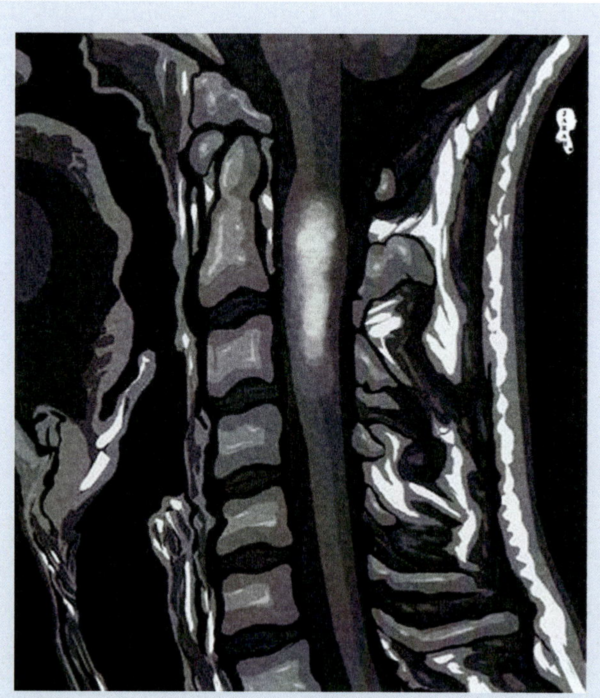

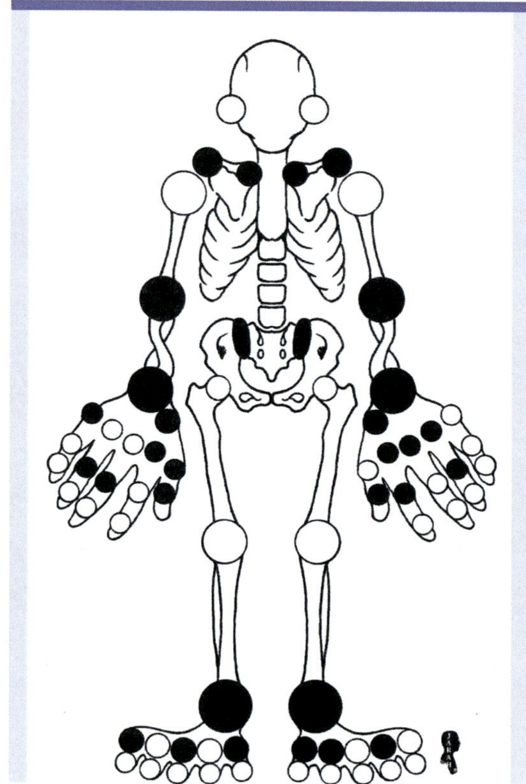



**Fig. 6.11.2** Sagittal T1W postcontrast cervical spine MR illustration demonstrates transverse myelitis as thickened spinal cord with

**Fig. 6.12.1** An illustration that demonstrates the body's geographic distribution of relapsing polyarthritis arthropathy

## Further Reading

Colombo A, et al. Mixed connective tissue disease (Sharp syndrome): description of two cases. Ital J Neurol Sci. 1983;2:203–5.

Malaviya AN, et al. Sharp's syndrome (mixed connective tissue disease) with extensive inflammatory panniculitis complicated with pyoderma gangrenosum–a case report. J Indian Rheumatol Assoc. 2003;11:45–50.

Matsui H, et al. Encephalopathy and sever neuropathy due to probable systemic vasculitis as an initial manifestation of mixed connective tissue disease. Neurol India. 2006;54:83–5.

## 6.12 Relapsing Polychondritis

Relapsing polychondritis (RP) is a rare, multisystemic, autoimmune disease characterized by recurrent, episodic inflammation and destruction of cartilaginous tissues.

The peak age for disease onset is the fifth decade. RP is associated with HLA class II DR4 and is frequently associated with autoimmune, rheumatologic, or hematologic disorders (>30%). Examples of diseases associated with RP include diabetes mellitus, Crohn's disease, rheumatoid arthritis, and lymphoma.

Patients with RP present with recurrent episodes of inflammation involving the elastic cartilage of the nose, and ears, hyaline cartilage of the peripheral joints, fibrocartilage of the vertebrae, tracheobronchial cartilage, and proteoglycan-rich structures like the blood vessels, eyes, and inner ear. Symptoms include fever, asymmetric polyarthritis, weight loss, and deformity of the ears and nose. Painful swelling of the cartilaginous part of the ears with violaceous discoloration is its characteristic. Hearing impairment may occur if the external auditory canal is closed due to serous otitis media or due to vasculitis of the internal auditory artery.

Arthritis in RP is usually asymmetric (Fig. 6.12.1), migratory, seronegative, and nonerosive, affecting most commonly the metacarpophalangeal, PIP, wrists, and knees with or without synovitis. In short, any joint with cartilage is affected or vulnerable. Symmetric involvement may be seen, sometimes mimicking rheumatoid arthritis.

Up to 25% of patients present with respiratory symptoms and symptoms due to laryngeal or tracheal cartilage inflammation like hoarseness of voice, persistent cough, stridor, and dyspnea. Mortality due to recurrent respiratory infections or tracheal collapse ranges between 10 and 50 %.

Nasal chondritis is seen in up to 50 % of cases and may lead to saddle nose deformity. Symptoms of nasal chondritis include nasal pain, swelling, nasal stuffiness, rhinorrhea, and maybe epistaxis. Dermatological manifestations are seen in 15–20 % of cases and resemble urticaria.

Ocular manifestations include recurrent scleritis, keratitis, and/or conjunctivitis. Cardiovascular manifestations include aortic aneurysm, aortic valve rupture, pericarditis, and complete heart block. Glomerulonephritis with proteinuria may occur.

Laboratory investigations are nonspecific and include elevated levels of C-reactive protein and ESR. Rheumatoid factor and ANA are negative unless RP coexist with SLE or rheumatoid arthritis. Antibodies against collagen type II, IX, and XI as well as matrilin I can be found.

Neurorelapsing polychondritis occurs as a rare manifestation of relapsing polychondritis and is characterized by fluctuating headache, confusion, gait deterioration and ataxia, memory loss, personality change, and paranoia. Neurological manifestations occur in up to 5 % of patients. The main pathological features on brain biopsy have been vasculitis and parenchymal inflammation. Other neurological manifestations include meningoencephalitis, cranial nerves palsies, seizures, ataxias, isolated cerebellar syndrome, and stroke-like episodes, all of which can be attributed to cerebral vasculitis. Uncommonly, limbic encephalitis may occur with neurorelapsing polychondritis.

## Diagnostic Criteria for Relapsing Polychondritis

1. Recurrent chondritis of both auricles
2. Nonerosive seronegative inflammatory polychondritis
3. Inflammation of ocular structures (*uveitis, keratitis, scleritis, and/or episcleritis*)
4. Chondritis of the respiratory tract involving laryngeal or tracheal cartilage
5. Cochlear and/or vestibular damage causing sensorineural hearing loss, tinnitus, and/or vertigo

Diagnosis is established if (1) the patient has three of the above clinical criteria, (2) the patient has one criteria with cartilage biopsy conformation, or (3) chondritis at two or more separate anatomical locations with respond to steroid therapy.

## Differential Diagnoses and Related Diseases

### ■ MAGIC Syndrome

MAGIC syndrome is a disease characterized by *Mouth And Genital* ulcers with *Inflamed Cartilage*. MAGIC syndrome is simply a combination of both relapsing polychondritis and Behcet's disease (◘ Fig. 6.12.2).

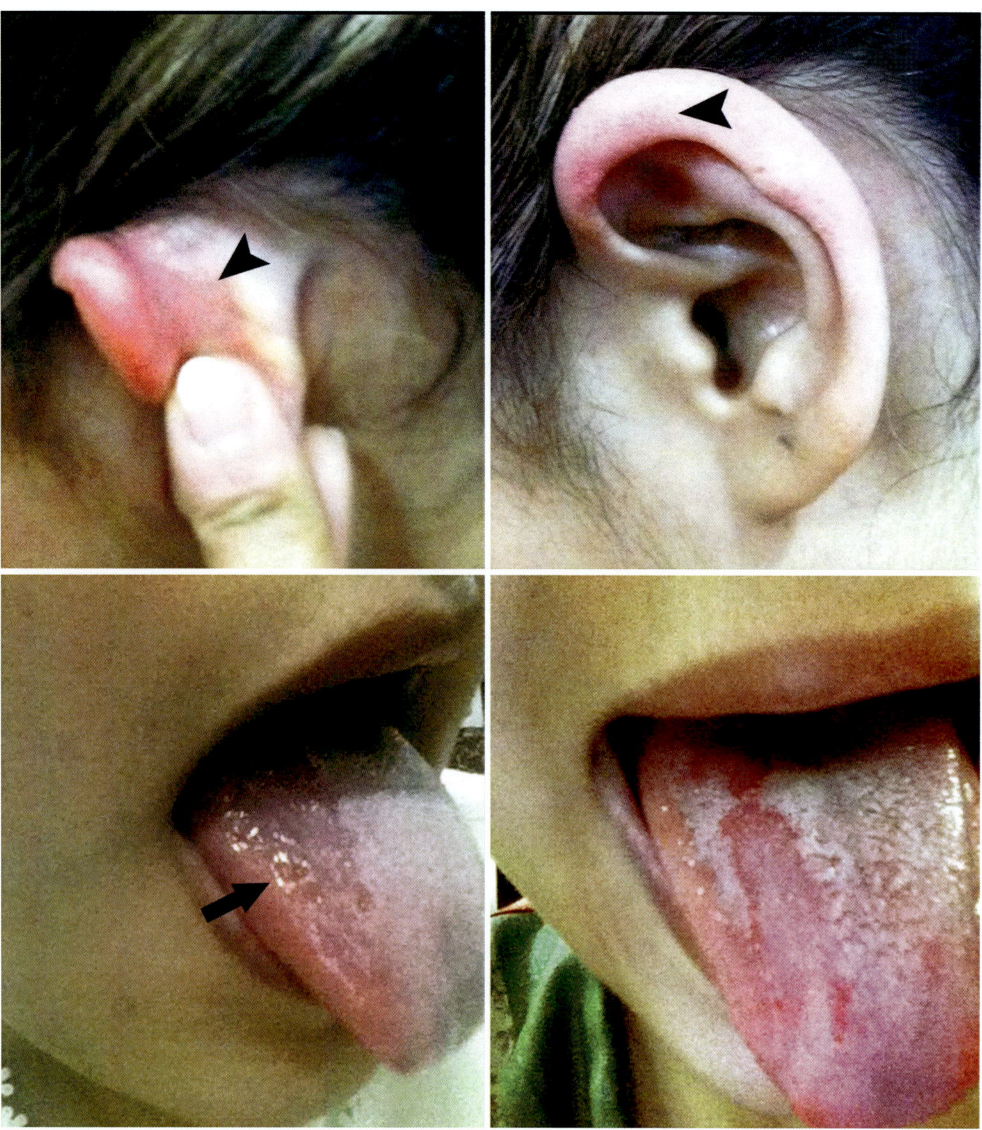

**Fig. 6.12.2** Multiple images of a 43-years-old female patient with MAGIC syndrome that shows the classical clinical signs of ear pinna redness (*arrowhead*) and mouth ulcers seen in the tongue (*arrow*)

### Signs on Radiographs

On plain radiography, patients with relapsing polychondritis present with calcified ear pinna and/or nasal cartilage (pathognomonic) (Fig. 6.12.3).

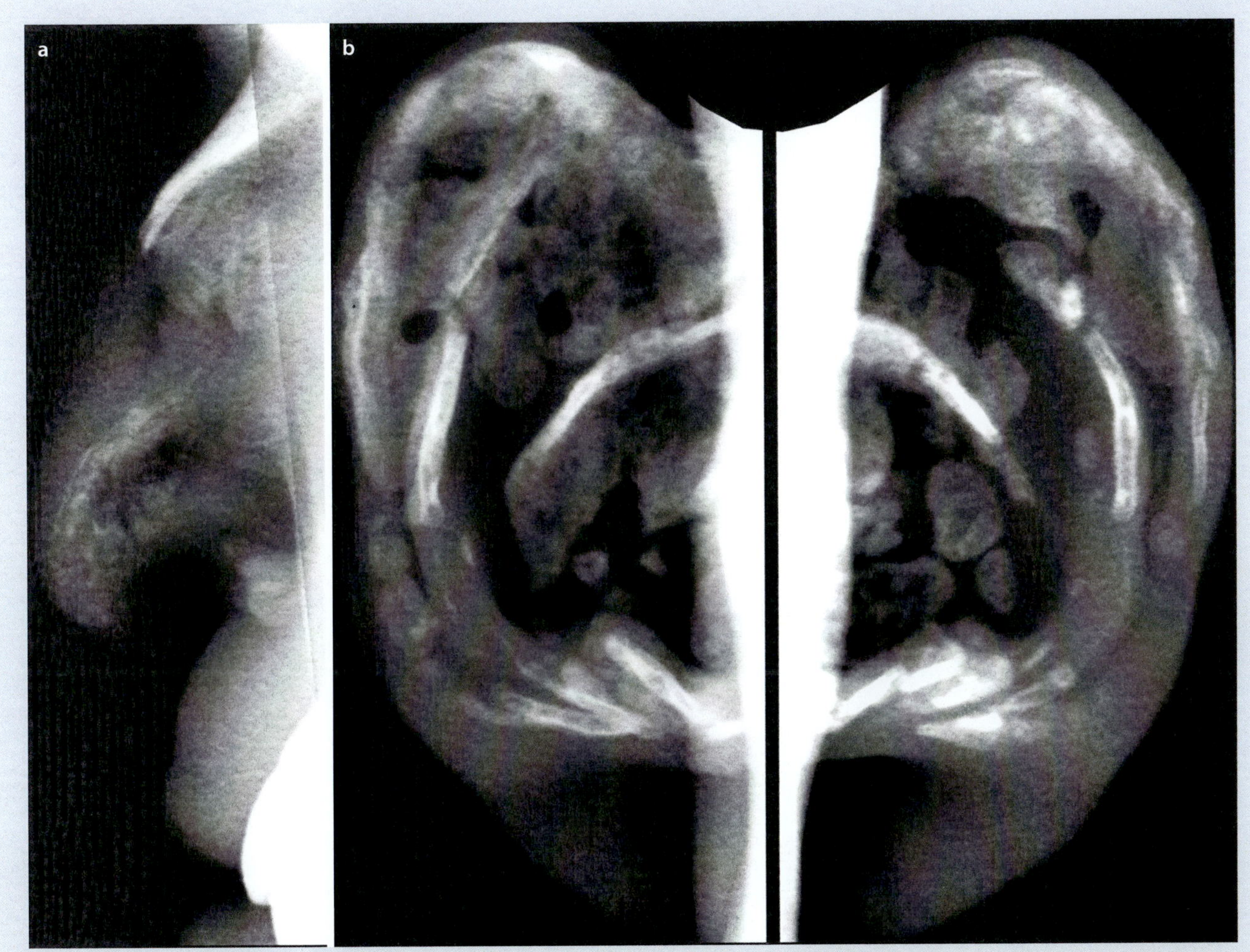

**Fig. 6.12.3**    Plain radiographs of the nose and the ears of a patient with relapsing polychondritis shows the classical feat of calcified ear pinnae bilaterally and the nasal cartilage

#### ▪▪ Signs on US

1. Ear pinna chondritis or perichondritis can be detected by ear pinna US. The ear pinna is a highly specialized structure that serves to collect sound and conduct it to the middle ear. On sonograms, it is possible to distinguish two different zones of the ear pinna: an upper region and a lower region. The anatomic difference is mainly the presence or absence of cartilage inside the layers. The upper region corresponds to the higher two thirds of the ear pinna and consists of three layers: anterior and posterior, each depicted as echoic thin skin layers, and a middle layer containing cartilage, which is represented as a completely hypoechoic regular thin band that follows the different concavities and convexities of the ear pinna (▪ Fig. 6.12.4). The lower region is depicted by the ear lobule, which is a 1-layer structure and consists of only skin because of the absence of cartilage in this area. The normal mean thickness of the hypoechoic cartilage at the antihelix boarder is 0.7–0.9 mm, and the normal mean thickness of the lobule is 6–8 mm. Ear pinna chondritis is detected as thickened, echogenic, and beaded-shaped cartilage. A dissecting fluid collection may be seen, dividing the normally uniform 1-layer hypoechoic cartilage into a 2-layer structure.

2. On musculoskeletal ultrasound, the cartilage surface of the metacarpophalangeal joint, seen as completely hypoechoic circular layer over the metacarpal heads, can show increased signal on power Doppler sonography, reflecting the hyperemia of chondritis (▪ Fig. 6.12.5).

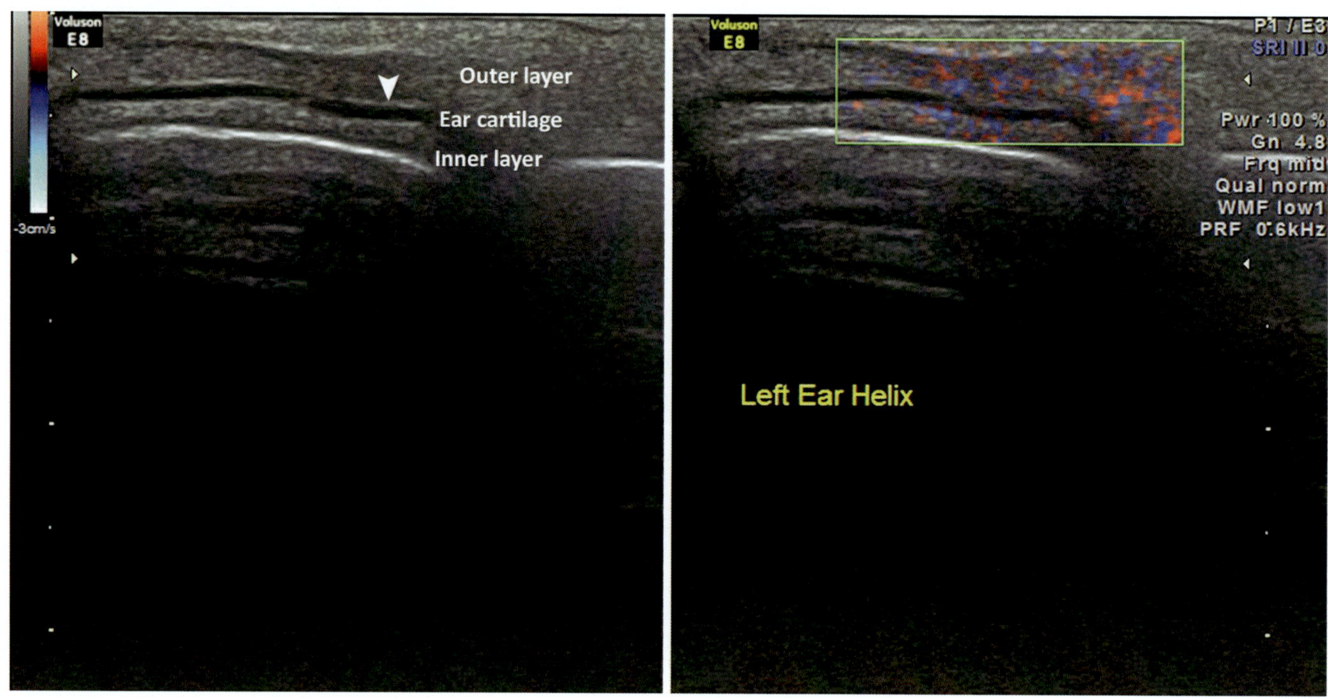


▪ **Fig. 6.12.4**   Ear helix ultrasound image of a patient with relapsing polychondritis that demonstrates the sonographic anatomy of the ear helix with the cartilage layer seen as a hypoechoic layer (*arrowhead*)

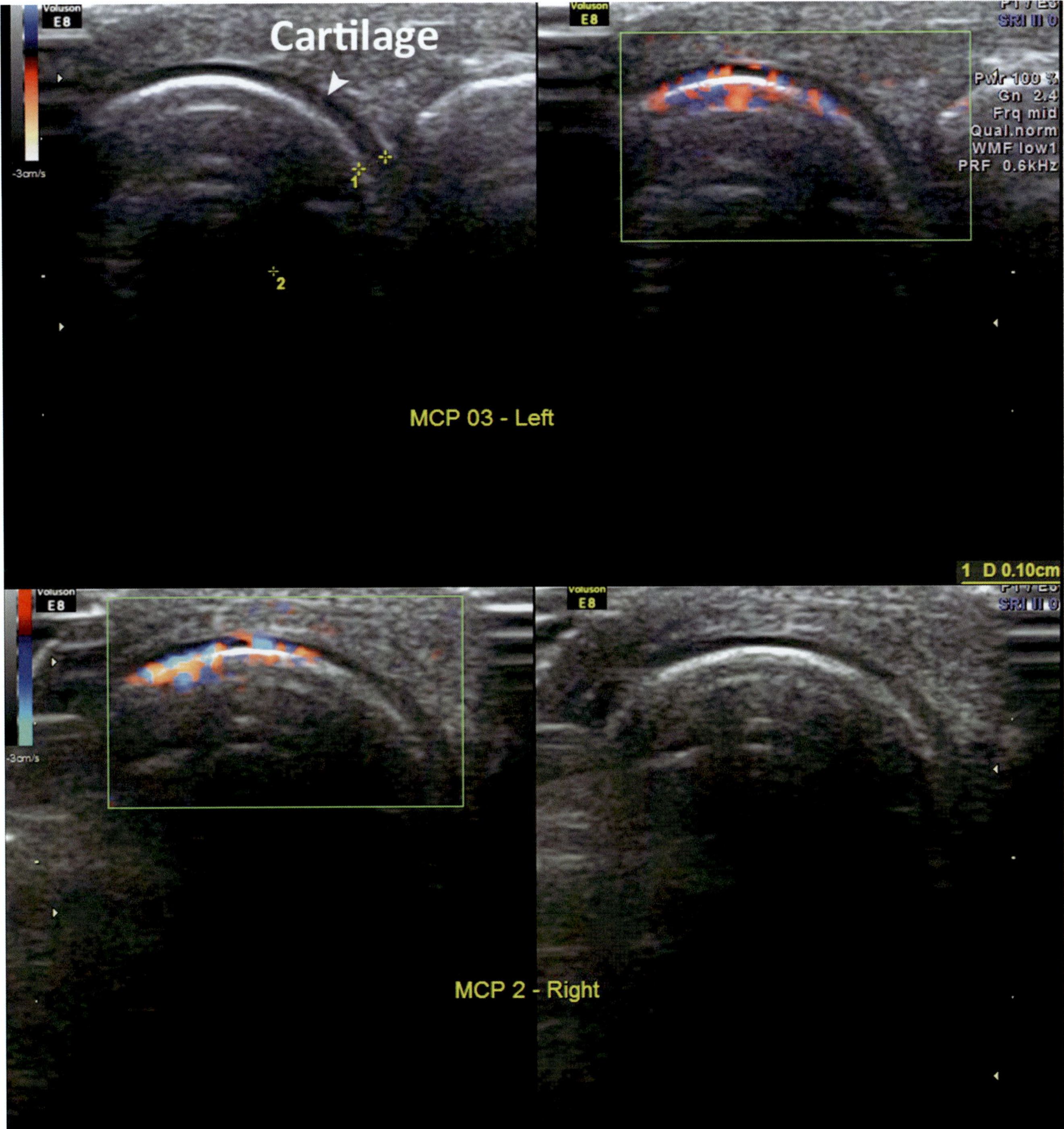


**Fig. 6.12.5** Two musculoskeletal ultrasound images of the metacarpal bones of a patient with relapsing polychondritis demonstrating increase signal of the power Doppler signal of the cartilage over the metacarpal head (*arrowhead*), which denotes inflammation (chondritis)

**Signs on CT and MRI**

1. The same radiographic features of cartilage calcification can be seen on CT images detected in the ear pinnae, nose, and trachea.
2. On MRI, tracheal stenosis with circumferential increased signal intensity, and contrast enhancement is detected when tracheal chondritis is present.
3. Brain MRI, especially angiographic time-to-flight (TOF) images, can show stenotic and beading of the circle of Willis if vasculitis is present (◘ Fig. 6.12.6).

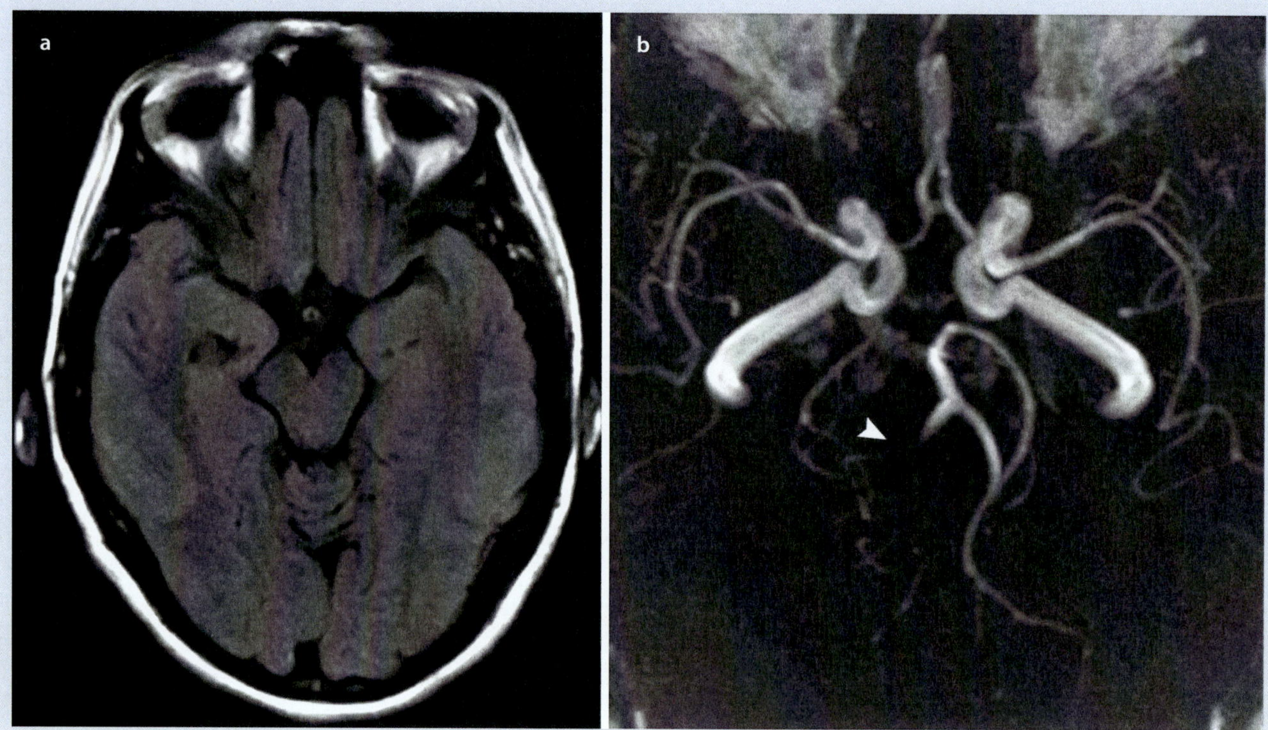

◘ **Fig. 6.12.6**   Axial FLAIR-T2W MR-image (**a**) and TOF MR-image (**b**) of a patient with relapsing polychondritis; the patient presented with severe headache for MR investigation. Although the FLAIR-T2W image shows no brain injury, the TOF image shows stenosis of the right vertebral artery (*arrowhead*)

## Selected References

Ananthakrishna R, et al. Relapsing polychondritis-case series from south India. Clin Rheumatol. 2009;28 Suppl 1:S7–10.

Caceres M, et al. Transverse aortic arch replacement associated with MAGIC Syndrome: case report and literature review. Ann Vasc Surg. 2006;20:395–8.

Coppola M, et al. Relapsing polychondritis: an unusual cause of painful auricular swelling. Ann Emerg Med. 1992;21:81–5.

Fornadly JA, et al. The role of MRI when relapsing polychondritis is suspected but not proven. International Journal of Pediatric Otorhinology. 1995;31:101–7.

Gergely P. Relapsing polychondritis. Best Pract Res Clin Rheumatol. 2004;18(5):723–38.

Giordano M, et al. Relapsing polychondritis with aortic arch aneurysm and aortic arch syndrome. Rheumatol Int. 1984;4:191–3.

Hidalgo-Tenorio C, et al. Magic syndrome and true aortic aneurysm. Clin Rheumatol. 2008;27:115–7.

Irani SR, et al. Relapsing "encephalo" polychondritis. Pract Neurol. 2006;6:372–5.

Kumakiri K, et al. A case of relapsing polychondritis preceded by inner ear involvement. Auris Nasus Larynx. 2005;32:71–6.

Oddone M, et al. Relapsing polychondritis in childhood: a rare observation studied by CT and MRI. Pediatr Radiol. 1992;22:537–8.

Wortsman X, et al. Sonography of the Ear Pinna. Ultrasound Med. 2008;27:761–70.

## 6.13   Reflex Sympathetic Dystrophy

The complex regional pain syndromes (CRPS I and CRPS II), also known as *reflex sympathetic dystrophy (CRPS I)* and *causalgia (CRPS II)*, are diseases characterized by discrete sensory, motor, and autonomic findings. Nerve supply to any limb can be divided into three main neuronal supplies: sensory, motor, and autonomic.

Injury to the sensory supply results in paresthesia and numbness, with complete loss of sensation in extreme irreversible sensory neuronal damage. Injury to the motor neuronal supply results in paraparesis or paralysis depending on the degree of neuronal loss. In contrast to both sensory and motor neuronal injury, autonomic injury results in CRPS I. CRPS I is also called *Sudeck's atrophy* and *hand-shoulder syndrome* in some medical literatures.

CRPS II, or causalgia, is defined as a limb pain that is always preceded by a partial injury to a peripheral nerve or one of its major branches. This syndrome is not always progressive and can persist for years without any clinical changes.

Patients with CRPS I diffuse pain in a limb that affects the autonomic and maybe the motor innervation of that limb (*commonly affecting the upper limbs compared to the lower limbs*).

CRPS I has a female predominance, with a normal age distribution with a peak of 50 years of age. The disease can be suspected and differentiated from other causes of neuropathy by the following typical features:

A. *History of a noxious event preceding the pain*: typically, the pain is preceded by a noxious even such as minor trauma, sprains, bone fractures, surgery (*e.g., carpal tunnel, Dupuytren's contracture*), and other lesions such as shoulder trauma, myocardial infarction, or even contralateral stroke. However, CRPS I is idiopathic in 35 % of cases. CRPS I can be transiently produced in healthy individuals by immobilizing a limb for 1 month.

B. *Exaggerated pain*: the pain is typically disproportionate to the inciting event (*a small trauma not mentioned, followed later by severe limb pain*) and is felt deep within the limb. Pain can be felt even due to water or air exposure, known in the neurological literature as *allodynia*, which is defined as pain that arises due to non-painful stimuli.

The pain is typically described as burning, throbbing, pressing, shooting, or aching. In nearly all cases, the continuous pain is felt deeply inside the distal part of the affected extremity. It always shows a diffuse distribution that is unrelated to territories of individual nerves.

C. *Pain that does not follow a specific dermatom*: The signs and symptoms of CRPS I are not confined to the innervation zone of an individual nerve and show a distally generalized distribution (95 % of cases).

D. *Complain that shows sensory, motor, and autonomic affection*: CRPS I pain has a triad of sensory, motor, and autonomic symptoms that are present in 90 % of cases of CRPS I; however, there appears to be no fixed combinations.

E. *Limb swelling*: typically, the affected limb shows swelling due to loss of the autonomic control of the microvasculature of that limb causing localized vascular shunting at the site of trauma.

F. *Mirror image syndrome*: in CRPS I, the pain extend along the limb or migrates to other body parts in nearly 70 % of patients. The pain becomes bilateral, producing a "mirror image" of pain in up to 50 % of cases. In rare cases, the pain can even encompass the entire body. Mirror-image pain arises from the healthy body region contralateral to the actual site of trauma or inflammation. Mirror-image pain is generally characterized as mechanical allodynia.

CRPS I clinically can be divided into three stages: acute phase, which is marked by pain, edema, warm skin, and increased sweating; dystrophic phase, which is marked by cold, dry skin, and trophic changes; and atrophic phase, which is marked by atrophied skeletal muscles and bones, joint contractures, progressive loss of function, and persistent pain.

**Signs on Plain Radiographs**

Plain radiographs often show a diffuse and spotty distal distribution of demineralization (osteopenia) of small bones with periarticular dominance at the longer bones (◘ Fig. 6.13.1). These radiologic findings (*which are called Sudeck's atrophy*) are generally not evident until the syndrome has been established for several months. The pathophysiological explanation for the bone demineralization is due to the vascular shunting that causes autonomic bone marrow edema and inflammation, which in the end will boost the osteoclastic activity over the osteoblastic one. It should be remembered that the radiographic manifestations of CRPS I means that the patient has been suffering for years without proper therapy.

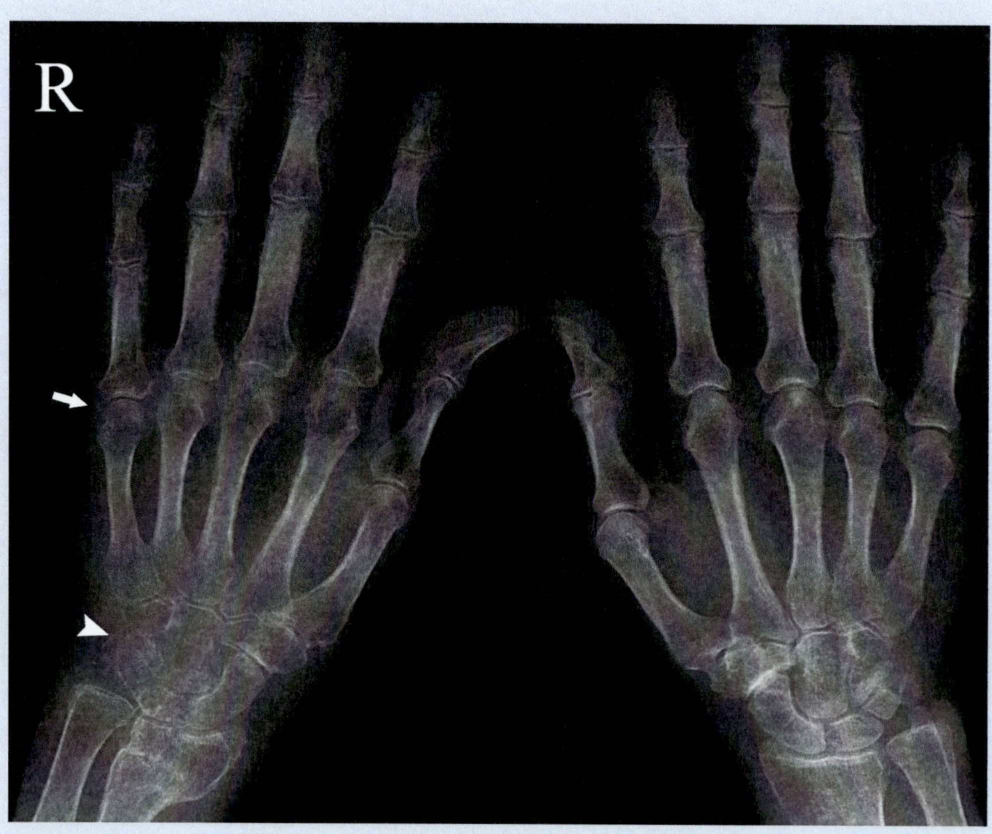



**Fig. 6.13.1**    Plain radiograph of both hands of a patient with CRPS I that shows right-sided, bone osteopenia compared to the left hand that affects the metacarpal heads (*arrow*) and the carpal bones (*arrowhead*), with old fracture of the distal radius

### Signs on Doppler Sonography

1. In the acute phase, arterial Doppler of the arteries in the affected limb above the area of pain (or injury) shows mono- to biphasic waveform spectrum, compatible with the arterial shunting which occurs due to autonomic disturbance (**Fig. 6.13.2**). In comparison, the same artery on the contralateral arm or leg shows normal triphasic waveform spectrum. After treatment, the mono- to biphasic waveform spectrum can return to normal (triphasic).

2. On musculoskeletal US, the affected nerve will show a *hypo*echoic texture (**Fig. 6.13.3**); a normal nerve will show a *hyper*echoic texture due to the fatty nature of the myelin sheath. The hypoechoic texture seen in neuropathies is suggested by the medical literature to be seen due to lipid peroxidation.

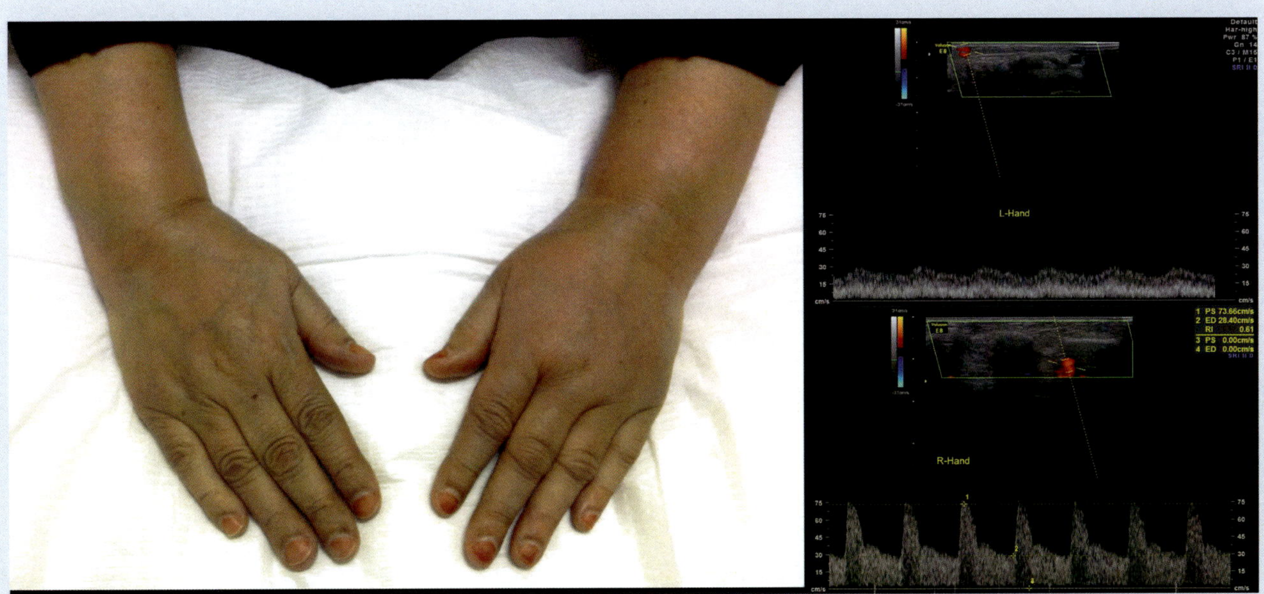

**Fig. 6.13.2** Doppler sonographic images of a 53-year-old female patient presented with 3 months history of left-sided pain and allodynia due to CRPS I. Doppler sonography of the deep palmar arch revealed a classical sign of mild "arteriovenous shunting" in Doppler sonography, detected as a mixture wave pattern that merges the arterial and venous waves together (*upper image*). In comparison, the right-sided Doppler wave sonography (*lower image*) shows biphasic Doppler waveform, not the normal peripheral, arterial triphasic pattern, which denotes a mild arterial shunting present, but not as severe as the left hand (mirror syndrome)

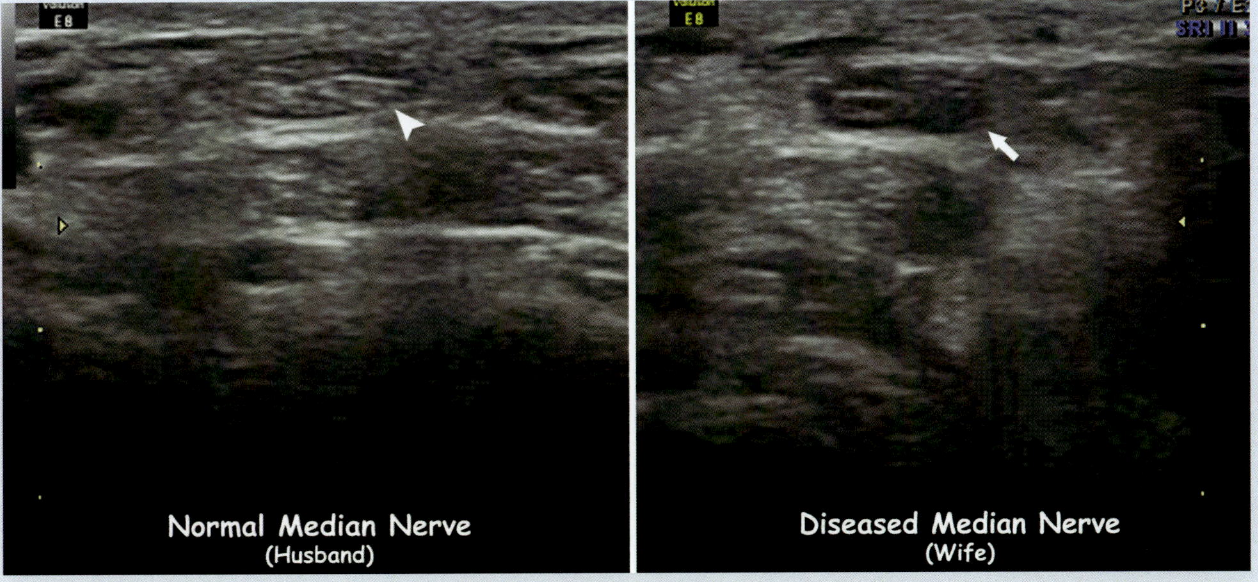


**Fig. 6.13.3** Nerve ultrasound image of a 47-year-old female patient presented with CRPS I for 1-month duration. The median nerve ultrasound showed hypoechoic texture (*arrow*), while her husband's median nerve shows normal iso- to hyperechoic texture (*arrowhead*)

## Signs on MRI

The distal bones of the limb affected by CRPS I can show nonspecific, patchy bone marrow edema; any bone can be affected. In the medical literature, CRPS I commonly affects the hip joint in pregnant women, a condition known as *hip bone marrow edema syndrome*, a variant of CRPS I.

## Selected References

Bennett DS, et al. Complex regional pain syndromes (reflex sympathetic dystrophy and causalgia) and spinal cord stimulation. American Academy of Pain Medicine. 2006;7:S64–96.

Crozier F, et al. Magnetic resonance imaging in reflex sympathetic dystrophy syndrome of the foot. Joint Bone Spine. 2003;70:503–8.

Oyen WJG, et al. Reflex sympathetic dystrophy of the hand: an excessive inflammatory response? Pain. 1993;55:151–7.

Pekindil G, et al. Doppler sonographic assessment of post-traumatic reflex sympathetic dystrophy. J Ultrasound Med. 2003;22:395–402.

## 6.14  Polymyalgia Rheumatica

Polymyalgia rheumatica (PR) is an inflammatory condition with unknown origin characterized by morning stiffness and aching sensation in the cervical region, shoulder, and pelvic girdles. It has been considered in the past as a variant manifestation of giant cell arteritis, until it has been redefined by Bird et al. (1979) as a separate rheumatic entity. Although PMR is considered a disease of unknown origin, it has been found to have a close concurrence with some infections like *Mycoplasma pneumonia*, *Chlamydia pneumonia*, and parvovirus B19.

The diagnostic criteria of PR include (*according to Healey; 1984*):

(a) Bilateral pain persisting for at least one month and involving one of the following areas: neck, shoulders, and pelvic girdles.

(b) Morning stiffness lasting more than one hour.

(c) Rapid response to low-dose steroid (10–15 mg in the morning).

(d) Absence of other diseases explains the current symptoms.

(e) Age more than 50 years.

(f) Erythrocytes sedimentation rate and C-reactive protein serum levels are raised.

(g) Ultrasonographic features of bursitis and/or synovitis in the shoulder and/or hip joints.

Patients with PR present with bilateral discomfort in the upper limbs that interfere with the daily activities. The pain in the shoulder and pelvic girdles often radiates to the elbows and the knees. Symmetric peripheral arthritis affecting the knees and wrists, carpal tunnel syndrome, and pitting edema of the dorsum of the hands may be seen (☐ Fig. 6.14.1). Due to the absence of specific laboratory serological tests for this condition, radiological investigations are important to assist in investigating the clinical diagnostic criteria.

### ■ Unusual Presentations of Polymyalgia Rheumatica

1. *Peripheral joint synovitis*: affecting typically the shoulder and the hip joints, symmetrically or asymmetrically.

2. *Sternoclavicular synovitis*: the sternoclavicular joint is not usually affected in inflammatory diseases, but it is sometimes involved in polymyalgia rheumatica.

3. *Distal swelling with pitting edema*: another unusual syndrome is known as RS3PE (*remitting seronegative symmetrical synovitis with pitting edema*).

4. *Aortic dissection*: due to giant cell aortitis.

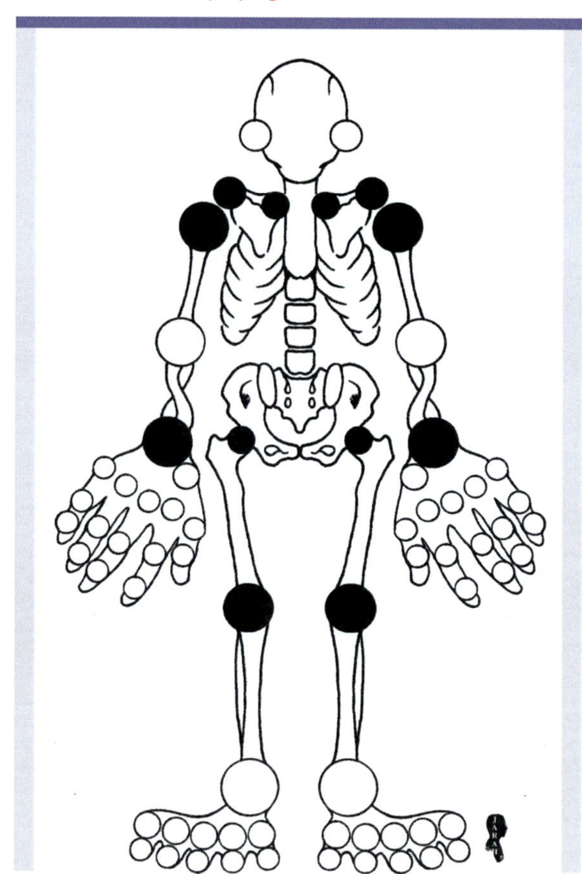


☐ **Fig. 6.14.1**   An illustration that demonstrates the body's geographic distribution of polymyalgia rheumatica arthropathy

## Signs on US

Shoulder US shows hip effusion (68 %), shoulder subacromial bursa fluid collection (96 %), and biceps tendon tenosynovitis with peritendinous fluid collection (Figs. 6.14.2 and 6.14.3), all attributed to bursitis and/or synovitis of these joints

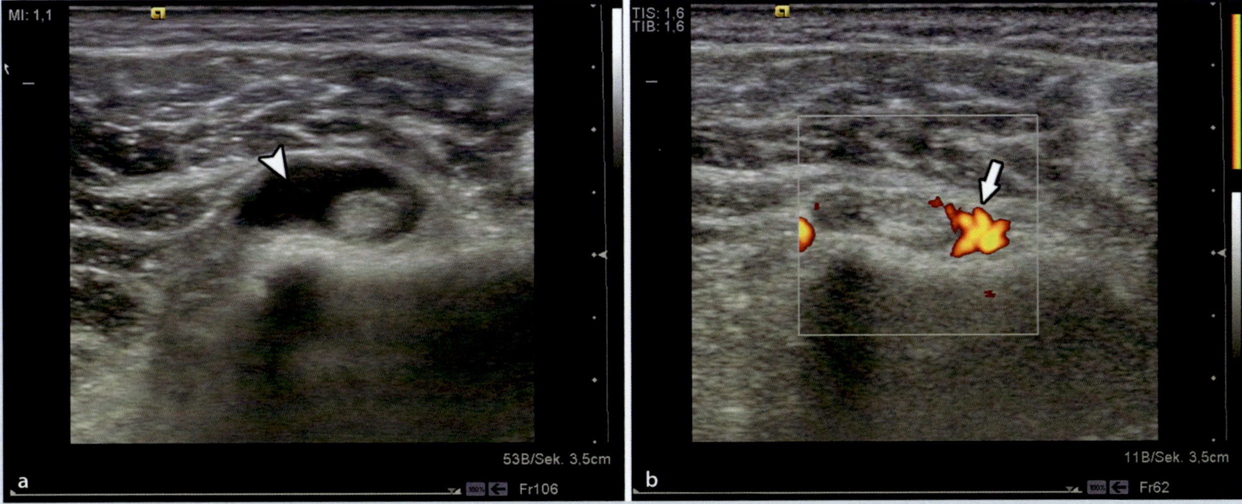

**Fig. 6.14.2** Musculoskeletal sonographic images of the right shoulder of a patient with polymyalgia rheumatic showing fluid collection around the long head of biceps tendon (*arrowhead* in **a**), associated with hyperemia seen as increased power Doppler signal (*arrow* in **b**); the findings reflects tenosynovitis

## Signs on MRI

1. Shoulder MRI may show subdeltoid and subacromial bursitis, and biceps tendon tenosynovitis. Tenosynovitis is seen as an enlarged tendon with free fluid surrounding it due to inflammation and edema.
2. Subacromial bursitis is seen as free fluid located above the supraspinatus tendon with *intact* supraspinatus tendon (no signs of tears or tendinosis).
3. Hands and wrists tenosynovitis may be seen as abnormal tendon signal intensity on T2W images with surrounding free fluid.
4. A patient with chest pain should be investigated for aortic dissection.

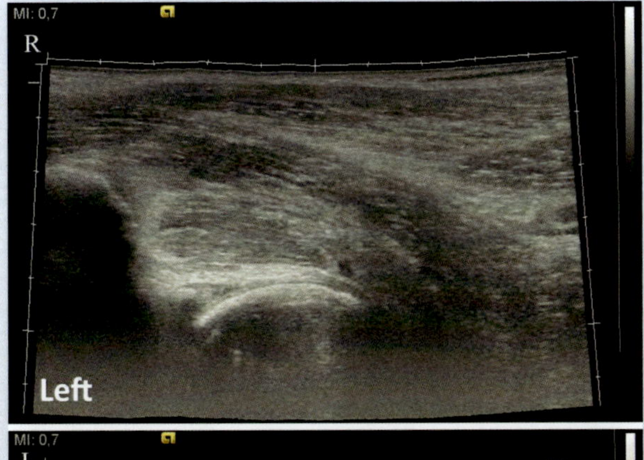

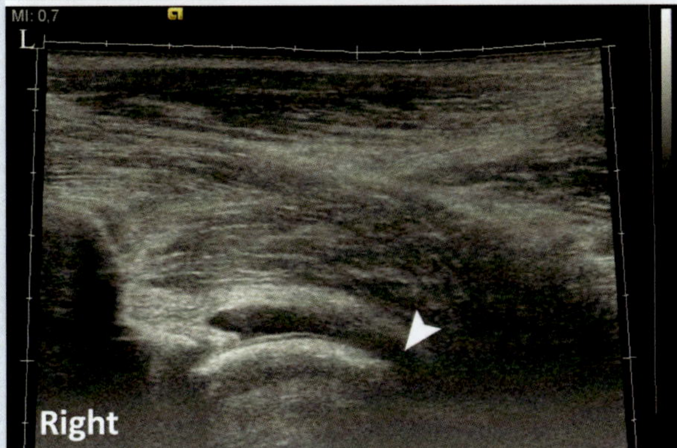

**Fig. 6.14.3** Musculoskeletal, panoramic sonographic images of the same patient in Fig. 6.14.2 showing fluid collection around the iliopsoas tendon at the right hip (*arrowhead*), reflecting iliopsoas bursitis

## Selected References

Mandell B. Polymyalgia rheumatic: clinical presentation is key diagnosis and treatment. Cleve Clin J Med. 2004;71(6):489–95.

Salvarani C, et al. Polymyalgia rheumatica and giant-cell arteritis. N Engl J Med. 2002;347:261–71.

Salvarani C, et al. Polymyalgia rheumatica. Best Pract Res Clin Rheumatol. 2004;18(5):705–22.

Soriano A, et al. Polymyalgia rheumatica in 2011. Best Pract Res Clin Rheumatol. 2012;26(1):91–104.

## 6.15   Systemic Lupus Erythematosus

Systemic lupus erythematosus (SLE) is a chronic, inflammatory, autoimmune systemic disorder of unknown origin characterized by the formation of autoantibodies that attack multiple organs. SLE has a female predominance, with periods of flares and remissions. SLE antibodies can be categorized into categories:

1. *Antibodies against nuclei (antinuclear antibodies)*: anti-DNA histone, anti-double-stranded DNA (dsDNA), and anti-single-stranded DNA antibodies
2. *Antibodies against cytoplasmic components*: mitochondrial and microsomal antibodies
3. *Organ-specific antibodies*: e.g., antithyroid antibodies
4. *Others*: rheumatoid factor (50 % of cases), cryoglobulins, and antiphospholipid antibodies

SLE pathology is characterized by widespread of vasculitis, affecting capillaries, arterioles, and venules. SLE can be localized to the skin without systemic manifestations (*chronic cutaneous lupus*), self-limiting due to certain medications (*drug-induced lupus*), and affecting neonates due to maternal anti-Rho antibodies crossing the placenta (*neonatal lupus*). SLE can be triggered by endogenous factors (e.g., sex hormones) or exogenous factors (e.g., sunlight exposure). Drugs that induce lupus-like reaction include alpha interferon and hydralazine.

Serological characteristics of SLE include high serum levels of antinuclear antibody (ANA), anti-double-strand DNA (anti-dsDNA), rheumatoid factor, and antiphospholipid antibodies. Patients with SLE have ANA-positive results in 95 % of cases. However, positive ANA results are not specific to SLE and can be seen in normal individuals > 65 years of age (15 %) at low titers, patients with Sjögren's syndrome, patients with scleroderma, and patients with autoimmune thyroid disease.

*Manifestations of SLE include (diagnosis is confirmed by fulfilling at least four systemic manifestations with positive serological tests)*:

1. *Cutaneous SLE*: this includes malar rash, photosensitivity, and discoid lupus
2. *Cardiopulmonary SLE*: this is seen mostly in the form of pleuritis, pericarditis, bilateral pleural effusion, and uncommonly noninfective (Libman–Sacks) endocarditis.
3. *Renal SLE*: these are ranges from mild asymptomatic proteinuria to rapidly progressing glomerulonephritis associated with end-stage renal disease. The main injury of the kidneys in SLE is related to glomerular lesions with or without injury to the tubules and interstitium. Rarely, isolated tubulointerstitial changes can be encountered in the presence of minimal glomerular abnormalities in SLE or so-called predominant tubulointerstitial lupus nephritis.
4. *Neuropsychiatric manifestations of SLE*: these manifestations include headaches, dementia, seizures (focal or diffuse), and psychoses.
5. *Pulmonary SLE*: this includes unilateral or bilateral pleural effusions, reticular interstitial lung disease, pleural thickening, alveolar lung disease, and shrinking lung syndrome. *Shrinking lung syndrome* (SLS) is a rare complication of SLE with unknown origin characterized by unexplained progressive dyspnea, pleuritic chest pain, fever, dry cough, small lung volumes, elevation of the diaphragm, and restrictive physiology on pulmonary function tests. It is suggested that SLS is caused by myositis of the diaphragm, phrenic nerve paresis, restrictive rib cage abnormality of unknown pathology, or pleural adhesions.
6. *Other systemic manifestations of SLE*: fever and anemia. There is increased frequency of midtrimester abortions (15 %), prematurity (20 %), and stillbirth (10 %) in pregnant women with SLE flares.
7. *Skeletal rheumatological manifestations of SLE include*:

I.   *Lupus arthritis*: arthritis affects 69–95 % of SLE patients in the form of symmetric, nonerosive polyarthritis that preferentially involves the small joints over the large joints, although any joint may be affected. The most common joints affected are the hand joints including the metacarpal phalangeal (MCP), proximal interphalangeal (PIP), and distal interphalangeal (DIP) as well as the knees (Fig. 6.15.1). Shoulders, ankles, and elbows are less commonly affected but can be involved. Swelling of the joints or synovial proliferation can be present, although the swelling is often not as prominent as it is with rheumatoid arthritis (RA). Other signs include morning stiffness, arthralgia, and joint erythema.

II.  *Sacroiliitis*: although sacroiliitis is typically thought of as a manifestation of the seronegative spondyloarthropathies, it has been reported in SLE in up to 50 % of cases.

III. *Atlantoaxial subluxation*: it is seen in 8.5 % of SLE patients, especially patients with Jaccoud's arthropathy.

IV.  *Deforming arthropathy (Jaccoud's arthritis)*: this is an uncommon form of deforming arthritis characterized by ligament laxity, joints deformity, which may be associated with joints erosions (◘ Fig. 6.15.2). It affects 3–13 % of SLE patients and is associated with high serum titers of anti-RNP antibodies. Jaccoud's

**SLE arthritis**

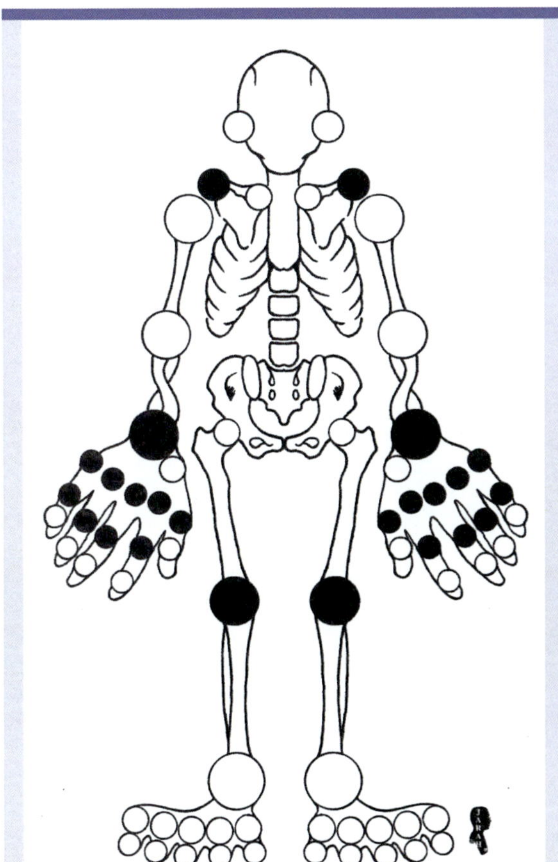



**Fig. 6.15.1** An illustration that demonstrates the body's geographic distribution of SLE arthropathy

**Jaccoud's arthropathy**

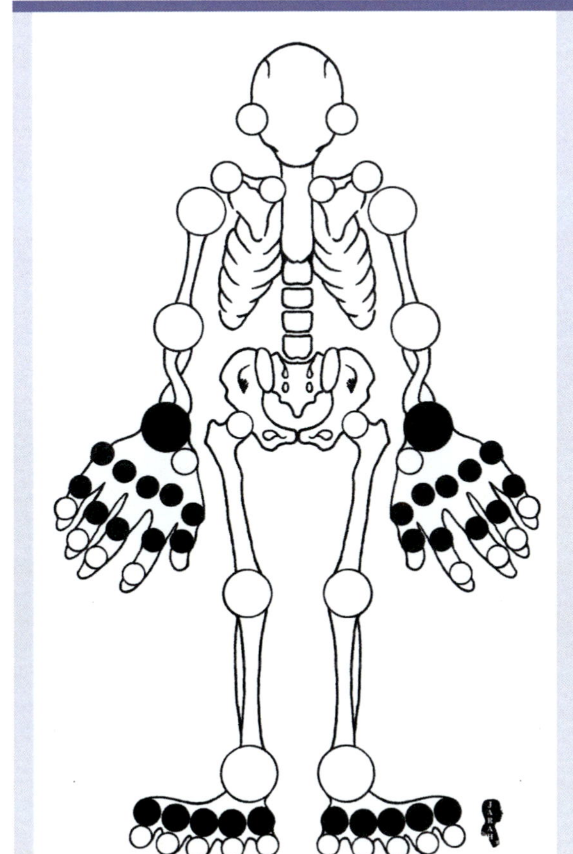



**Fig. 6.15.2** An illustration that demonstrates the body's geographic distribution of Jaccoud's arthropathy

arthropathy is not specific for SLE and can be seen on other conditions including scleroderma and dermatomyositis.

V. *Erosive arthritis (rhupus)*: SLE arthritis is typically nonerosive. However, erosive SLE arthritis can be seen in cases of SLE/RA overlap, also known as (rhupus). Rhupus has an incidence of 0.01–2 % of SLE patients and has been associated with high serum titers of anti-CCP and anti-RA33 antibodies in some studies.

VI. *Synovitis and tenosynovitis*: they are seen in up to 44 % of SLE patients typically symmetrical in distribution. Tendon rupture is a rare complication of SLE. The tendons that are more commonly involved include the Achilles, patellar, infrapatellar tendons, and tendons in the hand.

VII. *Avascular necrosis and bone infarction*: it is commonly seen in SLE patients who show high serum titers of antiphospholipid antibodies, especially in the femoral head.

VIII. *Others*: periarticular osteoporosis, acral sclerosis, soft-tissue calcification (calcinosis), and cystic bone lesions.

## Differential Diagnoses and Related Diseases

### ■ ■ Brown's Syndrome

Brown's syndrome is a disease characterized by intermittent diplopia due to congenital or acquired motility impairment of the superior oblique muscle. The disease is believed to be secondary to restriction of the superior oblique muscle in the trochlea/tendon complex, causing tethering of the muscle when the eye is adducted. Acquired Brown syndrome can be caused by paranasal sinuses infections, trauma, orbital inflammation, rheumatoid arthritis stenosing synovitis, SLE, scleroderma, and rarely psoriasis. Acquired Brown syndrome usually responds to corticosteroids therapy, especially when inflammation or systemic connective tissue disorders are the cause. Patients are presenting with intermittent diplopia when gazing upward, and the disease is characterized by inability to actively or passively elevate the affected eye in full adduction. Other features include widened palpebral fissure on adduction and divergence on midline eye elevation.

### Signs on Plain Radiographs

1. Pleura effusion unilaterally or bilaterally can be seen in SLE patients in 26 % of cases.
2. Cardiomegaly may be seen due to pericardial effusion (15 % of cases).
3. In *shrinking lung syndrome*, typically, chest radiographs will show elevated hemidiaphragms, with blunting of the costophrenic angles and platelike atelectasis at the lower lobes bilaterally.
4. *Femoral head avascular necrosis* is seen on radiographs with different signs depending on the stage: *stage I (normal X-rays), stage II (sclerotic or cystic lesions without fracture), stage III (crescent sign indicative of subchondral collapse),* and *stage IV (further progression with osteoarthritis and acetabular changes).*
5. *Jaccoud's arthropathy* is seen on radiographs as ulnar deviation, subluxation of the MCP, PIP and DIP joints, swan-neck deformities of fingers, localized osteoporosis, and absence of juxta-articular erosions (◗ Fig. 6.15.3).

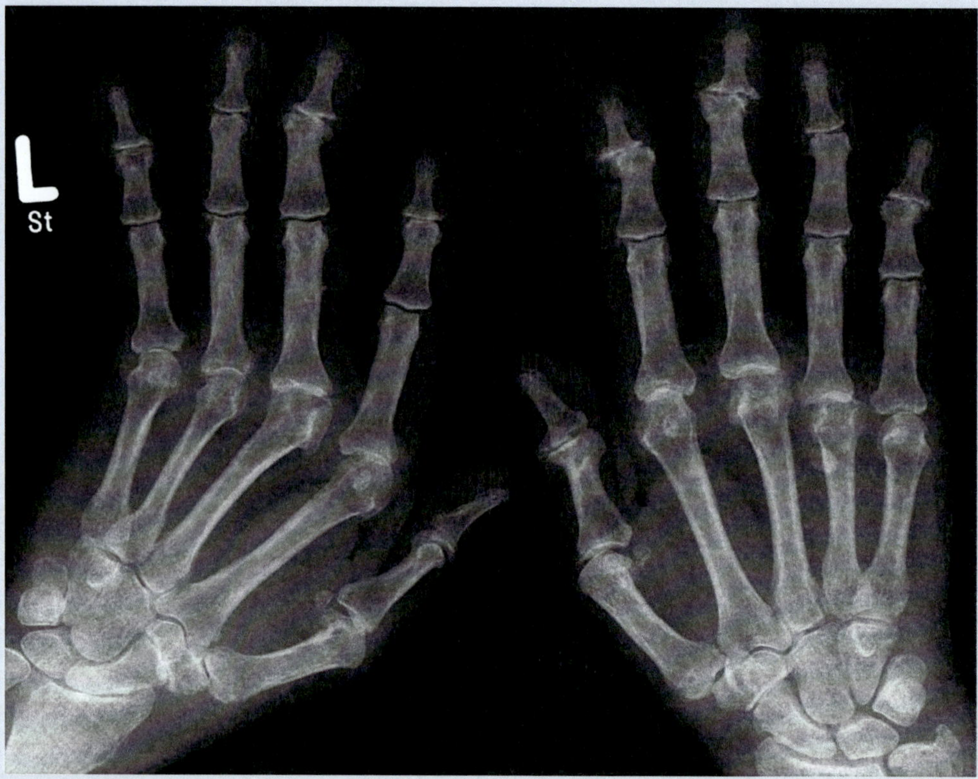

◗ **Fig. 6.15.3**    Plain radiography of the hands of a patient with Jaccoud's arthropathy that demonstrates diffuse subluxation deformities without bone erosions

### Signs on PD Sonography

1. Power Doppler (PD) sonography can differentiate between primary or secondary Raynaud's phenomenon in the fingers or toes. The patient is examined first by PD with the probe to gain the baseline images. The region of interest is examined; then, the patient is asked to place their fingers into cold water (7 °C) for 3 min, and then the region of interest is reexamined again with PD sonography. Primary Raynaud's phenomenon will show moderate to mark hyperemia with red-to-orange (PD) signal in the normal temperature and then show reduced PD signal after the cold challenge. In contrast, secondary Raynaud's phenomenon will almost always show reduced hyperemia with red-to-orange (PD) signal before and after cold challenge.

## Signs on CT

1. Retroperitoneal lymphadenopathy with lymph nodes > 15 mm in diameter (64 % of cases).
2. The kidneys may be enlarged due to nephrotic syndrome or shrunken due to long-term disease. Spontaneous subcapsular hematomas may occur and seen as renal masses with high attenuation values on noncontrast-enhanced scan (38–64 HU). Predominant tubulointerstitial lupus nephritis shows bilateral, multiple, wedge-shaped areas or streaky zones of low enhancement that extend from the papilla to the renal cortex with or without slight cortical atrophy. This CT sign is nonspecific to SLE predominant tubulointerstitial lupus nephritis, but is a common sign observed in tubulointerstitial nephritis for any cause.
3. Hepatosplenomegaly may be seen, especially with lymphadenopathy (11 % of cases).
4. Diffuse bladder wall thickening can be seen; however, exclusion of infectious cystitis is necessary.
5. Venous thrombosis may be seen, affecting the IVC or the femoral veins.
6. *Abscesses* may be seen within the pancreas (difficult to differentiate from pseudocyst), liver, small bowel, spleen, and kidneys. An abscess is seen as a cystic lesion with thick wall that enhances after contrast injection, with maybe intracystic air (*pathognomonic*).
7. *Infarctions* may occur within the intestine or the kidneys. Intestinal infarction shows bowel wall thickening with gas within the wall (pneumatosis intestinalis). In the kidneys, there is a wedge-shaped area that does not enhance after contrast injection. Differentiating focal pyelonephritis from renal infarction is difficult since both show the same radiological features; however, an enhancing rim around the low-density wedge may be seen in 46 % of renal infarctions, a feature that is not seen in pyelonephritis.
8. Pancreatitis may be seen due to steroid treatment, a common therapy for SLE.

9. Pulmonary manifestations include ground-glass alveolar opacities, pleural thickening, pleural effusion, and/or reticular interstitial patterns. In shrinking lung syndrome, the chest shows pleural thickening involving the diaphragmatic pleura bilaterally with an otherwise normal lung parenchyma.
10. In acquired Brown's syndrome, there is thickening of the superior oblique tendon of the affected eye compared to the normal side. Signs of inflammation and contrast enhancement affecting the trochlea/tendon complex may be seen in cases of inflammation or synovitis.

## Signs on MRI

1. Cortical hyperintensity lesions in the brain MRI may be seen on T2W and DW images due to thrombotic cerebral infarction. Multiples stroke episodes can be seen in SLE due to hypercoagulability especially when SLE is associated with positive anticardiolipin antibodies or due to embolic events related to Libman–Sacks endocarditis (■ Figs. 6.15.4 and 6.15.5).
2. *Acute lupus encephalopathy* is seen as reversible lacy areas of hyperintensity in cortical gray matter and subcortical white matter, particularly in occipital, temporal, and parietal lobes on T2 and FLAIR images. Long-standing neuro-SLE cerebral disease can show poroencephalic cysts formation due to old brain infarctions, diffuse brain atrophy, and/or intracranial hemorrhages due to SLE vasculitis affecting the circle of Willis (■ Figs. 6.15.6 and 6.15.7).
3. Cerebral calcinosis (*Fahr's disease*) has been reported to occur uncommonly as a severe, rare manifestation of neuropsychiatric SLE. Fahr's disease is seen as extensive calcification in the thalamus, putamen, caudate nucleus, white matter, and posterior gray matter.
4. In lupus arthritis, the MRI findings in the hand, including tenosynovitis, were nearly indistinguishable from early RA except that RA patients had more bone marrow edema of the MCP joints and more abnormalities of the right fourth extensor tendon.

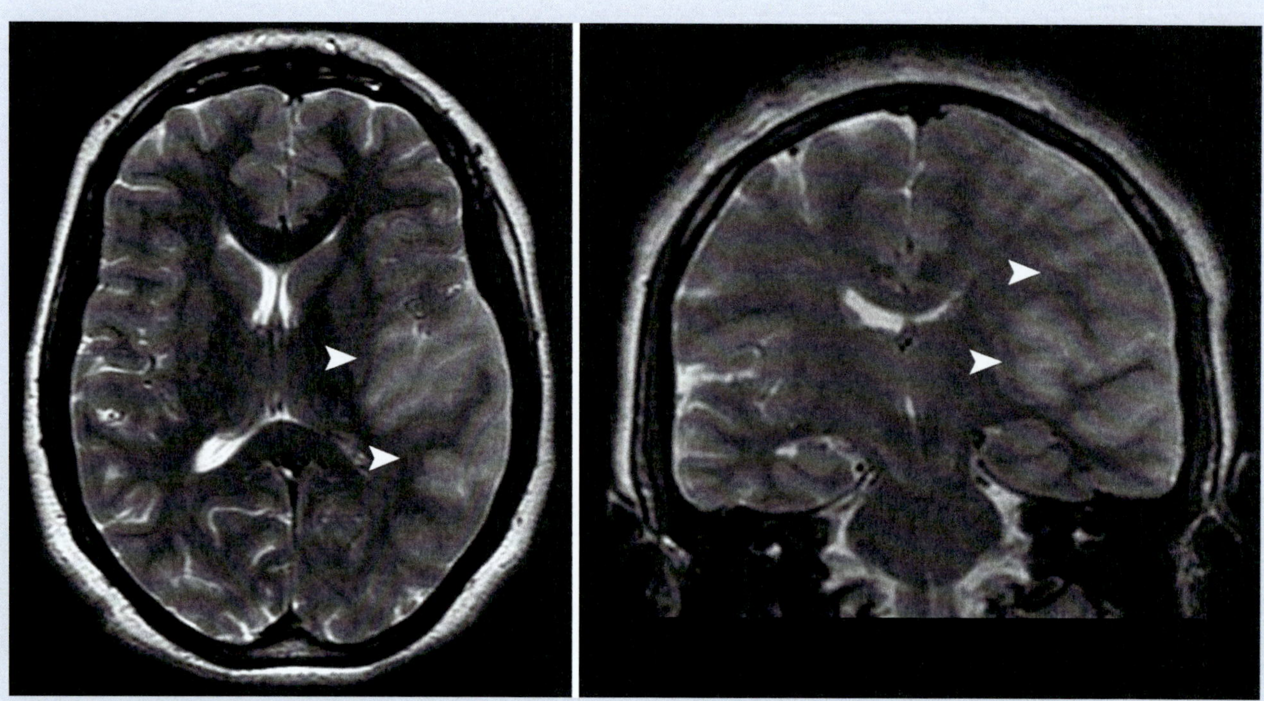

**Fig. 6.15.4** Axial and coronal T2W-MR images of a patient with neuro-SLE show infarction of the left hemisphere seen as hyperintense cortices at the parietotemporal regions (*arrowhead*)

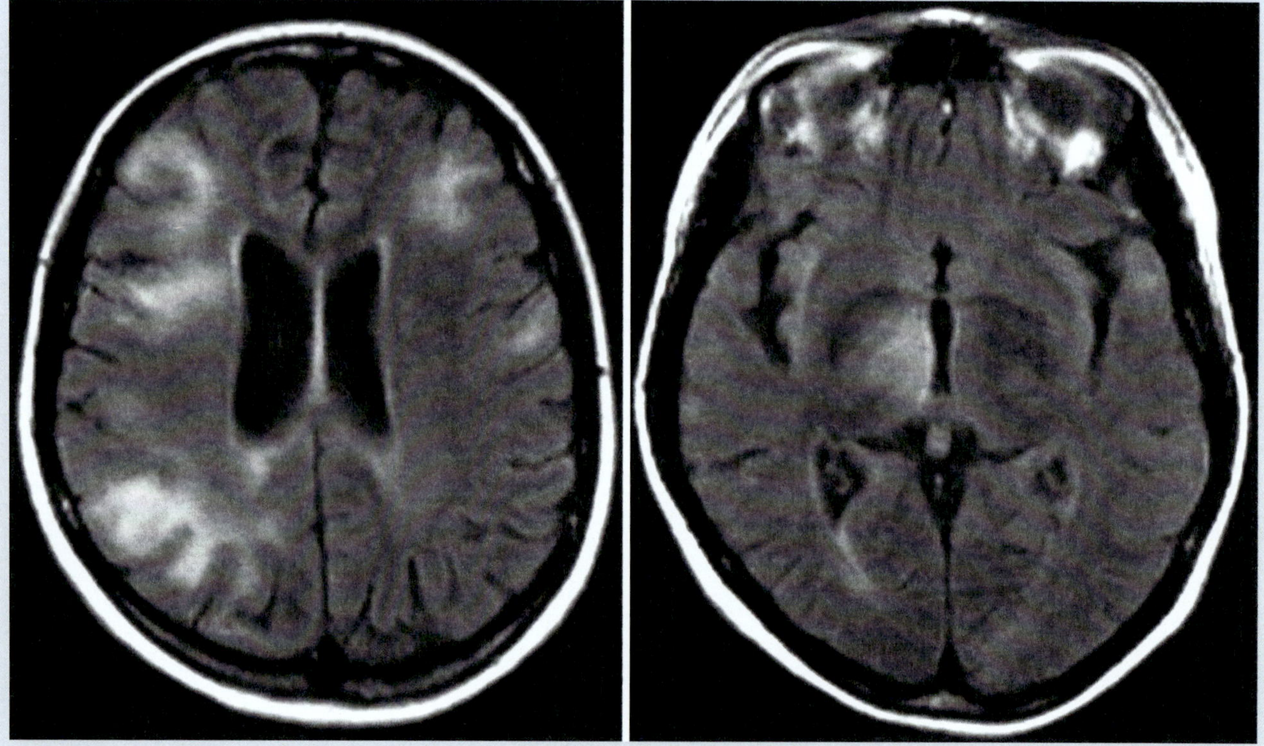

**Fig. 6.15.5** Axial and coronal FLAIR-T2W-MR images of a patient with neuro-SLE show ischemic, vasculitis insults to the brain seen as diffuse lesions affecting both hemispheres in the white matter's U-fibers and even including the right thalamus

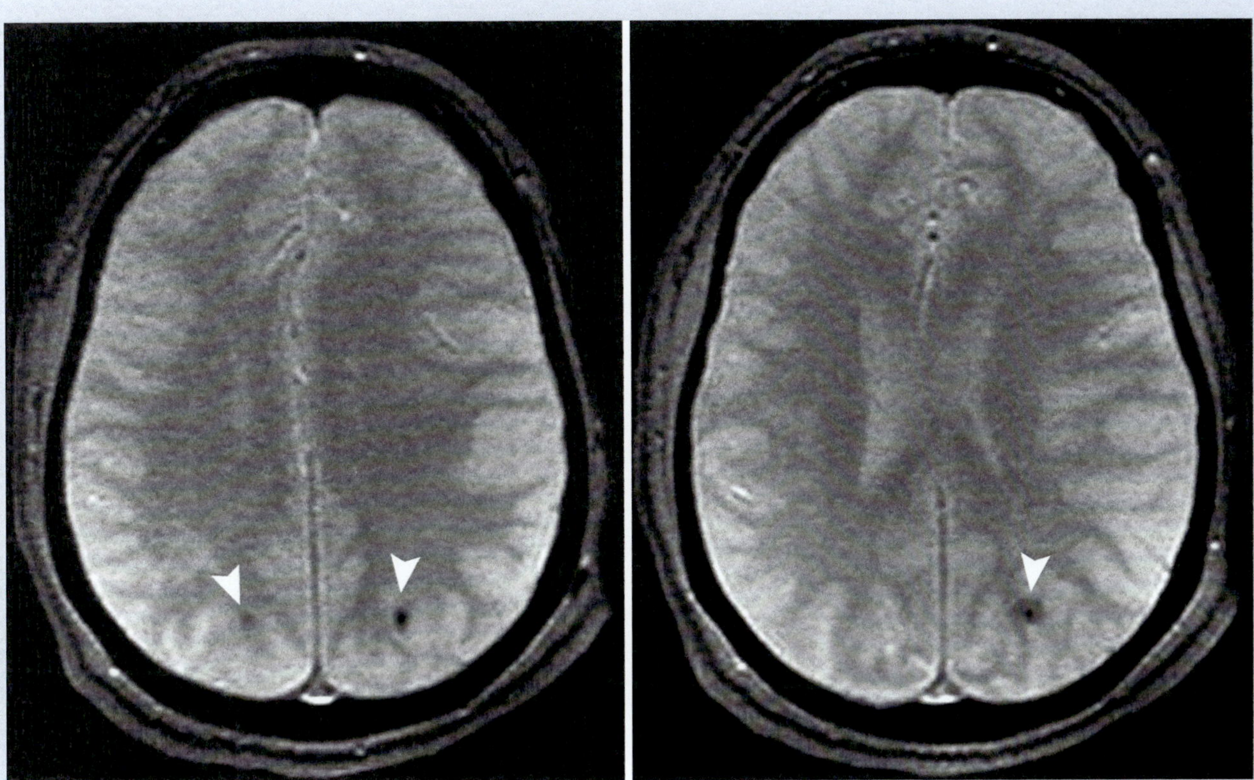

**Fig. 6.15.6** Axial gradient-T*MR images of a patient with neuro-SLE show multiple microbleedings (arrowheads) detected as hypointense foci in the occipital lobes bilaterally

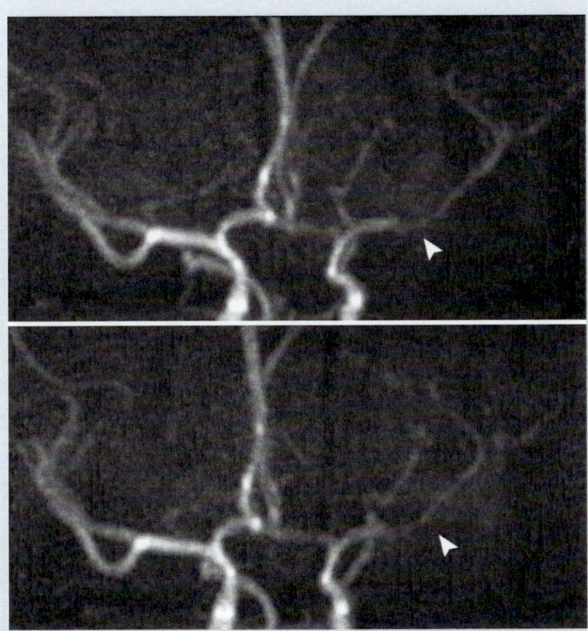

**Fig. 6.15.7** Time-to-flight (TOF) MR images of the same patient in Fig. 6.15.6 showing left-sided beading of the internal carotid artery (M2–M3) segments due to long-standing neurovasculitis (*arrowheads*)

## Selected References

Gezer A, et al. Bilateral acquired Brown syndrome in systemic scleroderma. J AAPOS. 2005;9:195–7.

Grossman JM, et al. Lupus arthritis. Best Pract Res Clin Rheumatol. 2009;23:495–506.

Heiberg E, et al. Body computed tomography findings in systemic lupus erythematosus. Journal of Computed Tomography. 1988;12:68–74.

Kakati S, et al. A clinical study of pulmonary manifestations in systemic lupus erythematosus with special reference to CT findings. Indian Journal of Rheumatology. 2007;2(4):133–6.

Kamishima T, et al. Predominant tubulointerstitial nephritis in a patient with systemic lupus erythematosus with an emphasis on CT and MR imaging findings. European Journal of Radiology Extra. 2009;72:e87–90.

Lee SI, et al. The usefulness of power Doppler sonography in differentiating primary from secondary Raynaud's phenomenon. Clin Rheumatol. 2006;25:814–8.

Mafee MF, et al. Computed tomography in the evaluation of Brown syndrome of the superior oblique tendon sheath. Radiology. 1985;154:691–5.

Rodnan GP, et al. Systemic lupus erythematosus. Dis Mon. 1964;10(8):1–38.

Sibbitt Jr WL, et al. Magnetic resonance imaging and brain histopathology in neuropsychiatric systemic lupus erythematosus. Semin Arthritis Rheum. 2010;40:32–52.

Sp T, et al. Association of the shrinking lung syndrome in systemic lupus erythematosus with pleurisy: A systematic review. Semin Arthritis Rheum. 2008;39:30–7.

Wilson ME, et al. Brown's syndrome. Surv Ophthalmol. 1989;34:153–72.

# Pulmonology



© Springer International Publishing Switzerland 2017
J.A. Al-Tubaikh, *Internal Medicine*, DOI 10.1007/978-3-319-39747-4_7

## 7.1    Pleural Diseases

The pleura are composed of two layers, parietal and visceral layers, separated by a pleural space. The parietal pleuron is supplied by systemic vessels and drains into the right atrium via the azygos, hemiazygos, and internal mammary veins. The visceral pleuron is supplied by bronchial and pulmonary vessels and drains into the pulmonary veins.

The pleural space normally contains interstitial fluid (1–5 mL) that is cleared by the parietal pleural lymphatic vessels. There is no direct communication between the visceral pleura lymphatics and the pleural space.

The pleura appear normally on radiographs only when the X-ray beam is tangentially set on the film. On radiographs, the pleura appear as fissures and junctional lines. Fissures are made up of two layers of visceral pleura. The normal parietal pleuron is never visualized on posteroanterior (PA) radiographs.

Different pathological conditions affecting the pleura can be diagnosed with confidence by PA chest radiographs alone. This topic discusses the main pathological pleural conditions with their typical radiologic manifestations.

### Pleural Effusion

*Pleural effusion* is a condition characterized by abnormal fluid collection between the parietal and visceral pleura (excess pleural space fluid). The pleural fluid can be *water* (edematous effusion), *blood* (hemothorax), *pus* (empyema), *tumor cells* (malignant pleural effusion), or *lymph* (chylothorax).

Pathologically, pleural effusion is divided into serous or exudative according to the protein content after lab analysis. *Serous plural effusion* contains little protein content (<2.5 g/dL) and usually arises due to systemic disease like cardiac failure, nephrotic syndrome, or liver failure. *Exudative pleural effusion* contains high protein count (>2.5 g/dL) and usually arises due to inflammatory or infectious process like tuberculosis, malignancy, and acute pancreatitis.

Disruption of the thoracic duct due to lymphoma or a tumor can cause lymphatic blockage and leakage into the pleural space causing chylothorax. Malignant effusion typically results from metastasizing of the malignant cells into the pleural cavity via the parietal pleura lymphatics, and it is often massive.

*Bronchopleural fistula* is a condition characterized by opening of a bronchus into the pleural space. It can develop occasionally following thoracic surgery, infection, medical intervention, or malignancy. Bronchopleural fistula is seen in 2–3 % of postpneumonectomy cases.



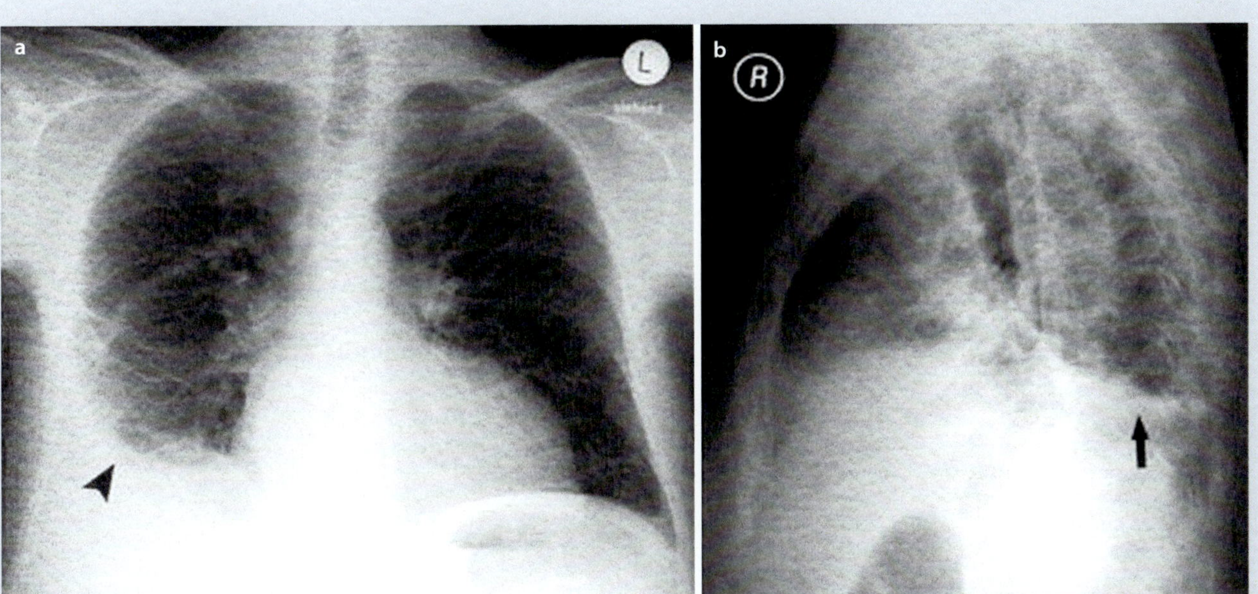

**Fig. 7.1.1** Posteroanterior (**a**) and lateral (**b**) chest radiographs in two different patients with pleural effusion show meniscus sign with right pleural effusion obliterating the lateral costophrenic angle (*arrowhead*) in (**a**) and pleural effusion obliterating the posterior costophrenic angle in (**b**) (*arrow*)

200 mL is necessary to obliterate the lateral costophrenic angle.

- *Subpulmonic pleural effusion (SPE)* is a pleural effusion that occurs below the lungs at the diaphragmatic surface. SPE does not obliterate the costophrenic angle, but it distorts the shape of the diaphragmatic dome, giving the impression of raised hemidiaphragm. You can suspect SPE in the left lung when the space between the gastric bubble and the lower lung margins increases up to 3 cm instead of usual few millimeters. Beside the raised hemidiaphragm, the lung appears to end early on PA radiographs (◘ Fig. 7.1.2).
- *Encysted (loculated) pleural effusion* is a localized encysted fluid at the fissures between lobes of the lung. It occurs usually at the right lung's minor fissure, and it has biconvex contour mimicking a mass (◘ Fig. 7.1.3). Very rarely, a benign form of mesothelioma can grow along the major or minor fissures mimicking encysted pleural effusion, a condition known as *pseudotumor*.
- *Parapneumonic effusion* is an effusion that develops adjacent to pneumonias (empyema). Almost 30 % of patients with pneumonia develop pleural effusion and usually resolve with antibiotic therapy.
- *Mediastinal pleural effusion* is a fluid collection around the mediastinum. It is an unusual

condition, and when it occurs, it forms silhouette sign along the mediastinal borders causing mediastinal widening. *Silhouette sign* is a term used to describe any opacity within the chest radiograph that obliterates a mediastinal border.

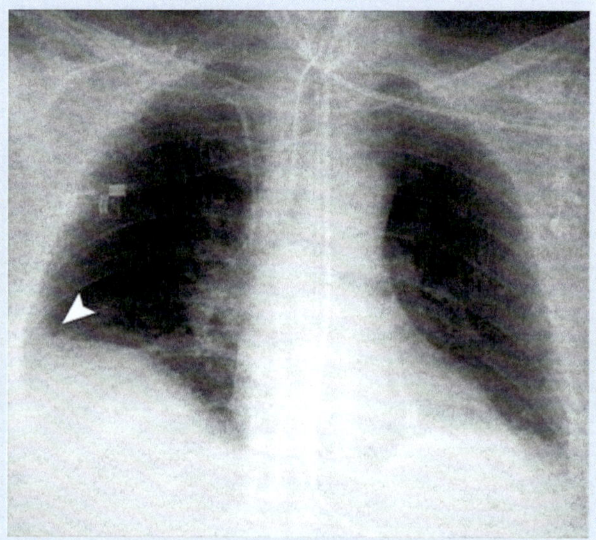

◘ **Fig. 7.1.2**  Posteroanterior chest radiograph of a patient with right subpulmonic pleural effusion (*SPE*) shows raised hemidiaphragm, and the lung seems to end early (*arrowhead*)

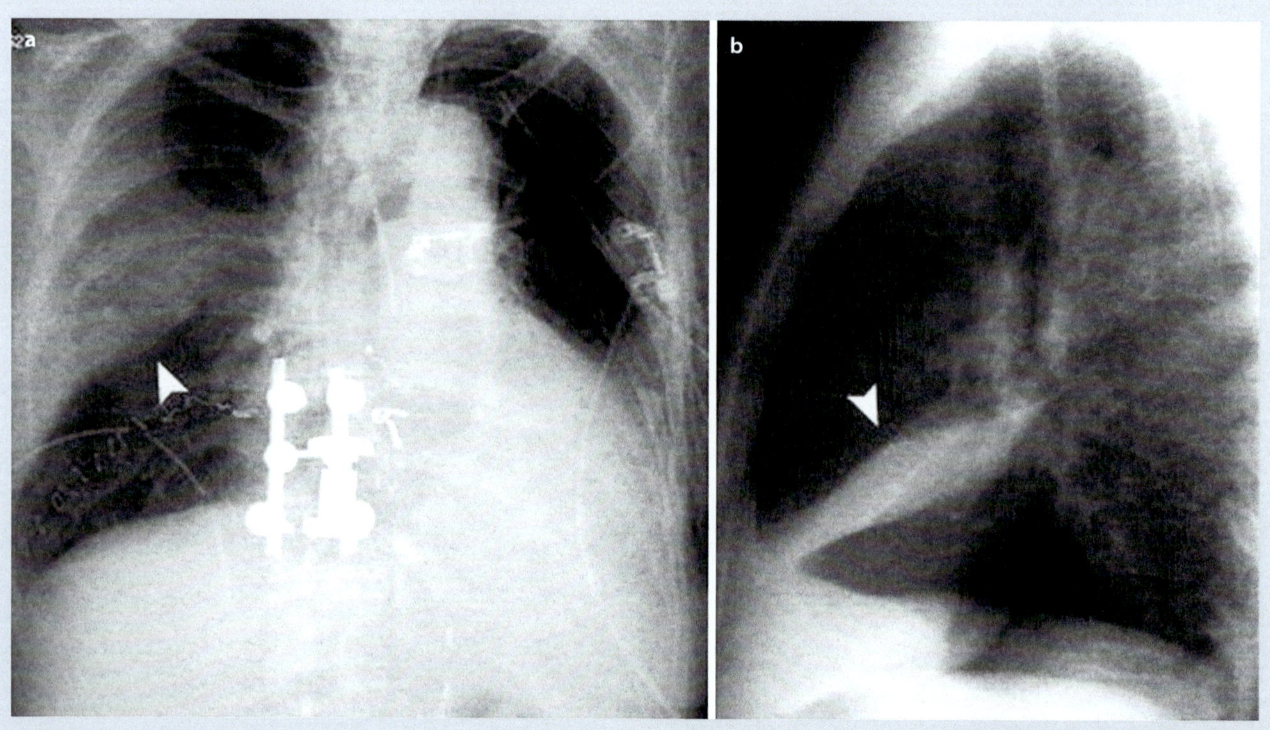

◘ **Fig. 7.1.3**  Posteroanterior (**a**) and lateral (**b**) chest radiographs show right-sided encysted pleural effusion (*arrowheads*)

## Signs on US

Pleural effusion appears as anechoic or hypoechoic collection that lies between the echogenic line of the visceral pleura and lung ( Fig. 7.1.4).

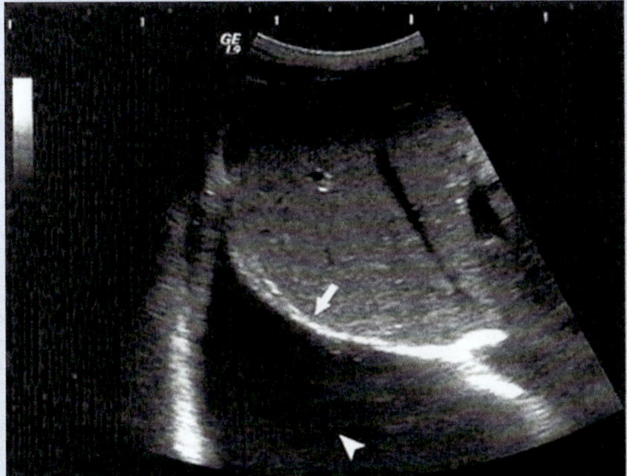

 **Fig. 7.1.4** Transverse ultrasound image shows right-sided pleural effusion (*arrowhead*). The diaphragm can be visualized as a hyperechoic line separating the right lung base from the liver (*arrow*)

## Signs on CT

- Serous pleural effusion is visualized as a crescent peripheral area with CT water density. Exudative effusion can be hyperdense.
- Empyema characteristically demonstrates thickened parietal/visceral pleura (e.g., > 2 mm) with effusion in between (split pleura sign) ( Fig. 7.1.5). Enhancement of both pleura occurs in 80–100 % cases after contrast injection. Multiple gas pockets within the empyema may be seen.
- Bronchopleural fistula occurs when a bronchus opens into the pleural space due to lung parenchymal destruction (e.g., pneumonia with empyema formation). It is seen as pleural effusion with air–fluid level on radiographs or HRCT ( Fig. 7.1.6).

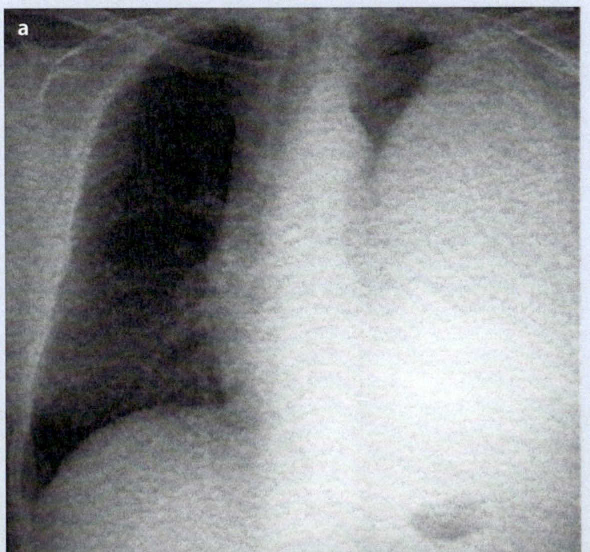


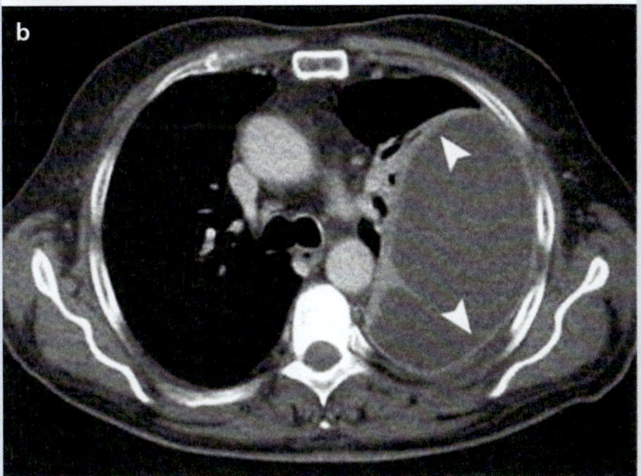

 **Fig. 7.1.5** Posteroanterior chest radiograph (**a**) and axial chest CT (**b**) of a patient with huge left-sided empyema show split pleura sign in (**b**), with thickened, enhanced pleura with effusion in between (*arrowheads*)

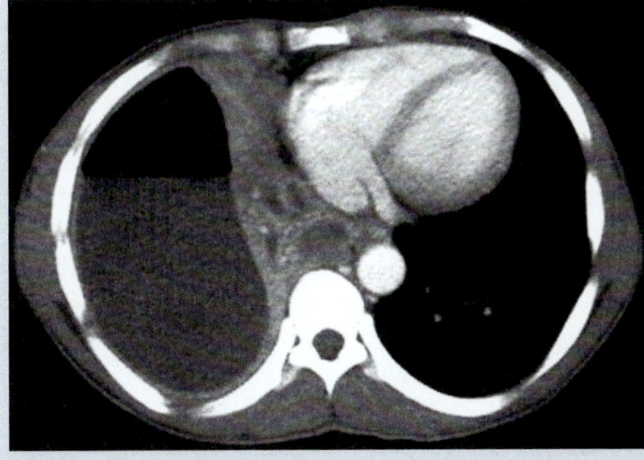

 **Fig. 7.1.6** Axial chest CT shows huge right bronchopulmonary fistula

## Differential Diagnoses and Related Diseases

— *Meigs' syndrome* is a disease characterized by ascites, pleural effusion, and one of the following ovarian tumors (fibroma, thecoma, granulose cell tumor, or Brenner's tumor). In contrast, *Pseudo-Meigs' syndrome* is defined as ascites, pleural effusion, and ovarian tumor other than the ones mentioned previously. The absence of malignant cells from the ascites or the pleural effusion is mandatory for the diagnosis of Meigs' syndrome. Typically, the ascites and the pleural effusions resolve after tumor resection. Meigs' syndrome often occurs in postmenopausal women.

— *Yellow nail syndrome* is a rare disease characterized by extremities lymphedema and thickened, slowly growing, yellowish-green nails that are excessively curved from side to side (Fig. 7.1.7). The disease is commonly accompanied by idiopathic pleural effusion, chronic bronchiectasis, chronic sinusitis, and lymphedema of the face. Yellow nail syndrome may be accompanied by rheumatoid arthritis or thyroid disease. The disease is believed to be caused by hypoplasia, atresia, or varicosity of the lymphatics.

## Pneumothorax

Pneumothorax is a condition characterized by the presence of air between the parietal and visceral pleura. There are three types of pneumothoraces:

— *Primary (spontaneous) pneumothorax*: this type occurs without a defined cause and mainly seen in young males who are tall, thin, and smokers. Primary pneumothorax is attributed to rupture of subpleuritic blebs at lung apices according to some investigators.

— *Secondary pneumothorax*: this type occurs usually after penetrating trauma, ruptured bulla, or an interventional thoracic procedure (e.g., lung mass biopsy).

— *Tension pneumothorax*: this type occurs when the air collection within the subpleural space is large enough to push the mediastinum to the other side, interfering with blood circulation within the major vessels.

Up to 40 % of pneumothoraces may not be detected by chest radiographs. CT is 100 % sensitive for detection of pneumothoraces. When pneumothorax opens into the mediastinum, a pneumomediastinum develops. Pneumomediastinum is characterized by the presence of air around the mediastinal structures.

### Sign on Radiograph

— Thin visceral pleural line: it is visible on radiographs. The line is outlined by air with the absence of the peripheral vasculature laterally and lung tissue with possible increased density due to collapse, medially (Fig. 7.1.8). Lung apices are the best sites checked for early detection of pneumothorax.

— Deep sulcus sign: the costophrenic angle deepens at the site of the pneumothorax (Fig. 7.1.9). It is seen in pneumothorax with large air collection.

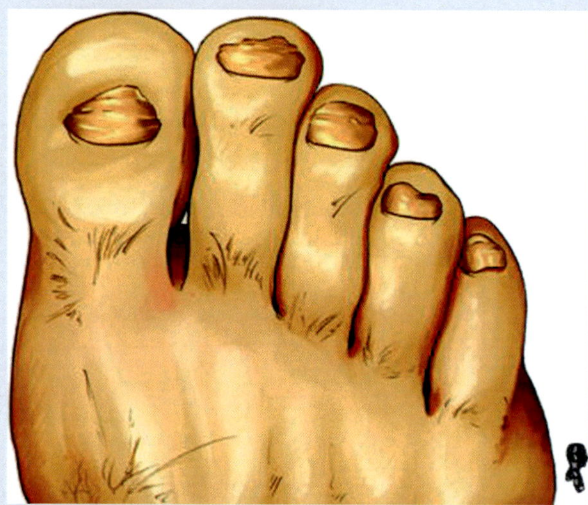

**Fig. 7.1.7**    An illustration demonstrates the yellowish-green nails of the yellow nail syndrome

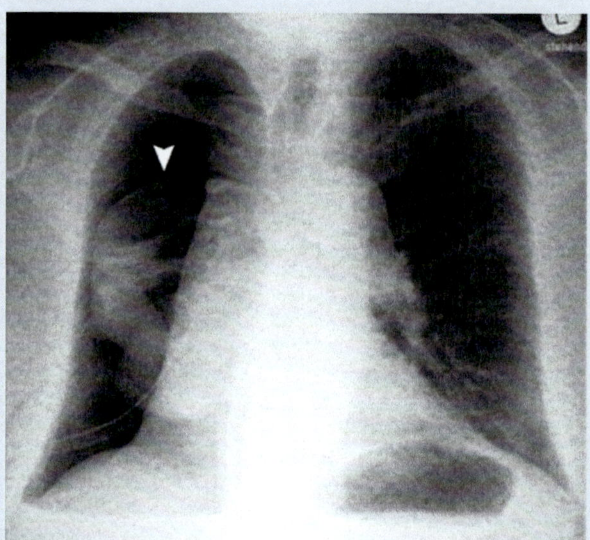

**Fig. 7.1.8**    Posteroanterior chest radiograph shows right pneumothorax with lung collapse (*arrowhead*)

- Tension pneumothorax: it is seen as complete collapse of the lung and shift of the trachea and mediastinum to the contralateral (other side) collapsed lung (Fig. 7.1.10).
- Pitfall: a skinfold and underlying clothing can mimic a pneumothorax (Fig. 7.1.11). Always correlate the radiological findings with the patient history and current status.
- Pneumomediastinum: it is detected when the mediastinal structures are surrounded by dark radiolucent line of air (Fig. 7.1.12).

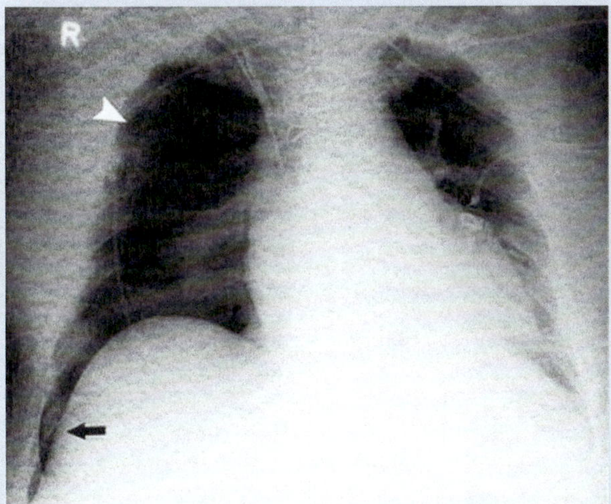

**Fig. 7.1.9** Posteroanterior chest radiograph shows right-sided pneumothorax (*arrowhead*) with right deep sulcus sign (*arrow*)

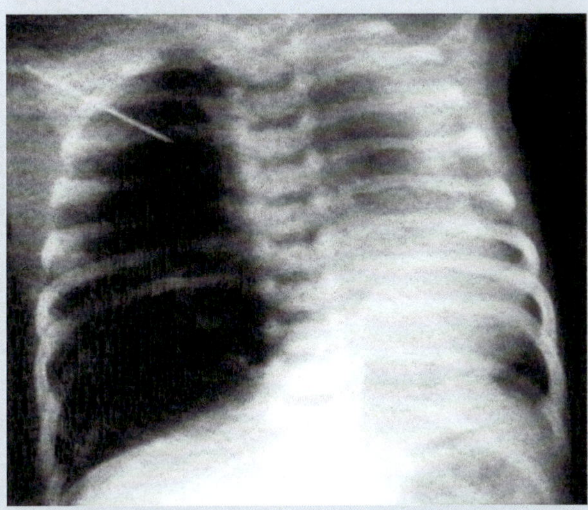

**Fig. 7.1.10** Posteroanterior chest radiograph of a child with right tension pneumothorax shows mediastinal shift toward the left side

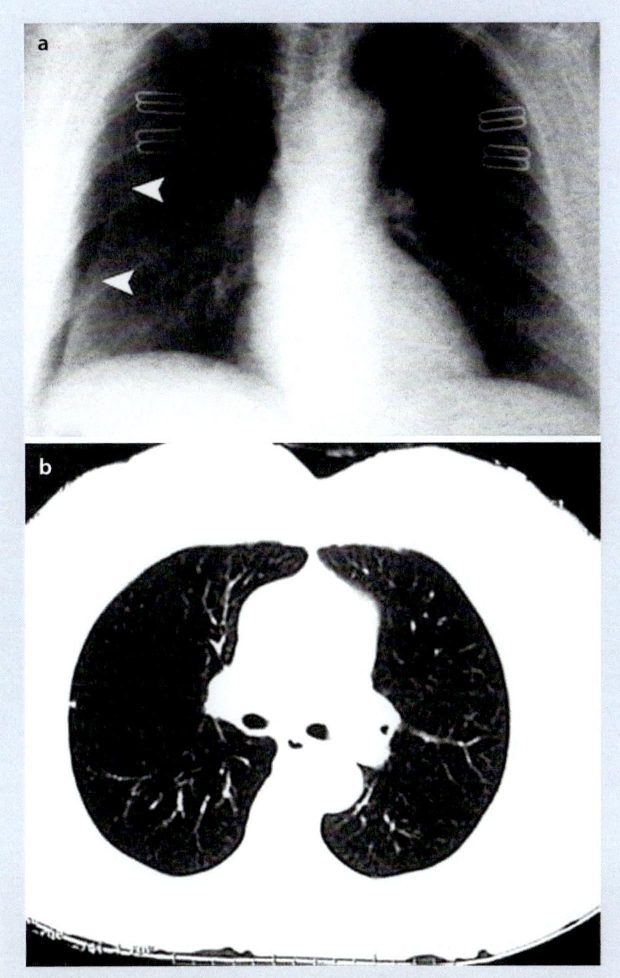

**Fig. 7.1.11** Posteroanterior chest radiograph (**a**) and axial chest CT (**b**) of a patient with skin flap that appears as right-sided pneumothorax on chest radiograph (*arrowheads*), while on the HRCT, no pneumothorax is detected

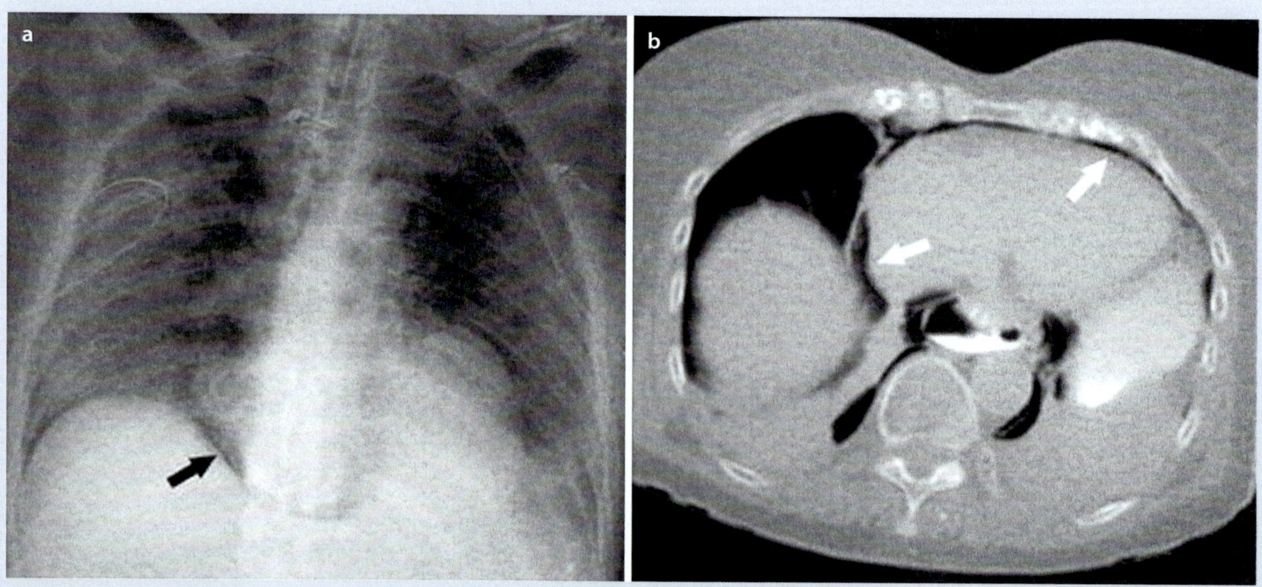



**Fig. 7.1.12** Posteroanterior chest radiograph (**a**) and axial chest CT (**b**) of a patient with pneumomediastinum show air around the heart and the mediastinal structures (*arrows*)

## Pleural Calcification

Pleural calcification can be seen following chronic pleural damage. Pleural calcification can be unilateral or bilateral. Unilateral pleural calcification occurs usually as a late complication of empyema, hemothorax, fungal infection, or tuberculosis. Bilateral pleural calcification is commonly caused by asbestosis

*Asbestosis* is a pathological condition that results from previous exposure to asbestos. Pleural plaques are the commonest manifestation of asbestosis, and they usually develop 20–30 years after the exposure to asbestosis. They are composed of focal areas of parietal pleural thickening with dense hyaline collagen. *Mesothelioma* is an uncommon primary tumor of the serosal lining of the pleura or peritoneum. Only 5–7 % of patients with asbestosis develop mesothelioma. Mesothelioma has poor prognosis, with survival rate of 12 months. Bronchogenic carcinoma develops in 25 % of cases of asbestosis, and it is the main cause of death.

- Pleural calcification is seen in 15–25 % of cases after a latency period of 30–40 years (**Fig. 7.1.13**). Diaphragmatic calcification is pathognomonic finding of asbestosis.
- Asbestos-related diffuse pleural thickening is a bilateral thickening involving at least 25 % of the chest or 50 % if unilateral, plus pleural thickness >5 mm at any site. The diffuse pleural thickening can affect the visceral layer and the parenchyma below, causing "fluffy fibrous strands."
- Round atelectasis is seen as a pleural mass (3–5 cm) that abuts over the pleura with a

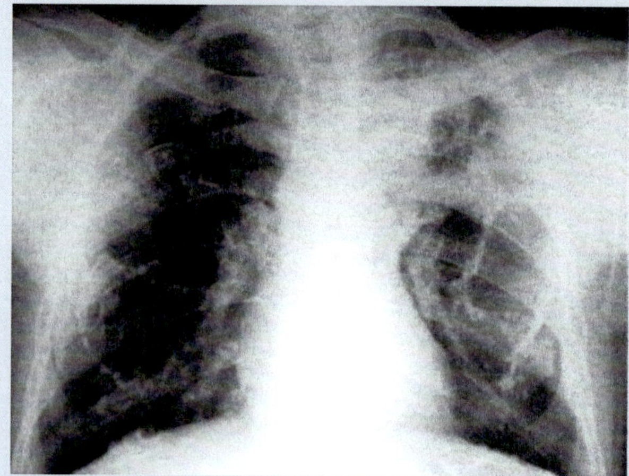

**Fig. 7.1.13** Posteroanterior chest radiograph of a patient with asbestosis shows bilateral calcified pleural plaques

### Signs on Chest Radiographs
- Pleural plaques are seen as smoothly demarcated, well-defined opacities (in profile) or faint, ill-defined plaques (en face), in a bilateral fashion. Unilateral pleural plaques may be seen in 25 % of cases and usually located on the left side. The plaques usually are <1 cm in thickness and seen parallel to the chest wall.

curvilinear tails entering the mass (comet tail sign). The curvilinear densities are composed of fibrosed vessels, and the mass is commonly visualized at the base of the lungs ( Fig. 7.1.14). Air bronchograms within the mass are common.

— Malignant mesothelioma is visualized as visceral or parietal pleural nodules that are indistinguishable from pleural metastases. The most common manifestation of malignant mesothelioma is a unilateral massive pleural effusion.

**Signs on HRCT**
— Pleural plaques appear as well-circumscribed areas of pleural thickening separated from the underlying ribs by thin layer of fat. The edges of the pleural plaque are typically thicker than its center.
— Malignant mesothelioma is visualized as nodular pleural thickening (94 %) that commonly involves the lung bases (50 %) ( Fig. 7.1.15). Diaphragmatic involvement (80 %), pleural calcification (20 %), and pleural effusion (80 %) are other common features.

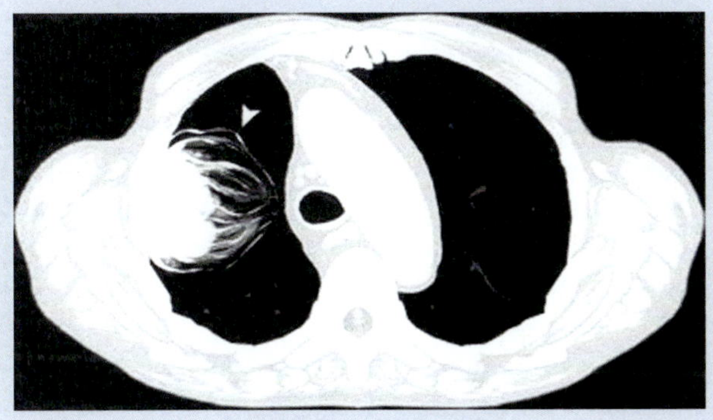

**Fig. 7.1.14** Axial chest HRCT illustration demonstrates round atelectasis with comet tail sign (*arrowhead*)

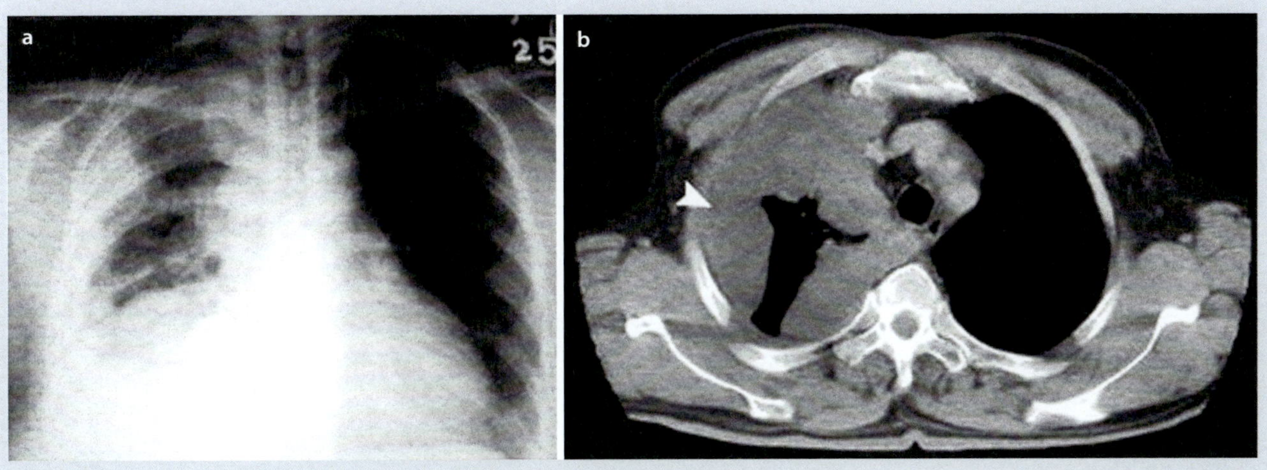

**Fig. 7.1.15** Posteroanterior chest radiograph (**a**) and axial chest CT (**b**) of a patient with malignant pleural mesothelioma show nodular thickening of the pleura in the right lung field with extension toward the apex in (**a**) and (**b**). Notice the nodular mass that follows the pleural distribution in (**b**) (*arrowhead*)

## Further Reading

Akira M, et al. Asbestosis: high-resolution CT-pathologic correlation. Radiology. 1990;176:389–94.

DeCoste SD, et al. Yellow nail syndrome. J Am Acad Dermatol. 1990;22:608–11.

Gallardo X, et al. Benign pleural diseases. Eur J Radiol. 2000;34:87–97.

Goyal M, et al. Malignant pleural mesothelioma in a 13-year-old girl. Pediatr Radiol. 2000;30:776–8.

Nicholas G, et al. Asbestosis and malignancy. AJR. 1967;100:597–602.

Nimkin K, et al. Localized pneumothorax with lobar collapse and diffuse obstructive airway disease. Pediatr Radiol. 1995;25:449–51.

O'Lone E, et al. Spontaneous pneumothorax in children: when is invasive treatment indicated? Pediatr Pulmonol. 2008;43:41–6.

Qureshi NR, et al. Imaging in pleural disease. Clin Chest Med. 2006;27:193–213.

Sacco O, et al. Yellow nail Syndrome and bilateral cystic lung disease. Pediatr Pulmonol. 1998;26:429–33.

Váuez JL, et al. Pneumomediastinum and pneumothorax as presenting signs in severe Mycoplasma pneumoniae pneumonia. Pediatr Radiol. 2007;37:1286–8.


## 7.2 Alveolar Lung Diseases

Alveolar lung diseases (ALD) are group of disorders characterized by pathological insult involving mainly the alveoli. The alveoli can be imagined as an empty cup, and alveolar diseases are classified according to the content of this cup. Alveolar diseases are characterized by filling of the alveoli with materials that impede its normal physiological function (ventilation). Alveolar diseases can be localized (focal) or diffuse. Names of the conditions depend upon the content of the material filling the alveoli.

## Types of Alveolar Lung Diseases

- Alveoli filled with *serous fluid*: cardiogenic and noncardiogenic edema
- Alveoli filled with *blood*: pulmonary hemorrhage, commonly due to vasculitis (e.g., Churg–Strauss syndrome)
- Alveoli filled with *pus*: pneumonia
- Alveoli filled with *proteins*: alveolar proteinosis and amyloidosis
- Alveoli filled with *malignant cells*: bronchoalveolar carcinoma
- Alveoli filled with *calcium*: alveolar microlithiasis

### Pulmonary Edema

The alveoli are the main units for respiratory–blood ventilation and oxygenation and normally are full of air on inspiration. You can think of the alveoli as an empty cup, and any pathological condition that fills this cup will form a pathological condition according to the cup content. Pulmonary edema arises due to alveolar filling with serous fluid (water).

Pulmonary edema can be either due to cardiac disease (cardiogenic) or other conditions (noncardiogenic). Most cases of noncardiogenic pulmonary edema are due to acute respiratory distress syndrome (ARDS).

Cardiogenic pulmonary edema is commonly seen with heart failure. It starts as an interstitial edema before it turns into alveolar edema, because the pulmonary veins lie in the interstitium. As the hydrostatic pressure within the veins rises, they leak into the interstitium first and then progress to fill the alveoli. This process is rapid, and only very early edema can be seen as a pure interstitial linear pattern in chest radiographs.

Noncardiogenic pulmonary edema has the same radiographic features as the cardiogenic pulmonary edema, but the causes are different: ARDS, chemical pneumonitis, drug-induced pulmonary edema, and transfusion reaction are the most common causes for noncardiogenic pulmonary edema. ARDS is a situation where an alveolar capillary injury occurs as a result of variety of causes (e.g., sepsis). *Chemical pneumonitis* is a pulmonary edema that occurs due to inhalation of noxious chemical substance such as ammonia, smoking inhalation, near-drowning situations, and gastric acid aspiration. The mechanism of pulmonary edema is the result of one of the three mechanisms: irritation of the tracheobronchial tree that leads to inflammation and pulmonary edema formation; absorption of the noxious material from the respiratory tract, which can affect the lungs directly by its metabolites; and asphyxiation due to inhalation of high concentration of the noxious material that will displace oxygen from the blood and cause tissue hypoxia. *Drug-induced and transfusion reactions pulmonary edema* arise due to anaphylactic lupus-like reaction formation. The radiographic picture cannot be differentiated from ARDS unless you have history of drug ingestion or recent transfusion reaction. Classic examples of drugs causing pulmonary edema are heroin, aspirin, and penicillin. *Negative pressure pulmonary edema* is a term used to describe noncardiogenic edema that arises due to acute airway obstruction (type 1) or after the relief of chronic airway obstruction (type 2).

### Signs on Radiograph

- There is a centrally located, bilateral, symmetrical diffuse alveolar opacities emitting from the helium and spares the periphery (butterfly or batwings sign) (□ Fig. 7.2.16). Usually, pulmonary edema causes homogenous opacities, but sometimes they can cause nodular or blotchy opacities.
- Cardiomegaly and signs of congestive heart failure (e.g., congested pulmonary vessels).
- Kerley lines represent thickening of the interlobar septae. Lung lymphatics and veins run in the interstitium, leakage of the veins (edema), or tumor infiltration of the lymphatics (lymphangitis carcinomatosis) can result in thickening of the interlobar septa, which are called Kerley lines. Kerley A lines are long lines located near the lung hilum and extend obliquely near the bronchoarterial bundle into the peripheries. Kerley B lines are short white lines seen perpendicular to the pleural surface at the lung bases, commonly near the costophrenic angles (□ Fig. 7.2.17). Kerley C lines are a mixture between the two lines resulting in a reticular pattern.
- Air-bronchogram sign is a sign seen when the alveoli are filled with fluid and the terminal

bronchioles and bronchi are devoid of fluid (filled with air). The bronchioles appear as radiolucent lines within whitish radio-opaque opacities (◘ Fig. 7.2.18). This sign is specific for alveolar disease, but nonspecific for the cause. Pulmonary edema, pulmonary hemorrhage, pneumonia, and alveolar carcinoma all look the same on radiographs. All appears as ALD with air bronchogram. The medical history plays a very important role in differentiating these conditions because the radiographic signs can be nonspecific.

— In blood diversion, normally, the upper lobe vessels are not visualized on radiographs, and the lower lobe vessels are mildly dilated and visible due to the gravity effect in upright posteroanterior (PA) radiographs. In cases of cardiac diseases and pulmonary hypertension, the upper lobe vessels will be as wide as the lower lobe vessels in upright radiographs. Note that the upper lobe vessels can be seen dilated normally in supine (lying) chest radiographs (e.g., in intensive care unit radiographs).Silhouette sign refers to a patchy, ill-defined radio-opaque shadow that obscures part of the normal mediastinal configuration.

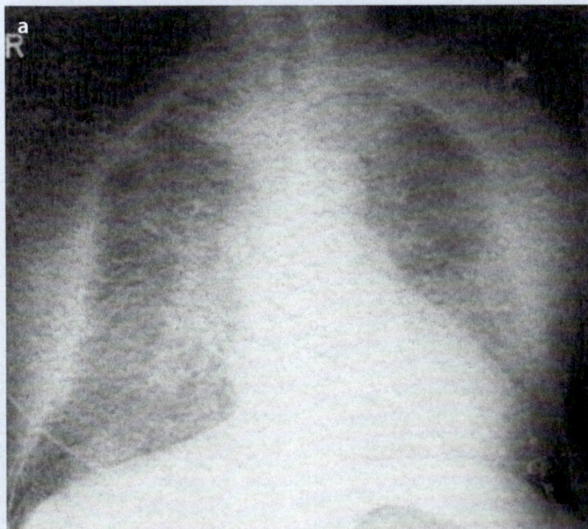

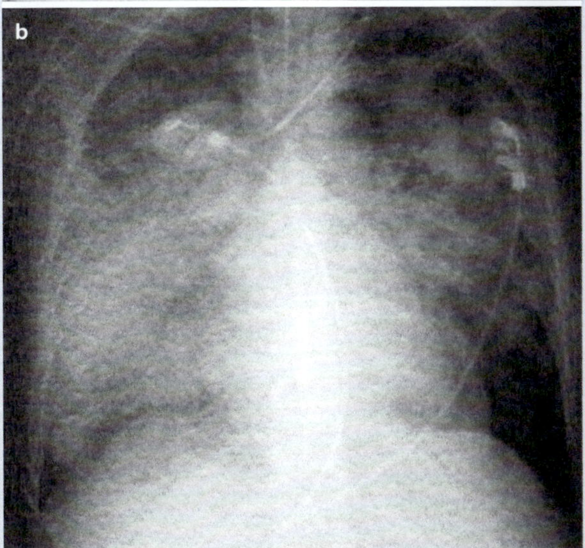

◘ **Fig. 7.2.16** Anteroposterior plain chest radiographs in two different patients show bilateral symmetrical pulmonary edema with bat wings appearance in (**a**), and bilateral, almost symmetrical pulmonary hemorrhage in (**b**). Notice that without history, you cannot differentiate pulmonary hemorrhage from pulmonary edema based on radiographic presentation alone

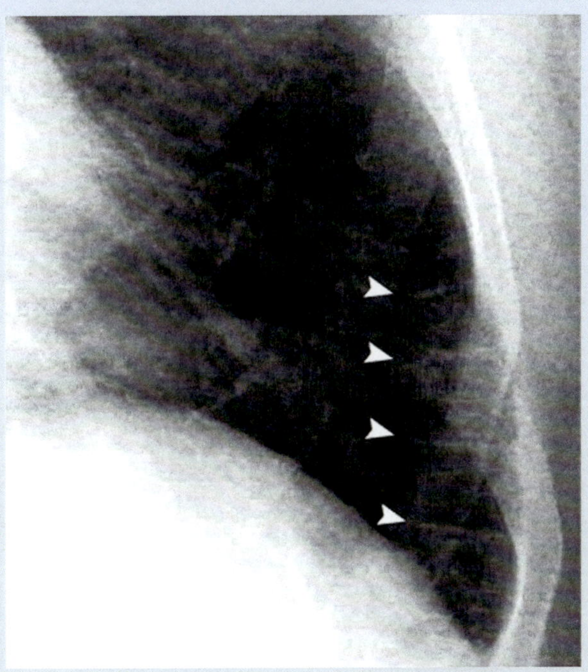

◘ **Fig. 7.2.17** Posteroanterior plain chest radiograph shows Kerley B lines (*arrowheads*)

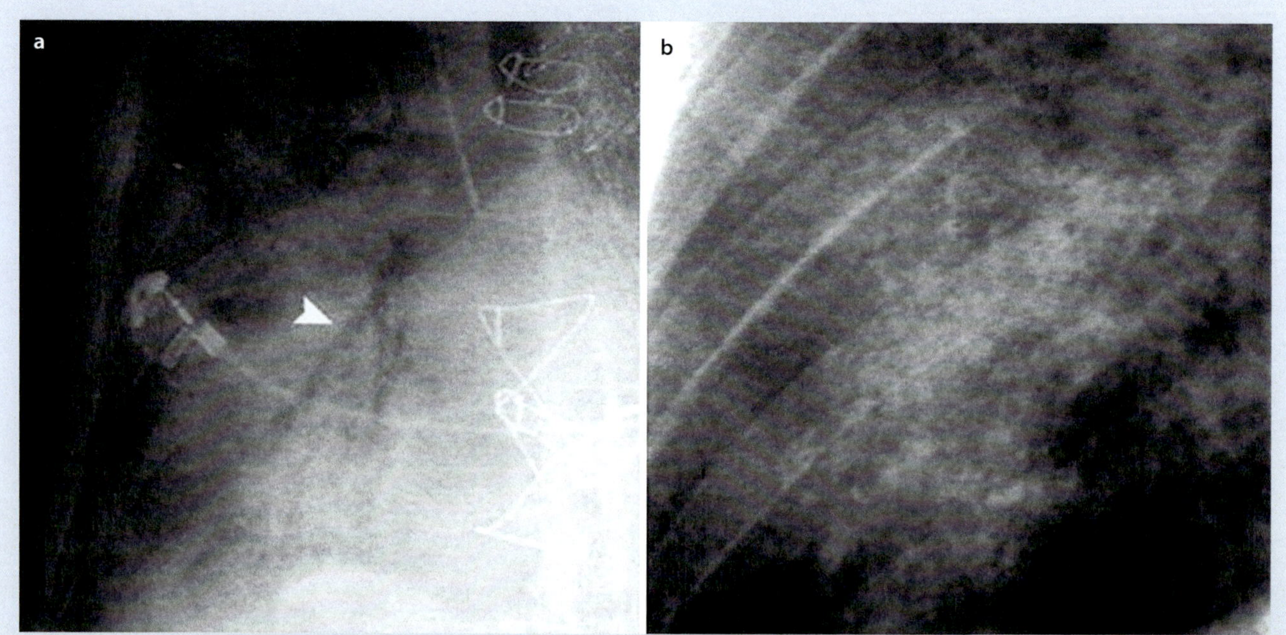

**Fig. 7.2.18** Posteroanterior plain chest radiographs in two different patients with pneumonia show pneumonic lung patch with air columns within the patchy due to unaffected bronchi in (**a**) (*arrowhead*) and pneumonic lung patch with no air-bronchogram sign in (**b**). Patient (**a**) presents with airspace pneumonia, whereas patient (**b**) presents with bronchopneumonia

## How to Differentiate Between Cardiogenic Edema from ARDS on Plain Chest Radiographs?

- ARDS usually has a normal heart size, while cardiogenic pulmonary edema shows signs of heart failure.
- ARDS usually affects peripheral lung field more than central, whereas cardiogenic edema typically starts from the center to the periphery.
- ARDS usually has no Kerley B lines.

### Pneumonia

Pneumonia is a condition characterized by an infectious inflammation of the lung parenchyma and deposition of pus within the alveoli. Pneumonia can be caused by bacteria (e.g., methicillin-resistant Staphylococcus aureus (MRSA)), fungi (e.g., *Pneumocystis carinii*), and viruses (e.g., *Cytomegalovirus* (CMV)).

Patients with pneumonia present with dyspnea, purulent sputum, fever, tachycardia, and maybe hemoptysis (e.g., tuberculosis). Complications of pneumonia include lung abscess formation, septicemia, and empyema. Rarely, arthritis and neurological symptoms may be encountered in atypical pneumonias (e.g., *Mycoplasma* pneumonia).

Pneumonias are divided into "typical pneumonia," which is caused by *Streptococcus pneumoniae* (*pneumococcus*), and "atypical pneumonia," which is caused by any pathogen that is not *pneumococcus*. Typical pneumonia is clinically dominated by respiratory symptoms, whereas atypical pneumonia clinically is dominated by symptoms of fever and malaise more than the respiratory symptoms.

## Types of Pneumonias

- *Airspace pneumonia* (*lobar pneumonia*): in this type, the infection is confined to a single lobe. There is usually one patch filling the whole affected lobe. This type is seen with *pneumococcus*, *Legionella*, *Pseudomonas*, and primary tuberculosis infection. Lobar pneumonia is characterized by an "air-bronchogram sign."
- *Bronchopneumonia*: this type is characterized by an infection that starts in the bronchioles and small bronchi walls and then spreads to the alveoli. This type is seen with *Staphylococcus aureus*, *Haemophilus influenza*, and *Mycoplasma* pneumonias.
- *Interstitial pneumonia*: this type is characterized by an infection that involves the interstitial septa and giving reticular interstitial pattern on chest radiograph. This type can be seen with viral infections like influenza virus and varicella-zoster virus (VZV) and *Mycoplasma* infections (30 % of cases).

*MRSA* is a serious infection with antibiotic-resistant staphylococci. MRSA is categorized as community-acquired, nosocomial, and healthcare-associated infection. MRSA is the leading cause of nosocomial and healthcare-associated bloodstream infection, globally. Also, it is responsible for 30–50 % of ventilator-associated pneumonia. MRSA causes metastatic foci of infections in 30 % of cases into the lungs, liver, kidneys, heart valves, and joints. Most community-associated MRSA strains carry the Panton–Valentine leukocidin (PVL) gene, which is rarely found in the hospital-acquired MRSA or the normal strain of *S. aureus*.

PVL toxin is a potent lethal factor to neutrophils, which causes tissue necrosis and severe necrotizing pneumonia. MRSA pneumonia is more frequently associated with sepsis, high-grade fever, hemoptysis, pleural effusion, and death compared to PVL-negative *S. aureus*. MRSA pneumonia can result in the formation of pulmonary cavitary infiltration due to the development of necrotizing pneumonia. The development of MRSA necrotizing pneumonia should be suspected in a young patient presenting with hypoxia, hemoptysis, and single or multiple cavitary lung lesions.

Viral pneumonias are characterized by several pathologies that include bronchiolitis, tracheobronchitis, and classical pneumonia. Viruses that attack immunocompetent patients include influenza viruses, Epstein–Barr virus, and adenoviruses. Viruses that attack immunocompromised patients include measles virus, VZV, and CMV. Measles virus attacks usually children due to immunosuppression or vaccine failure. VZV pneumonia is a common complication of VZV septicemia in children with a mortality rate of 9–50 %. Up to 90 % of VZV pneumonia cases are seen in patients with lymphoma or immunosuppression. CMV pneumonia is commonly seen in transplant patients and immunocompromised patients. Patients may develop severe necrotizing pneumonia in spite of antiviral therapy.

## Differential Diagnoses and Related Diseases

*Hyperimmunoglobulinemia E syndrome (Job's syndrome)* is a rare condition characterized by marked elevation of serum IgE levels against *S. aureus*, resulting in decreased production of antistaphylococcus IgG. The patient with this syndrome presents with frequent attacks of *S. aureus* pneumonia, pustular dermatitis, eczema, and sinusitis. Formation of chronic lung abscesses is a common feature on radiographs.

### Signs on Radiograph
- Radio-opaque patches with an air-bronchogram sign (◻ Fig. 7.2.18).
- For bulging fissure sign, some infections will increase the volume of the lobe involved, causing the adjacent fissure to bulge (commonly the transverse fissure) (◻ Fig. 7.2.19). This sign is classically seen in Klebsiella pneumonia.
- In bronchopneumonia, there are multiple patchy infiltrations of the lung with or without segmental lobe atelectasis (if the bronchus is totally obstructed) (◻ Fig. 7.2.18).
- Interstitial pneumonia shows nonspecific linear or reticular interstitial lung pattern. Correlation with history and laboratory findings is essential to establish the diagnosis.
- Viral pneumonias can appear as poorly defined nodules (4–10 mm in diameter), with lung hyperinflation due to bronchiolitis.
- Measles pneumonia shows mix pattern of reticular interstitial pattern with patchy pneumonia

(◻ Fig. 7.2.20). Hilar lymphadenopathy may be associated.
- VZV pneumonia appears as multiple, ill-defined micronodules (5–10 mm) (◻ Fig. 7.2.21). The lesions may calcify persisting as well-defined, randomly scattered, dense pulmonary calcification.
- CMV pneumonia is commonly seen as a mixed nodular interstitial pattern with ill-defined patchy lung infiltration. The patchy filling is caused

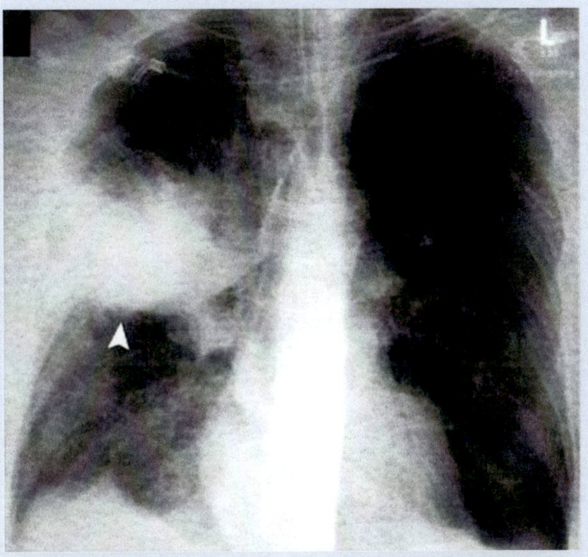

◻ **Fig. 7.2.19** Anteroposterior plain chest radiograph of a bedridden patient shows right upper lobe pneumonia with bulging of the transverse fissure (*arrowhead*)

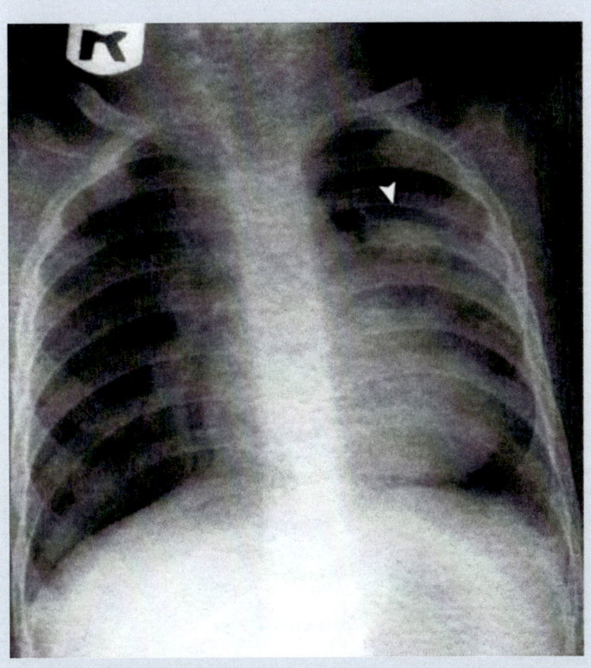

◻ **Fig. 7.2.20** Posteroanterior plain chest radiograph of a 5-year-old child with measles presenting with dyspnea shows ill-defined patchy pneumonia in the upper zone of the left lung (*arrowhead*)

pathologically by hemorrhage, neutrophilic and fibrinous exudates, and hyaline membrane formation ( Fig. 7.2.22).

— Chronic pneumonia can lead to fibrosis, traction bronchiectasis, and paracicatricial emphysema ( Fig. 7.2.23).

— In MRSA necrotizing pneumonia, a pneumonic patch or a pulmonary mass with central cavitary lesion can be found. The lesion can be single or multifocal. The same manifestations are observed in HRCT. Differential diagnoses of cavitary lung infiltrations include lung abscess, metastases, pulmonary lymphoma, and Wegener's granulomatosis.

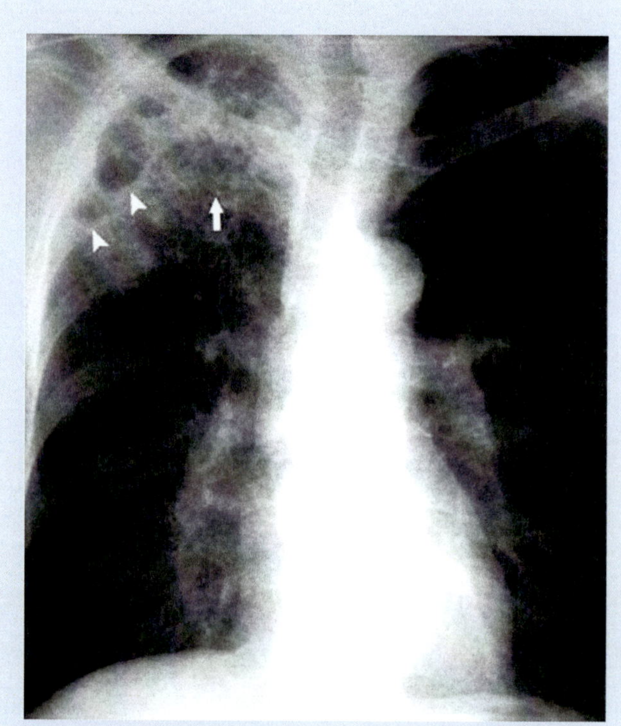

 **Fig. 7.2.23**   Posteroanterior plain chest radiograph of a patient with mycoplasma pneumonia shows right upper lobe fibrosis with honeycombing due to traction bronchiectasis (*arrow*) and paracicatricial emphysema (*arrowheads*)

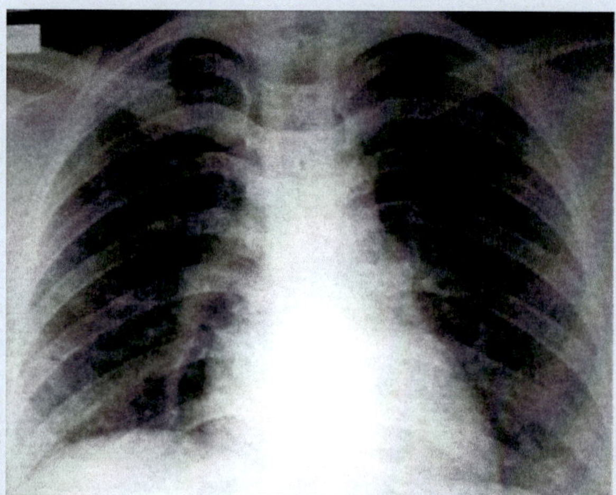

 **Fig. 7.2.21**   Posteroanterior plain chest radiograph of a patient with varicella-zoster virus (VZV) pneumonia shows diffuse micronodular interstitial lung pattern bilaterally

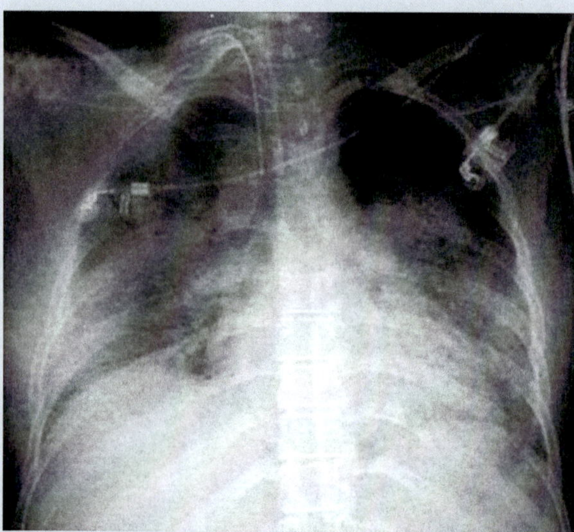

 **Fig. 7.2.22**   Posteroanterior plain chest radiograph of a patient with cytomegalovirus (CMV) pneumonia after heart transplant shows mixed patchy lung infiltration with micronodular interstitial lung pattern

## Further Reading


Anuradha G. Methicillin-resistant staphylococcus aureus bacteremia and pneumonia. Dis Mon. 2008;54:787–92.

Chuang YC, et al. Negative pressure pulmonary edema: report of three cases and review of the literature. Eur Arch Otorhinolaryngol. 2007;264:1113–6.

Connolly B, et al. Bronchial artery aneurysm in hyperimmuno-globulinemia E syndrome. Pediatr Radiol. 1994;24:592–3.

Corriere MD, et al. MRSA: an evolving pathogen. Dis Mon. 2008;54:751–5.

Decker CF. Pathogenesis of MRSA infection. Dis Mon. 2008;54:774–9.

Ebert MD, et al. Necrotizing pneumonia caused by community-acquired methicillin-resistant Staphylococcus aureus: an increasing cause of "mayhem in the lung". Emerg Radiol. 2009;16:159–62.

Fujinaga S, et al. Pulmonary edema in a boy with biopsy-proven poststreptococcal glomerulonephritis without urinary abnormalities. Pediatr Nephrol. 2007;22:154–5.

Gattinoni L, et al. The role of CT-scan studies for the diagnosis and therapy of acute respiratory distress syndrome. Clin Chest Med. 2006;27:559–70.

Kawamata M, et al. Acute pulmonary edema associated with transfusion of packed red blood cells. Intensive Care Med. 1995;21:443–6.

Kim EA, et al. Viral pneumonias in adults: radiologic and pathologic findings. Radiographics. 2002;22:S137–49.

## 7.3  Atelectasis (Lung Collapse)

Atelectasis is a condition characterized by lung collapse, which can be subtotal (25–50 % collapse) or total (100 % collapse).

Atelectasis can result due to air resorption (*resorptive atelectasis*), lung compression (*compression atelectasis*), or loss of the surfactant in *acute respiratory distress syndrome (ARDS) and hyaline membrane disease (respiratory distress syndrome)* in preterm infants (microatelectases). Pulmonary atelectasis is a recognized complication of general anesthesia.

Pulmonary surfactant is secreted by pneumocytes type II, which is composed of phospholipids and proteins. The surfactant stabilizes the lung by reducing the surface tension at the air–liquid interface in the alveoli. Therefore, deficiency of pulmonary surfactant could result in collapse of the alveolar spaces.

Patients with atelectasis commonly present with dyspnea, tachypnea, cough, and pleuritic chest pain on inspiration. Hypoxemia may result from atelectasis due to reduced ventilation–perfusion equilibrium.

## Types of Pulmonary Atelectases

- *Resorptive atelectasis* can arise due to intrinsic obstruction (e.g., mucus plug) or extrinsic obstruction (e.g., hilar lymphadenopathy). *Brock's syndrome* is a term used to describe right middle lobe (RML) atelectasis by enlarged hilar lymphadenopathy compressing the right main bronchi.
- *Passive atelectasis* results when the natural tendency of lung tissue to collapse due to elastic recoil goes unstopped. This condition can be seen in atelectasis due to pneumothorax.
- *Compressive atelectasis* is a variant of passive atelectasis and occurs when a space-occupying lesion abuts the lung causing atelectasis (e.g., massive pleural effusion).
- *Cicatrization atelectasis* is seen with fibrosis, where the scar tissue contracts and collapses the alveoli.
- *Adhesion atelectasis* occurs due to surfactant deficiency, which is classically seen in hyaline membrane disease in infants and ARDS and pulmonary embolism in adults.
- *Plate atelectasis* is composed of sheets of horizontal tissue collapse, which is commonly located 1–3 cm above the diaphragm. This type is commonly seen in conditions which impede normal respiration (e.g., inflammatory conditions in the chest or abdomen).
- *Congenital atelectasis* is seen in newborn infants due to failure to aerate the lung after pregnancy.
- *Round atelectasis* is seen in asbestosis, and it is characterized by atelectasis of parenchymal tissues near the pleura. It is best diagnosed by CT, which will show bronchovascular marks entering the mass (comet tail sign).
- *Segmental atelectasis* is an uncommon type of atelectasis characterized by an entire lung segment collapse. It is highly suggestive of a tumor blocking the bronchial feeding of that segment.

**Signs on Chest Radiograph**
- Diaphragmatic elevation due to reduced lung volume.
- Shift of the right horizontal fissure upward due to upper lobe collapse (◘ Fig. 7.3.24).
- RML and left lower lobe (LLL) atelectases are located behind the heart. They can be seen as dense radio-opaque triangles overlying the heart shadow (◘ Figs. 7.3.25 and 7.3.26). They can be easily missed if the atelectasis is examined in posteroanterior view only; lateral views are advised if RML or LLL atelectases are suspected.
- Left upper lobe (LUL) atelectasis is generally seen as increase in lung density on posteroanterior (PA) view. This is explained by the fact that the LUL collapses anteriorly. Lateral view is shown clearly as an anterior mediastinal radio-opaque shadow representing the collapsed lobe (◘ Fig. 7.3.27).
- Right upper lobe (RUL) atelectasis is seen as homogenous opacity located at the right upper lung zone and bounded inferiorly by the transverse fissure (◘ Fig. 7.3.28).
- Shift of the trachea and the mediastinum toward the collapse.
- For spine sign, normally the lower vertebrae on lateral view are less dense than the upper vertebra. The upper vertebrae appear denser due to the arm and axilla shadow overlying them. With progressive atelectasis of the lower lobes, the lobes will move more posteromedially, making the lower vertebra appears as dense as the upper vertebrae (◘ Fig. 7.3.26).
- Golden S sign is seen when the RUL is collapsed due to hilar mass blocking the right main bronchus (e.g., in Brock's syndrome).
- Plate atelectasis is detected on radiographs as linear horizontal radio-opaque lines commonly located 1–3 cm above the diaphragm (◘ Fig. 7.3.29).

7

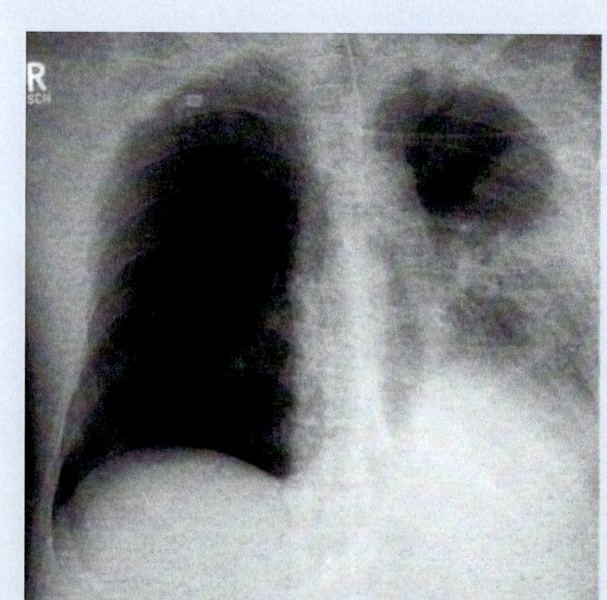

**Fig. 7.3.24** Anteroposterior plain chest radiograph of a bedridden patient shows mediastinal shift toward the left side due to collapse of the left lung

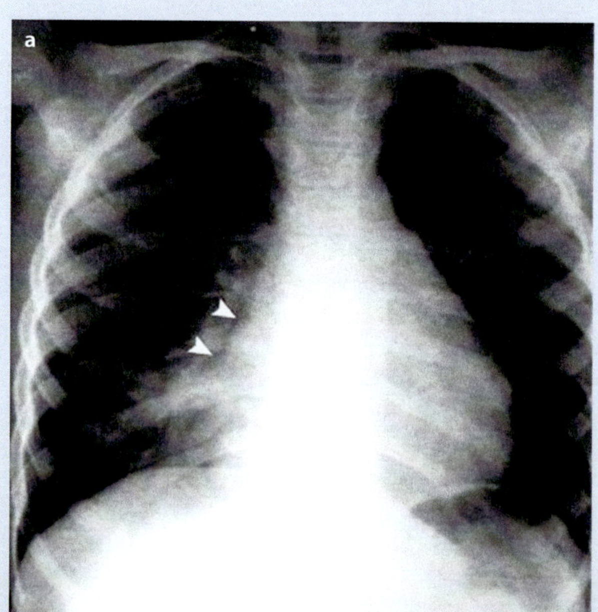

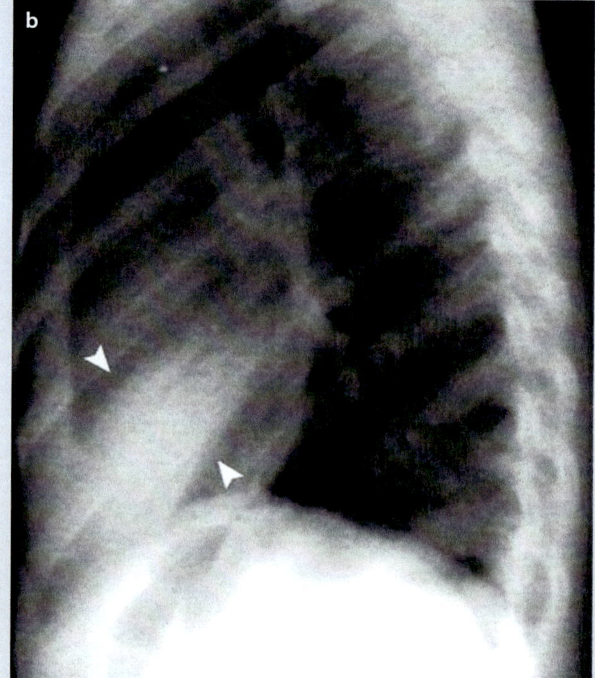

**Fig. 7.3.25** Posteroanterior (**a**) and lateral (**b**) plain chest radiographs show right middle lobe (RML) atelectasis (*arrowheads*)

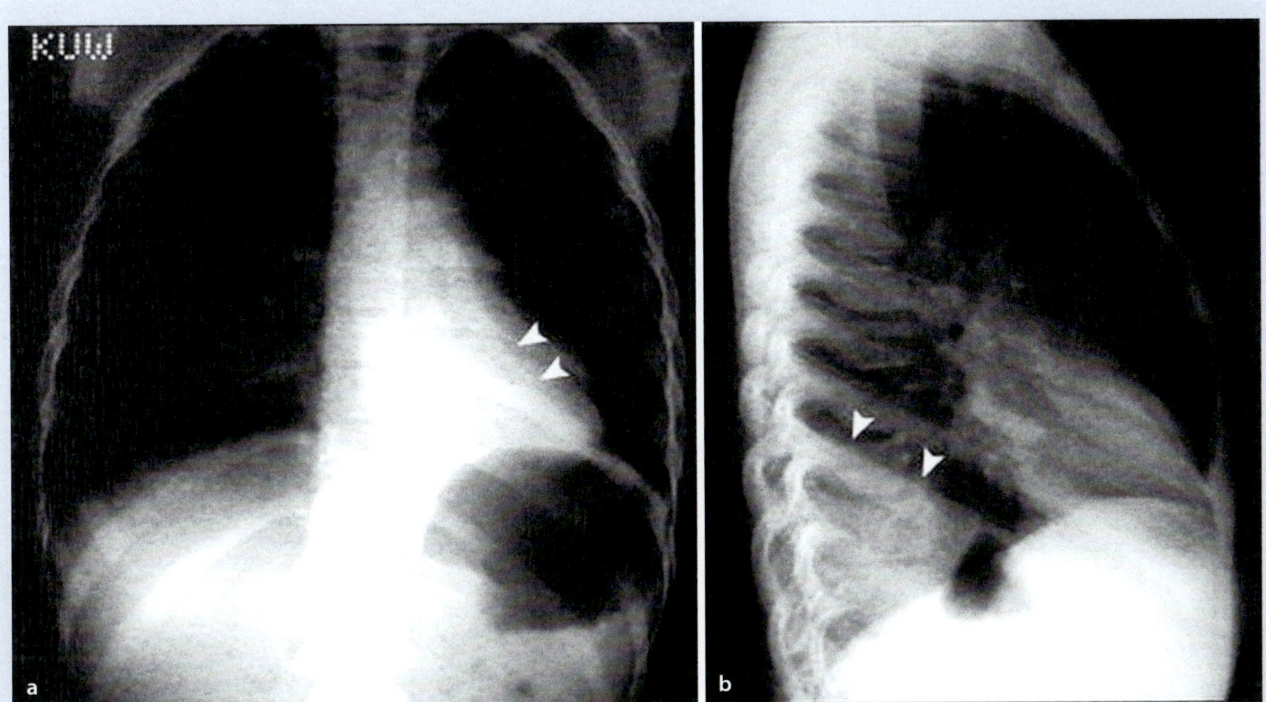

**Fig. 7.3.26** Posteroanterior (**a**) and lateral (**b**) plain chest radiographs show left lower lobe (LLL) atelectasis (*arrowheads*). Notice that the lower thoracic vertebrae appear denser than the upper thoracic vertebrae due to the shadow of the atelectatic lobe overlying them (*spine sign*)

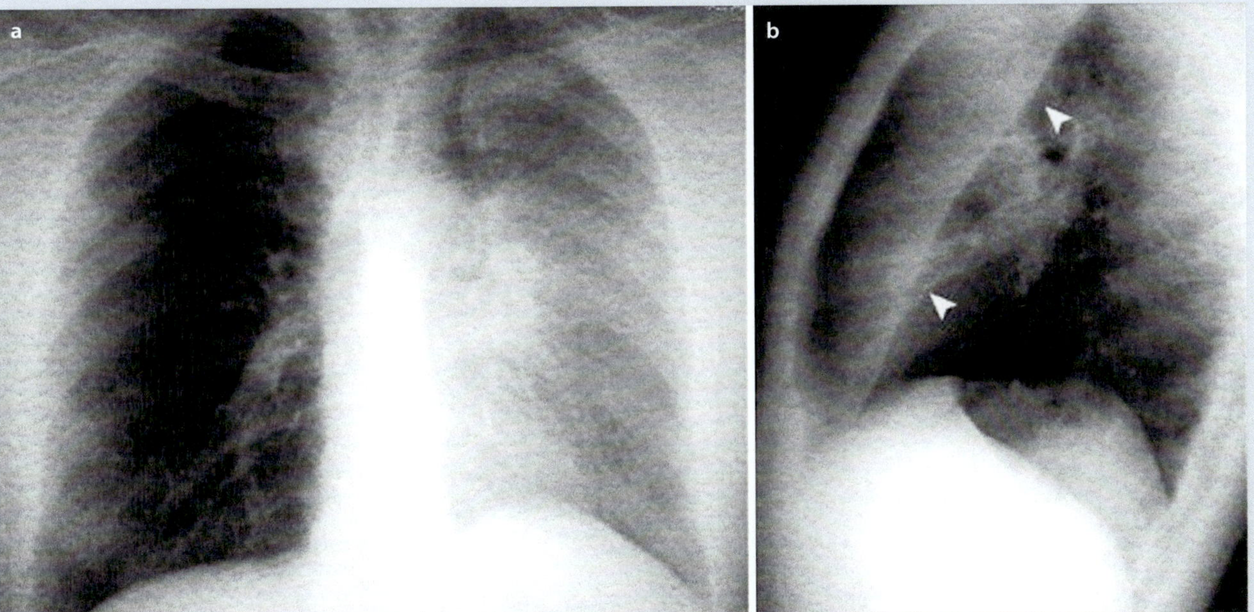

**Fig. 7.3.27** Posteroanterior (**a**) and lateral (**b**) plain chest radiographs show left upper lobe (LUL) atelectasis. Notice the high-density left lung field in (**a**), which is explained by atelectasis of the LUL anteriorly in (**b**) (*arrowheads*)

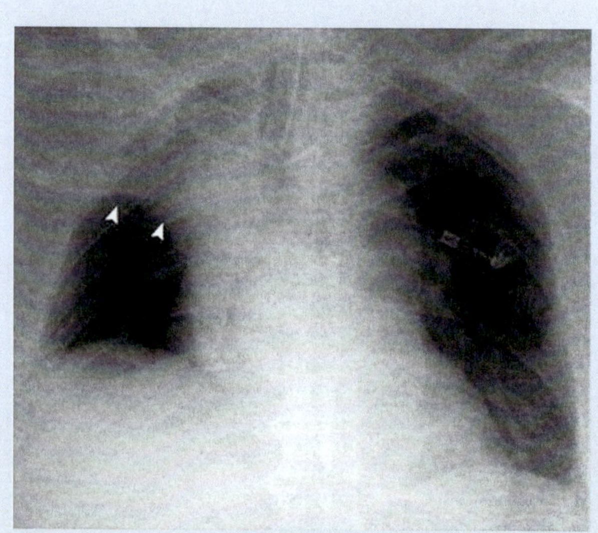

**Fig. 7.3.28** Posteroanterior plain chest radiographs show right upper lobe (RUL) atelectasis bounded inferiorly by the transverse fissure (*arrowheads*)

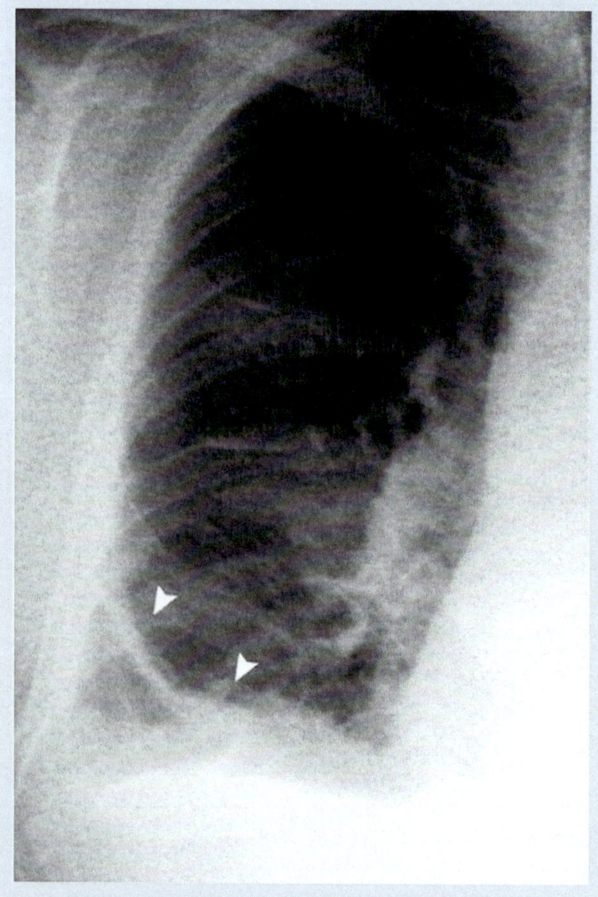

**Fig. 7.3.29** Posteroanterior plain chest radiograph shows plate atelectasis as thick radio-opaque shadow at the right costophrenic angle

## Further Reading


Glay J, et al. Unusual pattern of left lower lobe atelectasis. Radiology. 1981;141:331–3.

Sargent MA, et al. Atelectasis on pediatric chest CT: comparison of sedation techniques. Pediatr Radiol. 1999;29:509–13.

Tsai KL, et al. Pulmonary atelectasis: a frequent alternative diagnosis in patients undergoing CT-PA for suspected pulmonary embolism. Emerg Radiol. 2004;10:282–6.

Westcott JL, et al. Plate atelectasis. Radiology. 1985;155:1–9.

Zhao Y, et al. Atelectasis: an unusual and late complication of lung transplant. Clin Transplant. 2002;16:233–9.


## 7.4    Sarcoidosis

Sarcoidosis, also known as *Boeck's sarcoid*, is a multisystemic granulomatous disorder characterized by the formation of multiple epithelioid granulomas within more than one system. Sarcoidosis belongs to a large family of granulomatous disorders, which includes tuberculosis, leprosy, Langerhans cell histiocytosis, and more. All members of the granulomatous disease are characterized by the formation of granulomas within the body system.

*Granuloma* is a specific kind of chronic inflammation, and it is a term used to describe a nodular chronic inflammation that occurs in foci (granules), with collection of macrophages called epithelioid cells. *Epithelioid cells* are macrophages with abundant cytoplasm that is similar to the cytoplasm of epithelial cells. When multiple epithelioid cells fuse together, they form a bigger macrophage known as *giant cell*. Epithelioid cells define granulomatous inflammation. On histological specimens, granulomas show endarteritis obliterans, fibrosis, and chronic inflammatory cells (epithelioid cells). Granuloma can be due to an infection (e.g., tuberculosis) or due to an inorganic foreign body (e.g., silicosis).

Langerhans cells are characteristically found within the sarcoid granuloma, which develops by the fusion of epithelioid cells, resulting in a modified macrophage with nuclei arranged in an arc-like pattern. Langerhans cells secrete lysozyme, collagenase, calcitriol, angiotensin-converting enzyme (ACE), and varied cytokines.

No body tissue is spared from sarcoidosis. There are two forms of the disease, an acute form and chronic form. *Acute sarcoidosis* responds well to steroids with frequent spontaneous recovery. Moreover, it is characterized by serum elevation of ACE in two thirds of patients and abnormal calcium metabolism (high serum calcium levels). In contrast, the *chronic sarcoidosis* is persistent, and the serum levels of calcium and ACE are often normal.

Sarcoidosis is often seen between 20 and 40 years of age. However, juvenile form (pediatric sarcoidosis) with a smaller age peak at 13–15 years has been reported to occur rarely.

Sarcoidosis manifestations are seen in almost any part of the body. The definite diagnosis is based on histopathology examination. Radiological investigations play an important role in monitoring the therapy and the disease progression.

## Pulmonary Sarcoidosis

The pulmonary system is involved in up to 90 % of patients with sarcoidosis. Patients with sarcoidosis are classically young females presenting with nonspecific symptoms of a systemic disease (e.g., malaise). In pulmonary sarcoidosis, dyspnea and cough are common, whereas hemoptysis (coughing blood) is rare.

### Sarcoidosis Has Five Radiological Grades on Plain Chest Radiograph

*Grade 0*: Normal chest radiograph.

*Grade 1*: There are clear lung fields with bilateral hilar lymphadenopathy (85 % of cases). It is usually identified by accident, and the patient is asymptomatic (◘ Fig. 7.4.30).

*Grade 2*: There is reticulonodular interstitial pattern with hilar lymphadenopathy. The areas affected are usually located in the upper lobes.

*Grade 3*: There is reticulonodular interstitial pattern without hilar lymphadenopathy (◘ Fig. 7.4.31).

*Grade 4*: There is pulmonary parenchymal scarring and fibrosis (◘ Fig. 7.4.32).

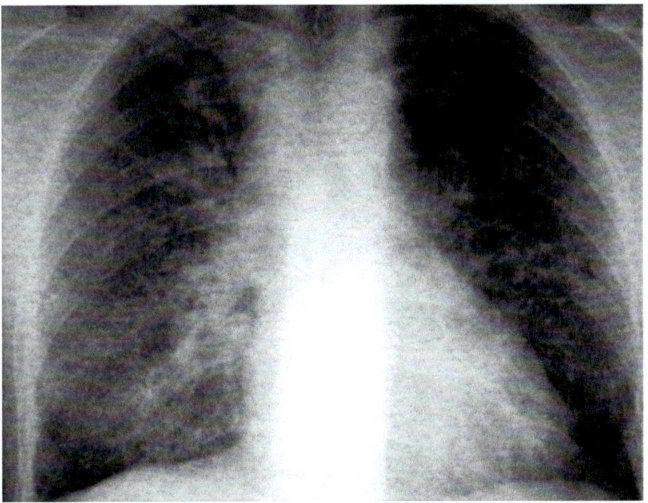

◘ **Fig. 7.4.31** Posteroanterior chest radiograph of a patient with grade 3 pulmonary sarcoidosis shows bilateral diffuse reticular interstitial pattern due to lung fibrosis

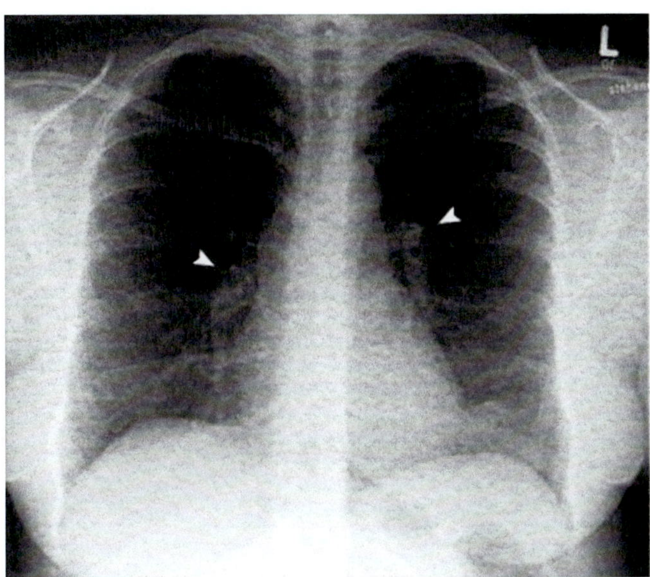

◘ **Fig. 7.4.30** Posteroanterior chest radiograph of a female patient with grade 2 pulmonary sarcoidosis shows bilateral hilar lymphadenopathy (*arrowheads*) with clear lung fields

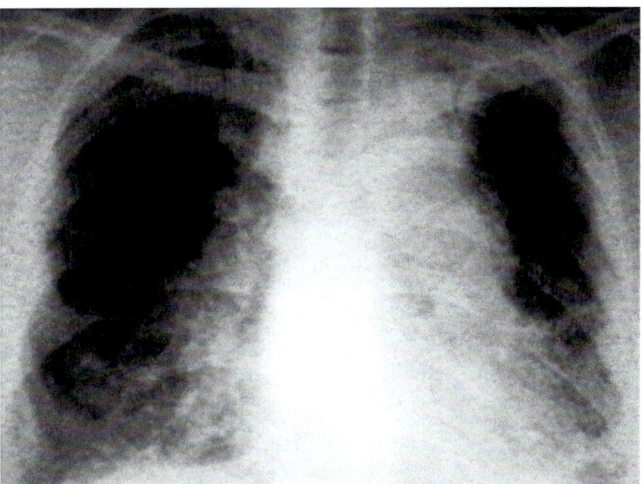

◘ **Fig. 7.4.32** Posteroanterior chest radiograph of a patient with chronic grade 4 pulmonary sarcoidosis shows bilateral lung fibrosis distorting the heart silhouette (shaggy heart appearance)

**Signs on HRCT**

- Sarcoid granulomas are typically distributed along the lymphatic vessels within the interstitium. Due to this fact, miliary nodules plus linear thickening of the interlobar septa can be found in a similar fashion to the interstitial disease seen in lymphangitis carcinomatosis and lymphoproliferative diseases.
- Bilateral hilar lymphadenopathy observed in grade 2 and 4. Punctuate, stippled, or egg shell calcification patterns may be seen.
- Occasionally, multiple granulomas may aggregate to form a mass-like nodule within the lungs that mimics metastasis (◘ Fig. 7.4.33). Lung nodule is a lesion <3 cm in diameter, whereas lung mass is a lesion >3 cm in diameter.
- Necrotizing sarcoid granulomatosis is a rare variant of sarcoid characterized by the formation of cavitating granulomas.

- Hilar lymphadenopathy with eggshell calcification and bilateral upper lobe fibrosis are typical findings in pulmonary silicosis. Sarcoidosis may mimic silicosis when it produces the same set of radiographic manifestations on plain chest radiograph.

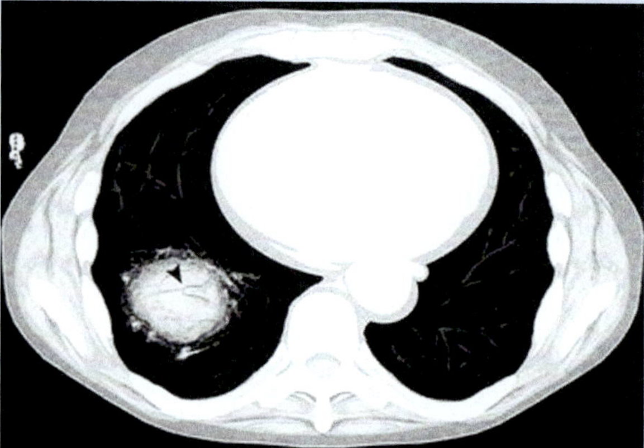

**Fig. 7.4.33** Axial thoracic lung-window HRCT illustration demonstrates a pulmonary mass that is composed of multiple aggregated sarcoid granulomas. Although it is a difficult diagnosis to confirm without biopsy, the presence of air bronchogram or areas of normal tissue lines within the mass (*arrowhead*) can differentiate this rare lesion from bronchogenic carcinoma

- Gastric sarcoidosis features range from ulceration mimicking peptic ulcer to mucosal thickening mimicking Menetrier disease. Diagnosis requires endoscopic biopsy to confirm the epithelioid granuloma.

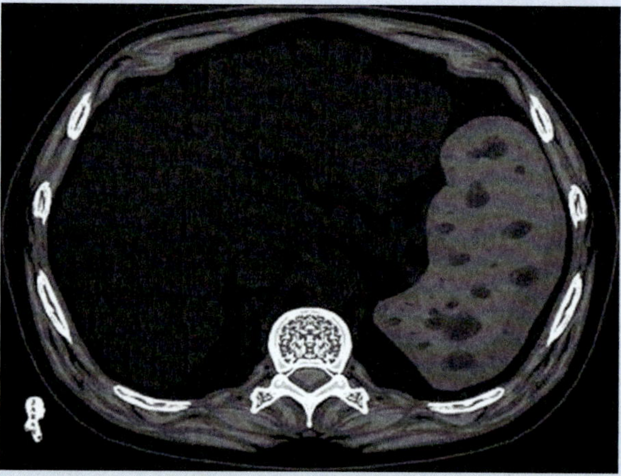

**Fig. 7.4.34** Abdominal nonenhanced CT illustration demonstrates multiple hypodense lesions within the spleen representing splenic sarcoid granulomas

## Hepatic, Splenic, and Gastric Sarcoidosis

Hepatic sarcoidosis is seen in 5–15 % of patients with high ACE levels (acute disease). There are multiple hepatic granulomas that can be easily mistaken on CT and MRI for metastasis or lymphoma. Simultaneous involvement of the spleen favors the diagnosis of sarcoidosis and lymphoma.

Splenic sarcoidosis classically affects the white bulb and the arterial circulation. The spleen is affected in 5–14 % of patients with sarcoidosis. Patients may suffer from symptoms of hypersplenism, anemia, thrombocytopenia, and leukopenia.

Gastric sarcoidosis is the most common feature of gastrointestinal involvement of sarcoidosis. It often involves the antrum. Massive retroperitoneal lymphadenopathy may be rarely encountered in sarcoidosis.

**Signs on CT**
- Hepatic sarcoidosis is seen as multiple hypodense lesions with irregular shapes on liver contrast-enhanced images.
- Splenic sarcoidosis is seen on contrast-enhanced images as multiple, irregularly diffuse, hypodense lesions within the spleen representing granulomas (**Fig. 7.4.34**). Hepatic lesions may be noticed in the same scan (50 % of cases). The same lesions are seen hypoechoic on US and hypointense on T1W and T2W images on MRI compared to the background.

## Dermatological Sarcoidosis

Skin lesions are seen in up to 25 % of patients with sarcoidosis. Skin lesions in sarcoidosis are divided into reactive and specific lesions. Reactive sarcoidosis skin lesions do not contain granuloma formation histologically (e.g., erythema nodosum). In contrast, specific sarcoidosis skin lesions are characterized by noncaseating granuloma formation (e.g., Darier–Roussy nodules).

In the acute reactive sarcoidosis, *erythema nodosum* is the most common finding, and it is seen as multiple patchy red lesions found over the shin, often in a bilateral fashion. Systemic manifestations like fever, malaise, and polyarthralgia occur in about 50 % of patients with erythema nodosum.

The chronic reactive sarcoidosis, on the other hand, is characterized by a specific lesion called "lupus pernio." *Lupus pernio* is a specific skin lesion in sarcoidosis characterized by dusky-red plaques formation on the nose, ears, lips, and face. Lupus pernio is classically seen in women with chronic sarcoidosis and extensive pulmonary infiltration, anterior uveitis, and bone lesions. The nose lesion is typically red to purple in color and seen on the tip of the nose, causing bulbous appearance (**Fig. 7.4.35**). The nose lesion infiltrates the mucosa and may destroy the underlying nasal bone.

In black patients, maculopapular eruptions are the most common skin manifestations of sarcoidosis. *Darier–Roussy nodules* are small painless subcutaneous nodules that arise within the dermis and the epidermis. They represent noncaseating granulomas.

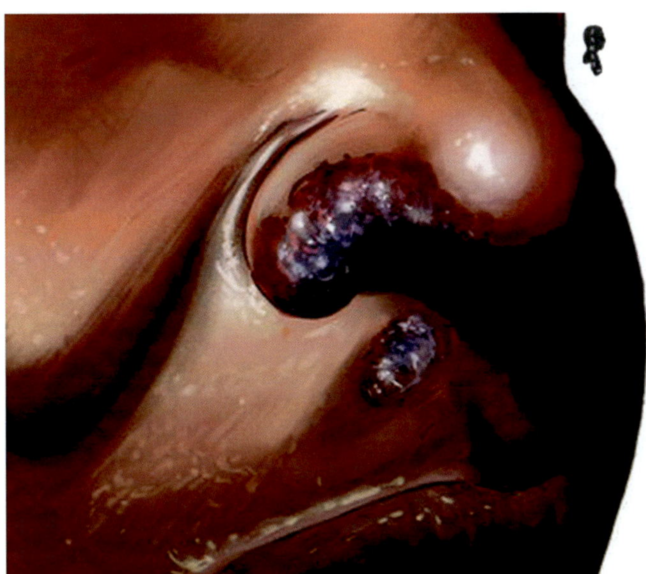

**Fig. 7.4.35** An illustration demonstrates lupus pernio on the ala of the nose

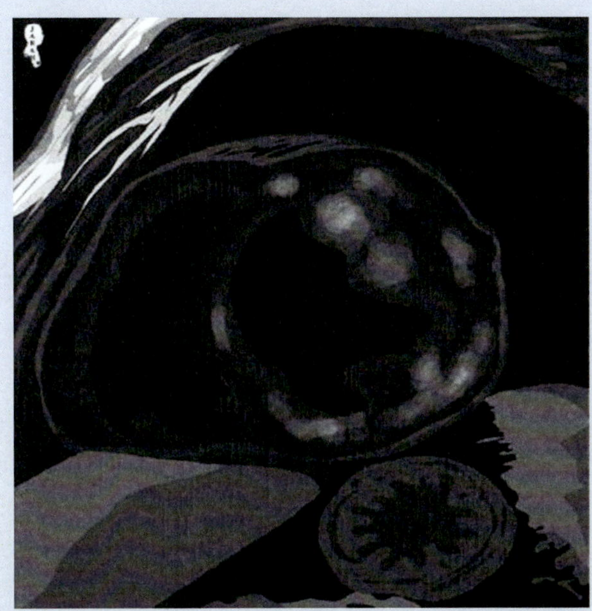

**Fig. 7.4.36** Short-axis dark-blood cardiac T2W MR-illustration demonstrates multiple high signal intensity lesions within the myocardium due to granuloma formation in a patient with sarcoidosis

## Differential Diagnoses and Related Diseases

*Löfgren syndrome* is a disease characterized by the combination of arthralgia, bilateral hilar lymphadenopathy, and erythema nodosum in a patient with sarcoidosis.

## Cardiac Sarcoidosis

Sarcoidosis affects the heart in the form of patchy infiltration of the myocardium by granulomas causing fibrosis and scarring. Patients with cardiac sarcoidosis are at risk of sudden cardiac death due to ventricular arrhythmias or conduction block. Most patients are asymptomatic, with only 5 % of cardiac sarcoidosis patients being symptomatic. Cor pulmonale may arise secondary to pulmonary hypertension as a consequence of pulmonary fibrosis.

> **Signs on Cardiac MRI**
> - The protocol of cardiac sarcoidosis should include T1W pre- and postcontrast images (there are multiple areas of contrast enhancement due to noncaseating granulomas), T2-STIR (to show edema or scar formation as low intensity areas), and CE-IR images to assess global function.
> - Inflammatory changes show myocardial high T2 signal intensity lesions (**Fig. 7.4.36**), with postcontrast enhancement and myocardial thickening. Postinflammatory changes include myocardial high T2 signal intensity lesions, with no contrast enhancement.

## Neurosarcoid

Involvement of the central nervous system by sarcoidosis (neurosarcoid) is noticed in <10 % of patients. There are three patterns of involvement: meningeal, parenchymal, and vascular.

In the brain, neurosarcoid has an affinity to involve the base of the brain and the cranial nerves. It commonly affects the hypothalamus, pons, meninges, spinal cord, basal ganglia, and cranial nerves (optic, facial, and vestibulocochlear). Neurosarcoid is the most common cause of bilateral facial nerve paralysis. Leptomeningeal thickening in the form of aseptic meningitis is commonly seen in neurosarcoid. When the lesion affects the hypothalamus, it leads to abnormal water balance and disturbance of thirst mechanism (sarcoid diabetes insipidus). Neurosarcoid can present in the absence of systemic sarcoidosis in 3 % of cases.

## Differential Diagnoses and Related Diseases

*Klein–Levin syndrome* is a disease that arises due to hypothalamic or medial thalamic lesions characterized by episodes of compulsive eating (bulimia), hypersexuality in adolescent males, and hypersomnolence. Patients with hypersomnolence sleep an excessive amount of time at night, take long naps during the day, and generally feel drowsy and distracted when awake. Each episode lasts days to weeks with a symptom-free interval of 3–6 months between attacks. Klein–Levin syndrome is reported to occur rarely due to neurosarcoidosis.

### Signs on MRI

- Within the brain parenchyma, multiple or solitary brain lesions with a ringlike appearance may be seen on T2W and FLAIR images.
- Thickening and enhancement of the meninges of postcontrast images are a classic finding in neurosarcoid in the area of the sellar diaphragm and the spinal cord (■ Fig. 7.4.37). Inflammation of basal meninges can lead to interference with cerebrospinal fluid (CSF) flow or aqueduct involvement leading to obstructive hydrocephalus.
- Cranial nerve neuritis is seen as enhancement of the nerves like the facial or the vestibulocochlear within the internal auditory canal on T1W postcontrast images (■ Fig. 7.4.38).
- When diabetes insipidus is present, thickening of the infundibulum and the optic chiasm with isointense T1/T2 high signal intensities and homogenous contrast enhancement is typically observed.

- Intramedullary spinal cord lesions on T2W images with enhancement after contrast injection may be found representing neurosarcoid granuloma.
- In Klein–Levin syndrome, hypothalamic T2 high signal lesions with leptomeningeal enhancement on postcontrast injection images may be seen.

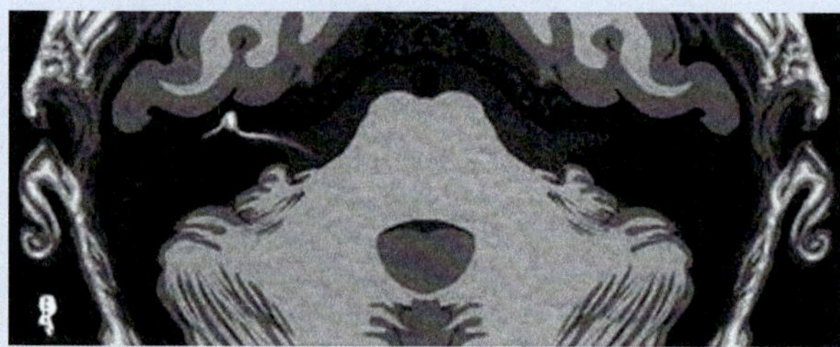

■ **Fig. 7.4.38**   Axial cerebellopontine angle T1W postcontrast MR-illustration demonstrates enhancement of the right facial nerve due to neuritis (the labyrinthine segment, the geniculate ganglion, and the proximal tympanic segment)

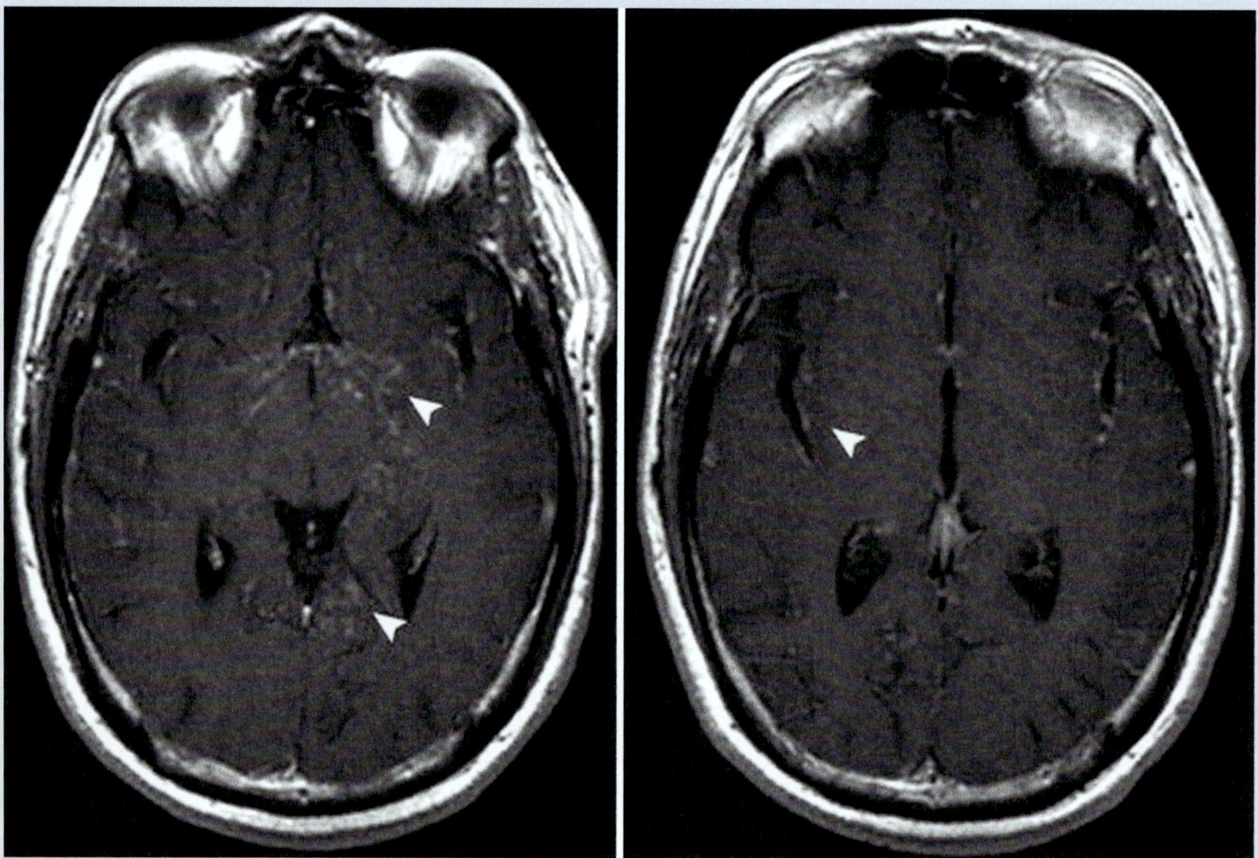

■ **Fig. 7.4.37**   Sequential axial T1W postcontrast brain images show nodular thickening and enhancement of the leptomeninges (*arrowheads*) in a patient with sarcoidosis (neurosarcoid)

## Musculoskeletal Sarcoidosis

The musculoskeletal system in sarcoidosis present in the form of arthritis (40 %), bony lesions, and muscular lesions. The musculoskeletal manifestations are commonly seen in chronic sarcoidosis, not in the acute form.

Sarcoid arthritis is migratory polyarthritis that involves usually the ankles and the knees, followed by the wrists and the interphalangeal joints. Early sarcoid arthropathy occurs in the first 6 months of symptoms, and it involves migratory polyarthritis (>4 joints). The second form occurs after 6 months or more and is characterized by oligoarthritis (2–3 joints) and inflammation of fingers or toes (dactylitis). Tenosynovitis may occur occasionally, causing a sausage-like finger similar to that seen in psoriatic arthritis.

Bony lesions in sarcoidosis are seen in 5–10 % of patients. They present as extensive bony erosions or cystic-like osteolytic lesions typically seen in the phalanges in the hands and feet (*osteitis multiplex cystica*). The same type of lesions can be seen in tuberculosis and classically known as *osteitis tuberculosa multiplex cystica*. Uncommonly, calvarial sarcoidosis may manifest as an expansile bony lesion.

Muscular sarcoidosis often presents as a nodular mass within the muscle due to granuloma formation.

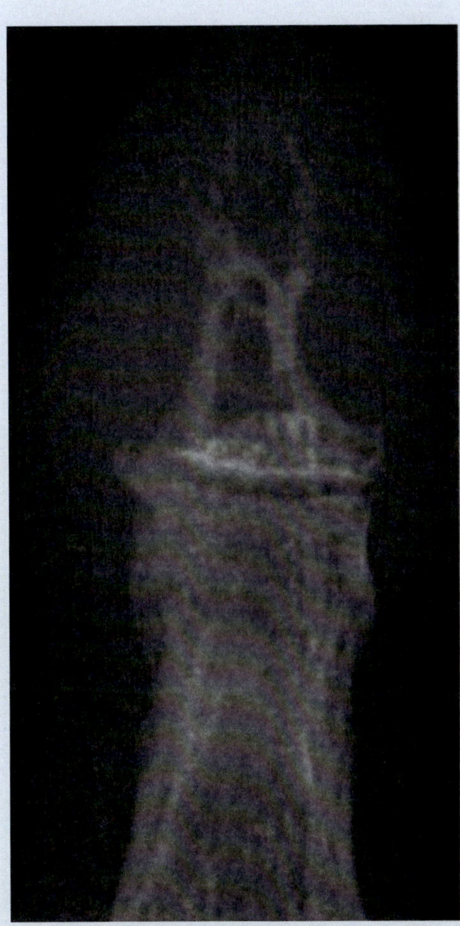

**Fig. 7.4.39** Plain radiograph of the index finger of a patient with chronic sarcoidosis shows multiple osteolytic cystic lesions located within the terminal phalanges (osteitis multiplex cystica)





## Head and Neck Sarcoidosis

Ocular manifestations of sarcoidosis occur in up to 80 % of patients in the form of bilateral uveitis and lacrimal duct inflammation. However, any structure of the eye may be involved. Conjunctival lesions are the second most common lesions seen in ophthalmic sarcoidosis after anterior uveitis. Keratoconjunctivitis sicca may occur in 5 % of cases when lacrimal gland infiltration occurs.

Parotid gland involvement in a bilateral fashion can be seen in up to 6 % of patients. The features resemble the parotid symptoms observed in Sjögren's syndrome and lymphoma.

In up to 30 % of cases, patients with sarcoidosis present with cervical, nontender, movable lymphadenopathy commonly located in the posterior triangle.

Hoarseness of voice may rarely arise in patients with sarcoidosis due to vocal cord thickening and granulomas formation. It is a rare manifestation affecting 1–3 % of patients.

Paranasal sarcoidosis may occur, especially with lupus pernio. It has an affinity to involve the mucosa of the inferior turbinate and the nasal septum, causing mucosal thickening and nasal septal destruction.

## Differential Diagnoses and Related Diseases

*Heerfordt syndrome* is a disease that occurs in a patient with sarcoidosis characterized by the triad of fever and anterior uveitis, bilateral parotid enlargement, and facial nerve palsy.

### Signs on CT and MRI
- Bilateral enlargement of the lacrimal glands with contrast enhancement is commonly seen in ophthalmic sarcoidosis.
- Bilateral parotid enlargement, with high signal T2 intensity, and enhancement on postcontrast images are seen in cases of parotid involvement.
- Inferior turbinate destruction with nasal septum erosion is seen in paranasal sinus CT ( Fig. 7.4.40).

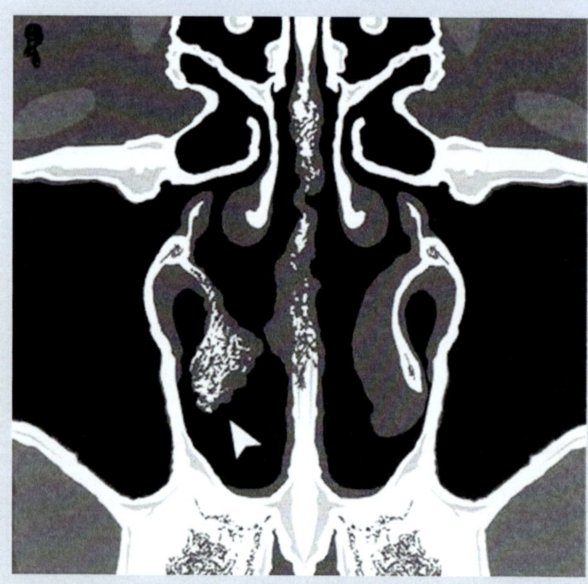

 **Fig. 7.4.40**  Coronal paranasal sinuses CT illustration demonstrates right inferior turbinate destruction (*arrowhead*) with nasal septum erosions due to sarcoidosis

## Genitourinary Sarcoidosis

Renal sarcoidosis manifestations are related to nephrocalcinosis due to hypercalcemia or granuloma formation within the cortex and the medulla (interstitial nephritis). Scrotal sarcoidosis is uncommon but can present in the form of bilateral epididymitis.

### Signs on Scrotal US
Epididymitis is seen as enlarged heterogeneous epididymis with marked increased signal flow on color Doppler and power Doppler due to hyperemia.

### Signs on CT
- Interstitial nephritis is seen on postcontrast images as striated nephrogram, usually on both kidneys.
- Rarely, renal sarcoidosis may present with bilateral hypodense tumorlike nodules on contrast-enhanced images that may be mistaken for lymphoma.

### Signs on MRI
Epididymitis is seen as bilaterally enlarged epididymis with high signal intensity on T2W images, with contrast enhancement in postgadolinium injection.

## Further Reading


Afshar A, et al. Sarcoidosis: a rare cause of Kleine-Levine-Critchley syndrome. Sarcoidosis Vasc Diffuse Lung Dis. 2008;25:60–3.

Burov EA, et al. Morpheaform sarcoidosis: report of three cases. J Am Acad Dermatol. 1998;39:345–8.

Cummings MM, et al. Sarcoidosis. Dis Mon. 1960;6:1–40.

Farman J, et al. Gastric sarcoidosis. Abdom Imaging. 1997;22:248–52.

Fodor D, et al. Dactylitis and bone lesions at the onset of sarcoidosis: a case report. Pol Arch Med Wewn. 2008;118:774–7.

Geraint JD, et al. Descriptive definition and historic aspects of sarcoidosis. Clin Chest Med. 1997a;18:663–79.

Geraint JD, et al. Descriptive definition and historic aspects of sarcoidosis. Clin Chest Med. 1997b;18:663–79.

Henry DA, et al. Multiple imaging evaluation of sarcoidosis. Radiographics. 1986;6:75–95.

Koyama T, et al. Radiologic manifestations of sarcoidosis in various organs. Radiographics. 2004;24:87–104.

Kuhlman JE, et al. The computed tomographic spectrum of thoracic sarcoidosis. Radiographics. 1989;9:449–66.

Moore SL, et al. Musculoskeletal sarcoidosis: spectrum of appearances at MR imaging. Radiographics. 2003;23:1389–99.

Pattishall EN, et al. Sarcoidosis in children. Pediatr Pulmonol. 1996;22:195–203.

Poyanli A, et al. Vertebral sarcoidosis: imaging findings. Eur Radiol. 2000;10:92–4.

Rosell A, et al. Lupus pernio with involvement of nasal cavity and maxillary sinus. ORL. 1998;60:236–9.

Sharma OP. Sarcoidosis. Dis Mon. 1990;36:474–535.

Spilberg I, et al. The arthritis in sarcoidosis. Arthritis Rheum. 1969;12:126–36.

Tamme T, et al. Sarcoidosis (Heerfordt syndrome): a case report. Stomatologija Baltic Dent Maxillofac J. 2007;9: 61–4.

Turkish M, et al. Osteitis tuberculosa multiplex cystica: its treatment with streptomycin and promizole. J Pediatr. 1949;35:625–9.

Warshauer DM. Splenic sarcoidosis. Semin Ultrasound CT MRI. 2007;28:21–7.

Yanardağ H, et al. Bone cysts in sarcoidosis: what is their clinical significance? Rheumatol Int. 2004;24:294–6.

## 7.5    Emphysema

Emphysema is a chronic obstructive airway disease characterized by an abnormal, irreversible, permanent enlargement of the air spaces distal to the terminal bronchioles, associated with destruction of the alveolar walls, and without obvious fibrosis.

The mechanism of emphysema is mainly mediated by the proteolytic enzymes (proteases) of the neutrophils and macrophages. The proteolytic enzymes dissolve the alveolar walls, creating holes that facilitate air leak from one alveolus to another, compromising gas exchange and trapping air within the acini. Normally, there are few small physiological holes between the alveoli that connect two adjacent alveoli together (pores of Kohn). In emphysema, the holes between the alveoli are numerous and much bigger than the normal Kohn's pores, resulting in reducing the surface area for gas exchange.

The enzyme α-1 antitrypsin is a proteinase inhibitor that counteracts the effect of the proteolytic enzymes produced by neutrophils and macrophages. Emphysema results from imbalance between the proteolytic enzymes (proteases) production and α-1 antitrypsin (antiproteases).

The first emphysema mechanism arises due to increased alveolar infiltration by neutrophils and macrophages, with increased proteolytic enzymes' production that exceeds the capacity of the normal circulating α-1 antitrypsin levels to counteract. This scenario is classically seen in emphysema due to cigarette smoking. The other mechanism of emphysema is seen due to congenital α-1 antitrypsin deficiency disease, where emphysema is produced with normal quantities of proteolytic enzymes.

Pathologically, emphysema is divided according to the level of alveolar destruction and the air trapping pattern within the secondary lobule (e.g., central or peripheral). Four major types of emphysema are described:

- *Centrilobular emphysema*: this type starts at the center of the secondary lobule (centrilobular), and it results from the destruction of the alveoli around the proximal respiratory lobule. This type is typically seen in chronic cigarette smokers, and it affects predominantly the upper lung lobes. The emphysematous spaces may coalesce into a lager *bulla*, which is defined as sharply demarcated area of air collection >1 cm in diameter and with a wall less than 1 mm in thickness (Fig. 7.5.41).

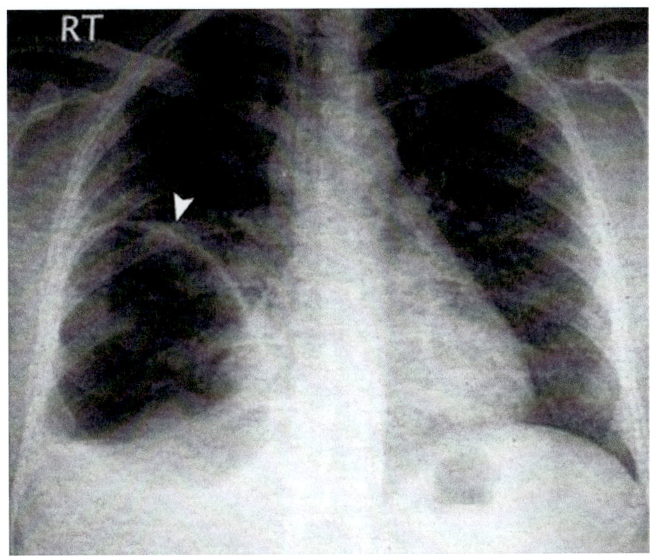


**Fig. 7.5.41** Posteroanterior plain chest radiograph shows large right lower zone bulla (*arrowhead*)

- *Panlobular (panacinar) emphysema*: this type of emphysema is diffuse and involves the whole secondary lobule. This type is classically seen in nonsmoker patients with congenital α-1 antitrypsin deficiency disease and in *Swyer–James syndrome* (unilateral hyperinflated lung with pulmonary vasculature atresia, and it may be accompanied by bronchiectasis). Panlobular emphysema can be seen in conjunction with centrilobular emphysema in chronic smokers. Panlobular emphysema involves mainly the lower lung lobes.
- *Paraseptal (distal lobular) emphysema*: this type is seen as air trapping at the periphery of the secondary lobule, especially adjacent to connective tissue septa. This type is typically seen at the periphery, at the subpleural spaces, and along the fissures and pleural reflections. It plays an important role in the development of spontaneous pneumothoraces.
- *Irregular (paracicatricial) emphysema*: this type is an air collection that occurs in an area of massive fibrosis (scar tissue). It is commonly found in the upper lobes in an area of old tuberculosis fibrosis.

Other types of emphysema include:
- *Emphysema due to old age*: it occurs due to the loss of lung volume (atrophy). It is panacinal type without airways obstruction.
- *Compensatory emphysema (postpneumonectomy syndrome)*: this type occurs when a lung lobe collapses or has been removed. The other lung will expand to occupy the space of lung deficiency. There is no airway obstruction with this type.
- *Giant bullous emphysema (vanishing lung syndrome)*: it is airways destruction due to extensive alveolar atrophy due to avascular necrosis of the lung parenchyma, resulting in hyperinflation of the affected lung. It is most commonly seen in young men with bilateral upper lobes bullae. It is a panlobular type affecting the upper lobes mainly and

commonly present in individuals in their 40s. Up to 20 % of patients have congenital α-1 antitrypsin deficiency disease.

- *Bronchial atresia emphysema*: this type arises due to developmental bronchial atresia. The segment with the atrophic bronchus receives its aeration by the "collateral air-drift mechanism" via "pores of Kohn" and "canals of Lambert." It is panacinar type and usually affects the left upper lobe.
- *Foreign body emphysema*: it is lung hyperinflation due to an obstructed bronchus. It's a reversible airway obstruction.
- *Subcutaneous (surgical) emphysema*: it is defined as collection of air at the level of subcutaneous tissues superficial to the deep fascia that covers the skeletal muscle plane. This type is commonly seen after trauma to the trachea or the esophagus in car accidents, stab wounds, or gunshot wounds. It can also be seen in intensive patients on a positive airway pressure ventilator. *Air-leak syndrome* is a term used to describe generalized thoracic air leak that includes subcutaneous emphysema, pneumomediastinum, and pneumopericardium, with or without pneumothorax.

### Signs on Chest Radiographs
- Lung hyperinflation, which is detected as posterior rib counts >10 ribs, anterior rib count >7 ribs, and increased intercostals spaces distance.
- Prominent hilar vessels with disappearance of the peripheral vessels.
- Increase in the retrosternal trans-radiant area size on lateral radiographs, which is the area behind the sternum where the two lungs come in contact. This space is usually up to 3 cm deep. An increase in this area above 3 cm might indicate emphysema (◘ Fig. 7.5.42).
- Deep sulcus sign: the costophrenic angle deepens due to lung hyperinflation (◘ Fig. 7.5.43).
- Flattening of the diaphragm with barrel (funnel-shaped) chest configuration (◘ Fig. 7.5.44).
- Bulla is visualized as a hyperlucent area surrounded by a thin wall.
- Compensatory emphysema: a hyperinflated lung with a part herniating into the other side of the chest to compensate an area of lung deficiency or atelectasis (◘ Fig. 7.5.43).
- Vanishing lung syndrome: bilateral upper zones giant bullae (◘ Fig. 7.5.45).
- Foreign body emphysema: unilateral hyperinflated lung usually with radio-opaque structure located at the areas of the main bronchi or trachea.
- Subcutaneous emphysema: radiolucent air is visualized under the skin and around the muscles (◘ Fig. 7.5.46).

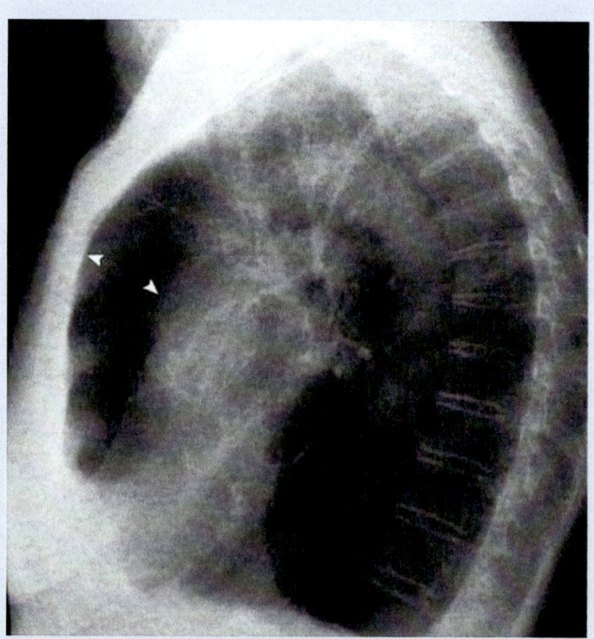

◘ **Fig. 7.5.42** Lateral plain chest radiograph of a patient with congenital α-1 antitrypsin deficiency disease shows increased retrosternal space due to emphysema (*arrowheads*)

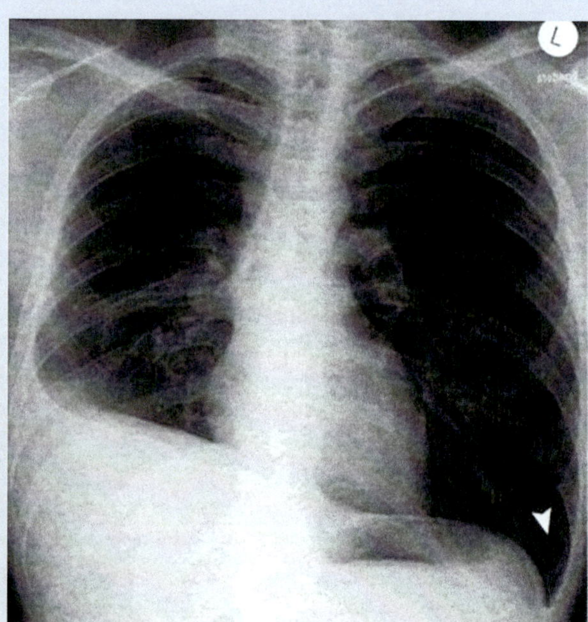

◘ **Fig. 7.5.43** Posteroanterior plain chest radiograph of a patient with postpneumonectomy of the right lower lung lobe shows compensatory emphysema of the left lung with deep sulcus sign (*arrowhead*)

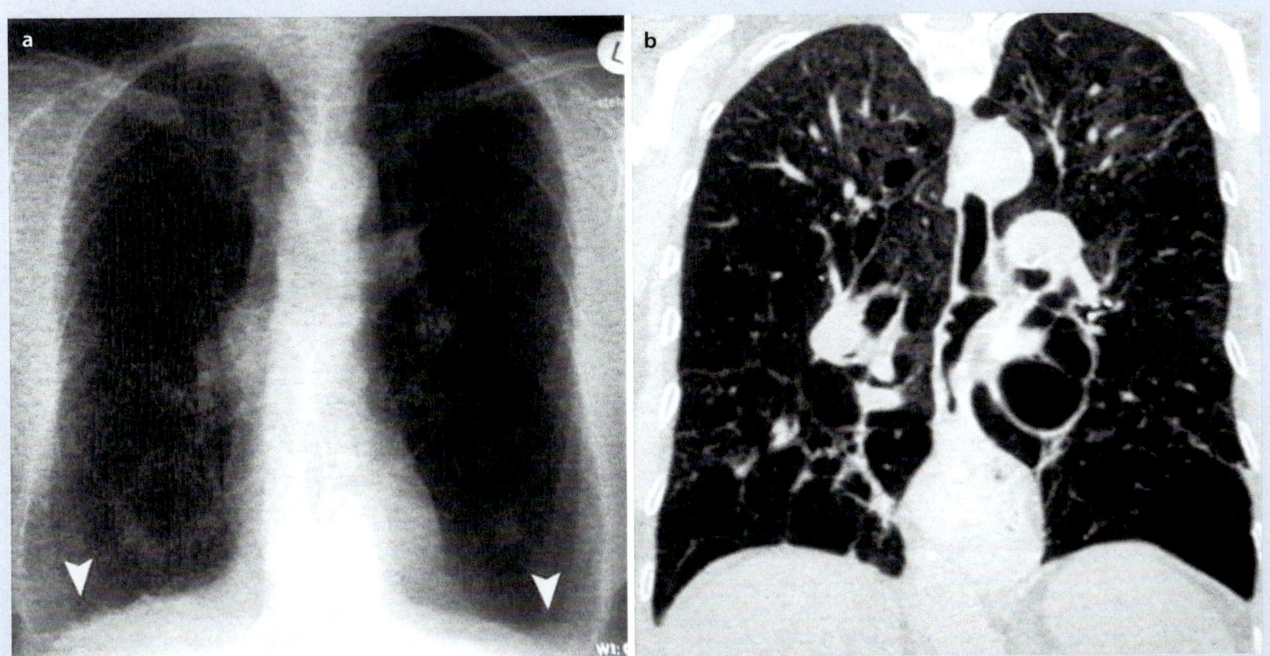

◨ **Fig. 7.5.44** Posteroanterior plain chest radiograph (**a**) and coronal chest HRCT (**b**) of two patients with congenital α-1 antitrypsin deficiency disease shows flattened diaphragm in (**a**) (*arrowheads*), and bilateral panlobular and centrilobular emphysema in (**b**)

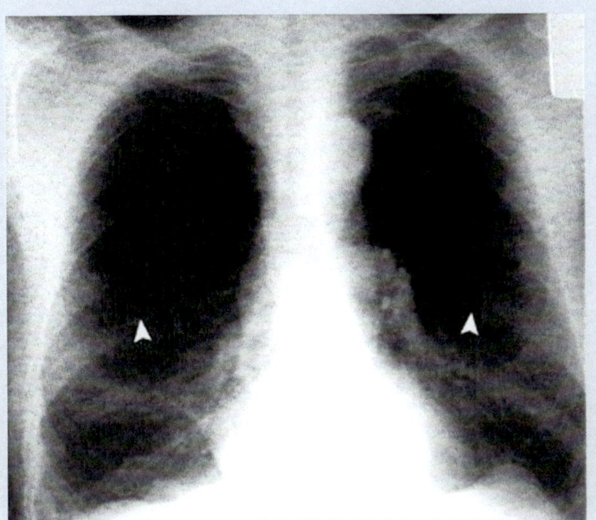

◨ **Fig. 7.5.45** Posteroanterior plain chest radiograph of a patient with vanishing lung syndrome shows bilateral giant upper lobes bullae (*arrowheads*)

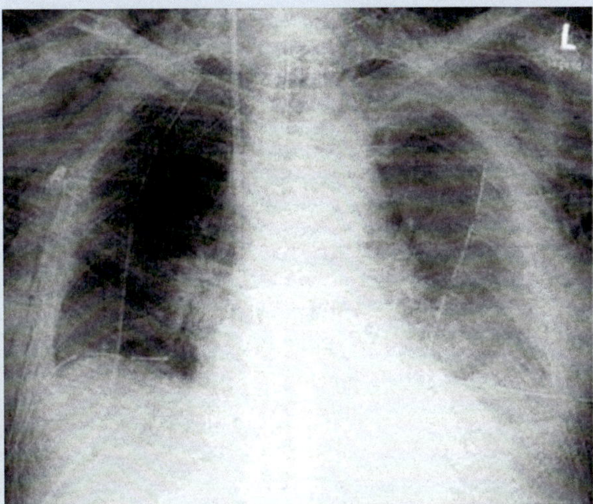

◨ **Fig. 7.5.46** Anteroposterior plain chest radiograph of a patient with subcutaneous emphysema shows air that surrounds the pectoralis muscle fibers bilaterally

### Signs on HRCT and Conventional CT

- Centrilobular emphysema appears as focal, oval, or round areas of low attenuation up to 1 cm in diameter, within a homogenous background of lung parenchyma (◨ Fig. 7.5.47), and not associated with fibrosis. It has a characteristic of upper lung zone predominance.

- Panlobular emphysema appears as large, uniform low-attenuation areas with characteristic lower lung zone predominance (◨ Fig. 7.5.47).
- Paraseptal emphysema appears as multiple small areas of low attenuation located typically at lung peripheries with subpleural location (◨ Fig. 7.5.47). It has thin walls and should not be confused with

honeycombing, which is characterized by thick wall bronchiectasis, with signs of fibrosis and architectural distortion.

- Irregular emphysema appears as air bullae trapped within areas of fibrosis.
- Congenital α-1 antitrypsin deficiency disease is typically associated with signs of liver cirrhosis, with risks of developing hepatocellular carcinoma. Patients are typically in their 40s presenting with dyspnea with signs of hepatic dysfunction.
- Air-leak syndrome is detected as generalized subcutaneous emphysema, pneumomediastinum, parenchymal emphysema, and pneumopericardium, with or without pneumothorax (◘ Fig. 7.5.48).

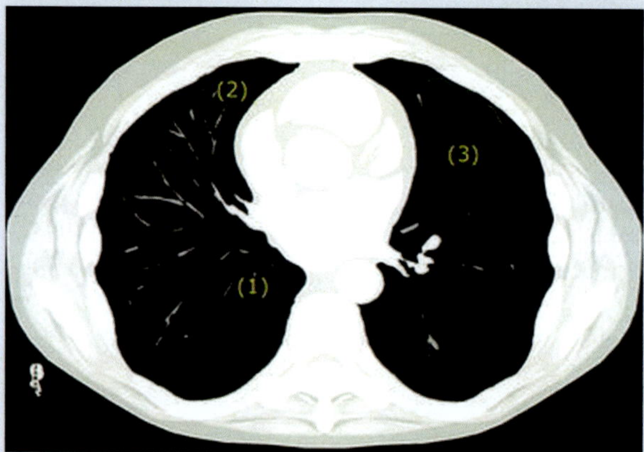

◘ **Fig. 7.5.47** Axial thoracic HRCT illustration demonstrates types of emphysema on HRCT: (*1*) centrilobular, (*2*) paraseptal, and (*3*) panlobular

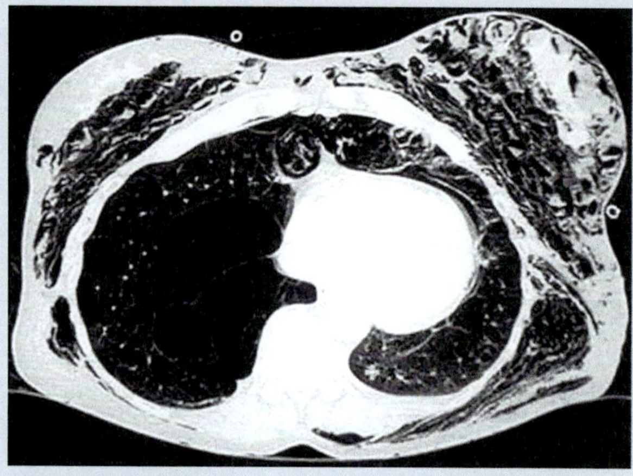

◘ **Fig. 7.5.48** Axial thoracic HRCT of a female patient with air-leak syndrome shows right panlobular emphysema, subcutaneous emphysema affecting the thoracic wall and breasts bilaterally, and mild pneumopericardium

## Further Reading


Bergin C, et al. The secondary pulmonary lobule: normal and abnormal CT appearance. AJR Am J Roentgenol. 1988;151:21–5.

Kazerooni EA, et al. Imaging of emphysema and lung volume reduction surgery. Radiographics. 1997;17:1023–36.

Marti de Gracia M, et al. Subcutaneous emphysema: diagnostic clue in the emergency room. Emerg Radiol. 2009;16:343–8. doi:10.1007/s10140–009–0794-x.

Stern EJ, et al. CT of the lung in patients with pulmonary emphysema: diagnosis, quantification, and correlation with pathologic and physiologic findings. AJR Am J Roentgenol. 1994;162:791–8.

Thurlbeck WM, et al. Radiographic appearance of chest in emphysema. AJR Am J Roentgenol. 1978;130:429–40.

Thurlbeck WM, et al. Emphysema: definition, imaging, and quantification. AJR Am J Roentgenol. 1994;163:1017–25.

Yamanoha A, et al. Air-leak syndrome associated with bronchiolitis obliterans after allogeneic peripheral blood stem cell transplantation. Int J Hematol. 2007;85:95–6.


## 7.6    Idiopathic Interstitial Pneumonias

Idiopathic interstitial pneumonias (IIPs) are a group of diseases characterized by parenchymal lung fibrosis. IIPs are classified by the American Thoracic Society (ATS) and the European Respiratory Society (ERS) into seven disease entities: idiopathic pulmonary fibrosis, nonspecific interstitial pneumonia (NSIP), cryptogenic organizing pneumonia (COP), respiratory bronchiolitis-associated interstitial lung disease (RB-ILD), desquamative interstitial pneumonia (DIP), lymphoid interstitial pneumonia (LIP), and acute interstitial pneumonia (AIP).

Although the ATS-ERS classification differentiates between the subtypes of IIPs based on histopathology findings, radiology can help in the diagnosis assessment based on the computed tomography findings of each disease. Lung extension can be characteristic for some IIP subtypes.

Patients with IIPs generally present with progressive dyspnea, cough, and other nonspecific respiratory symptoms.

## Idiopathic Pulmonary Fibrosis

Idiopathic pulmonary fibrosis (IPF), also known *usual pulmonary fibrosis*, is a disease characterized by lung fibrosis with unknown cause.

Patient with IPF is typically a 50-year-old patient presenting with progressive dyspnea and nonproductive cough. Clinical examination may show signs of chronic cyanosis, finger clubbing, and basal lung crepitation on auscultation. Diagnosis of IPF by histology is very important because IPF patients usually do not respond to high corticosteroid therapy, with a median survival time ranging from 2 to 4 years after starting symptoms.

History of smoking can be a risk factor for IPF. However, it does not affect the course of the disease.

### Signs on Radiographs and HRCT

- Typically, patients with IPF present with reticular interstitial pattern with reduced lung volume, subpleural reticular opacities, and macrocytic honeycombing (bronchiectatic changes). The distribution of the lung fibrosis characteristically involves the lung bases and decrease toward lung apices (apicobasal gradient) (■ Figs. 7.6.49 and 7.6.50).

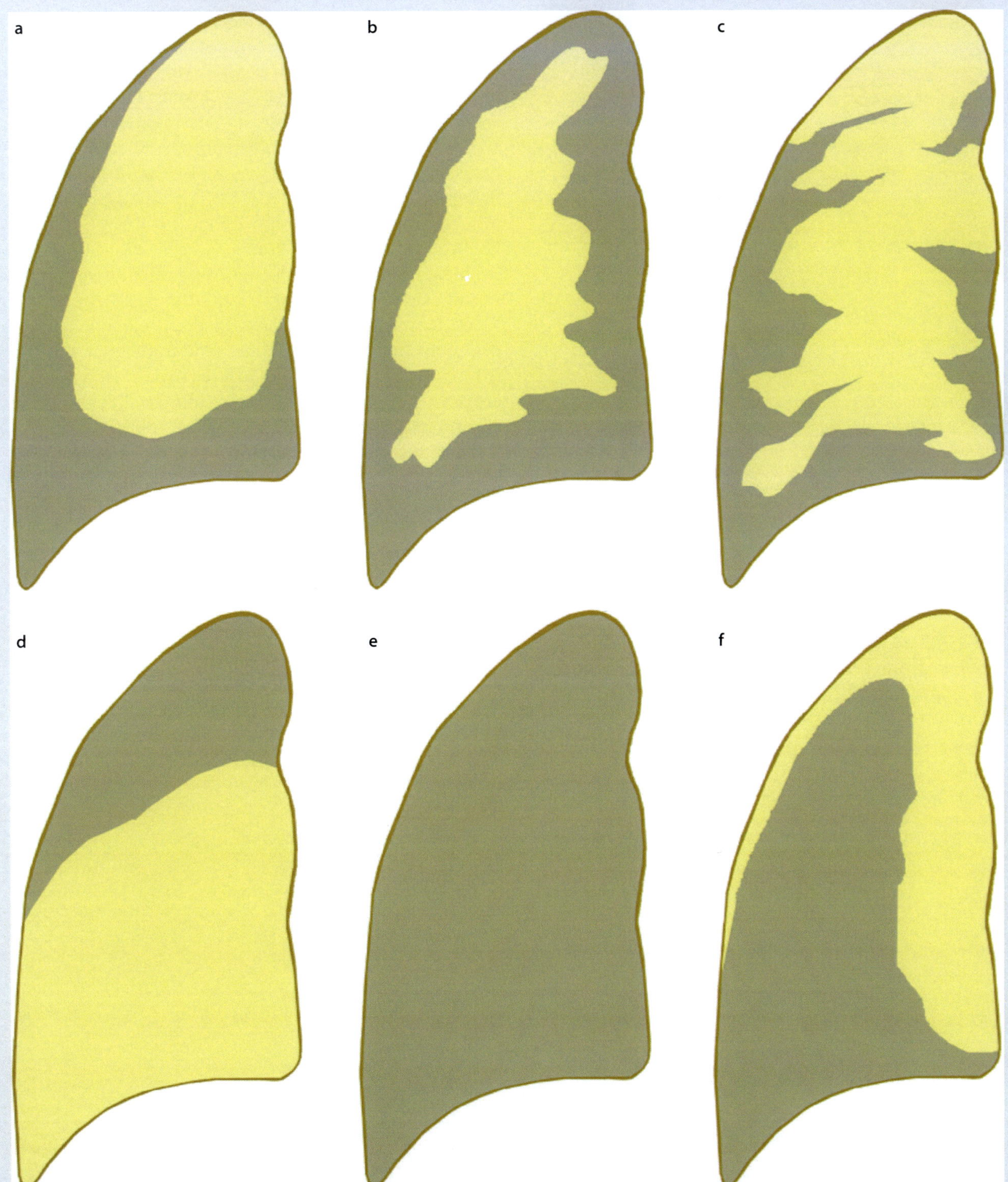

■ **Fig. 7.6.49** An illustration demonstrates the different types of idiopathic interstitial pneumonias (IIPs) and their pathological distribution patterns: (**a**) idiopathic pulmonary fibrosis, (**b**) nonspecific interstitial pneumonia (NSIP), (**c**) cryptogenic organizing pneumonia (COP), (**d**) respiratory bronchiolitis-associated interstitial lung disease (RB-ILD), (**e**) lymphoid interstitial pneumonia (LIP), and (**f**) acute interstitial pneumonia (AIP)

- Shaggy heart appearance is a term used to describe fibrosis silhouetting the heart borders (Fig. 7.6.50).

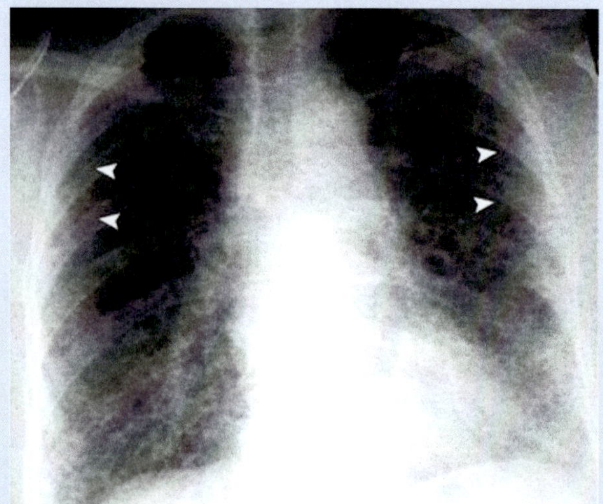

**Fig. 7.6.50**  Posteroanterior chest radiograph of a patient with idiopathic pulmonary fibrosis (IPF) shows bilateral reticular interstitial lung pattern located mainly at the base with gradient crawling toward the apices (*arrowheads*). Notice the shaggy heart appearance

## Nonspecific Interstitial Pneumonia

NSIP is a disease with lung fibrosis that is usually difficult to differentiate from IPF. However, differentiating IPF from NSIP is important, since the latter has a better response to high corticosteroid therapy.

Patients with NSIP are typically seen in their 40s with signs and symptoms similar to IPF. NSIP has no obvious relation with cigarette smoking. NSIP may be encountered with other systemic disorders (e.g., connective tissue disorders).

### Signs on Radiographs and HRCT

Patients with NSIP show patchy subpleural reticulonodular pattern, bilateral almost homogenous lung involvement, and microcytic honeycombing (Fig. 7.6.49). The main differences between IPF and NSIP are the lack of the apicobasal gradient involvement (seen in IPF) and the macrocytic honeycombing (also seen in IPF).

## Cryptogenic Organizing Pneumonia

COP, formerly known as *bronchiolitis obliterans with organizing pneumonia* (BOOP), is a chronic pulmonary disease characterized by bronchiolar inflammation (bronchiolitis) and obstruction by a polypoid plug of granulation tissue formation (obliterans). The granulation tissue blocks the small airways proximal to the alveoli resulting in patchy

parenchymal disease. Pneumonia often develops in bronchiolitis obliterans due to inflammation of the surrounding parenchyma as a consequence to the bronchiolitis (organizing pneumonia).

The bronchioles are classified into terminal bronchioles and respiratory bronchioles. A disease involving the terminal bronchioles will result in a clinical picture that resembles a conductive airways disease. In contrast, when the respiratory bronchioles are affected by a disease, a clinical picture resembles restrictive airway disease that arises because the adjacent alveoli are affected too. COP is a disease of the respiratory bronchioles.

Most cases of COP are unknown and seen in patients between 40 and 60 years of age. COP in adults can arise secondary to a variety of causes such as chronic aspiration pneumonia, radiation therapy, bone marrow transplant, medications (e.g., amiodarone), and connective tissue disorders (e.g., rheumatoid arthritis). Most patients with COP are nonsmokers or ex-smokers.

Patients usually present with persistent nonproductive dry cough that resists antibiotics for duration that can last up to months. Dyspnea, low-grade fever, malaise, and weight loss are other common features. Lab results usually show elevated erythrocyte sedimentation rate (ESR) and C-reactive proteins, with restrictive pattern on pulmonary function tests.

### Signs on Radiographs
- Chest radiographs show peripheral lung field patchy infiltration that can be unilateral or bilateral, often with basilar predominance (Figs. 7.6.49 and 7.6.51).
- Bilateral interstitial, reticulonodular pattern may be seen.

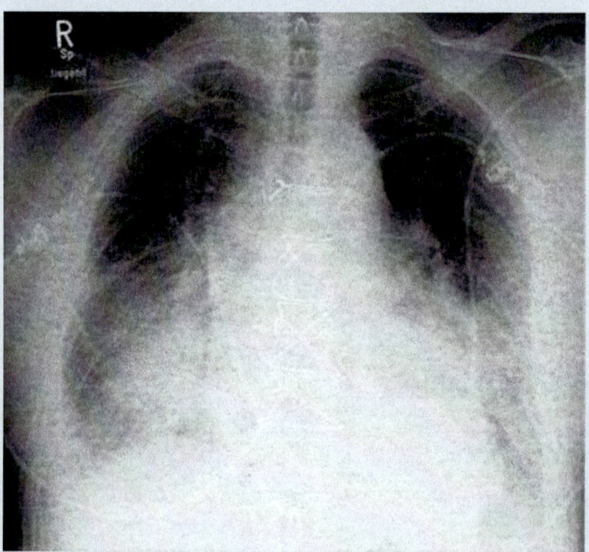

**Fig. 7.6.51**  Anteroposterior chest radiograph of a patient with bone marrow transplant due to leukemia who developed COP shows bilateral patchy infiltrations located at the lung bases with peripheral patchy infiltration

## Signs on HRCT

- The typical HRCT picture of COP is bilateral, patchy, triangular areas of consolidation located in the peripheral subpleural areas (60–90 % of cases) ( Fig. 7.6.52). Also, peribronchial patchy consolidations located in the lower lobes are also a common presentation.
- Bilateral, scattered ground-glass appearance opacities with thickened interlobular septa can be seen in up to 60 % of cases ( Fig. 7.6.52). These areas are hyperdense in cases of amiodarone toxicity due to the presence of iodine in the drug.
- Another uncommon presentation of COP is a focal parenchymal mass often located in the upper lobes in contact with the pleura and fissures (30 % of cases). This presentation cannot be differentiated from cancer by imaging alone; biopsy is needed to confirm the diagnosis.
- COP also can present as multiple, mass-like parenchymal lesions with speculated margins, another presentation that may mimic metastasis, infections, or lymphoma. Biopsy is needed to confirm the diagnosis. This pattern can be produced by therapy with bleomycin in cancer patients.
- Bronchocentric COP appears as areas of parenchymal consolidation around the bronchovascular bundle (33 % of cases). This pattern resembles the HRCT picture of patients with vasculitis (e.g., Churg–Strauss syndrome) ( Fig. 7.6.52).
- Atoll sign is seen as an area with ground-glass opacity surrounded by a ring of increased density parenchyma. This sign is typical of COP ( Fig. 7.6.52).
- Band-like opacities are threadlike opacities that run from the bronchi toward the pleura; they may show air-bronchogram sign.

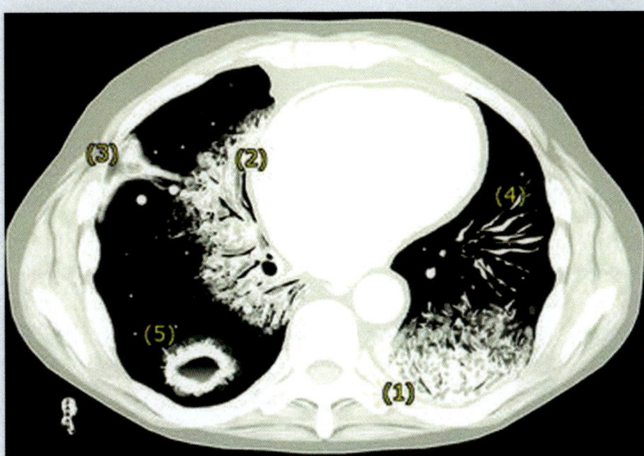

 **Fig. 7.6.52** Axial thoracic lung-window HRCT demonstrates the different manifestations of COP: (*1*) peripheral classical patchy infiltration of COP, (*2*) bronchogenic COP, (*3*) bronchocentric COP, (*4*) thickened interlobar septae, and (*5*) Atoll sign

## Respiratory Bronchiolitis-Associated Interstitial Lung Disease

RB-ILD is a disease that is considered as an exaggerated form of respiratory bronchiolitis, and it is a smoking-related condition. Also, RB-ILD is considered as the early stage of DIP.

Patients with RB-ILD are commonly males in their 30s or 40s with history of chronic smoking. Smoking cessation is an important element in the medical management of RB-ILD.

### Signs on Radiographs and HRCT

- Chest radiograph can be normal.
- On HRCT, the key findings in RB-ILD are centrilobular nodules in combination with ground-glass opacities and bronchial wall thickening predominantly located in the upper lung zones ( Fig. 7.6.49).

## Desquamative Interstitial Pneumonia

DIP is a condition that is considered as a severe form of RB-ILD, and it is strongly associated with cigarette smoking. However, it can arise in nonsmokers due to variety of conditions (e.g., exposure to organic dust). Patients with DIP are often between 30 and 40 years old.

### Signs on Radiographs and HRCT

- Radiographic findings are nonspecific.
- CT finding shows diffuse ground-glass opacity that is predominantly located peripherally and in the lower lobes. However, features overlapped with RB-ILD may be seen.

## Lymphoid Interstitial Pneumonia

LIP is a disease characterized by lymphoid tissue proliferation and infiltration of the pulmonary interstitium by lymphocytes.

The normal lymphoid system of the lung is composed of four components:

- *Bronchus-associated lymphoid tissue* (*BALT*): it consists of submucosal lymphoid follicles distributed along distal bronchi and bronchioles, usually at the bifurcation. This complex is analogous to other mucosa-associated lymphoid tissue (MALT) such as Peyer's patches in the intestine.
- *Hilar lymph nodes*: these are seen along the trachea and at the lung helium.
- *Intrapulmonary lymph nodes*: they are composed of noncapsulated lymphocytes clusters, usually located in the subpleural parenchyma.
- *Interstitial lymphocytes*: they are seen within the lung interstitium with the pulmonary venules.

LIP is a disease characterized by interstitial lymphocyte proliferation, resulting in an interstitial lung disease. It arises commonly secondary to systemic autoimmune disease (e.g., Sjögren's syndrome) and rarely as idiopathic disease. Most patients are middle aged, who often present with systemic symptoms, dyspnea, and cough. Almost all patients have dysproteinemia, usually polyclonal hyper- or hypogammaglobulinemia.

> **Signs on Radiographs and HRCT**
> ━ Radiographic signs are nonspecific reticulonodular interstitial pattern that is commonly diffuse.
> ━ On CT, LIP shows ground-glass opacities plus multiple fine lung cysts located mainly at the center of mid- and lower lung zones (◘ Fig. 7.6.49). The combination of systemic disease, ground-glass opacities, and small lung cysts at the mid- and lower zones are suggestive criteria of LIP.

## Acute Interstitial Pneumonia (Hamman–Rich Syndrome)

AIP is a rare fulminant form of lung disease that occurs in previously healthy individuals. Patients present with signs of acute respiratory distress syndrome (ARDS), fever, and cough with rapid deterioration suggesting pneumonia-like illness.

Patients with AIP are usually lung disease-free and are over 40 years old. Most patients develop severe dyspnea that requires mechanical ventilation. The condition is treated with corticosteroid, with a mortality rate that reaches >50 % of cases.

> **Signs on Radiographs and HRCT**
> Patients show the radiographic signs of ARDS with lower zone predominance bilaterally and may show spared costophrenic angles (◘ Fig. 7.6.49).

### If You Were Given One Investigation to Detect Lung Fibrosis Cause, What Would You Choose?

*Invasive test*: open lung biopsy
*Noninvasive*: HRCT

### Further Reading

Arakawa H, et al. Bronchiolitis obliterance with organizing pneumonia versus chronic esinophilic pneumonia: high resolution CT findings in 81 patients. AJR. 2001;176: 1053–8.

Desai SR, et al. Traction bronchiectasis is cryptogenic fibrosing alveolitis: associated computed tomographic features and physiological significance. Eur Radiol. 2003;13: 1801–8.

Fellrath JM, et al. Idiopathic pulmonary fibrosis/cryptogenic fibrosing alveolitis. Clin Exp Med. 2003;3:65–83.

Ghanei M, et al. Bronchiolitis obliterance following exposure to sulfur mustard: chest high resolution computed tomography. Eur J Radiol. 2004;52:164–9.

Gibson M, et al. Lymphocytic disorders of the chest: pathology and imaging. Clin Radiol. 1998a;53:469–80.

Gibson M, et al. Lymphocytic disorders of the chest: pathology and imaging. Clin Radiol. 1998b;53:469–80.

Katzenstein AA, et al. Diagnosis of usual intestitial pneumonia and distinction from other fibrosing interstitial lung diseases. Human Pathol. 2008;39:1275–94.

Mueller-Mang C, et al. What every radiologist should know about idiopathic interstitial pneumonias. Radiographics. 2007;27:595–615.

Polverosi R, et al. Organizing pneumonia: typical and atypical HRCT patterns. Radiol Med. 2006;111:202–12.

Sharief N, et al. Fibrosing alveolitis and desquanative interstitial pneumonitis. Pediatr Pulmonol. 1994;17:359–65.

Tempone V, et al. Bronchiolitis obliterance organizing pneumonia secondary to chronic aspiration of pharmaceutical tablets: radiologic-pathologic correlation. Eur J Radiol (Extra). 2008;67:e99–101.

## 7.7    Histiocytoses

Histiocytoses are a group of diseases characterized by abnormal proliferation and multiorgan infiltration by histiocytes. Different diseases and clinical presentations fall under the umbrella of histiocytoses.

Histiocytes are bone marrow-derived cells, and they fall into two main groups: the mononuclear phagocytes (macrophages) and dendritic cells. Macrophages are part of the immune system, and their main function is to engulf bacteria and damaged tissues (phagocytosis). They are found in all body organs like the liver (Kupffer cells), brain (microglial cells), etc. In contrast, dendritic cells are a cell family that includes Langerhans cells, interdigitating reticulum cells, and follicular dendritic cells. They are found in the reticuloendothelial system, and their main function is to activate the major histocompatibility complex (MHC)-restricted T cells by expressing high levels of MHC class II molecules. The reticuloendothelial system includes the liver, spleen, and lymph nodes.

Histiocytoses are classified into three main classes:

*Class 1 histiocytoses*: Langerhans cell histiocytosis (LCH).

*Class 2 histiocytoses*: Infection-associated hemophagocytic syndrome, Rosai–Dorfman's syndrome, and Omenn syndrome (OS).

*Class 3 histiocytoses*: True malignant proliferation and include acute monoblastic leukemia and true histiocytic lymphoma.

There are other diseases classified as non-LCH and include Erdheim–Chester disease (ECD) and xanthoma disseminatum (Montgomery syndrome).

## Langerhans Cell Histiocytosis

LCH is a disease of unknown origin characterized by proliferation and body infiltration by nonmalignant histiocytes (macrophages and dendrites cells).

The basic lesion in LCH is a granuloma composed of Langerhans cells and lymphocytes (proliferative stage). Next, the granuloma becomes necrotic, with admixture of eosinophils and sometimes multinucleated giant cells (granulomatous stage). Finally, fibrosis of the granuloma occurs with deposition of lipid-laden histiocytes (xanthogranulomatous stage). Electron microscopy reveals characteristic rod-shaped bodies in the cytoplasm of the cells (Birbeck granules).

LCH is a broad spectrum of overlapped syndromes with multiple systemic manifestations. Characteristic bone manifestations include sharply defined, punched-out lytic bony lesions and vertebra plana. Lung involvement is common and shows diffuse reticulonodular interstitial pattern of involvement, cystic bronchiectasis, and pneumothorax. Central nervous system (CNS) involvements mainly affect the hypothalamic–pituitary axis resulting in diabetes insipidus. Other CNS involvements include white matter lesions that are often seen in the cerebellum and the pyramidal tracts, causing ataxia in advanced stage of the disease. Skin involvement is characterized by reddish-brown thoracic and pelvic purperic papules. When these purperic papules are found in a newborn, the condition is called *blueberry muffin baby*, which is commonly seen in neonates with congenital infection (TORCH) and congenital leukemia (■ Fig. 7.7.53).

The disease can be seen in pediatric and adult patients in a localized or diffuse form. In pediatrics, the disease presents in three main forms: eosinophilic granuloma (EG, local form), Hand–Schüller–Christian's disease (HSCD, chronic form), and Letterer–Siwe disease (LSD, acute form). In adults, the most severe presentation is pulmonary LHC.

*Eosinophilic granuloma (EG)* is a solitary localized lytic lesion of the bone, which is typically seen in children <15 years of age. Children EG can be asymptomatic or present with pain, swelling, and fracture at the site of the lesion.

The bony lesions are classically found in flat bones, such as the skull, mandible, and pelvis. When EG affects long bones, the lytic lesions are typically seen in the diaphyses and maybe the metaphyses. ES affecting the epiphyses is rare.

*Hand–Schüller–Christian's disease (HSCD)* is a disease that is seen in children <10 years of age and characterized by a triad of exophthalmos, diabetes insipidus, and hepatosplenomegaly. Cases of HSCD may occur between 20 and 30 years of age. Other manifestations of HSCD include anemia, scaly seborrheic skin rash, restrictive lung diseases (fibrosis), and cerebellar ataxia. Osteolytic bony lesions like EG can be seen.

*Letterer–Siwe disease (LSD)* is a disease seen in children <2 years old and characterized by hepatosplenomegaly, lymphadenopathy, and sclerosing cholangitis. In LSD, the child grows normally from birth until 2 years of age, where the disease starts to manifest. LSD is the most aggressive form of LCH. Mental retardation, multiple bony fractures, hemorrhagic rash, anemia, and thrombocytopenia may be seen.

*Adult pulmonary Langerhans' cell histiocytosis (PLCH)* affects 1–2 cases per million, and it is often seen in young smokers. There is a strong association between PLCH and cigarette smoking. Cigarette smoking was found to increase the number and accumulation of dendritic cells and Langerhans' cells within the alveolar epithelium in smokers. Most patients with PLCH are asymptomatic. Symptomatic PLCH patients present with dyspnea (35–87 %), pleuritic chest pain (9–18 %), nonproductive cough (50–70 %), pneumothorax (25 %), and fever (15 %).

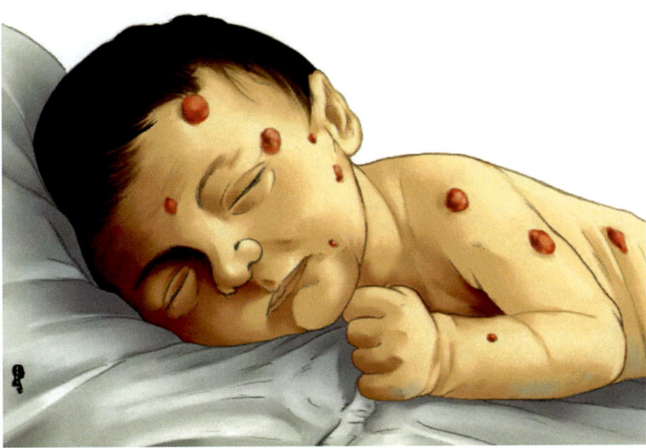

**Fig. 7.7.53** An illustration demonstrates the purpuric papules in a neonate with blueberry muffin baby condition

normal adjacent vertebral disks and sparing of the posterior elements.

- Jaw lesions in EG or HSCD (20 %) can present as radicular cysts, periodontal disease, osteomyelitis, and sharply, expansile, punched-out alveolar lesions that spare the roots, making the teeth appear as if they are "floating in air."

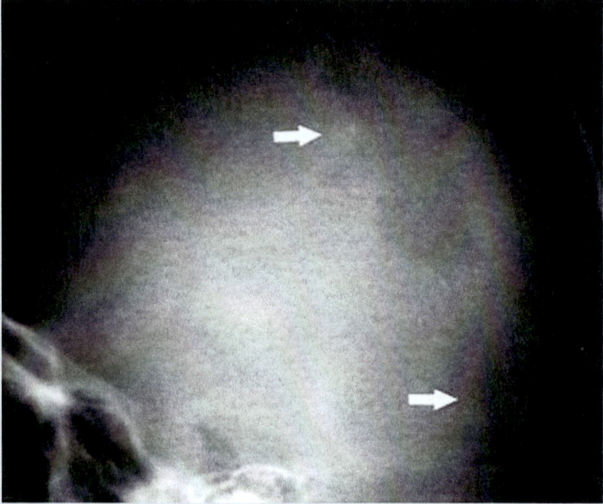

**Fig. 7.7.54**   Lateral plain skull radiograph shows two sharply lytic, punched-out lesions with geographic edges (*arrows*) in a child with eosinophilic granuloma

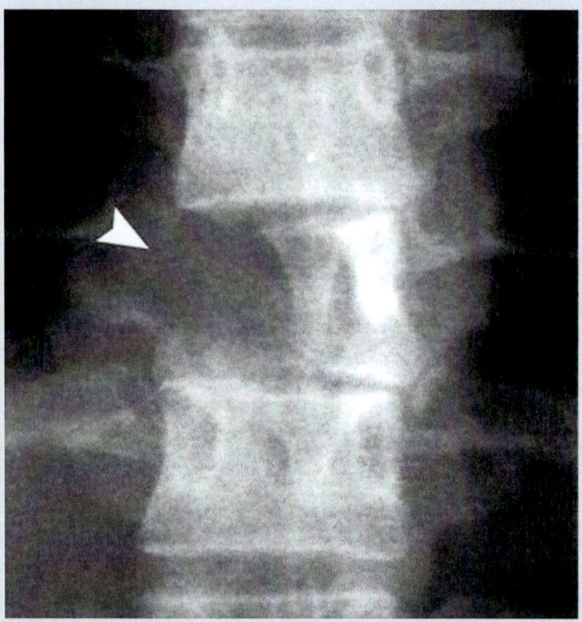

**Fig. 7.7.55**   Anteroposterior thoracic vertebral plain radiograph shows punched-out lytic lesion affecting the vertebral body in a patient with Langerhans cell histiocytosis (LHC) (*arrowhead*)

### Signs on Chest Radiographs and HRCT

- In early PLCH, lung fields show small nodules (1–10 mm in diameter) with irregular borders. The nodules are predominantly seen in the upper and mid-lung zones, sparing the lung bases (**Fig. 7.7.56**).
- Advanced PLCH shows reticulonodular interstitial pattern and cystic bronchiectasis. The cystic interstitial patterns mimic that of bullous emphysema or lymphangiomyomatosis; the latter is typically seen in tuberous sclerosis. The cysts usually measure 2–3 cm in diameter (**Fig. 7.7.57**).
- Pneumothorax can be seen in 25 % of cases (**Fig. 7.7.57**).
- Hilar lymphadenopathy can be seen in rare cases.

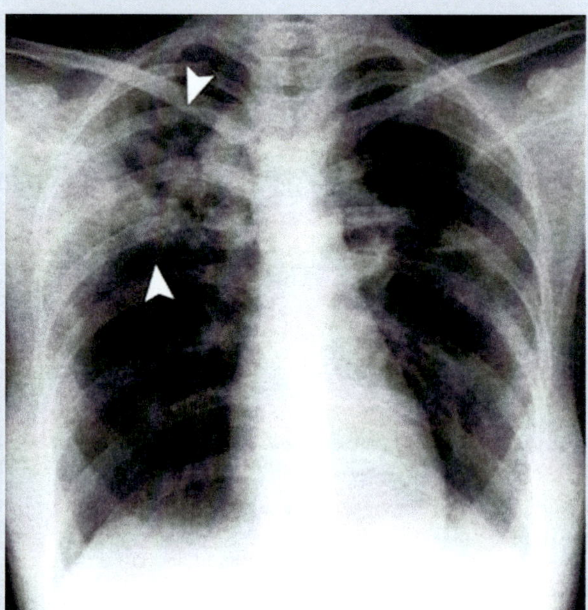

**Fig. 7.7.56**   Posteroanterior chest radiograph of a patient with adult pulmonary Langerhans' cell histiocytosis (PLCH) shows multiple pulmonary nodules with different sizes located at the right upper lung zone (*arrowheads*)

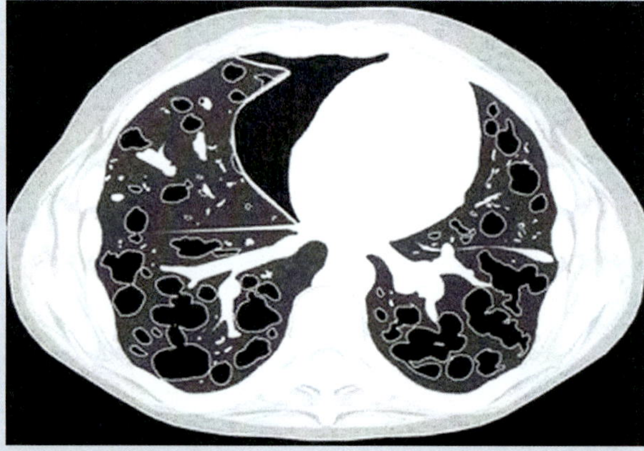

**Fig. 7.7.57**   Axial HRCT illustration of a patient with PLCH shows diffusely bronchiectatic, cystic changes of the lung parenchyma in a bilateral pattern with right pneumothorax

**Signs on MRI**

- In the sella, the pituitary stalk is typically thickened and shows contrast enhancement in cases of diabetes mellitus (HSCD).
- On MRCP, sclerosing cholangitis in LSD shows the absence of the peripheral biliary radicals with intrahepatic biliary tree stenosis. Notice that these findings are seen in a child.
- Vertebra plana is seen as severely flattened vertebral body (Fig. 7.7.58).

Fig. 7.7.58 Sagittal thoracic vertebral MRI shows vertebra plana (*arrowhead*)

## Infection-Associated Hemophagocytic Syndrome

*Infection-associated hemophagocytic syndrome* is a disease characterized by histiocytes hyperplasia (increased numbers), often due to viral infection (e.g., human immunodeficiency virus).

Patients present with high spiking fever, jaundice, lethargy, and generalized lymphadenopathy and hepatomegaly. Laboratory investigations show hemophagocytosis, hypertriglyceridemia, pancytopenia, and consumptive coagulopathy.

## Omenn Syndrome

*Omenn syndrome* (OS) is a rare, autosomal recessive, non-Langerhans cell histiocytosis disorder characterized by severe combined immunodeficiency (SCID), erythroderma, hepatosplenomegaly, lymphadenopathy, and alopecia.

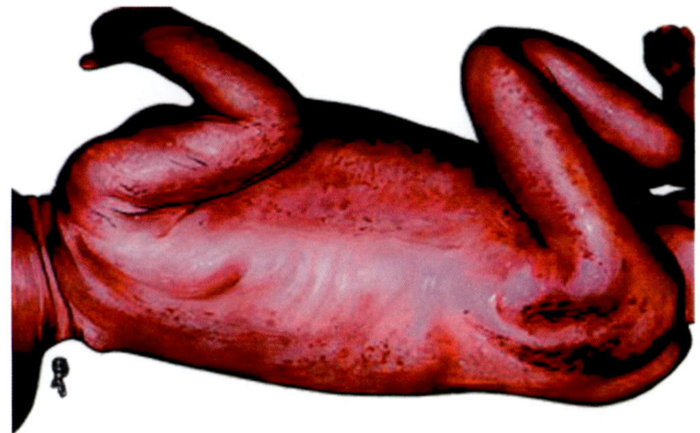

Fig. 7.7.59 An illustration demonstrates the features of Omenn syndrome in a neonate

Infants with OS typically present in the first few years of life with generalized cutaneous lesions composed of red, exfoliative dermatitis that involves almost the whole body (erythroderma) (Fig. 7.7.59). Erythroderma in infants combined with splenomegaly or lymphadenopathy is diagnostic of OS.

Laboratory investigations may show high serum levels of IgE and hypogammaglobulinemia.

## Chédiak–Higashi Disease

Chédiak–Higashi disease (CHD) is an autosomal recessive, rare disorder characterized by oculocutaneous albinism, increased susceptibility to infections due to immunodeficiency, silvery gray hair, photophobia, neurological impairment, and abnormal giant lysosomes in the leukocytes. Most patients with CHD develop lymphoma-like phase characterized by widespread lymphohistiocytic infiltrates in the lymphoreticular organs (85 %).

CHD presents in two main forms: childhood and adult forms. The childhood form is characterized by recurrent pyogenic infections and hepatosplenomegaly. In contrast, the adult form presents in early adulthood with various neurological manifestations that include Parkinsonism, dementia, spinocerebellar degeneration, and peripheral neuropathy.

Skin hyperpigmentation after exposure to sunlight is a characteristic initial feature of CHD. Increased susceptibility to infections in CHD patients is attributed to the defective function of neutrophils. Parental consanguinity is a common feature of CHD.

## Differential Diagnoses and Related Diseases

- *Griscelli disease* is a rare condition characterized by abnormal transfer of melanin granules resulting in light skin and silver hair (Fig. 7.7.60). Griscelli syndrome may be accompanied by neurological abnormalities (type 1), immunodeficiency and

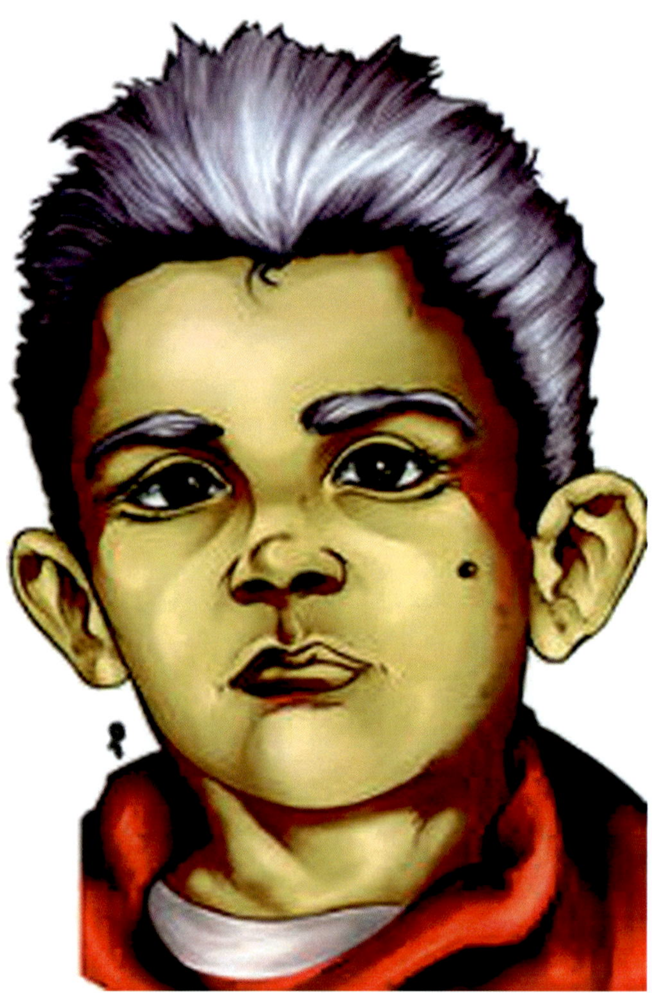



**Fig. 7.7.60** An illustration demonstrates the features of Griscelli disease

neutropenia (type 2), or no other abnormalities (type 3). Patients with Griscelli disease are typically children presenting with characteristic silver hair in addition to febrile episodes, lymphadenopathy, hepatosplenomegaly, anemia, and pancytopenia. Patients may develop seizures and hemiparesis. Brain CT may show brain atrophy. Griscelli disease can be initially mistaken with CHD.

- *Elejalde syndrome (neuroectodermal melanolysosomal syndrome)* is a very rare disease characterized by silvery gray hair, bronze-colored skin, profound CNS dysfunction, and a normal immune system. Neurological abnormalities in Elejalde syndrome include severe hypotonia or hyperreflexia, spastic hemi- or quadriplegia, ataxia, seizures, and profound developmental delay. Some investigators believe that Elejalde syndrome and Griscelli syndrome type 1 are the same disease. However, Elejalde syndrome lacks the immunological abnormalities commonly seen in patients with Griscelli and Chédiak–Higashi syndromes.

## Rosai–Dorfman's Disease (Sinus Histiocytosis)

Rosai–Dorfman's disease (RDD) is a rare benign disease characterized by idiopathic proliferation of the phagocytes within the lymph nodes sinuses.

Patients with RDD are typically male children presenting with bilateral massive cervical lymphadenopathy (■ Fig. 7.7.61) and low-grade fever, with or without exophthalmos. Extranodal manifestation like any other histiocytosis disease can involve any part of the body.

Pathologically, the enlarged lymph nodes show infiltration of the sinuses by large histiocytes. The histiocytes contain engulfed lymphocytes and plasma cells (emperipolesis), which is the hallmark of this disease. Laboratory investigations show leukocytosis, high erythrocyte sedimentation rate, and hypergammaglobulinemia. Burkitt's lymphoma should be ruled out before establishing the diagnosis of RDD. RDD generally resolves without treatment after several months. However, RDD transformation into true malignant lymphoma may occur.

## Xanthoma Disseminatum (Montgomery Syndrome)

Xanthoma disseminatum (XD) is a rare, nonmalignant form of non-Langerhans cells histiocytosis characterized by body xanthomata formation that includes the skin, trachea, and the larynx in a normal lipid profile patient. Other manifestations include hypopituitarism, diabetes insipidus (40 % of

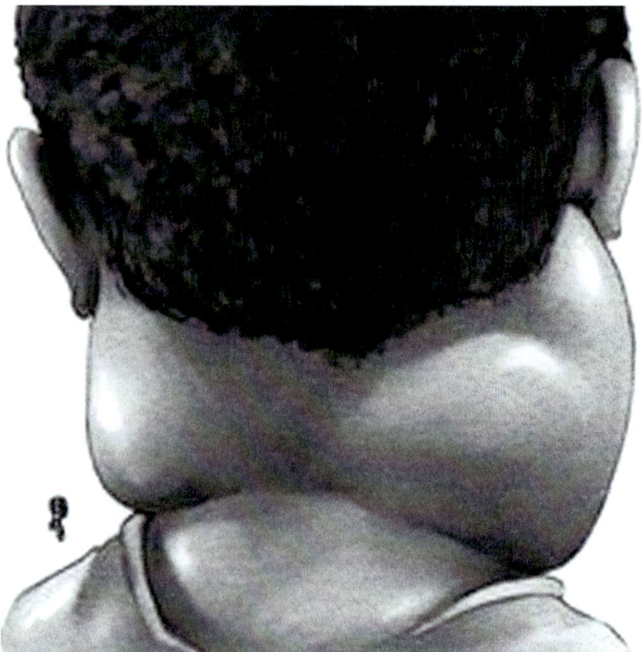

**Fig. 7.7.61** An illustration demonstrates the features of s's disease (RDD)

patients), multiple osteolytic lesions seen on plain radiographs, and expansile cystic lesions in the bones of the hands. Patient's brain MRI may show nongliotic brain mass with heterogeneous contrast enhancement. Moreover, multiple spinal cord lesions with heterogeneous high T2 signal intensities and intense contrast enhancement may be found. CT of the neck and the thorax may show laryngeal and tracheal wall thickening.

# Erdheim–Chester Disease (Lipogranulomatosis)

ECD is a rare, non-Langerhans cell histiocytosis characterized by almost constant bone lesions and extraosseous manifestations.

ECD affects patients with wide age range (7–78 years). Patients often present with painless bilateral exophthalmos, progressive cerebellar ataxia, diabetes insipidus, and bone pain. Bone involvement is found in 60 % of patients, and it is a diagnostic criteria. Diagnosis of ECD is based on the presence of characteristic bony lesions, visceral involvement (especially the retroperitoneal structures), and pathological findings.

### Signs on Plain Radiographs
- Bilateral symmetrical osteosclerotic lesions affecting the metaphyses (83 %) and the diaphyses of long bones (98 %), with relative sparing of the epiphyses. The corticomedullary junction is blurred, and the bone marrow is obliterated by dense bone. These lesions classically spare the axial skeleton, hands, and feet.
- Radiolucent bands separating the sclerotic metaphysis from the sclerotic diaphysis can be found.
- In <10 % of ECD cases, the bony lesions can be purely lytic with no osteosclerosis.

### Signs on MRI
- The affected long bones diaphyses and metaphyses exhibit low T1 and T2 signal intensities due to osteosclerosis. Periostitis may be seen in some cases. After contrast injection, enhancement of the periosteum is seen as a white line along the bone margin.
- In CNS, multiple contrast-enhanced lesions on T1W images affecting the meninges, eye, and pituitary are typically found (this combination is very characteristic of ECD).
- Orbital involvement in ECD is seen in the form of retro-orbital masses or diffuses infiltration of the retro-orbital fat (causing exophthalmos).

ECD is characterized by the formation of lipid granulomas. The cerebral manifestations of ECD are similar to other histiocytoses. Laboratory findings are usually unremarkable, and cerebrospinal fluid analysis is usually normal.

## How Can You Differentiate ECD from HSCD?
- ECD presents with osteosclerotic lesions, whereas HSCD presents with osteolytic lesions.
- ECD affects patients in the range of 7–78 years, whereas HSCD affects children <10 years old.
- Retroperitoneal lesions are almost a characteristic finding in ECD.
- On pathology, ECD shows lipid-laden histiocytes.

## Further Reading

Abbott GF, et al. Pulmonary Langerhans cell histocytosis. Radiographics. 2004;24:821–41.

Albayram S, et al. Spinal dural involvement in Erdheim-Chester disease: MRI findings. Neuroradiology. 2002;44:1004–7.

Alexander AS, et al. Xanthoma disseminatum: a case report and literature review. Br J Radiol. 2005;78:153–7.

Baron J, et al. Xanthoma disseminatum: a rare cause of upper airway narrowing. AJR. 2003;180:1180–1.

Burihan J, et al. Elejalde syndrome: report of a case and review of the literature. Pediatr Dermatol. 2004;21: 479–82.

Caparros-Lefebvre D, et al. Neuroradiologic aspects of Chester-Erdheim disease. AJNR. 1995;16:735–40.

Dion E, et al. Bone involvement in Erdheim-Chester disease: imaging findings, including periostitis and partial epiphyseal involvement. Radiology. 2006;238:632–9.

Doyle DJ, et al. Imaging of multisystem Langerhans cell histocytosis in an adult. Eur J Radiol (Extra). 2007;61:109–17.

Haraldsson Á, et al. Griscelli disease with cerebral involvement. Eur J Pediatr. 1991;150:419–22.

Hauser RA, et al. Adult Chediak-Higashi parkinsonian syndrome with dystonia. Mov Disord. 2000;15:705–8.

Hoover KB, et al. Langerhans cell histiocytosis. Skeletal Radiol. 2007;36:95–104.

Hurvitz H, et al. A kindred with Griscelli disease: spectrum of neurological involvement. Eur J Pediatr. 1993;152:402–5.

Ivanovich J, et al. 12-year-old male with Elejalde syndrome (neuroectodermal melanolysosomal disease). Am J Med Genet. 2001;98:313–6.

Jurić G, et al. Extranodal sinus histiocytosis (Rosai-Dorfman disease) of the brain parenchyma. Acta Neurochir. 2003;145:145–9.

Kaneda T, et al. Langerhans cell histiocytosis in the mandible: computed tomography and magnetic resonance imaging. Oral Radiol. 1997;13:109–14.

Kashihara-Sawami M, et al. Letterer-Siwe disease: immunopathologic study with a new monoclonal antibody. J Am Acad Dermatol. 1988;18:646–54.

Kumar P, et al. Chediak-Higashi syndrome. Indian J Pediatr. 2000;67:595–7.

Leatherwood DL, et al. Pulmonary Langerhans cell histocytosis. Radiographics. 2007;27:265–8.

Malhotra AK, et al. Griscelli syndrome. J Am Acad Dermatol. 2006;55:337–40.

Meyer JS, et al. Langerhans cell histiocytosis: presentation and evolution of radiologic findings with clinical correlation. Radiographics. 1995;15:1135–46.

Odell WD, et al. Xanthoma disseminatum: a rare cause of diabetes insipidus. J Clin Endocrinol Metab. 1993;76:777–80.

Pupo RA, et al. Omenn's syndrome and related combined immunodeficiency syndrome: diagnostic considerations in infants with persistent erythroderma and failure to thrive. J Am Acad Dermatol. 1991;25:442–6.

Scolozzi P, et al. Multisystem Langerhans' cell histiocytosis (Hand-Schüller-Christian disease) in an adult: a case report and review of the literature. Eur Arch Otorhinolaryngol. 2004;261:326–30.

Shaffer MP, et al. Langerhans cell histiocytosis presenting as blueberry muffin baby. J Am Acad Dermatol. 2005;53:S143–6.

Simanski C, et al. The Langerhans' cell histiocytosis (eosinophilic granuloma) of the cervical spine: a rare diagnosis of cervical pain. Magn Reson Imaging. 2004;22:589–94.

Stéphan JL. Histiocytoses. Eur J Pediatr. 1995;154:600–9.

Tamura T, et al. Congenital Letterer-Siwe disease associated with protein losing enteropathy. Eur J Pediatr. 1980;135:77–80.

Weidauer S, et al. Cerebral Erdheim-Chester disease: case report and review of the literature. Neuroradiology. 2003;45:241–5.

Young PM, et al. Rosai-Dorfman disease presenting as multiple soft tissue masses. Skeletal Radiol. 2005;34:665–9.

## 7.8    Hemoptysis

Hemoptysis is a term used to describe the pathological condition of coughing blood, typically due to lower respiratory tract disease. Hemoptysis can be a life-threatening condition, and the condition needs urgent evaluation.

The normal lung is supplied by pulmonary arterial system and bronchial arterial system. *The pulmonary arteries* supply the lungs and take part in gas exchange. In contrast, *the bronchial arteries* are small arteries (2 mm or less in diameter) that arise from the descending thoracic aorta and supply the trachea, the bronchial tree, the visceral pleura, the esophagus, and part of the mediastinal lymph nodes. Histologically, the two systems are connected by thin-walled capillary anastomoses.

The right bronchial artery arises at the level of the fifth or sixth thoracic vertebra posteriorly and usually forms a common trunk with the intercostals artery. The left bronchial artery arises from the descending thoracic aorta anteriorly, with a second left bronchial artery found in up to 70 % of population. On CT angiography scan, the right bronchial artery is seen as dots or lines of increased density located in the retrotracheal, retrobronchial, and retroesophageal regions (◘ Fig. 7.8.62). The left bronchial artery is identified typically as a linear or nodular hyperdensity in the space

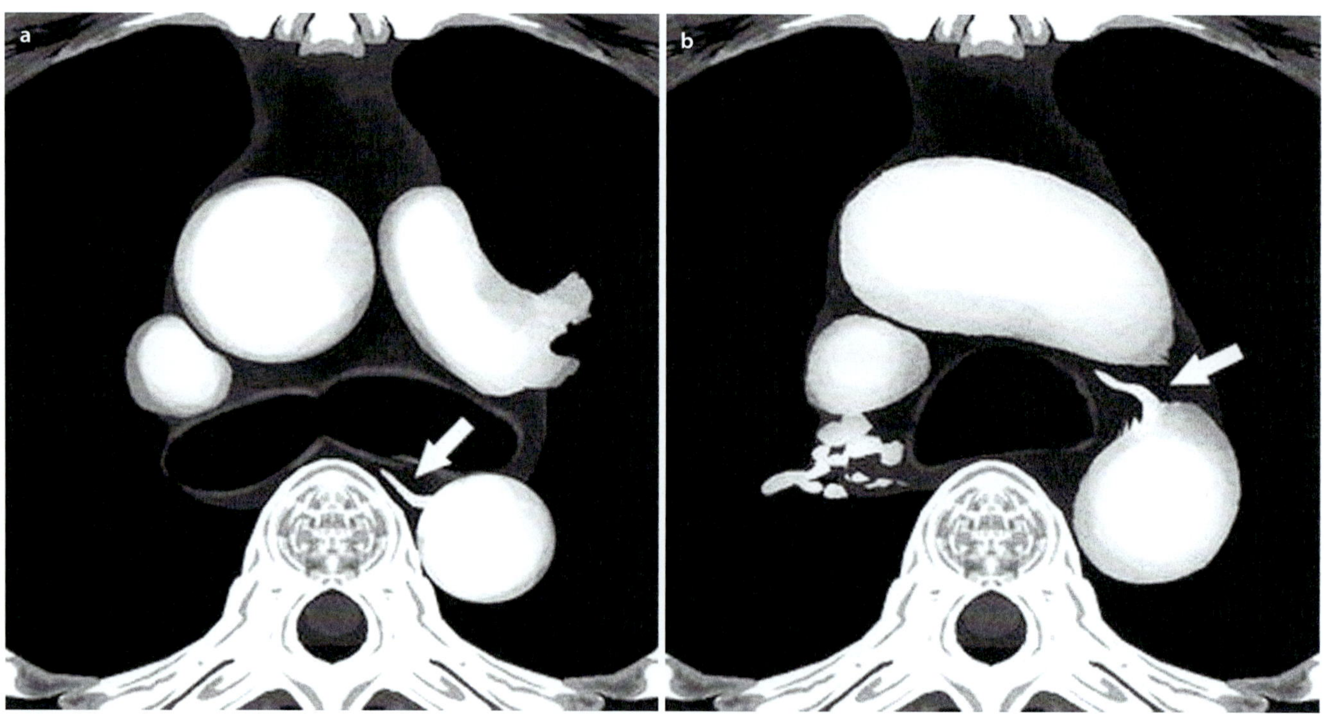

◘ **Fig. 7.8.62**    Sequential axial CTA illustration demonstrates the normal anatomy of the right bronchial artery (*arrow in* **a**) and the left bronchial artery (*arrow in* **b**)

below the aortic arch above the pulmonary artery (within the aortopulmonary window) (■ Fig. 7.8.62). Both bronchial arteries normally have highly tortuous course.

The differential diagnosis of hemoptysis is diverse and can occur due to pulmonary infection (e.g., tuberculosis), malignancy (e.g., bronchogenic carcinoma), vascular event (e.g., pulmonary embolism), and vascular anomaly (e.g., arteriovenous malformation). *Cryptogenic hemoptysis* is a term used to describe hemoptysis with no identifiable cause, and it is responsible for up to 42 % of hemoptysis episodes, especially in smokers. Cryptogenic hemoptysis is a diagnosis of exclusion, and patients are often recommended to perform another CT several months later to exclude small occult neoplasm formation.

This topic discusses some of the causes of hemoptysis, in which radiology plays an important role in establishing their diagnosis.

## Bronchopulmonary Sequestration

Bronchopulmonary sequestration (BPS) is a rare condition characterized by nonfunctioning lung parenchyma mass that is not in continuity with the tracheobronchial tree and is supplied by an anomalous systemic arterial vessel, typically arising from the abdominal aorta and ascending to the mass through the pulmonary ligament. The term sequestration describes disconnected lung tissue with its own anomalous systemic artery.

The primitive lung tissue mass of BPS has its own anomalous systemic vascular supply, usually from the aorta (not bronchial pulmonary circulation). Most cases are diagnosed before the age of 10 years, where the child presents with chronic cough, hemoptysis, and recurrent pneumonias. *Hybrid lesion* is a term used to describe a lesion, where the sequestered lung mass has a congenital cystic adenomatous malformation lesion within it. The definite diagnosis of hybrid lesion is by histopathology. BPS is divided into intralobar and extralobar forms.

In *intralobar BPS*, the mass is located inside the lung, surrounded by normal lung parenchyma, and shares the visceral pleura with the normal lung tissue. It accounts for 75 % of the sequestration cases. The mass is located on the left side in the posterior basal segment in 98 % of cases. The mass has its arterial supply from the descending aorta and its venous drainage from the azygos or systemic veins. In *extralobar BPS*, the mass usually lies within the pleura and has its own pleural layer and has the same radiological features as the interlobar sequestration. It accounts for 1–6 % of the sequestration cases. The mass receives its arterial supply from the thoracic or the abdominal aorta in 80 % of cases and is usually found between the lower lobes and the diaphragm. Most cases present within the first 6 months of life with dyspnea, cyanosis, and feeding difficulties.

### Signs on CT

The scan shows a hyperdense pulmonary mass that may contain cystic changes or air–fluid level. The mass may appear as a consolidation or atelectatic mass. After contrast injection, an anomalous vessel arises from the abdominal aorta, or the descending thoracic aorta is seen penetrating the mass, which is a pathognomonic finding (■ Fig. 7.8.63). The sequestered mass may show homogenous or inhomogeneous contrast enhancement.

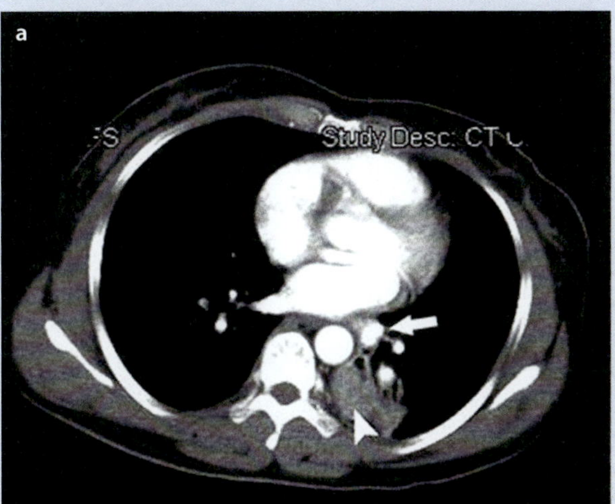
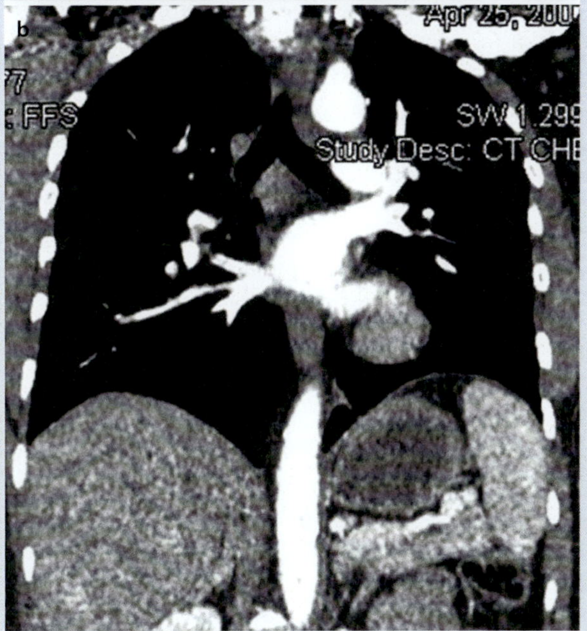

■ **Fig. 7.8.63** Axial (**a**) and coronal (**b**) chest CT shows left lower lobe intralobar bronchopulmonary sequestration mass (*arrowheads*) with its abnormal arterial supply arising from the descending thoracic aorta (*arrows*)

## Anomalous Systemic Artery Supplying Normal Lung Parenchyma

Anomalous systemic artery supplying normal lung parenchyma is a condition characterized by a normal lung parenchyma supplied by anomalous artery in the absence of congenital heart or lung disease. Unlike bronchopulmonary sequestration, there is no abnormal tissue mass, and the vessel is not typically arising from the abdominal aorta. The condition is sometimes referred to as *pseudosequestration*.

Adult patients with the anomalous systemic artery can be asymptomatic or present with recurrent hemoptysis. In contrast, pediatric patients with this condition often present with cardiac murmur.



**Signs on CTA**

- The normal bronchial arteries are <2 mm in diameter and arise directly from the descending thoracic aorta between the levels of T5 and T6 thoracic vertebrae (orthotopic origin). Anomalous bronchial arteries are defined as arteries that originate outside the range of T5 and T6 thoracic vertebrae (ectopic origin). Hypertrophied bronchial arteries are visualized as nodular or linear mediastinal or retrobronchial dilated vessels (>2 mm in size) with early enhancement and density similar to the aorta. The hypertrophied bronchial arteries are classically detected in the retrotracheal area, retroesophageal area, aortopulmonary window, or the posterior wall of the main bronchus.
- In anomalous systemic artery supplying normal lung parenchyma, a hypertrophied vessel is often identified in an area of normal lung parenchyma in the absence of signs of intra- or extrathoracic abnormal lung mass (differentiate it from bronchopulmonary sequestration) (◘ Fig. 7.8.64).

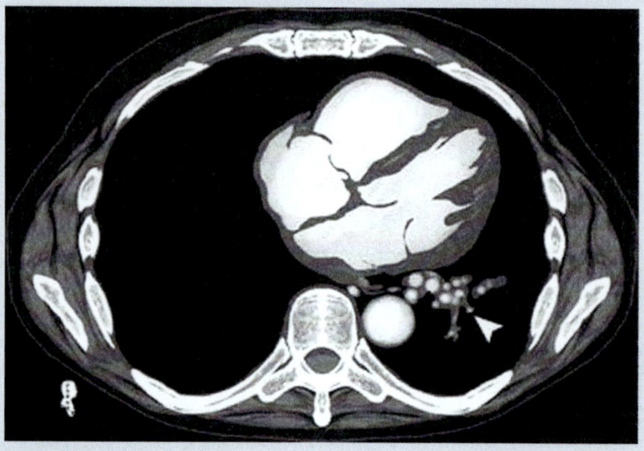

◘ **Fig. 7.8.64** Axial CTA illustration demonstrates left pseudosequestration seen as multiple dilated vascular nodules surrounded by normal lung parenchyma (*arrowhead*)

The anomalous systemic arteries usually are very tortuous and are not parallel to the bronchi (differentiate them from normal bronchial arteries).

- Nonbronchial systemic arteries enter the lung parenchyma through the pulmonary ligament or the adherent pleura. Identification of dilated vessels within extrapleural fat associated with pleural thickening (>3 mm) and lung parenchymal abnormalities may be regarded as nonbronchial systemic arteries responsible for hemoptysis.

## Pulmonary Vasculitis

Pulmonary vasculitis is a group of disorders characterized by inflammation of the pulmonary vessels with granuloma formation. Patients are typically middle aged presenting with recurrent attacks of fever, dyspnea, and hemoptysis.

The most recognized pulmonary vasculitis diseases are Wegener's granulomatosis (WG), Churg–Strauss syndrome (CSS) (allergic vasculitis and granulomatosis), and lymphomatoid granulomatosis.

*Wegener's granulomatosis* (*WG*) is a disease characterized by the triad of febrile sinusitis, glomerulonephritis, and pulmonary vasculitis. Patients often present with dyspnea, rhinitis, otitis media, pleuritic chest pain, and hemoptysis. The presence of cytoplasmic pattern of antineutrophil cytoplasmic autoantibody (c-ANCA) in the patient's serum is a high indicator of WG (96 % sensitive for active WG). The serum level of c-ANCA can be used to monitor the disease activity. Histopathologically, WG is characterized by chronic inflammation of the medium-sized and small pulmonary arteries, veins, and capillaries.

*CSS* is a disease characterized by the triad of asthma or allergic rhinitis, marked peripheral eosinophilia, and systemic vasculitis involving two or more extrapulmonary organs. *Asthma* is a disease characterized by reversible airways obstruction. Patients with CSS are presenting with pulmonary distress, hemoptysis, fever, gastrointestinal symptoms, and arthralgia occasionally. The typical laboratory findings include marked eosinophilia in the absence of parasitic disease and high levels of serum rheumatoid factor in 52 % of cases. Extrapulmonary vasculitis may be seen in the form of coronary vasculitis, renal-induced hypertension, glomerulonephritis, cerebral hemorrhage, and purpuric skin lesions. CSS can be differentiated from WG by the characteristic association with asthma (rarely encountered in WG), cardiac involvement (up to 47 % of CSS cases), and less severe paranasal sinus involvement in CSS. Moreover, patients with CSS show serological positivity of perinuclear antineutrophil cytoplasmic autoantibody (p-ANCA), while WG shows serological positivity of c-ANCA.

*Lymphomatoid granulomatosis* (*LG*) is a multisystemic disease characterized by lung manifestations (100 % of cases), skin and nervous system manifestations (up to 53 %), and renal disease (up to 40 %). It is characterized pathologically by angiocentric infiltration of the lymphoid tissues and the vessels by atypical lymphocytes, and a mixture of plasma cells and histiocytes, causing tissue destruction and necrosis. Patients typically present with severe generalized symptoms that can be confusing. There is no specific serological marker, and erythrocytes sedimentation rate can be normal in spite of active disease. The main diagnostic method is biopsy of the lesions.

**Signs on Radiographs and HRCT**
- In *WG*, the early stages of the disease show reticular or nodular interstitial lung pattern mainly located at the lung basis. As the disease progresses, diffuse alveolar lung disease may be seen bilaterally due to pulmonary hemorrhage (■ Fig. 7.8.65). WG may cause areas of consolidation or nodules with a cavity formation in the center.
- In *CSS*, the plain radiographs may be normal in 25 % of cases. The pathological signs are similar to WG, with the formation of multiple granulomatous nodules with or without central cavity likely to be seen (■ Fig. 7.8.66).
- In *LG*, there are typically large lung mass-like opacities located within the lung parenchyma (due to pulmonary infarcts). Up to 80 % of cases present as multiple, bilateral nodules located within the

middle and the lower lung lobes (■ Fig. 7.8.67). Unilateral involvement is unusual (21 % of cases). Subpleural nodules may be seen, with pleural effusion likely to be found in 40 % of cases. Mediastinal lymphadenopathy is unusual.

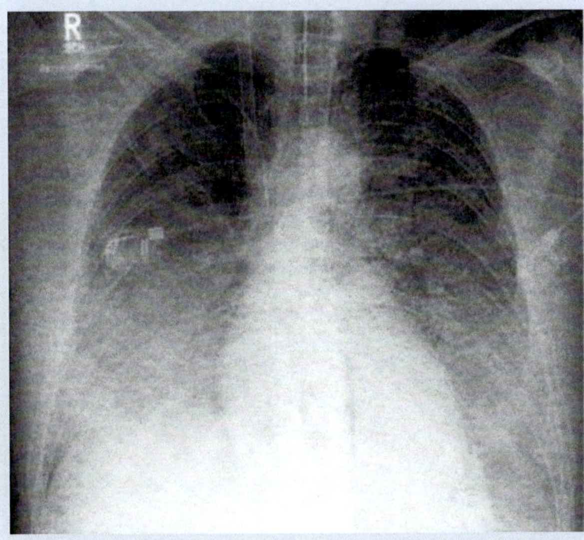

■ **Fig. 7.8.65** Anteroposterior plain chest radiograph of a Wegener's granulomatosis (WG) patient in the intensive care unit shows bilateral diffuse alveolar lung disease due to pulmonary hemorrhage

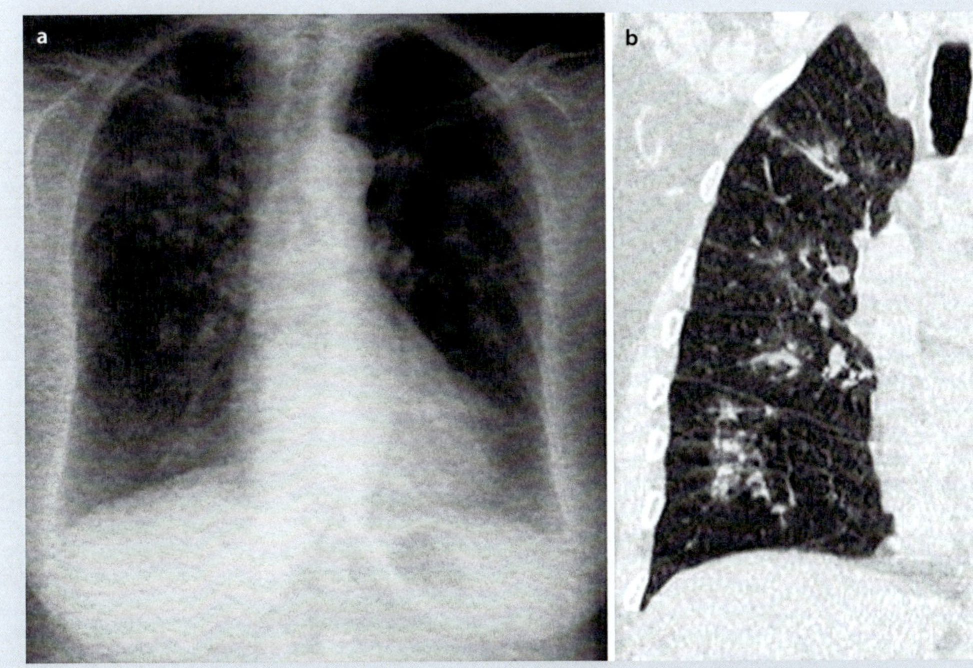
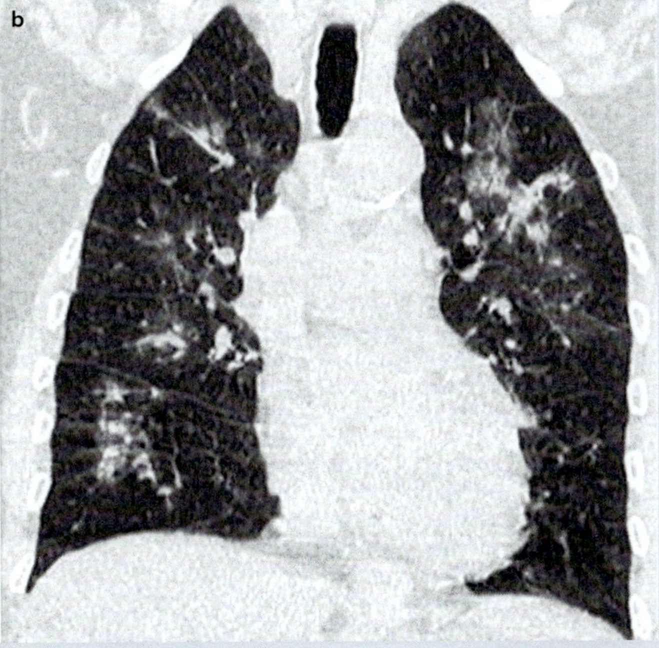

■ **Fig. 7.8.66** Posteroanterior plain chest radiograph (**a**) and coronal HRCT (**b**) of a patient with Churg–Strauss syndrome (CSS) show bilateral nodular patchy lung infiltration due to vasculitis and granulomatosis

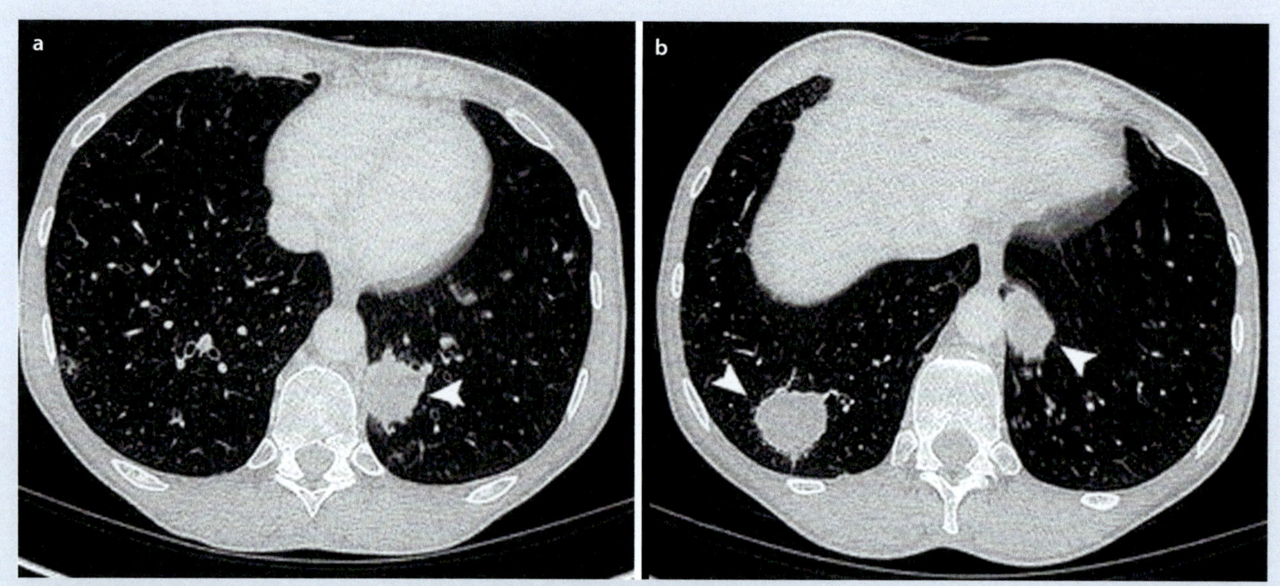

**Fig. 7.8.67**  Sequential axial HRCT of a patient with lymphomatoid granulomatosis (LG) shows multiple lung masses located at the lung bases in the left lung in (**a**) and bilaterally in (**b**) (*arrowheads*)

## Cardiac Bronchus

Cardiac bronchus is a rare congenital anomaly in which there is accessory bronchus that arises from the medial wall of the intermediate bronchus at its proximal third, but occasionally from the right main bronchus. The accessory bronchus runs medially and caudally toward the heart, hence the cardiac appellation.

Cardiac bronchus is not identified on plain chest radiographs and usually incidentally found on CT scans. The anomaly is asymptomatic; however, it may result in hemoptysis when it is infected.

### Signs on CT
The cardiac bronchus is typically identified as a small accessory bronchus medial to the intermediate bronchus on the right lung (■ Fig. 7.8.68).

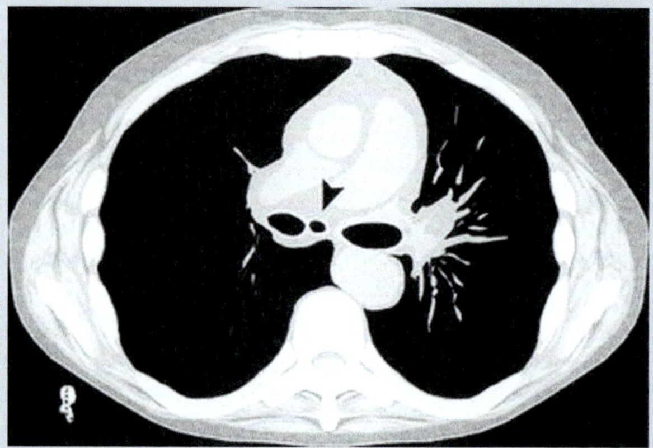

**Fig. 7.8.68**  Axial HRCT illustration demonstrates the typical radiographic sign and location of the cardiac bronchus on CT (*arrowhead*)

## Dieulafoy Disease

Dieulafoy disease is a very rare condition characterized by abnormally dilated submucosal vessels that are prone to bleed and classically described in the colon, small intestine, and the bronchi.

Dieulafoy disease can be seen with cases of chronic bronchitis. On bronchoscopy, the visualization of dilated submucosal blood vessels in the presence of mucosal dilatation should alert the bronchoscopist of the possibility of Dieulafoy disease. Dieulafoy disease can be the case of massive upper gastrointestinal bleeding in 1–2 % of cases.

### Further Reading


Ahmed M, et al. Multislice CT and CT angiography for non-invasive evaluation of bronchopulmonary sequestration. Eur Radiol. 2004;14:2141–3.

Bentala M, et al. Cardiac bronchus: a rare cause of hemoptysis. Eur J Cardiothoracic Surg. 2002;22:643–5.

Bolca N, et al. Bronchopulmonary sequestration: radiological findings. Eur J Radiol. 2004;52:185–91.

Bruzzi JF, et al. Multi-detector row CT of hemoptysis. Radiographics. 2006;26:3–22.

Chung MJ, et al. Bronchial and non-bronchial systemic arteries in patients with hemoptysis: depiction on MDCT angiography. AJR Am J Roentgenol. 2006;186:649–55.

Cooper C, et al. CT appearance of the normal inferior pulmonary ligament. AJR Am J Roentgenol. 1983;141:237–40.

Do KH, et al. Systemic arterial supply to the lung in adults: spiral CT findings. Radiographics. 2001;21:387–402.

Frazier AA, et al. Pulmonary angiitis and granulomatosis: radiologic-pathologic correlation. Radiographics. 1998;18:687–710.

Furuse M, et al. Bronchial arteries: CT demonstration with arteriographic correlation. Radiology. 1987;162:393–8.

Katayama K, et al. Adult case of accessory cardiac bronchus presenting with bloody sputum. Jpn J Thorac Cardiovasc Surg. 2005;53:641–4.

Khalil A, et al. Role of MDCT in identification of the bleeding site and the vessels causing hemoptysis. AJR Am J Roentgenol. 2007;188:W117–25.

Löschhorn C, et al. Dieulafoy's disease of the lung: a potential disaster for the bronchoscopist. Respiration. 2006;73: 562–5.

Son JS, et al. Anomalous systemic arterial supply to the basal segments of the right lower lobe in neonate. Pediatr Cardiol. 2008;29:1009–10.

Temes E, et al. Young patient with recurrent hemoptysis. Resp Med (Extra). 2006;2:64–6.

van der Werf TS, et al. Fatal hemorrhage from Dieulafoy's disease of the bronchus. Thorax. 1999;54:184–5.

Wilson SR, et al. CT visualization of mediastinal bronchial artery aneurysm. AJR Am J Roentgenol. 2006;187: W544–5.

Yoon YC, et al. Hemoptysis: bronchial and non-bronchial systemic arteries at 16-detector row CT. Radiology. 2005;234:292–8.

## 7.9 Cystic Fibrosis (Mucoviscidosis)

Cystic fibrosis (CF) is an autosomal recessive, systemic disorder characterized by abnormal function of the exocrine glands due to defect in the permeability of epithelium to chloride ions. The disease is caused by mutation in the cystic fibrosis transmembrane conductance regulator (CFTR) gene located on the long arm of chromosome 7.

CF affects between 1 in 4500 children of Caucasian origin. Orientals and blacks are rarely affected. Median survival age is 29 years, and up to 95 % of deaths are due to progressive pulmonary disease. Other areas affected by CF include the sweat glands, pancreas, liver, intestine, and Wolffian ducts in males.

## Pulmonary Manifestations of Cystic Fibrosis

Patients with cystic CF are prone to progressive pulmonary deterioration due to formation of bronchiectasis. The defective ciliary mechanism within the bronchial tree causes the pulmonary secretions to accumulate within the terminal bronchioles (mucus plugs).

The most frequently encountered pathologies in CF include mucus plugs, sacculations, emphysema, bronchiectasis, atelectasis, and lung fibrosis in terminal lung disease due to chronic inflammation. CF patients are susceptible to airway colonization with specific bacteria such as *Staphylococcus aureus*, *Hemophilus influenza*, allergic *bronchopulmonary aspergillosis* (*ABPA*), and *Pseudomonas* species. Hemoptysis is an unusual complication of CF and arises due to enlargement of the bronchial arteries.

*Burkholderia cepacia*, formerly known as *Pseudomonas cepacia*, is an anaerobic, catalase-positive, gram-negative rod that was first described by William Burkholder in 1950 as a plant pathogen capable of causing onion rot. *B. cepacia* emerges as a problematic cystic fibrosis pathogen almost 30 years ago. Unlike other pathogens affecting cystic fibrosis patients, *B. cepacia* causes rapid, uncontrolled, and fatal clinical disease in 10 % of cystic fibrosis patients, a condition known as *cepacia syndrome*. The infection is capable of transmission through social contact. *B. cepacia* uncommonly causes community-acquired infections in immunocompetent patients, causing chronic suppurative otitis media complicated by cerebellopontine abscesses.

### Signs on Pulmonary HRCT

1. The most frequent manifestations of CF in chest HRCT include emphysematous air trapping (100 %), peribronchial thickening (97 %), atelectasis, sacculations, bronchiectasis, and fibrosis in long-standing disease (◘ Fig. 7.9.69).
2. Mucus plugs appear as centrilobular densities, typically against isodense background of collapsed pulmonary lobule (◘ Fig. 7.9.70).
3. Sacculations are seen as excessively dilated bronchi (◘ Fig. 7.9.71).
4. On angiography, enlargement of the bronchial arteries may be seen in CF patients presenting with hemoptysis.
5. Pulmonary lobar atelectasis with high-density materials seen within the bronchi can be due to acute hemorrhagic aspiration or more commonly infection with aspergillosis (ABPA). Mucus plugs have typically low attenuation on HRCT; only 30 % of mucus plugs have high attenuation. The high attenuation is due to calcium oxalate crystal deposition within the plugs for unknown reason.

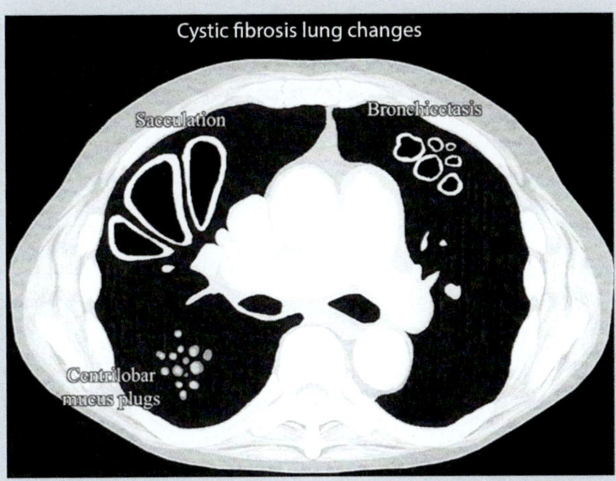


◘ **Fig. 7.9.69** Axial pulmonary HRCT illustration that demonstrates the most common manifestations detected on HRCT in patients with cystic fibrosis

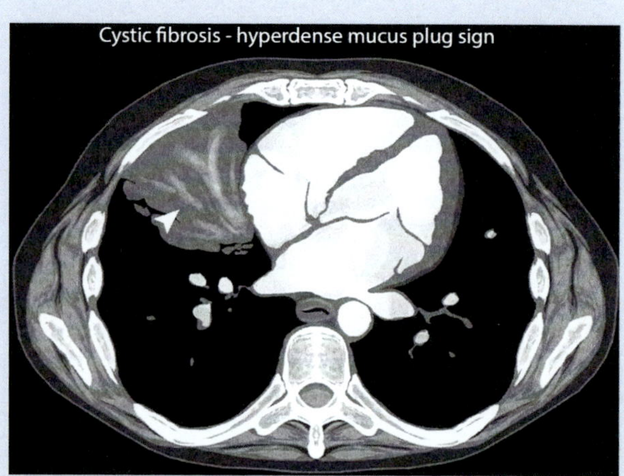



☐ **Fig. 7.9.70**   Axial pulmonary CT, postcontrast illustration that demonstrates hyperdense mucus plug sign in bronchial tree in patients with cystic fibrosis (*arrowhead*)

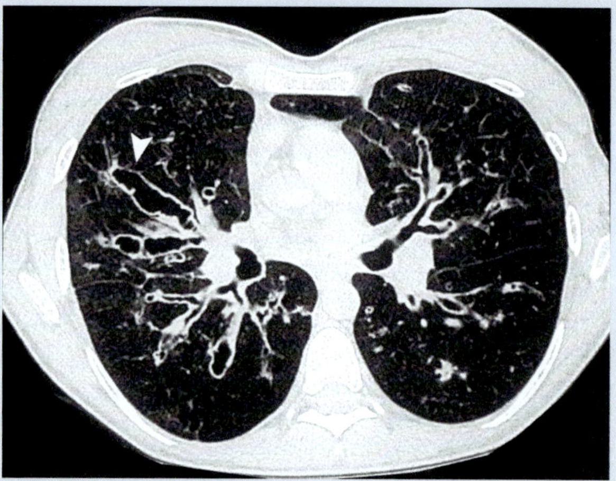

☐ **Fig. 7.9.71**   Axial pulmonary HRCT image of a patient with cystic fibrosis shows bilateral sacculations, seen as excessively dilated bronchi (*arrowhead*)

sage. Retention cysts in contrast are due to blockage of a mucous gland duct, not the sinus itself. Mucoceles may take years to grow large enough to cause symptoms. Up to 70 % of mucoceles are located in the frontal and the ethmoid sinuses (maxillary mucocele is rare). Patients with mucocele can present with proptosis and unilateral visual disturbance if the mucocele presses over the globe and the optic pathways. When the mucocele is infected, it is called *pyocele* and presents clinically with fever and pain. Lastly, hypoplasia or aplasia of the nasal sinuses has been reported in patients with CF.

> **Signs on Radiograph**
> 1. Polyps are seen as rounded, pedunculated mucosal swelling within the affected sinus (☐ Fig. 7.9.72).
> 2. Mucoceles are detected as complete sinus opacification with expansion of the affected sinus.

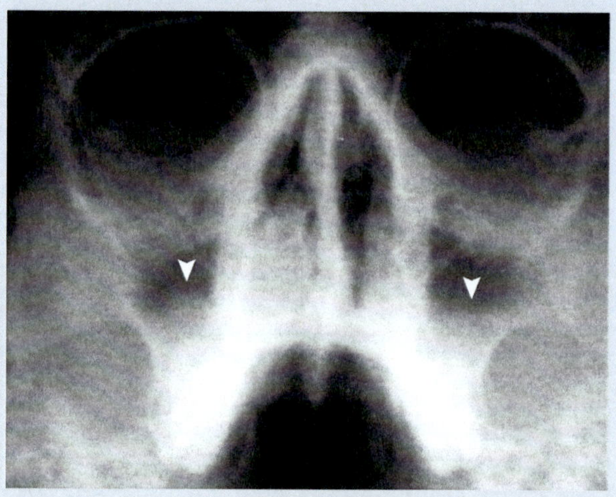

☐ **Fig. 7.9.72**   Plain radiograph of the sinuses (water-view) that shows bilateral maxillary sinus polyposis seen as radio-opaque, rounded shadows (*arrowheads*)

## Nasal and Sinus Manifestations of Cystic Fibrosis

Patients with CF suffer from sinonasal symptoms in 10 % of cases. Most complaints are due to unilateral or bilateral nasal blockage (81 %), rhinorrhea (50 %), daily headache (51 %), nasal polyposis (48 %), and anosmia (27 %). Up to 33 % of CF patients have broadening of the nasal bridge.

Nasal polyposis is seen in 48 % of CF patients with sinonasal symptoms. Polyps are circumferential, rounded, pedunculated swellings of the nasal and sinus mucosa with an unknown origin. They commonly arise secondary to chronic sinusitis.

Some patients with CF may develop mucoceles. A mucocele is a slow-growing, expansile, cyst-like mass within the paranasal sinus due to blockage of the normal drainage pas-

> **Signs on CT**
> 1. Nasal polyposis on CT is detected as complete or almost-complete opacification of the sinus without destruction of the fine air cell bony septations (differentiate it from mucocele). When polyps occur in the ethmoid sinus, bilateral bowing of the lamina papyracea occurring in the late stage can lead to acquired hypertelorism (lateralization of the total orbit).
> 2. Mucocele on CT is detected as a mass filling the sinus with thinning and expansion of the sinus walls. Erosion of the sinus wall can occur. The mass does not enhance after contrast injection. Pyocele can show hyperdense mass with air inclusions.

### Signs on MRI

1. Nasal polyps on MRI show low T1 and high homogenous T2 signal in MRI (the signal of normal sinus mucosa). After contrast injection, only the mucosa around the mass will enhance, while the center will not enhance as high as the normal mucosa.
2. Mucocele on MRI shows a signal that depends upon the content of the mass. Normal mucocele shows signal similar to normal mucosa (low T1 and high T2 signal intensities). If the mucocele contains hemorrhage, then it will show high signal intensity in all pulses. If the mucocele is filled with dry, inspissated material, then it will show low signal intensity in all pulses.

## Gastrointestinal (GI) Manifestations of Cystic Fibrosis

Patients with CF show GI abnormalities that are mainly located within the pancreas and the liver. Pancreatic abnormalities are seen in 85–90 % of CF patients below 30 years of age. Pancreatic insufficiency is common due to the inherent defect in epithelial chloride ion permeability, which is linked to bicarbonate and water secretion. Up to 30–50 % of patients suffer from exocrine dysfunction, fat malabsorption, and glucose intolerance. Pancreatic insufficiency arises due to pancreatic fatty replacement, cystic changes, and pancreatic cystosis. Up to 30 % of patients with CF have hepatic steatosis, biliary cirrhosis (30 %), portal hypertension, and splenomegaly. Other GI complications include cholelithiasis (10 %), appendicitis, and gastroesophageal reflux disease.

The intestines and colon are commonly affected in patients with CF. Complications affecting the intestine and colon include meconium ileus syndrome, distal intestinal obstruction syndrome, intussusception, fibrosing colonopathy, and colonic wall redundancy. *Meconium ileus syndrome* is seen in 10–15 % of CF infants, causing intestinal obstruction by sticky material that can cause colonic strictures and peritonitis. In older children, intestinal obstruction can occur due to fecal and colonic fecal impaction (*distal intestinal obstruction syndrome*). *Intussusception* occurs in 1 % of CF patients and is typically seen between the ages 4 and 10 years. *Fibrosing colonopathy* is a condition that arises in CF patients receiving high-strength pancreatic enzyme replacement to control intestinal malabsorption. The colon shows marked strictures, longitudinal shortening, and loss of the haustra due to mucosal fibrosis and thickening of the muscularis mucosa. *Colonic wall redundancy* (CWR) is a frequent condition in adult CF patients (39 % of cases). Patients with CWR can be asymptomatic or present with nonspecific GI symptoms.

Amyloidosis type-AA can develop in older CF patients due to systemic chronic inflammation. Patients with systemic amyloidosis can present with thyroid goiter, proteinuria, and hepatosplenomegaly.

### Signs on Plain Radiographs

1. Pancreatic calcifications may be seen due to liposclerosis and calcification of the intraductal secretions.
2. Abdominal punctuated or plaque-like calcifications that may extend along the processus vaginalis to the scrotum may be seen due to meconium peritonitis in meconium ileus syndrome.

### Signs on US

1. Hepatic steatosis is detected as highly echogenic liver.
2. Intussusception is seen as a "donut appearance" mass with hypoechoic rim and echogenic center. The Doppler signal is increased due to vascular congestion.
3. Focal cholestasis (intrahepatic biliary ducts >2 mm in diameter), periportal thickening (>2 mm wall thickness), with focal irregular liver contour can be seen in cases of liver cirrhosis due to CF (pathognomonic). This focal cirrhosis and cholestasis are caused by obstruction of small intrahepatic biliary ducts with ductal proliferation and hyperplasia.
4. Multiple scattered areas of fatty infiltration can be seen in the liver in CF patients, and these masses are called pseudomasses. Typically, they are visualized hyperechoic fatty masses with hypoechoic rim and can be easily mistaken for abnormal liver masses.
5. Colonic wall redundancy is detected as hypertrophic colonic wall folds (>4 mm) with overlapping.

### Signs on CT

1. In early stages of CF, the pancreas appears heterogeneous due to areas of fat attenuation and normal parenchymal attenuation. In advanced stages of CF with symptoms of pancreatic insufficiency, complete replacement of the pancreas with fat with high-attenuation pancreatic duct within it can be seen (*pancreatic lipomatosis*) (◨ Fig. 7.9.73). Similar case can be seen in obesity, old age, chronic pancreatitis, and Cushing's syndrome.
2. Micro- (<3 mm) or macrocysts (>3 mm) can be found within the pancreas due to inspissation of proteins in the acini and ductules, causing their dilatation and atrophy of the acinar tissue (◨ Fig. 7.9.74). *Pancreatic cystosis* is a term used to describe complete replacement of the pancreas by cysts (◨ Fig. 7.9.75). Similar case can be encountered in polycystic kidney disease, von Hippel–Lindau syndrome, lymphangiomas, and mucinous cystadenoma.
3. In the liver, signs of cholestasis may be seen with pseudomasses. Pseudomasses are seen as multiple

hypodense masses with fat attenuation surrounded by normal liver parenchyma.

4. On axial view, intussusception shows "target sign" with crescent hypodense area inside it representing the mesentery. Enhancing mesenteric vessels within the mass is frequently seen (very characteristic; ■ Fig. 7.9.76). On longitudinal axis, the intussusception is seen as an area of "sausage-shaped" mass. The contrast makes a rim around the area of the intussusception due to bowel invagination.

5. Colonic wall redundancy shows overlapping colonic folds, producing a double or triple appearance of the wall mimicking wrinkles (■ Fig. 7.9.77). Hyperdensity areas within the wall before contrast injection may be seen due to inspissated mucofeculent material. After contrast injection, the inner wall shows marked enhancement due to hypervascularity.

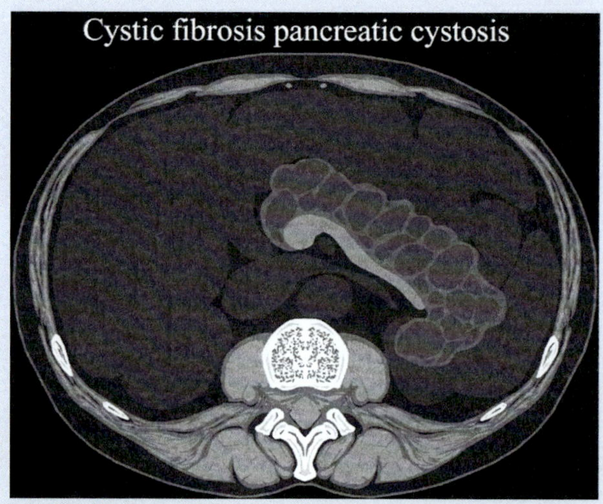


■ **Fig. 7.9.75**  Axial abdomen CT illustration that shows pancreatic cystosis

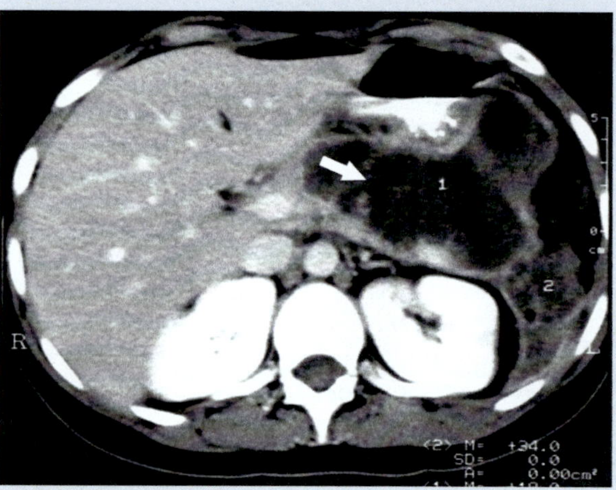

■ **Fig. 7.9.73**  Axial abdomen CT postcontrast image that shows complete fatty replacement of the pancreas in a patient with chronic cystic fibrosis (*arrow*)

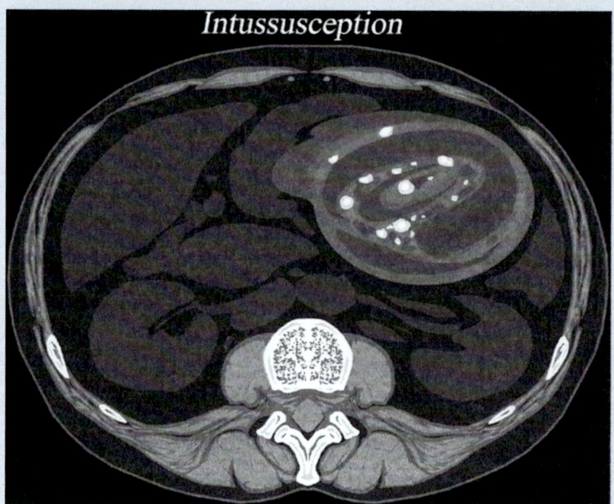


■ **Fig. 7.9.76**  Axial abdomen CT illustration that shows the classical "target sign" of intussusception

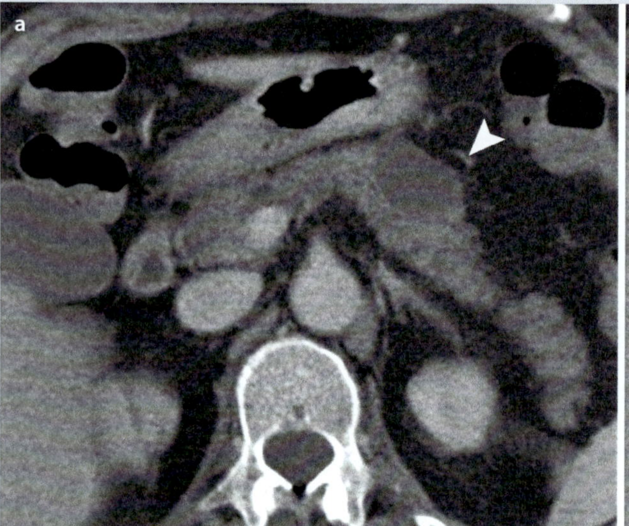

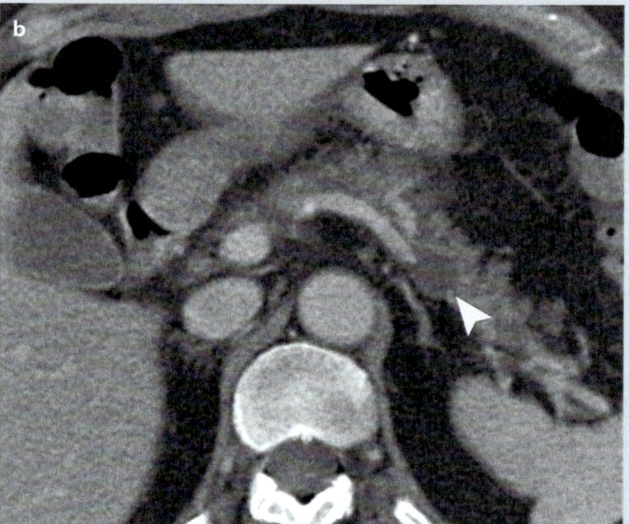

■ **Fig. 7.9.74**  Axial abdomen CT post-contrast image of a patient with cystic fibrosis that shows multiple cysts formation in the pancreas (*arrowheads* in **a** and **b**)

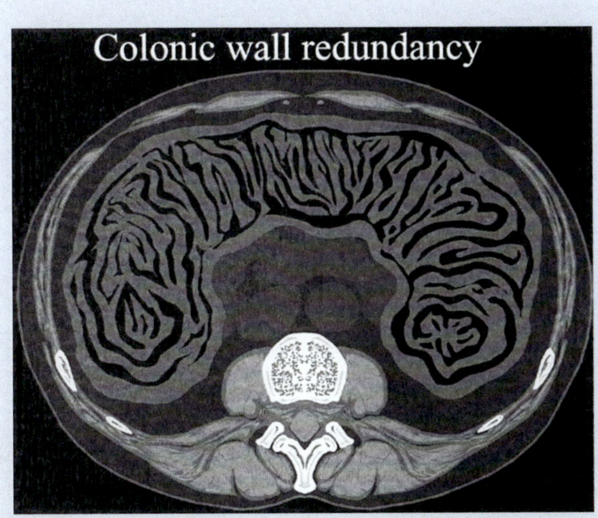


**Fig. 7.9.77** Axial abdomen CT illustration that shows colon wall redundancy CT features

## Signs on MRCP
1. Pancreatic cysts or pancreatic cystosis shows multiple pancreatic cysts that has no communication with the pancreatic duct or duct of Wirsung.
2. In the liver, dilatation of the intrahepatic biliary tree with focal areas of stenosis can be seen mimicking primary sclerosing cholangitis.

## Signs on MRI
1. In the liver, periportal wall thickening with high signal intensity on T1W images can be seen due to periportal fat deposition instead of cirrhosis.
2. Colonic wall redundancy shows the same overlapping colonic wall folds mimicking wrinkles in CT, with hyperintense signal intensity on T1W and T2W images before contrast injection, and inner wall enhancement after contrast injection due to hypervascularity.

## Genitourinary Manifestations of Cystic Fibrosis

About 97 % of males with CF are sterile due to congenital bilateral absence of the vas deference, which can be associated with the absence of the seminal vesicles and absence or atrophy of the distal portion of the epididymis. Testicular calcification or microlithiasis may be seen.

*Testicular microlithiasis* is a condition characterized by the presence of multiple punctuated 1–3 mm calcifications within the testicular parenchyma. The condition is usually bilateral and can be associated with conditions like Klinefelter syndrome, Down syndrome, Peutz–Jeghers syndrome, alveolar microlithiasis, cryptorchidism, and male infertility. The condition is premalignant, with 10 % of cases turning into germ cell tumors. Annual ultrasound screening is recommended for patients with testicular microlithiasis.

### Signs on Radiographs
Rarely, CF patients may show calcified scrotum due to meconium periorchitis (extension of meconium peritonitis into the scrotum).

### Signs on US
1. The epididymis may be absent, atrophic, or show internal cysts.
2. Testicular microlithiasis is seen as multiple echogenic foci 1–3 mm in size in a diffuse bilateral fashion.
3. Calcifications within the scrotum can be seen due to meconium periorchitis.

## Musculoskeletal Manifestations of Cystic Fibrosis

Cystic fibrosis arthropathy (CFA) is a poorly understood unique form of polyarthritis that occurs in CF patients. CFA arthropathy is characterized by recurrent painful attacks of mono- or polyarthritis associated with erythema nodosum-like rash and purpuric skin lesions ( Fig. 7.9.78). The flares of joint inflammation last from day 1 to several weeks (average 1–7 days). Most cases are self-limiting; however, active synovitis persists. Majority of the reported cases are negative for both serum rheumatoid factor and antinuclear antibodies.

**Cystic fibrosis arthitis**

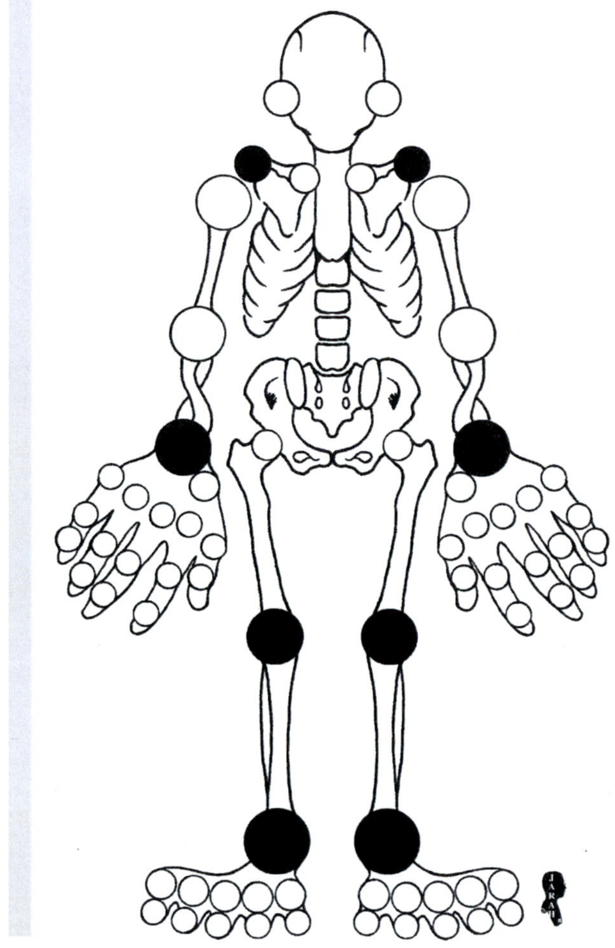



**Fig. 7.9.78** An illustration that demonstrates the body's geographic distribution of cystic fibrosis arthropathy

### Signs on Radiographs
In CFA, affected joints show effusion, osteoporosis, and hypertrophic osteoarthropathy.

## Selected References


Ablin DS, et al. Ulcerative type of colitis associated with the use of high strength pancreatic enzyme supplements in cystic fibrosis. Pediatr Radiol. 1995;25:113–6.

Akata D, et al. Hepatobiliary manifestations of cystic fibrosis in children: correlation of CT and US findings. Eur J Radiol. 2002;41:26–33.

Akata D, et al. Liver manifestations of cystic fibrosis. Eur J Radiol. 2007;61:11–7.

Brihaye P, et al. Pathological changes of the lateral nasal wall in patients with cystic fibrosis (mucoviscidosis). Int J Pediatr Otorhinolaryngol. 1994;28:141–7.

Cahill ME, et al. Pancreatic cystosis in cystic fibrosis. Abdom Imaging. 1997;22:313–4.

Carucci LR, et al. Focal fatty sparing of the pancreatic head in cystic fibrosis: CT findings. Abdom Imaging. 2003;28:853–5.

Chaudry G, et al. Abdominal manifestations of cystic fibrosis in children. Pediatr Radiol. 2006;36:233–40.

Chrispin AR, et al. The systematic evaluation of the chest radiograph in cystic fibrosis. Pediatr Radiol. 1974;2:101–6.

De Baets F, et al. Achromobacter xylosoxidans in cystic fibrosis: prevalence and clinical relevance. J Cyst Fibros. 2007;6:75–8.

De Gruchy S, et al. Pancreatic cystosis in a child with cystic fibrosis. Pediatr Radiol. 2008;38:1142.

Demirkazık FB, et al. High resolution CT in children with cystic fibrosis: correlation with pulmonary functions and radiographic scores. Eur J Radiol. 2001;37:54–9.

El-Laboudi AH, et al. Acute Burkholderia cepacia pyomyositis in a patient with cystic fibrosis. J Cyst Fibros. 2009;8:273–5.

Lang I, et al. Abdominal calcification in cystic fibrosis with meconium ileus: radiologic-pathologic correlation. Pediatr Radiol. 1997;27:523–7.

Ledesma-Medina J, et al. Abnormal paranasal sinuses in patients with cystic fibrosis of the pancreas. Radiological findings. Pediatr Radiol. 1980;9:61–4.

Lipnick RN, et al. Bone changes associated with cystic fibrosis. Skeletal Radiol. 1992;21:115–6.

Lugo-Olivieri CH, et al. Cystic fibrosis: spectrum of thoracis and abdominal CT findings in the adult patient. Clin Imaging. 1998;22:346–54.

Mahenthiralingam E, et al. Burkholderia cepacia complex bacteria: opportunistic pathogens with important natural biology. J Appl Microbiol. 2008;104:1539–51.

Marioni G, et al. Burkholderia cepacia complex nasal isolation in immunocompetent patients with sinonasal polyposis not associated with cystic fibrosis. Eur J Clin Microbiol Infect Dis. 2007;26:73–5.

Mc Laughlin AM, et al. Amyloidosis in cystic fibrosis: a case series. J Cyst Fibros. 2006;5:59–61.

Merkel PA. Rheumatic disease and cystic fibrosis. Arthritis Rheum. 1999;42(8):1563–71.

Monti L, et al. Pancreatic cystosis in cystic fibrosis: case report. Abdom Imaging. 2001;26:648–50.

Morozov A, et al. High-attenuation mucus plugs on MDCT in a child with cystic fibrosis: potential cause and differential diagnosis. Pediatr Radiol. 2007;37:592–5.

Paling MR, et al. Scoliosis in cystic fibrosis: an appraisal. Skeletal Radiol. 1982;8:63–6.

Quillin SP, et al. Hepatobiliary sonography in cystic fibrosis. Pediatr Radiol. 1993;23:533–5.

Rathaus V, et al. Sonographic findings of the genital tract in boys with cystic fibrosis. Pediatr Radiol. 2006;36:162–6.

Robertson JM, et al. Nasal and sinus disease in cystic fibrosis. Paediatr Respir Rev. 2008;9:213–9.

Ryan S, et al. Pancreatic replacement by cysts in cystic fibrosis. Pediatr Radiol. 2008;38:1141.

Sodhi KS, et al. Pancreatic lipomatosis in an infant with cystic fibrosis. Pediatr Radiol. 2005;35:1157–8.

Vergesslich KA, et al. Portal venous blood flow in cystic fibrosis: assessment by Duplex Doppler sonography. Pediatr Radiol. 1989;19:371–4.

## 7.10  Sleep Apnea Syndromes

Sleep apnea syndromes are group of diseases characterized by complete or partial cessation of breathing, lasting at least 10 s, which occurs repeatedly throughout the night. These conditions are defined by a respiratory disturbance index (RDI) >10, and the prevalence is 70 % in elderly men and 56 % in elderly women respectively.

Sleep apnea syndromes can arise due to abnormalities in the pharynx (obstructive), tracheal tree (obstructive), or the respiratory center within the medulla oblongata (central type).

*The most common subtypes of sleep apnea disorders:*
1. Obstructive sleep apnea/hypopnea syndrome
2. Upper airway resistance syndrome
3. Central alveolar hypoventilation syndrome (Ondine's curse)

## Obstructive Sleep Apnea Syndrome

Obstructive sleep apnea syndrome (OSAS) is a disease characterized by repeated episodes of pharyngeal wall collapse during sleep, causing apnea or hypopnea. The most common symptoms of OSAS patients include chronic loud snoring, excessive daytime sleepiness, personality changes, and deterioration of quality of life.

Patients with OSAS suffer from hypoxemia and hypercapnia with negative consequences in particular on the cardiorespiratory system (*pulmonary hypertension, systemic hypertension, cardiac arrhythmias, and myocardial ischemia*), central nervous system (*cerebral ischemia*), and decreased survival. OSAS is classified according to the respiratory distress index (RDI) into:

*Normal*: RDI <5 attacks per hour of sleep
*Mild*: RDI = 5–15 attacks per hour of sleep
*Moderate*: RDI = 16–30 attacks per hour of sleep
*Severe*: RDI >30 attacks per hour of sleep

### OSAS and Obesity

OSAS often coexists with obesity, with significant OSAS present in approximately 40 % of obese individuals and about 70 % of OSAS patients being obese. Many studies showed that increased levels of leptin in OSAS are due to leptin resistance. Also, the direct relationship between OSAS and leptin is supported by the fact that effective OSAS treatment with continuous positive airway pressure (CPAP) treatment also influences leptin levels.

Adiponectin is an adipocyte-derived cytokine with regulatory functions in glucose and lipid metabolism. It also has profound anti-inflammatory and antiatherogenic effects. Levels of plasma adiponectin are decreased in obesity and metabolic syndrome.

### OSAS and Endocrine–Metabolic Abnormalities

Men who suffer from OSAS may manifest decreased libido and a decline in morning serum testosterone levels. It is also accepted that obesity in men is associated with reduced androgen secretion, since increased leptin levels is known to cause impairment of testicular Leydig cell function.

Women with the polycystic ovary syndrome (*a condition associated with hyperandrogenism and insulin resistance*) were found to be much more likely than controls to have sleep-disordered breathing and daytime sleepiness, suggesting a pathogenetic role for insulin resistance in OSAS.

In OSAS, chronic hypoxia, hypercarbia, and respiratory acidosis associated with periodic upper airway obstruction stimulate peripheral and central chemoreceptors in the body that promote a cardiovascular and respiratory sympathetic reflex. This increase in sympathetic activity promotes hyperinsulinemia by stimulating glycogenolysis and gluconeogenesis and produces an increase in circulating free fatty acids via stimulation of lipolysis that promotes insulin resistance.

### OSAS and Cardiovascular Diseases

There are many evidences which suggest that cyclic intermittent hypoxia in OSAS patient causes hypercoagulability and disturbs nocturnal rennin and aldosterone secretion profiles and increases nighttime urine excretion.

**Signs on Plain Radiographs**
1. Cephalometry is a lateral plain radiograph of the head and neck that is used to obtain certain cephalometric parameters that describe the relations between the craniofacial structures. The lateral head and neck radiograph should be obtained after complete expiration to ensure standardization. A frontal plain radiograph can be obtained also to complete the measurements. The same measurements can be obtained from CT sinuses in coronal and sagittal planes (◘ Fig. 7.10.79).
2. The most common cephalometric parameters are the *same parameters applied to CT*:
   a. *Posterior pharyngeal wall (PPW)*: the thickness of the posterior pharyngeal wall in front of the tubercle of the atlas (normal MPH >3.7 mm).
   b. *Posterior airway space (PAS) at C3 level*: the measurement of the pharyngeal airway space at C3 (normal >5 mm).
   c. *Central incisor to the tongue base (TT-TB)*: OSA <90 mm (◘ Figs. 7.10.80 and 7.10.81).
   d. *Velum width (Vw)*: maximal velar width, i.e., thickness of the velum measured on cross section at the widest point (normal Vw >12 mm).
   e. *Posterior uvular space (PUS)*: (OSA <4.5 mm).
   f. *Medial orbit to medial orbit (MOMO) distance*: the medio-orbitale (MO) is the point on the medial

orbital margin that is the closest to the medial plane (left and right) (■ Fig. 7.10.79). The distance between the two MO points (MOMO) is normal MOMO <26 mm.

g. *Mandibular plane to hyoid (MPH)*: the distance in mm between the mandibular plane and the most anterior point on the hyoid (normal MPH <20.8 mm).

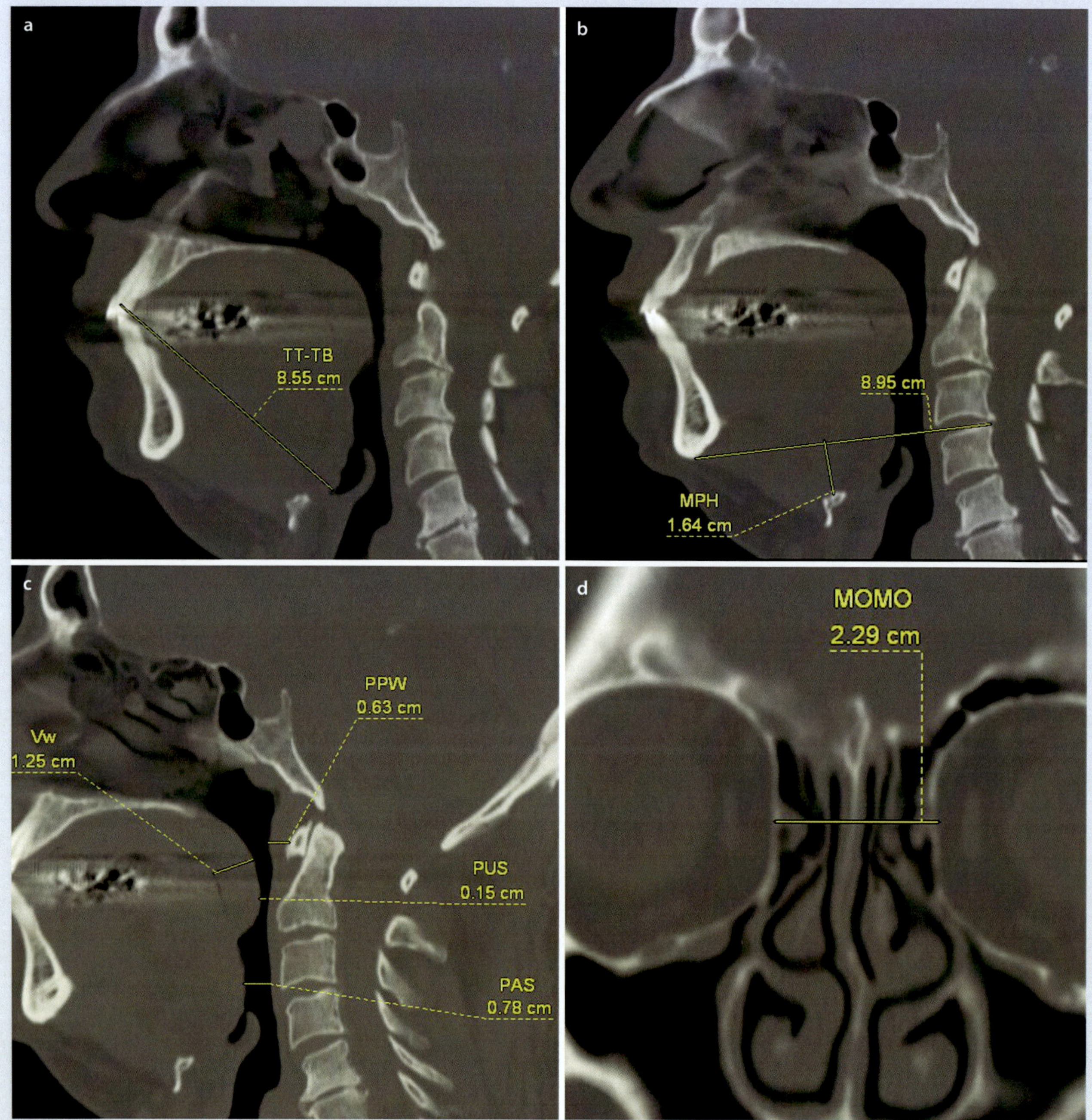


■ **Fig. 7.10.79**    Sagittal CT sinuses images (**a–c**) and coronal (**d**) that shows the cephalometric lines used to measure the degree of stenosis in OSA

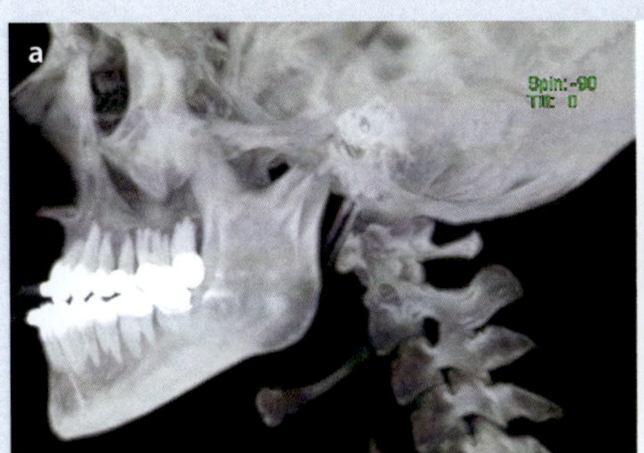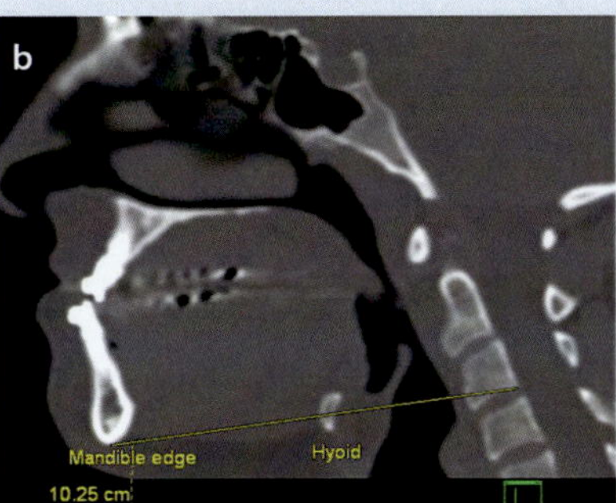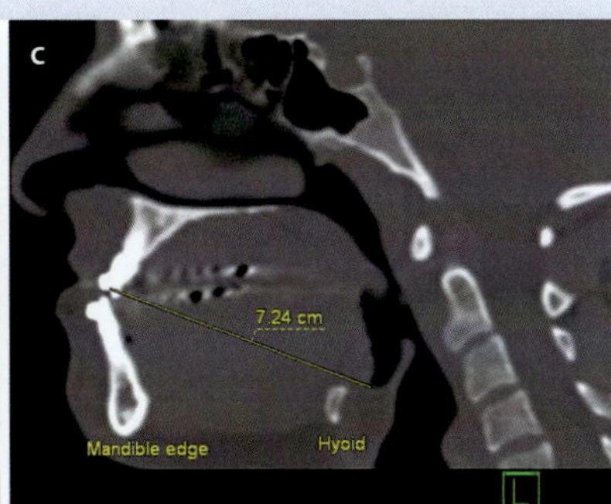

**Fig. 7.10.80** Sagittal CT sinuses images (**b**, **c**) with 3D reconstruction image of a patient with OSA due to prognathism shows reduced central incisor to tongue base (TT-TB) distance (**c**)

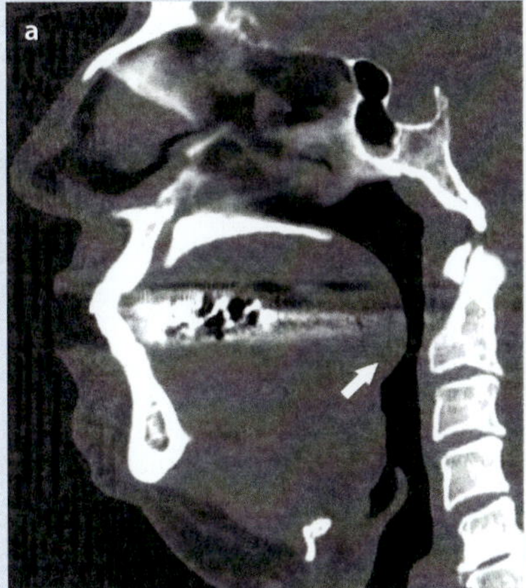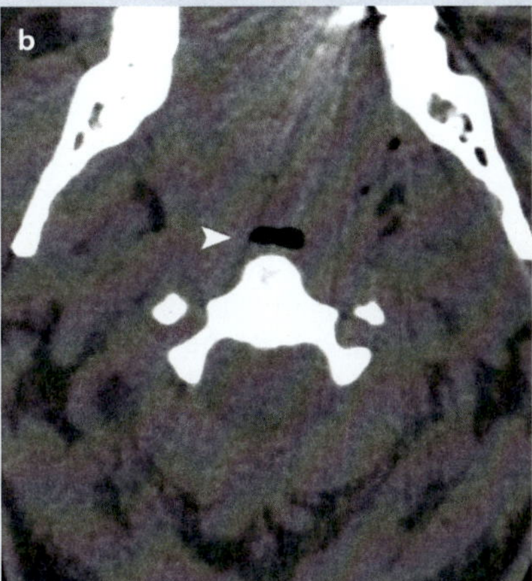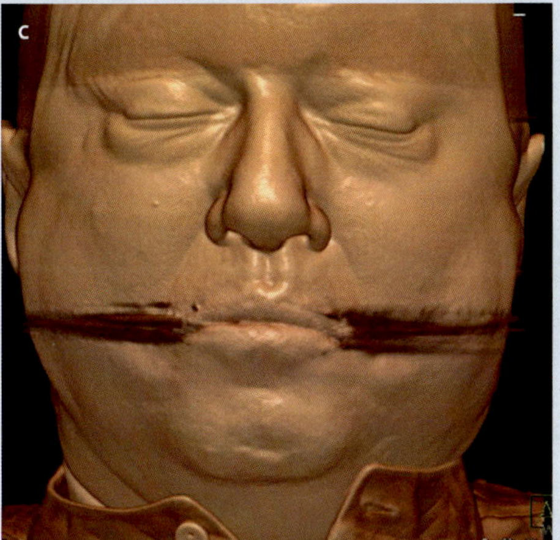

**Fig. 7.10.81** Sagittal (**a**) and axial (**b**) CT images of a patient with OSA and narcolepsy show thickened posterior uvula (*arrow*) and reduced oropharyngeal space (*arrowhead*)

### Signs on CT and MRI

1. The oropharynx provides a common pathway for both swallowing and respiration. There are three main factors that determine the balance between airway patency and collapse:

   a. *The tone in the dilator muscles of the upper airways:* these muscles are activated just before diaphragmatic contraction, and their tone is primarily dependent on the state of consciousness. As a result, prolonged obstruction occurs only during sleep.

   b. *The magnitude of the negative intra-airway pressure:* this negative force is generated by contraction of the diaphragm and is related to the total airway resistance. Narrowing of the nasopharyngeal airway increases total airway resistance and requires additional negative intra-airway pressure to maintain flow.

   c. *The cross-sectional dimension of the oropharynx:* the smaller the oropharyngeal airway, the greater the likelihood of closure at any level of negative intrapharyngeal pressure (**Figs. 7.10.81 and 7.10.82**).

2. Patients with obstructive sleep apnea have abnormally narrow airway (oropharynx) posterior to the tongue, which can be appreciated on dynamic CT imaging of the oropharynx.

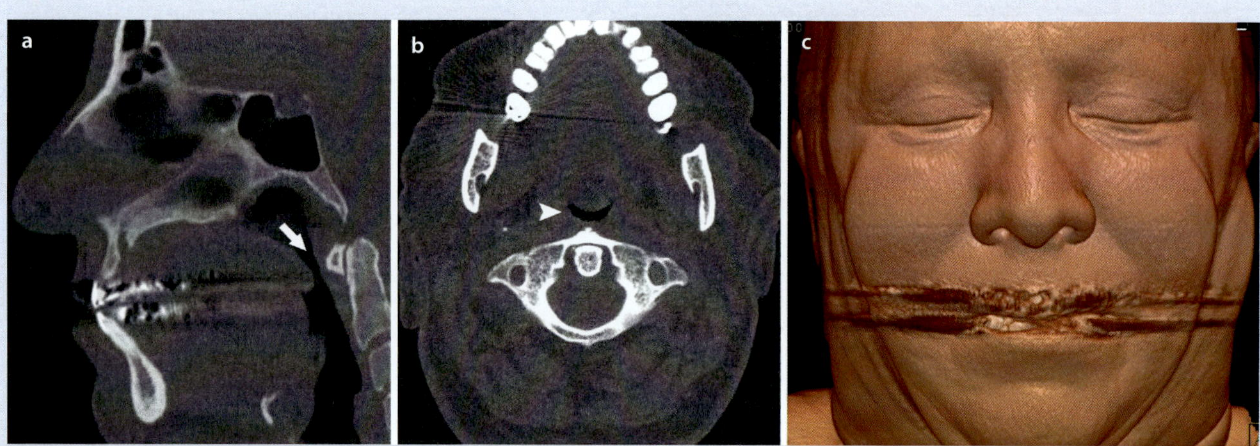

■ **Fig. 7.10.82**    Sagittal (**a**) and axial (**b**) CT images of a patient with OSA show severe retro-palatal nasopharyngeal stenosis by a hypertrophic soft palate (*arrow*) and retro-palatal nasopharyngeal space stenosis (*arrowhead*)

## Upper Airway Resistance Syndrome

Upper airways resistance syndrome (UARS) is a disease that lies in between primary snoring and obstructive sleep apnea syndrome in severity (OSAS). UARS is defined as intermittent attacks of sleep apnea associated with snoring and respiratory disturbance index (RDI) less than 5 with daytime sleepiness attacks. Unlike OSAS, UARS is characterized by the absence of frank sleep apneas or oxygen desaturation with daytime hypersomnolence.

UARS patients are typically nonobese (in contrast to OSAS) and have a mean age of 37 years and body mass index <25 kg/m presenting with snoring and daytime hypersomnolence. UARS arises due to retrolingual narrowing, low soft palates, long uvulas, and high, narrow hard palates as determined by cephalometry.

OSAS patients are typically obese (BMI >30) and have RDI >5 and daytime sleepiness (hypersomnolence). In contrast, primary snoring is defined as snoring at night, RDI <5, and no daytime sleepiness.

## Central Alveolar Apnea Syndrome (Ondine's Curse)

Central sleep apnea is defined as an absence of airflow and respiratory effort lasting at least 10 s. Central alveolar apnea syndrome, also known as Ondine's curse, is a disease characterized by failure of the automatic control of ventilation during sleep due to a lesion affecting the descending anterolateral medullocervical pathway of the reticular formation.

Ondine's curse is a mythological fairytale about a mermaid who exchanged into a human to marry the man she loves. She made an excellent wife; however, her husband cheated on her with another woman. Ondine was still retaining part of her magic power as a mermaid, so she cursed her husband with a curse that whenever he falls asleep, he suffocates. So he has to be awake forever; otherwise, he will die.

Ondine's curse can be congenital or acquired. Congenital Ondine's curse may be associated with Hirschsprung's disease (*known as Haddad syndrome*) or neuroblastoma. The disease arises due to mutation in the PHOX2B gene.

Neonates with Ondine's curse syndrome presents typically with hypotonia and apnea that needs continuous ventilation hours after birth. The pathological process is related to insensitivity to hypercarbia with raised serum $pCO_2$ levels (*may be up to 80–90 mmHg*), especially during sleep, when the respiration is maximally under chemical control.

Acquired Ondine's curse is an uncommon condition that arises in adults and has been reported in association with medullary tumors, infection (*particularly poliomyelitis*), upper cervical trauma with Duret hemorrhage, some mitochondrial diseases, degenerative diseases (e.g., *multiple system atrophy*), medullary capillary telangiectasias, demyelinating disease (e.g., *multiple sclerosis*), or nonspecific anoxic–ischemic insults.

Diaphragmatic pacing has been described in series, with reported success rates between 50 and 70 %. Candidates for diaphragmatic pacing must be severely incapacitated by chronic ventilatory insufficiency and are usually receiving ventilatory support before pacing is instituted.

**Signs on MRI**
1. Congenital Ondine's curse infants can show molar tooth sign due to cerebellar peduncle atrophy.
2. The brain in congenital Ondine's curse may show signs of ischemic encephalopathy due to hypoxia and hypercapnia.

## Cheyne–Stokes Respiration

Cheyne–Stokes respiration (CSR) is present in up to 50 % of patients with chronic heart failure (CHF) and left ventricular (LV) ejection fraction ≤45 %. CSR is characterized by repetitive apneas and arousal cycles induce sleep fragmentation followed by fatigue, daytime sleepiness, and neurohumoral activation including sympathoadrenergic stimulation.

## Uncommon and Rare Causes of Sleep Apnea

1. Arnold–Chiari malformation 1: usually associated with neurological manifestations
2. Atlantoaxial dislocation/subluxation
3. Olivopontocerebellar atrophy (Dejerine–Thomas syndrome)
4. Posterior fossa tumors (e.g., *medulloblastoma*)
5. Syringobulbia
6. Bulbar poliomyelitis

## Selected References

Block AJ. Sleep apnea and related disorders. Dis Mon. 1985;31(5):6–56.

Calvin JR, et al. Obstructive sleep apnea: diagnosis with ultrafast CT. Radiology. 1989;171:775–8.

Cartwright R. Obstructive sleep apnea: a sleep disorder with major effects on health. Dis Mon. 2001;47(4):109–47.

D'Souza S, et al. Haddad syndrome: congenital central hypoventilation associated with Hirschsprung's disease. Indian J Pediatr. 2003;70(7):597–9.

Fernbach SK, et al. Radiologic evaluation of adenoids and tonsils in children with obstructive sleep apnea: plain films and fluoroscopy. Pediatr Radiol. 1983;13:258–65.

Finkelstein Y, et al. Frontal and lateral cephalometry in patients with sleep-disordered breathing. Laryngoscope. 2001;111:634–41.

Gaisie G, et al. Coexistent neuroblastoma and Hirschsprung's disease: another manifestation of the neurocristopathy? Pediatr Radiol. 1979;8:161–3.

Galvin JR, et al. Obstructive sleep apnea: diagnosis with ultrafast CT. Radiology. 1998;171:775–8.

Hegstrom T, et al. Obstructive sleep apnea syndrome: preoperative radiologic evaluation. AJR. 1988;150:67–9.

Kerbl R, et al. Congenital central hypoventilation syndrome (Ondine's curse syndrome) in two siblings: delayed diagnosis and successful noninvasive treatment. Eur J Pediatr. 1996;155:977–80.

Lam B, et al. Arnold-Chiari malformation presenting as sleep apnea syndrome. Sleep Med. 2000;1:139–44.

Macpherson RI, et al. Upper airway obstruction in children: an update. Radiographics. 1985;5(3):339–76.

Pracharktam N, et al. Cephalometric assessment in obstructive sleep apnea. Am J Orothod Dentofac Orthop. 1996;109:410–9.

Randerath WJ. Treatment options in Cheyne-Stokes respiration. Ther Adv Respir Dis. 2010;4:341–51.

Roshkow JE, et al. Hirschsprung's disease, ondine's curse, and neuroblastoma-manifestations of neurocristopathy. Pediatr Radiol. 1988;19:45–9.

Stein MG, et al. Cine CT in obstructive sleep apnea. AJR. 1987;148:1069–74.

Susarla SM, et al. Cephalometric measurement of upper airway length correlates with the presence and severity of obstructive sleep apnea. J Oral Maxillofac Surg. 2010;68:2846–55.

Wiegand L, et al. Obstructive sleep apnea. Dis Mon. 1994;40(4):202–52.

Zamarron C, et al. Obstructive sleep apnea syndrome is a systemic disease. Current evidence. Eur J Intern Med. 2008;19:390–8.

# Dermatology

J.A. Al-Tubaikh, *Internal Medicine*, DOI 10.1007/978-3-319-39747-4_8

## 8.1 Scleroderma (Systemic Sclerosis)

Scleroderma is a systemic disease characterized by progressive fibrosis of the skin and multiple organs. The term "scleroderma" means literally "hard skin."

In scleroderma, the dermis is infiltrated by T lymphocytes, causing abnormal fibroblasts activation, which leads to increased production of extracellular collagen type I. This increase in collagen causes skin thickening and tightening, which is the main manifestation of this disease.

Scleroderma is divided into two major forms: diffuse and focal. In the generalized form, diffuse skin disease with organ involvement is typically seen. In the focal form, there is limited cutaneous involvement of the skin. Linear scleroderma and morphea are examples of focal scleroderma.

Females are affected by scleroderma seven times as often as males. Patients present classically with flexural contracture of the terminal phalanges (claw-hand like appearance), loss of the skin folds around the mouth (masklike appearance), atrophied nasal alae (mouse facies), reduced opening of the mouth with jaw fixation, pathological changes of minor salivary glands mimicking Sjögren's syndrome, and uncommonly trigeminal neuralgia (4 %). Laboratory investigations show positive antinuclear antibodies (70–90 %), rheumatoid factor (25 %), and hyperglobulinemia.

*CREST syndrome* is a variant of diffuse scleroderma characterized by *C*alcinosis cutis, *R*aynaud's phenomenon, *E*sophageal dysmotility with dysphagia, *S*clerodactyly, and *T*elangiectasia. *Calcinosis cutis* is deposition of calcium in the skin producing hard cutaneous nodules. *Raynaud's phenomenon* is a series of finger discoloration after exposure to either temperature alternation or emotional disturbance. First, fingers become pale (white) due to small vessels vasoconstriction, then turn blue as the vessels dilate to keep blood flow, and finally turn red as blood flow returns (◘ Fig. 8.1.1). *Sclerodactyly* means skin thickening of the fingers and toes that produces claw-hand deformity. *Telangiectasia* is dilatation of the small vessels over the skin and the mucus membranes ranging between 0.51 mm in diameter. They are commonly seen over the face and the neck as small red marks on the skin.

*Morphea* is a superficial-localized form of scleroderma characterized by a plaque of thickened skin, often with an active, violaceous border with a yellow to white center. It is commonly seen in children, with an incidence of 1 per 100,000 individuals. *Generalized morphea* is a term used to describe morphea lesions covering >30 % of the body surface. *Disabling pansclerotic morphea (deep morphea)* is a term used to describe morphea that extends deep into the soft tissues with fixation to the underlying structures.

*Nodular (keloid) scleroderma* is a rare form of cutaneous scleroderma that can occur in association with diffuse scleroderma or morphea. It is seen as keloidal hyperpigmented papules that develop early in the course of the disease. An inflammatory infiltrate is present during the period of active fibrosis.

*Linear scleroderma*, also known as *en coup de sabre*, is a localized form of scleroderma seen as a linear, ivory-colored, deforming depression on the scalp and the forehead mimicking a blow of a sword, which is described as "coup de sabre" (◘ Fig. 8.1.2). The lesion usually results in furrowing of the forehead, causing significant facial asymmetry and cosmetic deformity. Linear scleroderma lesions can be seen following *Blaschko's lines* (◘ Fig. 8.1.3). These lines determine the distribution of many congenital and acquired skin diseases (e.g., epidermal nevi). Many authors believe that these lines represent the pattern of embryonic migration of skin cells.

Linear scleroderma is usually seen in children and in the young population, and it can affect the limbs, especially the lower limbs, resulting in unilateral, atrophic limb. Linear scleroderma is usually confused with *Parry–Romberg syndrome* when it extensively affects half of the face. Brain involvement in linear scleroderma usually presents in the form of epilepsy, with or without brain abnormalities.

## Differential Diagnoses and Related Diseases

— *Hypothenar hammer syndrome* (HHS) is a rare condition characterized by episodic digital ischemia as a result of occlusion of the distal ulnar artery at the level of the hamate bone, typically due to repetitive blunt trauma to the ulnar artery at the hypothenar eminence. The ulnar injury usually results from thrombosis or aneurysms from the repetitive trauma. The distal ulnar artery is most vulnerable to trauma at the level of the hook of the hamate, which works as an anvil against the distal ulnar artery as the patient uses his/her hypothenar eminence of the hand. The disease usually occurs in males who engage in activities that expose the hypothenar eminence to repetitive hand injuries. Workers using vibrating hand tools are commonly affected. Sportsmen who use their hands extensively in sports activities such as baseball, handball, karate, and weightlifting or dumbbell training are also affected. Patients usually present with palm pain, paresthesia, and numbness with cold fingers and pallor, usually affecting the dominant hand. HHS can be mistaken for Raynaud's disease. Raynaud's disease is defined as episodic ischemia of the fingers and toes, clinically presenting as pallor (arterial vasospasm), cyanosis (deoxygenated static venous blood), and rubor (reactive hyperemia).

— *Eosinophilic fasciitis (Shulman's syndrome)* is a rare condition with scleroderma-like illness characterized clinically by inflammatory swelling and induration of the arms and legs. Patients with eosinophilic fasciitis are usually females presenting with painful thickening and induration of the skin and subcutaneous tissues of the affected limb. The disease may affect the upper limbs, trunk, and lower limbs but spares the face. Raynaud's phenomenon is usually not present, and organs are not affected. The skin is typically thickened with orange-peel appearance. Bilateral symmetrical muscle weakness and stiffness of the joint may occur. Pathologically, there is inflammation and infiltration of the superficial muscle

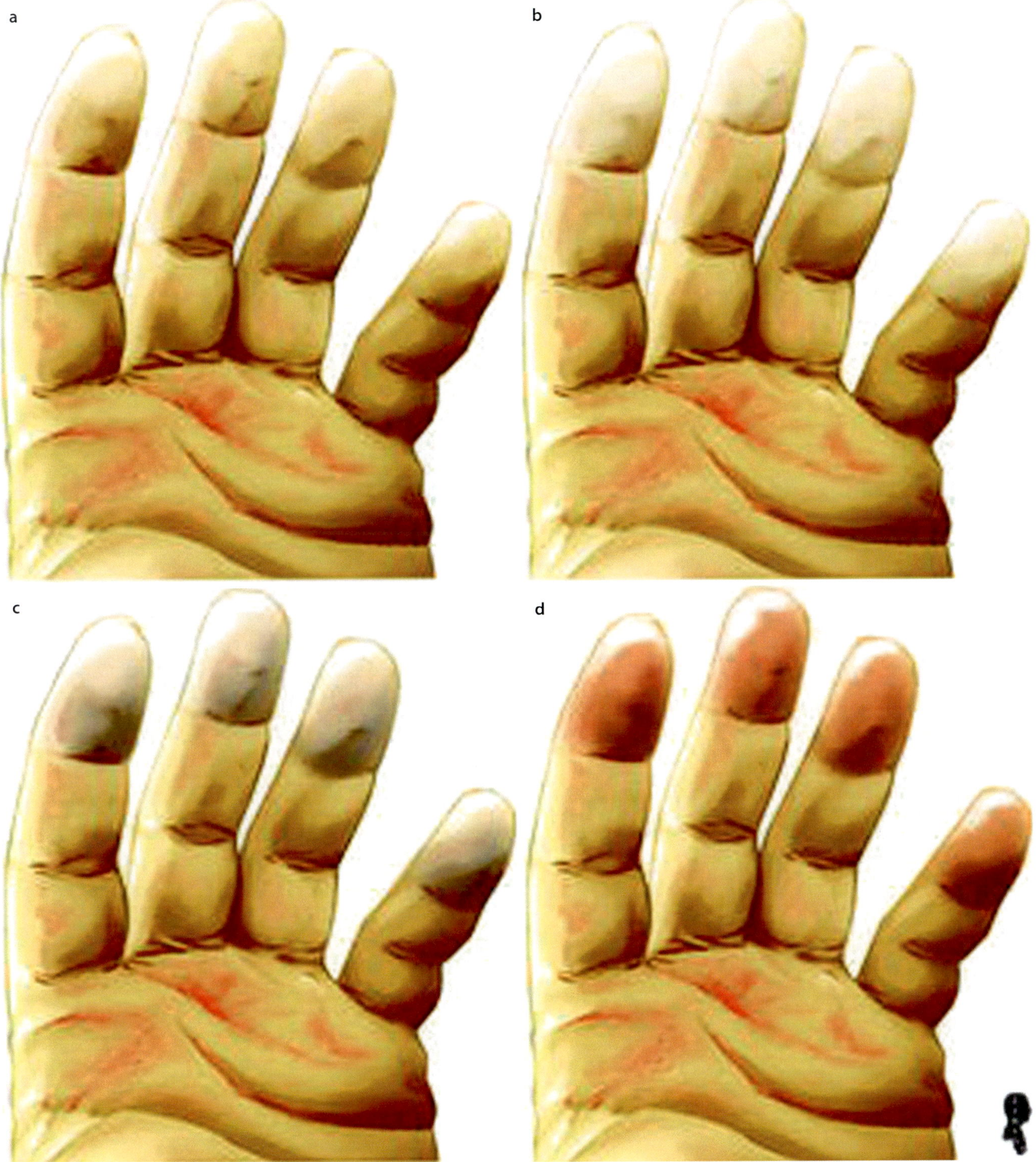

**Fig. 8.1.1** An illustration demonstrates the finger discoloration stages of Raynaud's phenomenon: (**a**) normal fingers, (**b**) pale fingers, (**c**) bluish discoloration due to ischemia, and (**d**) reddish discoloration due to postischemic hyperemia

fasciae by lymphocytes, plasma cells, and occasionally eosinophils. Laboratory findings show high ESR, blood eosinophilia (characteristic), and hyperglobulinemia. Diagnosis is usually based on MRI and laboratory findings; however, definite diagnosis requires full-thickness skin-to-muscle biopsy.

*How can you differentiate between hypothenar hammer syndrome and Raynaud's disease?*
- HHS has a male predominance, while Raynaud's disease has a female predominance.
- HHS is an occupational disease, while Raynaud's disease is a primary disease or secondary to systemic disease.

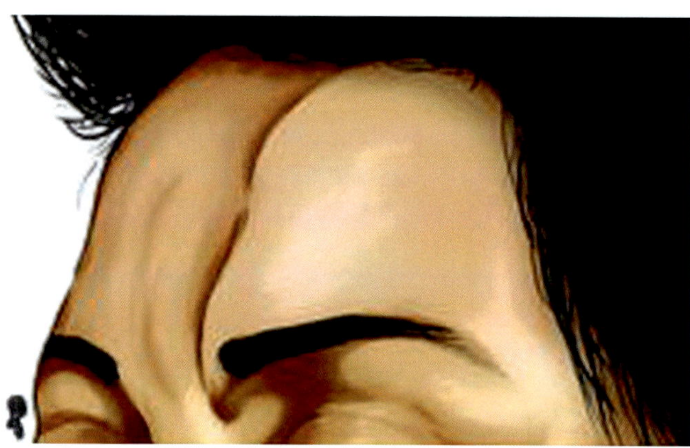

**Fig. 8.1.2**   An illustration demonstrates linear scleroderma affecting the left forehead

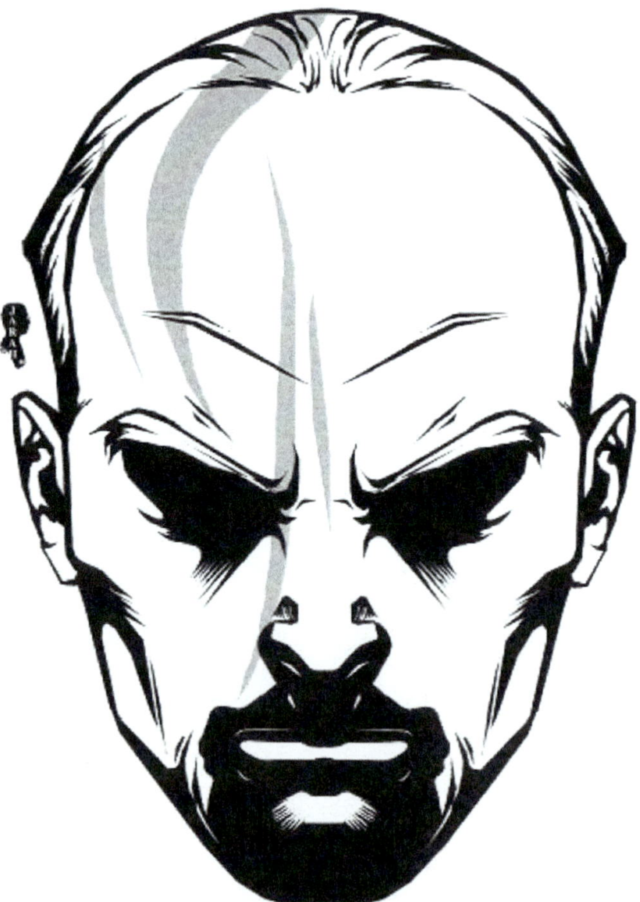

**Fig. 8.1.3**   An illustration demonstrates Blaschko lines over the right forehead. The same lines can be found on the left side

- HHS has an asymmetric distribution (affects one hand), while Raynaud's disease is typically symmetrical, affecting the hands or toes.

**Signs on Radiographs**
- Resorption of the terminal phalanges (acro-osteolysis) of the hands and the distal portion of the radius and ulna are the most common radiological features of scleroderma (80 %).
- Mandibular resorption resembling "Gorham syndrome osteolysis" may be seen.
- Soft-tissue calcinosis may be seen, especially in the digits ( Figs. 8.1.4 and 8.1.5).
- Widening of the periodontal space on dental radiographs may be seen.
- Pulmonary fibrosis can be seen in advanced chronic stages of scleroderma.

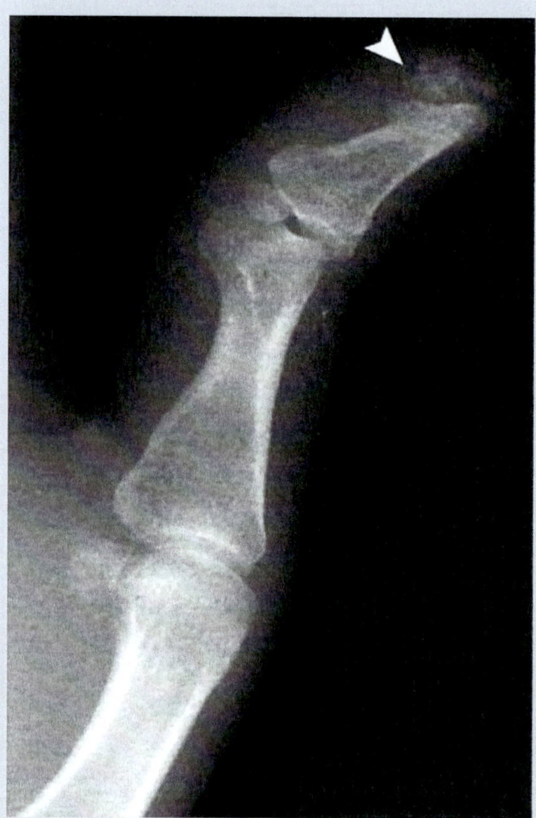

**Fig. 8.1.4**   Plain thumb radiograph of a patient with scleroderma shows fingertip calcinosis (*arrowhead*)

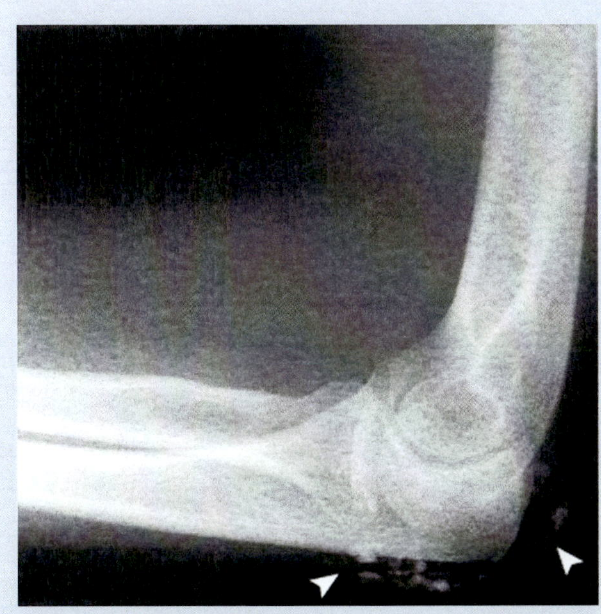

**Fig. 8.1.5** Lateral plain elbow radiograph of a patient with scleroderma shows calcinosis around the elbow joint (*arrowheads*)

### Signs on Barium Swallow
The esophagus in CREST syndrome shows weak peristalsis with no stripping waves (**Fig. 8.1.6**). The esophagus may show fine, wavy horizontal lines due to muscular contraction of the esophagus wall (*Feline esophagus*).

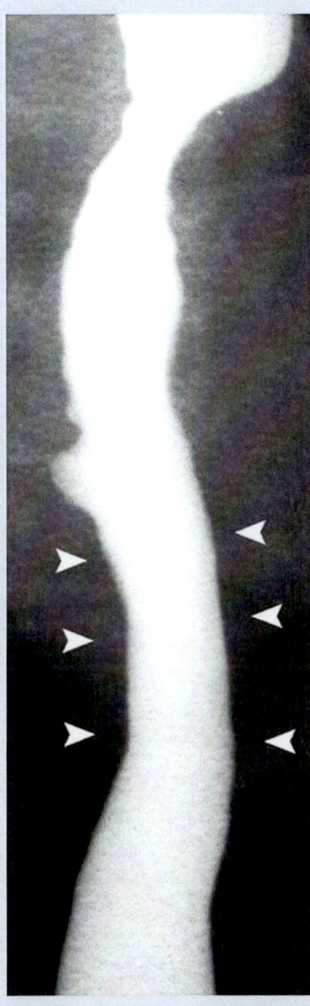

**Fig. 8.1.6** Anteroposterior barium swallow radiograph of the esophagus in a patient with scleroderma shows poor esophageal motility (*arrowheads*)

### Signs on MRI
- In *linear scleroderma*, there are intracranial parenchymal calcifications affecting mainly the thalami, and the basal ganglia ipsilateral to the skin lesion may be seen. Progressive multiple brain aneurysms can be seen in linear scleroderma.
- In *hypothenar hammer syndrome*, the axial wrist images will show hyperintense mass usually seen on T1W images located around the ulnar artery at the level of the hook of the hamate, representing hematoma or thrombus (**Fig. 8.1.7**).
- In *deep morphea*, there is T2 hyperintensity signal observed over the skin and subcutaneous tissue that may involve the muscles and the bone beneath. The bone shows bone marrow edema signal without bone erosions. Contrast

enhancement of the affected tissues reflects ongoing inflammatory reaction. Enhancement around the tendons may be observed due to inflammation of the synovial sheath (synovitis).

— In *eosinophilic fasciitis*, there is increased thickening and T2 signal intensity of the superficial muscle fasciae with marked contrast enhancement after contrast injection (◘ Fig. 8.1.8). Characteristically, there is little or no signal change within muscles, and the pathological changes are confined only to the superficial muscle fasciae and to a lesser degree to the deep muscle fasciae.

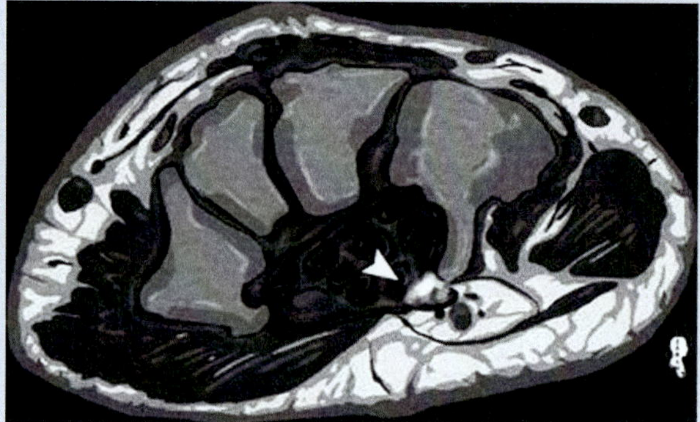

◘ **Fig. 8.1.7** Axial T2W wrist MR illustrations show high signal intensity at the tip of the hook of hamate within the Gyon's canal representing hematoma of the ulnar artery (*arrowhead*)

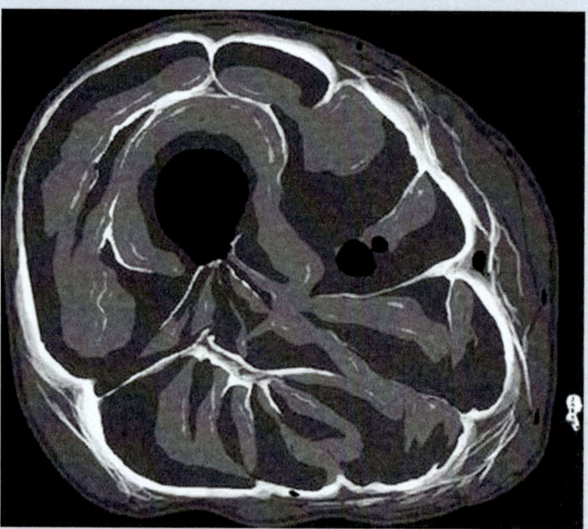

◘ **Fig. 8.1.8** Axial T1W postcontrast, fat-sat, thigh MR illustration demonstrates the typical findings in eosinophilic fasciitis. Notice the marked thickening and enhancement of the superficial and deep fascial planes with no signal intensity or contrast enhancement of the muscles of the subcutaneous tissues

**Further Reading**

Abudakka M, et al. Hypothenar hammer syndrome: rare or underdiagnosed? Eur J Vasc Endovasc Surg. 2006;32: 257–60.

Ahathya RS, et al. Systemic sclerosis. Indian J Dent Res. 2007;18:27–30.

Baumann F, et al. MRI for diagnosis and monitoring of patients with eosinophilic fasciitis. AJR Am J Roentgenol. 2005;184:169–74.

Bologina JL, et al. Lines of Blaschko. J Am Acad Dermatol. 1994;31:157–90.

Christen-Zaech S, et al. Pediatric morphea (localized scleroderma): review of 136 patients. J Am Acad Dermatol. 2008;59:385–96.

Genchellac H, et al. Hypothenar hammer syndrome: grayscale and color Doppler sonographic appearance. J Clin Ultrasound. 2008;36(2):98–100. doi:10.1002/jcu.

Grosso S, et al. Linear scleroderma associated with progressive brain atrophy. Brain Dev. 2003;25:57–61.

Horger M, et al. MRI findings in deep and generalized morphea (localized scleroderma). AJR Am J Roentgenol. 2008;190:32–9.

Jacobson L, et al. Superficial morphea. J Am Acad Dermatol. 2003;49:323–5.

James WD, et al. Nodular (keloidal) scleroderma. J Am Acad Dermatol. 1984;11:111–4.

Krell JM, et al. Nodular scleroderma. J Am Acad Dermatol. 1995;32:343–5.

Kreitner KF, et al. Hypothenar hammer syndrome caused by recreational sports activities and muscle anomaly in the wrist. Cardiovasc Intervent Radiol. 1996;19:356–9.

Mueller LP, et al. Hypothenar hammer syndrome in sports. Knee Surg Sports Traumatol Arthrosc. 1996;4:167–70.

Robitschek J, et al. Treatment of linear scleroderma "en coup de saber" with AlloDerm tissue matrix. Otolaryngol Head Neck Surg. 2008;138:540–1.

Soma Y, et al. Frontoparietal scleroderma (en coup de saber) following Blaschko's lines. J Am Acad Dermatol. 1998;38: 366–8.

## 8.2 Lipoid Proteinosis (Urbach–Wiethe Disease)

Lipoid proteinosis (LP) is a rare, autosomal recessive disease characterized by infiltration of the skin, oral cavity, larynx, vocal cords, and internal organs by a hyaline material composed of carbohydrates, proteins, and lipids.

LP is caused by defective basement membrane collagen metabolism. The patient commonly presents with hoarseness of voice since infancy due to deposition of the hyaline material within the vocal cords. Beaded, whitish papules along the margins of the eyelids (*Blepharosis moniliformis*) are classical

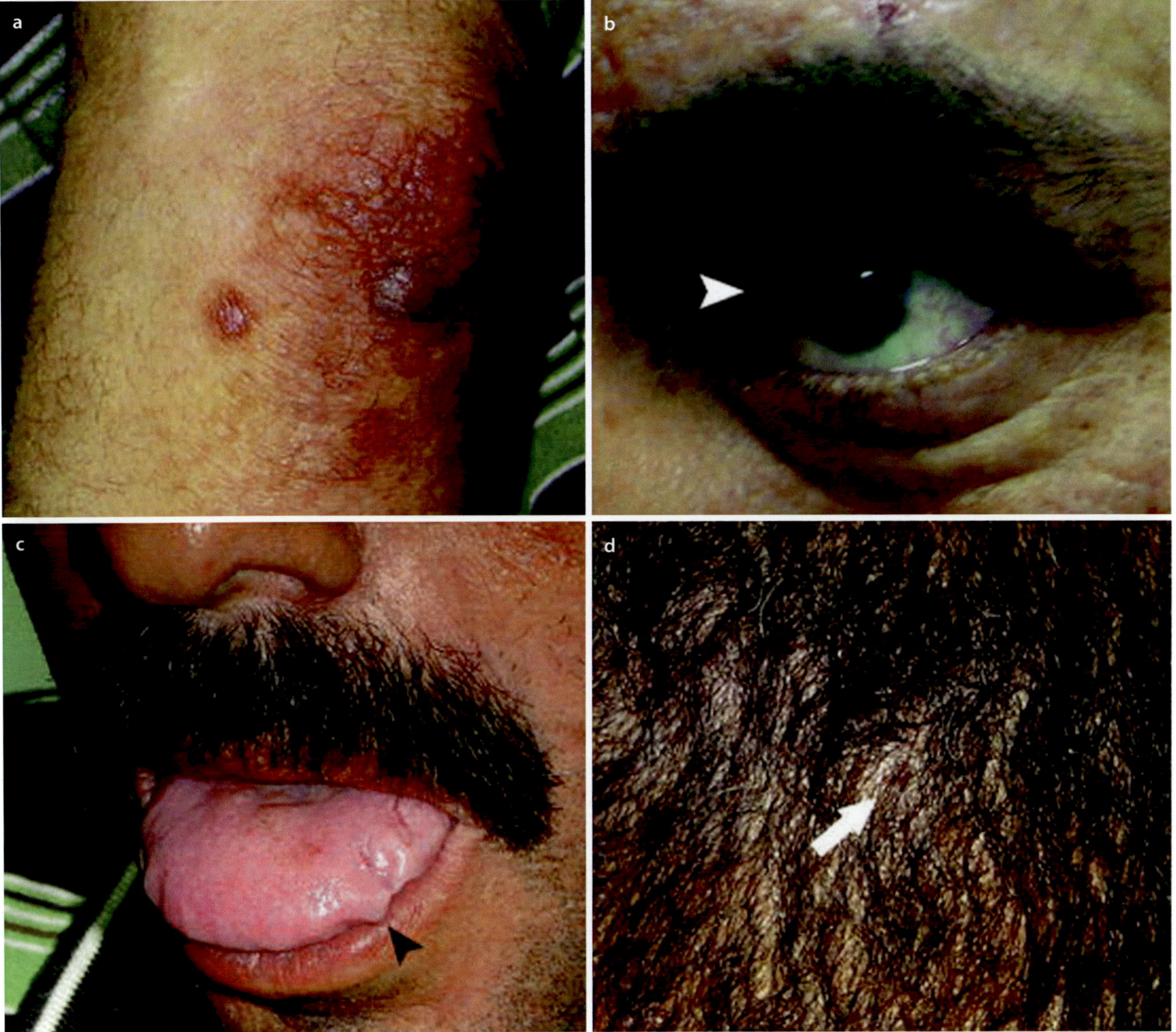

**Fig. 8.2.1** Multiple images from a 28-year-old patient with lipoid proteinosis show the dermatological features of this disease. In (**a**), there are multiple psoriatic-like lesions over the elbow. In (**b**), a whitish papule (blepharosis moniliformis) along the margin of the upper eyelid can be seen (*white arrowhead*). In (**c**), the tongue is thickened and shows multiple nodules (*black arrowhead*). In (**d**), there is a focal area with reduced hair on the scalp (*arrow*). The patient has a history of hoarseness of voice since the age of 3 years

features of this disease (**Fig. 8.2.1**). Pock-like scars over the face and the body, waxy papules, less mobile tongue, and thickened oral mucosa with yellowish tinges are other common findings. Deposition of the hyaline material in the scalp can lead to patchy loss of hair (*alopecia areata*).

Hyaline deposition can be found in some cases in the trachea, stomach, esophagus, testes, pancreas, and vagina. Diabetes mellitus, epilepsy, and calcified cerebral vessels can be seen associated with LP occasionally. Diagnosis can be confirmed by pathological skin biopsy. The hyaline material shows positive periodic acid–Schiff (PAS) stain result. Differential diagnoses of LP in adults include amyloidosis, lipoidoses, and myxoedema.

### Signs on Chest Radiographs
In severe cases, LP can present as a bilateral alveolar lung disease that mimics lung edema. This pattern is seen due to deposition of the hyaline material within the alveoli.

### Signs on CT
— Thickening and infiltration of the vocal cords by a hypodense hyaline material can be observed (■ Figs. 8.2.2 and 8.2.3).
— Calcification within the cerebral hemispheres can be seen when calcified vessels are present.

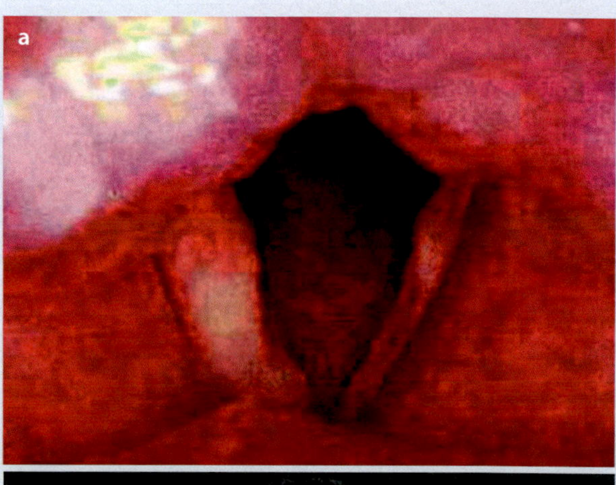

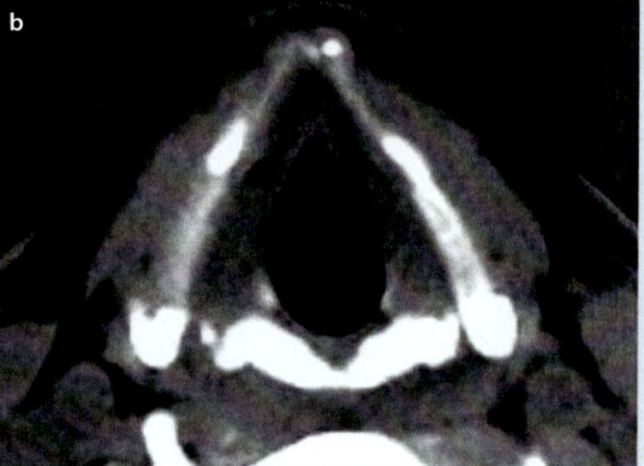

■ **Fig. 8.2.3** Bronchoscopic image (**a**) correlated with axial CT image (**b**) of the vocal cords of the same patient shows thickening of both vocal cords, with the right one markedly thickened compared to the left one in (**a**). In (**b**), the CT image shows hypodense areas found in the anterior aspect of both vocal cords bilaterally involving the anterior commissure (*arrowheads*), with subtle left vocal cord thickening anteriorly

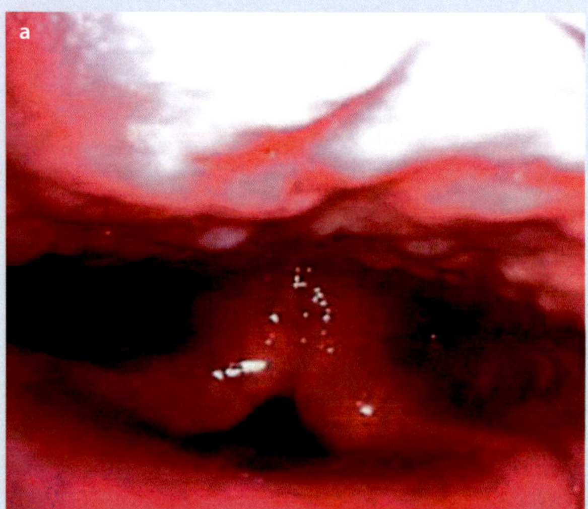

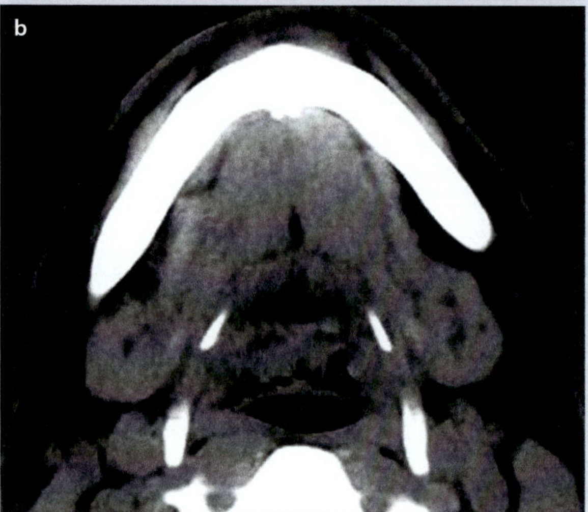

■ **Fig. 8.2.2** Bronchoscopic image (**a**) correlated with axial CT image (**b**) of the hypopharynx shows multiple submucosal nodules. After biopsy these lesions, the results stated that these nodules are composed of hyaline lipoid material deposited within the submucosa. The nodules in (**b**) are almost completely replacing the valleculae (*arrowheads*)

## Further Reading

Behera SK, et al. Lipoid proteinosis in two siblings. Indian J Dermatol. 2006;51(1):47–8.

Mirancea N, et al. Vascular anomalies in lipoid proteinosis (hyalinosis cutis et mucosae): basement membrane components and ultrastructure. J Dermatol Sci. 2006;42: 231–9.

Mukhija P, et al. Lipoid proteinosis. Indian J Dermatol. 2006;51(1):51–2.

Orton CI, et al. Lipoid proteinosis–The oro-facial manifestations. Br J Oral Surg. 1975;12:289–91.

Savage MM, et al. Lipoid proteinosis of the larynx: a cause of voice change in the infant and young child. Int J Pediatr Otorhinolaryngol. 1988;15:33–8.

Sen S, et al. Lipoid proteinosis. Indian J Dermatol. 2006;51(1):49–50.

Simpson HE. Oral manifestations in lipoid proteinosis. Oral Surg. 1972;33(4):528–31.

## 8.3    Dermatomyositis

Dermatomyositis (DM) is an inflammatory connective tissue disorder characterized by inflammation of the muscles and skin. DM is closely related to another inflammatory muscle disease called "polymyositis" (PM).

DM is diagnosed by specific criteria that include:

- *Proximal symmetrical muscle weakness*: the typical clinical presentation is bilateral symmetrical muscle weakness of the limb-girdle muscles, often affecting the shoulders and anterior neck flexors. Progressive weakness is experienced over weeks to months. Patients often first note an inability to groom their hair or to rise from a sitting position. Proximal dysphagia may be seen if the cricopharyngeus muscle and muscles of the pharynx are involved. Respiratory muscles of the chest wall can be affected.
- *Muscle biopsy*: muscle biopsy classically shows muscle necrosis and inflammatory changes; however, muscle biopsy can be normal in 10–15 % of cases.
- *Elevated muscle enzymes*: elevated muscle enzymes like creatine kinase (CK), serum transaminases, and lactic dehydrogenase (LDH) is a common finding in DM and PM. CK is a normal serum enzyme with three isoenzymes: CK-MM (found in skeletal muscles), CK-MB (found in cardiac muscles), and CK-BB (found in neural tissue). In PM and DM, CK-MM and CK-BB are often elevated. However, up to 40 % of DM cases have normal CK levels. CK is not so specific to muscular diseases, as it can be elevated in metabolic and neurological diseases as well.
- *Specific dermatological lesions*: two cutaneous lesions are very specific for DM, among other dermatological nonspecific manifestations. The first lesion is *Gottron's sign* (80 % of cases), which is characterized by erythematous papules and plaques that are found over bony prominences, particularly the metacarpal–phalangeal and proximal and distal interphalangeal joints (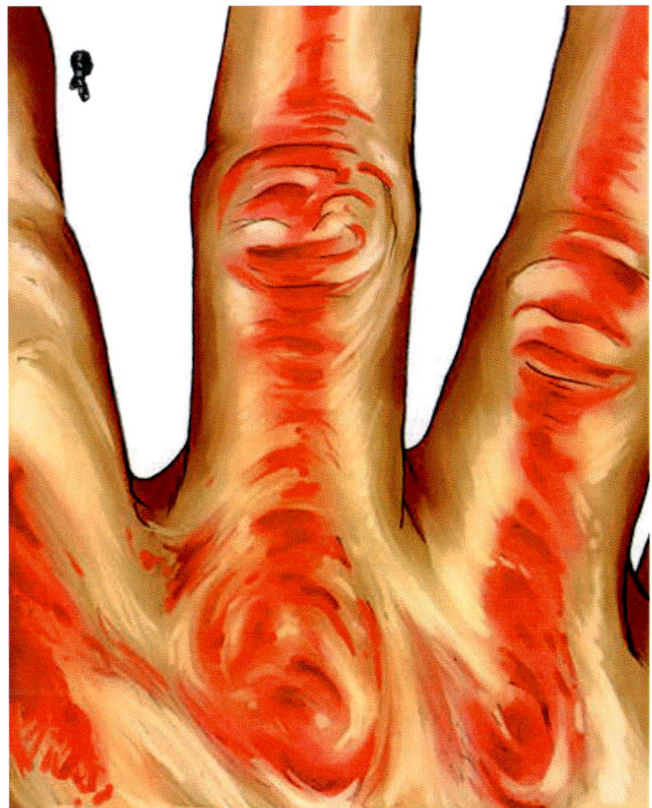 Fig. 8.3.1). They can also be found over the elbows and knees. The second lesion is *heliotrope rash* (60 % of cases), which is composed of violaceous to erythematous hue rash with or without edema located in the periorbital region (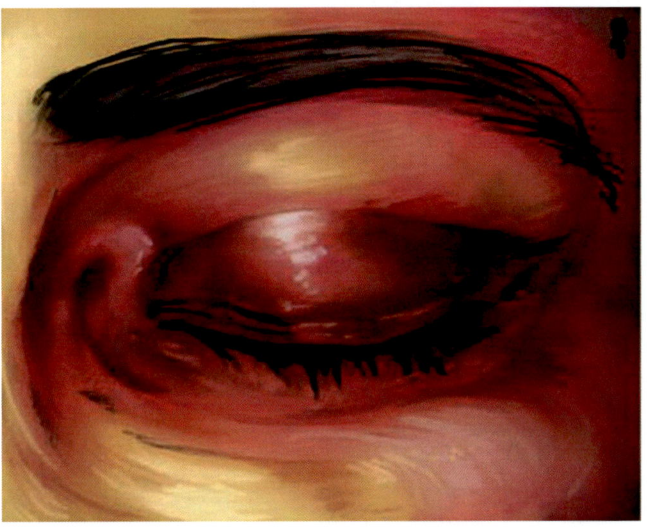 Fig. 8.3.2). Photosensitivity occurs in 75 % of patients with DM. Some patients with DM may develop poikiloderma of Civatte with Gottron's papules. *Poikiloderma of Civatte* is defined as a skin area with extra-pigmentation, demonstrating a variety of shades and associated with widened capillaries (telangiectasia).
- *Exclusion of other disorders causing a myopathy*: like endocrinopathies, neurological diseases, and muscular dystrophies.

DM can be precipitated by viral infections (e.g., retrovirus) or parasitic infections (e.g., toxoplasmosis). DM can also be associated with autoimmune disorders (e.g., scleroderma) and tumors. Arthralgia, Raynaud's phenomenon, and polyarthritis are seen with DM overlapped with autoimmune diseases. Cardiac symptoms are uncommonly seen in DM. When the heart is affected, atrioventricular (AV) conduction disturbance, arrhythmias, and mitral valve prolapse are commonly seen.

DM can be classified into four groups:
*Group 1*: pure PM
*Group 2*: PM with cutaneous lesions (DM)
*Group 3*: DM with autoimmune disease
*Group 4*: DM with malignant neoplasm

**Fig. 8.3.1**    An illustration demonstrates Gottron's signs

**Fig. 8.3.2**    An illustration demonstrates heliotrope rash

DM has a juvenile form that affects young adults <12 years old. It is often associated with high serum levels of Coxsackie B virus antibody titers. Patients show same signs and clinical manifestations as the adult form. Esophageal dysmotility occurs in 50 % of cases.

### Signs on Radiographs
- DM patients show soft-tissue calcifications in up to 40 % chronic cases. The calcifications can be superficial or deep and often located mainly within the girdle muscle areas. The calcifications are described as linear, reticular, or calcareal (■ Fig. 8.3.3).
- Pulmonary fibrosis is seen in the advanced stages of the disease.

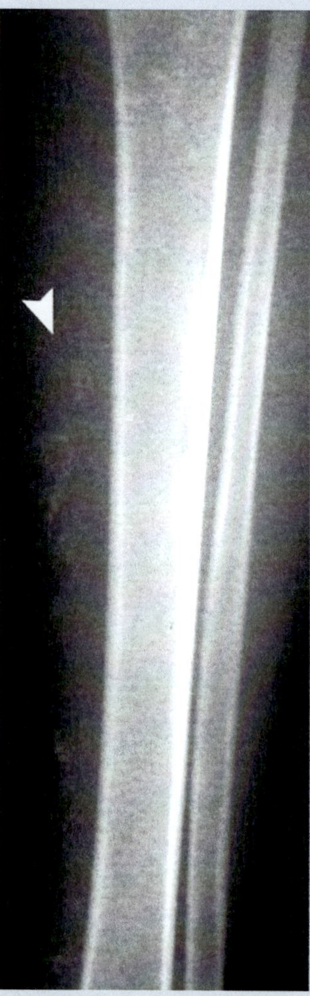

■ **Fig. 8.3.3**   Anteroposterior plain radiograph of the left leg shows multiple fine soft-tissue calcifications in a patient with dermatomyositis (*arrowhead*)

### Signs on MRI
- In the early stages of PM, there is tissue edema and high signal intensity of the muscles on T2W images.
- In chronic cases, the muscles are replaced by fat. There is high T1 signal intensity within the muscles due to fat replacement of the muscular tissue, with reduced muscle size due to chronic muscle wasting and inflammation.

*What is the difference between calcification and ossification?*
- *Calcification* is the presence of an area of calcium deposition within soft tissue that does not form a trabecular or cortical structure (no real bone formation within the soft tissue, only small area of calcium deposition).
- *Ossification* is the presence of an area of calcium deposition within the soft tissue that forms a trabecular or cortical structure (a real bone formation within the soft tissue).

*What are the types of calcifications and ossifications?*
- Calcification can be divided into *metastatic calcification* (calcium and phosphate metabolism disturbance that leads to ectopic calcification in normal tissues), *dystrophic calcification* (deposition of calcium in damaged tissues while the serum calcium level is normal), and *calcinosis* (deposition of calcium in soft tissue in the presence of normal calcium level). Dystrophic calcification is seen usually in posttrauma or after neoplastic therapy. Calcinosis is typically seen in rheumatic diseases and DM.
- Ossification is typically seen in cases like posttraumatic ligamentous ossification (e.g., *Pellegrini–Stieda disease*), neurogenic heterotopic ossification (soft-tissue ossification after long period of denervation), *myositis Ossificans traumatica (Sterner's tumor)*, and *fibrodysplasia ossificans progressiva (Munchmeyer disease)*. Pellegrini–Stieda disease is characterized by ossification of the medial collateral ligament of the knee, commonly after trauma. Myositis ossificans is a rare condition characterized by progressive skeletal muscles ossification, usually after a major trauma. Fibrous dysplasia ossificans is a rare disease characterized by disabling ossification of muscles, tendons, ligaments, and fascial planes (the normal soft tissues are transforming into bones).

## Further Reading
Agarwal V, et al. Calcinosis in juvenile dermatomyositis. Radiology. 2007;242:307–11.

Lee LA, et al. Lipodystrophy and metabolic abnormalities in a case of adult dermatomyositis. J Am Acad Dermatol. 2007;57:S85–7.

Magill HL, et al. Duodenal perforation in childhood dermatomyositis. Pediatr Radiol. 1984;14:28–30.

Marfatia YS, et al. Dermatomyositis in a human immunodeficiency virus infected person. Indian J Dermatol Venerol Leprol. 2008;74:241–3.

Stiglbauer R, et al. Polymyositis: MRI-appearance at 1.5 T and correlation to clinical findings. Clin Radiol. 1993;48:244–8.

## 8.4 Ochronosis (Alkaptonuria)

Ochronosis, also known as alkaptonuria, is a very rare autosomal recessive metabolic disease characterized by accumulation of homogentisic acid (HGA) in body tissues due to an inherited deficiency of the enzyme HGA oxidase. HGA is a main product of the amino acids tyrosine and phenylalanine. Acquired form of ochronosis can be seen after exposure to some chemicals like hydroquinone.

Ochronosis has an incidence of 1:1,000,000 in the general population. The urine of patients with ochronosis turns dark when it is exposed to air or alkaline environment because of HGA polymerization after its exposure to oxygen. The name "alkaptonuria" comes from Arabic and Greek words referring to the relationship between oxygen and urine kept standing.

Although HGA deposition may occur in any body tissue, the disease severity is mainly related to the musculoskeletal system. HGA accumulates particularly in the tendon ligament tissues and cartilage-rich joints. The tissues acquire black color grossly due to the HGA pigment.

Patients typically present in the third decade of life complaining of back pain and stiffness. Skin and soft-tissue lesions are seen in the fourth and fifth decades. HGA acts as a chemical irritant that leads to joint degeneration and inflammation. Patients develop osteoarthritis arthropathy in almost all large joints, but the main severity is classically observed in the vertebral column. The typical feature of this disease in the vertebral column involves intervertebral disk calcification.

Bluish-brownish discoloration of the skin is seen due to deposition of HGA in the subcutaneous tissues, and it is a pathognomonic finding of this disease. The skin pigment is observed in cartilage-rich tissue as the ear (70 %) and nose (◘ Fig. 8.4.1). The bluish pigment can also be seen in the cornea and the sclera (◘ Fig. 8.4.1). It may also be excreted in the sweat, causing changes of color in clothing.

Rarely, cardiac involvement of ochronosis may be seen in advanced stages. Mitral and aortic valve stenoses are the main pathologic complications seen. Renal function can deteriorate when the pigment accumulates in the prostate. Prostatic calcification causes obstructive renal uropathy and hydronephrosis.

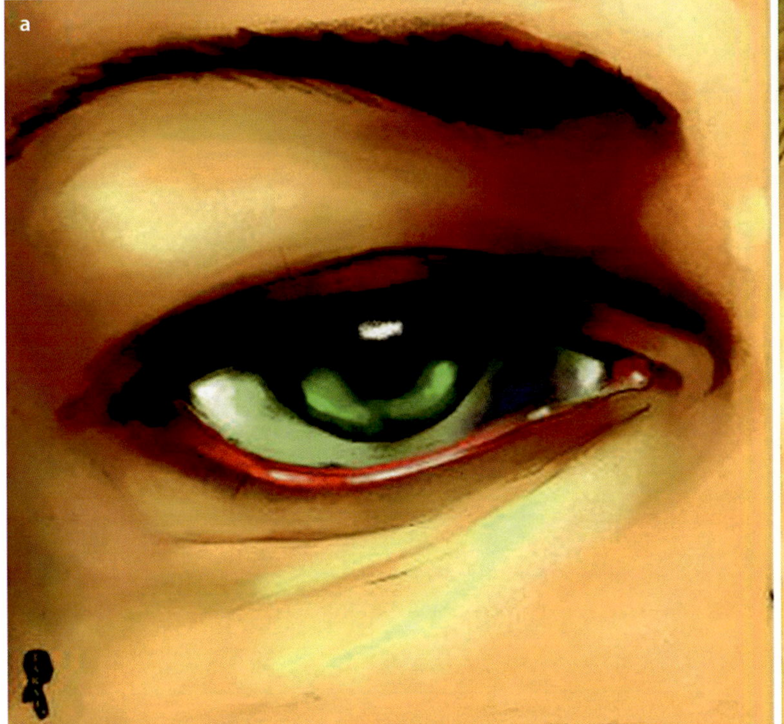
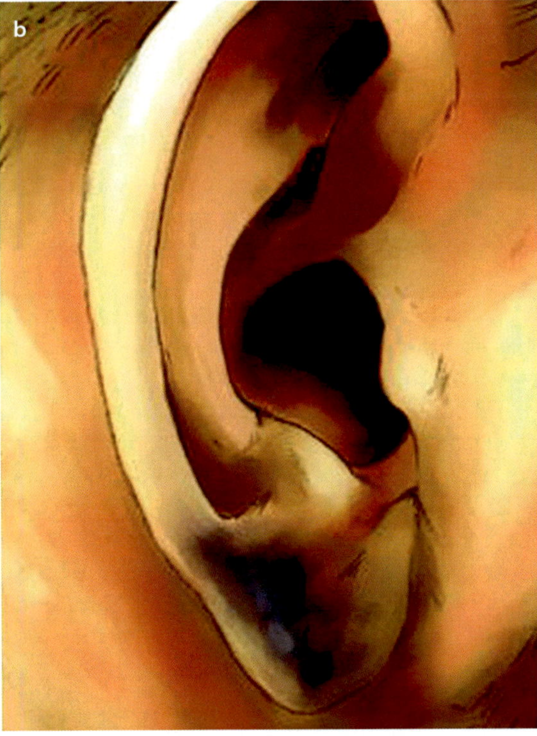

◘ Fig. 8.4.1 Two illustrations show bluish discoloration of the sclera (**a**) and the earlobe (**b**) in a patient with ochronosis

**Signs on Radiographs**
- Typically, the intervertebral disks are calcified in ochronosis, with severe intervertebral disk narrowing (Fig. 8.4.2). The disease affects the lumbar region first and then progresses to the thoracic and the cervical vertebrae.
- Osteoarthritic changes of the large joints with sclerosis and osteophytes formation.
- Progressive formation of marginal intervertebral bridges and obliteration of disk spaces resulting in "pseudo-block vertebrae."

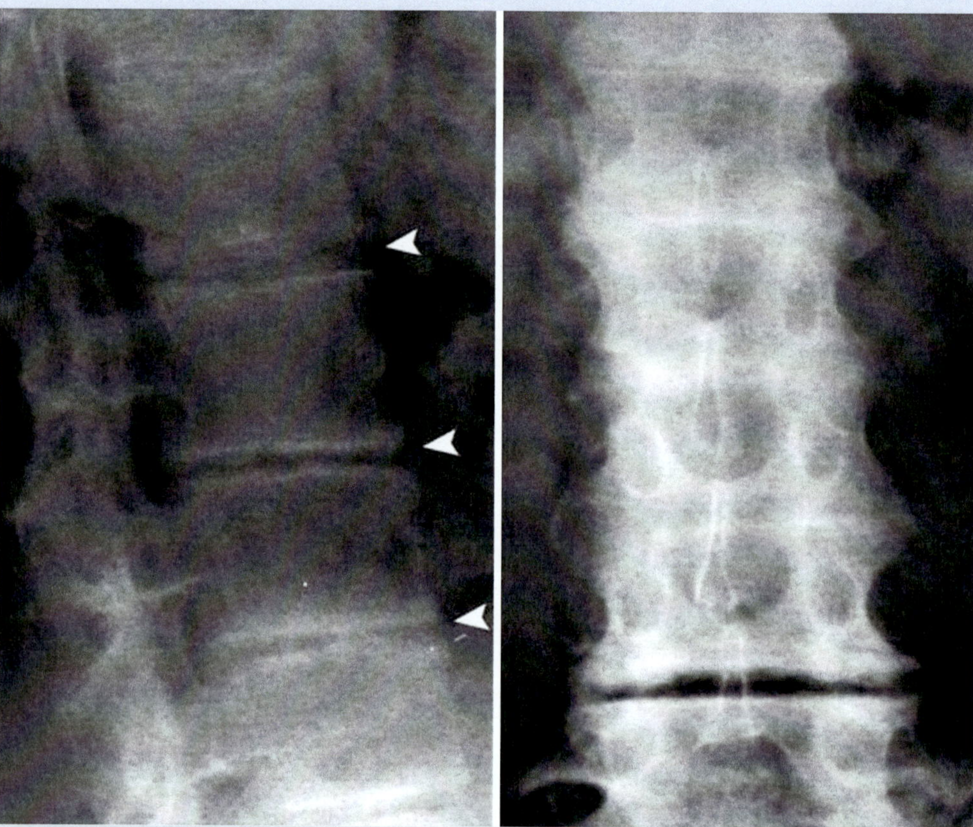

**Fig. 8.4.2**  Anteroposterior and lateral plain radiograph of the lower thoracic vertebrae in a patient with ochronosis shows severe intervertebral disk space narrowing (*arrowheads*)

*The main differential diagnosis of ochronotic changes of the vertebral column is ankylosing spondylitis. How can you differentiate between the two diseases?*
- Ankylosing spondylitis affects the sacroiliac joint in a bilateral symmetrical fashion, while sacroiliac joint affection is not necessarily observed in ochronosis.
- Ankylosing spondylitis shows syndesmophytes, bamboo spine appearance on radiographs, and positive HLA-B 27. All the past features are not part of ochronosis.
- Bluish skin pigmentation and calcification of the intervertebral disks are not features of ankylosing spondylitis.

**Further Reading**

Bal S, et al. Ochronosis with cardiovascular involvement: a case report. Rheumatol Int. 2008;28:479–82.

Çapkin E, et al. Ochronosis in differential diagnosis of patients with chronic back ache: a review of the literature. Rheumatol Int. 2007;28:61–4.

Demir S. Alkaptonuric ochronosis: a case with multiple joint replacement arthropathies. Clin Rheumatol. 2003;22: 437–9.

Güar D, et al. Ochronosis and lumbar disc. Acta Neurochir (Wien). 2006;148:891–4.

Lagier R, et al. Hip arthropathy in ochronosis: anatomical and radiological study. Skeletal Radiol. 1980;5:91–8.

Şahin G, et al. A case of ochronosis: upper extremity involvement. Rheumatol Int. 2001;21:78–80.

## 8.5 Lymphedema

Lymphedema is a pathological condition characterized by excessive, regional interstitial accumulation of protein-rich fluid, typically due to secondary lymph drainage failure in the presence of normal capillary filtration.

The lymph drainage system parallels the venous drainage system, and it moves through the lymphatic vessels in a one-way directional path to return protein, colloids, and particulate matter to the systemic venous circulation. Lymphedema usually involves abnormalities in the regional lymphatic drainage of the extremities (either upper or lower, or both), although visceral lymphatic abnormalities can also occur.

Lymphedema is caused by a reduction in lymphatic transport, and it can be either primary or acquired (secondary). In primary lymphedema, several anatomic problems can exist leading to lymphatic stasis, including lymphatic hypoplasia and functional insufficiency, absence of lymphatic valves, or impairment in the intrinsic contractility of the lymphangion (the segmentally contracting, functional vascular unit of the lymphatic circulation).

## Causes of Primary Lymphedemas

1. *Congenital lymphedema* (*Milroy's disease*): lymphedema that appears at birth or before 2 years of age. It is caused by a mutation that inactivates the VEGFR3 tyrosine kinase signaling mechanism that is felt to be specific to lymphatic vessels. The swelling often involves lower extremities, the genitalia, and even the face.
2. *Lymphedema praecox* (*Meige's disease*): lymphedema that appears between 1 and 35 years of age (mostly at the time of puberty). It is the most common form of lymphedema (94 %), and it typically involves one limb. Most cases involve the lower limbs, especially the foot and calf.
3. *Lymphedema tarda*: lymphedema that appears above 35 years of age. It is an uncommon form and constitutes less than 10 % of all lymphedema types.

## Causes of Secondary Lymphedemas

1. Post-breast cancer lymphatic axillary clearance (14 % of cases)
2. Posttraumatic or postsurgical
3. Infectious (e.g., *filariasis*)
4. Postradiation therapy
5. Due to advanced malignancy

Patients with lymphedema typically present with swelling in one limb (*lymphedema praecox or tarda*) with maximal increase in girth of the involved limb. Most patients with long-standing lymphedema have recurrent soft-tissue infection such as cellulitis, erysipelas, tinea pedis, and lymphangitis. Cutaneous changes of long-standing lymphedema include cutaneous and subcutaneous fibrosis (*peau d'orange skin changes*), hyperkeratosis, hyperpigmentation, and papillomatous or verrucous changes with increased skin turgor. The *Kaposi-Stemmer sign* is a clinical sign indicative of lymphedema, in which an examiner is unable to pinch a fold of skin at the base of the second toe on the dorsal aspect of the foot.

In very rare cases, chronic lymphedema can transform into cutaneous malignancy such as lymphangiosarcomata, angiosarcoma (*Stewart–Treves syndrome*), lymphoma, melanoma, squamous cell carcinoma, and Kaposi's sarcoma.

## Differential Diagnoses of Lymphedema

1. *Chronic venous insufficiency* (*postphlebitic syndrome/phlebedema*) is a condition characterized by limb swelling due to chronic venous thrombosis. Patients usually complain from aching discomfort in the lower extremities during sitting or standing and chronic pruritus. Limb examination often shows dusky-skin discoloration due to hemosiderin deposition within the dermis and cutaneous varicosities.
2. *Myxedema* is a special form of edema which arises when abnormal deposits of mucinous substances accumulate in the skin as a result of thyroid disease (e.g., hypothyroidism). It is characterized by roughening of the skin of the palms, soles, elbows, and knees; brittle, uneven nails; dull, thinning hair; yellow-orange discoloration of the skin; and reduced sweat production. However, it may be difficult to distinguish from lymphedema.
3. *Lipedema* is a syndrome characterized by bilateral symmetrical adipose deposition in the buttocks and lower extremities, causing subsequent enlargement, which stops abruptly at the malleoli, sparing the feet (*helpful in distinguishing this from lymphedema*). It is often associated with considerable aching and pain within the extremity, especially below the knee. Unlike lymphedema, lipedema is painful on touch, almost exclusively seen in females, and the skin can easily be bruised due to the blood vessels' fragility in the subcutaneous tissue. In contrast to lipedema, lipohypertrophy is a painless malfunction of the distribution of fat at the extremities. The absence of a Kaposi-Stemmer's sign is an additional clue. Most often, lipedema arises within 1–2 years after the onset of puberty.
4. *Armchair leg* is a descriptive term that results from sitting in a chair all day and night with one's legs in a dependent position. The immobility results in decreased lymphatic drainage and a functional lymphedema.
5. *Postoperative swelling* caused by femoropopliteal bypass grafting occurs as a result of disruption, or impaired lymphatic drainage, secondary to the surgical dissection in the thigh and popliteal areas. Swelling typically resolves within 3 months. Non-resolving edema after 3 months bares the risk of postoperative tibial or popliteal vein thrombosis.
6. *Podoconiosis* (*non-filarial elephantiasis*) is a rare condition typically seen in non-filarial regions of tropical Africa, Central America, and the Indian subcontinent. The condition is caused by long-term inoculation of microparticles of silica through the soles of barefoot walkers.

### Signs on US

Lymphedema shows thickened dermis with hypoechoic texture associated with loss of the normal cutaneo-myofascial layers distinction. Lymphatic vessels can be seen on duplex sonography within the thickened dermis and hypodermis as hypoechoic branches called *Marshall Clefts*. Dermal echogenicity is inversely proportional to its concentration in water; therefore, dermal edema results therefore in a loss of echogenicity of the skin in high-resolution cutaneous ultrasonography.

### *Signs* on Lymphoscintigraphy

Isotopic lymphoscintigraphy is the most commonly used test and is generally considered to be the gold standard for the diagnosis of lymphedema. A radiolabeled macromolecular tracer (e.g., sulfur colloid) is administered into the subdermal, interdigital region of the affected limb, and the typical abnormalities in lymphedema include absent or delayed transport of tracer, absent or delayed visualization of lymph nodes, crossover filling with retrograde backflow, and dermal back flow.

### *Signs* on CT and MRI

1. Typically in lymphedema, there is the absence of edema within the muscular compartment which helps to distinguish lymphedema radiographically from other forms of edema. The subcutaneous tissue shows thickening and characteristic epifascial plane honeycombing and thickening of the skin (◘ Fig. 8.5.1). The honeycombing appearance of the subcutaneous soft tissue in lymphedema is thought to be caused by pockets of fat surrounded by fluid or fibrous tissue. Phlebedema in CT will show the same features of lymphedema, but with thrombosed deep venous system (◘ Fig. 8.5.2).

2. In lipedema, the subcutaneous fat in CT shows thickening <u>without</u> the signs of honeycombing.

3. On MR lymphography, the lymphatic vessels are traced from the foot upward to the inguinal lymph nodes and then into the cisterna chyli in the abdomen at the level of L1 vertebra. The role of MR lymphography is to assess the level of lymphatic obstruction, seen as abrupt interruption of the gadolinium in the lymphatic vessels. T2W, fat-suppressed images often show subcutaneous edema affecting the soft tissues and the underlying muscles with subfascial fluid collections (◘ Figs. 8.5.3 and 8.5.4).

4. Lipedema is seen on MR-W1W images as diffuse subcutaneous fatty tissues that surrounds the lower limb (◘ Fig. 8.5.5).

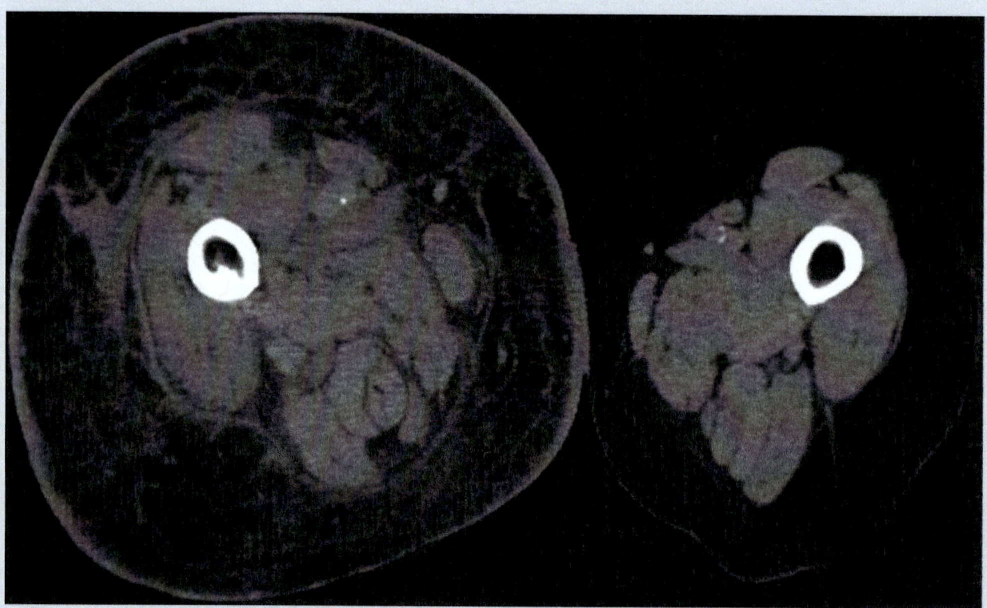

◘ **Fig. 8.5.1**   Axial CT image of a patient with right lower limb lymphedema shows marked subcutaneous edema with epifascial plane honeycombing

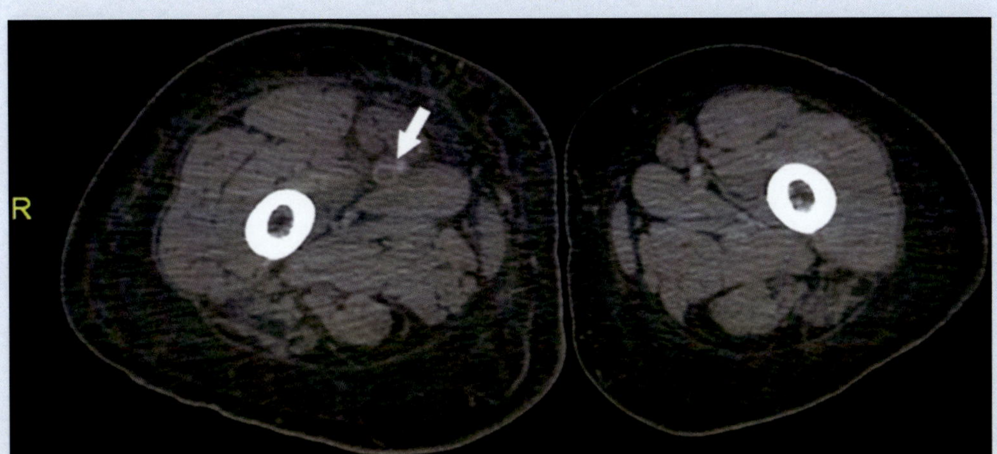

**☐ Fig. 8.5.2** Axial CT image of a patient with right lower limb phlebedema shows subcutaneous edema with epifascial plane honeycombing and thrombosis of the deep femoral venous system (*Arrow*)

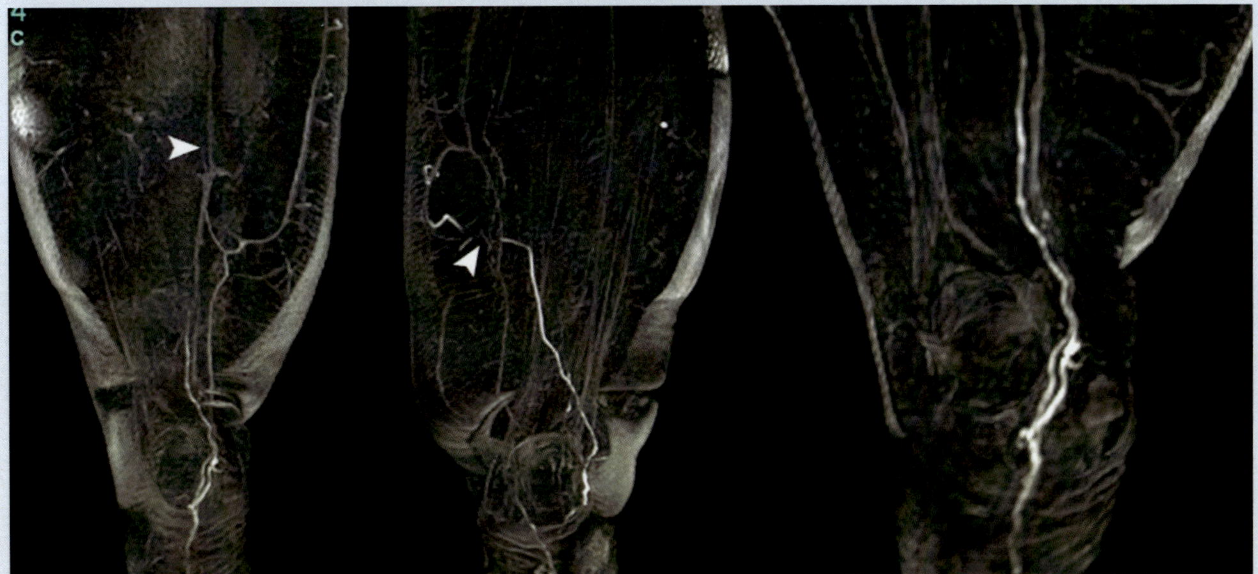

**☐ Fig. 8.5.3** Multiple coronal, T1W, postcontrast MR-lymphographic images that show lymphedema with areas of interruption of the gadolinium die in the lymphatic vessels (*arrowheads*)

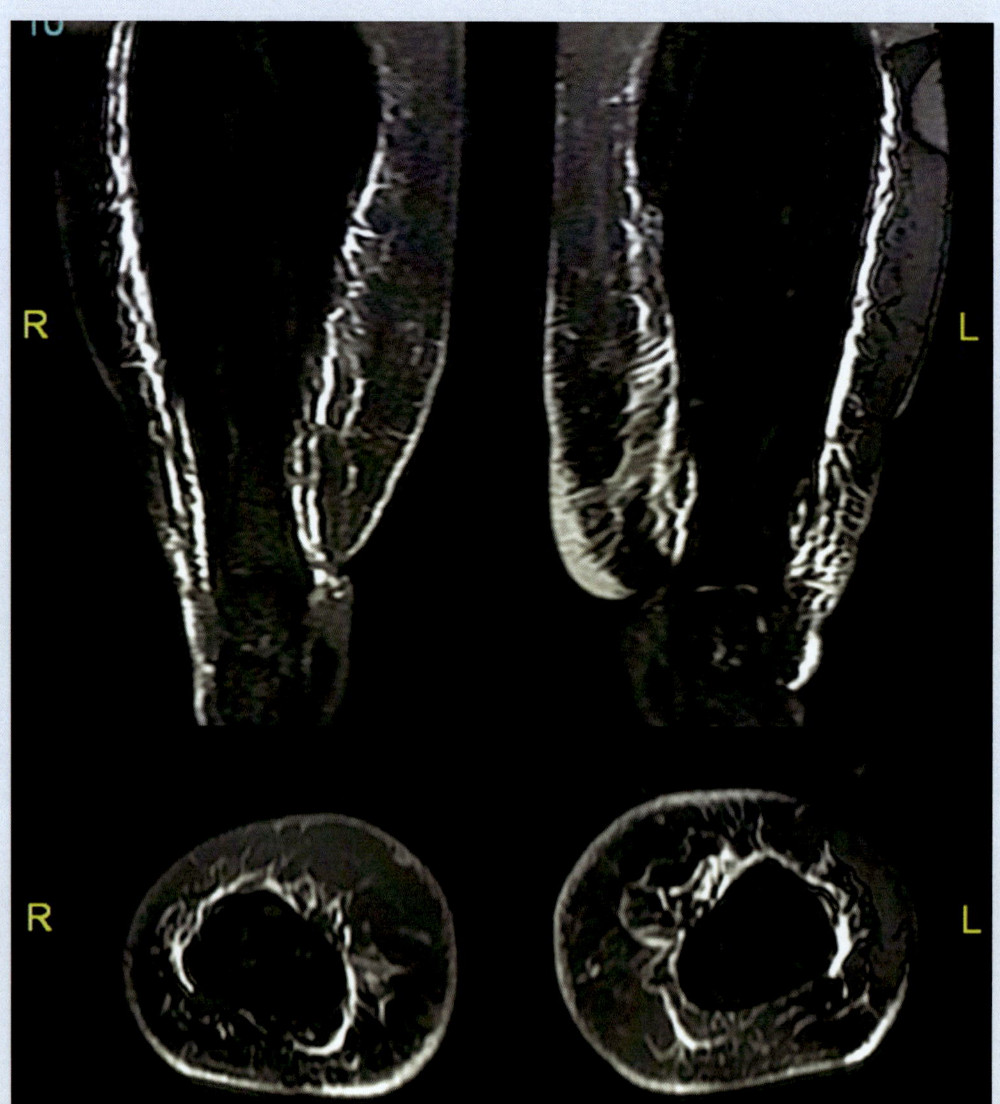

**Fig. 8.5.4** Coronal (*above*) and axial (*below*) T2W, fat-suppressed images of a patient with lymphedema that shows subcutaneous lymphatic congestion seen as high T2 signal intensity fluid in the subcutaneous tissues bilaterally

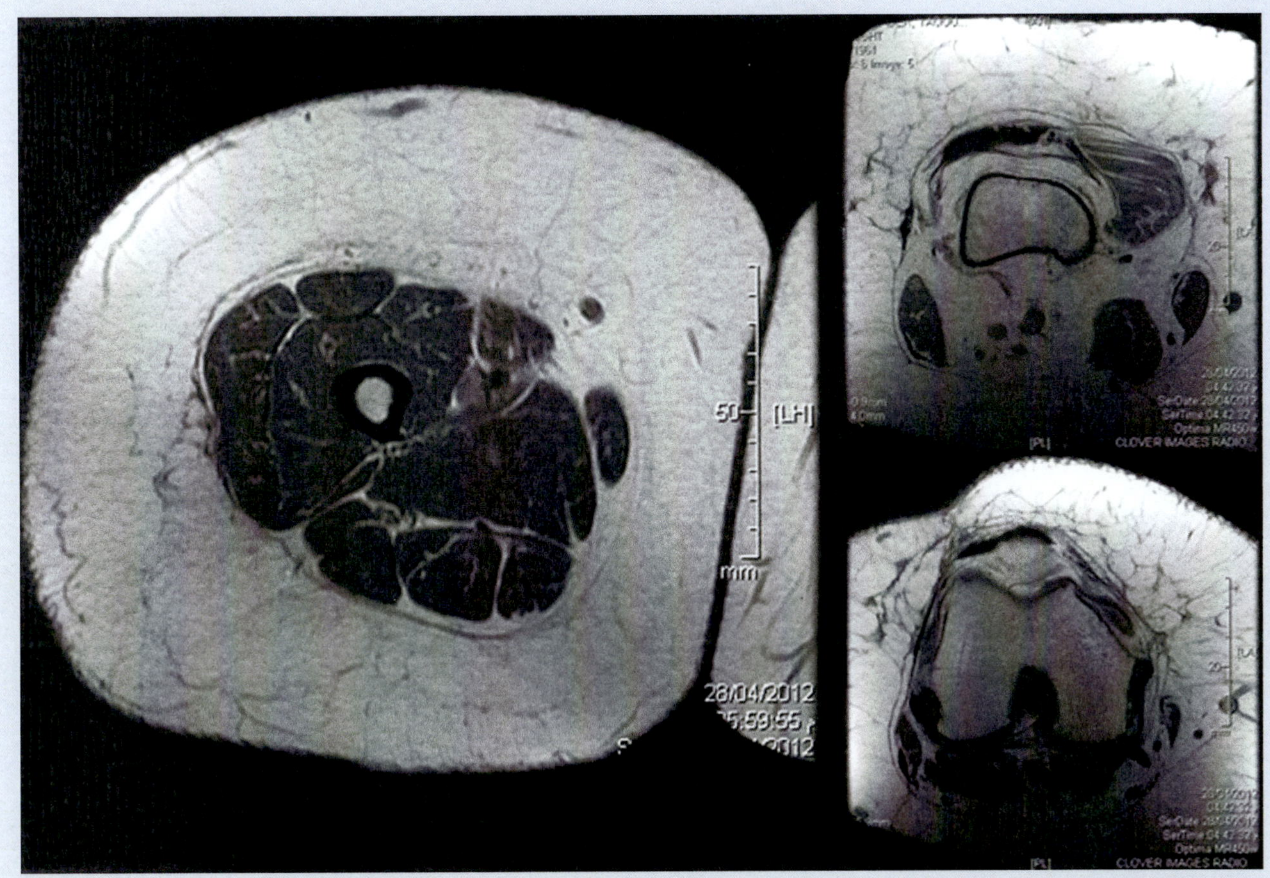

**Fig. 8.5.5** Multiple axial T1W-MR images of a patient with lipedema shows diffuse fatty infiltration of the subcutaneous tissue and around the muscular structures of the knee

## Selected References

Åström KGO, et al. MR imaging of primary, secondary, and mixed forms of lymphedema. Acta Radiol. 2001;42:409–16.

Child AH, et al. Lipedema: an inherited condition. Am J Med Genet Part A. 2010;152A:970–6.

Fonder MA, et al. Lipedema, a frequently unrecognized problem. J Am Acad Dermatol. 2007;57:S1–3.

Hadjis NS, et al. The role of CT in the diagnosis of primary lymphedema of the lower limb. AJR Am J Roentgenol. 1985;144:361–4.

Kerchner K, et al. Lower extremity lymphedema. Update: pathophysiology, diagnosis, and treatment guidelines. Am Acad Dermatol. 2008;59:324–31.

Lu Q, et al. Chronic lower extremity lymphedema: a comparative study of high-resolution interstitial MR lymphangiography and heavily T2-weighted MRI. Eur J Radiol. 2010;73:365–73.

Naouri M, et al. High-resolution cutaneous ultrasonography to differentiate lipoedema from lymphoedema. Br J Dermatol. 2010;163:296–301.

Rockson SG. Lymphedema. Am J Med. 2001;110:288–95.

## 8.6 Neuropathic Itch (Pruritus)

*Pruritus (itching)* represents a distinct sensation arising from the superficial layers of the skin, the mucous membranes (*including the upper respiratory tract*), and the conjunctivae. Itch can be classified into four main types:

1. *Pruritoceptive itch* arises in the skin because of dryness, inflammation, or other skin damage.
2. *Psychogenic itch* arises in patients with psychiatric disorders, such as "delusional parasitosis."
3. *Neurogenic itch* arises in the CNS without evidence of neural pathology; an example is the itch of cholestasis caused by the action of neuropeptides on opioid receptors.
4. *Neuropathic itch* is a pathological condition characterized by out of proportion itch that is completely independent of any pruritogenic stimuli and arises from a lesion in any point along the sensory pathway. This type of itch does not often respond to antihistamines, topical steroids, or other medications that are effective in treating of conventional itch.

The sensation of itching is linked with the motor response of scratching via a spinal reflex and can be inhibited by cortical centers. Scratching relieves itching for several minutes. Scratching is thought to stimulate large, fast conducting A-fibers adjacent to those conducting pruritus. The A-fibers synapse with the inhibitory interneurons and subsequently inhibit the C-fibers, thus reducing the pruritic sensation, according to the "gate control theory" of Melzack and Wall (1965).

The role of radiology in pruritus is to detect its non-dermatological differential diagnoses, especially those rare cases that arise from central nervous system causes, since both the skin and the neural tissues arise embryologically from the ectoderm.

## Neural Control Pruritus

1. *Higher centers*: cortical centers that modulate itch sensation include the "primary somatosensory cortex" and the "insula."
2. *Thalamus*: the "posterolateral ventral thalamic nucleus" acts as a relay station delivering sensation of pruritus coming from the spinal cord via the "anterolateral spinothalamic tract" to the "primary somatosensory cortex" and the "insula."
3. *Spinal cord*: itch impulses are conducted to the ipsilateral dorsal root ganglia and synapse there with secondary neurons. Afferents from these neurons immediately cross over to the opposite anterolateral spinothalamic tract. In the spinal cord, itch and pain processing can be sensitized such that touch stimuli evoke itch (*alloknesis*) or pain (*touch allodynia*).
4. *Pruriceptive receptors*: itch is mediated by small unmyelinated (C-fiber) axons that also transmit pain sensation. Pruriceptive receptors are activated by one of the itch mediators which are:
   (a) *Histamine*: it causes severe itching if applied to the superficially damaged skin or injected intradermally. If injected deeper, histamine produces pain. The majority of histamine released in the skin originates from the dermal mast cells, usually in response to an allergen.
   (b) *Serotonin*: it acts directly on peripheral serotonergic receptors inducing itch. Serotonin acts on the C-fibers via 5-HT3 receptors, which appear to be involved in the pathophysiology of both pruritus and pain.
   (c) *Opioids*: endogenous opioids exert a regulatory action on pain and itching through the CNS; opioids cause pruritus by acting directly on the $\mu$-opioid receptors and by releasing histamine from mast cells.

## Differential Diagnoses of Neuropathic Itch

1. *Psychogenic pruritus*: itching described by the patient as insects crawling over the skin (tactile hallucinations/delusional parasitosis).
2. *Malignancy pruritus*: it is described in multiple myeloma, leukemia, lymphoma, Hodgkin's disease, rectal or sigmoid cancer, and carcinoma of the cervix.
3. *Aquagenic pruritus*: it is a skin condition characterized by intense itching, sometimes accompanied by a burning or stinging sensation after contact with water, regardless of temperature, without any cutaneous alterations and skin or systemic disease. It may be an isolated symptom or accompany different proliferative disorders, like polycythemia vera. The discomfort appears 1–5 min after exposure to water and lasts for 10–120 min. The pathology is presumed to be caused by increased degranulation of the mast cells after the contact with water and the release of acetylcholine.
4. *Notalgia paresthetica* is an area of pruritus of the mid-back due to a form of peripheral neuropathy involving the T2–T6 thoracic nerves due to disk prolapse. It is characterized by focal, intense itching on a patch of the skin of the medial scapular border.
5. *Infectious causes*: herpes zoster (*shingles*) is the commonest cause of neuropathic itch. Postherpetic neuralgia is a chronic neuropathic pain persisting more than 3 months after the shingles rash resolves.
6. *Glossopharyngeal pruritus* is an itch that is felt in the throat or behind the angle of the jaw. Some patients with itch from CN 9 or CN 10 lesions report a *tickle* in their throat that causes chronic cough.
7. *Trigeminal trophic syndrome* is a rare disorder that arises due to destruction to the trigeminal (*Gasserian*) ganglion, resulting in ipsilateral nasal ala itch and trophic skin ulceration.
8. *Central pruritus* arises due to brain and/or spinal cord insult due to multiple sclerosis, neuro-Sjögren's syndrome, syrinx, Wallenberg syndrome, strokes (21 %), Creutzfeldt–Jakob disease, and intramedullary cavernoma.

## References

Carstens E. Scratching the brain to understand neuropathic itch. J Pain. 2008;9(11):973–4.

Cohen OS, et al. Pruritus in familial Creutzfeldt–Jakob disease: a common symptom associated with central nervous system pathology. J Neurol. 2011;258:89–95.

Curtis AR, et al. Holistic approach to treatment of intractable central neuropathic itch. J Am Acad Dermatol. 2011;64:955–9.

Ikoma A, et al. Anatomy and neurophysiology of pruritus. Semin Cutan Med Surg. 2011;30:64–70.

Krajnik M, et al. Understanding pruritus in systemic disease. J Pain Symptom Manage. 2001;21:151–68.

Lanotte M, et al. Central neuropathic itch as the presenting symptom of an intramedullary cavernous hemangioma: case report and review of literature. Clin Neurol Neurosurg. 2013;115:454–6.

Magrinelli F, et al. Neuropathic pain: diagnosis and treatment. Pract Neurol 2013;13(5):292–307.

Metz M, et al. Chronic pruritus – pathogenesis, clinical aspects and treatment. J Eur Acad Dermatol Venereol. 2010;24:1249–60.

Oaklander AL. Neuropathic itch. Semin Cutan Med Surg. 2011;30:87–92.

Sandroni P. Central neuropathic itch: a new treatment option? Neurology. 2002;59:778.

Schmelz M. Itch and pain. Neurosci Biobehav Rev. 2010;34:171–6.

Wiesner T, et al. Itch, skin lesions—and a stiff neck. Lancet. 2007;370:290.

Wood GJ, et al. An insatiable itch. J Pain. 2009;10(8): 792–7.

# Hematology



© Springer International Publishing Switzerland 2017
J.A. Al-Tubaikh, *Internal Medicine*, DOI 10.1007/978-3-319-39747-4_9

## 9.1　Hemosiderosis and Hemochromatosis

*Hemosiderosis*, or iron overload, is a pathological condition characterized by deposition of excess iron within the body tissues that normally do not contain iron. Hemosiderosis is usually secondary to a primary cause such as multiple blood transfusion, chronic hemodialysis, or hemolytic anemia (e.g., thalassemia).

When iron is released into the cytoplasm, it enters a cellular compartment called "labile iron pool" (LIP). Both ferrous ($Fe^{2+}$) and ferric ($Fe^{3+}$) iron forms are poorly bound with proteins and are highly toxic to the cells within this compartment. The unneeded iron from LIP is stored in the form of ferritin, which is organic and nontoxic. When the LIP iron content exceeds the ferritin capacity, hemosiderin is generated from ferritin denaturation. Iron in the form of hemosiderin is thought to be more toxic to the body tissues. Hemosiderin initially accumulates in the reticuloendothelial system (spleen, bone marrow, and Kupffer cells in the liver). When the reticuloendothelial system is saturated, deposition occurs in normal body tissues such as the hepatocytes, heart muscles, and the endocrine system. Chelation therapy (e.g., desferrioxamine) removes mainly the extracellular iron and only a fraction of the intracellular LIP iron.

Hemosideroses have different body manifestations according to the area of deposition:

- *Cardiac hemosiderosis*: myocardial iron deposition results in dilated cardiomyopathy that will lead to heart failure.

**◨ Fig. 9.1.1** Short-axis cardiac MRI illustration demonstrates a black ring within the myocardium, a sign of cardiac siderosis (*arrowhead*)

### Signs on Chest Radiograph

The heart appears larger than normal in cases of cardiac damage and development of dilated cardiomyopathy.

### Signs on MRI

MRI can detect early myocardial siderosis via obtaining T2* images, which show a dark, hypointense rim located within the myocardium in short-axis sequences, representing myocardial siderosis (◨ Fig. 9.1.1).

- *Hepatic hemosiderosis*: iron deposition in hepatocytes results in liver cirrhosis.

### Signs on CT and MRI

- On CT, the liver appears hyperdense compared to the spleen.
- On MRI, the liver appears extremely hypointense, with an almost black signal on all pulse sequences, depending on the severity of the iron overload.
- *Anterior pituitary gland hemosiderosis*: loss of the endocrine function of the anterior pituitary results in hypogonadism and loss of libido.

### Signs on MRI

The anterior pituitary shows a hypointense signal intensity area on both T1 and T2 images.

- *Pancreatic hemosiderosis*: deposition of iron in the pancreases results in impairment of both exocrine and endocrine functions. Diabetes mellitus may result due to pancreatic siderosis.

*Hemochromatosis* is a disease characterized by deposition of excess iron in the body as a result of genetic defect (primary hemosiderosis).

In hemochromatosis, iron deposition initially occurs in the hepatocytes and spares Kupffer cells (the reverse situation to hemosiderosis). The age of presentation is usually between 50 and 60 years of age. Menstruation blood loss in women has a protective effect against hemochromatosis due to iron loss.

Hemochromatosis is asymptomatic in early stages. As the iron deposition progresses, liver failure, skin hyperpigmentation, arthropathy (especially in the metacarpophalangeal joints), and cardiac failure may occur. Deposition of hemosiderin in the subcutaneous tissues results in increased skin tanning and darkening.

*Bronze diabetes* is a term used to describe maturity-onset diabetes seen in hemochromatosis. The term "bronze" is used because the diabetes is associated with skin tanning that mimics bronze coloring.

Diagnosis is confirmed by measuring serum ferritin level, transferrin saturation testing, liver biopsy, genetic testing, and MRI.

## Differential Diagnoses and Related Diseases

- *Bantu siderosis* a type of hemosiderosis only found in Africa. It is associated with liver cirrhosis, diabetes, and heart disease. The disease is linked with higher rates of tuberculosis infection.

- *Juvenile hemochromatosis* is a form of hemochromatosis present in the second decade of life. Patients often present with abdominal pain, cardiac arrhythmias, impaired glucose tolerance, and hypogonadotropic hypogonadism.
- *Ferroportin disease* is a genetic disease characterized by mutation in the gene responsible for the production of ferroportin, a protein that exports iron from body cells. Ferroportin is expressed mainly in Kupffer cells and splenic macrophages. Patients present with isolated hyperferritinemia and normal or slightly elevated transferrin saturation. In contrast to hemochromatosis, iron is mainly deposited within Kupffer cells.
- *Pulmonary hemosiderosis* is a rare condition that arises due to repeated episodes of bleeding within the lung alveoli. Iron overload within the lungs results in pulmonary fibrosis, anemia, and (rarely) death due to pulmonary hemorrhage. The disease has an incidence of less than 1:1,000,000 live births and occurs usually in children <7 years old (it is extremely rare in adults). Symptoms include coughing blood (hemoptysis) and iron-deficiency anemia.
- *Superficial brain siderosis* is a condition characterized by deposition of hemosiderin within brain tissues, often secondary to subdural hemorrhage and bleeding into the brain cisterns. When siderosis affects the vestibulocochlear nerve, tinnitus may result.

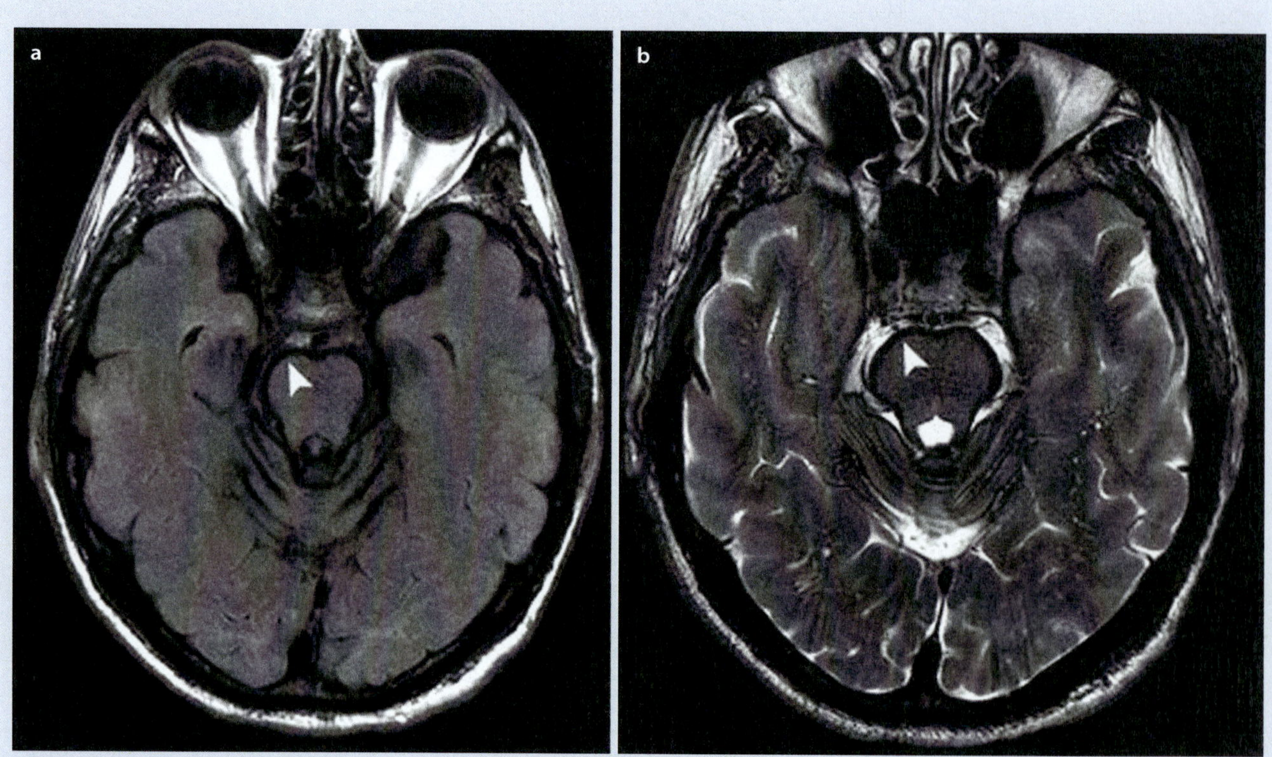

**Fig. 9.1.2**   Axial T1W (**a**) and T2W (**b**) brain MRI show a hypointense rim that surrounds the pons (*arrowhead*) due to superficial brain siderosis

## Further Reading

Argyropoulou MI, et al. MRI evaluation of tissue iron burden in patients with β-thalassemia major. Pediatr Radiol. 2007a;37:1191–200.

Bonetti MG, et al. Hepatic iron overload in thalassemic patients: proposal and validation of an MRI method of assessment. Pediatr Radiol. 1996;26:650–6.

Brasch RC, et al. Magnetic resonance imaging of transfusional hemosiderosis complicating thalassemia major. Radiology. 1984;150:767–71.

Chen CH, et al. Idiopathic pulmonary hemosiderosis: favorable response to corticosteroid. J Chin Med Assoc. 2008;71:421–4.

Deugnier Y, et al. Iron and the liver: update 2008. J Hepatol. 2008;48:S113–23.

Flyer MA, et al. Transfusional hemosiderosis in sickle cell anemia: another cause of an echogenic pancreas. Pediatr Radiol. 1993;23:140–2.

Koçak R, et al. The liver siderosis in beta-thalassemia intermedia and hemoglobin disease. J Islamic Acad Sci. 1993;6:42–5.

Positano V, et al. Improved T2* assessment in liver iron overload by magnetic resonance imaging. Magn Reson Imaging. 2008a;27:188–97. doi:10.1016/j.mri.2008.06.004.

Rosenberg W. Haemochromatosis Med. 2007;35:89–92.

Rosenberg W, et al. Haemochromatosis. Medicine. 2002;30:63–4.

## 9.2   β-Thalassemia Major (Cooley's Anemia)

β-thalassemia major is a hereditary hemolytic anemia, characterized by deficiency in the hemoglobin beta chain synthesis. Patients with β-thalassemia major are prone to repeated attacks of intravascular hemolysis that requires repeated hospitalization and blood transfusions.

Patients with β-thalassemia major present with microcytic hypochromic anemia with signs of fatigue and cardiac tachycardia.

Repeated blood transfusion predisposes to hemosiderosis and tissue iron burden, which is the most severe complication of this disease. Hemosiderosis causes cardiomyopathy, hepatic failure, hypogonadism (pituitary siderosis), and endocrinal abnormalities. *Bronze diabetes* is a term used to describe diabetes mellitus induced in a patient with thalassemia due to pancreatic hemosiderosis. The term "bronze" refers to skin darkening and hyperpigmentation that is seen in patients with chronic thalassemia, due to deposition of hemosiderin in the subcutaneous tissues. Hypoparathyroidism is one of the most important endocrinal complications of thalassemia.

Extramedullary hematopoiesis is commonly observed in these patients due to increased body demands. Extramedullary hematopoiesis can be appreciated on plain radiographs as abnormally widened, flat bones.

Within the past few years, MRI has emerged as a powerful diagnostic tool to detect hemosiderosis through the body. Techniques for tissue iron burden quantification are well established for the liver and the heart. Early treatment with chelating agents (e.g., desferrioxamine) reduces the severity of the iron burden complication. MRI iron burden quantification helps in monitoring chelation therapy.

### Signs on Skeletal Radiograph
- *Skull hair-on-end appearance*: increase of the trabeculae within the skull bones, due to extramedullary hematopoiesis that widens the calvarial flat bones (**Fig. 9.2.3**)
- Square-shaped metacarpals and thin cortex, due to bone marrow proliferation (**Fig. 9.2.4**)

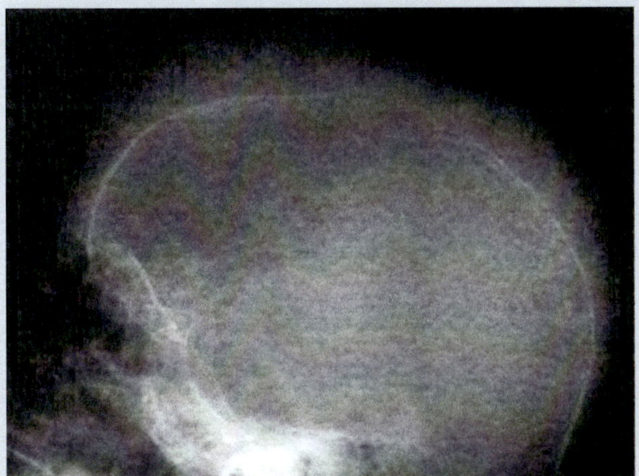

**Fig. 9.2.3** A plain radiograph of the lateral skull of a patient with thalassemia shows hair-on-end-appearance

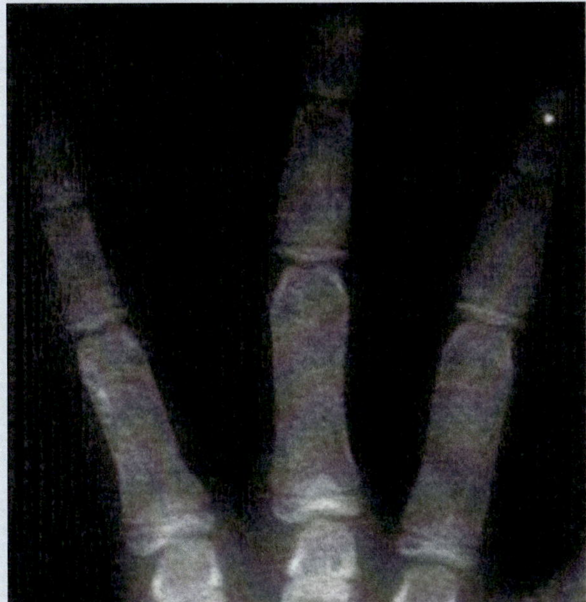

**Fig. 9.2.4** A plain radiograph of the hand shows squaring and expansion of the phalanges due to extramedullary hematopoiesis in a young patient with thalassemia

- Dilated ribs due to extramedullary hematopoiesis (**Fig. 9.2.5**)
- Splaying of the femoral metaphysis (Erlenmeyer flask deformity)

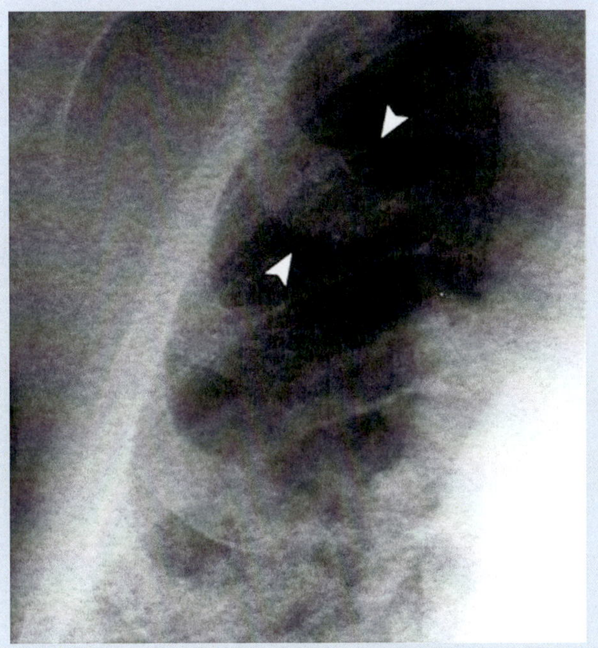

**Fig. 9.2.5** AP plain radiograph shows expansion of the ribs due to extramedullary hematopoiesis (*arrowheads*)

### Signs on CT
- Hepatic hemosiderosis is one of the main causes of high-density liver on nonenhanced CT images (**Fig. 9.2.6**). The liver density will show high HU difference compared to the muscles and the spleen, with a range of 80–140 HU. Other causes of

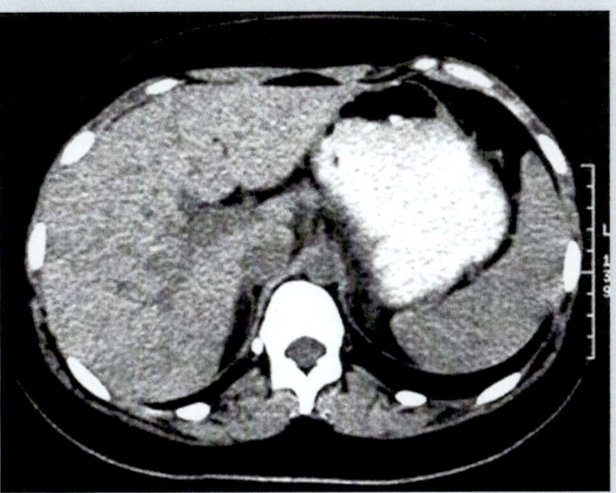

**Fig. 9.2.6** Axial nonenhanced CT of the abdomen shows high-density liver

nonenhanced CT high-density liver are Wilson's disease due to copper deposition, and hepatic iodine deposition, rarely seen in amiodarone toxicity.

— Hepatosplenomegaly often occurs due to extramedullary hematopoiesis (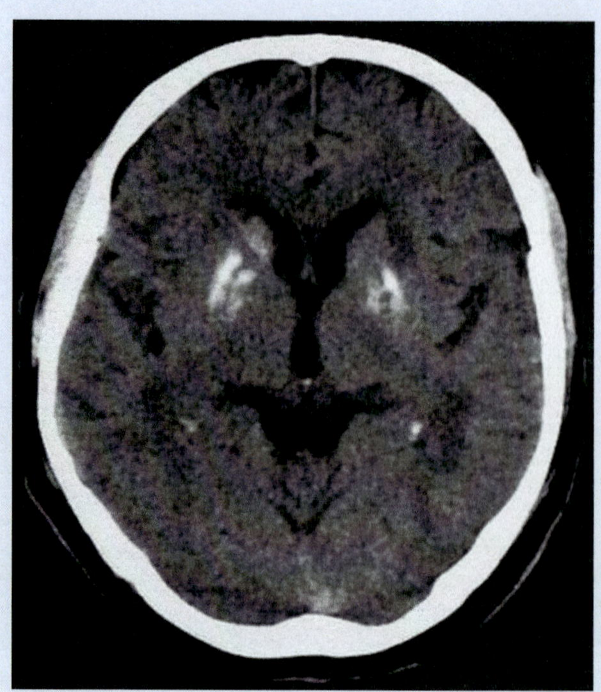 Fig. 9.2.7).
— Thoracic paraspinal masses and enlarged lymph nodes may be seen due to extramedullary hematopoiesis (Fig. 9.2.8).
— Cerebral calcification may be seen due to hypoparathyroidism in thalassemia patients. Patients may uncommonly show bilateral symmetrical basal ganglia calcifications (Fig. 9.2.9).

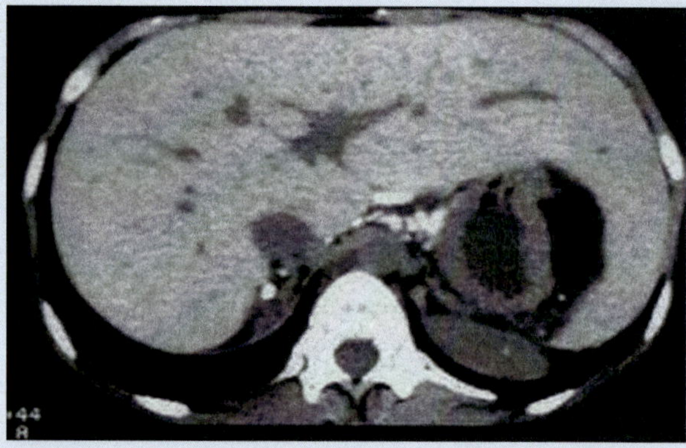

**Fig. 9.2.7** Axial nonenhanced CT of the abdomen shows hepatomegaly with left liver lobe hypertrophy

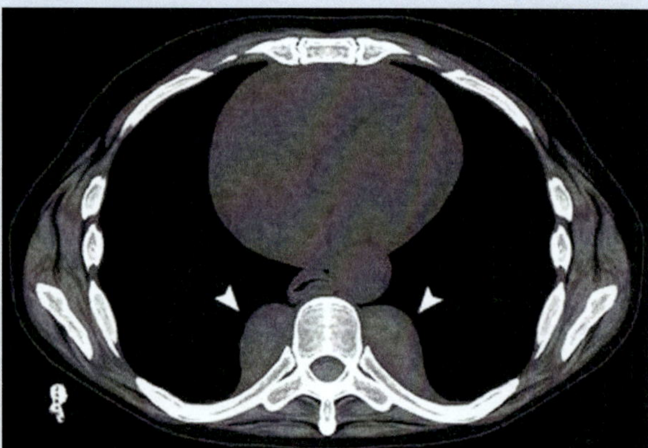

**Fig. 9.2.8** Axial nonenhanced CT illustration of the thorax shows bilateral paraspinal masses due to extramedullary hematopoiesis (*arrowheads*). These masses can be easily mistaken for tumors. Other signs of extramedullary hematopoiesis support the diagnosis

**Fig. 9.2.9** Axial nonenhanced brain CT shows bilateral, almost symmetrical, basal ganglia calcifications

### Signs on MRI

— Iron burden quantification is done with the use of T2* sequences (Fig. 9.2.10). The superparamagnetic properties of the iron deposited within the tissues cause decreased signal intensity of the tissues containing iron. As a result, hepatic parenchyma, splenic parenchyma, and cardiac muscles with siderosis appear hypointense compared to normal parenchyma.
— In mild liver siderosis, the liver appears hypointense only on T2* images, compared to muscles. In moderate to severe cases, the liver appears hypointense to spleen and muscles in all sequences. The spleen shows almost the same picture as the liver, due to iron deposition. In primary hemochromatosis, only the liver shows decreased signal intensity, while the spleen is spared.
— In the heart, iron overload appears as a dark ring on T1W, T2W, and T2* images.
— In bronze diabetes, the pancreas and sometimes the adrenals show low signal intensity due to iron deposition.
— In hypogonadism and signs of pituitary failure, the anterior pituitary shows low signal intensity on T1W, T2W, and T2* images, reflecting severe iron deposition.

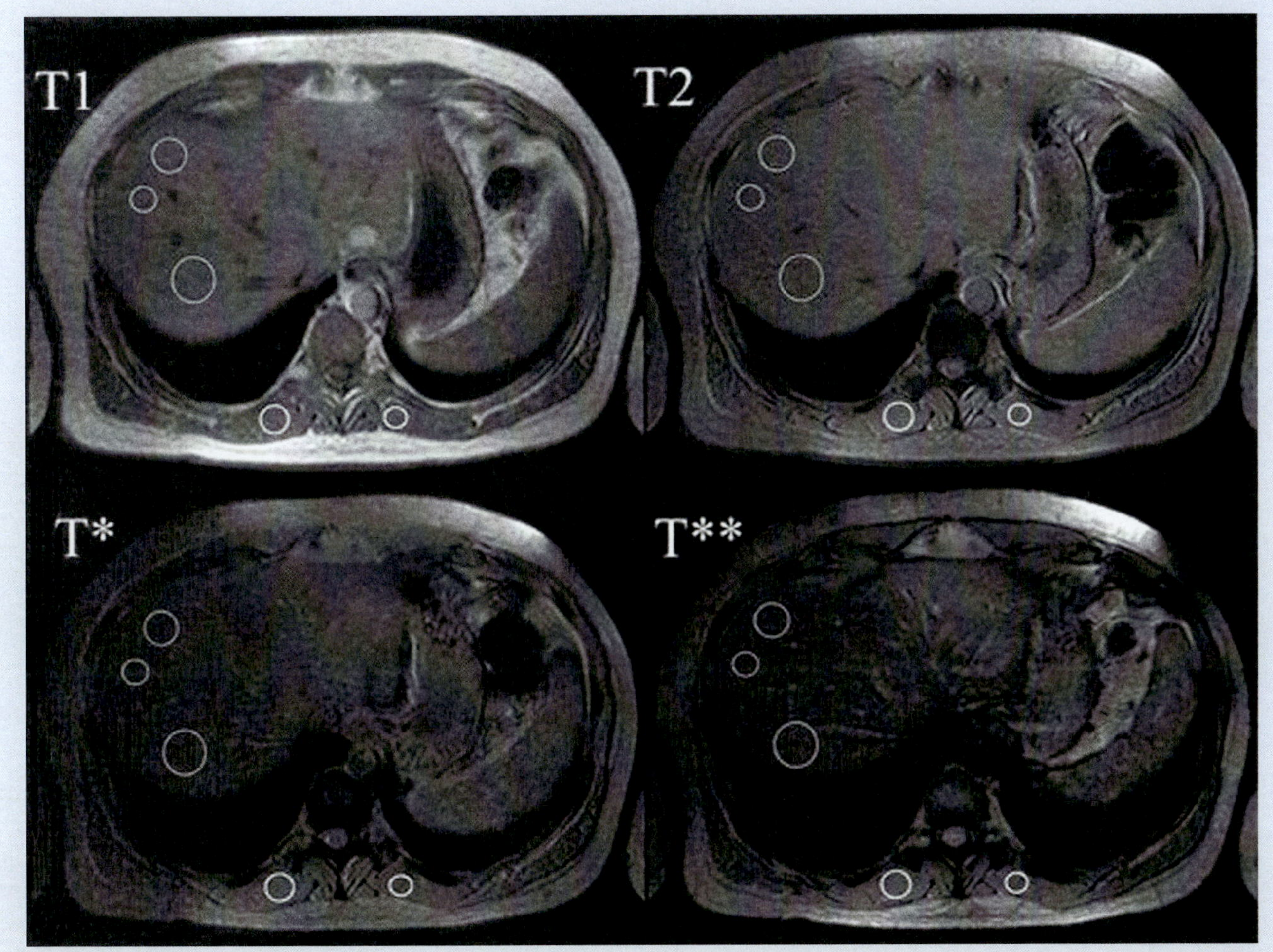


**Fig. 9.2.10** Axial abdomen section in different sequences illustrates the method of liver iron burden quantification in the liver and the paraspinal muscles

## Further Reading

Argyropoulou MI, et al. MRI evaluation of tissue iron burden in patients with β-thalassemia major. Pediatr Radiol. 2007b;37:1191–200.

Drakonaski E, et al. Adrenal glands in beta-thalassemia major: magnetic resonance (MR) imaging features and correlation with iron store. Eur Radiol. 2005;15:2462–8.

Karimi M, et al. Prevalence of hepatosplenomegaly in beta thalassemia minor subjects in Iran. Eur J Radiol. 2007;59:120–2. doi:10.1016/j.ejrad.2007.09.027.

Karimi M, et al. Hypoparathyroidism and intracerebral calcification in patients with beta-thalassemia major. Eur J Radiol. 2008;70:481–4. doi:10.1016/j.ejrad.2008.02.003.

Lal A, et al. Focal splenic lesions as a cause of extramedullary hematopoiesis in a case of thalassemia. Eur J Radiol Extra. 2008;68:e125–7.

Louis CK. Low growth of children with β-thalassemia major. Indian J Pediatr. 2005;72:159–64.

Mavrogeni S, et al. Magnetic resonance evaluation of liver and myocardium iron deposition in thalassemia intermedia and β-thalassemia major. Int J Cardiovasc Imaging. 2008;24:849–54.

Papakonstantinou O, et al. MR imaging of spleen in beta-thalassemia major. Abdom Imaging. 2006;40:2777–82. doi:10.1007/s00261.006.9138-4.

Positano V, et al. Improved T2* assessment in liver iron overload by magnetic resonance imaging. Magn Reson Imaging. 2008b;27:188–97. doi:10.1016/j.mri.2008.06.004.

## 9.3    Sickle Cell Disease

Sickle cell disease (SCD) is an autosomal recessive genetic disorder, characterized by episodic attacks of hemolytic anemia and vaso-occlusive attacks due to "sickling" of the red blood cells (RBCs) under certain body conditions that include dehydration, metabolic acidosis, and low oxygen saturation.

SCD results from abnormal production of hemoglobin (Hb-S). Sickle cell patients are homozygous (HbSS), while heterozygous patients have "sickle cell trait." SCD can also arise when Hb-S is combined with abnormal hemoglobin (e.g., Hb-S-thalassemia). Hb-S differs from the normal Hb-A only in the substitution of valine for glutamic acid in the sixth position of the β chain.

In SCD, the normal, discoid RBCs shape is transformed into a sickle-shaped, sticky mass during deoxygenation. These sickle cells can stick together, forming a hard mass that may lead to embolization and arterial infarction in different parts of the body.

Approximately 50 % of patients with SCD experience painful crises by the age of 5 years. Patients with sickle cell disease have natural protection against malaria; the reasons are unknown.

## The Lungs in SCD

Patients with SCD have greater susceptibility to pneumonia (100 times more than other children), due to impaired immune status. The infective agents are commonly *Streptococcus pneumoniae*, *Haemophilus influenzae*, and *Salmonella*. *Acute chest syndrome* (ACS) is a term used to describe newly developed pulmonary consolidation, accompanied by fever, chest pain, dyspnea, and cough. The underlying cause is known and presumably due to fat emboli. ACS is the second most common cause for hospital admissions in children with SCD, after painful crises. ACS is also seen in up to 10 % of SCD patients after general anesthesia.

## The Skeletal System in SCD

Skeletal manifestations in SCD range between vaso-occlusive crises, extramedullary hematopoiesis, osteomyelitis, and vertebral changes. Bone infarction is the most common cause of pain crises in SCD. However, silent infarctions do exist in patients with SCD. There are four zones seen in bone infarction by histology: the zone of cell death located in the center, the zone of ischemic tissue, the zone of hyperemia, and the outer zone of normal bony tissue.

*Osteomyelitis* means inflammation of the bone and the bone marrow. Osteomyelitis is commonly caused by *Salmonella* infection in sickle cell patients. In nonsickle cell patients, the most common cause of osteomyelitis is *Staphylococcus aureus*.

### Differential Diagnoses and Related Diseases

*Hand–foot syndrome* is an uncommon disease seen in sickle cell patients in up to 20 % of cases, characterized by bilateral inflammation and swelling of the fingers and toes (dactylitis). Patients present with fever, bilateral digital swelling in the hands and feet, leukocytosis, and pain. It can be mistaken for osteomyelitis in the initial presentation. Osteomyelitis is uncommonly known to cause bilateral infection in the hands and feet simultaneously. Also, osteomyelitis often involves the long bones, not the small bones of the hands and feet. Most

patients experience this syndrome before 4 years of age, and the disease has not been reported beyond 7 years. The condition is self-limiting, with a duration that varies from a week to a month.

*What Is the Difference Between Osteonecrosis, Avascular Necrosis, and Bone Infarction?*
*Osteonecrosis* is ischemic death of the bone and bone marrow.
*Avascular necrosis* is osteonecrosis that occurs in the epiphyses.
*Bone infarction* is osteonecrosis that occurs in the metaphyses or diaphyses.

## The Brain in SCD

In SCD, the brain may be damaged due to infarction from sickle cell emboli or from vasculitis. Up to 25 % of patients with SCD will have a neurological complication over their lifetime; 11 % of these complications will occur by the age of 20 years. *Silent infarction* is defined as MRI manifestation of cerebral infarction in the absence of clinical symptoms and occurs in up to 22 % of patients with SCD.

## The Spleen in SCD

Multiple spleen infarctions due to vaso-occlusive crises are a very common feature in SCD. With time, the spleen is replaced by fibrous tissue and by calcium and hemosiderin deposition (called *autosplenectomy*). Up to 94 % of patients are asplenic by the age of 5 years.

Patients with splenectomy are susceptible to infection with *Staphylococcus pneumoniae*, *Salmonella*, and *Haemophilus influenzae*. Pneumococcal vaccine is often started between 2 and 5 years of age.

*Sequestration syndrome* is another condition that commonly occurs in SCD patients, characterized by rapid pooling of the blood within the spleen, resulting in intravascular volume depletion and dropping hematocrit levels. When the sequestration is severe, patients present with abdominal fullness, thirst, tachycardia, and tachypnea that may rapidly progress into circulatory collapse. Up to 30 % of patients experience sequestration syndrome between the ages of 6 months and 3 years.

> **Signs on Chest Radiograph**
> - Pneumonia is seen as areas of patchy lung infiltration with air bronchogram. The airspace disease may be lobar or diffuse.
> - *Acute chest syndrome* is seen as single or multiple patchy areas of airspace disease, often confined to the middle and lower lobes. Up to 60 % of patients with ACS show normal chest radiograph.

### Signs on Skeletal Radiograph

- *Bone infarction*: it is seen as a radiolucent area surrounded by the sclerotic rim, typically in the epiphyses and the medullary cavity (Fig. 9.3.11). Later, sclerosis of the infarcted areas causes the appearance of dense bone within the affected bone (bone-in-bone appearance).
- *H-shaped vertebra*: there is central end plate depression, with sparing of the anterior and posterior margins due to previous infarctions of vertebral bodies. An H-shaped vertebra is a characteristic sign of SCD (Fig. 9.3.12).
- Expansion of the diploic medullary spaces of the skull due to increased hematopoietic demands (hair-on-end appearance).
- *Osteomyelitis*: the early changes seen radiographically are soft-tissue swelling or a mass, occasionally gas, periosteal reaction, and (later) cortical destruction. There are usually no signs on plain radiograph in the first 2 weeks of infection. The cortical destruction first appears as small lucent holes (permeative destruction), followed later by larger coalescent lesions (moth-eating destruction). Osteomyelitis can be difficult to differentiate from infarction.
- *Hand–foot syndrome*: the typical signs of dactylitis include soft-tissue swelling of the digits, cortical thinning, multiple intramedullary radiolucent deposits, and thick periosteal new bone formation (Fig. 9.3.13). The radiological manifestations are completely reversible after 8 months.
- Protrusio acetabuli: it may occur in SCD in up to 20 % of cases.

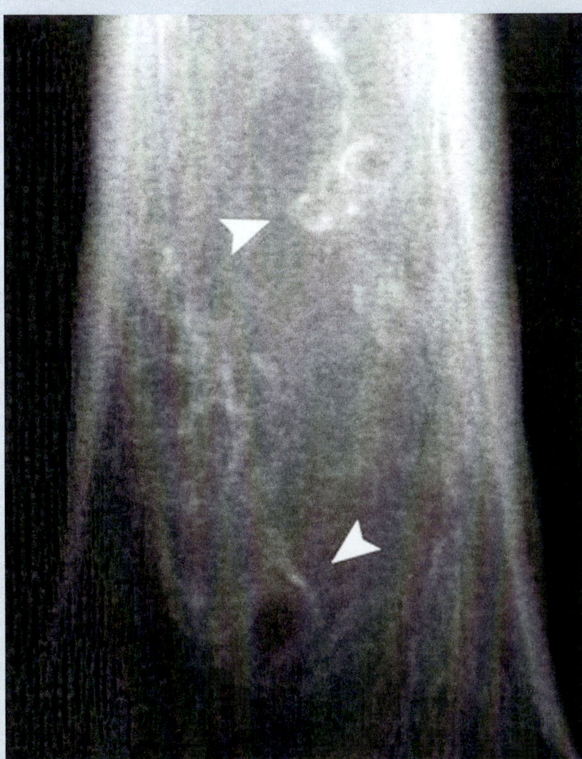

Fig. 9.3.11 Plain radiograph of the distal femur metaphysis shows radiolucent areas surrounded by sclerotic rims (*arrowheads*) due to old bone infarction in a patient with sickle cell disease (SCD)

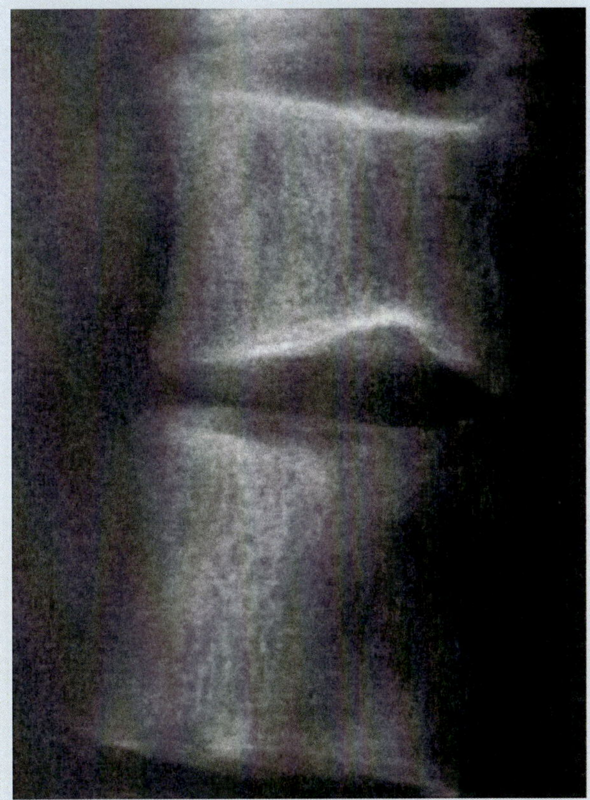

Fig. 9.3.12 Lateral vertebral plain radiograph of a patient with SCD shows H-shaped thoracic vertebra

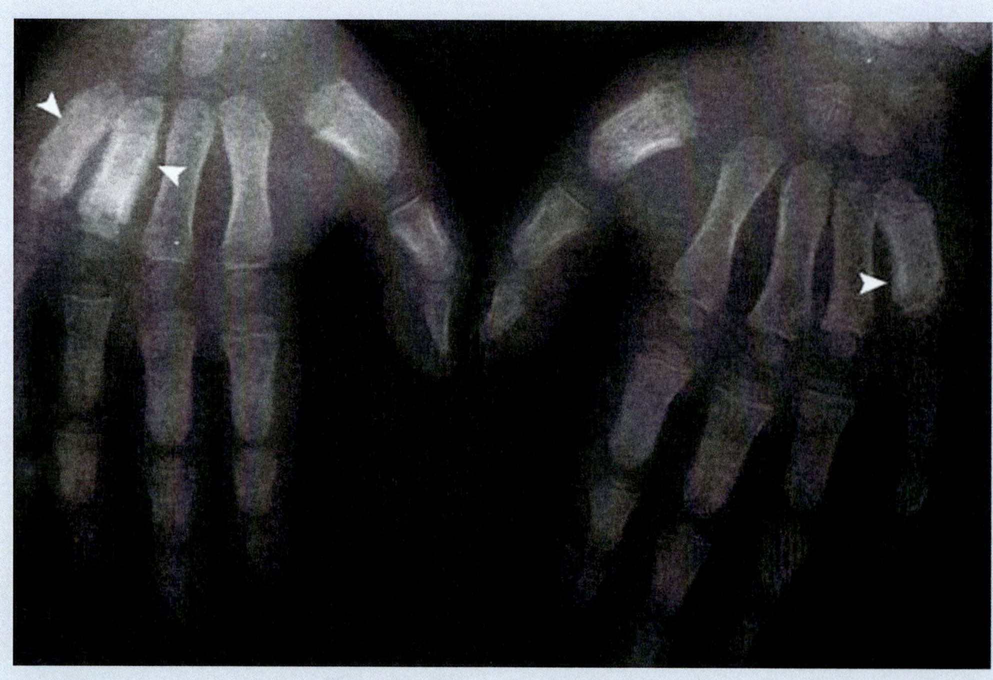

**Fig. 9.3.13**    Plain radiograph of both hands in a sickle-cell patient shows thick periosteal new bone formation affecting the fifth and fourth right metacarpal bones and the fifth left metacarpal bone (*arrowheads*), changes indicating hand-foot syndrome

### Signs on Chest CT

Extramedullary hematopoiesis may be found as bilateral or unilateral, smooth or lobulated paraspinal masses in the lower thoracic spine, without vertebral erosions. History of hematological disease is the key diagnosis to differentiate these masses from tumors.

### Signs on Abdominal CT

- *Spleen infarction* is seen on noncontrast-enhanced images as a hypodense, wedge-shaped area, which typically starts from the periphery toward the center, with no contrast enhancement (**Fig. 9.3.14**).
- *Sequestration syndrome* is seen as splenomegaly with hypodense peripheral areas.

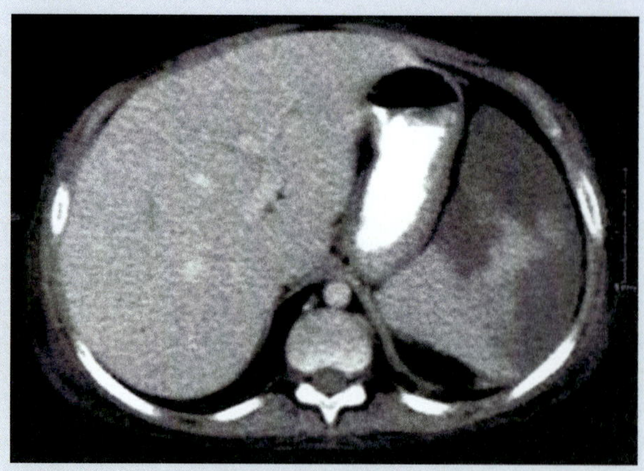

**Fig. 9.3.14**    Axial abdominal postcontrast CT shows multiple hypodense wedge-shaped areas within the spleen, due to multiple areas of infarction

### Signs on Skeletal MRI

- MRI is important in the early detection of bone infarction. On T2W images, there is an area surrounded by a hyperintense line and an outer hypointense line (*double-line sign*). The high-intensity line represents the zone of hyperemia. Double-line sign is found in up to 80 % of cases of bone infarction.
- The yellow marrow is made of 80 % fat, 15 % water, and 5 % proteins. On MRI, it gives high signal in T1W images. In contrast, the red marrow is made of 40 % fat, 40 % water, and 20 % proteins. This high water content gives low signal in both T1W and T2W images. Extracellular hematopoiesis, especially within the vertebrae, can be suggested by observation of the intervertebral disk signal. Normally, the vertebral bodies have higher signals than the intervertebral disks on T1W images, due to the fatty marrow. In extracellular hematopoiesis, the yellow marrow is reconverted into red marrow due to the hematopoietic demands, resulting in low signal intensity of the vertebral bodies compared to the intervertebral disks on T1W images (*high-density disk sign*). This sign is observed in any disease with bone marrow infiltration.

### Signs on Brain MRI

- *Silent infarction* is detected as a high signal intensity lesion within the white matter on T2W or FLAIR images.
- *Moyamoya disease* is detected by its classical "puff of smoke" appearance on MR angiography and occlusion of the ipsilateral internal carotid artery.

## Further Reading

Babhulkar SS, et al. The hand-foot syndrome in sickle-cell haemoglobinopathy. J Bone Joint Surg (Br). 1995;77-B:310–2.

Ejindu VG, et al. Musculoskeletal manifestations of sickle cell disease. Radiographics. 2007;27:1005–21.

Janet Watson R, et al. The hand-foot syndrome in sickle-cell disease in young children. Pediatrics. 1963;31:975–82.

Lonergan GJ, et al. Sickle cell anemia. Radiographics. 2001;21:971–94.

Lukens JN. Sickle cell disease. Dis Mon. 1981;27:1–56.

Lukens JN. Sickle cell disease. Dis Mon. 1981;27:1–56.

Schatz J, et al. Sickle cell disease as a neurodevelopmental disorder. Ment Retard Dev Disabil Res Rev. 2006;12:200–7.

## 9.4 Pernicious Anemia

Pernicious anemia (PA) is a disease characterized by the development of megaloblastic anemia due to destruction of the gastric parietal cells. *Megaloblastic anemias* are a subgroup of macrocystic anemias (large volume red blood cells), which most commonly arise due to vitamin $B_{12}$ and folate deficiencies.

Normally, the parietal cells in the gastric mucosa secrete an intrinsic factor, which is important for absorption of vitamin $B_{12}$ from the gastrointestinal tract. The fundus of the stomach contains parietal cells, the body contains the cells responsible for the secretion of pepsin and hydrochloric acid, and the antrum contains G cells. Patients with PA develop antigastric parietal cells (GPC) and anti-intrinsic factor antibodies (gastric parietal cells antibodies, or AGPA), which attack the parietal cells and cause autoimmune gastritis. Destruction of the gastric parietal cells leads to gastric mucosal atrophy and compromises the production of the intrinsic factor. Moreover, the atrophic gastritis also compromises the gastric acid pump, leading to deficiency in the secretion of gastric acids (hypo- or achlorhydria). Loss of vitamin $B_{12}$ causes defective synthesis of the bone marrow cellular activities, leading to the development of megaloblastic erythropoiesis and macrocytic anemia.

Chronic gastritis induces enterochromaffin-like cell hyperplasia, which may result in the development of gastric carcinoid tumors. Compared to the general population, gastric adenocarcinoma is 3–5 times more frequent among patients with PA. The activity of natural killer cells, which participate in immunosurveillance against tumor dissemination, is believed to be compromised in patients with PA.

Atrophic gastritis is divided into two types. Atrophic gastritis type (a) is characterized by mucosal atrophy affecting the fundus and the body of the stomach, with antral sparing. In contrast, atrophic gastritis type (b) is characterized by antral mucosal atrophy, with limited involvement of the fundus and body.

AGPAs are found in 20 % of patients with diabetes mellitus type 1 (DMT1). Researchers suggest that patients with DMT1 should be regularly screened for atrophic gastritis. PA is rare found in the general population, with an incidence of 0.1–2 % of the population. On the other hand, patients with DMT1 have a threefold increased incidence of PA, with a prevalence of 2.5–4 %.

Diagnosis is confirmed by detecting AGPA levels in the serum by the Schilling test.

### Signs on Barium Meal

- In a normal double-contrast barium meal examination, the stomach mucosal folds (rugae) are observed arranged in an irregular fashion through the fundus, body, and antrum (◘ Fig. 9.4.15). At the lesser curvature near the pylorus, the mucosal folds become longitudinal and are known as magenstrasse. *Area gastrica* is an area of nodular mucosal elevation located near the antrum ( Fig. 9.4.16).

— In Pernicious anemia, there is a tubular-shaped fundus <8 cm in diameter absent or reduced amount of the normal gastric rugae in the fundus of the body (bald fundus) and small or absent area gastrica ( Fig. 9.4.17).

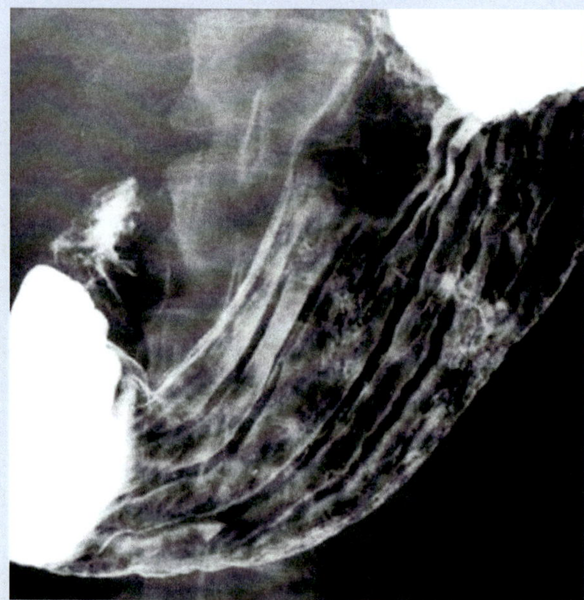

 **Fig. 9.4.15**   Double-contrast barium meal shows the normal configuration of the stomach with the mucosal folds (rugae) nicely demonstrated

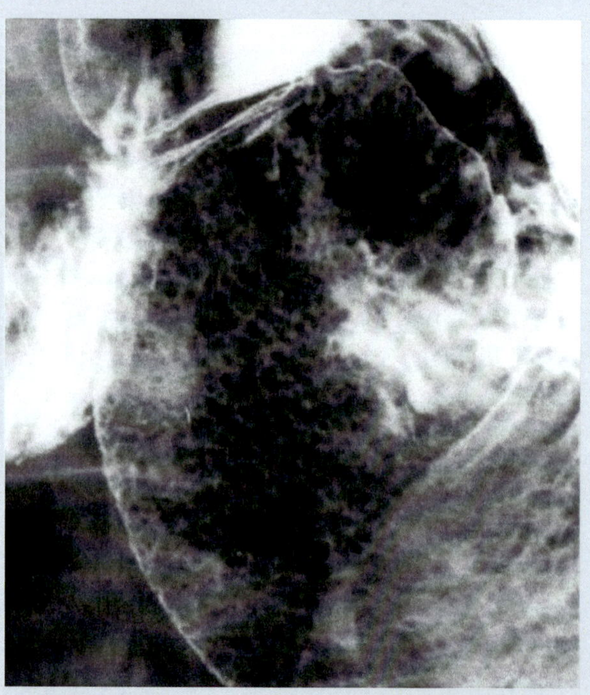

 **Fig. 9.4.16**   Double-contrast barium meal shows area gastrica, seen as an area with nodular mucosal pattern

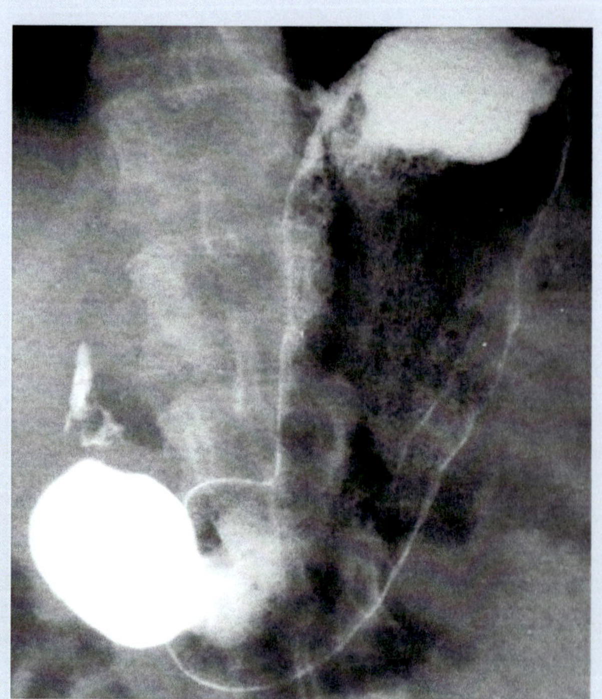

 **Fig. 9.4.17**   Double-contrast barium meal of a patient with pernicious anemia demonstrates severe atrophic gastritis with loss of the normal mucosal folds. Compare this image with  Fig. 9.4.15

## Further Reading

Levine MS, et al. Atrophic gastritis in pernicious anemia: diagnosis by double-contrast radiography. Gastrointest Radiol. 1989;14:215–9.

Tzellos TG, et al. Pernicious anemia in a patient with type 1 diabetes mellitus and alopecia areata universalis. J Diabetes Complications. 2009;23:434–7. doi:10.1016/j.jdiacomp.2008.o5.003.

Vargas JA, et al. Natural killer cell activity in patients with pernicious anemia. Dig Dis Sci. 1995;40:1538–41.

Varis K, et al. An appraisal of tests for severe atrophic gastritis in relatives of patients with pernicious anemia. Dig Dis Sci. 1979;24:187–91.

Wickramasinghe SN. Diagnosis of megaloblastic anemias. Blood Rev. 2006;20:299–318.

## 9.5    Hemophilia

Hemophilia is a rare, chronic X-linked genetic disease, characterized by the body's inability to form clotting factors necessary for the blood clotting cascade to occur, resulting in a tendency toward spontaneous bleeding or bleeding after minor body trauma.

The word *hemo* means bleeding, and the word *philia* means tendency toward something. Patients with hemophilia have a tendency for slow bleeding, at a constant rate and without clotting, into muscles, joint spaces, and body cavities.

Blood clotting is a complicated process that involves three primary steps. The first step involves immediate constriction of the blood vessels in the area of injury. The second step involves the formation of a platelet plug that stops the bleeding. The third step involves the activation of 12 clotting factors (identified by Roman numerals) that transform the platelet plug into a more stable clot by transforming it into fibrin. The activation of clotting factors is referred to as the "clotting cascade," because each factor stimulates the next factor in the series, until the formation of the fibrin. Deficiency of one factor will stop the cascade, and a stable clot will not form.

There are three types of hemophilia:
- *Hemophilia A* results from deficiency of clotting factor VIII, and it is the most common form of hemophilia (80 %). The incidence is 1:10,000 people.
- *Hemophilia B* (*Christmas disease*) results from deficiency of clotting factor IX and constitutes up to 23 % of hemophilia cases. The disease was named after a young boy, Stephen Christmas, who was the first patient identified with this disease. The incidence is 1:40,000 people.
- *Hemophilia C* results from deficiency of clotting factor XI. It is a much rarer form and constitutes less than 2 % of all cases of hemophilia.


Patients with hemophilia are prone to slow, steady, and continuous bleeding after minor trauma. Bleeding can also occur spontaneously without trauma. The most important complications include bleeding into joints (*hemarthrosis*), internal bleeding, intracranial bleeding, and susceptibility from hematological infections due to recurrent blood transfusions.

Bleeding into the joints can occur in any joint, but it commonly affects the knees and the elbows. *Target joint* is a term used in hemophiliacs to indicate a joint with more frequent bleeding than other joints, commonly the knee. The joint synovium is rich in blood vessels, causing it to bleed easily. Multiple bleeding within the joint causes synovium hypertrophy, which later causes articular joint destruction and osteoarthritis. Patients with joint bleeding experience severe pain, due to swelling of the affected joint with stretching of the intra-articular structures by the entrapped blood. Recurrent joint bleeding can stimulate the growth plate, resulting in bony hypertrophy.

Bleeding into the muscles (e.g., the psoas muscle), if not controlled, may lead to muscular swelling, nerve damage, and development of compartment syndrome. *Hemophilic pseudotumor* is a rare complication of hemophilia, occurring in 1–2 % of hemophiliacs. It results from a chronic, encapsulated, slow-growing intramuscular hematoma that displaces the surrounding tissues. Limb enlargement, bone resorption, and muscle and skin necrosis all can be seen in severe cases.

Internal bleeding can be seen as skin bruising, nose bleeding, or blood in the urine (hematuria). Moderate hemophiliacs

may bleed 5–6 times per year. Severe hemophiliacs may have 2–3 bleeding episodes per month.

Intracranial bleeding may occur within the brain parenchyma or within the subarachnoid space. Altered consciousness, headache, nausea, and vomiting in a patient with hemophilia after a minor head injury should be considered intracranial bleeding and investigated with a head CT without delay.

*Myositis ossificans* (*MO*), also known as "Sterner's tumor," is a rare, nonneoplastic condition characterized by formation of bone within muscles. The disease may be hereditary (fibrodysplasia ossificans progressiva, Munchmeyer disease), nontraumatic (e.g., in hemophilia), or traumatic, which is the most common form (e.g., after muscle trauma). The previous classification is applied to intramuscular MO; however, MO can arise against a bone (parosteal MO) or evolve as periostitis (periosteoma).

In the early stages of MO, there are richly vascularized fibroblastic cell proliferations with prominent mitotic activity that mimic malignancy (early pseudosarcomatous phase). As the cells mature, the lesion typically shows three distinct zones. The first zone is composed of rapidly proliferating fibroblasts with areas of hemorrhage and necrosis; the intermediate layer is composed of osteoblasts with osteoid matrix with islands of endochondral ossification; the third outer zone is composed of mature bone, separated from the surrounded tissue by myxoid-fibrous tissue. The peripheral zone usually calcifies at 6–8 weeks after lesion initiation, and complete lesion ossification can be seen 5–6 months from the onset of symptoms. Up to 30 % of lesions regress and resolve spontaneously with maturation.

Patients with MO typically present with painful swelling, commonly in the lower limbs (60–75 % of cases). Patients, especially children, may not recall the incidence of trauma. Diagnostic imaging approach for a patient with painful swelling, with suspicion of MO, should start with conventional radiography, US, CT, and later MRI, as the MRI appearance of MO is generally nonspecific unless the lesion starts to mature. History of trauma is important to suspect MO; however, the absence of history of trauma does not exclude it.

## Differential Diagnoses and Related Diseases

*Von Willebrand's disease* is a bleeding disorder that mimics hemophilia and results from deficiency of von Willebrand factor.

- *Genu recurvatum* is a disabling deformity condition, characterized by hyperextension of the knee to >5°. This deformity may occur in patients with hemophilia after recurrent knee hemarthrosis.
- Hemophilic pseudotumor is seen as an expanding limb with soft-tissue mass and lytic destruction of the bone within the mass. Bones that are often affected by pseudotumors are the femur, tibia, pelvis, and bones of the hands.

- MO is detected classically as bone within areas of soft tissue. The calcification is typically peripheral with a radiolucent center depending on the level of maturation. This pattern of ossification is important to differentiate MO from osteosarcoma, which typically shows a dense center and sunray peripheral edges. The ossification may appear as nonspecific flocculent areas of soft-tissue calcification called "dotted veil pattern" or may characteristically follow the course of muscle fibers (◘ Fig. 9.5.19).

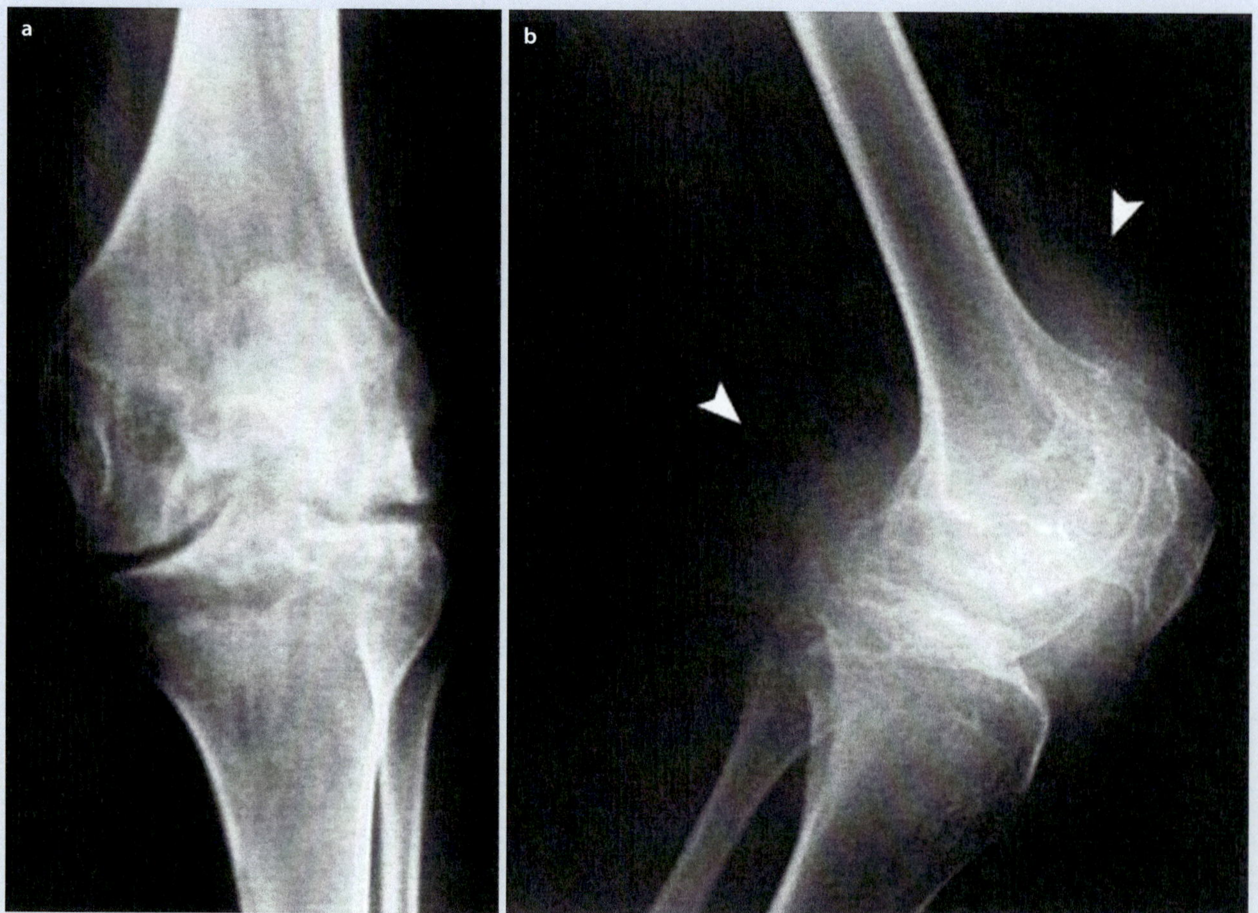

◘ **Fig. 9.5.18** Anteroposterior (**a**) and lateral (**b**) plain knee radiographs in a patient with hemophilic arthropathy. Notice the knee with obvious osteoarthritis, sclerosis, and joint effusion (*arrowheads*)

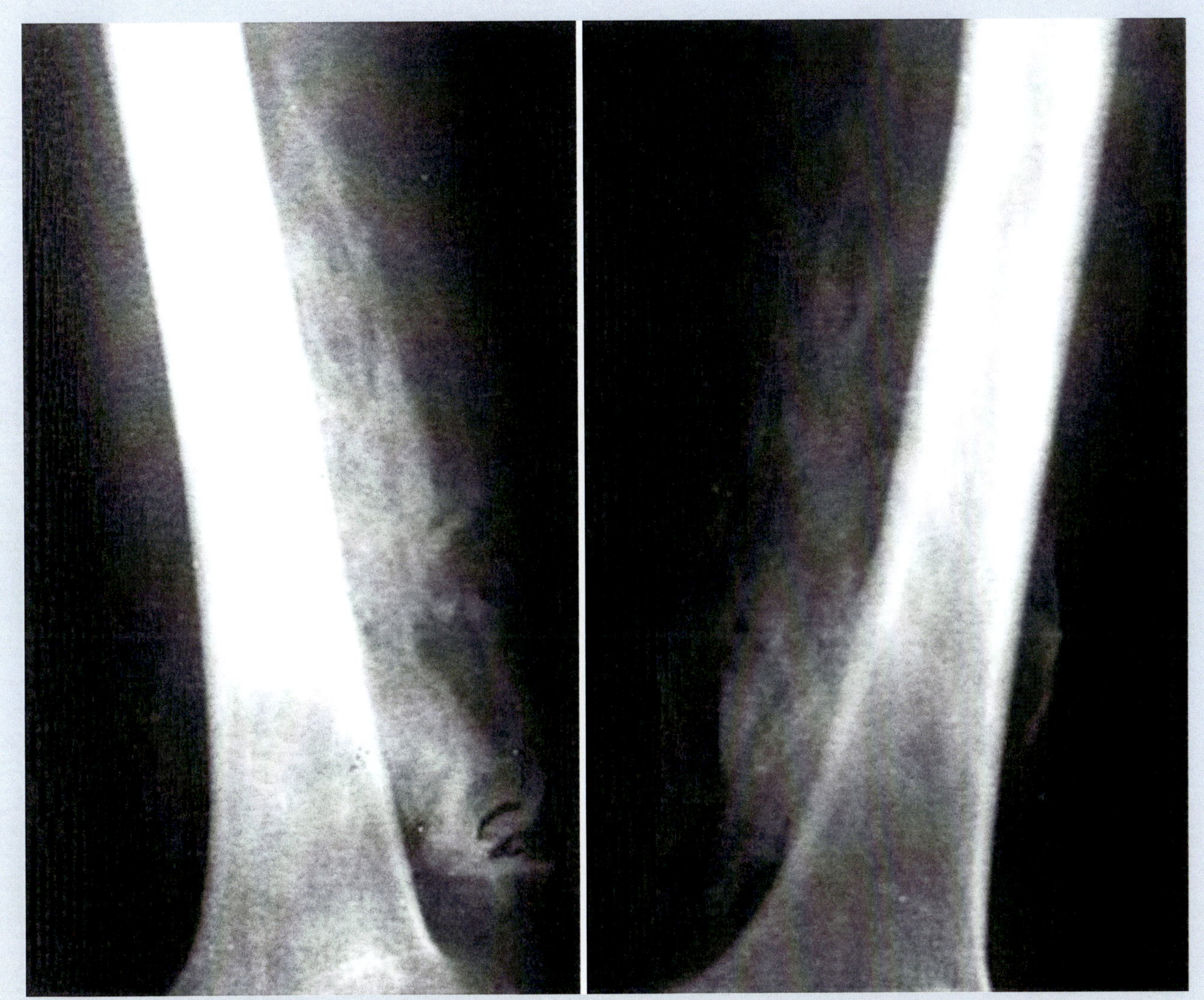

**Fig. 9.5.19** Anteroposterior bilateral radiograph of the legs and distal femur shows bilateral calcification that involved the vastus medialis and the rectus femoris muscles in a patient with myositis ossificans. Notice how the calcification follows the muscle fibers

**Signs on US**

In the early stage of myositis ossificans, the mass is detected as a hypoechoic mass with an outer hypoechoic zone enclosing a broader hyperechoic zone, which again encloses a central hypoechoic zone. After maturation, the outer layer becomes hyperechoic due to ossification.

**Signs on MRI**

- In general, the MRI findings of MO are nonspecific; however, a peripheral rim with low T1 and T2 signal intensities surrounding a heterogeneous intramuscular mass can be a clue for MO. The dark rim represents the calcified peripheral zone. It should be remembered that, at the initial stage, MO resembles musculoskeletal sarcomas, even when a biopsy is done.
- After contrast injection, MO shows peripheral rim enhancement in the early stages, which can lead to mistaking it for an abscess or a necrotic tumor.

## Further Reading

Bae DK, et al. Total knee arthroplasty in hemophilic arthropathy of the knee. J Arthroplasty. 2005;20:664–8. doi:10.1016/j.arth.2005.01.008.

Dauty M. Iliopsoas hematoma in patients with hemophilia: a single-center study. Joint Bone Spine. 2007;74:179–83.

Gindele A, et al. Myositis ossificans traumatica in young children: report of three cases and review of the literature. Pediatr Radiol. 2000;30:451–9.

Gupta AD, et al. Genu recurvatum in hemophilia: a case report. Arch Phys Med Rehabil. 2007;88:791–3.

Hatano H, et al. MR imaging findings of an unusual case of myositis ossificans presenting as progressive mass with features of fluid-fluid level. J Orthop Sci. 2004;9:399–403.

Kovacs CS. Hemophilia, low bone mass, and osteopenia/osteoporosis. Transfus Apher Sci. 2008;38:33–40.

Llauger J, et al. Nonseptic monoarthritis: imaging features with clinical and histopathologic correlation. RadioGraphics. 2000;20:S263–78.

Malhotra R, et al. Elbow arthropathy in hemophilia. Arch Orthop Trauma Surg. 2001;121:152–7.

Nguyen DD, et al. Evaluation and management of hereditary hemophilia in the emergency department. J Emerg Nurs. 2009;35:437–41. doi:10.1016/j.jen.2008.09.009.

Stafford JM, et al. Hemophilic pseudotumor: radiologic-pathologic correlation. Radiographics. 2003;23:852–6.

Yoon KH, et al. Arthroscopic synovectomy in haemophilic arthropathy of the knee. Int Orthop (SICOT). 2005;29:296–300.

## 9.6    Lymphomas

Lymphoma is a disease characterized by malignant transformation of lymphoid cells or other cells native to lymphoid tissues.

Lymphoma can be nodal (affecting lymph nodes) or extranodal (arising from lymphoid tissues within the organs). If left untreated, many lymphomas turn into leukemias. Not every lymphoma transforms into leukemia, but all lymphocytic leukemias are originally lymphomas. Lymphomas are divided into Hodgkin's and non-Hodgkin's diseases.

*Hodgkin's lymphoma (HL)*, also known as *Hodgkin's disease*, constitutes <1 % of all cancers worldwide and is a lymphoma with features of systemic inflammatory disease (33 % of cases). HL is characterized by fever, pruritus, fatigue, and loss of weight. It predominantly affects young men, except in its nodular sclerosis subtype, which predominantly affects young women. HL has a bimodal incidence curve, with the first incident occurring in young adulthood and the second at >50 years of age. HL is diagnosed pathologically based on identification of *Reed-Sternberg cells*, which are multinucleated giant cells with eosinophilic inclusion-like nucleoli. History of previous infection with infectious mononucleosis increases the risk of developing HL by up to three times the normal incidence rate.

*Non-Hodgkin's lymphoma (NHL)* is a diverse group of diseases with almost 40 distinct entities. NHL is divided into two main groups according to the cell of origin: either B-cell neoplasms (precursor B cell) or T-cell neoplasm (precursor T cell). Each type is made up of well-differentiated cells (low-grade lymphomas) or undifferentiated cells (high-grade lymphomas). In general, NHL has a worse prognosis than does HL. *Composite lymphoma* is a term used to describe simultaneous occurrence of two histologically different types of lymphomas situated in one location.

*T-cell lymphomas* are often related to previous viral infection with human T-cell leukemia virus-1 (HTLV-1) and Epstein–Barr virus (EBV). EBV can also be responsible for the development of B-cell lymphomas (e.g., Burkitt's lymphoma). T-cell lymphomas constitute 10–15 % of NHL, and they are commonly present with extranodal manifestations. Lymphomas and tuberculosis are generally more common in immunocompromised people than immunocompetent people.

*Extranodal marginal zone B-cell lymphoma of MALT type (MALToma)* is a form of lymphoma that develops in areas of chronic inflammation or autoimmune diseases. MALT stands for "mucosa-associated lymphoid tissue." This type of NHL is often seen in malignant transformation of chronic or autoimmune diseases like Hashimoto's thyroiditis, Sjögren's syndrome, and chronic gastritis caused by *Helicobacter pylori* infection.

NHL can be further divided into two groups based on growth rate: indolent lymphomas and aggressive lymphomas. Indolent lymphomas are slow-growing and have fewer symptoms (e.g., MALT lymphoma), whereas aggressive lymphomas are rapidly growing with multiple symptoms (e.g., Mantel cell lymphoma).

Gastric lymphoma develops from the neoplastic MALT transformation as a result of long-standing *Helicobacter pylori* gastritis. Intestinal lymphoma develops from Peyer's patches neoplasia. Most cases are seen in the ileum (62.7 %), followed by the jejunum (22 %). Low-grade NHL often presents as polyposis. Salivary gland lymphoma is seen in chronic cases of *sialadenitis* (obstruction of the salivary gland outflow with superimposed infection). Orbital lymphoma can arise due to chronic lachrymal gland inflammation, as in cases of Sjögren's syndrome (primary), or secondary to dissemination. Urinary bladder lymphoma is either primary MALT type or secondary to dissemination. Testes lymphomas are commonly due to disseminated acute lymphoblastic leukemia/lymphoma (ALL). Hepatic lymphoma is commonly secondary to primary lymphoma elsewhere and is associated with poor prognosis. Primary bone lymphomas are seen in <5 % of all bone tumors and commonly seen in male patients above 45 years of age.

Testicular NHL accounts for up to 7 % of all testicular neoplasms and 25–50 % of testicular neoplasms in patients >50 years of age. The testes are affected in <1 % of patients with lymphoma, and it is usually bilateral when it occurs

(40 % of cases). The testes may be the only site involved in NHL in 10 % of cases.

*Childhood lymphoma* is a lymphoma that occurs in a patient <15 years old. In children <15 years old, NHL is more common than HL, while in adults >15 years, HL is more common than NHL. Most childhood lymphomas present with gastrointestinal manifestations. Up to 70 % of childhood Burkitt's lymphoma cases present with an abdominal mass. Intussusception in childhood Burkitt's lymphoma is not uncommon. According to some investigators, childhood lymphoma staging is less important than in adults, because the disease is considered to be disseminated even if the radiological findings suggest localized disease.

## Cotswold Staging of Lymphoma

*Stage I*: involvement of a single lymph node region or lymphoid structure (e.g., spleen) or involvement of a single extralymphatic site

*Stage II*: involvement of two or more lymph node regions on the same site of the diaphragm

*Stage III*: involvement of lymph node regions on both sites of the diaphragm

*Stage IV*: distant metastases with disseminated involvement of one or more extranodal structures

## Criteria for Therapy Response Assessment

*Complete remission*: no signs or symptoms of disease

*Partial remission*: at least 50 % decrease in tumor size

*Stable disease*: neither partial remission nor progressive disease

*Progressive/relapse disease*: at least 50 % increase in disease or new lesions

*Cutaneous T-cell lymphoma (CTCL)* is a group of disorders characterized by proliferation of homing T cell in the skin. Almost all CTCLs have the potential to transform into high-grade T-cell lymphomas. CTCL is divided into mycosis fungoides (MF) CTCL (50 %) and non-MF CTCL.

*Mycosis fungoides (MF)* is a rare form of NHL, characterized by skin patches composed of dermal T-cell infiltrations. The name comes from the first description of this disease, which shows mushroomlike tumors developed on the skin of a patient with advanced disease. There are three common clinical presentations of MF. The first presentation is a skin plaque with hypopigmented and hyperpigmented areas. The second presentation is dermatosis that mimics psoriasis, lichen planus, vitiligo, or atopic dermatitis. The third presentations include pruritus or lichenification. *Lichen planus* is an inflammatory disease characterized by reddish-purple skin lesions that can be very itchy. The name *lichen planus* comes from the word "lichen," which refers to

the plant which grows on rocks or trees, and "planus" means flat.

Diagnosis of MF requires >5 cm skin lesions that show arcuate polymorphic hyperpigmented and hypopigmented areas, with the classical distribution that involves the hip, buttocks, and the inguinal area (bathing suit distribution). The breasts, face, palms, and soles may be affected atypically. Biopsy classically shows Pautrier microabscesses and epidermal lymphocytes larger than dermal lymphocytes.

## Differential Diagnoses and Related Diseases

— *Sézary syndrome* is a rare variant of MF, characterized by a triad of erythroderma, lymphadenopathy, and neoplastic atypical lymphocytes with cerebriform nuclei (Sézary cells) in the peripheral circulation and in the skin infiltrates. *Erythroderma* is defined as diffuse reddish infiltration of the skin that lacks the sharp demarcation from the normal skin as seen in patch or plaque type MF. When erythroderma involves the skin on the face, it can produce markedly exaggerated facial lines producing the finding of "leonine facies" or the face of a lion. Rarely, Sézary syndrome can present with white, vitiligo-like skin lesions, a leukemic variant of MF referred to as *leukoderma*.

— *Pseudolymphoma (anticonvulsant hypersensitivity syndrome)* is a rare drug-induced reaction characterized by an infectious mononucleosis-like reaction that is characterized by fever, rash, lymphadenopathy, hepatitis, and nephritis. Phenytoin is the most common drug to cause this reaction, which is typically seen 3–4 weeks after initiation of therapy. Laboratory investigations often show leukocytosis, eosinophilia, lymphocytosis, positive rheumatoid factor, and anti dsDNA antibodies. Dermal biopsy of the skin eruptions often shows lymphocytic infiltration of the dermis. Rarely, biopsy shows changes that are indistinguishable from MF.

— *Tolosa–Hunt syndrome* is a disease characterized by painful ophthalmoplegia caused by a nonspecific, granulomatous inflammatory condition within the cavernous sinus or the superior orbital fissure. This ophthalmoplegia is attributed to the involvement of the cranial nerves by the inflammatory process. The cavernous sinus contains the cranial nerves (third, fourth, sixth, and the maxillary and ophthalmic divisions of the fifth cranial nerve). Many diseases can infiltrate the cavernous sinus producing ophthalmoplegia; therefore, Tolosa–Hunt syndrome is a diagnosis of exclusion when all other possible pathologies are excluded. Pathologies that can infiltrate the cavernous sinus and cause Tolosa–Hunt syndrome-like symptoms include chondrosarcoma of the bone, lymphoma, metastasis, cavernous sinus thrombosis, and infectious diseases such as aspergillosis.

### Signs on Plain Radiographs

- Bilateral symmetrical hilar lymphadenopathy is a common feature of lymphoma ( Fig. 9.6.20).
- Pleural thickening with malignant effusion can be seen. Malignant effusion is usually massive and caused by lymphatic or venous obstruction.
- Linear interstitial lung pattern is noticed more in HL than in NHL patients, due to lymphangitis carcinomatosis.
- Bone lymphomas are classically seen as metaphyseal osteolytic lesions with a permeative appearance and layered (onion skin) periostitis.
- Complete sclerosis of the vertebral body (ivory vertebra) can be seen in cases of vertebral body infiltration by lymphoma ( Fig. 9.6.21).

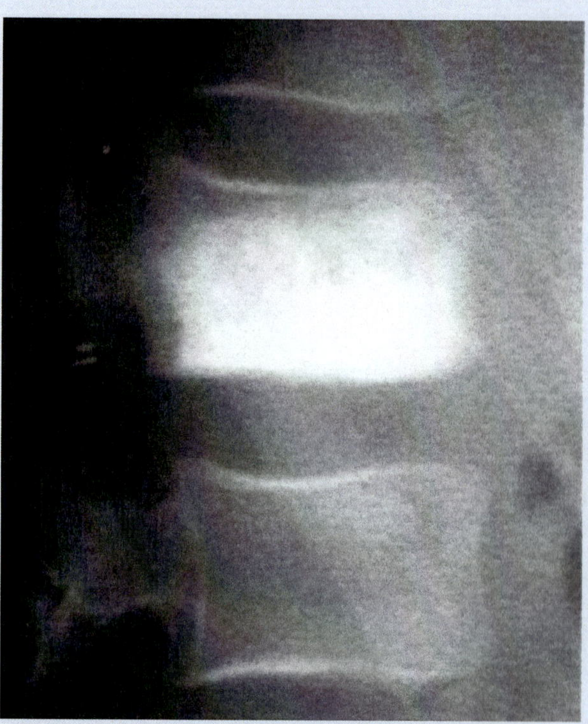

 **Fig. 9.6.21**   Lateral plain thoracic vertebral radiograph shows complete sclerosis of a single vertebra (ivory vertebra). The differential diagnosis of ivory vertebra includes lymphoma infiltrating the vertebral body, Paget's disease, and metastases infiltrating the vertebral body

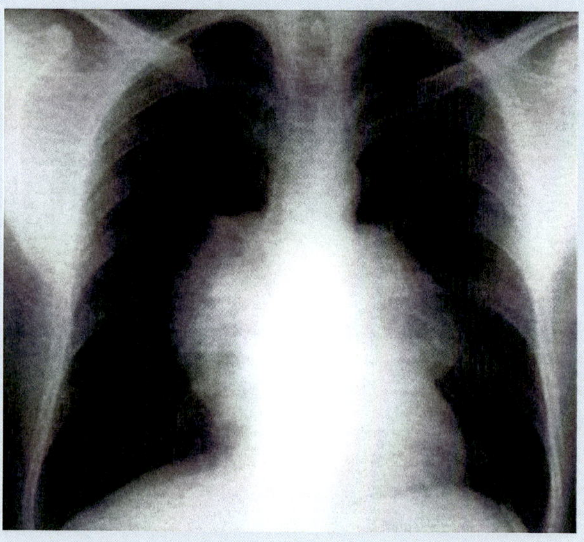

 **Fig. 9.6.20**   Posteroanterior plain chest radiograph of a patient with NHL shows bilateral enlarged, potato-like hilar lymphadenopathy

### Signs on US

- Lymphoma of the spleen appears as splenomegaly or multiple focal splenic parenchymal lesions. US is more sensitive than CT in detecting splenic lesions in lymphoma. The majority of the lymphoma's foci are hypoechoic compared to the normal splenic tissue. Only 6 % of lymphomas show hyperechoic lesions.
- Intestinal lymphoma (e.g., Burkitt's lymphoma) is visualized as thickened, ringlike bowel loops with a "doughnut sign" on axial sections. A layered, thickened wall is often demonstrated, with the outer hypoechoic layer corresponding to the bowel wall layers and an inner hyperechoic layer due to intraluminal air or mucus.
- Testicular lymphoma is detected as hypoechoic, focal, or diffusely enlarged testes with a preserved oval shape. Intratesticular hemorrhage, necrosis, and calcification are rare. Extension to the epididymis and the spermatic cord is common (60 % of cases). The same sonographic picture can be seen in infiltrative hematologic neoplasms such as leukemia and (rarely) plasmacytoma.

- **Signs on CT**
- More than 80 % of patients with HL present with cervical and hilar lymphadenopathy. Involvement of the Waldeyer's ring is common (50 % of cases). The Waldeyer's ring is an anatomical ring of lymphoid composed of the pharyngeal tonsils, palatine tonsils, lingual tonsils, and tubal tonsils (◘ Fig. 9.6.22). It is located at the back of the oral cavity and the pharynx. A lymphoma is considered extranodal when its main bulk of disease is located at an extranodal site.
- Splenomegaly (30 % in HL and 70 % in NHL). Focal splenic lesions <1 cm are common in HL, whereas large focal splenic lesions are more commonly seen in NHL. The lesions are isodense to the normal splenic tissue density on noncontrast-enhanced CT. After contrast injection, the lesions appear hypodense compared to the normal contrast-enhanced splenic tissues. Infarction of the spleen is a rare complication of lymphoma and can typically be seen as a hypodense, peripheral, wedge-shaped area with no contrast enhancement. Lymphoma infiltrates the splenic white pulp follicles (Malpighian corpuscles).
- *Orbital lymphoma*: a lymphoma usually present as a well-defined, soft-tissue mass within the orbit that may involve the lachrymal glands, the retrobulbar fat, or the muscles. Moreover, the soft-tissue mass has a tendency to coat the globe. The mass enhances homogenously after contrast injection. Orbital muscles will be diffusely enlarged with their tendons when infiltrated (lymphoma commonly involves the superior rectus muscle).
- In the *kidneys*, lymphomas can present as solitary or multiple hypodense solid masses (60 %) with homogenous contrast enhancement. In 20 % of cases, lymphoma can present with diffuse renal infiltration that causes nephromegaly without renal distortion. Retroperitoneal lymphadenopathy is commonly found, and it is a useful clue to lymphoma (◘ Fig. 9.6.23). After contrast administration, lymphoma enhances homogenously, but always lower than the normal renal parenchyma (◘ Fig. 9.6.24).

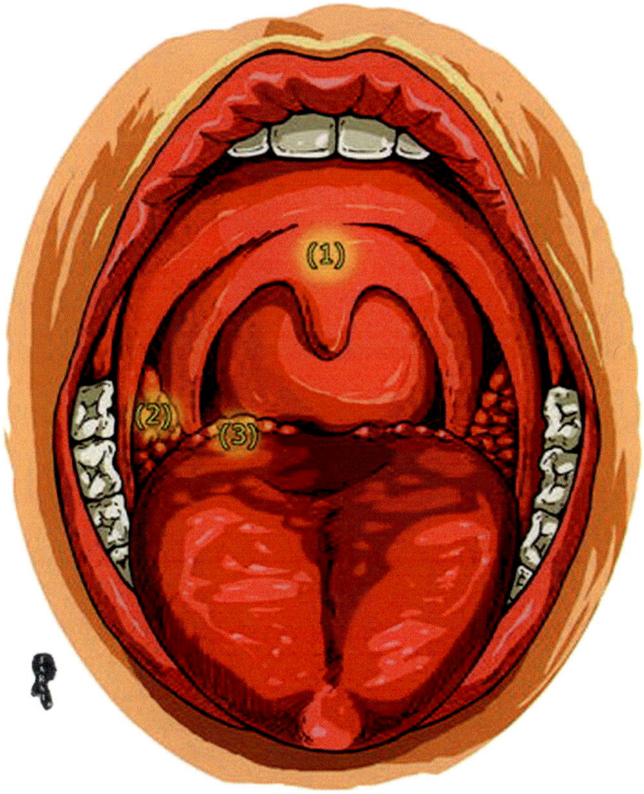

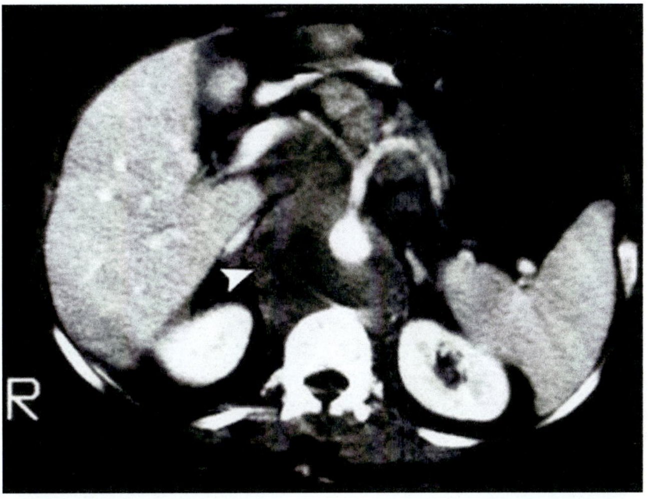

◘ **Fig. 9.6.23** Axial postcontrast CT of a patient with retroperitoneal lymphoma shows a homogenous hypodense mass surrounding the aorta (*arrowhead*)

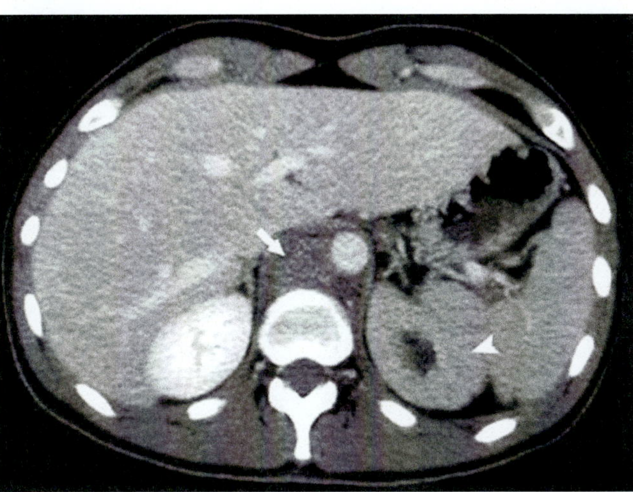

◘ **Fig. 9.6.24** Axial postcontrast CT of a patient with left renal lymphoma shows renal contrast enhancement (*arrowhead*) that is less than the normal right kidney enhancement due to diffuse parenchymal infiltration of the left kidney by lymphoma. Notice the enlarged retroperitoneal para-aortic lymph nodes, which are a good clue for lymphoma (*arrow*)

◘ **Fig. 9.6.22** An illustration of the mouth cavity demonstrates the region of the lymphatic components of Waldeyer's ring: (*1*) pharyngeal tonsils (behind the soft palate), (*2*) palatine tonsils, and (*3*) lingual tonsils

- In the *central nervous system*, lymphomas can present as solitary or multiple supratentorial lesions with hyperdense attenuation on noncontrast-enhanced CT. This native CT hyperdensity is attributed to the highly packed malignant cells within the lesion. After contrast injection, lymphomas show homogenous contrast enhancement (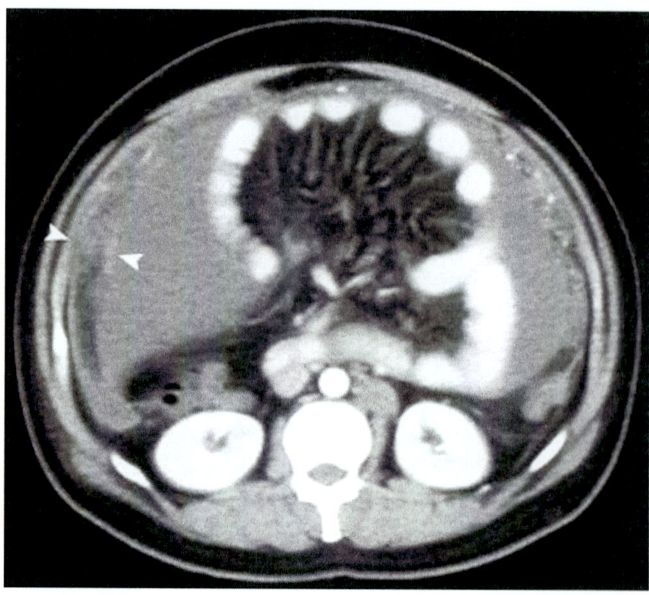 Fig. 9.6.25). Lymphoma does not show calcification unless treated, and it can cross from one hemisphere to the other via the corpus callosum in a butterfly pattern resembling glioblastoma multiforme. Moreover, CNS lymphoma shows minimal brain edema and no mass effect over the adjacent structures. In immunocompromised patients, lymphoma grows fast and can have central necrosis with ring enhancement mimicking a brain abscess.
- *Omental or peritoneal lymphoma* usually presents with diffusely thickened peritoneum and thickened omentum with contrast enhancement (omental cake sign). This presentation can be seen in abdominal manifestations of tuberculosis, especially in immunocompromised patients. The presence of abdominal septations near the thickened peritoneum favors tuberculosis over lymphoma (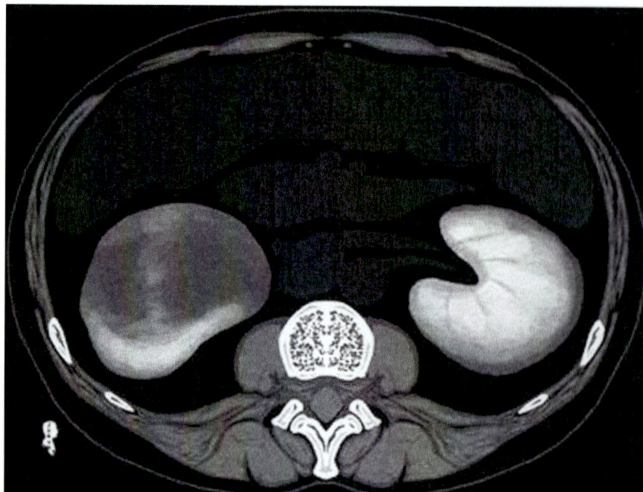 Fig. 9.6.26).
- *Faceless kidney* is an uncommon feature of lymphoma where the renal parenchyma is diffusely infiltrated by lymphoma while lacking its typical familiar features of the central renal sinus structures (◘ Fig. 9.6.27).

**Fig. 9.6.26** Axial postcontrast abdominal CT of a patient with TB peritonitis shows thickened peritoneum and enhanced omentum (*arrowheads*) representing the "omental cake sign," with massive abdominal ascites. The same radiological picture can be caused by lymphoma

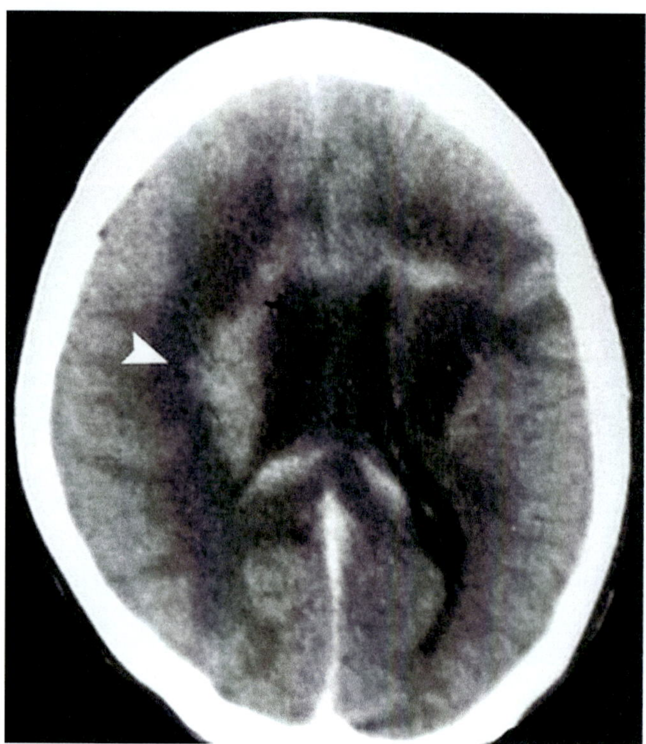

**Fig. 9.6.25** Axial postcontrast brain CT of a patient with CNS lymphoma shows right-sided homogenously-enhanced sub-ependymal mass (*arrowhead*)

**Fig. 9.6.27** Axial postcontrast abdominal CT illustration demonstrates right faceless kidney

**Signs on MRI**
- Brain lymphoma often shows hypointense T1 signal intensity and slightly hypointense signal intensity on T2W images. This again is attributed to the highly packed cells within the tumor.
- Orbital lymphoma shows low T1 signal intensity, relatively hypointense on T2W images, with moderate contrast enhancement (◘ Fig. 9.6.28).
- The classical *Tolosa–Hunt syndrome* shows a nonspecific mass lesion within the cavernous sinus that enhances mildly after contrast enhancement (◘ Fig. 9.6.29). The lesion shrinks in size after therapy is initiated.

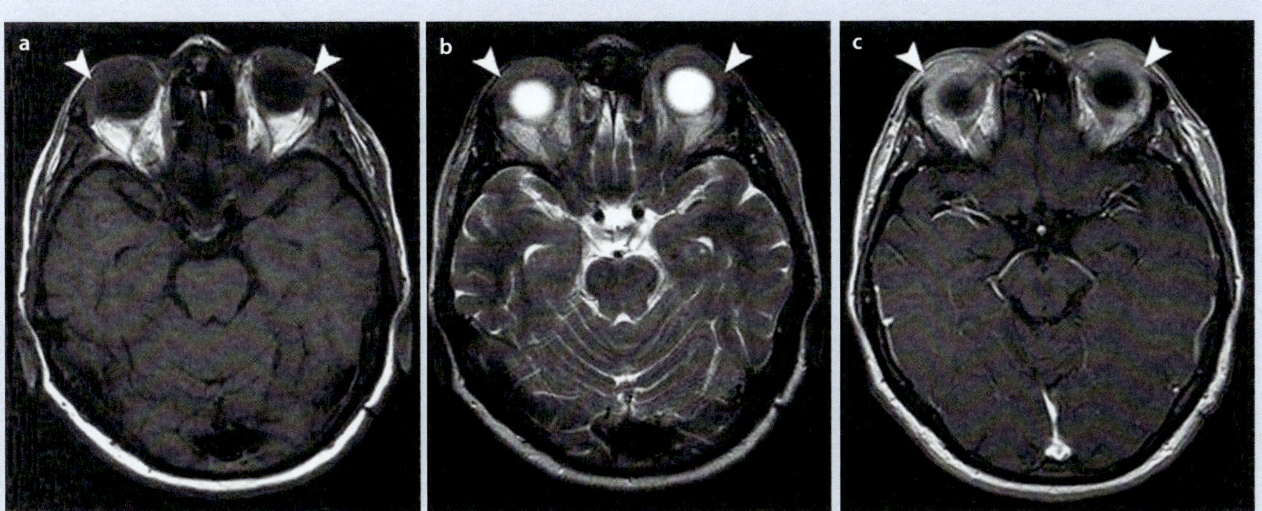

■ **Fig. 9.6.28** Axial T1W (**a**), T2W (**b**), and T1W postcontrast MRI of a patient with orbital lymphoma shows bilateral hypointense T1, relatively hypointense T2 lesions with homogenous contrast enhancement on postcontrast image in (**c**) (*arrowheads*). Notice how the lymphoma tends to coat the globe

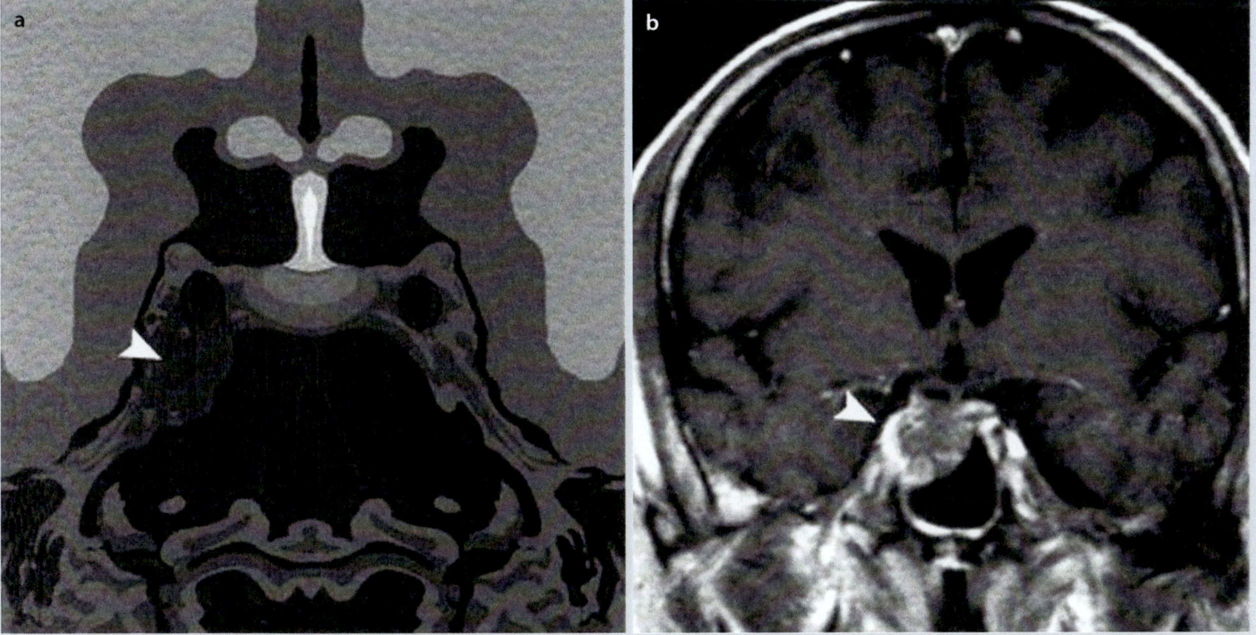

■ **Fig. 9.6.29** Coronal native T1W magnified MR illustration of the cavernous sinus (**a**) and T1W postcontrast sellar mass on MRI show Tolosa-Hunt syndrome. In (**a**), the right cavernous sinus is infiltrated by an inflammatory mass, which often affects the cranial nerves resulting in ophthalmoplegia. In (**b**), brain lymphoma infiltrating the right cavernous sinus resulting in a Tolosa-Hunt syndrome such as ophthalmoplegia (*arrowheads*)

## Further Reading

Bhatia K, et al. Lymphoma of the spleen. Semin Ultrasound CT MRI. 2007;28:12–20.

Chua SC, et al. Imaging features of primary extranodal lymphomas. Clin Radiol. 2009;64:574–88. doi:10.1016/j.crad.2008.11.001.

Dyer RB, et al. Classic signs in uroradiology. Radiographics. 2004;24:S247–80.

Hinds GA, et al. Cutaneous T-cell lymphoma in skin of color. J Am Acad Dermatol. 2009;60:359–75.

Jacobs P. Hodgkin's disease and the malignant lymphomas. Dis Mon. 1993;39:217–97.

Karaosmanoglu D, et al. CT findings of lymphoma with peritoneal, omental and mesenteric involvement: peritoneal lymphomatosis. Eur J Radiol. 2008;71:313–7. doi:10.1016/j.ejrad.2008.04.012.

Mengiardi B, et al. Primary lymphoma of bone: MRI and CT characteristics during and after successful treatment. AJR Am J Roentgenol. 2005;184:185–92.

Naik KS, et al. Staging lymphoma with CT: comparison of contiguous and alternate 10 mm slice techniques. Clin Radiol. 1998;53:523–7.

Nathan DL, et al. Carbamazepine-induced pseudolymphoma with CD-30 positive cells. J Am Acad Dermatol. 1998;38:806–9.

Panda S. Mycosis fungoides: current trends in diagnosis and management. Indian J Dermatol. 2007;52:5–20.

Rademaker J. Hodgkin's and non-Hodgkin's lymphomas. Radiol Clin North Am. 2007;45:69–83.

Turner RB, et al. Anticonvulsant hypersensitivity syndrome associated with bellamine S, a therapy for menopausal symptoms. J Am Acad Dermatol. 2004;50:S86–9.

Weissman DE, et al. A case of large cell CNS lymphoma associated with a systemic small cell lymphocytic lymphoma. J Neuro Oncol. 1990;9:171–5.

## 9.7    Leukemia

The bone marrow manufactures the white blood cells (myeloid tissues) and the lymphocytes (lymphoid tissues), but the majority of bone marrow is myeloid tissue. Leukemia is a term used to describe a group of malignancies of either lymphoid or myeloid origin, which are characterized by malignant transformation of the leukocyte-forming tissue. The bone marrow is diffusely infiltrated with the leukemic cells that often inhibit the normal hematopoietic cell proliferation and development. Leukemias represent 30 % of malignancies diagnosed in children <15 years and 25 % in young adults <20 years.

If the leukemia is myeloid in origin, it will involve the myeloid tissue mainly (e.g., bone marrow), whereas if leukemia started in the lymphoid tissue, it will involve both the lymph nodes and the bone marrow lymphoid tissue. Lymphadenopathy in leukemia is seen when the leukemia is lymphocytic in origin or the leukemic patient develops lymphoma.

Leukemia is described as "acute" when the malignant cells are immature blasts with a rapid cell proliferation rate. In contrast, leukemia is described as "chronic" when the malignant cells are more mature than those of acute leukemias. Chronic leukemias have a less devastating clinical course than do acute leukemias, but they are less responsive to treatment in comparison with acute leukemias.

### Acute Lymphoblastic Leukemia

Acute lymphoblastic leukemia (ALL) is characterized by proliferation and predominance of lymphoblasts in the blood circulation and in the bone marrow. ALL is the most common type of leukemia (80 %), and it has a sharp peak incidence among children 2–3 years old, which decreases by the age of 8–10 years.

Patients with leukemia classically present with fatigue, pallor, anemia, sneezing blood (epistaxis), and bruising easily (ecchymosis). Lymphadenopathy is seen in 50 % of patients, and bone pain is a common complaint due to bone marrow stretching and expansion by the infiltrating leukemic cells. Cough and respiratory symptoms that mimic pneumonia may be seen in cases of mediastinal infiltration. Uncommonly, ALL can present as an isolated testicular mass.

Laboratory investigation shows anemia, thrombocytopenia, and pancytopenia. Diagnosis is essentially established by bone marrow biopsy. The presence of more than 25 % blasts in the bone marrow is diagnostic of acute leukemia. Cerebrospinal fluid analysis by lumbar puncture is often included in the diagnostic workup to exclude central nervous system (CNS) infiltration. In boys with ALL, testicular ultrasound should be performed to exclude testicular enlargement.

*Aleukemic leukemia* is a term used to describe leukemia where the malignant blasts are not found in the peripheral blood.

### Acute Myeloblastic Leukemia

Acute myeloblastic leukemia (AML) is characterized by predominance of myeloblasts and promyelocytes in the blood circulation and in the bone marrow. AML has a high incidence rate within the first 2 years of life, thereafter decreasing in incidence with a nadir at 9 years of age and then a slow increase in incidence again during adulthood. AML is often seen in adults.

Patients present with classical symptoms as ALL. *Congenital AML* is leukemia that present in the first few years of life, often with skin infiltration (*leukemia cutis*). There is a high incidence of AML in children with Down's syndrome. AML is characterized by extramedullary manifestation called chloroma. *Chloroma (granulocytic sarcoma)* is a solid soft-tissue mass of leukemic cells that occurs anywhere in the body, and it represents extramedullary myeloblastic leukemia. The name is derived from the Greek word *chloros* meaning green, due to the green hue that these tumors demonstrate on gross specimens. The green color is due to the increase levels of the enzyme myeloperoxidase in the tumor cells.

Chloromas are rare, occurring in 2.5 % of AML cases and mostly in children <15 years of age (60 %). A chloroma can be the primary presentation of AML, and the classic leukemia develops later (up to 2 years). Most cases of chloromas are seen in the head and neck region. However, any part of the body can be affected. Diagnosis of chloroma is essentially established by biopsy. Recurrence rate after excision is up to 23 %.

*Hyperleukocytosis syndrome* is an uncommon condition that is seen in AML and (rarely) ALL due to increased white blood cell count (>100,000/µL), which will lead to sludging of the leukemic blasts in tissue microvasculature. Patients present with neurologic or pulmonary manifestations due to blockage of the microcirculation by the leukemic cells.

*Tumor lysis syndrome* is another clinical condition commonly seen in patients with AML due to rapid tumor cell death and release of the intracellular contents into the circulation. Patients present with hyperkalemia, hyperuricemia, and secondary uric acid nephropathy and acute renal failure.

## Differential Diagnoses and Related Diseases

- Shwachman–Diamond syndrome (SDS) is an autosomal recessive disorder of infancy, characterized by exocrine pancreas insufficiency, metaphyseal dysostosis (50 %), and bone marrow dysfunction. The bone marrow dysfunction results in neutropenia (the most constant feature) and occasionally in pancytopenia (10–25 %). Most infant deaths in the first year of life are due to recurrent bacterial infections. There is increased risk of leukemic transformation in these patients. SDS is the second most common cause of exocrine pancreatic insufficiency in children, after cystic fibrosis.
- Bloom syndrome is a rare autosomal recessive disease characterized by a triad of lupus-like erythematous telangiectasias of the face, stunted growth with dwarfism, and sun sensitivity. Other manifestations include characteristic facies, immunodeficiency, azoospermia and infertility in men and subfertility in women, and well-circumscribed dermal hypo- and hyperpigmentation. The major complications in Bloom syndrome include the development of different kinds of cancers, late-onset diabetes mellitus, and chronic lung disease. The most common cancers that arise in patient with Bloom syndrome are leukemia, lymphoma, and Wilm's tumor.

## Chronic Lymphocytic Leukemia

Chronic lymphocytic leukemia (CLL) is characterized by proliferation of lymphoid cells, almost always B cells.

CLL primarily affects adults between 65 and 70 years of age. Up to 50 % of patients are asymptomatic at presentation, and the disease is incidentally discovered following a routine blood investigation. Symptomatic presentations include autoimmune hemolytic anemia, lymphadenopathy, and hepatosplenomegaly. Diagnosis is essentially established by bone marrow biopsy and immunophenotyping.

## Differential Diagnoses and Related Diseases

Richter's syndrome is a type of lymphoma that occurs in a patient with CLL who develops large-cell lymphoma (leukemia transforms into lymphoma). It is seen in 5–10 % of CLL cases, and the survival rate is very short (2–8 months).

## Chronic Myelogenous Leukemia

Chronic myelogenous leukemia (CML) is characterized by leukemia that arises from chromosomal translocation between chromosome 9 and 22 (Philadelphia chromosome), generating an aberrant tyrosine kinase. The aberrant tyrosine kinase fuels proliferation of a malignant clone of myeloid cells.

Up to 50 % of CML cases are diagnosed incidentally. Patients are between 40 and 60 years of age and present with malaise, weight loss, and splenomegaly. Laboratory investigations show neutrophil leukocytosis with basophilia and occasional eosinophilia. Diagnosis is essentially established by bone marrow biopsy and immunophenotyping.

In CML, the peripheral blood shows marked leukocytosis. Differential diagnosis of such leukocytosis includes a reactive, nonneoplastic peripheral blood leukocytosis due to an infection (e.g., infectious mononucleosis). This infectious, reactive, nonneoplastic leukocytosis is sometimes referred to as *leukemoid reaction.*

In all types of leukemia, chemotherapy and immunosuppressive medications are used for therapy. Brain toxicity from cytotoxic agents such as methotrexate is a common complication of the medication, because methotrexate is capable of crossing the blood–brain barrier. In patients treated for leukemia, methotrexate can induce diffuse white matter lesions with demyelination and necrosis (leukoencephalopathy). *Disseminated necrotizing leukoencephalopathy* is a fatal complication of methotrexate, characterized by multifocal areas of white matter necrosis. An insult to the tissue microvasculature and oligodendrocytes are the most likely mechanisms of injury to explain this condition. Hyperviscosity from the cytotoxic medications can lead to dural sinus thrombosis.

### Signs on Plain Radiographs
- Leukemic infiltration of the bone often presents with osteopenia and linear bands of osteoporosis, observed mainly in the metaphyses of long bones (leukemic lines). However, leukemic lines can be seen normally in neonates.
- Chloroma of the bones is seen as pure lytic lesions affecting the sacrum, cranium, sternum, ribs, and spine. The lesions are typically located in the subperiosteal areas and progress internally.

### Signs on CT
- Chloroma is commonly found in the head and neck region as a solid mass with density similar to the skeletal muscle, and the mass shows homogenous contrast enhancement. Regional lymphadenopathy is commonly found (◘ Fig. 9.7.30). If the bone is affected, lytic rather than sclerotic lesions are demonstrated.

- CNS chloroma is seen as an intermediate to hyperdense lesion (60–80 HU), with typically homogenous enhancement after contrast injection (nonspecific pattern). Mild to moderate hypervascularity can be seen on CT angiography.
- Small parenchymal brain calcifications can be seen after episodes of intracranial radiation therapy.

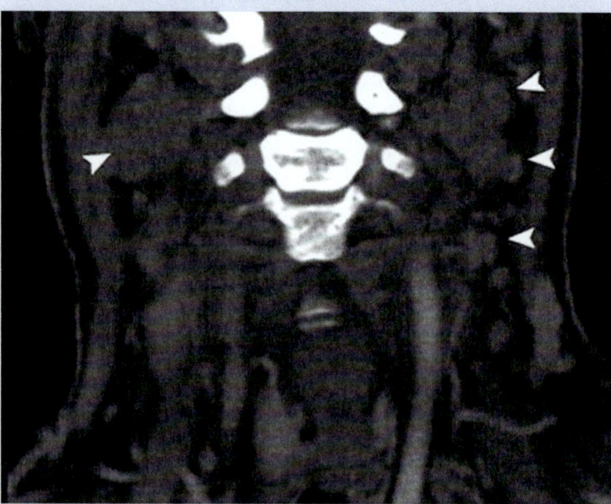

**◘ Fig. 9.7.30**　Coronal postcontrast neck CT of a patient with neck chloroma shows bilateral lymphadenopathy (*arrowheads*)

**Signs on MRI**

- Diffuse vertebral bone marrow leukemic infiltration results in low signal intensity of the vertebral bodies in relation to the intervertebral disks (*bright disk sign*) (◘ Fig. 9.7.31). Hematopoietically active marrow is referred to as "red marrow." Red marrow is composed of water (40 %), fat (40 %), and proteins (20 %). In contrast, hematopoietically inactive marrow is referred to as "yellow marrow." Yellow marrow is composed of fat (80 %), water (15 %), and proteins (5 %). The normal yellow marrow is hyperintense on T1W images. Normal red marrow is generally hypointense on MRI compared to yellow marrow, but its signal is generally greater than that of muscle. It is perhaps difficult to distinguish red marrow from infiltrative marrow processes. Infiltrative bone marrow pathology is any pathology that replaces the normal bone marrow contents. This pathological process can be diffuse or focal; neoplastic disease (e.g., leukemia) represents the most common etiology for vertebral bone marrow infiltration.
- *CNS chloroma* shows low T1 and high T2 signal intensities with marked homogenous enhancement after contrast injection (◘ Fig. 9.7.32).
- *Methotrexate leukoencephalopathy* is seen as areas of high signal intensities with no contrast enhancement after contrast injection (◘ Fig. 9.7.33).
- In *disseminated necrotizing leukoencephalopathy*, there are multiple areas of high T2 signal intensities with small irregular low T2 signal foci due to coagulative necrosis. The small low T2 signal foci show enhancement after contrast injection.
- *Superior sagittal sinus thrombosis* is seen as a triangular filling defect on sagittal images (*empty delta sign*). Sinus thrombosis can also be seen on T2W images as a hyperintense vessel (◘ Fig. 9.7.34). The vessel loses its void signal and appears clearly due to the thrombosed intravascular blood. The thrombus can show contrast enhancement if it is old and organized.

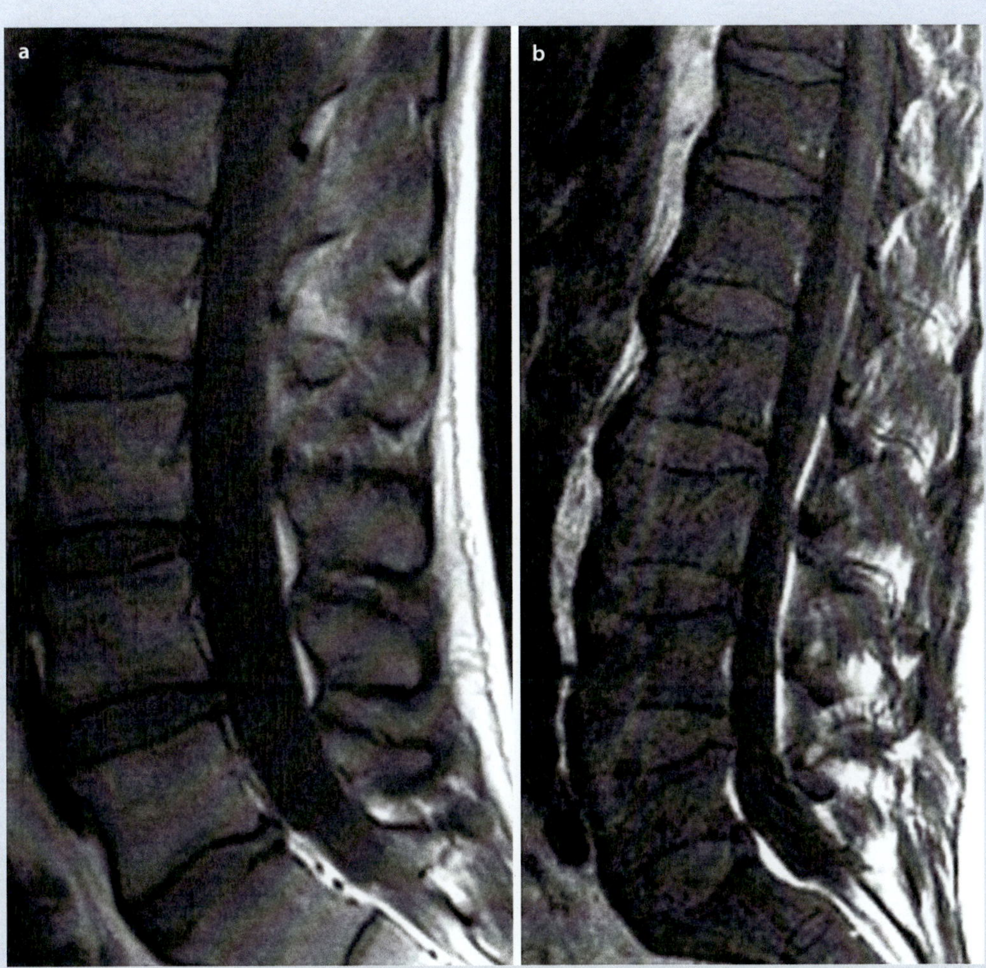

**Fig. 9.7.31** Sagittal T1W thoracolumbar MRI in a normal patient (**a**) and a patient with leukemia, with diffuse vertebral bone marrow infiltration, shows the classic bright disk sign in (**b**). Notice how the vertebral body shows higher signal intensity than the intervertebral disk in (**a**) due to the presence of yellow marrow. In (**b**), the vertebral body shows lower signal intensity than the intervertebral disk, which is described as the bright disk sign

9

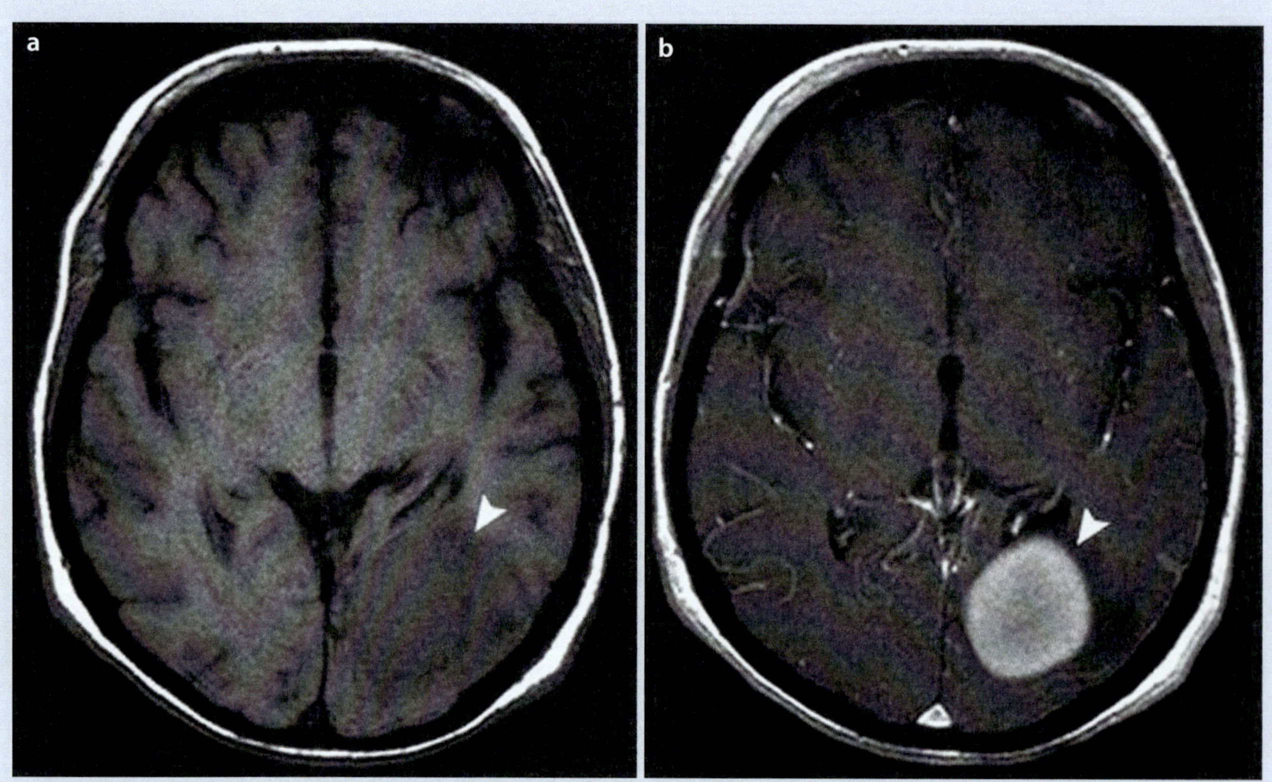

**Fig. 9.7.32** Axial native T1W (**a**) and T1W postcontrast (**b**) brain MRI of a patient with biopsy-proved chloroma shows a large occipital mass with a relatively hypointense signal on the left of the T1W image, with homogenous marked enhancement (*arrowheads*)

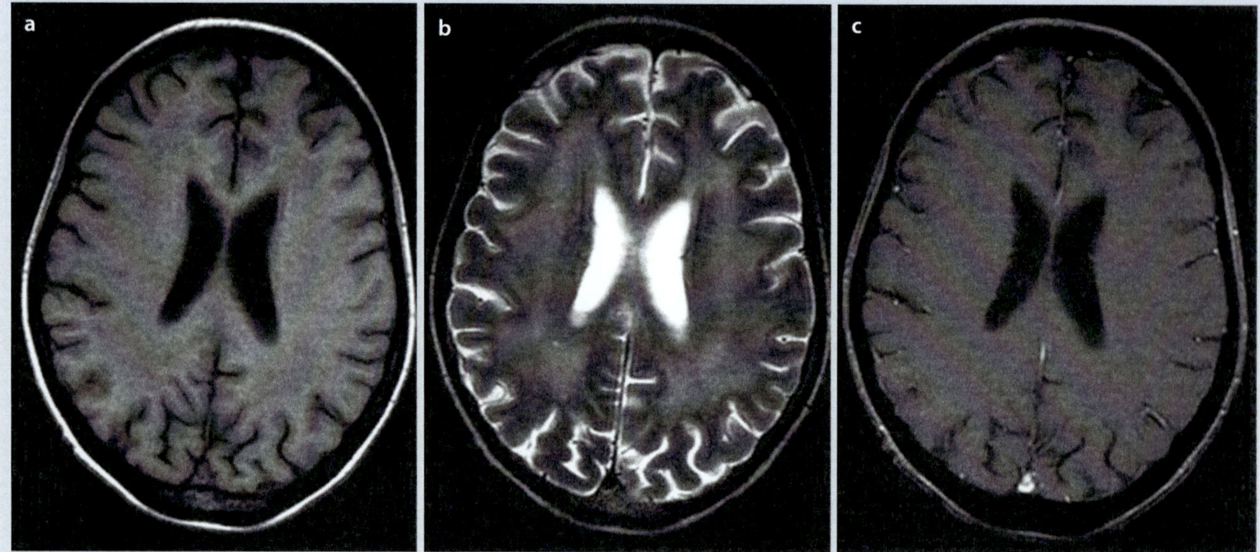

**Fig. 9.7.33** Axial T1W (**a**), T2W (**b**), and T1W postcontrast brain MRI of a patient with ALL treated with methotrexate show diffuse leukoencephalopathy of the centrum semi-ovale bilaterally (**b**), with no contrast enhancement in (**c**)

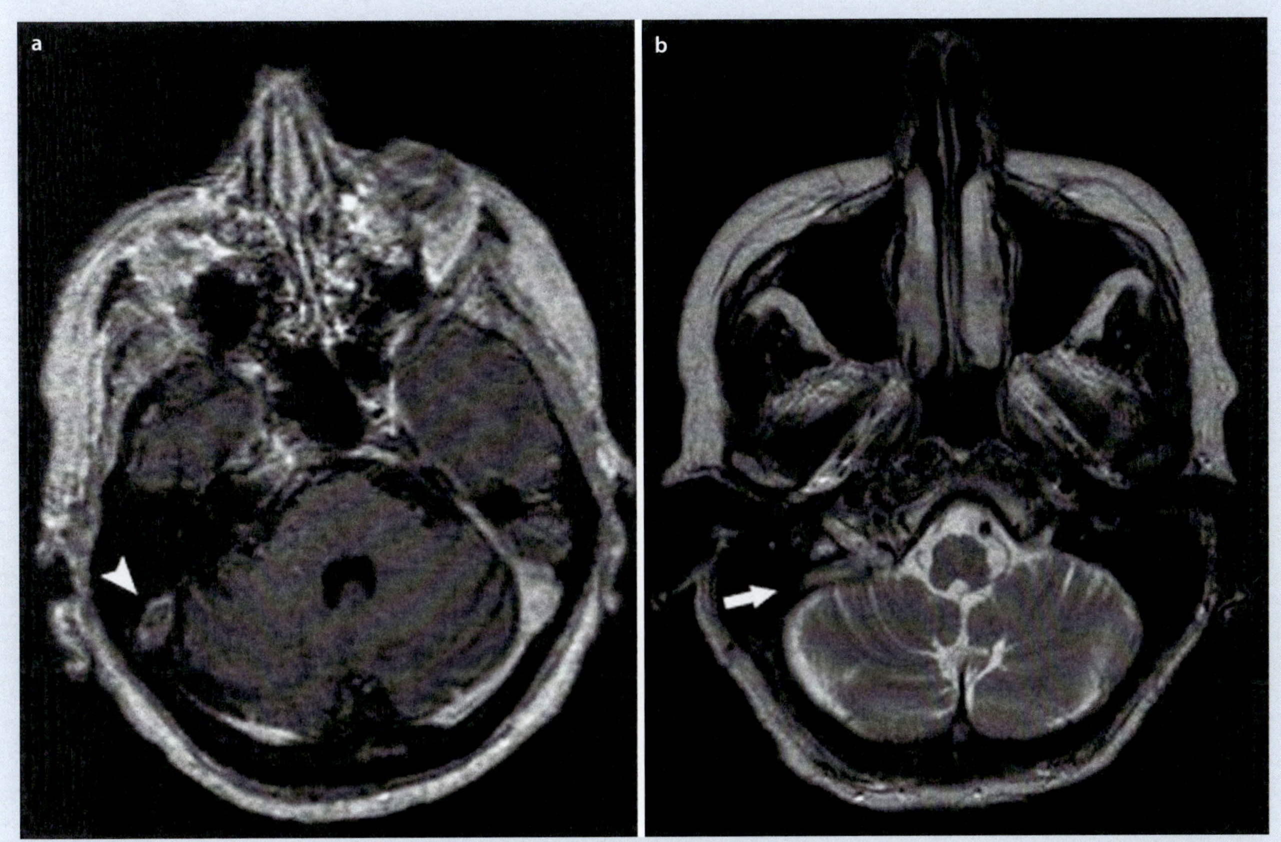

**Fig. 9.7.34** Axial T1W postcontrast (**a**) and T2W (**b**) brain MRI of a patient with ALL treated with chemotherapy, who developed right transverse sinus thrombosis, show filling defect in (**a**) (*arrowhead*), and hyperintense vessel in (**b**) due to the intravascular thrombus (*arrow*)

## Further Reading

Alkubaidan FO, et al. Granulocytic sarcoma (chloroma) of the shoulder in Shwachman-Diamond syndrome. Eur J Radiol Extra. 2007;64:107–10.

Carroll KW, et al. Useful internal standards for distinguishing infiltrative marrow pathology from hematopoietic marrow at MRI. J Magn Reson Imaging. 1997;7:394–8.

Cretzula JC, et al. Bloom's syndrome. J Am Acad Dermatol. 1987;17:479–88.

Enright H, et al. Chronic leukemias. Dis Mon. 2008;54: 242–55.

Faber J, et al. Shwachman-diamond syndrome: early bone marrow transplantation in a high risk patient and new clues to pathogenesis. Eur J Pediatr. 1999;158:995–1000.

Frohna BJ, et al. Granulocytic sarcoma (chloroma) causing spinal cord compression. Neuroradiology. 1993;35:509–11.

Hermann G, et al. Skeletal manifestations of granulocytic sarcoma (chloroma). Skeletal Radiol. 1991;20:509–12.

Jacobs P. Myelodysplasia and leukemias. Dis Mon. 1997;43:505.

Jain D, et al. Bloom syndrome in sibs: first report of hepatocellular carcinoma and Wilms tumor with documented anaplasia and nephrogenic rests. Pediatr Dev Pathol. 2001;4:585–9.

Kolitz JE. Acute leukemia in adults. Dis Mon. 2008;54: 226–41.

Laningham FH, et al. Childhood central nervous system leukemia: historical perspectives, current therapy, and acute neurological sequelae. Neuroradiology. 2007;49: 873–88.

Lee YH, et al. Granulocytic sarcoma (chloroma) presenting as a lateral neck mass: initial manifestation of leukemia: a case report. Eur Arch Otorhinolaryngol. 2006;263:16–8.

O'Brien MM, et al. Acute leukemia in children. Dis Mon. 2008a;54:202–25.

O'Brien J, et al. An unusual cause of persistent headache: chloroma (2008:2b). Eur Radiol. 2008b;18:1071–2.

Pande AR, et al. Disseminated necrotizing leukoencephalopathy following chemoradiation therapy for acute lymphoblastic leukemia. Radiat Med. 2006;24:515–9.

## 9.8    **Multiple Myeloma (Kahler's Disease)**

Multiple myeloma (MM) is a malignant disease characterized by neoplastic proliferation of plasma cell precursors in the bone marrow. The disease can arise diffusely or focally in any region in the body. The focal form of multiple myeloma is called *plasmacytoma*. MM is a disease of older age groups and typically found in patients between 40 and 70 years of age.

The cardinal features of MM are osteolytic lesions found on plain X-rays, anemia, proteinuria, and bone pain. Other features include weight loss, anorexia, hepatosplenomegaly (25%), high serum alkaline phosphatase level, and high erythrocyte sedimentation rate (ESR). Peripheral blood smears show characteristic stacking of the red blood cells (Rouleaux formation).

Anorexia in MM has been attributed to the toxic effects from breakdown products, and pain is often intense, requiring narcotics. Pain in MM can arise due to different mechanisms such as bone pain due to expansion of the bone marrow by the myelomatous tissue, root pain caused by compression or direct invasion of the nerve roots, periarticular pain mimicking arthritis, and pathologic bone fractures. Back pain commonly arises due to vertebral pathologic fractures and collapse. Back pain in MM is made worse by turning or twisting and is aggravated by coughing or sneezing.

In MM, signs of amyloidosis may be seen in the form of macroglossia, skin papules, and alopecia. Raynaud's phenomenon, cold urticaria, and necrosis of the skin may be seen due to cryoglobulinemia. *Cryoglobulinemia* is a condition characterized by the presence of large amounts of proteins that become insoluble at reduced temperature (e.g., 4 °C). Increased plasma osmolarity due to the high plasma cell content in the blood may cause impairment of cerebral circulation due to increased plasma viscosity, a rare condition known as *paraproteinemic coma*.

One of the most dramatic complications of MM is the sudden compression of the spinal cord by collapsed vertebra or plasmacytoma. Vertebral plasmacytoma arises from the bone marrow and tunnels through the cortex until it spreads outside the vertebra as a soft-tissue mass arising from the vertebral body.

Renal disease in multiple myeloma often arises due to amyloidosis, causing proteinuria in 60–90% of cases and uremia in terminal stages, which is known as *myeloma kidney*. Renal failure in MM patients commonly arises due to infections, calculi, or nephrocalcinosis, rather than the classic myeloma kidney. In myeloma kidney, there is deposition of an abnormal globulin of small molecular weight as droplets in the cytoplasm of renal tubular epithelium. Later, fibrosis and degeneration of the renal tubules occur, resulting in replacement of the nephron by fibrous tissue. Identifying *Bence Jones protein* in the urine is diagnostic of MM. Signs of uremia in MM are similar to those of uremia due to other causes, except that hypertension is rarely present. Intravenous urography should not be used in patients with MM to assess the renal function, as it can result in renal failure and death in some MM patients.

Rarely, multiple myeloma of the mandible may present with paresthesia of the chin and the lower lip due to infiltration of the mental nerve, a branch of the third division of trigeminal nerve, when the mandible is affected by multiple myeloma. The condition is known as *numb chin syndrome*, and it is seen in malignancy that involves the mandible (e.g., leukemia).

*POEMS syndrome*, also known as *Crow–Fukase syndrome*, is a rare plasma cell disease with multisystemic involvement characterized by *p*olyneuropathy, *o*rganomegaly, *e*ndocrinopathy, *m*onoclonal gammopathy, and *s*kin changes. Patients with POEMS syndrome initially present with typical symptoms of connective tissue disorder, such as scleroderma-like skin thickening. Other manifestations include hepatosplenomegaly, Castleman's disease lymphadenopathy, hypothyroidism, hypogonadism, peripheral sensory-motor polyneuropathy, hypertrichosis, hyperpigmentation, scleroderma, and osteosclerotic plasmacytoma. POEMS syndrome has been linked to infection with human herpes-virus type 8.

*How Can You Differentiate POEMS Syndrome from Multiple Myeloma with Different Body Manifestations?*

- The osteolytic lesions of plasmacytoma and MM are "purely" lytic, with punched-out appearance on skeletal radiographs. In contrast, POEMS syndrome lesions are seen as well-defined fluffy sclerotic lesions or osteolytic lesions with sclerotic margins.
- Bone pain attributed to osteolytic lesions is common in MM, whereas bone pain is unlikely to occur due to bony lesions in POEMS syndrome.
- Patients with MM are typically elderly, >60 years of age, while patients with POEMS syndrome are usually younger.
- The monoclonal band in MM shows predominance of a kappa light chain, while in POEMS syndrome, it is a lambda light chain.
- The presence of Bence Jones protein in the serum and/or urine of classic MM patients is absent in POEMS syndrome.
- Bone scintigraphy is typically negative in MM, while it is positive in POEMS syndrome.

---

**Signs on Plain Radiographs**

- The classical appearance of MM is that of punched-out, sharply circumscribed, small osteolytic bone lesion that can be solitary or multiple. The osteolytic lesions are often found in the skull (◘ Fig. 9.8.35), vertebrae, ribs, pelvis, and long bones. Without the clinical picture, relying on radiographs alone to diagnose MM is not always possible, as multiple osteolytic bony lesions can be also seen in metastatic cancer and other tumors.
- Diffuse osteoporosis is commonly encountered in MM.

- Pathologic fractures may be seen, especially in the vertebrae.
- Acute myeloma presents as multiple lytic lesions (Fig. 9.8.36), while chronic myeloma can present as a dense and thick bone, mimicking Paget's disease.
- Although multiple osteolytic lesions are found in myeloma, bone scan is typically negative in MM.
- POEMS syndrome lesions are seen as well-defined fluffy sclerotic lesions or osteolytic lesions with sclerotic margins.
- Severe complication of diffuse infiltration of the vertebral body includes vertebral collapse due to pathological fracture. Severe collapse of the vertebral body (vertebra plana) can be seen (Fig. 9.8.37).

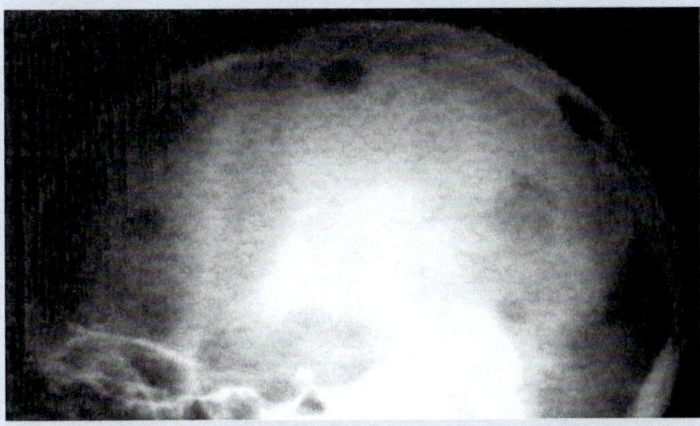

**Fig. 9.8.35**  Lateral plain skull radiograph of a patient with multiple myeloma shows multiple, osteolytic, sharply defined lesions affecting the calvarium

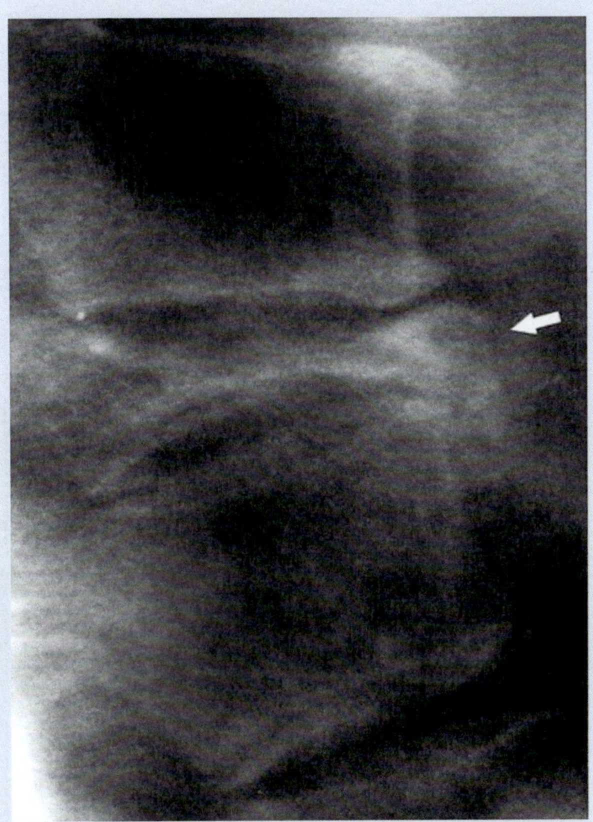

**Fig. 9.8.37**  Lateral plain thoracic vertebral radiograph of a patient with multiple myeloma shows vertebra plana (*arrow*)

### Signs on CT

- In *numb chin syndrome*, there is an expansile bony lytic lesion that destroys the mandibular ramus and infiltrates the masticator space (Fig. 9.8.38).
- *Vertebral plasmacytoma* is seen as an osteolytic lesion with soft-tissue mass that grows externally into the adjacent surrounding tissues (Fig. 9.8.39).

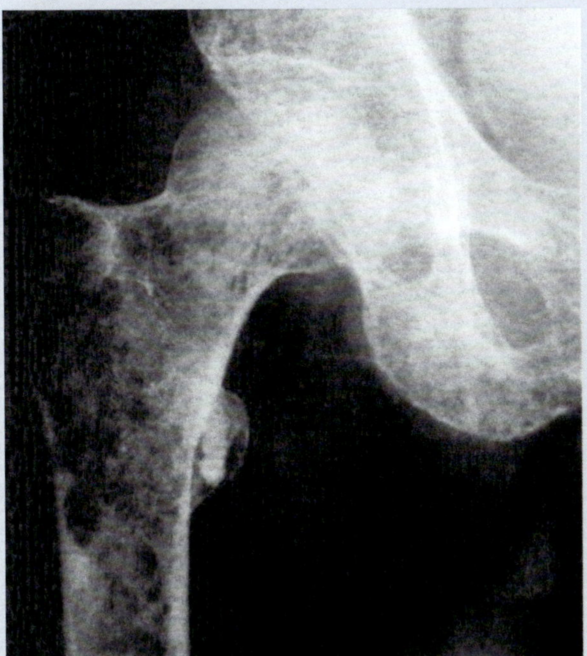

**Fig. 9.8.36**  Anteroposterior plain radiograph of the right hip joint shows diffuse small osteolytic lesions affecting the femur and the pelvis in a patient with acute multiple myeloma

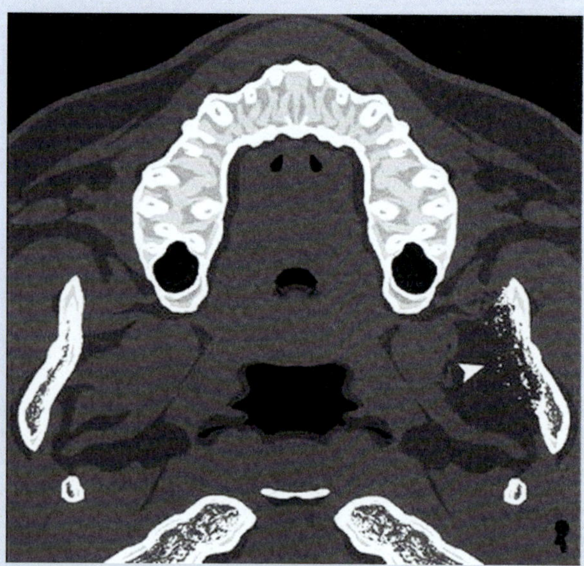

**Fig. 9.8.38**    Axial upper jaw dental CT illustration of a patient with numb chin syndrome due to multiple myeloma shows soft-tissue mass destroying and violating the right mandibular ramus integrity (*arrowhead*)

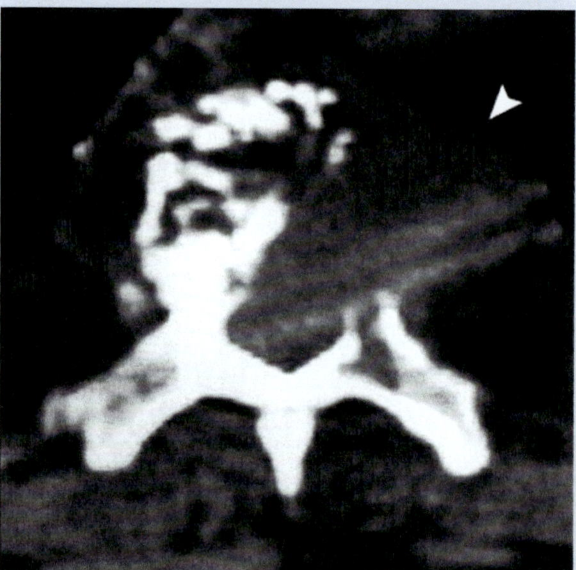

**Fig. 9.8.39**    Axial thoracic vertebral CT of a patient with plasmacytoma shows osteolytic soft-tissue mass with external and intraspinal canal extensions (*arrowhead*)

### Signs on MRI

- The MR appearance of lesions of MM, often in the vertebral column, is staged into four main types: normal, focal, variegated, and diffuse. The normal pattern shows no signs marrow infiltration of vertebral bodies, which is a very good sign for prognosis. The focal pattern shows localized areas

of low T1 and high T2 signal intensities within the vertebral bodies.
- The presence of multiple scattered small foci results in a variegated appearance (■ Fig. 9.8.40). The diffuse infiltration of the vertebral bodies results in reducing the total signal intensity of the vertebral column compared to the vertebral disks on T1W images (*positive disk sign*). In the normal vertebral MRI scan, the vertebral bodies have higher signal intensity than the vertebral disks on T1W images, due to the fatty bone marrow. The positive disk sign is commonly also found in patients with leukemia, when leukemic cells diffusely infiltrate the vertebral column.
- Infiltration of the meninges may be seen as nodular or thickened meninges with contrast enhancement (*Meningiosis carcinomatosis*).
- The degree of vertebral body bone marrow infiltration can be assessed by measuring the enhancement difference. On T1W images, this is done by applying a region of interest to the vertebral body and measuring the signal intensity (e.g., 240) and then copying the circle on the same section that was measured and applying it to the T1W postcontrast images to get the signal intensity of the vertebral body postcontrast (e.g., 320). Signal intensity (SI) difference is calculated by the following formula: (SI after contrast − SI before contrast/SI before contrast) × 100. Normal SI signal difference should be <18 %. An SI difference of >24 % reflects low-grade infiltration, while an SI difference of >49 % reflects high-grade infiltration (■ Fig. 9.8.41).

**Fig. 9.8.40** Sagittal T1W thoracic vertebral MRI shows the variegated appearance of multiple myeloma bone marrow infiltration

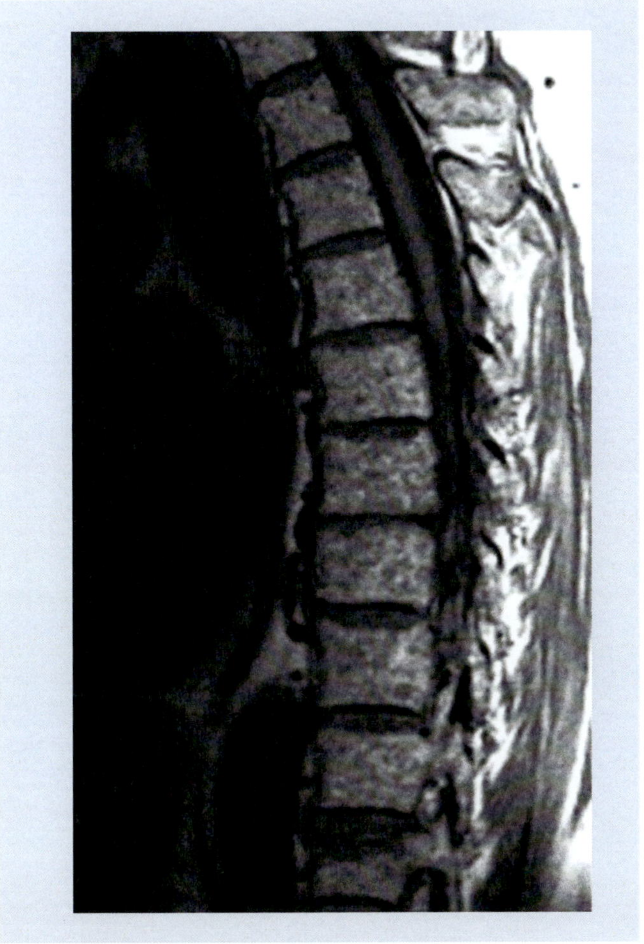

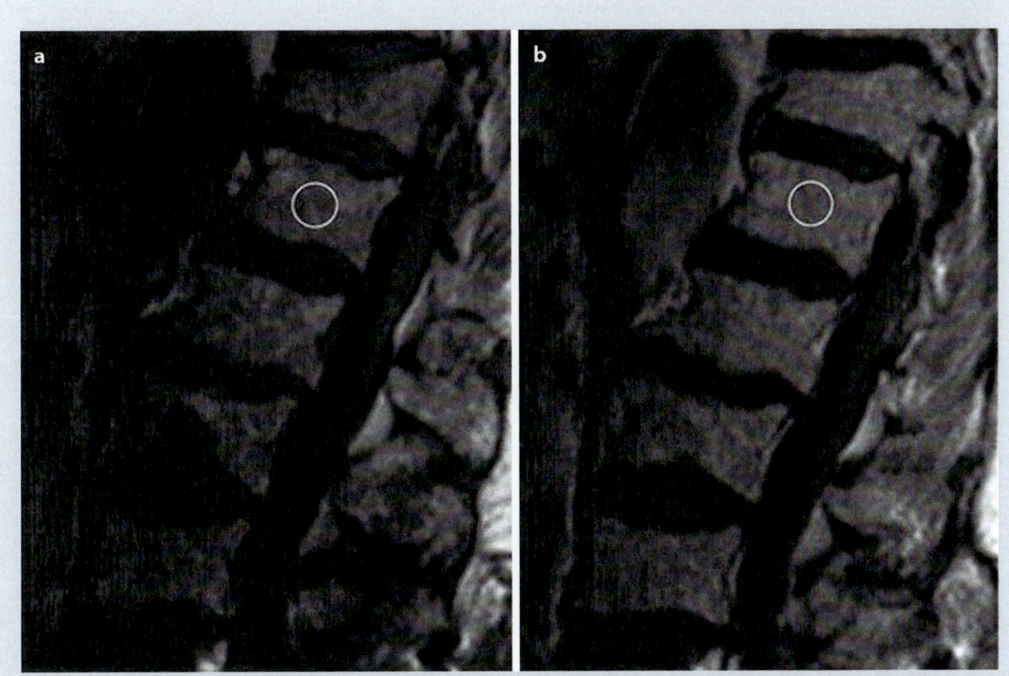

**Fig. 9.8.41** Sagittal T1W (**a**) and T1W postcontrast (**b**) of a patient with multiple myeloma shows two *circles* that measure the signal intensity in the region of interest. By applying the formula, the signal intensity difference was 26 %, reflecting low-grade diffuse vertebral bone marrow infiltration

## Further Reading

Angtuaco EJC, et al. Multiple myeloma: clinical review and diagnostic imaging. Radiology. 2004;231:11–23.

Attwell A, et al. Multiple myeloma involving the porta hepatic and peritoneum causing biliary obstruction and malignant ascites. Dig Dis Sci. 2005;50:1068–71.

Bauer A, et al. Neovascularization of bone marrow in patients with multiple myeloma: a correlation study of magnetic resonance imaging and histopathologic findings. Cancer. 2004;101:2599–604.

Chong ST, et al. POEMS syndrome: radiographic appearance with MRI correlation. Skeletal Radiol. 2006;35:690–5.

Eidner T, et al. Clinical manifestations of POEMS syndrome with features of connective tissue disorders. Clin Rheumatol. 2001;20:70–2.

Hess T, et al. Atypical manifestations of multiple myeloma: radiological appearances. Eur J Radiol. 2006;58:280–5.

Jacobs P. Myeloma Dis Mon. 1990;36:323–71.

Lecouvet FE, et al. Stage III multiple myeloma: clinical and prognostic value of spinal bone marrow MR imaging. Radiology. 1998;209:653–60.

Leonard RCF, et al. Multiple myeloma: radiology or bone scanning? Clin Radiol. 1981;32:291–5.

Libshitz HI, et al. Multiple myeloma: appearance at MR imaging. Radiology. 1992;182:833–7.

Magnusson S, et al. Multiple myeloma. Dis Mon. 1960;6:1–32.

Narváez JA, et al. POEMS syndrome: unusual radiographic, scintigraphic and CT features. Eur Radiol. 1988;8:134–6.

Patriarca F, et al. Meningeal and cerebral involvement in multiple myeloma patients. Ann Hematol. 2001;80:758–62.

Sugawara Y, et al. Paresthesia of the lower lip as a first manifestation of multiple myeloma – a case report. Oral Radiol. 2003;19:158–66.

Winterbottom AP, et al. Imaging patients with myeloma. Clin Radiol. 2009;64:1–11.

### 9.9 Amyloidosis

Amyloidosis is a systemic disease characterized by amyloid protein depositions in the extracellular matrix components such as blood vessel walls, the epithelial basement membrane, and the connective tissue matrix.

Amyloid is a term used to describe any protein with a "beta-pleated sheet" configuration. Amyloid proteins stain brown with iodine stain, from which the name was derived (amyloid means "starch-like"). Characteristically, amyloid proteins stain dark red with Congo red stain. When viewed under polarized light, amyloid stained with Congo red stain displays an apple-green birefringence. Any fibrillar protein with a "beta-pleated sheet" configuration will stain as amyloid.

Amyloid protein deposition in the extracellular matrix causes thickening and narrowing of the small vessel walls, destruction of the epithelial basement membrane, and mass effect over the cells, causing cellular ischemia and destruction over time. Any tissue can be affected by amyloid deposition. Amyloidosis can be systemic, affecting all body tissues, or localized to a certain organ.

## Classification of Amyloidosis (Clinical-Based Classification)

*Systemic amyloidosis* is a type of amyloidosis characterized by widespread body tissue disease and amyloid presence in the blood. The systemic form is divided into four major types:

- *B-cell dyscrasia (primary amyloidosis)*: this form arises due to defect in the B-cell function. The B cells produce amyloid precursor protein into the blood called "light-chain amyloid" and referred to as amyloid (AL). The monocytes engulf these AL amyloid precursors and then resecrete them in the blood in the form of the classic amyloid proteins. This type of amyloidosis is typically seen in patients with multiple myeloma and plasmacytoma (B-cell malignancies).

- *Reactive systemic amyloidosis (secondary amyloidosis)*: this form arises due to abnormal chemical signaling that evokes the liver to manufacture amyloid precursors and secretes them into the blood. The abnormal signaling can be initiated by different diseases. The liver forms "amyloid-associated protein," which is referred to as amyloid (AA). Like amyloid AL, monocytes play a major role in transforming amyloid AA precursor into complete amyloid protein form. This type of amyloidosis can be seen associated with diseases like ulcerative colitis, Crohn's disease, systemic vasculitis, tuberculosis, Hodgkin's disease, and rheumatoid arthritis.

- *Dialysis-associated amyloidosis*: this is a special form of systemic amyloidosis that occurs in patients on hemodialysis (up to 70 % of cases). It is believed that this form arises due to aggregation of $\beta_2$-microglobulins within the filtration machine, which will form amyloid protein, and then these amyloid proteins reenter the body via the machine when the clear blood returns to the body. This type of amyloid has an affinity to precipitate in the joints, ligaments, tendons, and synovial membranes.

- *Hereditary familial amyloidosis*: this form is rare, and it is seen in families and rare syndromes. An example of hereditary amyloidosis is *Muckle–Wells syndrome*, which is a rare autosomal dominant disease characterized by chronic recurrent urticaria, often combined with fever, chills, rigors, arthralgia, progressive sensorineural hearing loss, and AA-type amyloidosis in 30 % of cases. Another example of hereditary amyloidosis is familial Mediterranean fever. *Familial Mediterranean fever (Familial paroxysmal polyserositis)* is a genetic disease with autosomal recessive mode of inheritance, characterized by episodes of fever, abdominal pain, arthritis, and amyloidosis. The disease is common among Iraqi Jews, Armenians, Turks, and Middle Eastern Arabs. Patients experience multiple attacks of fever that last 12–72 h and resolve spontaneously. Recurrent attacks of abdominal pain that mimics acute abdomen are common, with constipation and diarrhea. The abdominal attack typically improves spontaneously in 24–72 h. Arthritis, including large-joint mono- and polyarthritis, is a common feature. Seronegative HLA-B27 sacroiliitis and ankylosing spondylitis are reported among patients with familial Mediterranean fever.

#### ■ ■ Localized Amyloidosis

This type of amyloidosis is characterized by deposition in a specific tissue (e.g., renal parenchyma). In this type, the amyloid proteins are manufactured in the affected tissue. Examples of localized amyloidosis include:

- *Amyloidoma*: this is a rare form of deposition of amyloid in a certain tissue, forming a solid mass in the absence of B-cell disease (dyscrasia) or elevation of serum proteins. Amyloidoma can occur in any body tissue and cannot be differentiated from other tumors except by biopsy.
- *Hormonal amyloidosis*: an example of this type is seen in endocrine cancerous cells that secrete amyloid proteins rather than normal hormones (e.g., thyroid medullary carcinoma).
- *Senile amyloidosis*: deposition of amyloid proteins due to the aging process in the choroids plexus, brain, and heart.

Up to 30% of patients with B-cell dyscrasia progress to multiple myeloma, while multiple myeloma is associated with systemic amyloidosis in 15% of cases. The median survival rate in patients with AL-type amyloidosis is 1.5 years, whereas the median survival rate in patients with AA-type amyloidosis is 4.5 years.

Although the features of amyloidosis are not specific, radiologists need to be familiar with the disease manifestations in different body organs, especially in secondary amyloidosis. Secondary amyloidosis can be suspected in patients with systemic diseases that present with body manifestations that cannot be explained by the original disease symptoms.

*Renal amyloidosis* can be divided into early and late stages. In the early stage, the kidney is normal in size and shape, after which it starts to progressively increase in size, due to the amyloid deposition. The enlarged amyloid kidney is firm in consistency and has a waxy appearance on postmortem gross examination. In later stages, chronic parenchymal ischemia occurs due to amyloid deposition within the renal vessels, which causes irreversible cell damage and fibrosis. The end result of renal amyloidosis is renal failure. Patients with kidney amyloidosis commonly present with *nephrotic syndrome*, a syndrome characterized by generalized edema, hyperlipidemia, hematuria, and gross proteinuria (>3 g/L). Bladder amyloidosis is often seen as a solitary mass (amyloidoma), which presents clinically with hematuria.

*Hepatic amyloidosis* can occur, but usually does not progress into liver failure. Normally, the liver parenchymal reservation is 85% of its mass, and the renal parenchymal reservation is 75% of the kidneys' mass. Due to these facts, most patients with systemic amyloidosis rarely develop hepatic failure, because they may die from renal failure before developing complete hepatic failure. However, hepatic dysfunction is observed, but hepatic failure is rare. The amyloid proteins are deposited in the arterioles, the extracellular compartments, and the hepatic sinusoids (space of Disse) until they fill the sinusoids and exert back pressure on the hepatocytes, causing pressure atrophy.

*Splenic amyloidosis* is detected clinically in the form of splenomegaly. The spleen is made of white pulp (15%) and red pulp (85%). Amyloidosis of the spleen may affect the white pulp or the red pulp. When amyloidosis affects the white pulp, it results in a moderately enlarged spleen, with a patchy, waxy appearance in postmortem gross examination (sago spleen). When it affects the red pulp, it causes diffuse enlargement, with diffuse waxy appearance in postmortem gross examination (diffuse amyloid spleen).

*Cardiac amyloidosis* is generally a rare condition. It can arise due to senility or due to chronic systemic disease. Amyloidosis of the heart can affect the atria more than the ventricles, for unknown reasons, and it may cause restrictive cardiomyopathy. Cardiac amyloidosis is usually caused by AL-type amyloidosis and rarely by AA-type amyloidosis.

*Endocrine amyloidosis* may occur and is classically seen in the form of endocrine insufficiency of the pituitary gland (hypopituitarism) or adrenal gland insufficiency (Addison's disease).

*Gastrointestinal tract amyloidosis* is detected as a disease of hollow organs. The colon is the most frequently affected organ. In the intestine, amyloid accumulates within the arterioles of the intestinal villi, resulting in malabsorption and diarrhea (due to failure of the villi to function), and mucosal ulceration and bleeding (due to villi ischemia and necrosis). Esophageal and gastric involvement results in dysmotility, wall thickening, and gastroesophageal reflux disease.

*Pulmonary amyloidosis* is a relatively rare condition, with patients often presenting with recurrent pneumonias, which characteristically occur in the same distribution that correspond to previous antibiotic treatment, but recurs at a later time. Features of pulmonary amyloidosis include diffuse interstitial nodular pattern, tracheal and bronchial wall thickening, and (rarely) a solitary mass (amyloidoma).

*Central nervous system amyloidosis* is often present in the form of cerebral amyloid angiopathy (CAA) with spontaneous nontraumatic intracranial bleeding or (rarely) as leptomeningeal thickening.

*Musculoskeletal amyloidosis* generally causes muscular hypertrophy, weakness, and chronic pain. Muscular amyloidosis preferentially involves the shoulder girdle. Deposition of amyloids within the periarticular tissues of the shoulder girdle resulting in shoulder enlargement is called the "shoulder pad sign" (◘ Fig. 9.9.42).

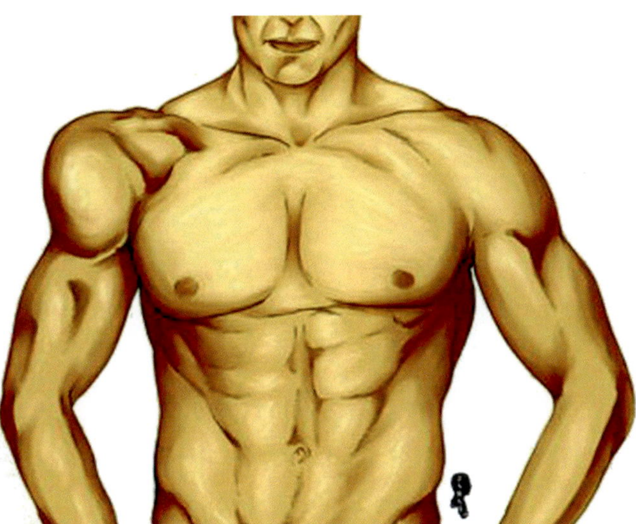

◘ **Fig. 9.9.42** An illustration demonstrates the shoulder pad sign (right shoulder)

*Amyloidosis in the head and neck region* usually manifests as vocal cord thickening causing hoarseness of the voice, tongue intrinsic muscles deposition causing macroglossia, supra- and subglottic larynx, and periorbital deposition causing bleeding and ecchymoses (the raccoon sign). Amyloidosis of the paranasal sinuses can be seen as a sinusoidal mass with "fluffy-bone appearance" of the adjacent bone.

### Signs on Plain Radiographs
- Pulmonary amyloidosis can be seen as a diffuse interstitial nodular pattern or (rarely) as a single solitary mass (amyloidoma) (◘ Fig. 9.9.43).
- When an amyloidoma involves a bone, it is usually visualized as an osteolytic mass lesion.
- Dialysis-related amyloid arthropathy is detected as periarticular bony cysts or erosions.

### Signs on US
- Amyloidosis is one of the rare cases of enlarged kidneys with high echogenicity.
- Hepatic amyloidosis may appear as multiple foci of increased liver parenchymal echogenicity.

### Signs on CT and MRI
- The affected kidney is normal or larger than normal in early stages of amyloidosis. In later stages, renal fibrosis shrinkage with parenchymal calcification is often seen.
- Hepatic amyloidosis can be seen on nonenhanced CT as a diffusely enlarged liver with hypoattenuation. Other radiological signs are nonspecific.
- Splenic manifestations of amyloidosis include splenomegaly, calcification, and lack of enhancement after contrast injection. The lack of contrast enhancement is thought to be due to vascular amyloid angiopathy and diffuse parenchymal infiltration by amyloid proteins.
- Small and large bowel involvement results in diffuse or nodular wall thickening.
- Cardiac amyloidosis can show many nonspecific findings, such as biventricular hypertrophy that mimics hypertrophic cardiomyopathy (◘ Fig. 9.9.44), thickening of the papillary muscles and the valvular leaflets, and pleural or pericardial effusion. Biatrial enlargement and enhancement is a characteristic sign, but unfortunately not always seen. On MRI, a relatively characteristic pattern of myocardial amyloidosis seen on postgadolinium injection consists of strong subendocardial and subepicardial late enhancement (zebra enhancement pattern) (◘ Fig. 9.9.45).

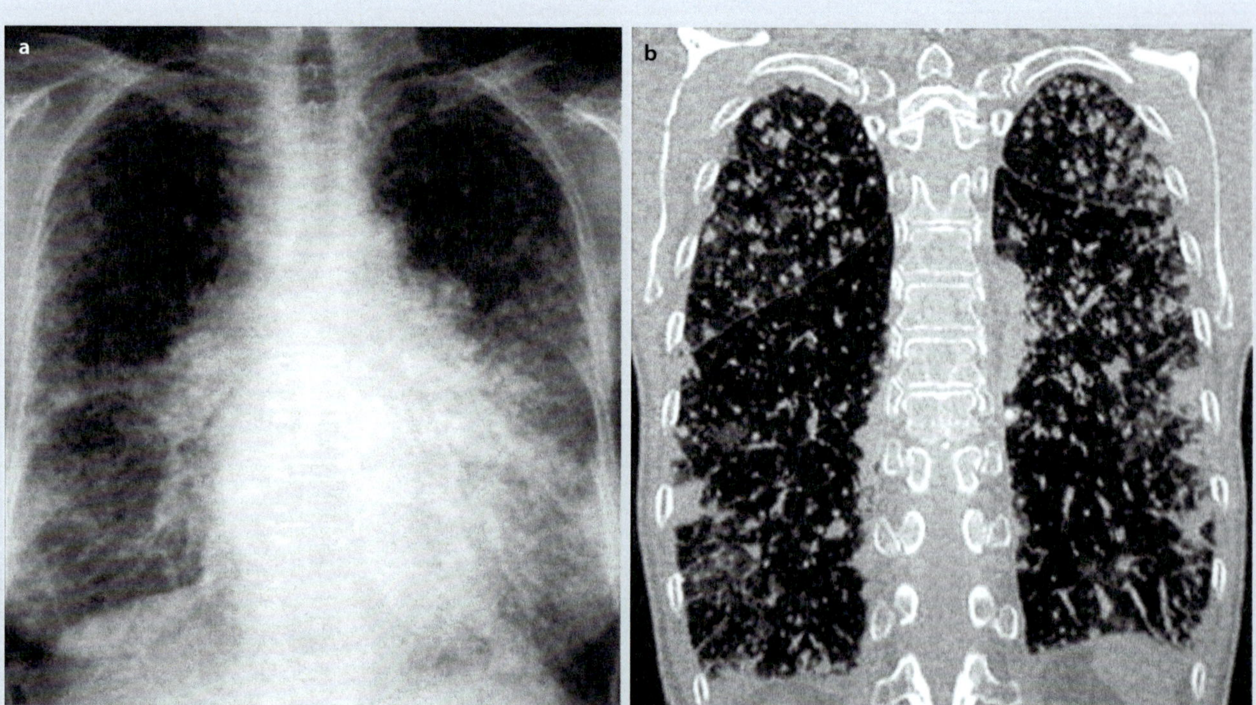

◘ **Fig. 9.9.43**  Posteroanterior plain radiograph (**a**) and coronal HRCT (**b**) of a patient with multiple myeloma who developed pulmonary amyloidosis shows diffuse bilateral nodular interstitial pattern lung disease

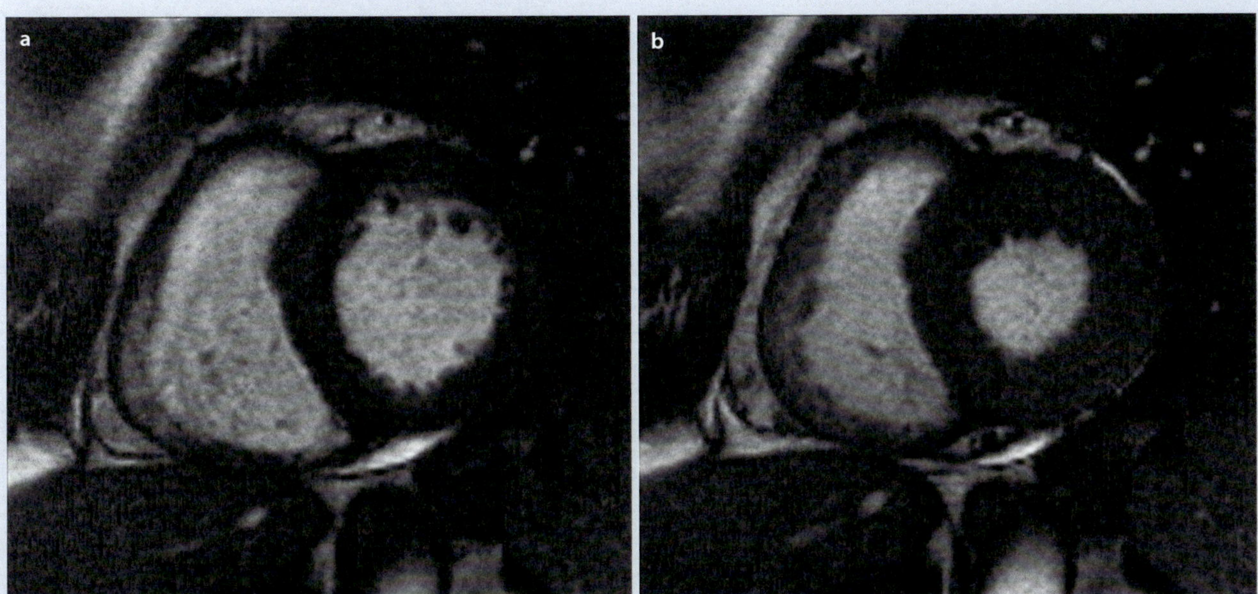

**Fig. 9.9.44** Short-axis white blood pool cardiac MRI in diastolic (**a**) and systolic (**b**) phases show hypertrophy of the right and left ventricles in a patient with systemic amyloidosis

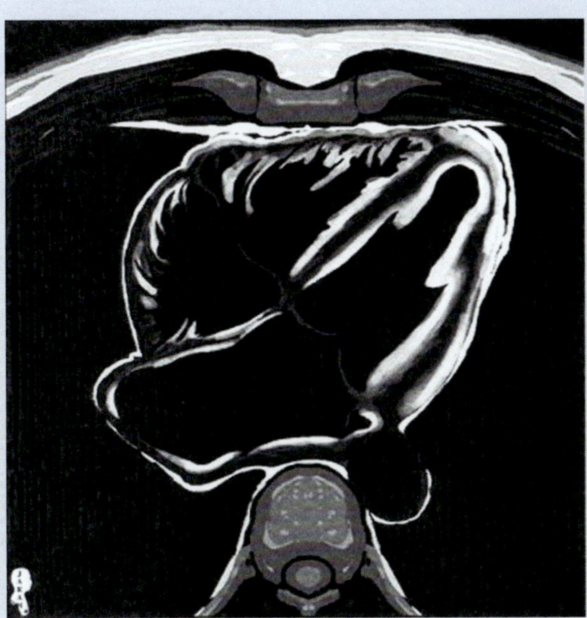

**Fig. 9.9.45** Axial, four-chambers postcontrast cardiac MR illustration of a patient with cardiac amyloidosis shows subendocardial and subepicardial enhancement that is described as a zebra enhancement pattern

- Pulmonary amyloidosis on HRCT may resemble the features of bronchiolitis obliterans, may diffuse interstitial nodular pattern (nodules <15 mm in diameter) which may cause a "budding tree" appearance, or may (rarely) present as a solitary solid mass with calcification (amyloidoma) (**Fig. 9.9.43**). Tracheal and bronchial wall thickening are other characteristic signs of amyloidosis of the bronchial tree.
- Paranasal sinuses amyloidoma is seen as a mass with "fluffy-bone appearance" of the adjacent bone. However, a biopsy is required to confirm diagnosis.
- On MRI, synovial thickening that resembles pigmented villonodular synovitis can be seen, which characteristically lacks the chronic hemorrhage and hemosiderin T1 and T2 hypointense signal intensities.
- Amyloid proteins on MRI typically show low T1 and T2 signal intensities and contrast enhancement. Therefore, signs of high signal intensity on T2W images in amyloidosis are usually due to the inflammatory reaction evoked by the amyloidosis, not by the amyloid proteins themselves.
- Cerebral amyloidosis may present on noncontrast-enhanced CT as intracranial hemorrhage due to CAA or (rarely) diffuse leptomeningeal thickening and enhancement.
- Amyloidoma in any body region is usually seen as a solid tissue mass that may cause bone osteolysis and contains calcification. However, this appearance is nonspecific, and biopsy is crucial to establish the diagnosis.
- Dialysis-related amyloid arthropathy is detected on CT as bony erosions and as formation of bony cysts. On MRI, the amyloid changes are detected as thickening and irregularity of the supraspinatus tendon, thickening of the iliofemoral portion of the hip joint capsule, and fluid collection within the bursae of the joints. Soft-tissue amyloid deposition can be seen in the spine, carpal tunnel, and knee synovium as typical low signal intensity on both T1W and T2W images.

## Further Reading

Arslan A, et al. Laryngeal amyloidosis with laryngocele: MRI and CT. Neuroradiology. 1998;40:401–3.

Asaumi J, et al. CT and MR imaging of localized amyloidosis. Eur J Radiol. 2001;39:83–7.

Q11 Chin SC, et al. Amyloidosis concurrently involving the sinusoidal cavities of the larynx. AJNR Am J Neuroradiol. 2004;25:636–8.

El-Darouti MA, et al. Muckle-Wells syndrome: report of six cases with hyperpigmented sclerodermoid skin lesions. Int J Dermatol. 2006;45:239–44.

Escobedo EM, et al. Magnetic resonance imaging of dialysis-related amyloidosis of the shoulder and hip. Skeletal Radiol. 1996;25:41–8.

Fonnesu C, et al. Familial Mediterranean fever: a review for clinical management. Joint Bone Spine. 2008;76:227–33. doi:10.1016/j.jbspin.2008.08.004.

Fujita Y, et al. Nail dystrophy and blisters as sole manifestations in myeloma-associated amyloidosis. J Am Acad Dermatol. 2006;54:712–4.

Geluwe FV, et al. Amyloidosis of the heart and respiratory system. Eur Radiol. 2006;16:2358–65.

Georgiades CS, et al. Amyloidosis: review and CT manifestations. Radiographics. 2004;24:405–26.

Gilad R, et al. Severe diffuse systemic amyloidosis with involvement of the pharynx, larynx, and trachea: CT and MR findings. AJNR Am J Neuroradiol. 2007;28:1557–8.

Guerreiro de Moura CG, et al. "Shoulder pad" sign. N Engl J Med. 2004;351(25):e23.

Hidalgo E, et al. Amyloidoma of the skull: plain radiographs, CT and MRI. Neuroradiology. 1996;38:44–6.

Keles I, et al. Familial Mediterranean fever and ankylosing spondylitis in a patient with juvenile idiopathic arthritis: a case report and review of the literature. Rheumatol Int. 2006;26:846–51.

Matsumoto K, et al. Primary solitary amyloidosis of the lung: findings on CT and MRI. Eur Radiol. 1997;7:586–8.

Metzler JP, et al. MRI evaluation of amyloid myopathy. Skeletal Radiol. 1992;21:463–5.

Motosugi U, et al. Localized nasopharyngeal amyloidosis with remarkable early enhancement on dynamic contrast-enhanced MR imaging. Eur Radiol. 2007;17:852–3.

Rafal RB, et al. MRI of primary amyloidosis. Gastrointest Radiol. 1990;15:199–201.

Singh SK, et al. Localized primary amyloidosis of the prostate, bladder, ureters. Int Urol Nephrol. 2005;37:495–7.

Sueyoshi E, et al. Cardiac amyloidosis: typical imaging findings and diffuse myocardial damage demonstrated by delayed contrast-enhanced MRI. Cardiovasc Intervent Radiol. 2006;29:710–2.

Touart DM, et al. Cutaneous deposition diseases. Part I. J Am Acad Dermatol. 1998;39:149–71.

Urban BA, et al. CT evaluation of amyloidosis: spectrum of diseases. Radiographics. 1993;13:1295–308.

Urban PP, et al. Leptomeningeal familial amyloidosis: a rare differential diagnosis of leptomeningeal enhancement in MRI. J Neurol. 2006;253:1238–40.

## 9.10    Evans' Syndrome

Evans' syndrome (ES) is a disease characterized by simultaneous development of autoimmune thrombocytopenia (AITP) and autoimmune hemolytic anemia (AIHA).

Patients with ES develop autoantibodies against erythrocytes, platelets, and neutrophils. ES often presents with a wide variety of clinical manifestations that include lymphoid tissue hyperplasia, interstitial nephritis, eczema, and insulin-dependent diabetes mellitus. AITP and AIHA can be also the first signs of systemic lupus erythematosus.

Uncommonly, ES patients may present with progressive dyspnea due to the formation of cryptogenic organizing pneumonia. Neurological symptoms due to sagittal vein thrombosis may occur.

Investigations show low platelet count, low hemoglobin, neutropenia, and positive Coombs test. Radiology investigations are requested mainly to detect complications of the disease (◘ Fig. 9.10.46).

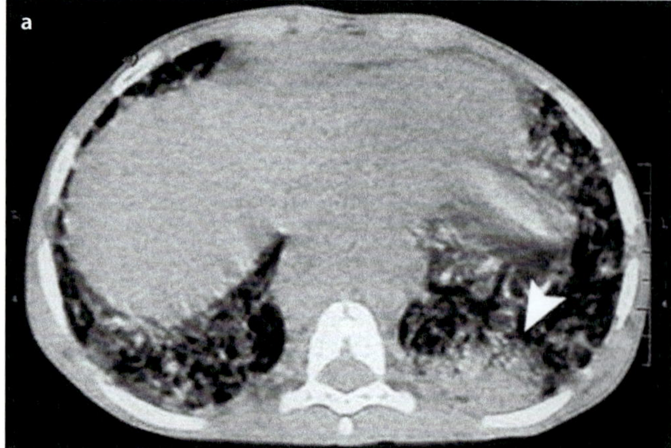

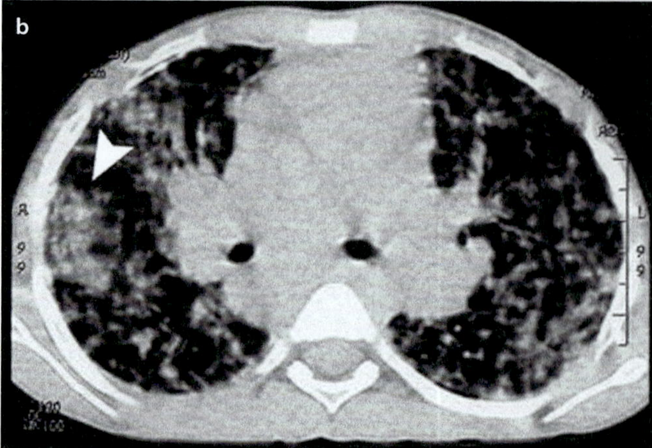

◘ **Fig. 9.10.46**    Axial lung window HRCT of the lungs show bilateral patchy lung consolidation with a mass of consolidation located at the subpleural, peripheral, posterior lung lobe (*arrowhead in* **a**) and the right subpleural area in the right middle lobe (*arrowhead in* **b**) due to cryptogenic organizing pneumonia

## Further Reading

Garcia-Muñoz R, et al. Splenic marginal zone lymphoma with Evans' syndrome, autoimmunity, and peripheral gamma/delta T cells. Ann Hematol. 2009;88:177–8. doi:10.1007/s00277-008-0555-z.

Máiz L, et al. Bronchiolitis obliterans organizing pneumonia associated with Evans syndrome. Respiration. 2001;68:631–4.

Miyamae T, et al. An infant with γ-globulin-induced hypersensitivity syndrome who developed Evans' syndrome after a second γ-globulin treatment. Mod Rheumatol. 2004;14:314–9.

Savasan S, et al. The spectrum of Evans' syndrome. Arch Dis Child. 1997;77:245–8.

Shiozawa Z, et al. Superior sagittal sinus thrombosis associated with Evans' syndrome of haemolytic anaemia. J Neurol. 1985;232:280–2.

Tsang KWT, et al. Rhodococcus equi lung abscess complicating Evans' syndrome treated with corticosteroid. Respiration. 1998;65:327–30.

Ucci G, et al. A case of Evans' syndrome in a patient with ulcerative colitis. Dig Liver Dis. 2003;35:439–41.

## 9.11  Other Lymphatic Disorders

This topic discusses some of the uncommon lymphatic disorders occasionally encountered in radiology and that can be mistaken initially for lymphoma or inflammatory conditions causing lymphadenopathy.

## Castleman's Disease (Angiofollicular Lymph Node Hyperplasia)

Castleman disease (CD) is a rare benign process of unknown cause, characterized by lymph nodes hyperplasia.

CD is liable to be misdiagnosed as other hypervascular tumors by radiology and pathology examinations. Lymph node hyperplasia may occur anywhere along the lymphatic chain within the body; however, it is commonly described in the mediastinum, abdomen, and pelvis.

The main pathology in CD concerns lymph nodes hyperplasia and the related small blood vessels. The lymph nodes are enlarged with high blood vessel proliferation and hypervascularity. CD is divided into two types: localized type and diffuse type.

The localized type is characterized by proliferation of the lymph nodes in a certain region within the body. Differential diagnoses of the localized type include tuberculosis lymphadenitis (ruled out by TB serology) and pheochromocytoma due to its hypervascularity (rules out by biochemistry investigations). CD diagnosis should be considered in differential diagnosis of hypervascular tumor in the retroperitoneum.

The diffuse type is characterized by lymph node proliferation through the body. The main differential diagnosis is lymphoma. Lymph node biopsy is the gold standard method to diagnose CD.

### Signs on CT

- There are enlarged lymph nodes located within the mediastinum or the retroperitoneum (◘ Figs. 9.11.47 and 9.11.48).
- The lymph nodes in CD are characterized by homogenous high-contrast enhancement in the early phase of dynamic enhancement that can exceed the enhancement of pheochromocytoma due to the hypervascularity of the lymph nodes. The high enhancement persists in the delayed phases.
- Typically, there is absence of necrosis or cystic changes within the enlarged lymph nodes, due to the abundant vascular supply. However, cystic changes may be found in 22 % of cases, especially when the lymph node is >5 cm in diameter.
- Punctuate or coarse calcification may be seen in 30 % of cases (lymphomas do not calcify unless treated).
- A thin rim-like enhancement sign may be noticed in the arterial phase, with several enhancing feeding vessels that surround the nodes.
- To differentiate CD from *pheochromocytoma* in the retroperitoneum, MRI should be done. Pheochromocytoma show higher signal intensity on T2W images compared to CD. Contrast-enhanced images may be similar due to the high vascular blood supply of the lymph nodes in CD.
- CD shows higher contrast enhancement than any other retroperitoneal sarcoma.

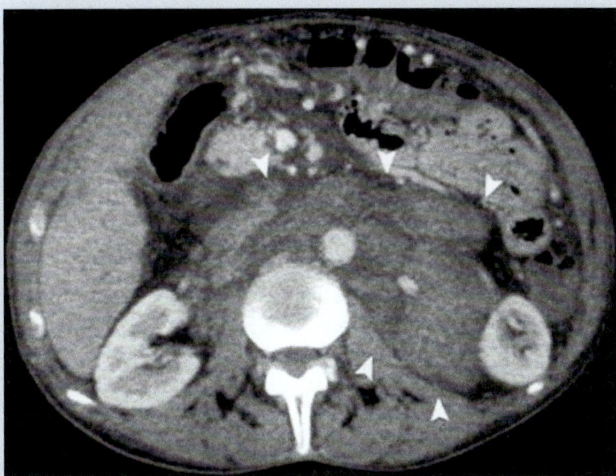

◘ **Fig. 9.11.47**   Axial abdominal portal phase, contrast-enhanced CT shows diffuse lymphadenopathy in the retroperitonium around the aorta and the inferior vena cava (*arrowheads*) in a patient with Castleman's disease

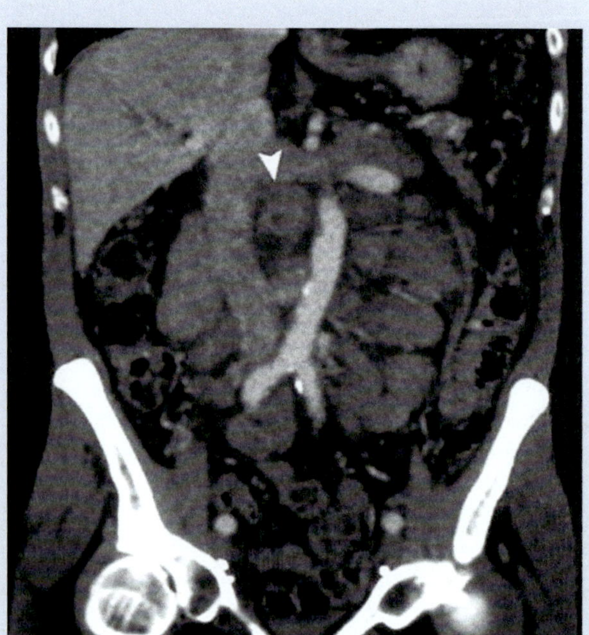

**Fig. 9.11.48** Coronal abdominal portal phase, contrast-enhanced CT of the same patient shows the enlarged lymph nodes separating the inferior vena cava from the aorta (*arrowhead*)

## Kikuchi–Fujimoto Disease (Histiocytic Necrotizing Lymphadenitis)

Kikuchi–Fujimoto disease (KFD) is a rare, self-limiting condition, characterized by the development of fever, weight loss, malaise, and lymphadenitis (commonly cervical).

KFD is often mistaken for tuberculous lymphadenitis, lymphoma, systemic lupus lymphadenitis, and infectious lymphadenitis. The misdiagnosis rate is up to 40 % of cases.

The disease is self-limiting and benign, with a course lasting 6–8 weeks. The recurrence rate is 3 % of cases. Laboratory findings are not specific and usually show high C-reactive protein and erythrocyte sedimentation rate, mild lymphocytosis, leukopenia, and atypical lymphocytes. Definite diagnosis is done by fine-needle lymph node biopsy.

The disease is of unknown origin, affects mainly females (mean age of 30 years), and may be associated with Epstein–Barr virus activation and systemic lupus erythematosus.

**Signs on CT**
Neck and mediastinal CT often show lymphadenopathy similar to the picture seen in lymphoma and tuberculous adenitis. History, laboratory investigations, and the biopsy report are the main elements for establishing the diagnosis.

## Kimura's Disease

Kimura's disease (KD) is a chronic inflammatory disease characterized by tumor-like soft-tissue swelling and lymphoid tissue hyperplasia (Fig. 9.11.49).

KD is characterized histopathologically by lymphoid hyperplasia with soft-tissue infiltration by eosinophils, which is a constant finding in this disease. The cause of this disease is unknown, but it is thought to be caused by chronic allergic reaction due to the eosinophilia and high serum immunoglobulin E in patients with KD.

KD has predominance in young males and is usually seen in Asian populations, especially in Japan and China (80 %). Patients often present with asymptomatic, unilateral soft-tissue swelling involving lymph nodes or salivary glands (e.g., the parotid glands). Regional lymphadenopathy is found in 66 % of cases. The head and neck region is affected in 70 % of cases. Atopic disorders can be seen in patients with KD. Rare manifestations include masses formation in the external auditory meatus, tongue, orbits, epiglottis, larynx, groin (15 %), and extremities (12 %). Nephrotic syndrome is found in 12 % of cases.

Definite diagnosis requires mass biopsy with laboratory evidence of eosinophilia that is not related to parasitic infection.

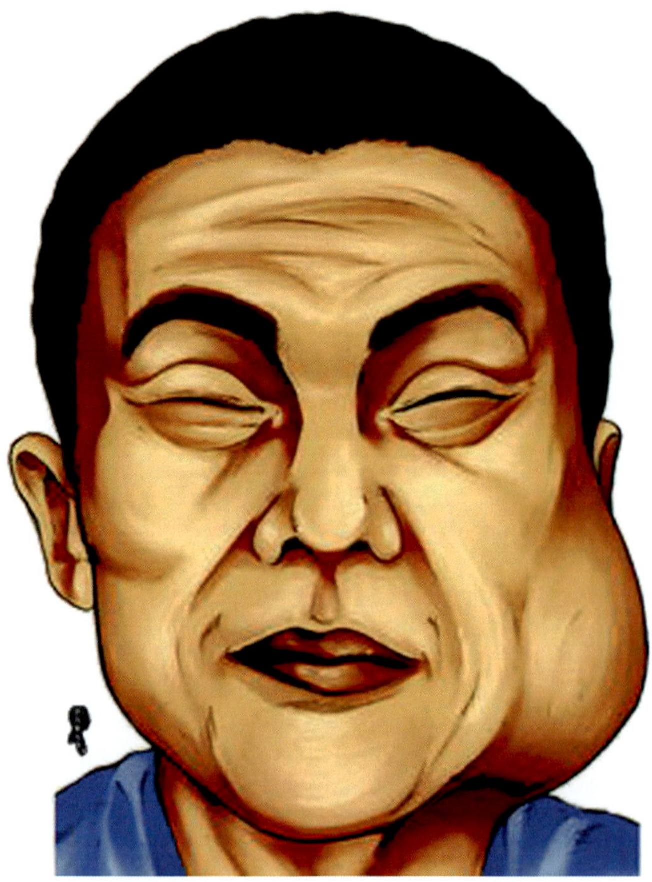

**Fig. 9.11.49** An illustration demonstrating left parotid enlargement in a patient with Kimura disease

## Further Reading

Chen HC, et al. Systemic lupus erythematosus with simultaneous onset of Kikuchi-Fujimoto's disease complicated with antiphospholipid antibody syndrome: a case report and review of the literature. Rheumatol Int. 2005; 25:303–6.

Chidambara Murthy S, et al. Kikuchi's disease associated with systemic lupus erythematosus. Indian J Dermatol Venereol Leprol. 2005;71:338–41.

Ching ASC, et al. Extranodal manifestations of Kimura's disease: ultrasound features. Eur Radiol. 2002;12:600–4.

Hiwatashi A, et al. Kimura's disease with bilateral auricular masses. Am J Neuroradiol. 1999;20:1976–8.

Hrycek A, et al. Kikuchi-Fujimoto disease: a case report. Rheumatol Int. 2005;26:179–81.

Irsutti M, et al. Castleman disease: CT and MR imaging features of a retroperitoneal location in association with paraneoplastic pemphigus. Eur Radiol. 1999;9: 1219–21.

Jeong YY, et al. Imaging of Kimura's disease involving teh abdomen. AJR Am J Roentgenol. 2006;187:W131–2.

Kaicker S, et al. PET-CT scan in patient with Kikuchi disease. Pediatr Radiol. 2008;38:596–7.

Kodama T, et al. Kimura's disease of the lacrimal gland. Acta Opthalmol Scand. 1998;76:374–7.

Liu PI, et al. Kimura's disease in upper arm: a case report and imaging findings. Chin J Radiol. 2007;32:153–6.

Ortak T, et al. Kimura disease: a brief clinical report. Eur J Plast Surg. 2008;31:253–7.

Zheng X, et al. Localized Castleman disease in retroperitoneum: newly discovered features by multi-detector helical CT. Abdom Imaging. 2008;33:489–92.

Zhou LP, et al. Imaging findings in Castleman disease of the abdomen and pelvis. Abdom Imaging. 2008;33:482–8.

## 9.12 Mastocytosis

Mastocytosis is a group of diseases characterized by abnormal proliferation of mast cells both in the bone marrow and the peripheral tissues such as the skin, gastrointestinal tract, liver, and spleen. Mastocytosis not only affects predominantly children (75 %) but also adults with more severe manifestations (25 %). Mastocytosis is classified into four clinical categories based on their clinical manifestations, prognosis, and pathological findings:

1. *Indolent mastocytosis*: this type generally has a good prognosis. It is subdivided into patients with isolated skin mastocytosis (*type IA, urticaria pigmentosa*) and systemic mastocytosis with visceral and bone involvement (*type IB*).
2. *Mastocytosis with hematologic disease*: this type is characterized by mastocytosis associated with myeloproliferative/myelodysplastic disorders. The prognosis is determined based on the severity of the hematologic disease.
3. *Aggressive mastocytosis*: this type is characterized by rapidly deteriorating clinical course with increase mastocytes burden. The patient develops eosinophilia with generalized lymphadenopathy; prognosis is poor.
4. *Mast cell leukemia*: this type is extremely rare and carries the worst prognosis.

Patients with urticaria pigmentosa present classically with small, yellow-tan to reddish brown macules. Nodules or plaque-like lesions may be seen. These skin lesions are seen in the upper and lower limbs sparing the palms, soles, face, and scalp. The thorax and the abdomen may be affected. The skin lesions are also found in 90 % of patients with systemic mastocytosis and 50 % in mastocytosis with hematological disorders.

*Darier's sign* is a term used to describe erythematous skin lesion that rises after rubbing or scratching lesions of cutaneous mastocytosis. The erythema appears 2–5 min after rubbing the skin and lasts from 30 min to several hours. Mast cells contain histamine, heparin, and prostaglandin. When the skin is rubbed, there is degranulation of mast cells with the release of mast cell contents within the dermis. Darier's sign is caused by the effect of histamine. Darier's sign can be also seen in leukemia cutis, lymphoma, and Langerhans cell histiocytosis. *Mastocytomas* are rare skin lesions that typically occur before 6 months of age as solitary or multiple skin nodules.

Patients with systemic mastocytosis present often with abdominal pain, diarrhea, nausea, peptic ulcers, and gastrointestinal bleeding. Symptoms can be precipitated by narcotics, nonsteroidal anti-inflammatory drugs, penicillin, cold or hot temperature, exercise and emotions, and alcohol. Other features include malabsorption, hepatosplenomegaly (50 %), and lymphadenopathy (60 %). Laboratory investigations classically show anemia (50 %) and eosinophilia (25 %). Bleeding tendency may occur due to high levels of heparin released by mast cells or vitamin K deficiency due to malabsorption.

Diagnosis is established by measurement of serum concentration of both mature and α-tryptase, which reflects mast cell numbers (normal level up to 11 ng/mL). Systemic mastocytosis is strongly suspected if serum tryptase level is >20 ng/mL. This test is best done during acute events caused by mastocytosis. The other method to detect mastocytosis is to measure 24-h urinary histamine concentration. The latter method is used when serum tryptase level measurement is unavailable.

### Signs on Chest Radiographs
Pulmonary mastocytosis is rarely detected in systemic mastocytosis as bilateral diffuse interstitial nodular pattern.

### Signs on Skeletal Radiographs
1. Classically, mastocytosis is seen as multiple nodular mixed osteolytic/osteosclerotic lesions that diffusely affects the skeleton (◘ Figs. 9.12.50 and 9.12.51). The osteolytic lesions are caused by granulomatous formation. In contrast, sclerotic lesions are caused by the effect of histamine which is known to stimulate the formation of fibrous tissue. Fibrous tissue will be later converted into osteoid, which will be converted into bony sclerotic lesions.
2. Osteoporosis may be seen due to the high heparin effect or the bone resorption effect of prostaglandin produced by mast cells.

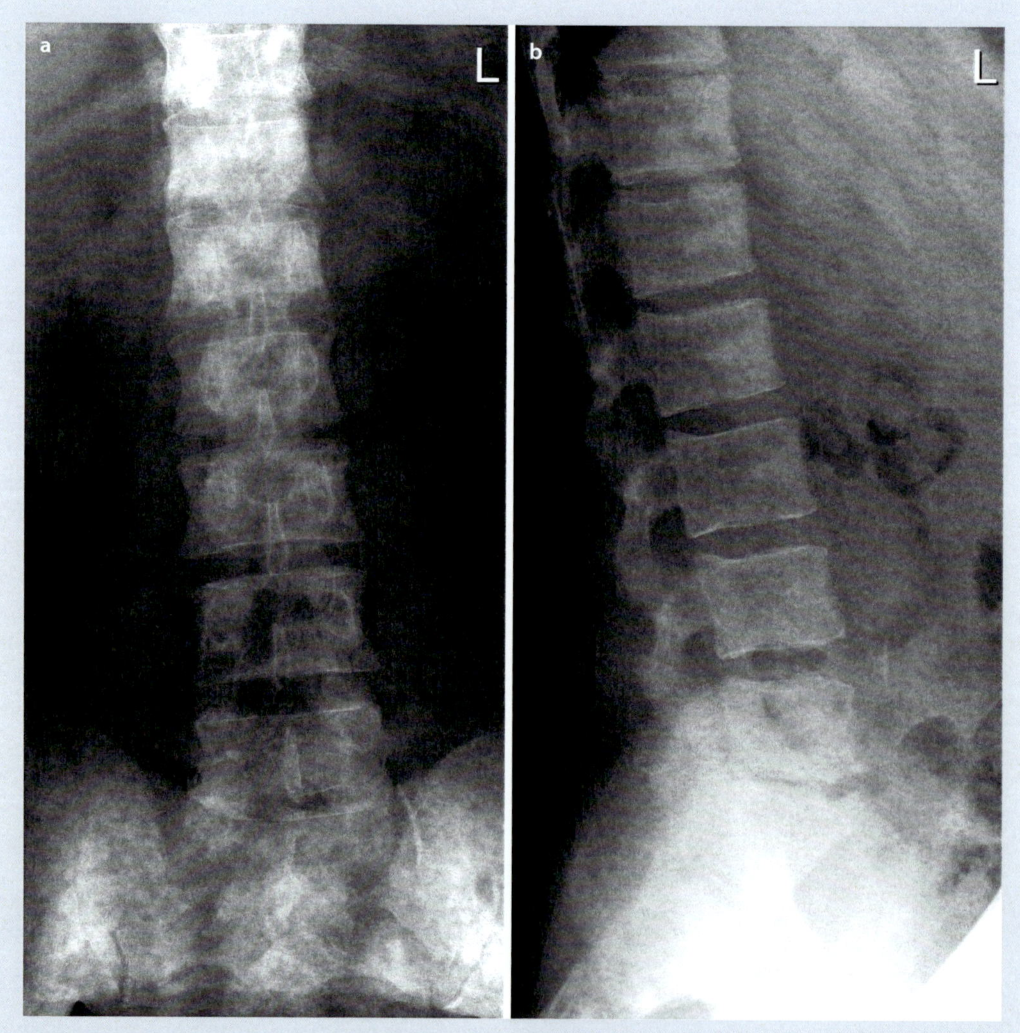


◘ **Fig. 9.12.50**   Anteroposterior and lateral plain radiographs of the lumbar spine of a patient with systemic mastocytosis show the classical, military, osteolytic/osteosclerotic pattern (both **a** & **b**)

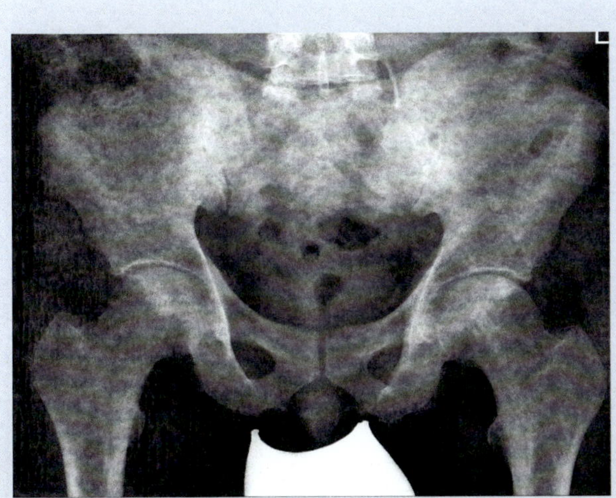



**Fig. 9.12.51** Anteroposterior pelvic radiograph of the same patient in **Fig. 9.12.50** show the classical, military, osteolytic/osteosclerotic pattern of mastocytosis

reaction causing collagen fibrosis, osteosclerosis, and angiogenesis of the bone marrow. MMM is accompanied by widespread extramedullary hematopoiesis. MMM is typically seen in patients >65 years of age. Death usually occurs 2–3 years after the first onset of the disease. Clinical presentation is divided to myeloproliferation, cytopenia, and constitutional symptoms.

Myeloproliferative symptoms include splenomegaly, hepatomegaly, lymphadenopathy bone pain, portal hypertension (10 %), risk of leukemia, and extramedullary hematopoiesis. Cytopenic symptoms include fatigue, thrombosis, and bleeding. Constitutional symptoms include fatigue, weight loss, night sweat, and hyperuricemia that can lead to gout (5–20 %), arthralgia, and fever. Rare CNS manifestations due to meningeal hematopoiesis include headache, seizures, altered consciousness, and hemiplegia.

Diagnosis is confirmed by laboratory investigations which will show anemia, thrombocytopenia, and characteristic teardrop red blood cells. The white blood count is initially high and then drops (leukopenia). Bone marrow aspiration histological results are nondiagnostic.

### Signs on Barium Follow-Through
1. There is diffuse bowel wall thickening with nodular mucosa due to infiltration of the intestinal lamina propria by mast cells. Differential diagnoses include Whipple's disease, amyloidosis, and lymphangiectasia.
2. Multiple, large bull's eye lesions may be detected. Differential diagnoses of intestinal bull's eye lesions include lymphoma, metastases, Kaposi sarcoma, and aberrant pancreas.

### Signs on Radiographs
1. There is diffuse bone sclerosis that can be patchy mimicking Paget's disease or fluorosis with sandwich vertebrae. Unlike Paget's disease, serum alkaline phosphatase levels are normal in myelofibrosis.
2. Periostitis can be seen along the diaphyses of long bones mimicking osteosarcoma.

### Signs on MRI
There is mosaic bone marrow pattern with high T2 signal intensity surrounded by hypointense rim, best to be seen in the vertebral column.

### Signs on CT
1. Lymphadenopathy, massive splenomegaly, and hepatomegaly are usually present.
2. Bilateral paraspinal masses may be seen in the mid-thoracic segment due to extramedullary hematopoiesis.
3. Bilateral symmetrical nephromegaly without signs of hydronephrosis can be seen due to hematopoiesis. This sign is usually seen in infiltrative processes affecting the kidneys like nephroblastomatosis, Beckwith–Wiedemann syndrome, acute glomerulonephritis, type I glycogen storage disease, and nephritic syndrome.

### Selected References
Avila NA, et al. Pulmonary and ovarian manifestations of systemic mastocytosis. AJR. 1996;166:969–70.

Avila NA, et al. Mastocytosis: magnetic resonance imaging patterns of marrow disease. Skeletal Radiol. 1998;27:119–26.

Haney K, et al. MRI characteristics of systemic mastocytosis of the lumbosacral spine. Skeletal Radiol. 1996;25:171–3.

Jabbour SA, et al. Rare syndromes. Clin Dermatol. 2006;24: 299–316.

Quinn SF, et al. Bull's-eye lesion: a new gastrointestinal presentation of mastocytosis. Gastrointest Radiol. 1984;9:13–5.

## 9.13  Myelofibrosis and Myeloid Metaplasia

Myelofibrosis with myeloid metaplasia (MMM) is a rare disease characterized by abnormal stem cell proliferation within the bone marrow that is accompanied by intense bone marrow

### Signs on MRI
1. The bone marrow contains multiple patchy low T1–T2 signal intensity areas representing fibrosis (**Fig. 9.13.52**); however, low T1–T2 signal intensity lesions within the bone marrow can be seen in MRI in infiltrative processes like leukemia.
2. Extramedullary hematopoiesis masses can be seen in the paraspinal muscles in the mid-thoracic segments

extending into the spinal canal compressing the spinal cord or extending into the neural foramina compressing the spinal nerves. Characteristically, the masses show low signal in T1W images, high signal intensity on T2W images, and diffuse homogenous contrast enhancement after contrast injection (◘ Fig. 9.13.53).

3. CNS meningeal hematopoiesis is a rare complication of MMM that presents as intracranial masses located within the meninges or the falx cerebri and enhances homogenously after contrast injection similar to meningiomas. The history and clinical presentation is important to differentiate between the two. Extramedullary hematopoiesis masses are sensitive to radiotherapy.

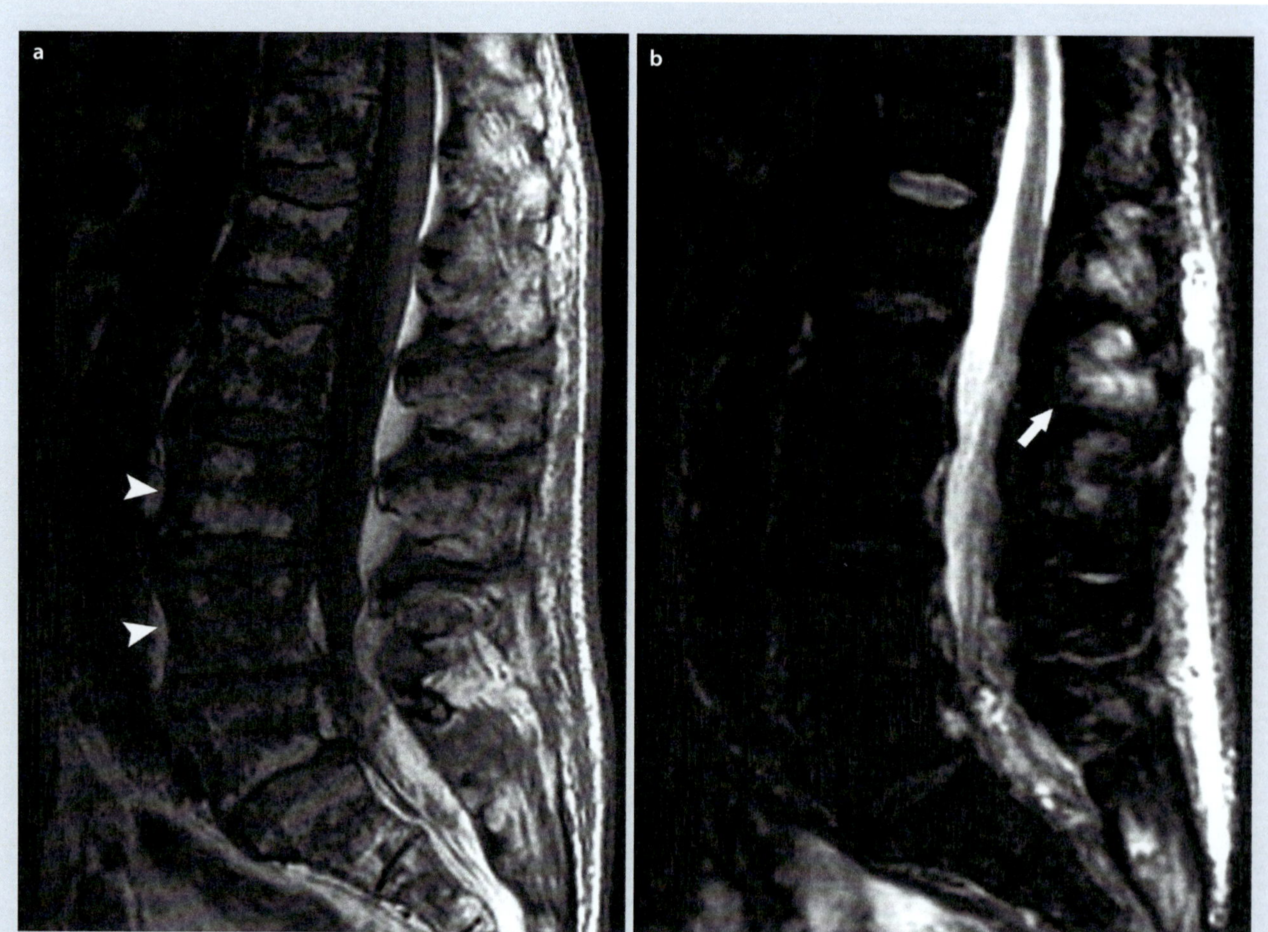

◘ **Fig. 9.13.52**   Sagittal T1W & STIR-W MR images of a patient with myelofibrosis showing reduced signal intensity of the bone marrow in the lumbar vertebrae (*arrowheads* in **a**) with increased T2 signal intensity of the posterior vertebral elements due to active extramedullary hematopoiesis (*arrow* in **b**)

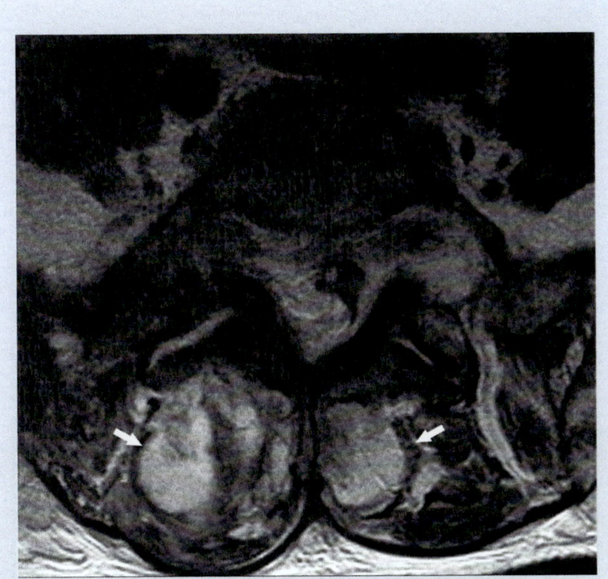

**Fig. 9.13.53** Axial T2W image of the same patient in Fig. 9.13.52 shows paraspinal muscle masses with high T2 signal intensity due to extramedullary hematopoiesis (*arrows*)

## Selected References

Fernback SK, et al. Extramedullary hematopoiesis in the kidneys in infants siblings with myelofibrosis. Pediatr Radiol. 1992;22:211–2.

Guermazi A, et al. Imaging of spinal cord compression due to thoracic extramedullary haematopoiesis in myelofibrosis. Neuroradiology. 1997;39:733–6.

Guermazi A, et al. Imaging findings in patients with myelofibrosis. Eur Radiol. 1999;9:1366–75.

Mesa RA, et al. Myelofibrosis and myeloid metaplasia: disease review and non-transplant treatment options. Best Pract Res Clin Haematol. 2006;19(3):495–517.

# Diabetology




© Springer International Publishing Switzerland 2017
J.A. Al-Tubaikh, *Internal Medicine*, DOI 10.1007/978-3-319-39747-4_10

## 10.1   Diabetic Hand and Diabetic Foot

Diabetes mellitus (DM) is a chronic metabolic disease that arises due to insulin deficiency (type 1 DM) or insulin receptor insensitivity (type 2 DM). Type 2 DM is more common than type 1.

Diabetic complications arise due to cellular ischemia, angiopathy, peripheral neuropathy, osteopathy, infections, skin changes, and atherosclerosis. The hands and feet are uncommonly affected in diabetes, but when they are affected, it may be severe enough to cost the patient loss of a limb.

Radiology offers great tools for early detection of diabetic complications by ultrasound and MRI. For diabetic foot screening, a Doppler scan is performed to detect arterial flow anomalies. If the Doppler scan shows abnormalities in the vessels, MRI can be done to detect hidden signs of diabetic foot complications. Adults with long-term DM should be annually examined for lower limb vascular abnormalities.

## Diabetic Angiopathy

Diabetic angiopathy is divided into two types: microangiopathy and macroangiopathy. Microangiopathy arises due to chronic hyperglycemia that impairs the walls of the microvessels, causing leakage of exudates and blood. Later, these exudates may lead to obstruction of the microvessels causing ischemia. This type is typically seen in diabetic retinopathy and diabetic nephropathy. Macroangiopathy, on the other hand, damages the arterial vessels due to atherosclerosis affecting the coronary, cerebral, and lower limb vessels. Arteriosclerosis occurs 10 years earlier in diabetics than in normal people.

Chronic limb ischemia and compromised vascular supply can lead to tissue necrosis and dry gangrene. This is often complicated by bacterial infection that may cause wet gangrene; this scenario is often seen in the feet. Amputation is the tragic end of severe limb osteomyelitis, extensive lower limb calcifications, and uncontrolled diabetes that suppresses the immune system. Within 2 years of amputation of one leg, the other leg has a 50 % chance of complications that might lead to a 50 % chance of contralateral amputation.

Gangrene can be divided into dry, wet, and infected. *Dry gangrene* arises due to an occluded artery with a patent vein; tissue liquefaction occurs at a very slow rate. It is seen in senile gangrene (due to atherosclerosis and vascular stasis) and Buerger's disease (thromboangiitis obliterans). Senile gangrene is seen in 50 % of elderly patients wearing tight shoes and commonly affects the big toe. *Wet gangrene* arises due to an occluded artery and vein, with rapid tissue liquefaction and sever toxemia. This type is classically seen in DM, crush injuries (accidents), and bedsores. *Infected gangrene* arises due to bacterial infection and is typically seen in lung abscess, necrotizing fasciitis, synergistic gangrene, and gas gangrene (due to muscular lesion with anaerobic fermentation of the tissues with *Clostridium difficile*).

As previously mentioned, patients with gangrene are treated by amputation of the gangrenous part of the lower extremity, which can be above or below the knee, depending on the extension of the compromised vascular supply. The amputee may develop stump pain after surgery, which can be attributed to stump infection, inflammation, impaired vasculature, or development of neuromas. A *neuroma* is a focal, nodular, noncapsulated soft-tissue mass that forms at the distal segment of peripheral nerves after surgery or traumatic avulsion injury. Schwann cells regenerate the peripheral nervous system axons and myelin sheath after trauma. In an amputated limb, regeneration of the nerve axon is unstoppable, because there is no distal end pathway for the regenerated nerve axon to fuse with, resulting in aggregation of the Schwann cells at the stump end, forming a mass of nerve tissue. Postamputation neuromas are usually multiple and may appear 1 month after amputation. Patients typically present with stump pain, usually in the absence of inflammation or stump infection.

### Signs on Radiographs

Calcification of pedal vessels occurs in 24 % of diabetic patients, and it is seen radiologically as classic "tramline" or "pipestem" calcification (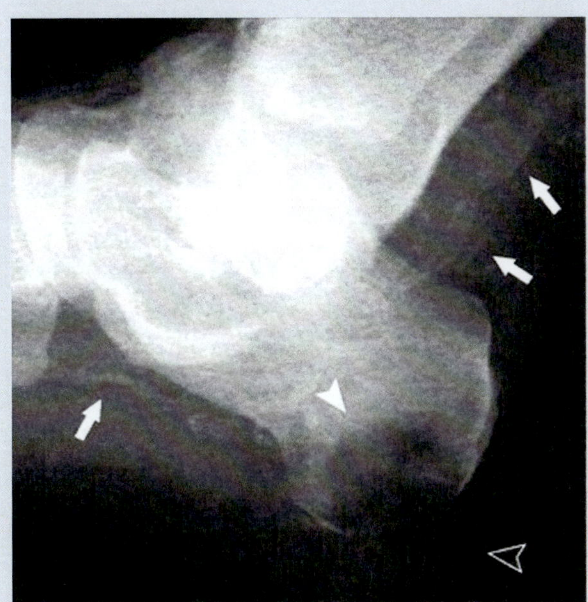 Fig. 10.1.1).

**Fig. 10.1.1**  A lateral plain radiograph of a patient with severe diabetic foot shows calcaneal ulcer (*hollow arrowhead*), osteomyelitis causing bone resorption and necrosis (*solid arrowhead*), and calcified arteries due to macroangiopathy (*arrows*)

## Diabetic Peripheral Neuropathy, Osteopathy, and Infections

Diabetic peripheral neuropathy often affects both hands and feet in a bilateral symmetrical fashion (*glove and stocking phenomenon*). Loss of the deep knee tendon reflex is the earliest sign of diabetic neuropathy, even before any sensory or motor disturbances manifest. Diabetic neuropathy is attributed to metabolic abnormalities affecting Schwann cells, the myelin-forming cells of the peripheral nervous system.

In the neuropathic diabetic foot, sympathetic denervation is the main pathological injury. Somatic and autonomic denervation causes numbness and loss of heat and pain sensation, along with reduction in the sensation of touch and vibration. Sympathetic denervation causes arteriovenous shunts within hands and feet, causing abnormal increase in the venous flow within the limbs. Moreover, the intracutaneous pressure causes the development of calcification within the medial layer of the arterial vascular wall (*Monckeberg's sclerosis*).

There are two types of neuroarthropathies in DM: atrophic and hypertrophic (*Charcot's joint*). Atrophic neuroarthropathy is characterized by osteoporosis, bone resorption, and dislocation. In contrast, Charcot's joint is characterized by the 5Ds: *dis*tention, *d*islocation, *d*isorganization, *d*ebris, and increased bone *d*ensity. In the absence of diabetes, atrophic neuroarthropathy is commonly caused by syrinx in the cervical spine, while Charcot's joint is commonly caused by neurosyphilis of the posterior columns of the spinal cord (*tabes dorsalis*). A syrinx is also the commonest cause of Charcot's joint of the shoulder.

Diabetic peripheral neuropathy affects 10–15 % of patients, and it can be diffuse or focal. The diffuse form presents in the form of bilateral, symmetrical denervation and sensory deficits of the hands and feet (glove and stocking phenomenon). In contrast, the focal form presents in the form of "mononeuritis," commonly affecting the cranial nerves CN III, CN IV, CN VI, and CN VII. Involvement of both sympathetic and sensory fibers leads to mechanical overuse, loss of the protective joint pain, proprioceptive sensation, and active hyperemia due to loss of vasoconstrictive neural impulses, which all result in atrophic neuroarthropathy. In contrast, sensory fiber denervation in the absence of sympathetic fiber involvement results in the development of Charcot's joint. The atrophic joint tends to involve the forefoot, while Charcot's joint tends to affect the mid- or hindfoot.

*Diabetic lumbosacral radiculoplexus neuropathy (DLRPN)*, also known as *Bruns–Garland syndrome*, is an uncommon condition, characterized by asymmetric lower extremity pain, weakness, and muscle atrophy commonly affecting the thigh muscles. The mechanism of injury is thought to be a result of microvasculitis and resultant ischemic injury to the sacral plexus and/or peripheral nerves. Patients with DLRPN are commonly between 46 and 71 years of age, often presenting with acute or subacute onset of severe asymmetric lower limb pain and paresthesia involving the anterolateral thigh region. The pain is described as aching and burning and tends to be worse at night or in contact with cloths or bed sheets (contact allodynia). DLRPN pain is usually followed by limb weakness, evolving over weeks or months, and commonly affects the quadriceps and iliopsoas muscles. Wasting of the quadriceps muscle and absence or reduction in the knee jerk reflex are classic features. DLRPN is commonly preceded by unintentional weight loss. Laboratory findings in DLRPN include high erythrocytes sedimentation rate, occasional positive rheumatoid factor (RF) and antinuclear antibody (ANA), and elevated cerebrospinal fluid protein content.

Osteomyelitis occurs in up to 90 % of cases in the diabetic foot, due to neurotropic pedal ulcers. Diabetic ulcers tend to occur at the sites of pressure over bony or joint protuberance (e.g., metatarsal heads or the calcaneus).

The diabetic foot can be rarely associated with tarsal tunnel syndrome. *Tarsal tunnel syndrome* is a condition characterized by entrapment of the posterior tibial nerve as it passes beneath the flexor retinaculum. The condition is analogous to carpal tunnel syndrome in the wrists. Patients often present with a burning sensation and paresthesia in the toes, sole of the foot, or medial heel, aggravated by weight bearing.

Uncommonly, Freiberg's disease may arise in patients with diabetic foot. *Freiberg's disease* is a disease characterized by infarction of the metatarsal heads. The disease typically develops 3–4 times more frequently in women than men, during late childhood or adolescence. Patients present clinically in the acute phase with local foot pain with tenderness, confined to the area of the metatarsal heads. In the chronic phase, which is characterized by osteonecrosis and repair, patients are typically asymptomatic.

- Osteomyelitis is seen as cortical bone destruction with a moth-eaten appearance of the affected bone (◘ Figs. 10.1.1 and 10.1.3).
- *Lisfranc fracture* is a clinical condition where the entire forefoot is displaced laterally. Lisfranc fracture is diagnosed radiographically when the second metatarsal bone is displaced laterally >2 mm from its articulation with the intermediate cuneiform bone (◘ Fig. 10.1.4).
- Charcot's joint of the hip can result in osteolysis of the acetabulum with loss of its boarders (*wandering acetabulum*) and hypertrophic sclerosis of the femoral head resulting in a "drumstick" appearance.
- The talonavicular joint is a preferred site for Charcot's joint in the hindfoot.

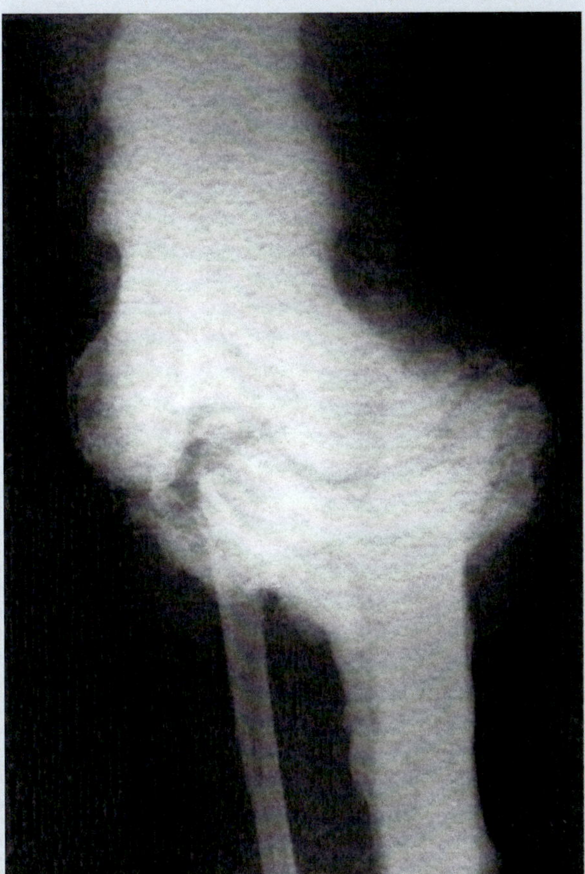

◘ **Fig. 10.1.2**  Anteroposterior plain knee radiograph of a patient with sever Charcot's knee joint demonstrates disorganization, debris, and increased bone density

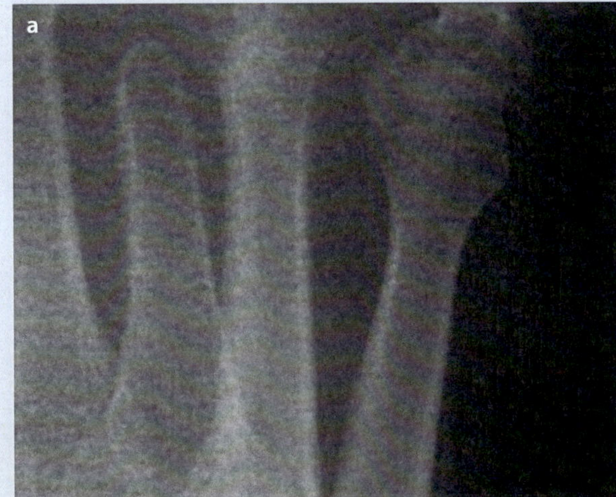

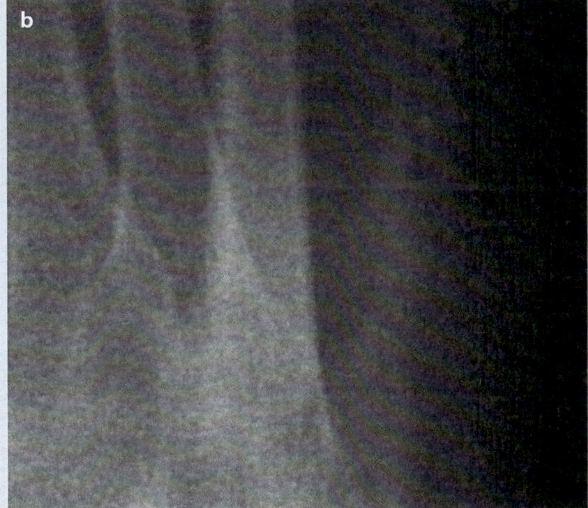

◘ **Fig. 10.1.3**  Plain foot radiographs of a patient with diabetic foot show acute osteomyelitis. In (**a**), the patient was investigated for a pain in the fifth toe, which shows mild osteoporosis compared to the rest of the metatarsals (note the third toe amputation). After 3 months (**b**), the patient showed moth-eaten osteomyelitis bone destruction of the fifth metatarsal bone, with complete cortical destruction

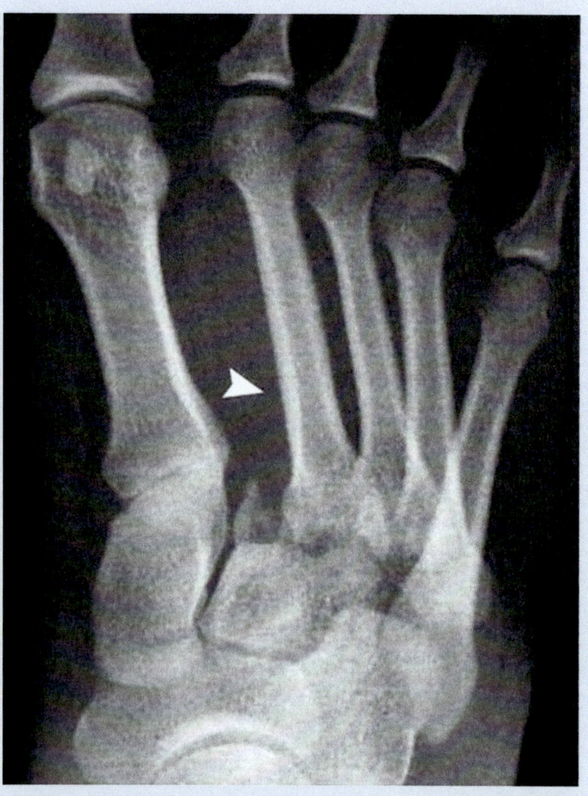



**Fig. 10.1.4**   Plain radiograph of the forefoot show Lisfranc fracture, with lateral displacement of the metatarsals (*arrowhead*)

**Signs on MRI**
- In DLRPN, the scan show enhancement of the lumbosacral nerve roots and plexus after contrast injection.
- In *Freiberg's infarction*, the metatarsal head shows low T1 signal intensity and high T2 signal intensity, with contrast enhancement (**Fig. 10.1.5**).

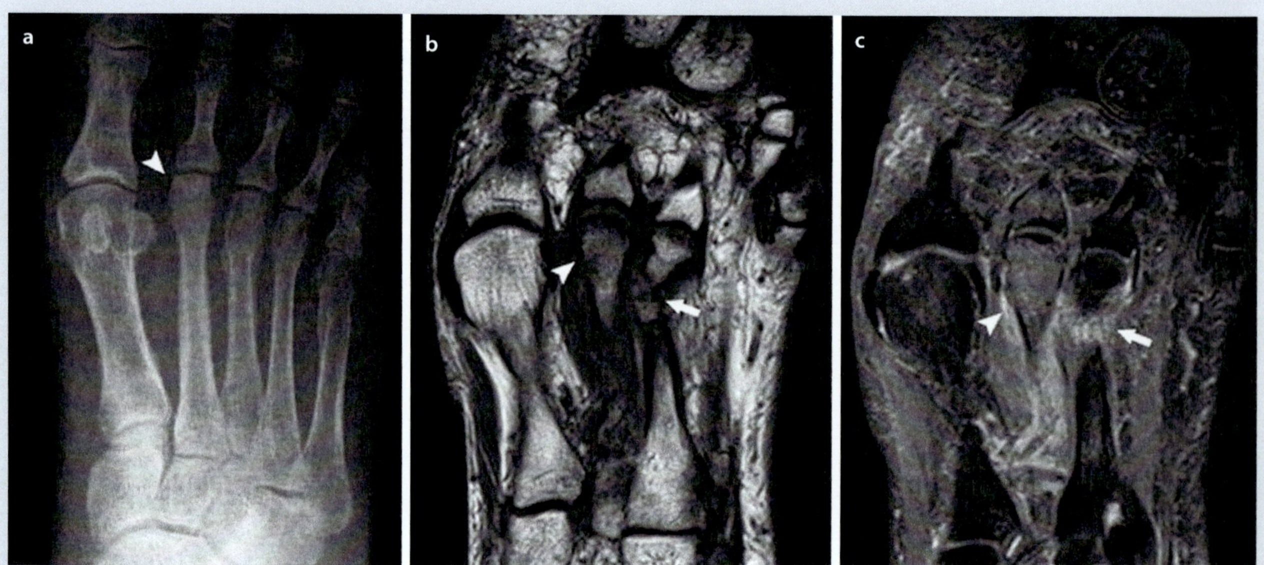



**Fig. 10.1.5**   Plain foot radiograph (**a**), T1W (**b**), and sagittal short tau inversion recovery (STIR) (**c**) foot MRI of a patient show the signs of Freiberg's infarction. In (**a**), there is mild flattening and sclerosis of the second metatarsal head (*arrowhead*). Later, the patient underwent a foot MRI that confirmed bone infarction of the second metatarsal head seen as low T1 signal intensity in (**b**) and high signal intensity in (**c**). The MRI shows also fracture of the third metatarsal neck (*arrows*), which was not well appreciated in the plain radiograph (**a**)

## Diabetic Myonecrosis

Diabetic myonecrosis is a rare complication of diabetes, characterized by muscle infarction. Most patient affected with diabetic myonecrosis are patients with type 1 DM (74 %) and type 2 DM (26 %) or patients with prolonged poorly controlled diabetes. Diabetic myonecrosis occurs in association with diabetic retinopathy (60 %), nephropathy (80 %), or neuropathy (64 %). It almost always occurs in the lower extremities and often affects the quadriceps muscles.

Patients with diabetic myonecrosis commonly present with a painful limb, swelling, and resting pain that is aggravated by walking. If one limb is affected by diabetic myonecrosis, the contralateral limb may be involved up to 2 years after the initial manifestation.

The main differential diagnosis of diabetic myonecrosis includes deep venous thrombosis (DVT) and pyomyositis. DVT can be ruled out by Doppler sonography. Pyomyositis is a severe muscle infection with formation of an intramuscular abscess. In 90 % of cases, it is caused by *Staphylococcus*. In contrast, diabetic myonecrosis does not show positive culture of *Staphylococcus*, because it is mostly caused by ischemia and infarction rather than infection.

> **Signs on MRI**
> The affected muscle shows extensive edema and swelling, with high signal intensity on T2W images involving the muscle and the subcutaneous tissues.

## Diabetic Skin Changes and Infections

Diabetic hand lesions are not as common as diabetic foot lesions, perhaps due to the stress load on the feet compared to the hands. The main lesions of the hands in diabetes are related to dermatological diseases rather than neuro-osteopathic diseases such as those of the feet.

*Diabetic dermopathy* is characterized by the formation of multiple skin thickening on the back of the fingers (finger pebbles), scleroderma-like skin and stiff joints of the fingers and dorsum of the hand, and brown atrophic macules over the shin. *Acanthosis nigricans* is hyperpigmentation and velvety brown thickening of the major skin flexures, which is often seen with type 2 DM and obese patients.

*Diabetic hand syndrome* refers to a condition of neuropathy denervation of the hand. It is characterized by intrinsic wasting of the hand muscles and atrophy of the palmar tissues, with flexion contractures of the fingers that may mimic Dupuytren's contracture. Patients with diabetic hand syndrome often complain of *carpal tunnel syndrome*, with paresthesia in the palmar distribution of the median nerve (the first three fingers) and positive *Tinel's sign* (pain and paresthesia initiated in the palmar sensory distribution of the median nerve by tapping over the palmar aspect of the wrist). Moreover, sever neuropathic denervation may lead to

Sudeck's atrophy (*shoulder–hand disease*). Sudeck's atrophy is a disease characterized by osteoporosis and swelling in one limb, especially the ankles, wrists, and elbows, after a minor trauma. It results from abnormal sympathetic innervations and secondary vascular changes after minor trauma and typically affects the distal part of a limb below the trauma.

*Tropical diabetic hand syndrome*, a terminology used to describe a specific infection of the hands in diabetics, usually occurs in tropical areas and is characterized by progressive synergistic gangrene (*Meleney's gangrene*) of the hand following minor trauma. The cause of this syndrome is a progressively severe form of cellulitis caused by multibacterial infection, usually after a history of minor trauma or a scratch (◘ Fig. 10.1.6).

*Necrobiosis lipoidica diabeticorum (NLD)* is a rare, degenerative, granulomatous skin disease that often affects the lower extremities in diabetic patients (0.3 % of diabetics). Lesions are red papules or oval plaques that grow peripherally and become atrophic and yellowish at the center, with elevated and erythematous edges (◘ Fig. 10.1.7). With time, these lesions become more brownish-yellow, telangiectatic, and porcelain-like. In most cases they are bilateral. Ulceration, the most common complication of NLD (35 %), usually arises after a minor trauma. Lesions in NLD are granulomatous, mainly affecting the subcutaneous tissues and the dermis, and the epidermis is often normal or atrophic. NLD is classically found in young Caucasian diabetic patients, with female predominance (80 %); however, it may occur also with sarcoidosis, rheumatoid arthritis, and inflammatory bowel disease.

When normal skin is stroked with a dull object, it rises and swells to assume the shape of the stroke, due to edema and

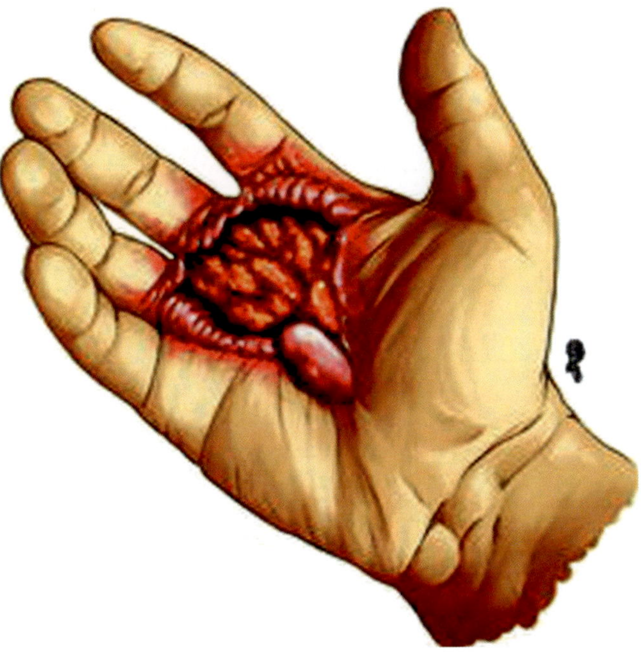

◘ **Fig. 10.1.6** An illustration demonstrates severe synergistic gangrene of tropical diabetic hand syndrome

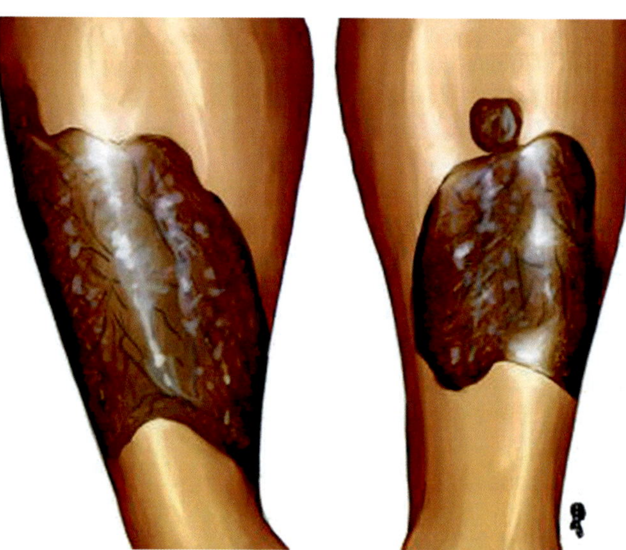



local erythema. In rare situations, exaggeration of this response may be seen in diabetic patients, a condition known as *dermatographism (mechanical urticaria)*. Skin stroke erythema in normal skin develops and subsides in less than 5–10 min, whereas in dermatographism, it can last up to 30 min.

*Fournier's gangrene*, also known as necrotizing fasciitis of the scrotum, is a medical emergency that is characterized by rapidly progressing gangrene of the penis and scrotum, usually in diabetic males aged 50–70 years. Fournier's gangrene is commonly seen after perineal trauma, urinary tract infection, or urological surgical procedures. Fournier's gangrene is initiated by perianal, perirectal, and ischiorectal abscesses, fissures, or urinary extravasation. Systemic findings include leukocytosis, fever, hypoglycemia, tachycardia, and dehydration.

The skin of the back of the neck is surrounded by tough deep fascia that attaches to the epidermis layer by fibrous bands, creating separated compartments. In diabetics, subcutaneous infection on the back of the neck is localized by these fibrous bands laterally and inferiorly, forcing the abscess to spread to the surface via a sinus. Multiple intercommunicating abscesses that open into the surface via multiple sinuses in diabetic patient is a special type of abscess called "*carbuncle.*"

### Signs on Plain Radiographs

Changes in the hand due to Sudeck's atrophy are typically seen as severe osteoporosis, which occurs at the ends of all the phalanges and up to 70 % of metatarsal heads ( Fig. 10.1.8). Pseudoperiostitis may be seen as striation of the cortices due to new bone formation. Severe subluxation of the phalangeal joints may occur later in the course of the disease.

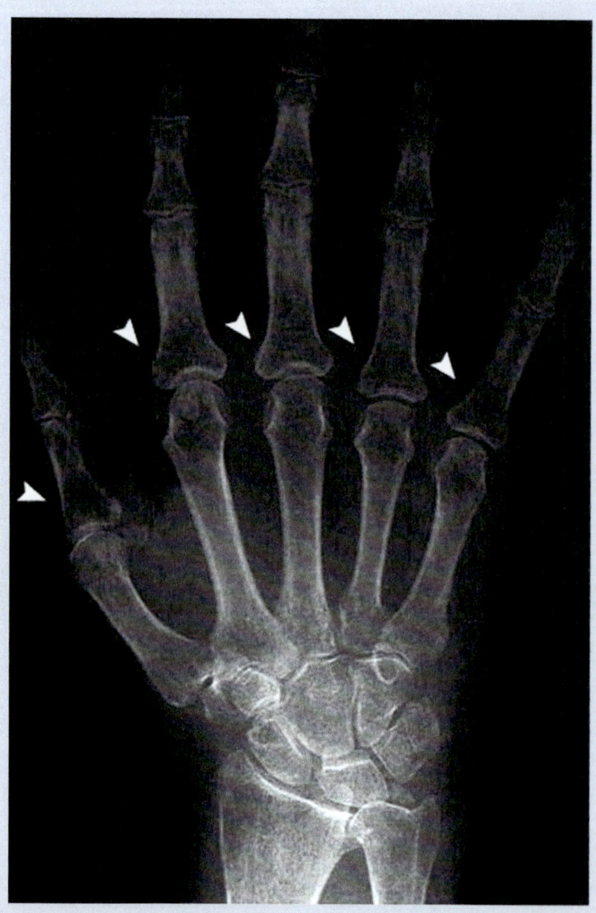

 Fig. 10.1.8   Plain hand radiograph of a patient with Sudeck's atrophy shows marked osteoporosis of the hand that is localized to the phalanges and the metatarsal heads (*arrowheads*)

### Signs on US

— Carpal tunnel syndrome can be diagnosed with wrist ultrasound by identifying the nerve below the flexor retinaculum. Diagnosis of nerve entrapment is achieved when the nerve transverse diameter exceeds 10 mm due to edema or when the nerve fails to return to its normal position when performing the flexion pinch maneuver ( Fig. 10.1.9).

— Fournier's gangrene is characterized by thickening of the scrotal skin, with gas formation within the subcutaneous skin, seen as hyperechoic foci surrounded by dirty shadowing.

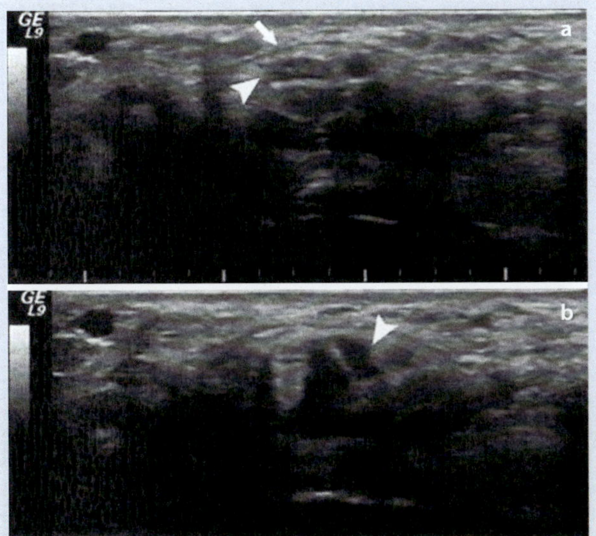

**Fig. 10.1.9**  Median nerve ultrasound in a healthy volunteer shows the normal median nerve (*arrowhead*) seen below the flexor retinaculum (*arrow*) as a hypoechoic structure in (**a**) and (**b**). The median nerve transverse diameter was 4 mm. In the flexion pinch maneuver, the patient is asked to flex his wrist, forcefully oppose the thumb to the index finger, hold the position for 3–5 s, and then release. In this maneuver, the median nerve moves in a sagittal motion deep into the carpal tunnel (*arrowhead* in **b**) and then returns to its normal position. Failure of the nerve to return to its normal position or to move deep into the carpal tunnel with this maneuver is a sign of entrapment

### Signs on CT

Fournier's gangrene is seen as thickened scrotal and/or penile skin with hypodense soft-tissue fluid collection surrounded by rim contrast enhancement (abscess). Air within the mass and the subcutaneous tissues is a typical sign of necrotizing fasciitis (◘ Fig. 10.1.10).

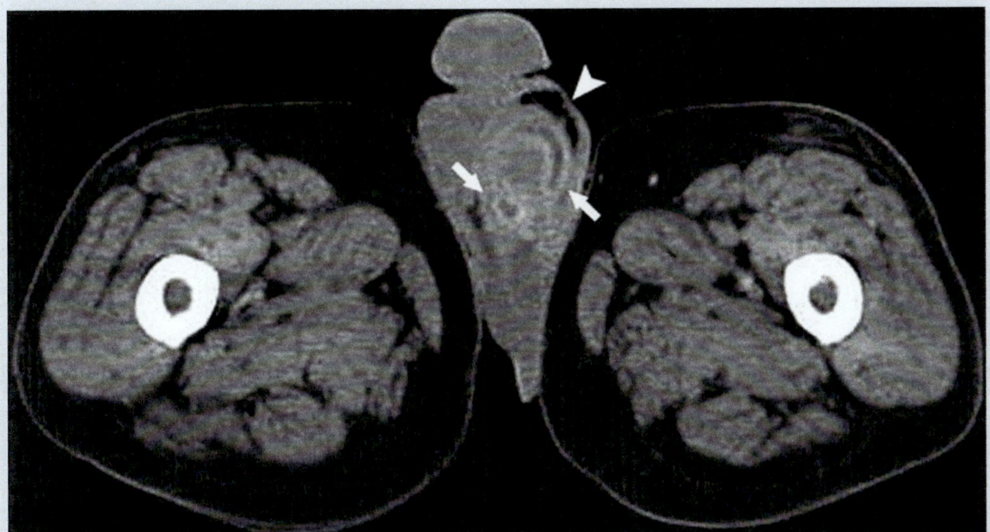

**Fig. 10.1.10**  Axial postcontrast CT of the scrotum and the upper thighs shows scrotal abscess with areas of ring contrast enhancement (*arrows*) and gas formation (*arrowhead*); a radiological stigma of Fournier's gangrene

**Signs on MRI**

**Signs on MRI**

In patients with carpal tunnel syndrome, there is a typical flattening of the median nerve, with high signal intensity in T2W images with contrast enhancement, due to inflammation.

## The Role of Doppler Sonography in DM

Doppler sonography is used to detect stenosis within the arterial system of the lower extremities. Arteriosclerosis is the most common cause of arterial stenosis with the formation of atheromas and calcium plaques within the arterial walls. Analysis of the Doppler wave spectrum is essential to detect the hemodynamic abnormalities of circulation in the lower limbs. Different spectral waves are observed, according to the degree of stenosis.

**Signs of Peripheral Vascular Disease on Doppler Scan (Can Be Detected Even Before the Appearance of Clinical Symptoms)**

- Medial arterial wall calcification with acoustic shadowing *string of beads sign* (◘ Fig. 10.1.11).
- Increased diastolic flow with reduced resistance index (RI) in the spectral flow analysis (◘ Fig. 10.1.12). The increase in diastolic flow is due to arteriovenous shunting.
- Spectral flow abnormalities.

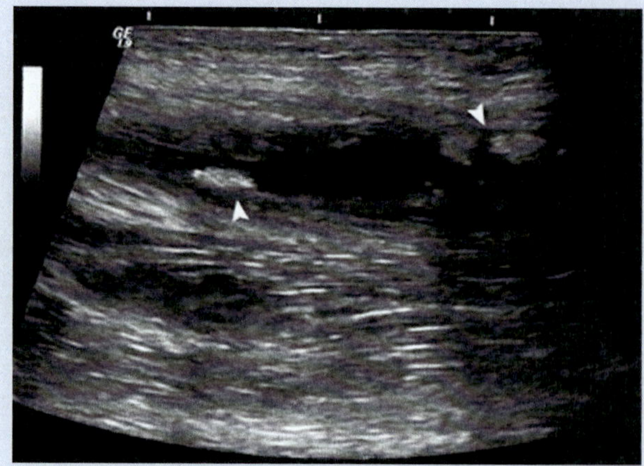

◘ **Fig. 10.1.11** Sagittal ultrasound image of the superficial femoral artery in a diabetic shows multiple dense calcifications of the arterial wall (*arrowheads*)

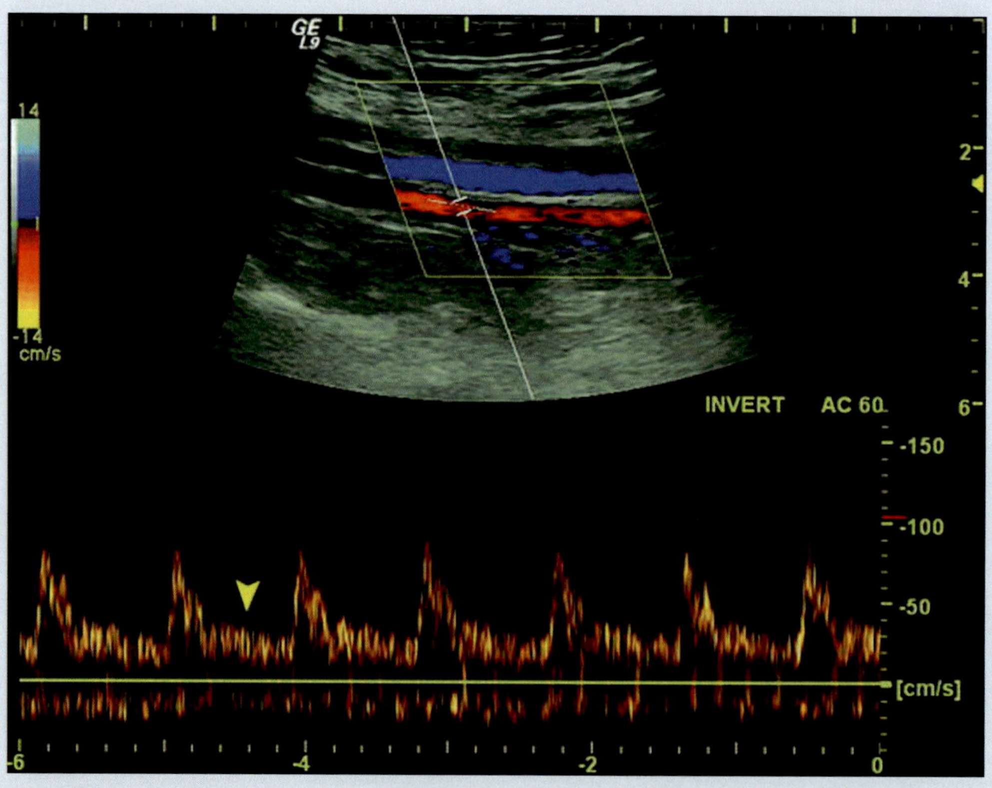

◘ **Fig. 10.1.12** Sagittal ultrasound image of the superficial femoral artery in a patient with peripheral vascular disease due to diabetes mellitus (DM) shows monophasic arterial spectral wave with increased diastolic flow (*arrowhead*)

## Spectral Flow Abnormalities on Doppler Scan of the Lower Limbs

- The normal arterial spectrum is triphasic, with peak systolic velocity (PSV) ~120 cm/s.
- 0–50 % stenosis: shows triphasic or biphasic arterial spectrum (due to loss of the reversal flow pattern), with PSV <180 cm/s.
- 50–75 % stenosis: shows biphasic or monophasic arterial spectrum, with PSV >180 cm/s (◘ Fig. 10.1.13).
- 75–99 % stenosis (high grade): shows biphasic or monophasic arterial spectrum, with PSV >250 cm/s.
- As the stenosis becomes generalized and affects a long segment of the artery, the flow spectrum becomes biphasic or monophasic, the acceleration upstroke is reduced, and the systolic peak becomes rounded (◘ Fig. 10.1.14).



## The Role of MRI in DM

MRI is a powerful tool to detect early bone changes that may not be seen on plain radiographs or evoke complaints – unless they are severe and destructive. Contrast-enhanced studies should be done to detect signs of soft-tissue inflammation, abscess formation, sinus tract detection, and devitalization.



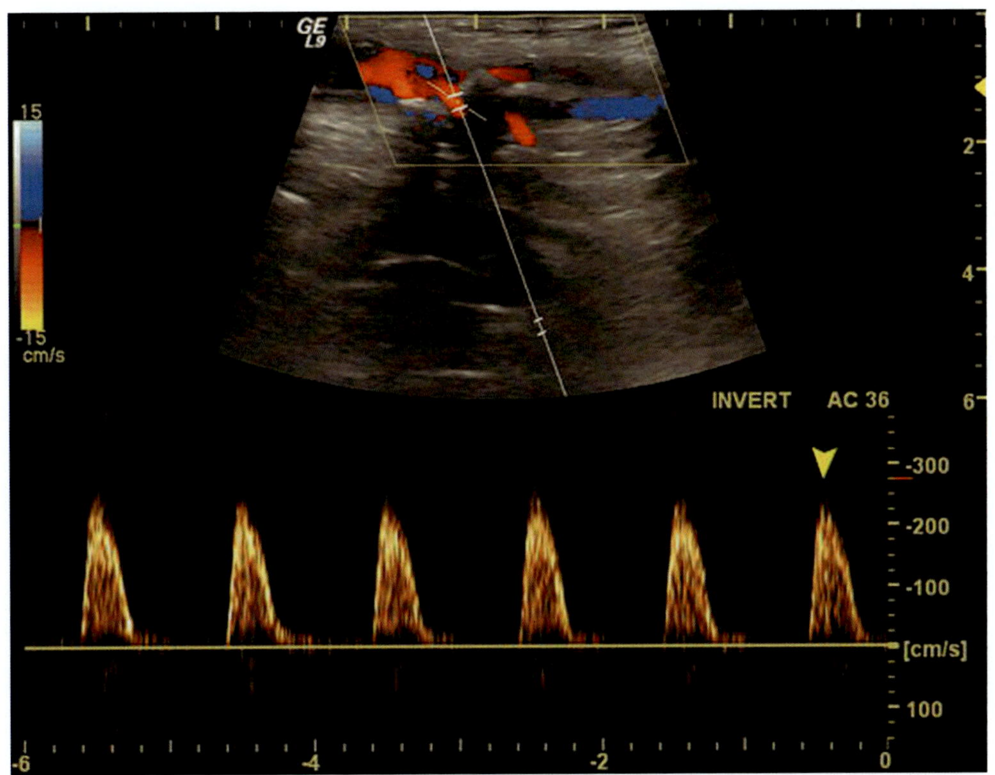

◘ Fig. 10.1.13 Sagittal ultrasound image of the superficial femoral artery in a patient with peripheral vascular disease due to DM shows monophasic arterial spectral wave with PSV >250 cm/s (*arrowhead*), representing >75–99 % arterial stenosis

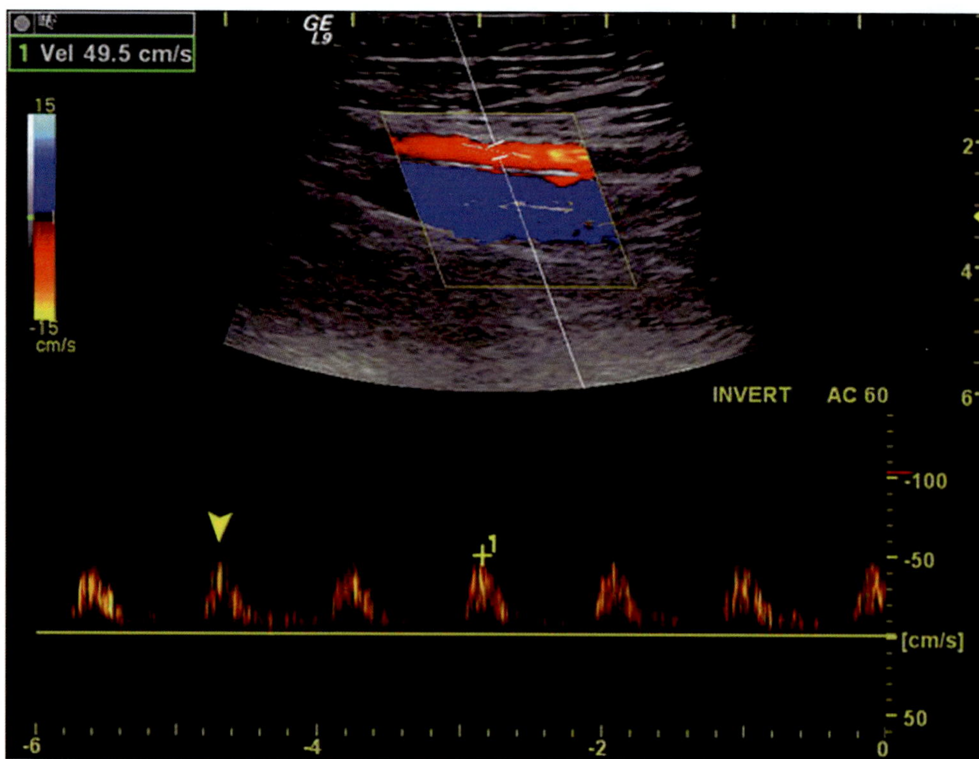

**Fig. 10.1.14** Sagittal ultrasound image of the superficial femoral artery in a patient with peripheral vascular disease due to DM shows monophasic arterial spectral wave with PSV <50 cm/s (*arrowhead*). As mentioned earlier, the normal peripheral arterial spectral wave for the superficial femoral artery is triphasic, with PSV <120 cm/s

- *Cellulitis* is an area of soft-tissue inflammation and is detected on MRI as an ill-defined area of soft tissue with low T1 and high T2 signal intensities, with ill-defined enhancement after contrast administration (**Fig. 10.1.16**).
- An *abscess* is a localized area of pus collection and typically detected as acystic area of low T1 and high T2 signal intensities, with ring enhancement after contrast administration (**Fig. 10.1.17**).
- *Reactive bone marrow* is detected as a normal (isointense) signal intensity of the bone marrow on T1W images, with high signal intensity on T2W images (**Fig. 10.1.18**).
- *Osteomyelitis* is inflammation of the bone and the bone marrow. It is detected on MR as areas of cortical bone defect characterized by the following characteristics: it diffuses bone marrow edema, may show sequestrum, shows no bone deformities (unless complicated by neuropathic joint), usually underlies an ulcer (e.g., metatarsal heads), and may show sinus formation into the skin surface, and the soft tissue around it is usually inflamed and shows marked contrast enhancement (**Fig. 10.1.19**). Signs of periostitis may be found, which is seen as linear contrast enhancement surrounding the outer cortical margin. An intraosseous abscess may occur in subacute osteomyelitis (*Brodie's abscess*), which is characterized by the *penumbra sign*. The penumbra sign is detected on MRI as a discrete zone of

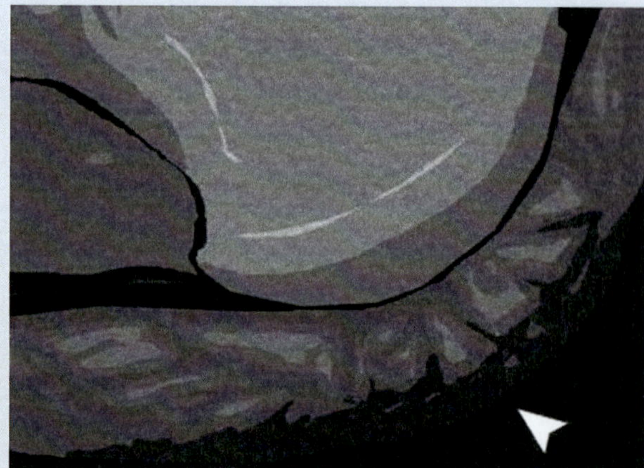
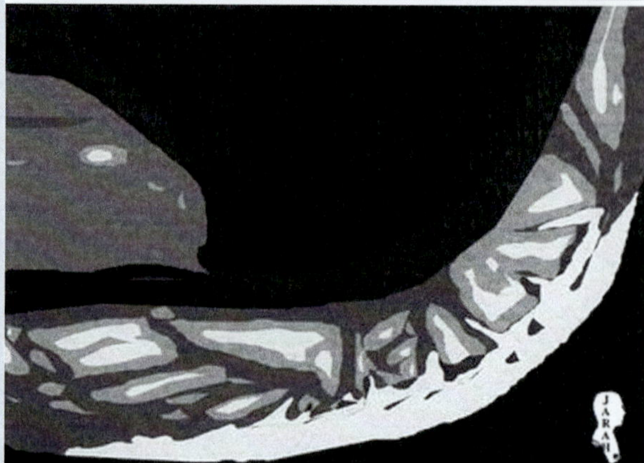

**Fig. 10.1.15** Sagittal T1W (**a**) and STIR (**b**) ankle MR illustrations demonstrate callus seen as an area of soft tissue with low T1 signal intensity in (**a**) and with high T2 signal intensity in (**b**) (*arrowheads*)

peripheral T2 hyperintensity signal surrounding a high T2 signal intensity intraosseous abscess (◨ Fig. 10.1.19). Osteomyelitis is classically located in a single focus. However, multiple lesions may be seen in 20 % of cases.

— *Septic arthritis* is inflammation of a joint due to infection. It is detected on MRI as high T2 signal intensity within a joint and its surrounded soft tissue, with signs of joint effusion and cartilage destruction. There is intense enhancement of the joint and its surrounding soft tissue after contrast administration (◨ Fig. 10.1.20).

— A *foreign body* is detected on MRI as an object of low T2 signal intensity, surrounded by a high-intensity signal in the soft tissues on T2W images (due to edema around the foreign body) (◨ Fig. 10.1.21).

— *Neuroarthropathic joint* (*Charcot's joint*) has the same presentation and signal intensities as osteomyelitis, with destruction of the subchondral cortices. Neuropathic joint is characterized by midfoot predominance, subchondral cyst formation, normal surrounding tissue with intact overlying skin, juxta-articular edema, signs of joint disorganization and deformity (5Ds), and no signs of fluid collection or abscess (◨ Fig. 10.1.22). Osteomyelitis, in contrast to neuropathic joint, predominates in pressure areas such as the metatarsal heads in the forefoot and the calcaneus in the hindfoot. The only common location for osteomyelitis in the midfoot is in the cuboid bone, which occurs in severe midfoot neuropathic joint. However, bone biopsy remains the definite diagnostic method to differentiate osteomyelitis from neuropathic joints in diabetics.

— *Tenosynovitis* is detected as normal tendon size, surrounded by high T2 fluid-signal intensity on T2W images.

— *Calcaneal insufficiency avulsion fracture* is an extra-articular fracture affecting the posterior third of the calcaneus (◨ Fig. 10.1.23). It is seen almost exclusively in diabetics. Sinus tract is detected as a hypodense line extending from an area of bone destruction to the adjacent soft tissues (◨ Fig. 10.1.19). It is best detected on postcontrast fast-suppressed T1W images.

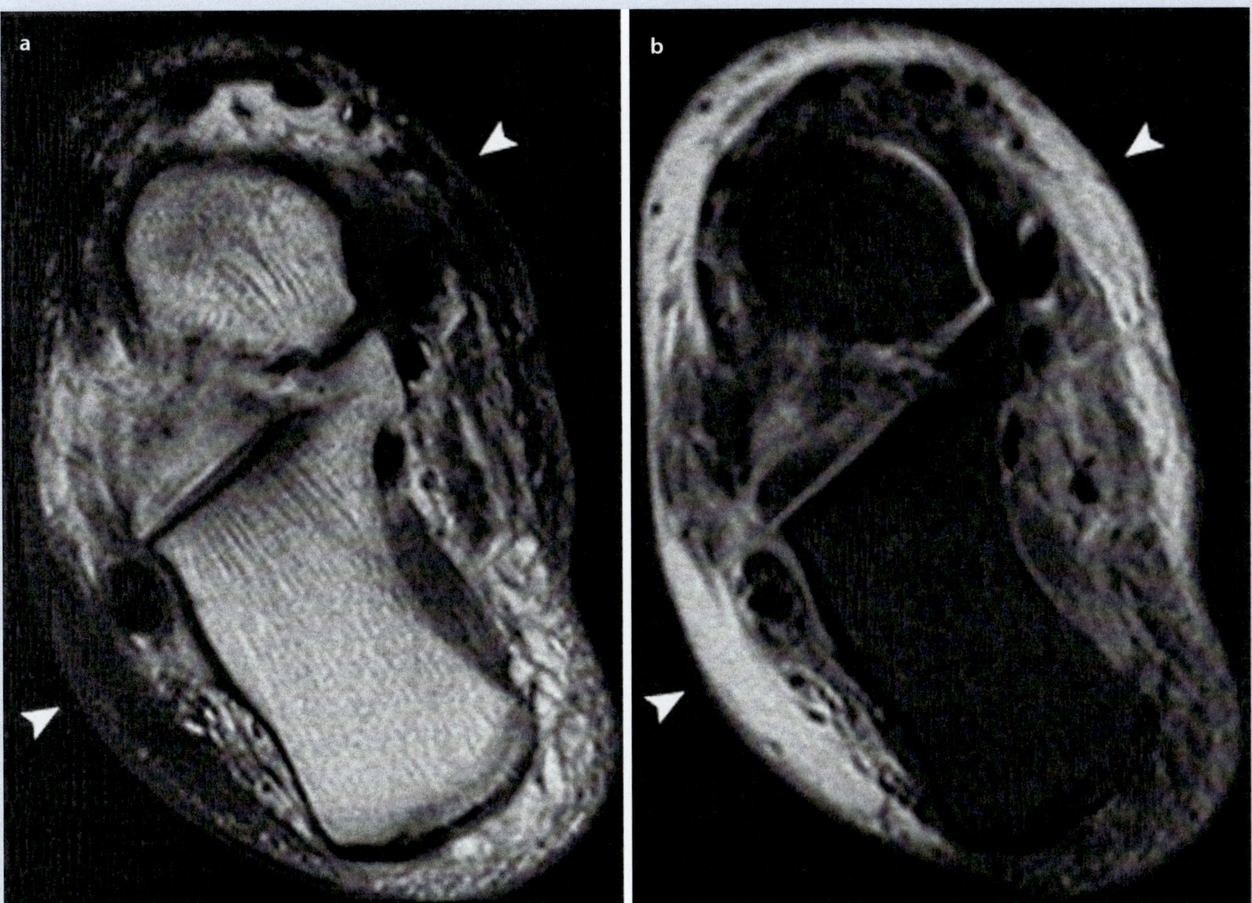

◨ **Fig. 10.1.16**   Sagittal T1W (**a**) and STIR (**b**) ankle MRI show areas of low T1 and high T2 signal intensity lesions confined to the skin and the subcutaneous tissue, without signs of bone marrow edema or joint effusion (*arrowheads*), representing cellulites

10

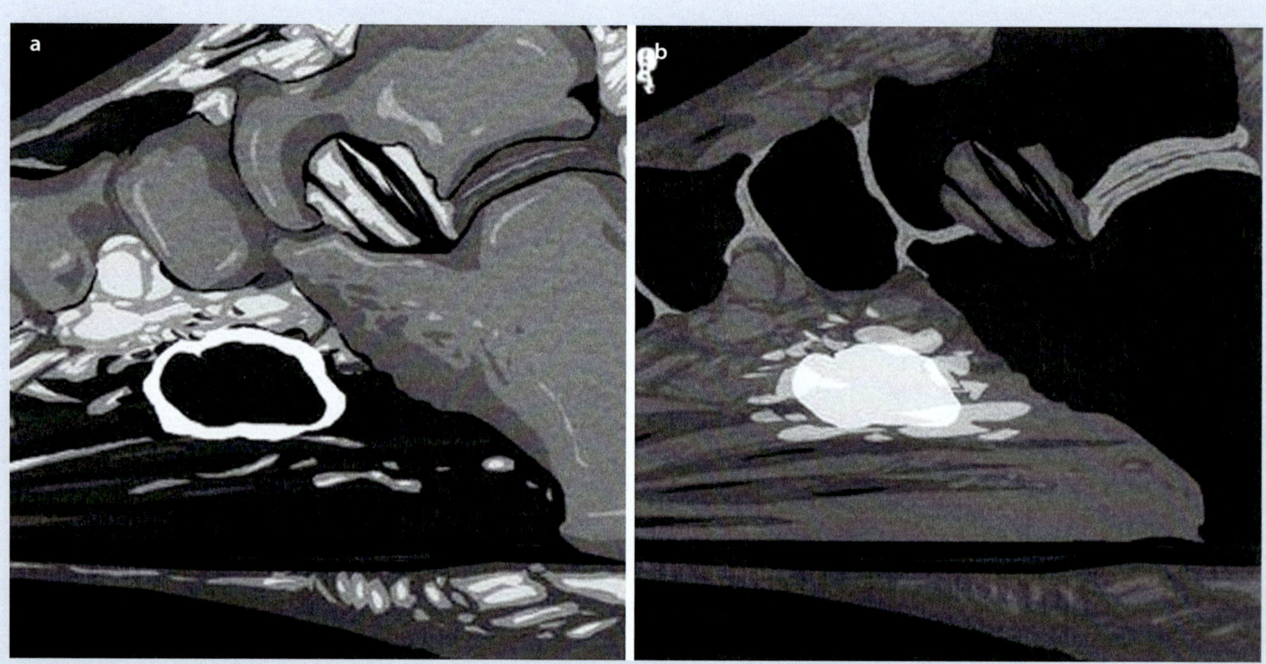

■ **Fig. 10.1.17** Sagittal T1W postcontrast (**a**) and STIR (**b**) ankle MR illustrations demonstrate abscess formation, seen as a cystic area surrounded by rim contrast enhancement in (**a**) and seen as an area of cystic fluid collection in (**b**)

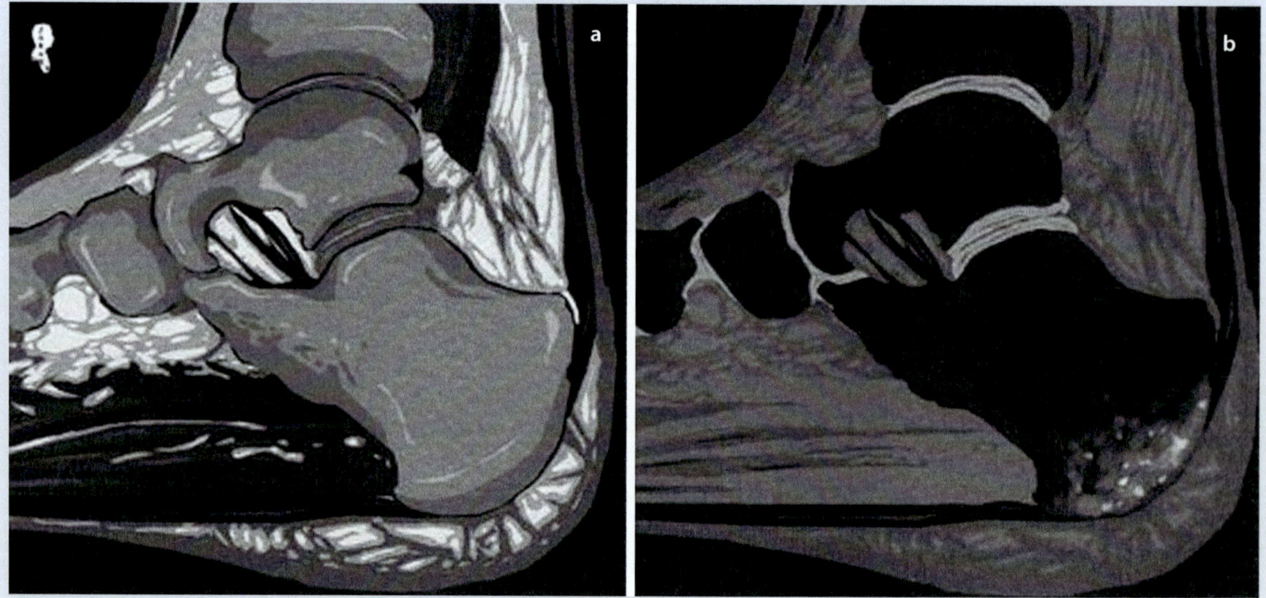

■ **Fig. 10.1.18** Sagittal T1W (**a**) and STIR (**b**) ankle MR illustrations demonstrate reactive bone edema affecting the posterior third of the calcaneus

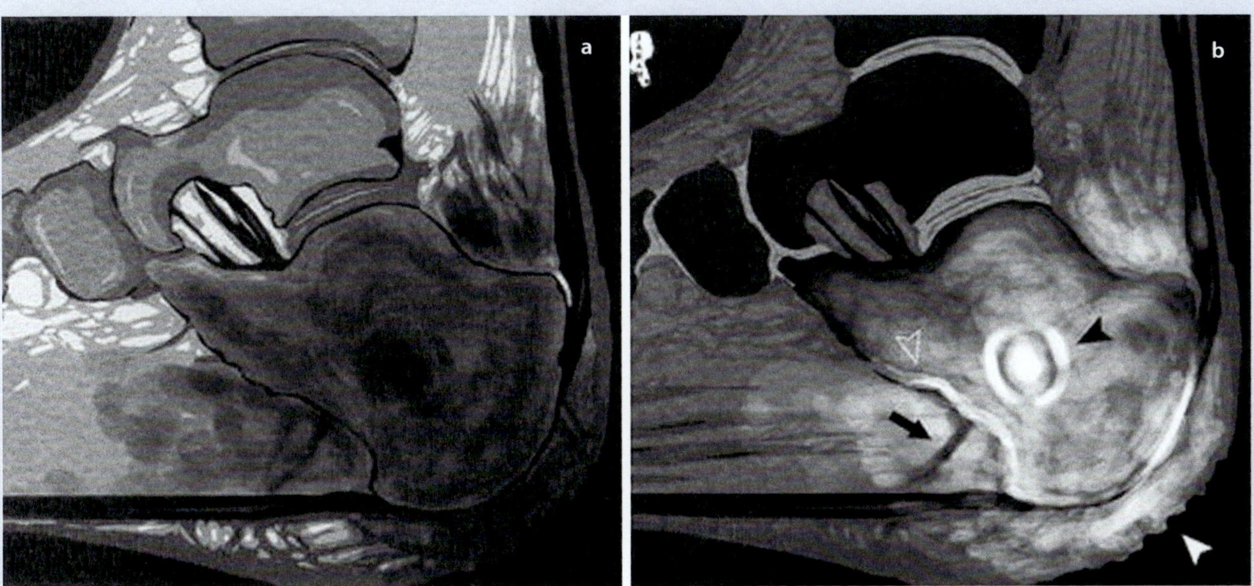

■ **Fig. 10.1.19** Sagittal T1W postcontrast (**a**) and STIR (**b**) ankle MR illustrations show signs of osteomyelitis. Notice the calcaneal ulcer with edema (*white arrowhead*), the penumbra sign (*black arrowhead*), sinus tract from the osteomyelitis spreading infection to the nearby soft tissues (*arrow*), and signs of periostitis seen as linear high signal intensities located around the cortex of the calcaneus (*hollow arrowhead*)

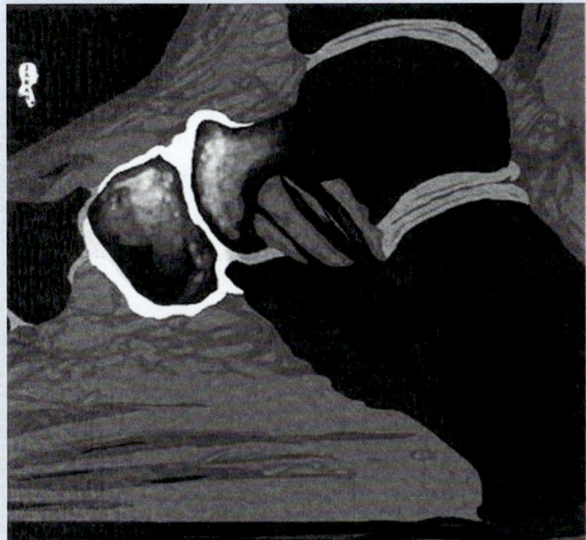

■ **Fig. 10.1.20** Sagittal STIR ankle MR illustration demonstrates talonavicular joint septic arthritis, seen as bone marrow edema affecting the articular bones with joint effusion

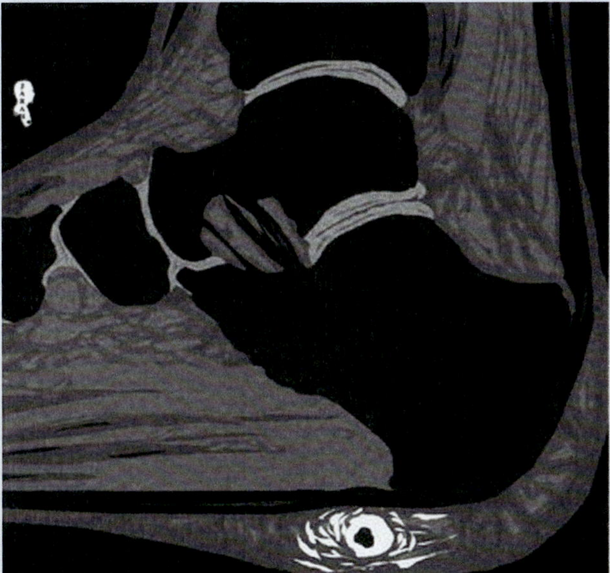

■ **Fig. 10.1.21** Sagittal STIR ankle MR illustration demonstrates a foreign body surrounded by tissue edema located within the infracalcaneal soft-tissue region

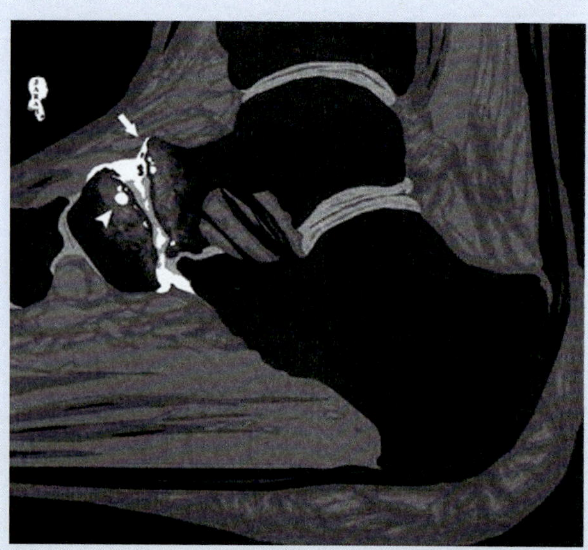

**Fig. 10.1.22** Sagittal STIR ankle MR illustration demonstrates talonavicular Charcot's joint. Notice the midfoot location, the joint deformity (*arrow*), the subchondral cysts (*arrowhead*), and the mild joint effusion due to reactive inflammation

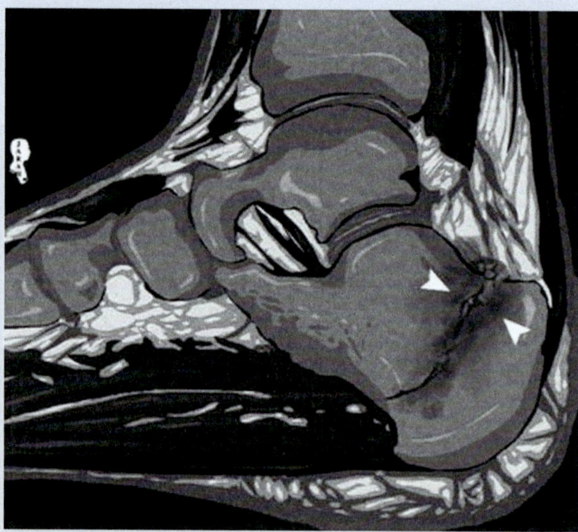

**Fig. 10.1.23** Sagittal T1W ankle MR illustration demonstrates avulsion fracture of the posterior third of the calcaneus (*arrowheads*)

## Differential Diagnoses and Related Diseases

*Congenital insensitivity to pain (CIPA)*: CIPA, also referred to as *hereditary sensory and autonomic neuropathy type IV*, is a rare disorder characterized by the inability to perceive pain stimuli due to peripheral autonomic nervous system demyelination and reduced fiber caliber. CIPA patients respond to normal pain stimuli but not to painful stimuli. Early symptoms include decreased sweating (anhidrosis), which causes episodes with extreme hyperpyrexia, multiple healed tongue bites since infancy, and multiple missing teeth due to auto-extraction (50 % of cases). Characteristically, CIPA patients present with multiple bony features at varying stages of the healing process. Interestingly, patients with CIPA develop aseptic necrosis and osteochondritis in the juxta-articular regions of the weight-bearing long bones (hip, knees, and ankles). Joint radiographs of CIPA patients show changes similar to those of chronic Charcot's joint and osteomyelitis.

## Further Reading


Abdel-Hafez HZ, et al. Congenital insensitivity to pain with anhidrosis (CIPA). Egypt Dermatol Online J. 2007;3(1):5.

Beltran J, et al. The diabetic foot: magnetic resonance imaging evaluation. Skeletal Radiol. 1990;19:37–41.

Bhanushali MJ, et al. Diabetic and non-diabetic lumbosacral radiculoplexus neuropathy. Neurol India. 2008;56(4):420–5.

Bhute D, et al. Dermatographism. Indian J Dermatol Venerol Leprol. 2008;74:177–9.

Biswal N, et al. Congenital indifference to pain. Indian J Pediatr. 1988;65:755–69.

Chantelau E, et al. "Silent" bone stress injuries in the feet of diabetic patients with polyneuropathy: a report on 12 cases. Arch Orthop Trauma Surg. 2007;127:171–7.

Chatha DS, et al. MR imaging of the diabetic foot: diagnostic challenges. Radiol Clin North Am. 2005;43:747–59.

Chuter V, et al. Limited joint mobility and plantar fascia function in Charcot's neuroarthropathy. Diabet Med. 2001;18:558–61.

Erickson SJ, et al. MR imaging of the tarsal tunnel syndrome and related spaces: normal and abnormal findings with anatomic correlation. AJR Am J Roentgenol. 1990;155:323–8.

Gefen A, et al. Integration of plantar soft tissue stiffness measurements in routine MRI of the diabetic foot. Clin Biomech. 2001;16:921–5.

Glauser SR, et al. Diabetic muscle infarction: a rare complication of advanced diabetes mellitus. Emerg Radiol. 2008;15:61–5.

Gold RH, et al. Imaging the diabetic foot. Skeletal Radiol. 1995;24:563–71.

Jung Y, et al. Diabetic hand syndrome. Metabolism. 1971;20(11):1008–15.

Marcus CD, et al. MR imaging of osteomyelitis and neuropathic osteoarthropathy in the feet of diabetics. Radiographics. 1996;16:1337–48.

McGuinness M, et al. Necrobiosis Lipoidica diabeticorum. Foot. 1997;7:47–51.

Naderi ASA, et al. Diabetic muscle necrosis. J Diabet Complications. 2008;22:150–2.

Nguyen VD, et al. Freiberg's disease in diabetes mellitus. Skeletal Radiol. 1991;20:425–8.

Nguyen K, et al. Necrobiosis Lipoidica diabeticorum treated with chloroquine. J Am Acad Dermatol. 2002;46:S34–6.

Peyri J, et al. Necrobiosis lipoidica. Semin Cutan Med Surg 2007;26(2):87–9.

Piedra T, et al. Fournier's gangrene: a radiologic emergency. Abdom Imaging. 2006;31:500–2.

Purewal TS. Charcot's diabetic neuroarthropathy: pathogenesis, diagnosis and management. Pract Diab Int. 1996;13(3):88–91.

Puttemans T, et al. Diabetes: the use of color Doppler sonography for the assessment of vascular complications. Eur J Ultrasound. 1998;7:15–22.

Reinhardt K. The radiological residua of healed diabetic arthropathies. Skeletal Radiol. 1981;7:167–72.

Singson RD, et al. Postamputation neuromas and other symptomatic stump abnormalities: detection with CT. Radiology. 1987;162:743–5.

Singson RD, et al. Postamputation neuromas. Skeletal Radiol. 1990;19:259–62.

Tan PL, et al. MRI of the diabetic foot: differentiation of infection from neuropathic change. Br J Radiol. 2007;80:939–48.

Tiwari S, et al. Tropical diabetic hand syndrome. Int J Diab Dev Ctries. 2008;28(4):130–1.

## 10.2  Diabetic Brain and Nervous System

In advanced stages, diabetes mellitus (DM) can affect the brain, due to microangiopathy and prolonged exposure to hypoglycemia. Over the past decade, many researches have evaluated the anatomical and functional status of the brain in diabetics compared to the normal population. This topic presents the most common, well-documented brain changes in diabetics, as reported in the medical and radiological literature.

DM type 1 can be associated (rarely) with chorea-ballismus episodes due to nonketotic hyperglycemia (NKH). The cause of these chorea-ballismus episodes is unknown, but it is believed that they are vascular in origin.

*Chorea* is defined as involuntary, continuous, random, fast, jerking, dance-like movements in the distal parts of the limbs. *Ballismus* shows a picture similar to chorea, but the movements are more irregular, of large amplitude, and violent, affecting the proximal portion of limbs.

*Nonketotic hyperglycemia (NKH)* is a severe form of hyperglycemia with hyperosmolarity and intracellular dehydration, with little or no ketoacidosis. It is typically observed in diabetic patients >50 years of age. NKH is characterized by partial insulin deficiency with enough insulin to inhibit ketoacidosis but not enough to transport glucose into the cells. Hyperglycemia causes an osmotic diuresis, with progressive dehydration, resulting in NKH. Up to 40 % of patients with NKH develop seizures beside the chorea-ballismus episodes.

The incidence of stroke is six times higher in patients with DM than in nondiabetics. This high stroke risk can be explained by the high incidence of atherosclerosis of the internal carotid artery in diabetics.

Many researchers reported high cerebral brain atrophy among long-term diabetics. Patients with DM type 2 were found to have an increased risk of Alzheimer's disease (AD) and vascular dementia. AD in diabetics is believed to be due to the increase in advanced glycation end products, which increase aggregation of proteins involved in AD development.

Furthermore, dysfunction of insulin signaling in the brain has been implicated in the pathogenesis of AD. Subcortical arteriosclerosis encephalopathy can develop in diabetics due to brain vessel atherosclerosis.

Cranial nerve involvement in DM is a rare complication. A single cranial nerve (*diabetic mononeuritis*) or multiple cranial nerves (*mononeuritis multiplex*) can be involved. DM classically affects the cranial nerves CN III, CN IV, CN VI, and CN VII. Cranial nerve involvement in diabetes is thought to be a result of microvasculitis and resultant ischemic injury to the nerves.

Patients with *diabetic ketoacidosis (DKA)* can develop subclinical cerebral edema for unknown reasons. The brain edema can start before or after treatment initiation. Patients with DM type 1 are most commonly affected, and it occurs in > 1 % of cases. Typically, patients present with severe headaches that can progress (rarely) into brain herniation. Other manifestations of symptomatic brain edema due to DKA include a drop in heart rate, altered mental status that ranges from dizziness to coma, and increased blood pressure.

**Signs on CT and MRI**

- Stroke is seen as a hypodense area on CT or a hyperintense area on T2W MR images. Focal neurological deficits and the clinical picture suggest the diagnosis.
- In *NKH–ballismus episode*, CT scan of the basal ganglia (caudate and putamen) is hyperdense compared to the rest of the brain parenchyma (◘ Fig. 10.2.1). Normal basal ganglia attenuation is between 33 and 36 HU. In diabetic chorea, the basal ganglia show attenuation between 40 and 51 HU. This finding is believed to be caused by multiple petechial hemorrhages within the basal ganglia. On MRI, the basal ganglia show hyperintense signal intensity on both T1W and T2W images (◘ Fig. 10.2.1). This sign is not specific and can be observed in cases of hepatic encephalopathy, carbon monoxide toxicity, Wilson disease, and neurofibromatosis.
- Generalized brain atrophy is seen in diabetics with signs of dementia. The hippocampus and the amygdale volume are reduced in diabetics who develop signs of dementia.
- Signs of subcortical arteriosclerosis encephalopathy may be seen when the clinical status of the patient suggests dementia.
- *Diabetic mononeuritis* is detected as enhancement of the affected cranial nerve after contrast injection ipsilateral to the site of cranial nerve clinical deficits. Multiple cranial nerve enhancements are seen in mononeuritis multiplex.
- *Diabetic ketoacidosis* brain edema often shows signs of loss of gray-white matter differentiation, effacement of the sulci, and decrease in ventricular size.

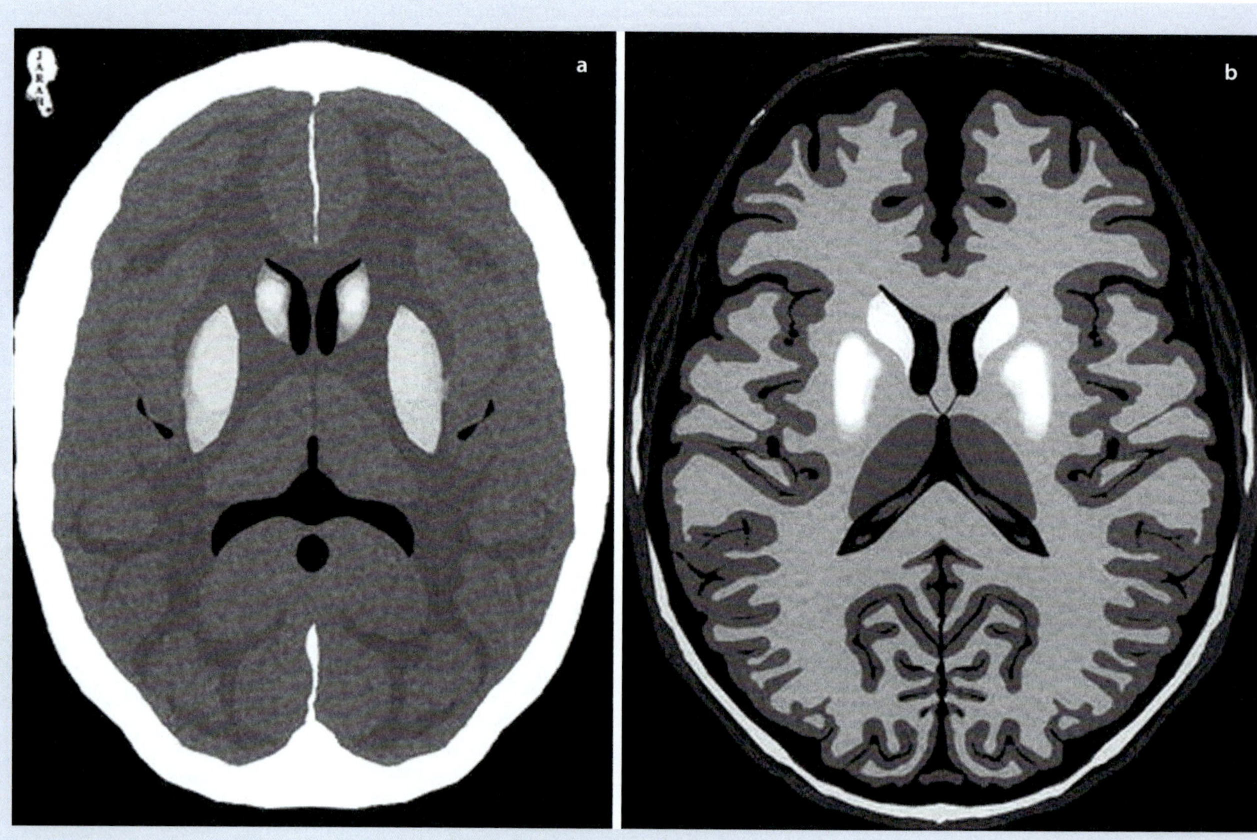

**Fig. 10.2.1** Axial nonenhanced brain CT (**a**) and MR (**b**) illustrations demonstrate high-density basal ganglia (**a**) and high-intensity signal of the basal ganglia (**b**), which is a sign detected in patients with ballismus episodes and in patients with nonketotic hyperglycemia

## Further Reading


Araki Y, et al. MRI of the brain in diabetes mellitus. Neuroradiology. 1994;36:101–31.

Brands AMA, et al. Cognitive functioning and brain MRI in patients with type 1 and type 2 diabetes mellitus: a comparative study. Dement Geriatr Cogn Disord. 2007;23:343–50.

Harten BV, et al. Brain imaging in patients with diabetes. A systematic review. Diabetes Care. 2006;29(11):2539–46.

Kelkar P, et al. Mononeuritis multiplex in diabetes mellitus: evidence for underlying immune pathogenesis. J Neurol Neurosurg Psychiatry. 2003;74:803–6.

Lai PH, et al. Chorea-ballismus with nonketotic hyperglycemia in primary diabetes mellitus. AJNR Am J Neuroradiol. 1996;17:1057–64.

Lavin PJM. Hyperglycemic hemianopia: a reversible complication of non-ketotic hyperglycemia. Neurology. 2005;65:616–9; den Heijer T, et al. Type 2 diabetes and atrophy of medial temporal lobe structures on brain MRI. Diabetologia. 2003;46:1604–10.

Pacheco E, et al. Pathophysiology and computed tomography findings in a case of diabetic ketoacidosis. Int Pediatr. 1999;14(2):118–20.

Witzke KA, et al. Diabetic neuropathy in older adults. Rev Endocr Metab Disord. 2005;6:117–27.


## 10.3    Diabetic Syndromes

Diabetic syndromes are a group of diseases characterized by the development of diabetes mellitus (DM) in childhood. Most of these diseases are originally syndromes, with DM constituting a major manifestation of these syndromes. This topic describes the most common pediatric syndromes associated with DM.

## Alström Syndrome

Alström syndrome (AS) is a very rare genetic disease, characterized by infantile dilated cardiomyopathy, diabetes mellitus, pigmentary retinal dystrophy causing blindness, sensorineural hearing loss, and obesity.

The disease has an autosomal recessive mode of inheritance, and it is linked to mutation in the short arm of chromosome 2. Dilated cardiomyopathy is the earliest manifestation of this syndrome and classically starts in the third to fourth week of life. Blindness and sensorineural hearing loss in an obese child should trigger the suspicion of AS.

Diagnostic and key features of AS include:

## Ophthalmologic Clinical Findings
- Atypical pigmentary retinopathy without classical bone spicules is a constant finding (*diagnostic criterion*).
- Nystagmus usually appears during the first 1–2 years of life.
- Visual deterioration occurs during the first decade of life.
- Loss of the papillary reactions appears during the second decade of life.

## Auditory Clinical Findings
Progressive, bilateral sensorineural hearing loss is found within the first decade of life (*diagnostic criterion*).

## Metabolic and General Clinical Findings
- Obesity with hypertriglyceridemia from birth (*diagnostic criterion*).
- Hyperinsulinemia and noninsulin-dependent DM (*diagnostic criterion*).
- Hepatic failure and hypogonadism are found occasionally.

## Renal Clinical Findings
Renal deterioration is a constant finding, and it is age related, often starting within the second decade of life.

## Dermatological Clinical Findings
Areas of hyperpigmentation and papillary hypertrophy on the neck and flexor creases (acanthosis nigricans) may be found occasionally.

> **Signs on Chest Radiographs**
> Increased cardiaothoracic ratio and signs of dilated cardiomyopathy can be seen in advanced stages.

> **Signs on US and CT**
> Multiple hyperechoic or hypodense liver lesions may be found with heterogeneous contrast enhancement. The lesions are usually due to hepatocellular adenoma with pericellular fibrosis.

## Bardet–Biedl Syndrome

Bardet–Biedl syndrome (BBS) is a rare, genetically heterogeneous disease, characterized by noninsulin-dependent DM in adulthood, ocular abnormalities, mental retardation, obesity, polydactyly, and renal dysfunction.

BBS has an autosomal recessive mode of inheritance, with prevalence of 1 in 125,000 live births. Key features of BBS include pigmentary (rod-cone) retinal dystrophy in the second decade of life (95 % of cases), truncal obesity with normal appetite (85 % of cases), genital hypoplasia (74 % of cases), mental retardation (70 % of cases), postaxial polydactyly (80 % of cases), and renal anomalies. Chronic end-stage renal failure is a constant feature (100 % of cases). Renal anomalies are the main cause of mortality in BBS patients.

> **Signs on IVU**
> - Bilateral small kidney size
> - Multiple calyceal clubbing and blunting, with medullary cysts in the absence of reflux on voiding cystourethrogram
> - Persistent fetal lobulation

> **Signs on US**
> - Loss of differentiation between the medulla and the cortex
> - Hyperechogenic parenchyma with multiple cysts
> - Moderately dilated renal pelvis

> **Signs on Plain Radiographs**
> Postaxial polydactyly and cutaneous syndactyly are classically found.

*The main differential diagnosis of BBS is AS. How can you differentiate between the two conditions?*
- Dilated cardiomyopathy is a feature of AS, not a feature of BBS.
- Mental retardation is a feature of BBS, not a feature of AS.
- Bilateral sensorineural hearing loss is found in AS, but not in BBS.

## Leprechaunism (Donohue Syndrome)

Leprechaunism (Donohue syndrome) is a very rare genetic metabolic disease, characterized by insulin-resistant DM with fasting hypoglycemia due to severe insulin receptor mutation. Infants with leprechaunism exhibit severe DM at birth, postnatal growth retardation, atrophy of the subcutaneous fat, characteristic facial features, and acanthosis nigricans.

Leprechaunism is a fatal disease, and most afflicted infants die before the age of 1 year. The disease has an incidence of 1: 4 million live births. The term "leprechaunism" is derived from "leprechaun," a green, manlike creature with magical powers, according to Irish folklore. The infant's features are acclaimed to be similar to the features of this mythical creature.

The key features of leprechaunism include hirsutism, severe failure to thrive (that might lead to death in the early months of life), growth retardation and failure to thrive, and areas of hyperpigmentation and papillary hypertrophy on the neck and flexor creases (acanthosis nigricans). Notice that all these features are seen in an infant. Laboratory investigations typically show hyperinsulinemia, hyperandrogenism, and elevated cord human chorionic gonadotropin (hCG).

## Prader–Willi Syndrome

Prader–Willi syndrome (PWS) is an autosomal dominant, multisystemic disease, characterized by multiple features that are almost all related to hypothalamic dysfunction. PWS has a prevalence rate of 1 in 15,000 live births.

PWS is characterized by hyperphagia and obesity, starting in the teens. Obesity is the major cause of morbidity and mortality in PWS. DM (19%), hypertension, obstructive sleep apnea, lower limb edema, and varicosity all can be explained by the morbid obesity caused by this disease.

Key features of PWS include almond-shaped palpebral fissures, dolichocephalic (wide) skull, micropenis, hypoplastic scrotum and hypogonadism, and history of fetal hypotonia and poor sucking. Body habitus features include sloping shoulders, genu valgum, and heavy midsection. Patients with PWS have high serum levels of "ghrelin," a peptide released from the stomach that can stimulate food intake.

> **Signs on Plain Radiographs**
> Lateral skull radiograph shows small sella turcica with prominent posterior clinoid process.

## Wolcott–Rallison Syndrome

Wolcott–Rallison syndrome (WRS) is a rare disease characterized by neonatal permanent DM, with multiple epiphyseal dysplasia causing short stature (dwarfism).

WRS has an autosomal recessive mode of inheritance, and the affected child has tendency to long bone fractures. WRS patients have a waddling gait and lordotic posture, with genu valgum.

Other abnormalities of WRS include hypoplastic pancreas, blue sclera, brown mottling of the teeth, mental retardation, seizures, and renal, hepatic, and cardiac abnormalities. Mild chronic neutropenia is reported in many cases but without immune deficiency.

*Multiple epiphyseal dysplasia (Fairbank disease)* is a genetic disease with autosomal dominant mode of inheritance, characterized by abnormalities in maturing epiphyses, resulting in dwarfism and stubby digits. The disorder is almost always bilateral. The disease is divided into a severe form (Fairback subtype) and a milder form. Patients usually present with severe flexion contractures, juvenile osteoarthritis, limb deformities, and limping during early childhood, with a duckling gait.

> **Signs on Radiograph**
> - Multiple epiphyseal dysplasia is characterized by bilateral hypoplastic epiphyses with irregular contour in the Fairbank form. Flattening of the epiphyses may be seen in the mild form (**D** Figs. 10.3.1 and 10.3.2). The most common

joints affected are the hips (100%), knees, and ankles. There is no epiphyseal sclerosis. Hands and wrists are involved in the severe form. The fingers and toes are short and thick. Hypoplastic tarsal and carpal bones may be seen. Persistent calcified cartilage within the bone may be found.
- Osteoporosis.

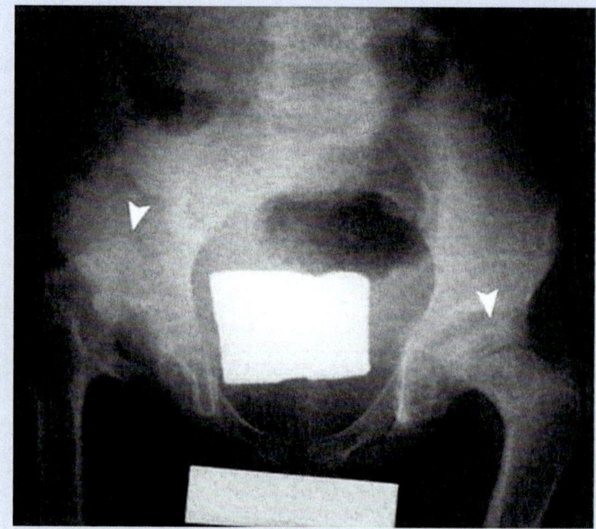

**D Fig. 10.3.1** Anteroposterior plain hip radiograph of a child with multiple epiphyseal dysplasia shows bilateral femoral epiphyses fragmentation and flattening (*arrowheads*), with right hip dislocation

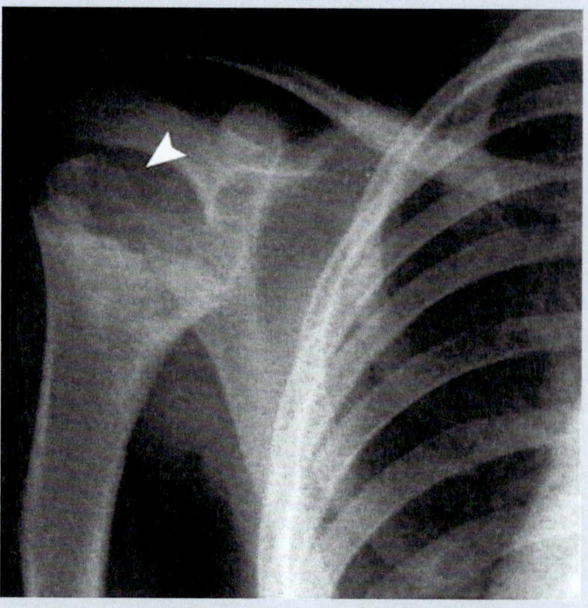

**D Fig. 10.3.2** Plain right shoulder radiograph of the same patient shows severe humeral epiphysis hypoplasia and dysplasia (*arrowhead*)

## Wolfram Syndrome (DIDMOAD)

Wolfram syndrome (WS) is a rare disease characterized by *diabetes insipidus, diabetes mellitus, optic atrophy,* and *sensorineural deafness,* making the acronym DIDMOAD.

WS has an autosomal recessive mode of inheritance, and it is caused by mutation in chromosome 4. Incidence of WS is estimated to be 1 in 100,000 live births.

Diagnostic and key features of DIDMOAD include:

### Ophthalmologic Clinical Findings

Bilateral progressive optic atrophy (98 % of cases) (*diagnostic criterion*)

### Auditory Clinical Findings

Bilateral sensorineural hearing loss is found in up to 12 % of cases (*diagnostic criterion*).

### Metabolic and General Clinical Findings

- Diabetes insipidus (35 % of cases) (*diagnostic criterion*)
- DM (99 % of cases) (*diagnostic criterion*)
- Hypogonadism (occasionally)

### Renal Clinical Findings

- Dilatation of the urinary tract with unknown cause (diagnostic criterion)
- Testicular atrophy (occasionally)

### Neurological Clinical Findings

- Ataxia due to cerebellar atrophy.
- Short-term memory loss and dementia.
- The mean age at death is 30 years, most commonly due to brain stem atrophy and central respiratory failure.

> **Signs on Brain MRI**
> - Generalized brain atrophy, especially in the cerebellum, medulla, and pons.
> - Loss of the posterior pituitary signal.
> - Atrophy of the optic nerves, tracts, and radiations.
> - Patchy areas of white matter demyelination may be seen occasionally.

## Rabson–Mendenhall Syndrome

Rabson–Mendenhall syndrome (RMS) is a rare genetic disease with various somatic abnormalities, characterized by noninsulin-dependent DM due to severe insulin resistance, caused by insulin receptors mutation. The disease has an autosomal recessive mode of inheritance.

Diagnostic and key features of RMS include:

### Metabolic and General Clinical Findings

- Noninsulin-dependent DM, postprandial hypoglycemia, and hyperinsulinemia (*diagnostic criterion*)
- Dysmorphic facial features, with large ears (diagnostic criterion)
- Generalized hypertrichosis, with coarse head hair
- Genital (phallic) enlargement (diagnostic criterion)
- Premature dentition

### Renal Clinical Findings

- Bilateral renal enlargement with medullary sponge kidney may be found. *Medullary sponge kidney* is a congenital disease characterized by dilatation of the collecting tubules in one or more renal papillae, affecting one or both kidneys. There is a high incidence of renal calculi formation in medullary sponge kidney, with hypercalciuria found in up to 50 % of patients. Gross hematuria can be found in 10–20 % of patients.
- Nephrocalcinosis.

### Dermatological Clinical Findings

Typically, there are areas of hyperpigmentation and papillary hypertrophy on the neck and flexor creases (acanthosis nigricans).

> **Signs on IVU**
> Sponge kidney is diagnosed by the presence of typical cystic collection of contrast material in the collecting ducts in a form of "bouquet of flowers or paintbrush appearance" ( Fig. 10.3.3).

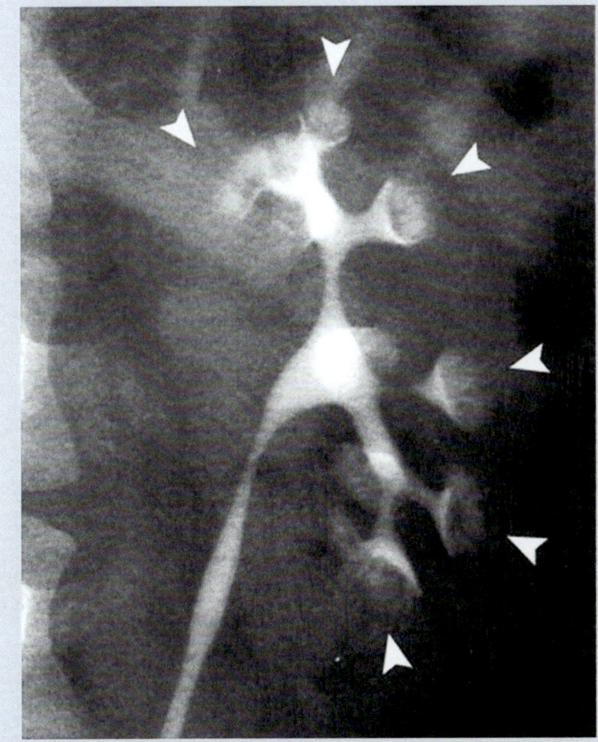

 **Fig. 10.3.3** Intravenous urography radiograph of a patient with sponge kidney shows the classical collecting duct paintbrush appearance (*arrowheads*)

## Further Reading

Barrett TG. Mitochondrial diabetes, DIDMOAD and other inherited diabetes syndromes. Best Prac Res Clin Endocrinol Metab. 2001;15(3):325–43.

Benso C, et al. Three new cases of Alström syndrome. Graefe's Arch Clin Exp Opthalmol. 2002;240:622–7.

Bin-Abbas B, et al. Wolcott-Rallison syndrome: clinical, radiological, and histological findings in a Saudi child. Ann Saudi Med. 2001;21(1–2):73–4.

Cohen Jr MM. Syndromology: an updated conceptual overview. V. Aspects of aneuploidy. Int J Oral Maxillofac Surg. 1998;18:333–8.

Dippell J, et al. Early sonographic aspects of kidney morphology in Bardet-Biedl syndrome. Pediatr Nephrol. 1998;12:559–63.

Donohue WL, et al. Leprechaunism. A Euphuism for a rare familial disorder. J Pediatr. 1954;45(5):505–18.

Fralick RA, et al. Early diagnosis of Bardet-Biedl syndrome. Pediatr Nephrol. 1990;4:264–5.

Galluzzi P, et al. MRI of Wolfram syndrome (DIDMOAD). Neuroradiology. 1999;41:729–31.

Genis D, et al. Wolfram syndrome: a neuropathological study. Acta Neuropathol. 1997;93:426–9.

Gupta S, et al. Medullary sponge kidney. Indian J Pediatr. 2002;69(12):1091–2.

Harris AM, et al. Rabson-Mendenhall syndrome: medullary sponge kidney, a new component. Pediatr Nephrol. 2007;22:2141–4.

Hatori M, et al. Multiple epiphyseal dysplasia – report of two families. Arch Orthop Trauma Surg. 2000;120:372–5.

Makaryus AN, et al. A rare case of Alström syndrome presenting with rapidly progressing severe dilated cardiomyopathy diagnosed by echocardiography. J Am Soc Echocardiogr. 2003;16:194–6.

Miller J, et al. Neurocognitive findings in Prader-Willi syndrome and early-onset morbid obesity. J Pediatr. 2006;149:192–8.

Morgan J, et al. US, CT, and MRI imaging of hepatic masses in Alström syndrome: a case report. Clin Imaging. 2008;32:393–5.

Papavramidis ST, et al. Prader-Willi syndrome-associated obesity treated by biliopancreatic diversion with duodenal switch. Case report and literature review. J Pediatr Surg. 2006;41:1153–8.

Parveen BA, et al. Rabson-Mendenhall syndrome. Int J Dermatol. 2008;47:839–41.

Rubin EL, et al. Cystic disease of the renal pyramids ('sponge kidney'). J Fac Radiol. 1959;10(3):134–7.

Sebik A, et al. The orthopaedic aspects of multiple epiphyseal dysplasia. Int Orthopaed (SICOT). 1998;22:417–21.

Shannon P, et al. Evidence of widespread axonal pathology in Wolfram syndrome. Acta Neuropathol. 1999;98:304–8.

Stöß H, et al. Wolcott-Rallison syndrome: diabetes mellitus and spondyloepiphyseal dysplasia. Eur J Pediatr. 1982;138:120–9.

Summitt RL, et al. Leprechaunism (Donohue's syndrome): a case report. J Pediatr. 1969;74(4):601–10.

Tekgül S, et al. Urological manifestations of the observation in 14 patients. J Urol. 1999;161:616–7.

Tobin JL, et al. Bardet-Biedl syndrome: beyond the cilum. Pediatr Radiol. 2007;22:926–36.

Urben SL, et al. Otolaryngologic features of Laurence-Moon-Bardet-Biedl syndrome. Otolaryngol Head Neck Surg. 1999;120:571–4.

Verri A, et al. A case of Wolfram syndrome: neurological features. Ital J Neurol Sci. 1982;4:351–3.

## 10.4    Diabetes Insipidus

Diabetes insipidus (DI) is a disease characterized by increased frequency of urination (polyuria), with increased fluid intake (polydipsia) secondary to inappropriate secretion of the antidiuretic hormone (ADH) vasopressin from the posterior pituitary gland.

ADH is secreted by the supraoptic and paraventricular hypothalamic nuclei and stored in the terminals within the posterior pituitary. *Neurohypophysis* is a term used to describe the posterior pituitary, the infundibular stalk, and the supraoptic and paraventricular hypothalamic nuclei. ADH regulates fluid and electrolytes balance within the body by promoting water reabsorption in the distal tubules in the kidneys.

According to its origin, DI is classified into three types:

- *Neurogenic DI* can be idiopathic (50 %), genetic (5 %), secondary to tumor (e.g., craniopharyngioma), or secondary to inflammatory reactions (e.g., Langerhans cell histiocytosis).
- *Nephrogenic DI* can be due to primary renal disease or secondary to chronic renal failure or hypercalcemia.
- *Dipsogenic DI* arises due to compulsive polydipsia or due to hypothalamic disorders affecting the thirst center.

DI has a prevalence of 1:25,000 of the population. Patients typically present with polyuria and polydipsia. The polyuria is not reduced by cessation of fluid intake. Signs of dehydration, such as dry skin, hypotension, and tachycardia, are often found. Serum electrolyte investigations show high plasma osmolarity, hypernatremia, hypokalemia, hyperglycemia, and hypercalcemia.

The most common hypothalamic tumors associated with DI are metastases, germinoma, and craniopharyngioma. *Craniopharyngioma* is a benign, slow-growing tumor that arises from the remnant of *Rathke's pouch* (craniopharyngeal duct). It can occur in children between 6 and 15 years of age and adults between 50 and 60 years of age. Up to 50 % of suprasellar lesions in children are craniopharyngiomas. Patients usually present with visual disturbance (bitemporal quadrantanopia), headache, and hypothalamic dysfunction.

As previously mentioned, the neurohypophysis is composed of the posterior pituitary lobe, the infundibular stalk, and the median eminence of the hypothalamus. The normal posterior pituitary shows high signal intensity on native T1W images (◖ Fig. 10.4.1). It is thought that this

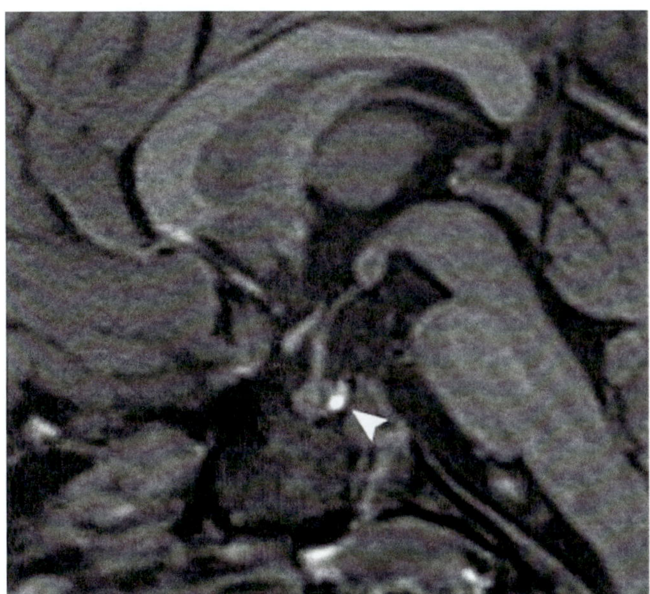



— *Craniopharyngioma*: on CT, the main bulk of the lesion is located in the suprasellar region and has cystic (90 %) and solid components with rim-like or nodular calcifications in up to 80 % of cases (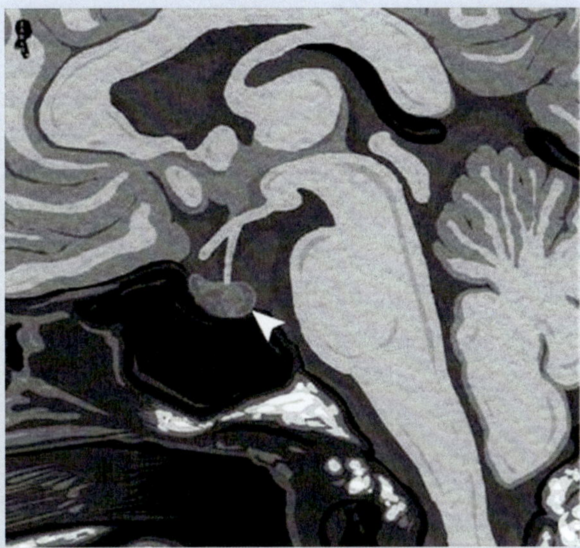Fig. 10.4.3). The solid component enhances after contrast administration. On MRI, the lesion has high T1 signal and high/low T2 signal according to the fat and thick protinaceous (motor oil) consistency within the lesion. The solid component enhances after contrast administration.

— *Langerhans cell histiocytosis*: there is typical enlargement of the central part of the infundibulum (>2.5 mm) when Langerhans cell histiocytosis is the main cause of DI (Fig. 10.4.4).

— Bilateral, symmetrical brain calcifications within the basal ganglia and the subcortical area have been reported as unusual manifestations of DI. These findings are best evaluated on CT.

— *Ectopic posterior pituitary* is seen as a bright spot, typically located in the hypothalamic eminence (Fig. 10.4.5).

bright spot is due to the macrogranules composed of the ADH neurophysin complex. *Ectopic posterior pituitary* is a condition where the posterior pituitary bright signal spot on MR imaging is not located in the posterior pituitary lobe but is typically seen in the median hypothalamic eminence.

The anterior pituitary gland (*adenohypophysis*) normally shows the same signal characteristic as the rest of the brain on T1W images. However, the adenohypophysis can show a bright signal on native T1W images during the first 2 years of life, due to secretory activity, or in preterm babies during the first 2 months of life. The bright signal of the adenohypophysis is best demonstrated with the magnetization transfer MR sequence.

### Signs on Brain MRI (Done in Patients with Suspected Neurogenic DI)

— *Genetic cause*: there is loss of the typical posterior pituitary hyperintensity signal on T1W contrast-enhanced images (Fig. 10.4.2). However, the neurohypophysis bright spot can be absent in 10–20 % of normal individuals.

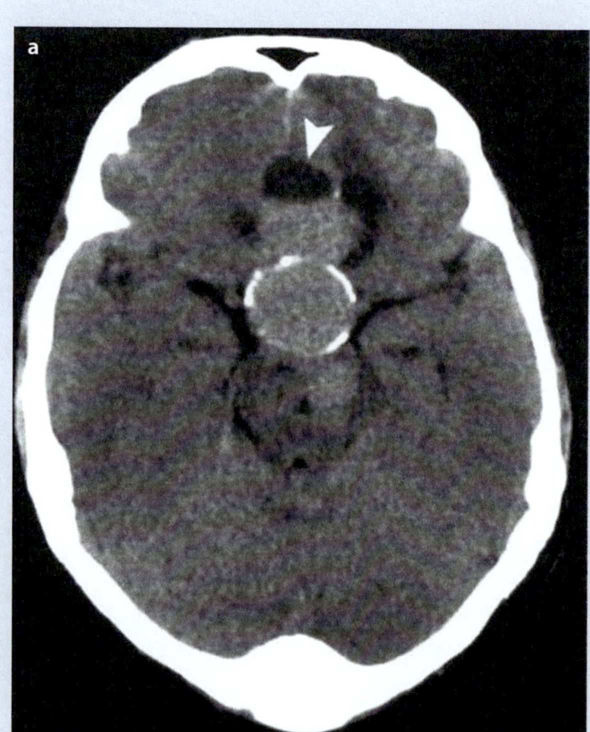

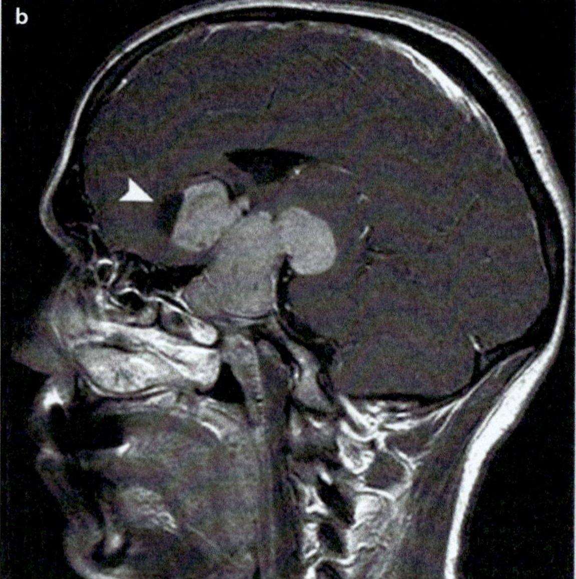

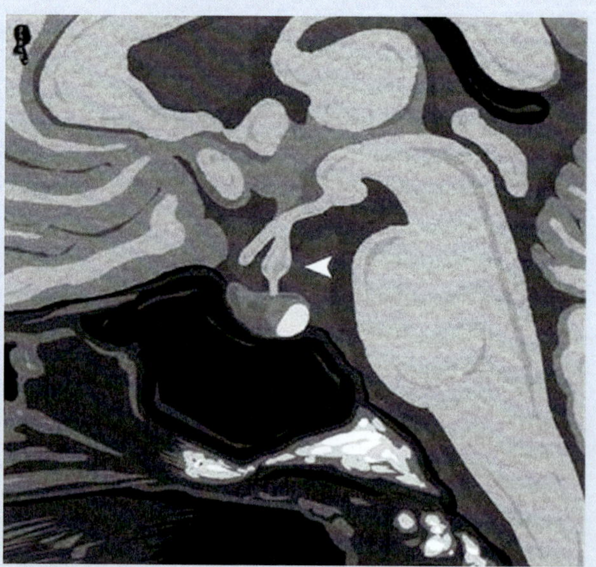

■ **Fig. 10.4.4**   Sagittal nonenhanced T1W MR illustration of the sella shows thickened infundibulum due to Langerhans cell histiocytosis (*arrowhead*)

■ **Fig. 10.4.3**   Axial nonenhanced brain CT (**a**) and sagittal contrast-enhanced T1W MRI of the sella show craniopharyngioma in a 40-year-old patient. In (**b**), the main bulk of the lesion is located in the suprasellar area, with infiltration of the sella turcica and the sphenoid sinus. The lesion is mostly solid, with anterior cystic component located in the inferior frontal region (*arrowhead*). In (**a**), a calcified rim that surrounds the lesion is nicely illustrated

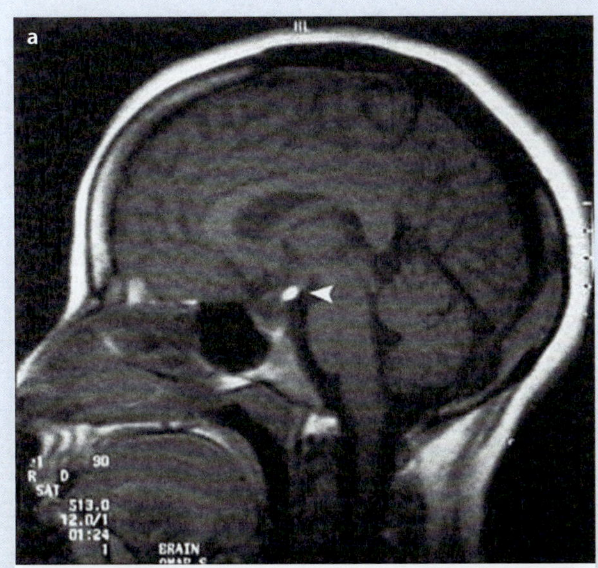

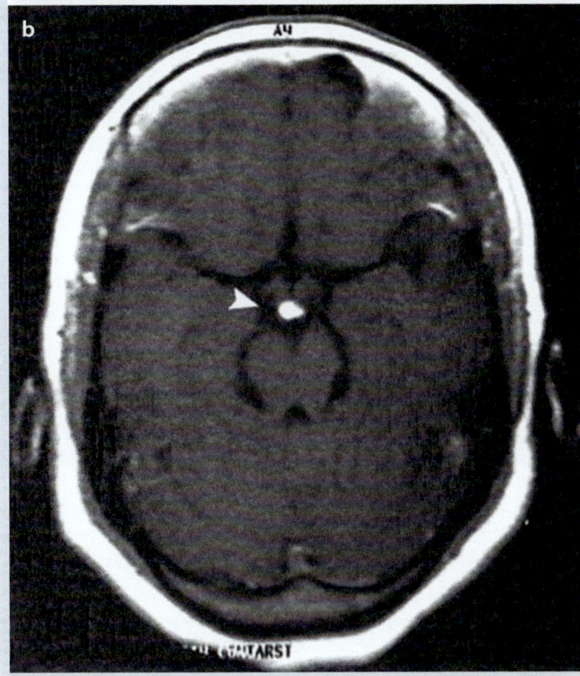

**Fig. 10.4.5** Sagittal (**a**) and axial (**b**) T1W MRI shows an ectopic high signal intensity spot located at the proximal part of the infundibulum (ectopic posterior pituitary)

### Further Reading

Al-Kandari SR, et al. Intracranial calcification in central diabetes insipidus. Pediatr Radiol. 2008;38:101–3.
Hadjizacharia P, et al. Acute diabetes insipidus in severe head injury: a prospective study. J Am Coll Surg. 2008;207:477–84.
Jane Jr JA, et al. Neurogenic diabetes insipidus. Pituitary. 2006;9:327–9.
Kassebaum N, et al. Diabetes insipidus associated with propofol anesthesia. J Clin Anesth. 2008;20:466–8.
Maghnie M, et al. Central diabetes insipidus in children and young adults. N Eng J Med. 2000;343:998–1007.
Maria IA. MRI of the hypothalamic-pituitary axis in children. Pediatr Radiol. 2005;35:1045–55.
Mavrakis AN, et al. Diabetes insipidus with deficient thirst: report of a patient and review of the literature. Am J Kidney Dis. 2008;51(5):851–9.
Mitchell LA, et al. Ectopic posterior pituitary lobe and periventricular heterotopia: cerebral malformation with the same underlying mechanism. AJNR Am J Neuroradiol. 2002;23:1475–81.
Saeki N, et al. MRI of ectopic posterior pituitary bright spot with large adenomas : appearances and relationship to transient postoperative diabetes insipidus. Neuroradiology. 2003;45:713–6.
Schmitt S, et al. Pituitary stalk thickening with diabetes insipidus preceding typical manifestations of Langerhans cell histiocytosis in children. Eur J Pediatr. 1993;152:399–401.

## 10.5 Obesity, Gastric Banding, and Liposuction

Obesity is a disease characterized by an increase in the size and number of fat cells. Fat cell size differs from region to region within the body, and the number of fat cells may increase three- to fivefold during adolescence. Overweight is defined as a body weight of 101–120 % of the ideal, while obesity is defined as fat accumulation >120 % of the ideal.

Obesity is defined by the World Health Organization (WHO) as the ratio of body mass to body height ($kg/m^2$), the so-called *body mass index* (BMI). A BMI of 25–30 $kg/m^2$ is considered "overweight," >30 $kg/m^2$ is defined as "obesity," and >40 $kg/m^2$ is defined as "morbid obesity." BMI is used as a marker for estimating the risks for diseases such as diabetes mellitus and cardiovascular diseases. Women usually have gynecoid fat distribution around the hips, while men have android fat distribution where adiposity is predominantly central.

Patients with obesity suffer from many systemic diseases such as diabetes mellitus and insulin insensitivity, cardiovascular diseases, obstructive sleep apnea, osteoarthritis, venous stasis and varicosities, and gout.

There are different causes of obesity. Apart from a sedentary lifestyle and high-carbohydrate food intake, hormonal, syndromic/pathologic, and drug-induced lipomatoses are other common causes of obesity. Each cause induces obesity by a different mechanism.

### Hormonal Obesity

- *Hypothalamic obesity*: obesity that arises after paraventricular ventromedial hypothalamic injury, causing hyperphagia due to loss of the serum leptin level sensitization.
- *Cushing's syndrome*: obesity is a cardinal sign of Cushing's syndrome. Patients classically present with truncal (android) obesity.
- *Hypothyroidism*: obesity in hypothyroidism is mainly due to a slow metabolic rate. The weight gain is often modest, without marked obesity.

- *Polycystic ovary disease*: up to 50 % of patients with polycystic ovary disease are overweight with insulin resistance.
- *Growth hormone deficiency*: growth hormone deficiency causes a reduction in lean body mass and an increase in fat body mass.

## Syndromic/Pathologic Obesity

- Lipoma is defined as the localized, encapsulated accumulation of fat. It can be single or multiple and can be seen in any part of the body (Fig. 10.5.1). Multiple lipomas can be seen in Maffucci syndrome and neurofibromatosis type 1 (*von Recklinghausen disease*).
- *Lipomatosis* is a condition characterized by proliferation of nonencapsulated fat cells (Fig. 10.5.2).
- *Liposarcoma* is a rare malignant tumor characterized by neoplastic proliferation of fat cells (Fig. 10.5.3).
- *Lipodystrophy* is a condition characterized by loss of body fat in one or more areas. It can be genetic or acquired (e.g., HIV drug-induced lipodystrophy).
- *Binge-eating disorder* is a psychiatric disorder, characterized by uncontrolled episodes of eating, usually in the evening.
- *Night-eating syndrome* is a psychiatric disorder, characterized by consumption of at least 25 % of daily energy between the evening meal and the next morning. Patients often awake at night to eat, three or more times per week.
- *Dercum's disease* (*lipomatosis dolorosa*) is a rare disease, characterized by painful subcutaneous fatty tissue with inflammatory characteristics. Patients are typically young obese women 25–40 years of age, presenting with vague pain that can be focal or generalized. Many patients live with this disease while being unaware of it, either

because the disease sometimes shows mild symptoms or because patients receive a wrong diagnosis.

Lipomatosis dolorosa can be mistaken for fibromyalgia rheumatica. Unlike fibromyalgia rheumatica, the pain in lipomatosis dolorosa increases with body weight gain. The pain often has insidious onset and progresses with time. The pain in lipomatosis dolorosa is chronic (>3 months duration), aching, stabbing, or burning and usually symmetrical (Fig. 10.5.4). However, localized pain may be seen in the upper limbs or around the knee. The face and hands are typically not involved.

The pain characteristically arises from the subcutaneous fat. The pain may worsen on any light touch or pressure (allodynia), wearing tight clothes, or taking a shower. Also, the pain is temperature and humidity dependent and usually reduces when the weather is hot and dry. Hot baths may reduce the pain but only temporarily. The pain is thought to be caused by

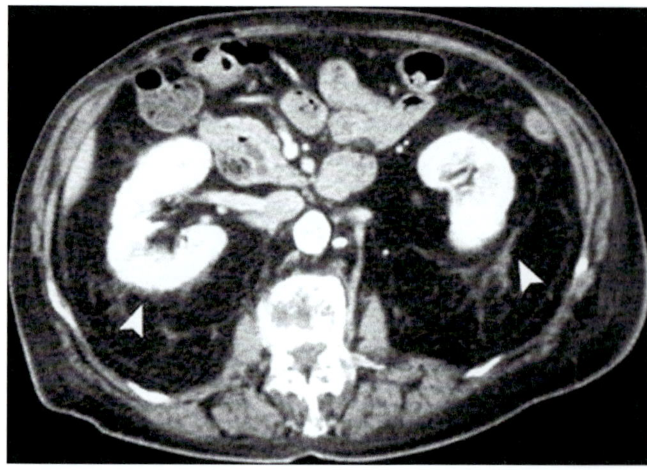

**Fig. 10.5.2** Axial abdominal postcontrast CT shows retroperitoneal lipomatosis, with increased fat content of the retroperitoneum pushing the kidneys anteriorly in a bilateral fashion (*arrowheads*)

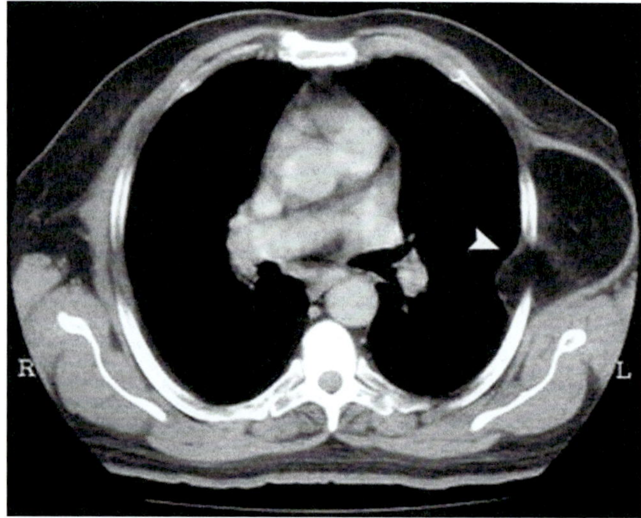

**Fig. 10.5.1** Axial nonenhanced chest CT shows left chest wall lipoma, seen as a typically well-circumscribed mass with fat attenuation (*arrowhead*)

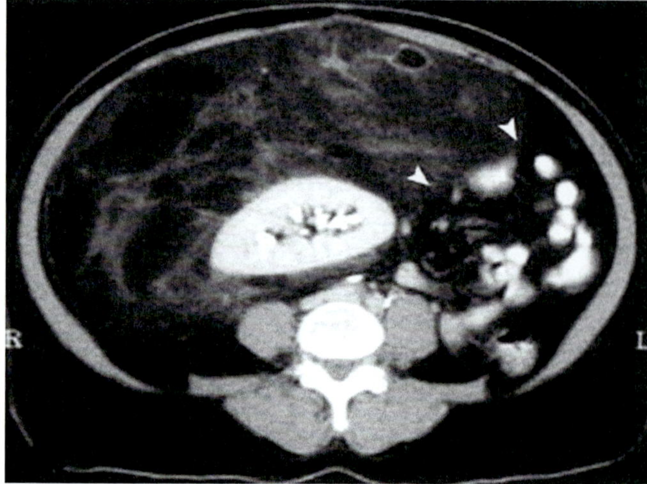

**Fig. 10.5.3** Axial abdominal postcontrast CT shows severe abdominal fatty proliferation that pushes the left kidney and the intestines to the left abdominal cavity region (*arrowhead*) due to proliferating retroperitoneal liposarcoma

fat masses pressing upon the nerve root endings or by releasing cytokines that induce pain (e.g., tumor necrosis factor-α).

Three types of lipomatosis dolorosa are described: *type 1 (juxta-articular)*, with painful subcutaneous folds around the knees or the hips; *type 2 (diffuse)*, which affects the whole body symmetrically; and *type 3 (nodular)*, characterized by intense pain around lipomas.

— *Weber–Christian disease* (WCS) is a disease characterized by painful subcutaneous nodules found mainly on the trunk and the extremities, with constitutional symptoms like fever, fatigue, polymyalgia, and arthralgia. The subcutaneous nodules are composed of lobular panniculitis (subcutaneous tissue inflammation). When the panniculitis is systemic, WCS can be fatal in up to 10 % of patients. Patients commonly show elevated erythrocyte sedimentation rate and C-reactive protein levels.

— *Madelung's disease (benign symmetric lipomatosis/Launois–Bensaude syndrome)* is a rare condition, characterized by massive symmetric deposits of nonencapsulated adipose tissue in the head, the neck, and the upper trunk.

Madelung's disease (MD) is typically seen in middle-aged males of Mediterranean origin with a history of excessive alcohol consumption (90 % of cases). Patients with MD typically consume more than 80 g of alcohol per day for more than 10 years. MD is considered a "sight diagnosis" because of the typical patterns of fat distribution in the head and neck region. Lipomatosis is typically seen accumulating in both parotid regions (hamster cheek appearance), cervical region (horse collar appearance), and the posterior neck region (buffalo hump appearance) (◘ Fig. 10.5.5). The disease is divided into two types: *type 1 MD* is characterized by symmetric body lipomatosis that gives the patient a "pseudo-athletic" appearance (◘ Fig. 10.5.5). *Type 2 MD* is characterized by diffuse lipomatosis that gives the patient a generalized obese appearance.

Sensory, motor, or autonomic polyneuropathy is seen in up to 85 % of patients with MD. Rarely, the tongue or the mediastinum is involved in lipomatosis, resulting in dysphagia and dyspnea.

— *Metabolic syndrome (syndrome X)* is defined by the WHO as the presence of impaired glucose regulation or

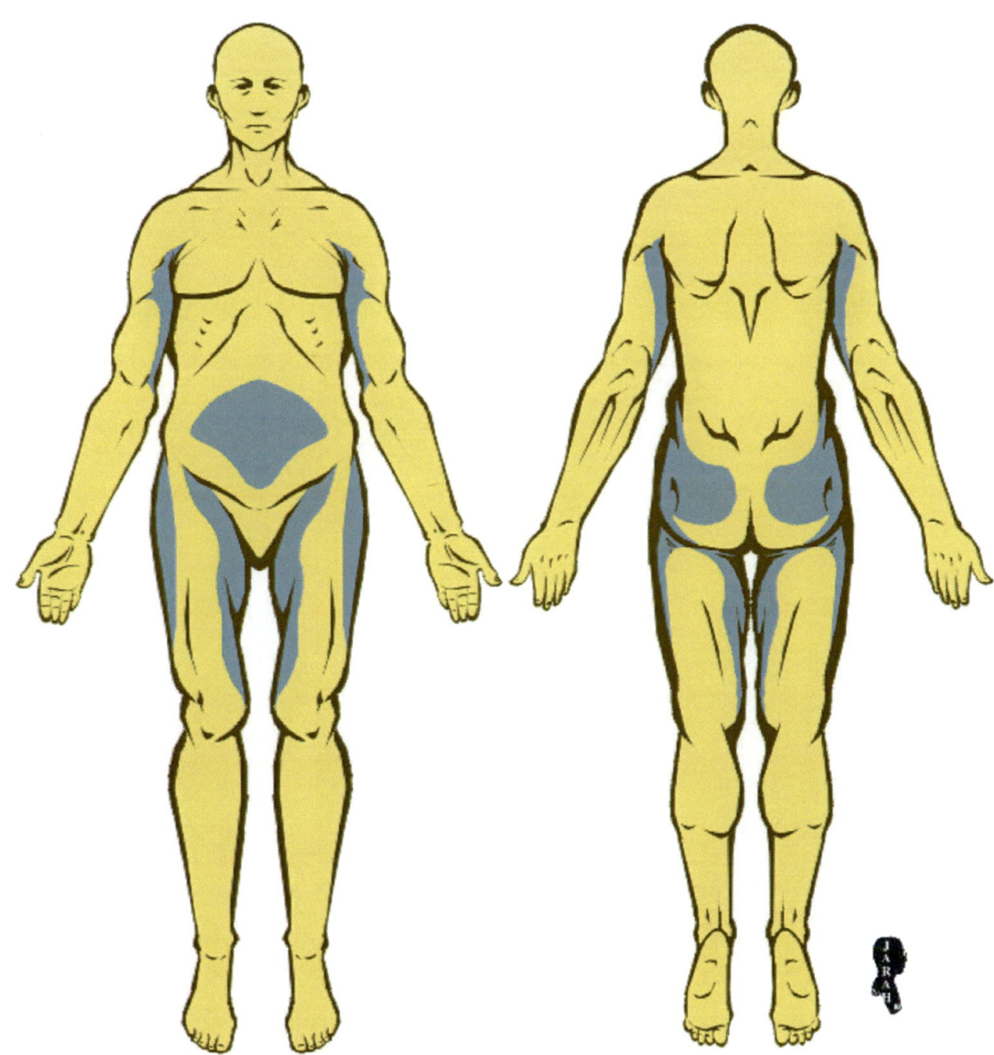

◘ Fig. 10.5.4  An illustration demonstrates the typical pain distribution in dercum dolorosa

diabetes, with two of the following risk factors: hypertension, dyslipidemia, central obesity, and microalbuminuria. There is a strong association between the development of metabolic syndrome and increase in visceral adipose tissue (VAT).

— *Fröhlich syndrome* is a rare hypothalamic disorder, characterized by obesity, stunned growth, and genital hypoplasia.

— *Obesity hypoventilation* (*Pickwickian*) *syndrome* is a disease characterized by the triad of morbid obesity, hypoventilation, and irresistible hypersomnolence (drowsiness). Hypoventilation in Pickwickian syndrome is defined clinically by an arterial blood gas as a $PaCO_2 > 45$ and/or a $PO_2 < 55$ in the presence of morbid obesity. This hypoventilation is attributed to obstructive sleep apnea in these patients and by the ventilation/perfusion mismatch that results from the irregular shallow breathing with or without compression by a thick chest wall.

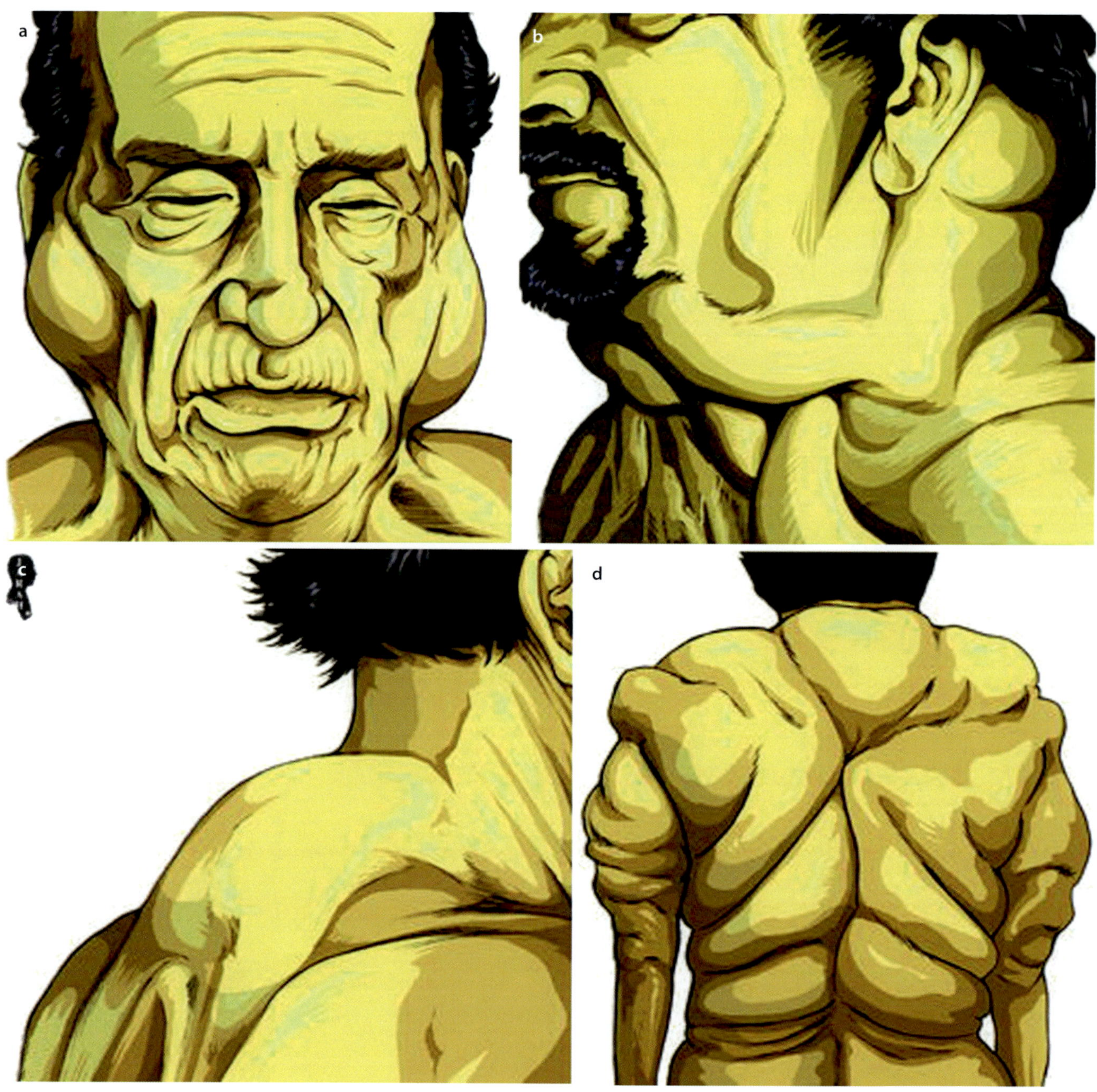

**Fig. 10.5.5**   An illustration demonstrates the typical clinical signs of Madelung's disease: (**a**) hamster cheeks appearance, (**b**) horse collar appearance, (**c**) buffalo hump appearance, and (**d**) pseudo-athletic appearance

## Drug-Induced Obesity

- *Glucocorticoids use*: glucocorticoids cause fat accumulation in the body in a similar fashion to people with Cushing's syndrome. Glucocorticoid obesity is seen in patients with chronic prednisolone intake >10 mg/day or its equivalent.
- *Cessation of smoking*: patients who quit smoking can gain up to 4–5 kg on average, and it is partly mediated by nicotine withdrawal.

## Evaluation of Fat Within the Body

There are several techniques used to estimate body fat. Anthropometry is a technique used to estimate BMI by measuring waist circumference and skinfold thickness. BMI is a good indicator of obesity, but it provides indirect measurement of body fat and is unable to differentiate lean body mass from body fat. The inability of BMI to discriminate lean body mass from fat body mass leads to defining lean, muscular individuals as obese.

The metabolism of adipocytes varies with fat sites. Fat deposits in the abdomen and flank are more metabolically active than fat deposits in the buttocks or thighs. Upper-body obesity is more associated with hypertension, glucose intolerance, and serum cholesterol levels than is lower-body obesity. Recent research emphasizes the high risks of cardiovascular diseases and metabolic abnormalities associated with increased intra-abdominal VAT. VAT is defined as the fatty tissue that accumulates beneath the abdominal muscle wall and surrounding the abdominal viscera. VAT mass is pathologically more important than subcutaneous fat thickness over the trunk. Also, visceral fat is a major determinant of whole body insulin resistance.

Adipose tissue is a specialized loose connective tissue that is laden with adipocytes. It works as a source of energy, thermal insulation (e.g., brown fat), and as a mechanical cushion in mammals. A 70-kg man normally has 15 kg of adipose tissue, representing 21 % of body mass. In contrast, fat is a term used to describe the chemical lipid component in the form of triglycerides. It can be found within adipocytes or in pathological conditions like fatty liver. Modern methods use ultrasound, CT, and MRI as useful and accurate tools for VAT quantification.

### Quantitative Assessment of Visceral Fat by US

Ultrasound can be used as a fast and easy method to quantify visceral and subcutaneous fat. Although it is not as standard as CT quantification, it is reported by many investigators to be an accurate method to quantify the abdominal wall fat thickness and preperitoneal fat thickness.

### Quantitative Assessment of Visceral Fat by CT and MRI

An axial body section is taken at the level of the navel or (L4/L5), and assessment is done via a computer software program to calculate the percentage of visceral fat distribution

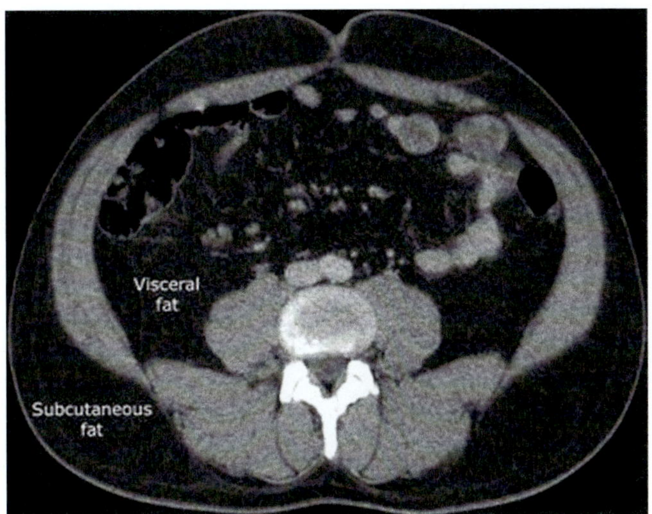


□ **Fig. 10.5.6**  An axial CT section obtained at the level of L4/L5 vertebra

(□ Figs. 10.5.6 and 10.5.7). Excess visceral fat typically separates the intra-abdominal structures. The drawbacks of the CT method are the use of radiation and the limited gantry diameter to patients less than 70 cm wide (the standard CT gantry diameter). MRI, on the other hand, is radiation-free but more expensive in its use as a regular monitoring method. The MRI method uses the same procedures as the CT method of quantification.

## Gastric Banding

Gastric banding is a widely performed surgical procedure as a surgical therapy for morbid obesity. The procedure consists of placing a silicon band around the upper part of the stomach to create a small gastric pouch that works as a stomach (neostomach). The pouch is connected to the rest of the stomach via a narrow stoma. The silicon band contains an adjustable inner balloon that can be inflated with air or fluid up to 5 cm³, and it is connected to a reservoir that is typically sutured to the anterior rectus sheath. The stoma width normally should be within 3–4 mm.

The gastric banding procedure controls obesity by restricting food administration to the stomach into a small gastric pouch and narrow stoma, which creates early satiety when the pouch is full. Although gastric banding is a relatively safe procedure, several complications may arise later in up to 35 % of cases. Additional surgery may be required in up to 11 % of cases.

Early complications of gastric banding include esophageal perforation (0.5 % of cases), dysphagia (14 % of cases), gastroesophageal reflux disease, and early slippage of the band (1 % of cases). Late complications include eccentric pouch dilatation (25 %), slippage of the band (24 %), intragastric band migration, and gastric necrosis (<0.3 %). Patients with diabetes show early gastric dilatation due to diabetic gastroparesis.

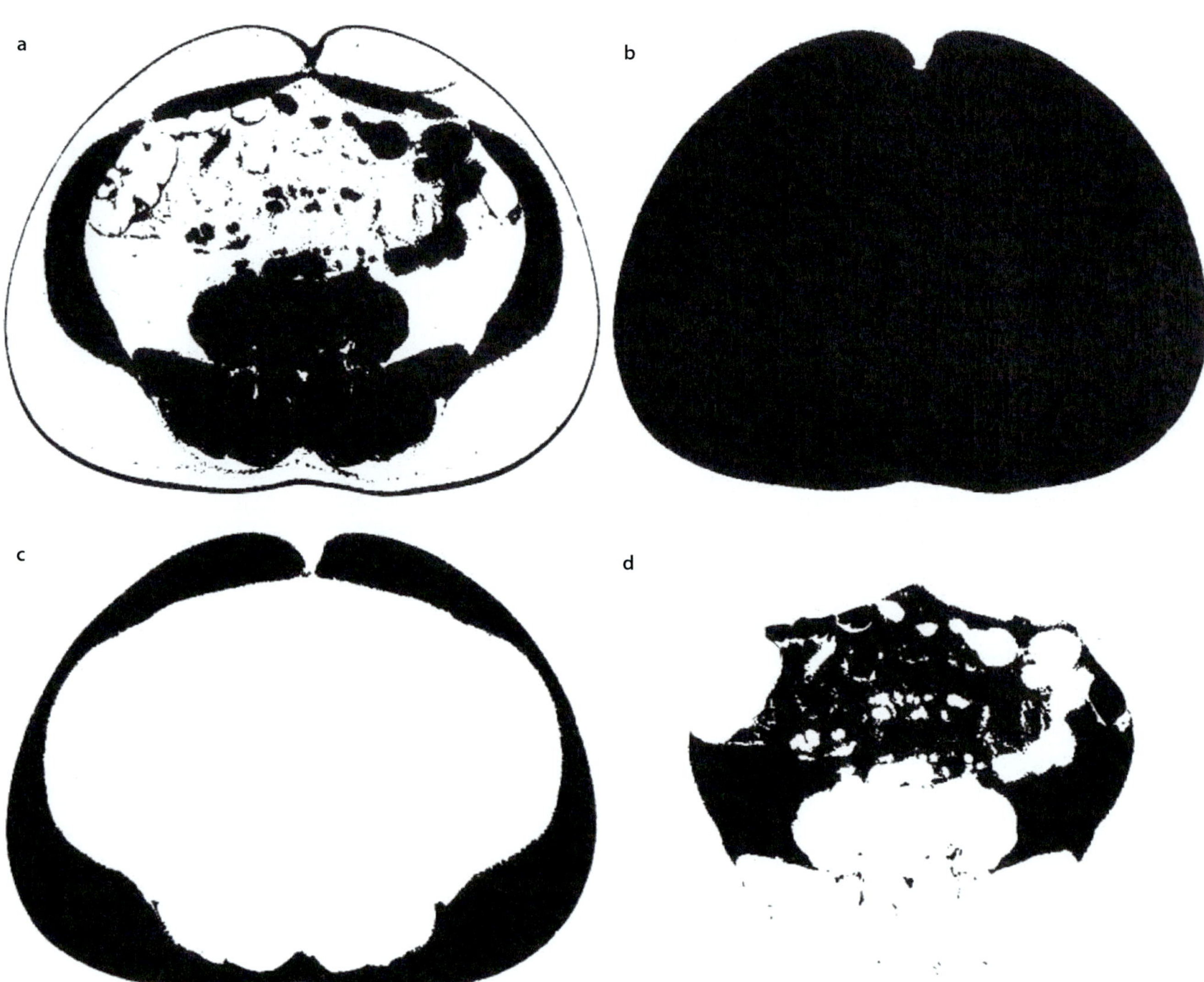

**◘ Fig. 10.5.7** Computer-generated histogram segmentation of the same CT section as (◘ Fig. 10.5.6) done by using image analysis software (Image J). The image in (**a**) reflects fat density (represented in *white*), and the other nonfatty tissues are removed (represented in *black*). Image (**b**) represents total body volume, image (**c**) represents subcutaneous tissue volume (in back after inversion of the original *white color*), and image (**d**) represents VAT volume (in *black*). The volume of VAT or subcutaneous tissue in this image is gained in cm$^2$. The volume must be multiplied by the slice thickness of the original image to get the fat volume in cm$^3$

Fluoroscopic barium meal examination is performed to detect abnormalities and complications of gastric banding. Initially, a scout supine abdominal image is taken to identify the place of the band and the reservoir. Water-soluble contrast media is initially administered in the early stages to confirm the absence of leakage. The normal images should reveal a small upper gastric pouch, a narrow stoma extending through the gastric band, and opacification of the rest of the stomach (◘ Fig. 10.5.8). CT can be performed after the fluoroscopic examination to detect other abnormalities.

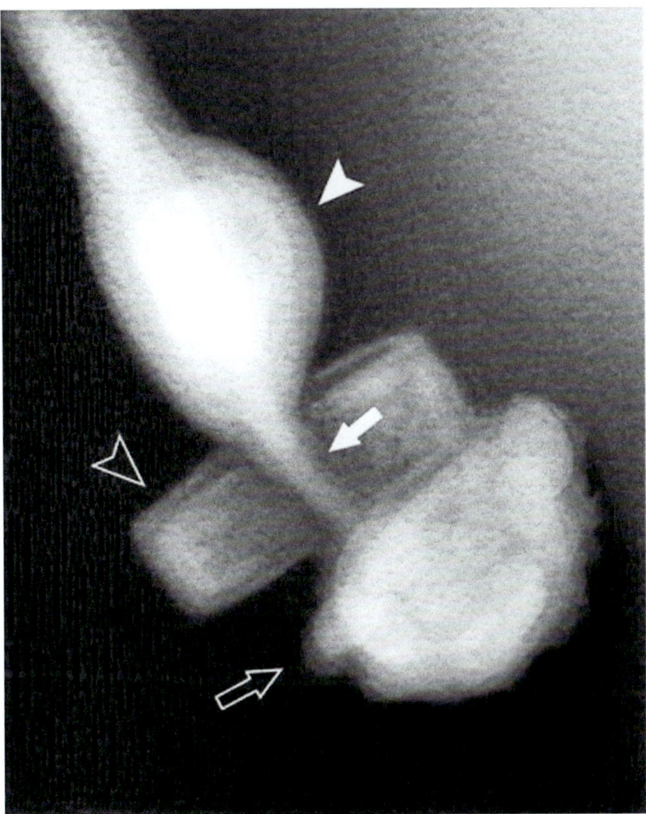

**Fig. 10.5.8** Barium meal illustration shows the normal radiographic findings in gastric banding: the gastric pouch (*solid arrowhead*), the stoma (*solid arrow*), the gastric band (*hollow arrowhead*), and the gastric fundus (*hollow arrow*)

### Signs on Barium Meal

- Eccentric pouch dilatation is seen as an abnormally dilated gastric pouch. It is usually seen in patients with dietary noncompliance (**Fig. 10.5.9**). The gastric pouch is dilated due to chronic overfilling. The stoma is usually in its normal position.
- Pouch dilatation may also occur due to narrow stoma (**Fig. 10.5.10**). The scan shows pouch dilatation, with narrow stoma (2–3 mm). Patients with this kind of obstruction often present with esophageal dysmotility, vomiting, and pseudoachalasia.
- Band slippage is seen as stomach herniation above the band, resulting in pouch dilatation (**Fig. 10.5.11**). Patients may be asymptomatic (20 %) or may present with epigastric pain, vomiting, and progressive gastroesophageal reflux disease. If not corrected, band slippage can lead to gastric volvulus and gastric necrosis.
- Intragastric migration of the band is a serious complication, in which the band gradually erodes into the gastric wall until it perforates the stomach. It is a rare complication, seen in 0.2–2 % of cases. Patients present with nonspecific gastric pain,

gastrointestinal bleeding, and peritonitis when perforation occurs. The herniated band edge is seen as a barium filling defect within the stomach on barium examination (pathognomonic).

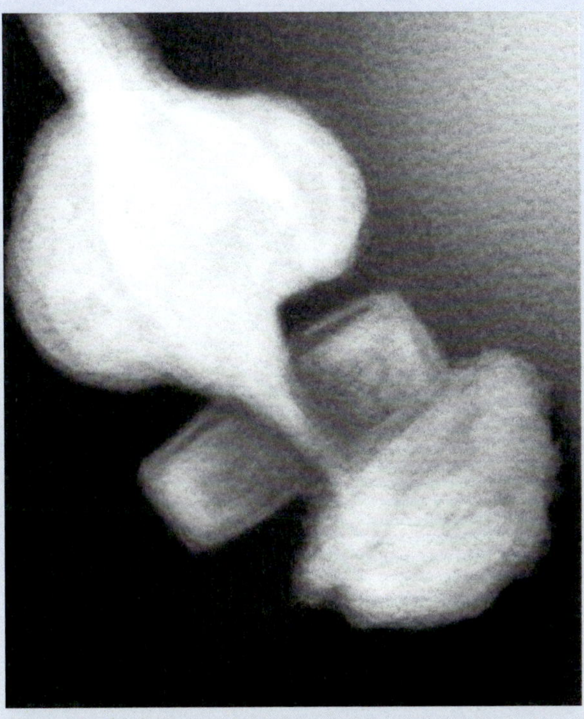

**Fig. 10.5.9** Barium meal illustration shows eccentric pouch dilatation

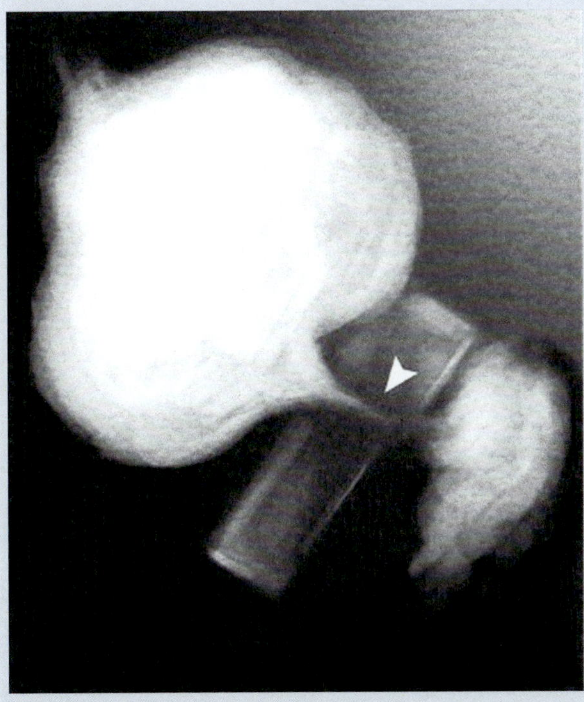

**Fig. 10.5.10** Barium meal illustration shows pouch dilatation due to narrow stoma (*arrowhead*)

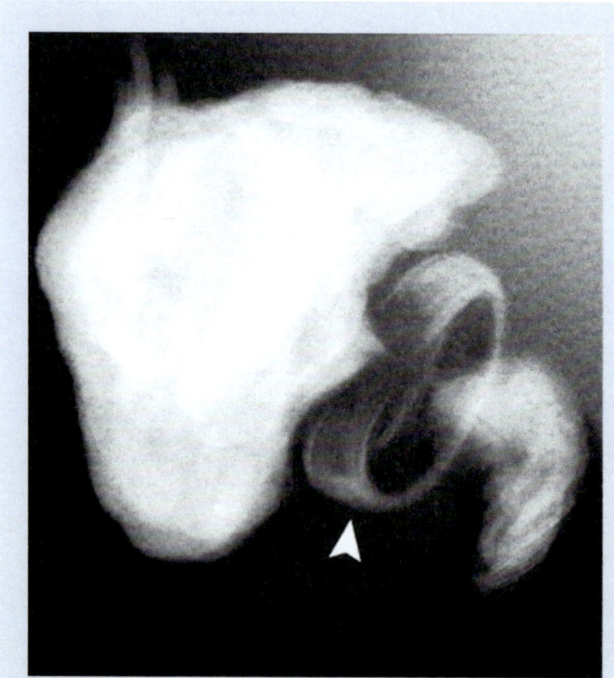

**Fig. 10.5.11** Barium meal illustration shows band slippage into the dilated gastric pouch (*arrowhead*)

## Liposuction

Liposuction is a procedure that allows surgical removal of excess adipose fat in healthy individuals. It is a very common and popular aesthetic surgical procedure that is performed in many countries around the world.

The main complications in fat removal procedures lies in the degree of hemostasis achieved after detachment of the subcutaneous fat layer from the skin in the area of desired fat removal. Poor hemostasis results in the formation of hematoma, seroma, infection, necrosis, and even shock and death, which was commonly seen in the old fat removal techniques that used cutting instruments. In modern liposuction techniques, the detachment of subcutaneous fat is accomplished by injecting fluid under the skin in the desired region through a blunt-edged cannula (hydrodissection). The cannula is used to create multiple tunnels within the subcutaneous fat, inject the dissecting fluid, and then pulled (rather than cut) from the neighboring structures. The liquefied dissected fat is then sucked into a container via the same cannula that injects the dissecting fluid. Classically, the amount of injected fluid equals the amount of fat to be removed (Illouz technique). The dissecting fluid is composed of isotonic saline, hyaluronidase, and perhaps lidocaine, epinephrine, and sodium bicarbonate.

Liposuction is a relatively safe procedure, with overall complications occurring in approximately 5–10 % of patients. Most of these complications include the formation of hematoma, seroma, edema, and skin pigmentation problems. Removal of more 3,000 mL of fat may carry the risk of severe systemic complications that require resuscitation and blood transfusion. The amount of fat removed should not exceed 6–8 % of the patient's body weight and 30 % of patient's body surface area. Also, blood loss should not exceed 1–1.5 units. Causes of severe complications and death in liposuction include the development of crush syndrome and fat embolism syndrome (FES). *Crush syndrome* is a pathological condition characterized by severe shock and hypotension, anuria, coma, and death. Classically, the disease is caused by muscle disintegration that releases myoglobin into the circulation, which has toxic effect over the renal glomerulus. During liposuction, the numerous tunnels created through the fat create a mechanism of subcutaneous injury similar to crush syndrome. Also, uncontrolled cannula movements may cause muscle injury, creating crisscrossed tunnels that may produce large cavities. These large cavities result in third space fluid loss, which produces severe symptoms. *FES* is a pathological situation characterized by the development of metastatic fat emboli in multiple body organs, resulting in a triad of pulmonary insufficiency, cerebral involvement, and petechial rashes. FES can result due to fat droplets leaking into the systemic circulation via ruptured veins at the site of cannula tunneling (mechanical theory) or due to the liberation of free fatty acids such as "chylomicrons" from the detached adipocytes. These free fatty acids are toxic to the pneumocytes and the capillary epithelium, producing chemical pneumonitis. FES typically manifests within 24–72 h after trauma or liposuction procedure. Neurological manifestations due to fat emboli to the brain include seizures, altered level of consciousness, focal neurological deficits, and even coma. Patients develop petechial skin rash on the head and neck region and on the upper body, which is believed to be the only pathognomonic feature (seen in 50 % of cases). Laboratory findings show decreased hematocrit level, increased serum lipase level, hypoxemia, and hypokalemia. These findings are observed during the first 24–72 h. Fulminant FES is a term reserved for severe manifestations of cardiopulmonary obstruction by fat produced by a sudden intravascular liberation of a large amount of fat. Severe heart failure, shock, and even death occur within the first 1–12 h of injury.

**Signs on Radiographs**

Pulmonary edema may be seen on chest radiograph if a large amount of fluid is injected subcutaneously or intravenously or if the patient develops ARDS due to multiple pulmonary fat emboli. When pulmonary manifestations develop, the radiological signs may remain for up to 3 weeks.

**Signs on US**

Seromas are detected as localized fluid (anechoic) collections below the skin, whereas hematoma is seen as hypoechoic to hyperechoic masses, depending on the age of the hematoma.

**Signs on MRI**

When FES affects the brain, it usually results in multiple diffuse foci of hyperintensity located in the white matter of the subcortical, periventricular, and centrum semiovale regions. Characteristic multiple hyperintense foci lesions in the centrum semiovale may be seen in DWI, resulting in a "starfield pattern" (Fig. 10.5.12).

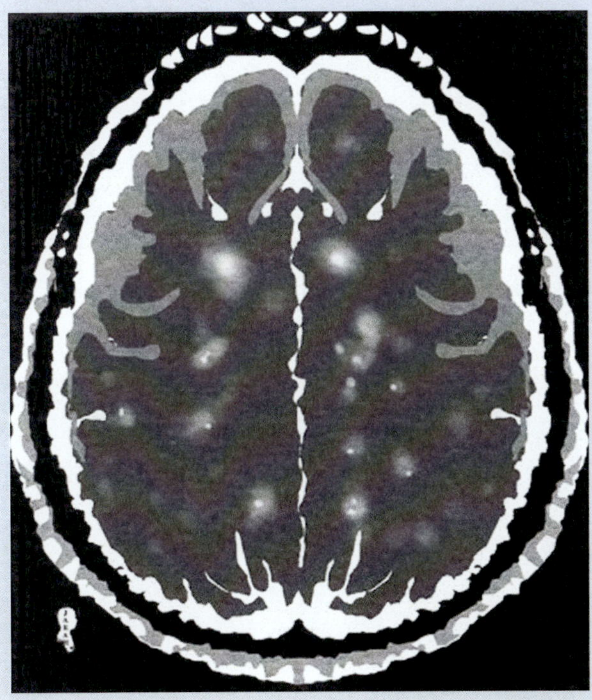

**Fig. 10.5.12** Axial brain DW illustration of a patient with fat embolism syndrome shows the starfield pattern

## Further Reading

Adami GF, et al. Metabolic syndrome in severely obese patients. Obes Surg. 2001;11:543–5.

Bray GA. Obesity Dis Mon. 1979;26(1):1–85.

Buckley O, et al. European obesity and radiology department. What can we do to help? Eur Radiol. 2009;19:298–309.

Bulum T, et al. Madelung's disease: case report and review of the literature. Diabetologia Croatica. 2007;36:25–30.

Carucci LR, et al. Adjustable laparoscopic gastric banding for morbid obesity: imaging assessment and complications. Radiol Clin North Am. 2007;45:261–74.

Chen JJS, et al. MR imaging of the brain in fat embolism syndrome. Emerg Radiol. 2008;15:187–92.

Illouz YG. Complications of liposuction. Clin Plast Surg. 2006;33:129–63.

Koda M, et al. Sonographic subcutaneous and visceral fat indices represent in the distribution of body fat volume. Abdom Imaging. 2007;32:387–92.

Landen S, et al. Complications of gastric banding presenting to the ED. Am J Emerg Med. 2005;23:368–70.

Lange U, et al. Dercum's disease (lipomatosis dolorosa): successful therapy with pregabalin and manual lymphatic drainage and a current overview. Rheumatol Int. 2008;29:17–22.

Nakai M, et al. Weber-Christian disease presenting with retroperitoneal panniculitis. Eur J Radiol Extra. 2006;60:89–92.

Pomerri F, et al. Radiological assessment of complications after laparoscopic suprabursal adjustable gastric banding for morbid obesity. Obes Surg. 2009;19:146–52.

Raguse JD, et al. Benign symmetric lipomatosis (Madelung's disease) complicated by involvement of the facial nerve. Eur J Plast Surg. 2004;27:306–8.

Reddix Jr RN, et al. Crush syndrome presenting three days after injury. Injury Extra. 2004;35:73–5.

Shen W, et al. Adipose tissue quantification by imaging methods: a proposed classification. Obes Res. 2003;11(1):5–16.

Trekner SW, et al. Imaging of morbid obesity procedures and their complications. Abdom Imaging. 2008;34(3):335–44. doi:10.1007/s00261-008-9389-3.

Valchos IS, et al. Sonographic assessment of regional adiposity. AJR Am J Roentgenol. 2007;189:1545–53.

Verna G, et al. Launois-Bensaude syndrome: an unusual localization of obesity disease. Obes Surg. 2008;18:1313–7.

Wang HD, et al. Fat embolism syndromes following liposuction. Aesth Plast Surg. 2008;32:731–6.

Wiesner W, et al. Adjustable laparoscopic gastric banding in patients with morbid obesity: radiographic management, results, and post-operative complications. Radiology. 2000;216:389–94.

Yoshida T, et al. Weber-Christian disease presenting with ocular manifestations. Clin Rheumatol. 2003;22:339–42.

## 10.6 Lipoatrophic–Lipodystrophic Syndromes

Lipoatrophy syndromes are a wide group of disorders, characterized by diffuse or focal paucity of fatty tissue within the body.

Loss of fat is known as *lipoatrophy*, whereas abnormal fat distribution is known as *lipodystrophy*. When diabetes mellitus occurs with lipoatrophy, it is called *lipoatrophic diabetes*.

Patients with lipoatrophy syndromes are clinically characterized by focal or diffuse loss of fatty tissue, diabetes mellitus, acanthosis nigricans, hyperandrogenism and amenorrhea in females, cardiomyopathy and muscular hypertrophy, increased appetite and high basal metabolic rate, and nonalcoholic liver steatosis or cirrhosis.

*Focal lipoatrophy* refers to a condition where the loss of fat involves a single region in the body. An example of focal lipoatrophy is loss of fat in the gluteal area, usually following intramuscular injection (Fig. 10.6.1).

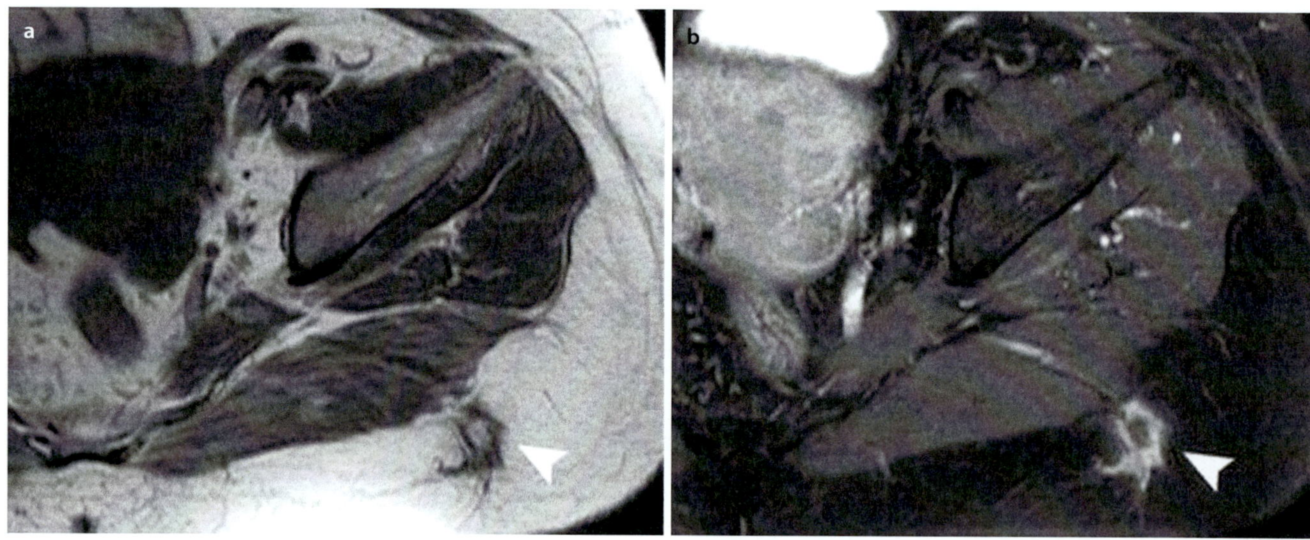

**Fig. 10.6.1** Axial T1W (**a**) and T1W postcontrast fat saturation (**b**) images show focal fatty necrosis with enhancement due to previous intramuscular injection (*arrowhead*)

Laboratory investigations in lipoatrophy syndromes typically show hyperinsulinemia, hyperglycemia, hypertriglyceridemia, abnormal cholesterol profile, elevated free fatty acids, and low leptin and other adipocytes hormones.

In general, radiological features show normal bone mineral density on DEXA scan and hepatic steatosis on ultrasound. However, the conventional radiographic and MRI features depend on the syndrome. Different lipoatrophy syndromes and their characteristic radiological features are discussed below.

## Congenital Generalized Lipodystrophy (Seip–Berardinelli Syndrome)

Seip–Berardinelli syndrome (SBS) is a disease characterized by generalized absence of fat within the first year of life (primarily affects neonates).

As neonates grow up, they develop diabetes mellitus type 2 before the teenage years. Acanthosis nigricans, hypertriglyceridemia, and frequent bouts of pancreatitis are other common features.

The syndrome has an autosomal recessive mode of inheritance, with females showing more severe lipid profile abnormalities than males. Features of gigantism are often found in patients with SBS.

Talon cusp has been reported in cases with SBS. *Talon cusp*, also known as "eagle cusp," is an extra cusp of an anterior tooth. In the premolar teeth, an extra tooth cusp is referred to as *dens envaginatus*. When dens envaginatus occurs in an anterior tooth such as an incisor or a canine, it is referred to as a talon cusp (**Fig. 10.6.2**).

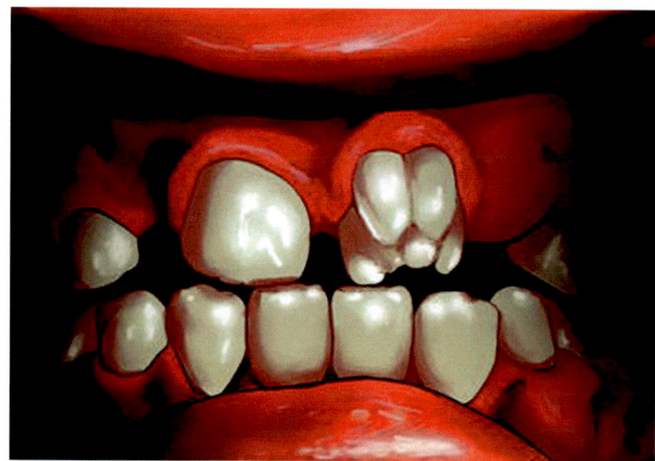

**Fig. 10.6.2** An illustration demonstrates talon cusp

**Signs on Plain Radiographs**
– Skeletal radiographs usually show advanced bone age plus loss of subcutaneous fat.
– Craniosynostosis may be seen in some patients (e.g., dolichocephaly).

**Signs on CT and MRI**
– Transverse sections of the torso at the level of the fifth lumbar vertebra often show markedly deficient subcutaneous fat and loss of the visceral fat.
– Liver cirrhosis or steatosis is a common feature of SBS.

## Familial Partial Lipodystrophy (Dunnigan–Kobberling Syndrome)

Dunnigan–Kobberling syndrome (DKS) is a rare autosomal dominant disease, characterized by normal fat distribution at birth, with progressive loss of subcutaneous fat, mainly that located in the extremities and the trunk, as the patient reaches puberty. The loss of subcutaneous fat from the extremities and the trunk is associated with increased fat deposition in the face and the neck as puberty is complete.

Like SBS, DKS shows a more severe course in females than in males. Diabetes and dyslipidemia are seen in much earlier ages in females compared to males. Polycystic ovary disease is often seen in females with DKS.

The presentation of DKS may be clinically mistaken for Cushing's syndrome. The absence of fat and the well-reserved muscles in the extremities enable establishing the correct diagnosis.

> **Signs on CT and MRI**
> - The patient's body shows loss of the subcutaneous fat in the extremities and increased subcutaneous fat in the head and neck region.
> - Transverse sections of the torso at the level of the fifth lumbar vertebra often show markedly reduced subcutaneous fat and increased visceral fat ( Fig. 10.6.3).

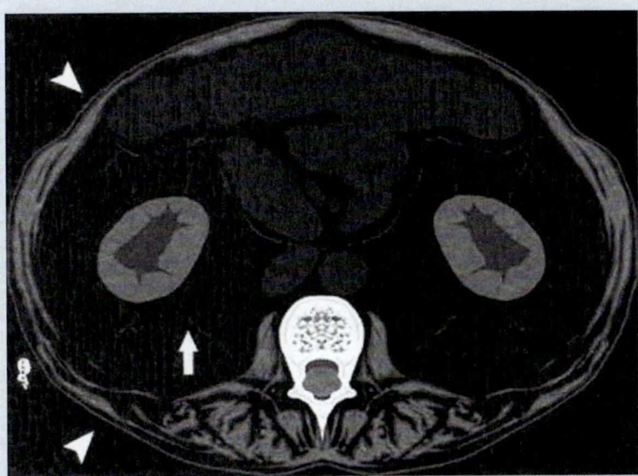

 **Fig. 10.6.3** Axial abdominal CT illustration demonstrates profound proliferation of the visceral fat in the retroperitoneum (*arrow*), with almost complete absence of subcutaneous fatty tissue (*arrowheads*), which is a typical finding in a patient with familial partial lipoatrophy

## Mandibuloacral Dysplasia

Mandibuloacral dysplasia (MAD) is a very rare, multisystemic, autosomal recessive disease, characterized by mandibular and clavicular hypoplasia ( Fig. 10.6.4), joint

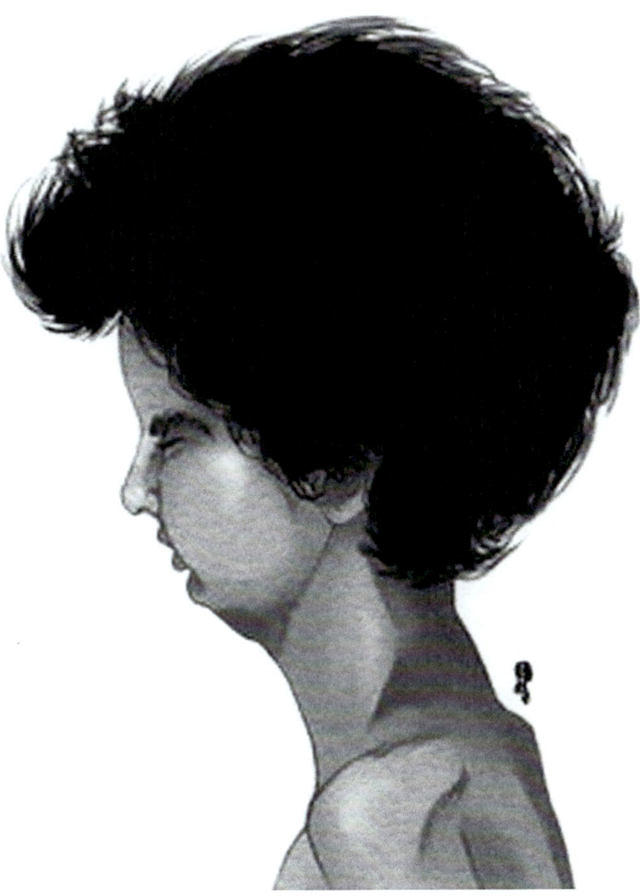

 **Fig. 10.6.4** An illustration demonstrates the clinical findings in a patient with mandibuloacral dysplasia. Notice the hypoplastic mandible (micrognathia)

contractures, acro-osteolysis, joint and skin problems, and lipodystrophy.

Patients with MAD present with loss of the subcutaneous fat of the extremities with increased visceral fat deposition.

> **Signs on Plain Radiographs**
> - Hypoplastic clavicle and mandible (micrognathia)
> - Loss of the terminal phalangeal tufts (acro-osteolysis)
> - Widened skull sutures

## Acquired Generalized Lipoatrophy (Lawrence–Seip Syndrome)

Lawrence–Seip syndrome (LSS) is an acquired generalized lipodystrophy disorder. Its clinical features are similar to SBS (congenital form), but it often arises after a triggering event (e.g., infection). The key diagnosis between the two conditions is the age of presentation. SBS typically starts in neonates, while LSS starts in much older patients after a triggering event.

Fat loss in LSS is usually severe and may lead to a dramatic change in the physical appearance. Patients often develop diabetes mellitus within 4 years from the time they started losing fat. The fat loss is profound, and it may affect the retro-orbital fat, hands, feet, the genital area, and the bone marrow. Nephrotic syndrome is often seen in patients with LSS.

**Signs on Plain Radiographs**
Skeletal radiographs usually show advanced bone age plus loss of subcutaneous fat.

**Signs on CT and MRI**
Almost the same radiological features as SBS

## Acquired Partial Lipoatrophy (Barraquer–Simons Syndrome)

Barraquer–Simons syndrome (BSS) is a disease with a wide range of variations, with a few shared features. Patients with BSS are typically women in their second or third decade of life, who also have autoimmune disorder (e.g., scleroderma), presenting with partial loss of fat.

The loss of fat in BSS typically starts from the face and descends downward until the gluteal line, with increased fat deposition in the lower extremities. Not all patients with BSS develop diabetes mellitus and dyslipidemia (only 50 %).

**Signs on CT and MRI**
A body section of the upper abdomen shows marked reduced subcutaneous fat compared to the lower pelvis and the lower extremities (◘ Fig. 10.6.5).

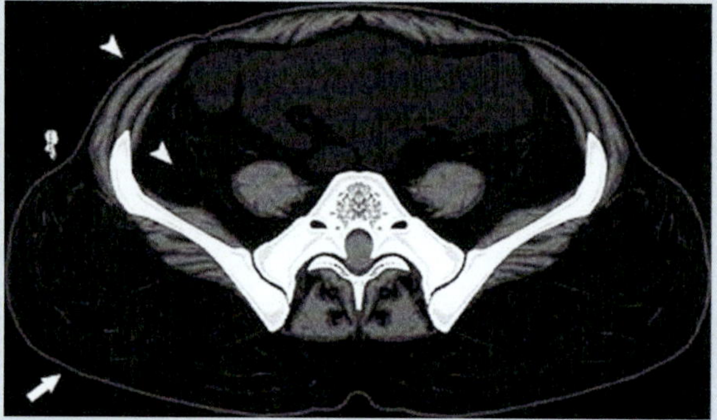

◘ **Fig. 10.6.5** Axial abdominal CT illustration demonstrates profound proliferation of the subcutaneous fat in the buttocks (*arrow*) compared to the visceral fat and the anterior abdominal wall subcutaneous fat (*arrowheads*), which is a characteristic finding in acquired partial lipoatrophy

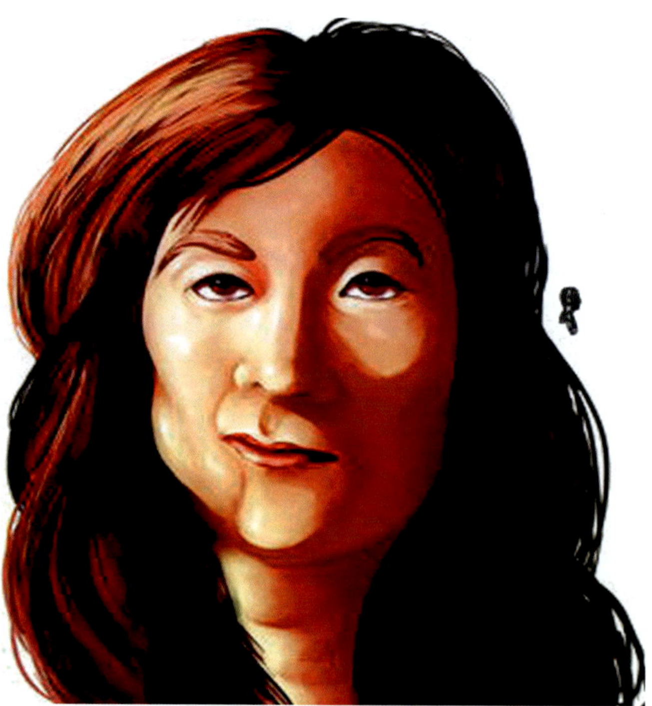

◘ **Fig. 10.6.6** An illustration demonstrates the facial features in Parry–Romberg syndrome (PRS). Notice the hypoplasia of the right side of the face with mouth deviation, reduced mandible size, and eye size compared to the normal, unaffected left side of the face

## Parry–Romberg Syndrome (Progressive Facial Hemiatrophy)

Parry–Romberg syndrome (PRS) is a sporadic disease of unknown origin, characterized by slow, progressive atrophy of the face with all its components, involving the skin, subcutaneous tissues, muscles, cartilage, and bones (◘ Fig. 10.6.6). Some authors consider PRS a focal form of lipoatrophy affecting the face, while other authors consider it a form of phakomatosis.

PRS starts at a young age and slowly progresses as the patient gets older. Patients commonly present with epilepsy and brain abnormalities ipsilateral to the facial atrophy. Bilateral facial atrophy is seen in 5–10 % of cases, and atrophy of the ipsilateral eye or enophthalmos is seen in 10–35 % of cases.

Histological examinations of the facial specimens of the disease reveal proliferative interstitial neurovasculitis. PRS may be mistaken for an extensive form of linear scleroderma.

**Signs on MRI**
The MRI in PRS usually shows cerebral hemiatrophy, cortical calcifications, focal areas of white matter abnormalities, and meningeal enhancement, all ipsilateral to the atrophic side of the face.

## Further Reading

Babu P, et al. Berardinelli Seip syndrome in a 6-year-old boy. Indian J Dermatol Venerol Leprol. 2008;74:644–6.

Garg A, et al. Lipodystrophies: rare disorders causing metabolic syndrome. Endocrinol Clin North Am. 2004;33:305–31.

Goldberg-Stern H, et al. Parry-Romberg syndrome: follow-up imaging during suppressive therapy. Neuroradiology. 1997;39:873–6.

Janaki VR, et al. Lawrence-Seip syndrome. Br J Dermatol. 1980;103:693.

Kobashi Y, et al. Berardinelli Seip lipodystrophy. Skeletal Radiol. 2007;36:999–1003.

Lt Col Prasad AN. Berardinelli Seip syndrome. MJAFI. 2006;62:83–4.

Mako SB, et al. Parry-Romberg syndrome: intracranial MRI appearances. J Cranio-Maxillofacial Surg. 2003;31:321–4.

Mazzeo N, et al. Progressive hemifacial atrophy (Parry-Romberg syndrome), case report. Oral Surg Oral Med Oral Pathol Oral Radiol Endod. 1995;79:30–5.

Novelli G, et al. Mandibuloacral dysplasia is caused by a mutation in *LMNA*-encoding lamin A/C. Am J Hum Genet. 2002;71:426–31.

Oral EA. Lipoatrophic diabetes and other related syndromes. Rev Endocr Metab Disord. 2003;4:61–77.

Owen KR, et al. Mesangiocapillary glomerulonephritis type 2 associated with familial partial dystrophy (Dunnigan-Kobberling syndrome). Nephron Clin Pract. 2004;96:c35–8.

Premkumar A, et al. Lipoatrophic-lipodystrophic syndromes: the spectrum of findings on MR imaging. AJR Am J Roentgenol. 2002;178:311–8.

Sheh JJ, et al. Mandibuloacral dysplasia caused by homozygosity for the R527H mutation in lamin A/C. J Med Genet. 2003;40:854–7.

Solanski M, et al. Talon cusps, macrodontia and aberrant tooth morphology in Berardinelli Seip syndrome. Oral Surg Oral Med Oral Pathol Oral Radiol Endod. 2008;105:e41–7.

Spranger S, et al. Barraquer-Simon syndrome (with sensorineural deafness): a contribution to the differential diagnosis of lipodystrophy syndromes. Am J Med Genet. 1997;71:397–400.

## 10.7 Diabetic Nephropathy

Diabetes mellitus (DM) microangiopathy effects are seen mainly in the retina and the kidneys (*capillary diseases*). Multiple genitourinary conditions are known to occur in the population but with a higher incidence in diabetics. Also, many genitourinary diseases are known to be almost exclusively seen in diabetes mellitus. This topic discusses the radiological features of some genitourinary conditions that are known to be seen among diabetics.

## Diabetic Nephropathy

Diabetic nephropathy is defined as the presence of persistent proteinuria (>0.5 g of albumin per 24 h) in a patient with concomitant diabetic retinopathy and high blood pressure but without renal or cardiac diseases. This is seen in up to 45 % of patients with DM type 1 and in less than 20 % in DM type 2.

The main histological changes in diabetic nephropathy are due to focal intercapillary glomerulosclerosis. Early in the course of diabetes, the kidney appears enlarged on intravenous nephrograms or ultrasound images due to glomerular hyperfiltration (>150 mL/min). Glomerular hyperfiltration is seen in about 25 % of patients after initiation of insulin therapy. Later in the course of the disease, the kidneys show progressive reduction in size and change in deteriorating functions.

In DM type 1, microalbuminuria (0.03–0.3 g of albumin per 24 h) can be seen within the first 5 years from clinical manifestations. Between 5 and 10 years of diabetes, microalbuminuria (>0.5 g of albumin per 24 h) is observed, and hypertension may be present at this time. After 17–35 years of diabetes, there is fall in the glomerular filtration rate with development of nephritic syndrome, which is complicated later by end-stage renal disease.

In radiological examinations, the use of contrast agents for CT and MRI in patients with DM type 1 may induce renal failure in patients without diabetic nephropathy. Renal failure due to contrast agents is manifested as raise in serum creatinine level 1–5 days after exposure to contrast agents with development of oliguria within 48 h from exposure. Persistent nephrogram 24–48 h after administration of contrast agent is characteristic but not specific finding. Renal failure due to contrast agents can be avoided by ensuring that the patient is well hydrated after the radiological examination.

### Signs on US

1. In newly diagnosed diabetics, the kidney size is normal or enlarged (>13 cm in diameter) due to glomerular hyperfiltration.
2. In diabetic nephropathy, the cortex shows hyperechogenicity with loss of the cortical-medullary differentiation according to the degree of disease damage (*revise the topic of renal failure in* Chap. 5).
3. In end-stage renal disease, the kidney is hyperechogenic and shrunken in size.

### Signs on Doppler Sonography

1. In normal healthy adults, the interlobar arteries resistance index (RI < 0.7). In patients with DM, there is increased resistance index (RI > 0.7) in diabetic nephropathy especially when there is high serum creatinine with low creatinine clearance.
2. Glomerular hyperfiltration is diagnosed when (RI < 0.5), which is highly specific (89 %).

## Renal Papillary Necrosis

Renal papillary necrosis (RPN) is a condition characterized by infarction of the renal medullary pyramids and papilla due to ischemia. RNP can be caused by nonsteroidal anti-inflammatory drug (NSAID) abuse, pyelonephritis, DM, sickle cell disease, and tuberculosis. DM causes up to 50 % of RNP cases and arises due to both vascular occlusion and nephrocalcinosis.

Patients with RPN present with signs and symptoms that mimics urinary tract infection (UTI) such as chills, renal colic, fever, and oliguria due to acute renal failure. Other features include microhematuria, pyuria, and proteinuria (<2 g/24 h).

### Signs on Ultrasound

1. Chronic renal papillary necrosis shows calcifications at the renal pyramids (medullary calcinosis – a typical finding).

### Signs on IVU

1. There are two kinds of RPN, papillary and medullary. In the papillary form, clefts originate from the fornices and extend into and dissect the medullary pyramids and papillae, causing sloughing of the papilla. This is seen as deepened medullary fornices that can extend to make a full contrast circle around the papilla (◼ Fig. 10.7.1).
2. In the medullary form of RPN, a central necrosis takes place at the tip of renal pyramid. This is seen as contrast filling that extends centrally into the pyramid causing a balloon-like inflation extending into the renal pyramid (◼ Figs. 10.7.1 and 10.7.2).
3. Nephrocalcinosis can be seen especially if the cause is NSAID abuse.

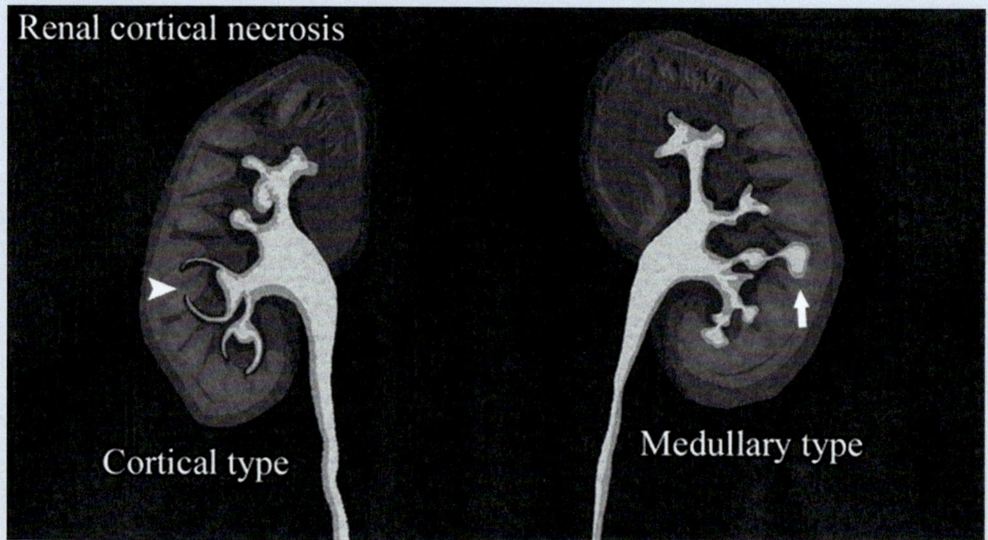


◼ **Fig. 10.7.1**    Coronal MR urographic illustration that demonstrates the radiological sign of cortical papillary necrosis (*arrowhead*) and medullary papillary necrosis (*arrow*)

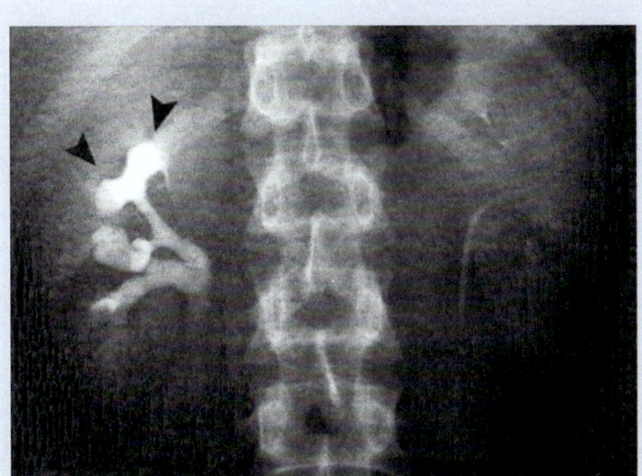

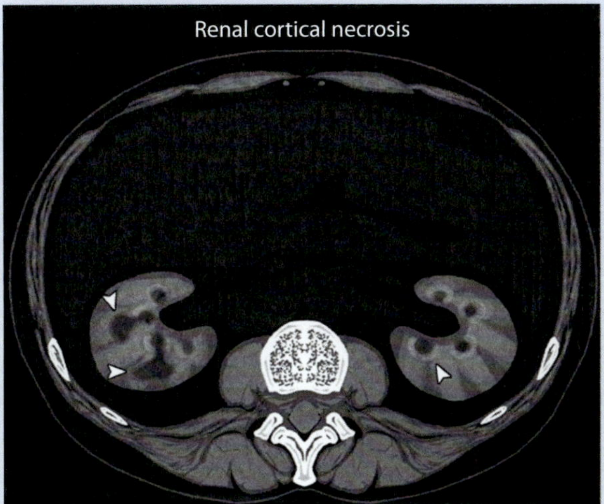


3. A pocket of contrast filling extends into the renal cortex and originating from the renal medullar may be seen due to central papillary necrosis seen in RPN medullary type.

**Fig. 10.7.2** Radiographic intravenous pyelographic image that demonstrates the findings of medullary-type renal papillary necrosis (*arrowheads*)

### Signs on CT
1. There are multiple hypodense lesions may be seen located at the renal papillae that fails to enhance after contrast injection due to infarction (**Fig. 10.7.3**).
2. When the RPN is old, calcification of the infracted renal papillae may be seen on nonenhanced CT with typical location along the renal papillae (**Fig. 10.7.4**).

**Fig. 10.7.3** Axial CT postcontrast illustration that shows the findings in case of acute medullary papillary necrosis seen as areas of no contrast enhancement surrounded by rings of mild contrast uptake due to renal parenchymal infarctions at the acute stage of cortical papillary necrosis (*arrowheads*)

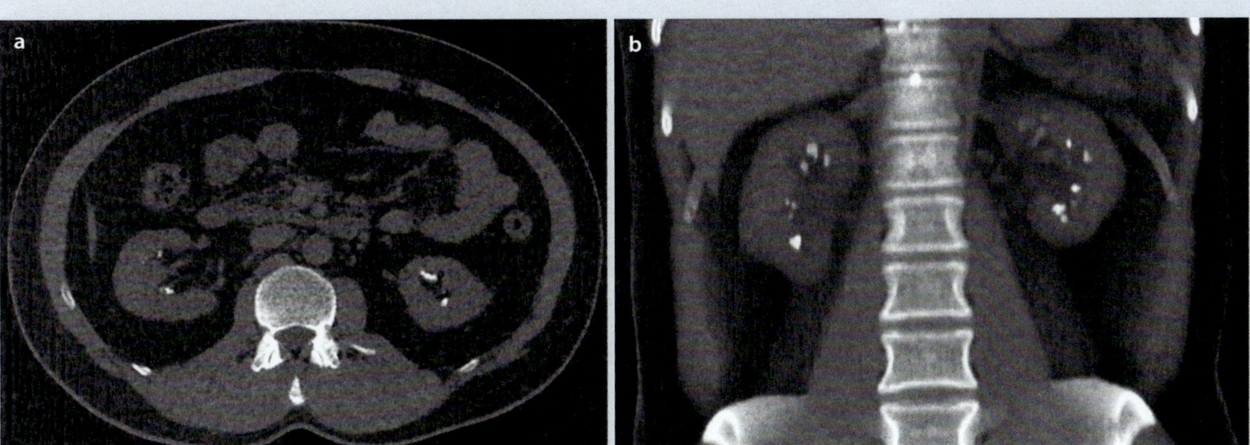

**Fig. 10.7.4** Axial and coronal-3D-MIP reconstruction plain CT images of a patient with history of NSAIDs abuse due to low back pain for 6 months showing calcified foci at the renal medullae bilaterally due to calcified papillary necrosis, a common complication of long-term NSAIDs abuse

## Diabetic Cystopathy (Neurogenic Bladder)

Diabetic cystopathy arises because of partial bladder denervation as a consequence of diabetic peripheral neuropathy affecting the pudendal nerve. There is decreased sensation of bladder overdistension with large residual urine volume after micturition. In chronic cases, vesicoureteric reflux and hydronephrosis may develop with recurrent attacks of pyelonephritis.


Neurogenic bladder is characterized by dilated, atonic bladder with multiple wall cystic formations due to dilated bladder wall trabeculation. The appearance in cystography is classically described as *Christmas tree* (◘ Fig. 10.7.5). The same features can be observed in MRI (◘ Fig. 10.7.6).

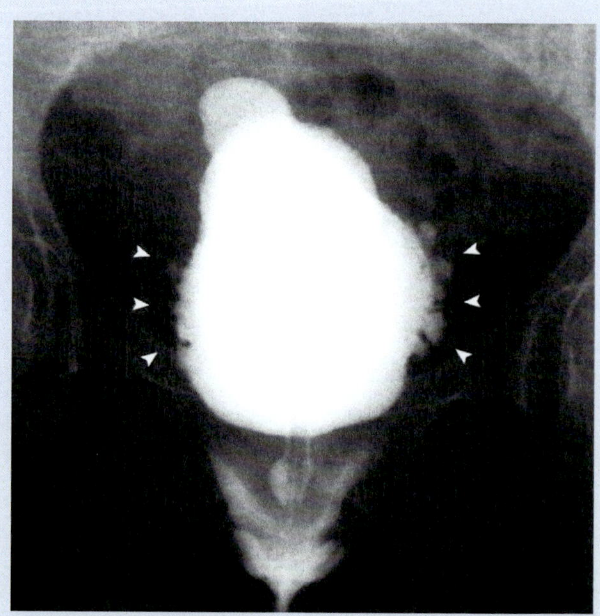

◘ **Fig. 10.7.5**   Cystographic image of a patient with neurogenic bladder demonstrating the *Christmas tree appearance* with the bladder dilated looking like a tree with its leaves are seen as dilated bladder wall trabeculations (*arrowheads*)

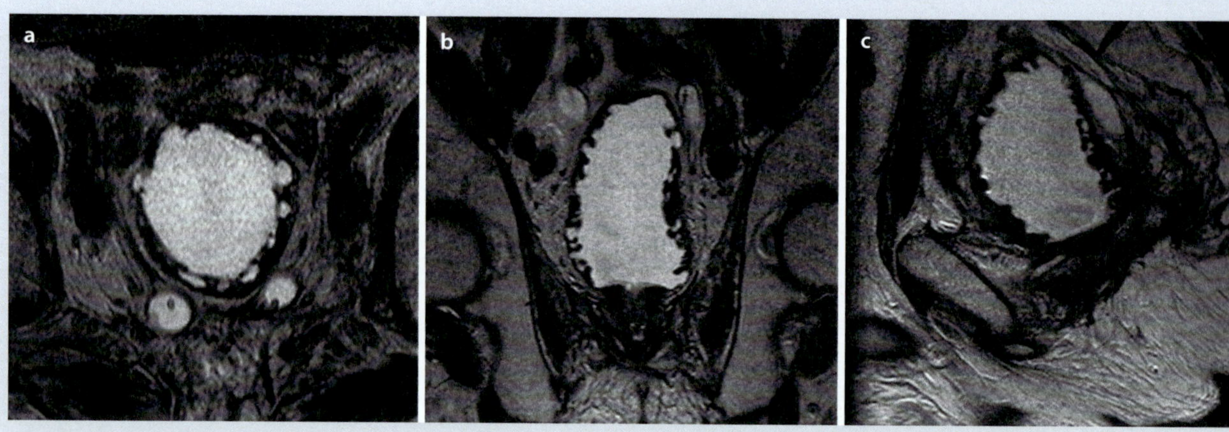

◘ **Fig. 10.7.6**   Axial (**a**), coronal (**b**), and sagittal (**c**) images of a patient with neurogenic bladder showing the *Christmas tree appearance* like in ◘ Fig. 10.7.5; however, the wall trabeculations here are much clearer and explain the cystographic appearance of ◘ Fig. 10.7.5

## Calcification of the Vas Deferens

Vas deferens calcification can occur due to old aging or due to DM in younger males with chronic noncontrolled DM. It can lead to infertility.


There are bilateral symmetrical parallel calcified lines that extend to each side of the midline above the symphysis pubis.

## Emphysematous Cystitis

Emphysematous cystitis is a rare condition characterized by the presence of gas within the bladder wall or the bladder lumen. This condition is almost pathognomonic for poorly controlled DM in patients > 50 years of age.

Emphysematous cystitis arises due to urinary tract infection (UTI) with *E. coli*, *Staphylococcus aureus*, *Nocardia*, and *Clostridium perfringens*. The gas within the bladder lumen or walls is due to urinary glucose fermentation by the invading bacteria. Symptoms are nonspecific and related to bladder irritation. Laboratory findings show pyuria, microhematuria, and even gross hematuria.

### Signs on Plain Radiographs and CT

The bladder shade is seen surrounded by radiolucent line due to air within the wall that may give cobblestone appearance due to the wall trabeculation (pathognomonic; ◘ Fig. 10.7.7).

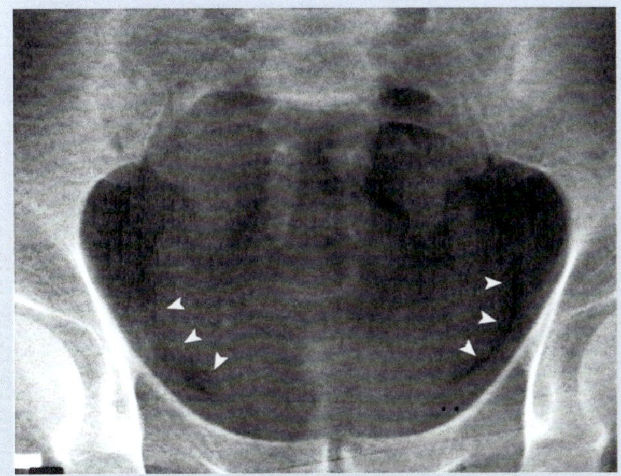

◘ **Fig. 10.7.7** Plain radiography of the bladder of a patient with emphysematous cystitis that shows radiolucent air within the bladder wall (*arrowheads*)

## Emphysematous Pyelonephritis

Pyelonephritis is a bacterial infection of the renal parenchyma that results in tubulointerstitial inflammation and usually results from ascending infection of the bladder (e.g., *via vesicoureteric reflux*). Emphysematous pyelonephritis is an acute necrotizing pyelonephritis characterized by gas formation within the renal parenchyma and the perirenal tissues. Emphysematous pyelonephritis is a surgical emergency that is seen almost exclusively in poorly controlled diabetic female > 50 years of age (90 % of cases). If medical intervention is delayed, mortality can reach up to 80 %. The causative organisms include *E. coli*, *Klebsiella pneumoniae*, and *Pseudomonas* species.

### Signs on Radiographs

Plain radiographs show signs of radiolucent air within the renal shades (pathognomonic).

### ▪▪ Signs on US

1. Classical pyelonephritis is seen as an area of parenchymal hyperechogenicity with low vascular flow (checked by Doppler and power Doppler sonography). Thickening of the renal edges can be seen, with loss of differentiation between the cortex and the medulla.
2. Emphysematous pyelonephritis will show signs on classical pyelonephritis plus multiple intraparenchymal echogenic foci due to the presence of gas. The condition is bilateral in 10 % of cases.
3. Multiple hypoechoic intraparenchymal lesions may be seen due to abscesses formation.

### Signs on CT

1. In classical pyelonephritis, there is enlarged edematous kidney, delayed renal enhancement, wedge-shaped areas of decreased attenuation, Gerota's fascia thickening, and obstruction of the renal tubules by debris impairing contrast excretion that results in "striated" appearance of the kidney (◘ Figs. 10.7.8 and 10.7.9).
2. In emphysematous pyelonephritis, there are gas-density lesions within the renal parenchyma with or without multiple abscesses that are seen as cystic lesions with rim contrast enhancement.

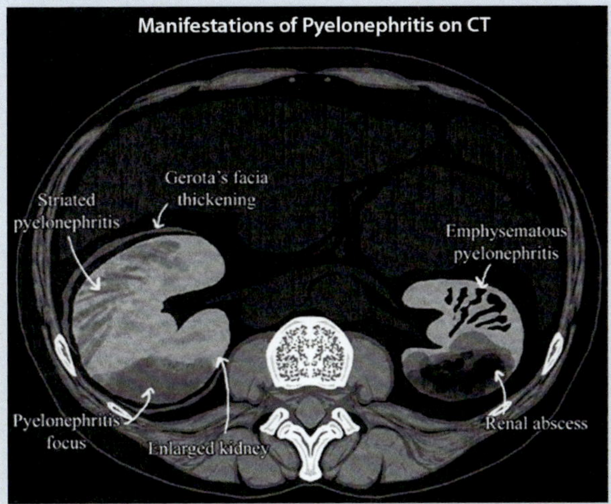


◘ **Fig. 10.7.8** Axial CT postcontrast illustration that shows the different manifestations of pyelonephritis on CT postcontrast images

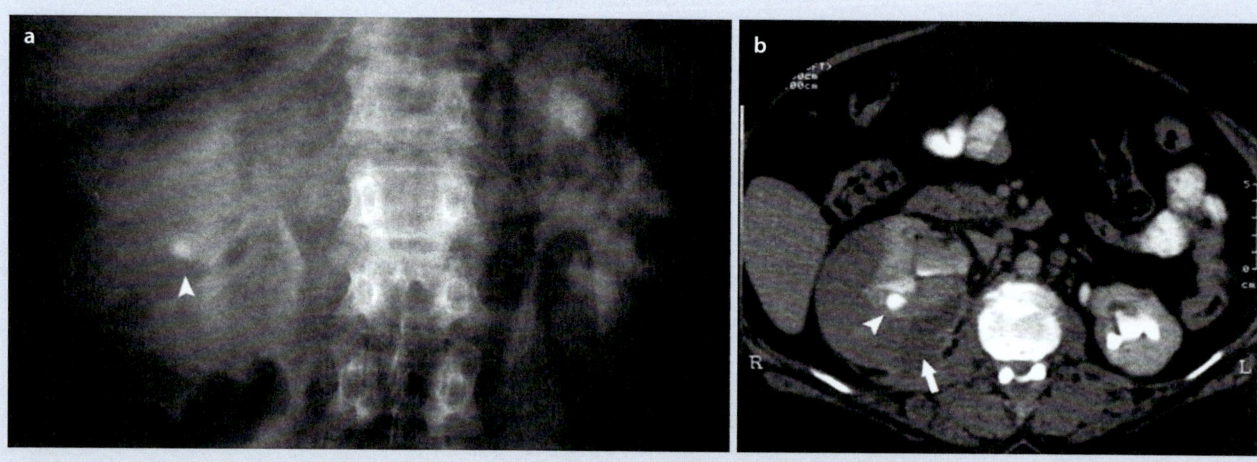



**Fig. 10.7.9**  Plain (**a**) and axial CT image postcontrast (**b**) of a patient with xanthogranulomatous pyelonephritis showing a stone impacted in the renal pelvic (*arrowhead* in **a** and **b**) and fatty infiltration of the renal parenchyma (*arrow* in **b**)

## Xanthogranulomatous Pyelonephritis

Xanthogranulomatous pyelonephritis is a rare condition characterized by chronic UTI that causes replacement of the renal parenchyma by lipid-filled microphages due to inflammation and renal calculus (80 % of cases). The causative organisms of xanthogranulomatous pyelonephritis include *Proteus* species (most common) and *Staphylococcus aureus*. Patients usually complain of multiple genitourinary symptoms more than 6 month in duration (40 % of cases), which include renal colic, fever, malaise, weight loss, anorexia, and persistent urosepsis.

### Signs on Plain Radiographs
Radiographs typically show staghorn calculus with enlarged renal shade (**Fig. 10.7.8a**).

### Signs on Ultrasound
Xanthogranulomatous pyelonephritis has a diffuse and a focal form. In the *diffuse form*, the kidney shows nephromegaly (<12 cm in diameter), multiple calyceal dilatation (multiple cystic formations), renal pelvis dilatation, and stone formation within the kidney. In the *focal form*, a lesion is confined to one part or pole of the kidney, usually occurring in women and children, and may not present findings similar to those of the diffuse form.

### Signs on CT
Typically, there is a stone in the ureter of the affected kidney (often staghorn), with signs of fatty lesions within the renal parenchyma (*you must see these two combinations before you diagnose xanthogranulomatous pyelonephritis*) (**Fig. 10.7.8b**).

### Selected References

Browne RFJ, et al. Imaging of urinary tract infection in the adult. Eur Radiol. 2004;14:E168–83.

Demertzis J, et al. State of the art: imaging of renal infections. Emerg Radiol. 2007;14:13–22.

Jung DC, et al. Renal papillary necrosis: review and comparison findings at multi-detector row CT and intravenous urography. Radiographics. 2006;26:1827–36.

Marzano MA, et al. Early renal involvement in diabetes mellitus: comparison of renal Doppler US and radioisotope evaluation of glomerular hyperfiltration. Radiology. 1998;209:813–7.

Rodriguez-de-Velasquez A, et al. Imaging the effects of diabetes on the genitourinary system. Radiographics. 1995;15:1051–68.

## 10.8  Lipomatosis

Lipomatosis is a benign condition characterized by proliferation of noncapsulated mature adipocytes. Similar conditions include lipoblastomatosis, which is defined as proliferation of noncapsulated immature adipocytes, and liposarcoma which is defined as proliferation of neoplastic adipocytes. Differentiation between the three clinical entities requires histopathological conformation.

Lipomatosis, lipoblastomatosis, and liposarcoma can arise from any part of the body. Lipomatosis of certain areas within the body can present with significant clinical symptoms, which radiological modalities can identify efficiently. This topic discusses some of the well-known symptomatic lipomatosis conditions within the body.

## Intestinal Lipomatosis

Intestinal lipomatosis is a rare benign condition characterized by the formation of multiple polypoid masses within the interior intestinal lumen composed of mature fatty tissues (lipomas).

Intestinal lipomas can be seen as normal variant commonly affecting the ileocecal valve, duodenum, or the cecum. Most cases of intestinal lipomatosis lesions involve solitary lipoma; multiple intestinal lipomatosis is a very rare condition. When multiple intestinal lipomatosis occurs, they are frequently involving the ileum (39%) and the jejunum (13%). Simultaneous presence of diverticulosis is a frequent feature.

Patients with intestinal lipomatosis typically present with recurrent attacks of abdominal pain, melena, anemia, and lower GI bleeding Abdominal pain is attributed to recurrent attacks of intussusception, while melena and lower GI bleeding are attributed to ulceration of the lipomas caused by intussusception. Laboratory investigations often show anemia and hypercholesterolemia.

■■ Signs on Barium Enteroclysis
1. Typically, there are multiple, sharply demarcated, intraluminal filling defects confined to the wall of the intestinal lumen caused by the lipomas (◘ Fig. 10.8.1).
2. Multiple intestinal diverticula may be seen.

■■ Signs on CT
1. Single or multiple intraluminal intestinal lipomas with typical fat density can be detected in any part of the gastrointestinal tract (◘ Figs. 10.8.1 and 10.8.2).

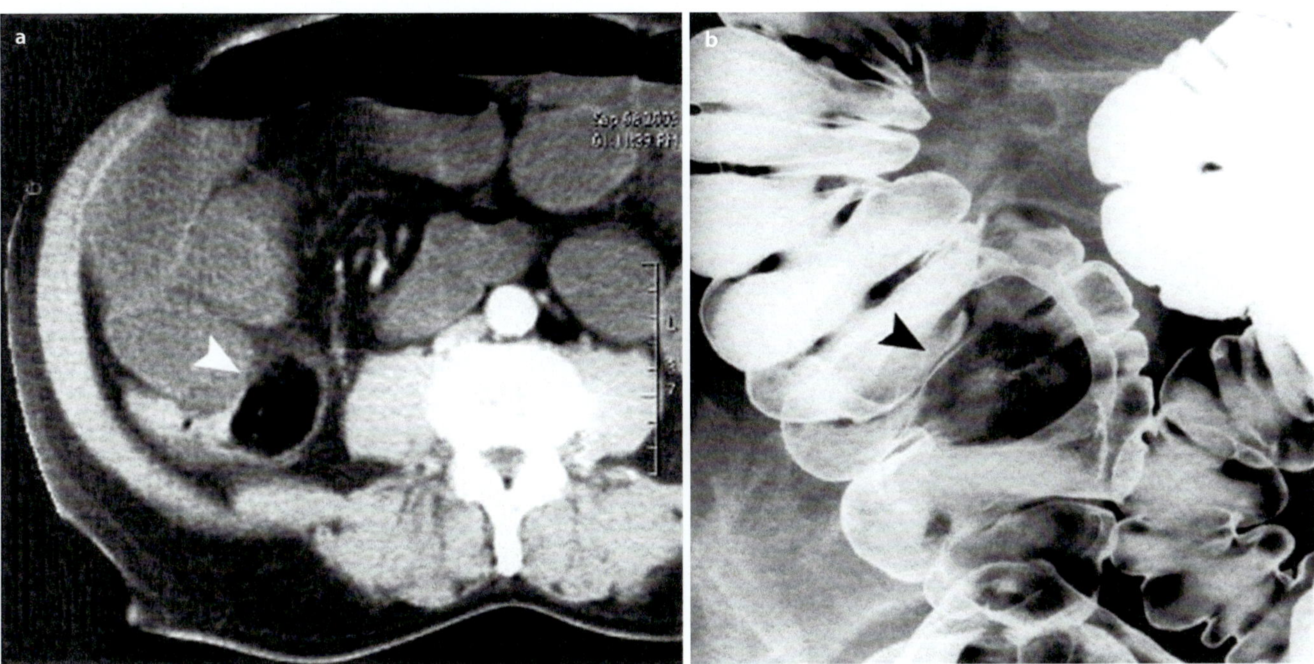

◘ Fig. 10.8.1 Axial CT image (**a**) and colonic enema image (**b**) that shows ileocecal lipoma (*white arrowhead* in **a**) and cecal lipoma (*black arrowhead* in **b**)

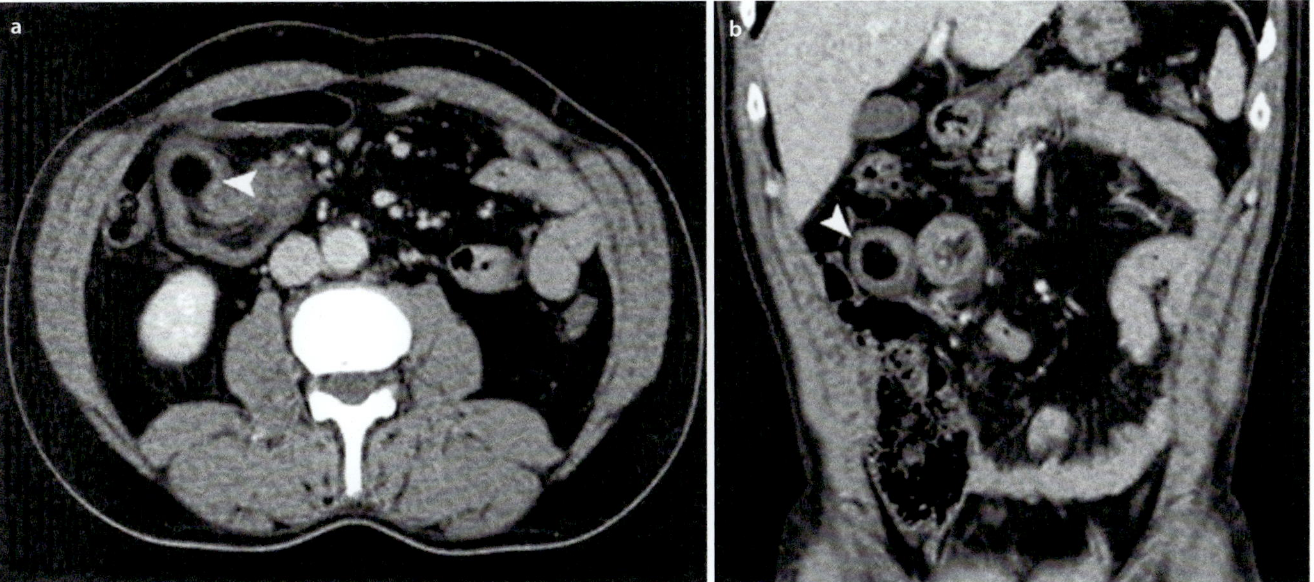

◘ Fig. 10.8.2 Axial (**a**) and coronal (**b**) abdominal CT postcontrast images that show duodenal intraluminal lipoma (*arrowhead* in **a** and **b**)

2. Intussusception may be found, especially if the CT is performed during the acute attack.

## Pelvic Lipomatosis

Pelvic lipomatosis is a rare benign condition characterized by fat proliferation around the bladder, prostate, and rectum producing characteristic radiographic appearance that simulates a pelvic neoplasm. The incidence of pelvic lipomatosis is 0.6–1.7 cases per 100,000 populations. The condition has a male predominance, affecting males of black origin (60 %) in their fourth and fifth decades. Symptoms are relatively mild and include urinary frequency, constipation, and occasionally low-grade fever.

> **Signs on IVU and CT**
> The bladder shows a banana shape with displacement anterosuperiorly out of the true pelvis due to the fat proliferation around it and below it (◘ Fig. 10.8.3). Differential diagnoses include pelvic hematoma and psoas muscle compression.

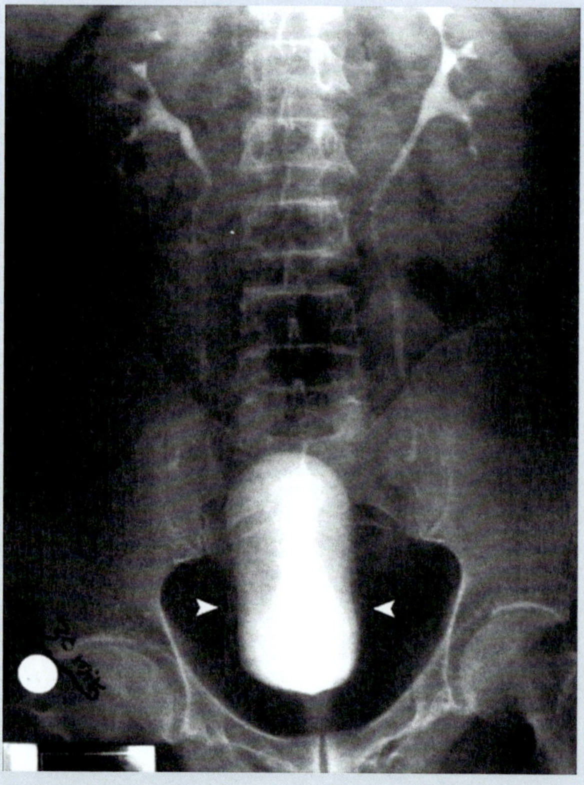

◘ **Fig. 10.8.3**   Intravenous pyelogram that shows elongated bladder shape due to pelvic lipomatosis (*arrowheads*)

## Epidural Lipomatosis

Epidural lipomatosis is a rare condition which is characterized by proliferation of the fat in the epidural space leading to cord compression and displacement within the spinal canal. When the proliferation occurs at the end of the spinal cord, cauda equina syndrome can develop. Patients often present with radicular pain and spinal claudication due to cord compression. There is often a history of chronic systemic steroid therapy or Cushing's syndrome.

> **Signs in CT and MRI**
> There is hypertrophic epidural fat pressing and flattening of the spinal cord. On axial images, Y-shaped compressed dural sac (very characteristic).

## Encephalocraniocutaneous Lipomatosis Syndrome (Haberland Syndrome)

Encephalocraniocutaneous lipomatosis (ECCL) is nonhereditary, congenital, neurocutaneous (phakomatosis) syndrome characterized by unilateral cutaneous hamartoma of the scalp with ipsilateral ophthalmologic and neurological malformations. Most reported cases are sporadic.

Cutaneous lesions of ECCL include nevus psiloliparus; multiple small, popular, or polypoid cutaneous lipomatous nodules usually present on the face and eyelid in a unilateral distribution; a scar-like lesions; and café au lait spots. Nevus psiloliparus is a term used to describe a lipomatous scalp lesion causing head asymmetry. The lipomatous scalp hamartoma is always devoid of hair (alopecia areata). Jaw odontomas can be found.

Ocular abnormalities are always present and include epibulbar choristoma, desmoids tumor of the sclera, persistent hyaloids vessels, ectopia lentis, cataract, and colobomas.

Cerebral manifestations include porencephalic cysts ipsilateral to the lipomatous scalp (major manifestation), causing hydrocephalus and brain atrophy. Seizures may be found, with spasticity of the contralateral limb.

*The diagnostic features of ECCL include*:
1. Unilateral lipomatous hamartoma of the scalp with ipsilateral ocular abnormalities
2. Ipsilateral porencephalic cysts with cerebral atrophy
3. Cranial asymmetry
4. Marked developmental delay and mental retardation
5. Seizures
6. Spasticity of the contralateral limb

> **Signs on Plain Radiographs**
> 1. Skull asymmetry
> 2. Jaw odontomas

### Signs on MRI

1. Scalp lipoma with ipsilateral porencephalic cyst and brain atrophy. The porencephalic cyst is classically located in the parieto-occipital region.
2. Cerebral calcifications.
3. Hydrocephalus.
4. Partial agenesis of the corpus callosum may be seen.
5. Intracranial lipoma (especially in the CP angle) may be found.

## Lipomatous Hypertrophy of the Interatrial Septum

Lipomatous hypertrophy of the interatrial septum (LHIS) is a rare condition defined as fatty deposits within the interatrial septum with a thickness more than 2 cm.

Although the LHIS is detected incidentally and usually asymptomatic, it can rarely cause atrial fibrillation, atrial premature contractions, and atrioventricular block as a consequence of involvement of the atrial wall and atrioventricular conduction pathway. An abnormal P wave configuration in leads II and III and aVF named "dome and dip" have been described in some patients with LHIS.

Differential diagnosis of LHIS in CT and MRI includes interatrial lipoma and atrial myxoma. Atrial myxoma is gelatinous tumors with 90 % of cases are seen in adult women between 30 and 60 years of age. It is the most common primary cardiac neoplasm in adults (50 % of cardiac neoplasms). Most cases are sporadic, and patients usually present with CNS symptoms, fatigue, arthralgia, fever, anemia, and weight loss; however, 20 % of myxomas are asymptomatic.

### Signs on CT and MRI

1. The interatrial septum is seen diffusely replaced by fatty tissue (hypodense in CT and high T1 signal intensity on MRI; 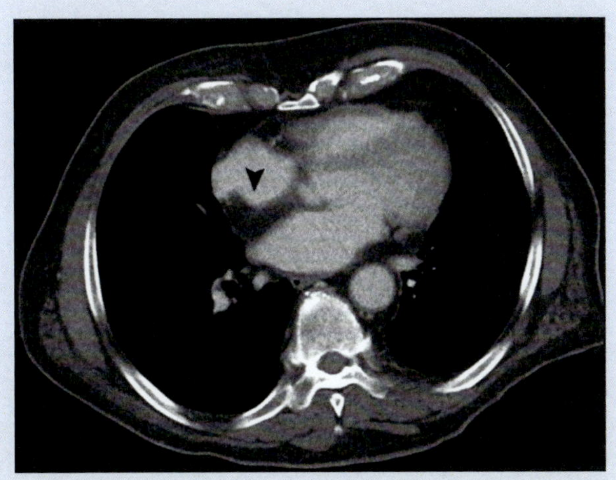 Fig. 10.8.4). The fatty tissue derives from the upper and/or lower part of the interatrial septum with typical sparing of the foramen ovale, giving the lesion a characteristic *dumbbell shape*.
2. Associated features include increased pericardial and mediastinal fat.
3. On CT, cardiac myxoma typically appears as a heterogeneous mass with a narrow base attachment located in the interatrial septum at the area of fossa ovalis (90 % of cases). Eighty percent of cases arise in the left atrium and 10 % in the right atrium. Calcification is frequently seen. On MRI, myxoma is seen as a high signal intensity lesion on T2W images. Heterogeneous enhancement is seen on both CT and MRI.
4. Unlike LHIS, interatrial septum lipoma is seen as localized well-defined (capsulated) fatty lesion.

**Fig. 10.8.4** Axial CT image of the heart shows lipomatosis of the interatrial septum (*arrowhead*)

## Selected References

Al-Mefty O, et al. The multiple manifestations of the Encephalocraniocutaneous lipomatosis syndrome. Child's Nerv Syst. 1987;3:132–4.

Andaç N, et al. Fat necrosis mimicking liposarcoma in a patient with pelvic lipomatosis. CT findings. J Clin Imaging. 2003;27:109–11.

Ayan K, et al. Lipomatous hypertrophy of the interatrial septum. Int J Cardiovasc Imaging. 2005;21:659–61.

Bodas A, et al. Intestinal lipomatosis in a 10-year-old girl. Eur J Pediatr. 2008;167:601–2.

Bogaert J, et al. Esophageal lipomatosis: another consequence of the use of steroids. Eur Radiol. 2000;10:1390–4.

Church PA, et al. Computed tomography and ultrasound in diagnosis of pelvic lipomatosis. Urology. 1979;14(6):631–3.

Fitoz S, et al. Intracranial lipoma with extracranial extension through foramen ovale in a patient with encephalocraniocutaneous lipomatosis syndrome. Neuroradiology. 2002;44:175–8.

Gawel J, et al. Encephalocraniocutaneous lipomatosis. J Cutan Med Surg. 2003;7(1):61–5.

Haloi AK, et al. Facial infiltrative lipomatosis. Pediatr Radiol. 2006;36:1159–62.

Hauber K, et al. Encephalocraniocutaneous lipomatosis: a case with unilateral odontomas and review of the literature. Eur J Pediatr. 2003;162:589–93.

Heyer CM, et al. Lipomatous hypertrophy of the interatrial septum: a prospective study of incidence, imaging findings, and clinical symptoms. Chest. 2003;124:2068–73.

Komagata T, et al. Extensive lipomatosis of the small bowel and mesentery: CT and MRI findings. Radiat Med. 2007;25:480–3.

Parazzini C, et al. Encephalocraniocutaneous lipomatosis: complete neuroradiologic evaluation and follow-up of two cases. AJNR Am J Neuroradiol. 1999;20:173–6.

Pugliatti P, et al. Lipomatous hypertrophy of the interatrial septum. Int J Cardiol. 2008;130:294–5.

Soles R, et al. MR of laryngeal and scrotal involvement in multiple symmetrical lipomatosis. Eur Radiol. 1997;7:946–8.

Türkavtan A, et al. Diffuse infiltrating abdominal lipomatosis. Eur J Radiol Extra. 2008;67:15–7.

Xanthos T, et al. Lipomatous hypertrophy of the interatrial septum: a pathological and clinical approach. Int J Cardiol. 2007;121:4–8.

Yakabe S, et al. Jejunal lipomatosis with diverticulosis: report of a case. Jpn J Surg. 1998;28:846–9.

## 10.9  Hypoglycemia

Hypoglycemia is defined as plasma glucose concentration less than 45 mg/dL and commonly develops when rate of glucose uptake by peripheral tissue exceeds the capacity of the liver glucose output.

Patients with hypoglycemia typically presents with features due to low glucose supply to the brain (*neuroglycopenia*) and increased catecholamine secretion (*counter-regulatory response*). Neuroglycopenia manifestations include altered mental status, aggressiveness, seizures, diplopia, and maybe coma. In contrast, counter-regulatory response manifestations include anxiety, tachycardia, and sweating. The most common causes of hypoglycemia include:

1. *Brittle diabetes*: it is a pathological condition characterized by recurrent sever hypoglycemia and/or ketoacidosis. It is seen mostly in type 1 diabetics who have had diabetes more than 10 years. Brittle diabetes is characterized by negligible insulin secretion and absent glucagon and adrenalin response to hypoglycemia.

2. *Endocrine and metabolic diseases*: like Addison's disease, congenital adrenal hyperplasia, familial fructose and galactose intolerance (*Dormandy's syndrome*), pluriglandular insufficiency syndrome (*Falta syndrome*), and pituitary insufficiency. *Pluriglandular inefficiency syndrome* is a disease characterized by failure of more than one gland, usually the thyroid and pituitary.

3. *Medications*: like weight gain-reducing agents, sulfonylurea, and alcohol. Alcohol induces hypoglycemia especially postprandial due to stimulation of beta cells to produce insulin. Also, alcohol can inhibit gluconeogenesis especially in fasting people or malnourished individuals.

4. *Autoimmune hypoglycemia*: this is uncommon cause of hypoglycemia that arises due to autoantibodies that bind and activate insulin receptors.

5. *Paraneoplastic syndrome*: this is seen with tumors that secret insulin-like growth factor (e.g., *hepatoma*).

6. *Insulin autoimmune syndrome (Hirata disease)*: this is a relatively rare disease characterized by recurrent attacks of postprandial and/or fasting hypoglycemia without evidence of exogenous insulin administration due to the presence of high titers of IgG insulin autoantibodies (IAA). Hirata disease is seen between 60 and 70 years of age and has a striking association with HLA-DR4. The disease has a high incidence among Asian population compared to the rest of the world. Patients present with hypoglycemic attacks more than 1 month and less than 3 month in duration. Eighty-five percent of patients have spontaneous remission. Up to 43 % of patients of Hirata disease develop the disease after intake of medications that contains sulfhydryl compounds for a period of time. Examples of medications that predispose to Hirata disease include glutathione, captopril, methimazole, penicillamine, α-interferon, and loxoprofen sodium.

7. *Late dumping syndrome*: this is a pathological situation seen after gastric or intestinal surgeries. The patient presents with signs of hypoglycemia 1 to 3 h after eating due to inappropriate high insulin secretion stimulated by secretin hormone, which is released from the gut due to the presence of hyperosmolar food form the stomach.

8. *Insulinoma*: this is a benign pancreatic islet cell tumor that secretes insulin and arises from beta cells of islets of Langerhans. The peak age of onset is in young adulthood. Most cases are sporadic; however, it may occur in multiple endocrine neoplasia (MEN) syndrome type 1. Insulinoma is classically suspected by *Whipple's triad*, described as symptoms associated with fasting or exercise; the symptoms are associated with hypoglycemia (serum glucose level <50 mg/dL), and the symptoms are relieved by glucose intake or administration.

Hypoglycemic symptoms of insulinoma falls into two main categories: reactive (acute) hypoglycemia and symptoms of prolonged hypoglycemia. Acute hypoglycemic symptoms include nervousness, palpitation, trembling, and weakness. Symptoms of prolonged hypoglycemia, on the other hand, include disturbances in consciousness, headache, visual disturbance, convulsions, and behavioral disturbances. The behavioral disturbances include manic episodes, personality change, negativism, and severe depression that may cause the patient to seek psychiatric help. Characteristically, the acute and chronic hypoglycemic symptoms are interspersed with symptom-free periods but tend to increase in frequency and severity. Exercise and fasting usually intensify the symptoms, although the patient is frequently unaware of the relationship. Late morning or early afternoon attacks are common.

Laboratory diagnosis can be confirmed by demonstrating hypoglycemia by measuring fasting blood glucose on three mornings, high levels of serum proinsulin levels, and elevated concentration of serum C-peptide (a peptide that connects alpha and beta chains of proinsulin). Ultrasound and MRI represents the first radiological approach for insulinoma detection. CT and angiography should be reserved for negative and/or doubtful cases.

9. *Congenital hyperinsulinism (persistent hyperinsulinemic hypoglycemia of infancy)*: this is a rare disorder characterized by excessive, glucose-independent insulin secretion in the neonatal period, causing severe attacks of recurrent hypoglycemia. Congenital hyperinsulinemia (CHI) is formerly known as *nesidioblastosis*, and it has an annual incidence of 1/30,000 live births.

There are two forms of CHI: focal and diffuse. Focal CHI is characterized by the presence of small endocrine lesion in the pancreas composed of hyperplastic but apparently normal islets of Langerhans. This lesion should not be confused with insulinoma, because the cells are hyperplastic not neoplastic. In contrast, diffuse CHI is characterized by diffuse proliferation of hyperplastic islets within the pancreas.

Symptoms are nonspecific and include feeding problems, irritability, and lethargy; if the condition is not treated properly or the diagnosis is delayed, permanent brain damage and atrophy may result. Laboratory investigations typically show hypoglycemia, hyperinsulinemia, hypoketosis, and hypofatty acidemia. The hypoglycemia is persistent and recurrent. Hypertrophic cardiomyopathy and gastroesophageal reflux are common in patients with CHI for unknown cause. Diagnosis of CHI can be further confirmed by $^{18}$F-fluorodopa PET scan. Surgery is reserved for medically uncontrolled hypoglycemia and involves local excision in focal CHI or subtotal pancreatectomy in diffuse CHI.

## Differential Diagnoses and Related Diseases

1. *Doege-Potter syndrome*: this is a term used to describe recurrent attacks of hypoglycemia in a patient with malignant solitary fibrous tumor due to secretion of insulin-like growth factor 2 by the tumor cells. Solitary fibrous tumor (SFT) is a relatively rare tumor that arises typically from the pleura and the upper respiratory tract. The tumor is locally aggressive, usually is > 8 cm in size, and with a broad base of attachment to the pleura. Distant metastases may be seen. Patients with SFT usually present with chest pain, shortness of breath, hemoptysis, and attacks of hypoglycemia with nervousness and irrational behavior. The hypoglycemia associated with SFT is seen in < 5 % of cases and is attributed to the secretion of insulin-like growth factor 2 (IGF-2). IGF-2 is a peptide hormone primarily made in the liver, while insulin is synthesized as a prohormone from beta cells in the pancreas. IGF circulate at nanomolar concentrations bound to IGF binding proteins, which are also manufactured by the liver. Free IGFs constitute up to 1 % of the circulating pool and have a half-life of approx. 10 min. Some tumors, like SFT, produce excessive amount of a prohormone form of IGF-2 often referred to as "Big IGF-2." Big IGF-2 causes hypoglycemia mainly by transporting glucose into muscles, inhibiting gluconeogenesis in the liver and lipolysis in adipose tissues. The optimal time to detect high serum levels of IGF-2 is during the hypoglycemic attack.
2. *Somogyi effect*: it is a condition characterized by nocturnal hypoglycemia that is followed by morning hyperglycemia due to counter-regulatory hormonal response. Somogyi effect arises due to high insulin or oral hypoglycemic medications therapy. It is diagnosed by detecting hypoglycemia mainly 2 to 3 a.m. in the morning in a patient on diabetes medications.

enhance in a lesser degree, causing the tumor to appear less enhanced against an enhanced tissue background. However, chronic pancreatitis fibrosis and pseudotumor lesions of the pancreas may also show low signal intensity, so interpretation with clinical data is essential to establish the correct diagnosis.

3. Brain MRI in children with neurological deficits or abnormalities due to hypoglycemia typically show bilateral hyperintense signal intensity lesions seen on T2W, FLAIR, and DW images in the parieto-occipital region, known as *hypoglycemia–occipital syndrome* (◘ Fig. 10.9.2). Central pontine myelinolysis, delayed myelination, leukomalacia, and ulegyria are also reported to occur in diabetics and children with congenital hyperinsulinemia.

4. Solitary fibrous tumor is detected on chest CT as a dense lobulated mass with homogenous contrast enhancement due to its rich vascular supply (◘ Fig. 10.9.3). The mass is typically attached to the pleura. Large masses may show areas of necrosis and inhomogeneous enhancement.

5. PET/CT scan with $^{18}$F-fluorodopa is used to detect the hyperplastic islets in congenital hyperinsulinemia. The sensitivity of $^{18}$F-fluorodopa PET in diagnosing focal CHI is 92 % with specificity of 100 %.

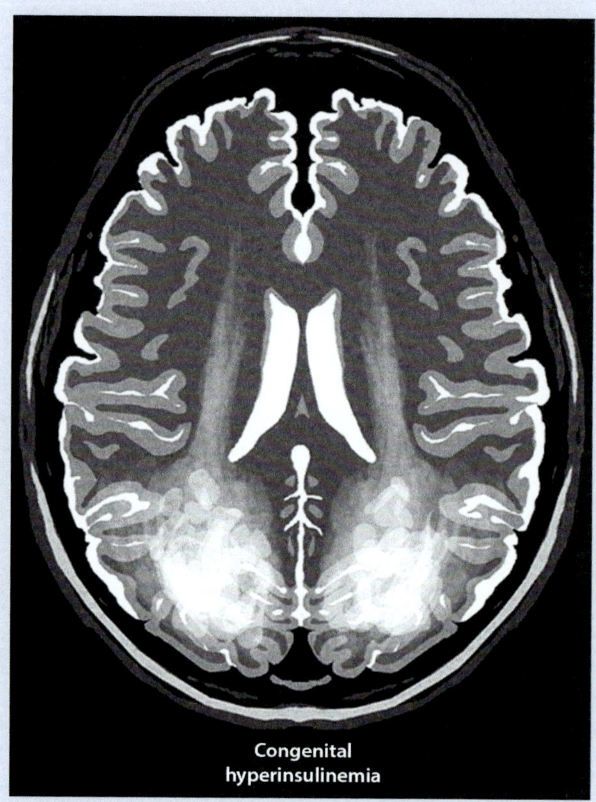


◘ **Fig. 10.9.2**   Axial, T2W-MR illustration that demonstrates the MR findings of patients with hypoglycemia–occipital syndrome

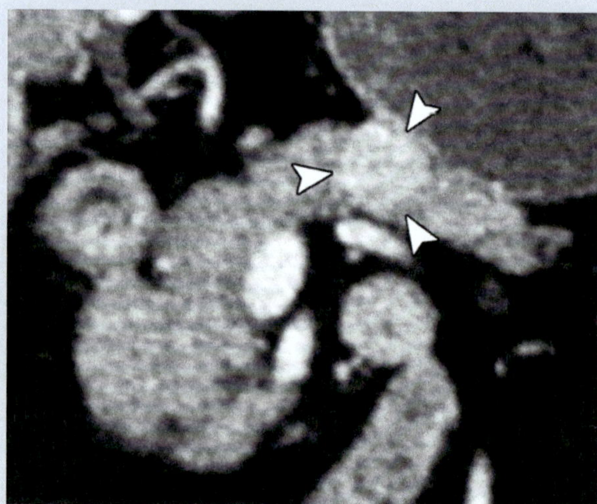

◘ **Fig. 10.9.1**   Coronal CT, arterial postcontrast image that shows insulinoma detected as a highly enhanced tumor in the body of the pancreas (*arrowheads*)

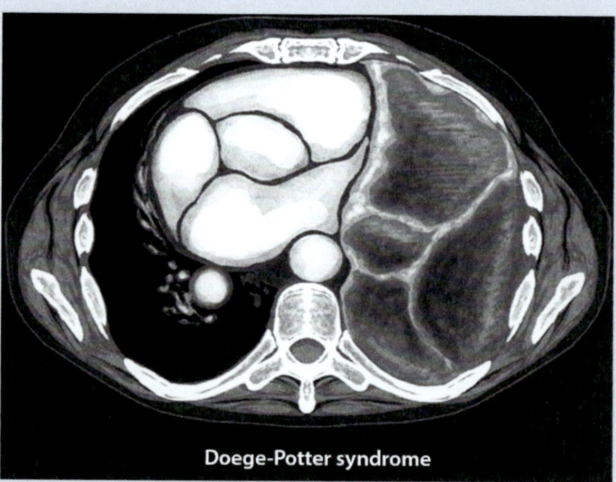


◘ **Fig. 10.9.3**   Axial, postcontrast CT illustration that demonstrates the CT findings of patients with solitary fibrous tumor

## Selected References

Aliefendioglu D, et al. Long-term MRI findings of a case with persistent hyperinsulinemic hypoglycemia of infancy (nesidioblastosis). Eur J Radiol Extra. 2006;60:79–84.

Bertolotto M, et al. Ultrasonography of the pancreas. 3. Doppler imaging. Abdom Imaging. 2007;32:161–70.

Chamberlain MH, et al. Solitary fibrous tumor associated with hypoglycemia: an example of the Doege-Potter syndrome. J Thorac Cardiovasc Surg. 2000;119:185–7.

Das CJ, et al. MR imaging appearance of insulinoma in an infant. Pediatr Radiol. 2007;37:581–3.

De Visschere PJL, et al. Brain injury due to persistent hyperinsulinemic hypoglycemia of infancy. Eur J Radiol Extra. 2007;62:35–8.

Eser G, et al. Mangafodipir trisodium-enhanced magnetic resonance imaging for evaluation of pancreatic mass and mass-like lesions. World J Gastroeneterol. 2006;12(10):1603–6.

Hamoud AK. Mangan-enhanced MR, imaging for the detection and localization of small pancreatic tumors. Eur Radiol. 2004;14:923–5.

Hardy OT, et al. Diagnosis and localization of focal congenital hyperinsulinism by [18]F-fluorodopa PET scan. J Pediatr. 2007;150:140–5.

Hassan K. Congenital hyperinsulinism. Semin Fetal Neonatal Med. 2005;10:369–76.

Noone TC, et al. Imaging and localization of islet-cell tumors of the pancreas on CT and MRI. Best Pract Res Clin Endocrinol Metab. 2005;19(2):195–211.

Otonkoski T, et al. Physical exercise-induced hyperinsulinemic hypoglycemia is an autosomal-dominant trait characterized by abnormal pyruvate-induced insulin release. Diabetes. 2003;52:199–204.

Pakhetra R, et al. Insulinoma: reversal of brain magnetic resonance imaging changes following resection. Neurol India. 2008;56(2):192–4.

Rieber A, et al. MRI with mangafodipir trisodium in the detection of pancreatic tumors: comparison with helical CT. Br J Radiol. 2000;73:1165–9.

Sempoux C, et al. Focal and diffuse forms of congenital hyperinsulinism: the key for differential diagnosis. Endocr Pathol. 2004;15(3):241–6.

Tamm EP, et al. Imaging of neuroendocrine tumors. Hematol Oncol Clin North AM. 2007;1:409–32.

Uchigata Y, et al. Insulin autoimmune syndrome (Hirata disease): clinical features and epidemiology in Japan. Diabetes Res Clin Pract. 1994;22:89–94.

Uchigata Y, et al. Worldwide difference in the incidence of insulin autoimmune syndrome (Hirata disease) with respect to the evolution of HLA-DR4 Alleles. Hum Immunol. 2000;61:154–7.

Uchigata Y, et al. Drug-induced insulin autoimmune syndrome. Diabetes Res Clin Pract. 2009;83:e19–20.

Wagner S, et al. Retroperitoneal malignant solitary fibrous tumor of the small pelvis causing recurrent hypoglycemia by secretion of insulin-like growth factor 2. Eur Urol. 2009;55:739–42.

Wang C, et al. Sequence optimization in Mangafodipir trisodium-enhanced liver and pancreas MRI. J Mag Reson Imaging. 1999;9:280–4.

Zafar H, et al. Doege-Potter syndrome. Hypoglycemia associated with malignant solitary fibrous tumor. Med Oncol. 2003;20(4):403–7.

# Infectious Diseases and Tropical Medicine



© Springer International Publishing Switzerland 2017
J.A. Al-Tubaikh, *Internal Medicine*, DOI 10.1007/978-3-319-39747-4_11

## 11.1 Fever

Fever is a condition characterized by elevation of body temperature above the normal daily variation, along with an increase at the hypothalamic thermal set point. A substance that induces fever is called a pyrogen.

Some infections produce exogenous toxins that induce the synthesis of endogenous pyrogenic cytokines such as interleukin-1, interleukin-6, and tumor necrosis factor. These endogenous pyrogens induce the synthesis of prostaglandin $E_2$ ($PGE_2$), which elevates the hypothalamic core temperature set point. When the hypothalamic set point is raised, vasoconstriction occurs, decreasing heat loss from the skin.

Fever can be caused by infections (e.g., abscess and septicemia), neoplasms (e.g., lymphoma), inflammatory diseases (e.g., collagen vascular disease), and other causes (e.g., Kawasaki syndrome).

*Pyrexia of unknown origin (PUO)* is defined as an illness of more than 3 weeks' duration, fever >38.3 °C on three occasions, and necessary initial investigations that fail to reveal the cause of the fever. The necessary initial investigations include detailed history and physical examination, complete blood count, antinuclear antibodies, rheumatic factor, urinalysis, three blood cultures, urine culture, chest radiograph, abdominal sonography, and tuberculin skin test. In 25–35 % of PUO patients, a diagnosis cannot be made.

*Central fever* is a term used to describe fever that arises after intracerebral hemorrhage, in the absence of infection, inflammation, or a tumor explaining the fever. This fever has been attributed to cytokine-related elevation of the hypothalamic set point.

**Signs on CT and MRI**
In patients with suspected central fever, the examination classically shows bleeding into the thalamus and the hypothalamus (◘ Fig. 11.1.1).

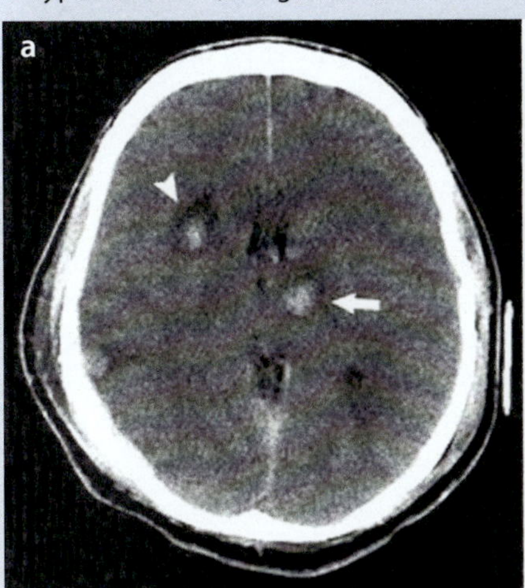
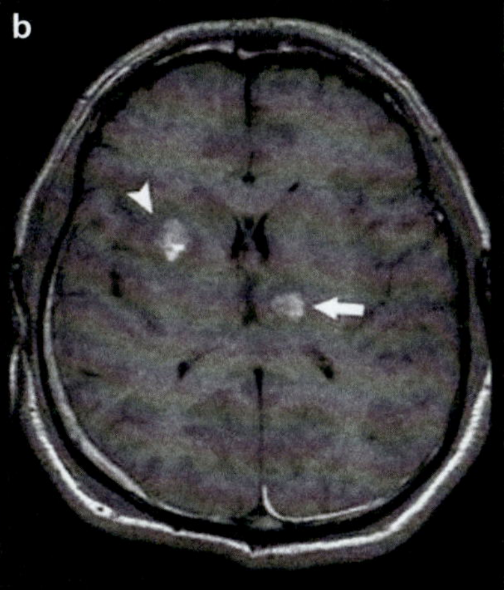
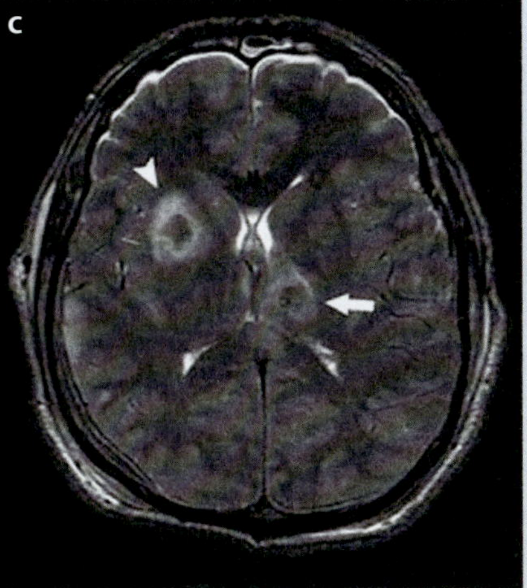

◘ **Fig. 11.1.1**  Axial CT (**a**), MR-T1W (**b**), and MR-T2W (**c**) images of a 26-year-old patient with intracranial bleeding after a car accident show multiple foci of intracranial bleeding. The patient developed high-grade fever, with no signs of infection detected in the serum or the cerebrospinal fluid. The scans showed focal intracranial hemorrhage involving the right lentiform nucleus (*arrowhead*) and the left thalamus (*arrow*). The patient was finally diagnosed as having central fever and was managed accordingly

*What is the difference between fever and hyperthermia?*
- Hyperthermia is a condition characterized by uncontrolled increase in body temperature that exceeds the body's ability to lose heat, in conjunction with a normal hypothalamic thermal set point.
- Hyperthermia does not involve pyrogens and does not respond to antipyretics.

### Further Reading

Chantal PBR, et al. Fever. Medicine. 2009a;37(1):28–34.
Chantal PBR, et al. Pyrexia of unknown origin. Medicine. 2005;33(3):33–6.
Deogaonkar A, et al. Fever is associated with third ventricle shift after intracerebral hemorrhage: pathophysiological implications. Neurol India. 2005;53(2):202–7.
Rudd P. Pyrexia of unknown origin (PUO). Curr Paediatr. 1996;6:105–7.

## 11.2 Giardiasis

Giardiasis is an infectious disease inducing fatty diarrhea caused by the intestinal protozoa *Giardia lamblia*. Protozoa are single-celled living organisms with two cell layers: an outer layer (ectoplasm) and an inner layer (endoplasm). In cases of environmental changes, the protozoa secrete a protective coat and shrink into a round, armored, infectious form called a "cyst." When humans ingest the cyst, it transforms again into the motile form and is called "trophozoite."

Giardiasis outbreak often occurs after sewage contamination of drinking water or after drinking from clear mountain streams contaminated with *G. lamblia*. After ingestion of the cysts, the parasites transform into trophozoites in the duodenum and jejunum and adhere to the intestinal wall. The parasites coat the duodenal and jejunal walls and interfere with fat absorption from the gut, resulting in fatty diarrhea. The parasites do not invade the intestinal wall, only coat it. The ileum is rarely affected by giardiasis.

Most patients with giardiasis are asymptomatic. Children and patients with low immunity may show mild abdominal discomfort, along with fatty diarrhea resembling celiac sprue or celiac disease diarrhea. Rarely, *G. lamblia* may invade the gallbladder, causing cholecystitis and jaundice. A concomitant infection with *Entamoeba histolytica* may be overlooked in cases of infection by a large number of *G. lamblia*.

There is an increased incidence of giardiasis in patients with hypogammaglobulinemia. Intestinal lymphoid hyperplasia (*Peyer's patches hyperplasia*) may be found in cases of giardiasis infecting a patient with hypogammaglobulinemia. Diagnosis of giardiasis is confirmed by identifying the cysts in the stool.

### *Differential* Diagnoses and Related Diseases

*Gay bowel syndrome*: there is an increased incidence of giardiasis in male homosexuals with diarrhea. Active male homosexuals may show cysts in the stool in up to 20 % of cases.

---

**Signs on Barium Enteroclysis**
As giardiasis mainly affects the duodenum and jejunum, bowel fold thickening, edema, and barium filling defects are usually seen in the duodenum and jejunum.
Occasional barium segmentation or fragmentation may be seen (◘ Fig. 11.2.1).

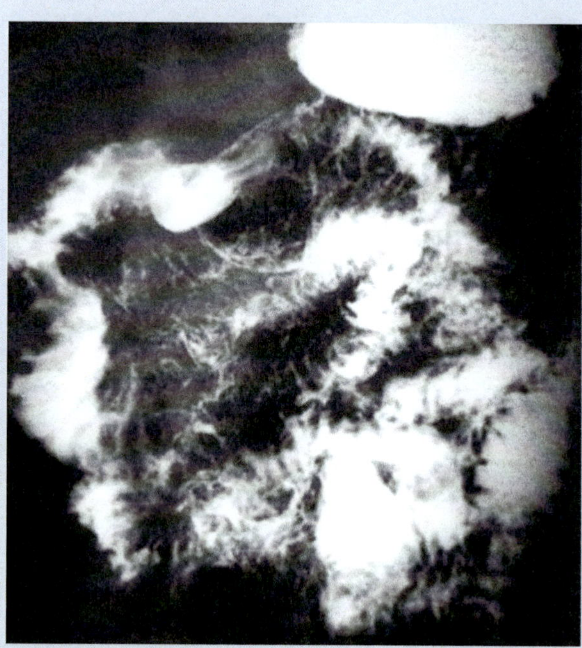

◘ **Fig. 11.2.1**   Barium enteroclysis examination in a patient with giardiasis shows some irregularity and mucosal thickening of the second part of the duodenum. The proximal jejunum loops show edema, irritability, and poor filling, with thickening and separation of mucosal folds

### Further Reading

David BH, et al. An update review on Cryptosporidium and Giardia. Gastroenterol Clin N Am. 2006;35:291–314.

Heymans HSA, et al. Giardiasis in childhood: an unnecessarily expensive diagnosis. Eur J Pediatr. 1987;146:401–3.

Maurice MR. Radiological diagnosis of giardiasis. Semin Roentgenol. 1997;32(4):291–300.

## 11.3 Amebiasis

Amebiasis is a parasitic infectious disease caused by the protozoan *Entamoeba histolytica*. It is the second most common cause of deaths from parasitic diseases after malaria.

Amebiasis is endemic in Mexico, India, Central and South America, and East and South Africa. There is a high incidence of amebiasis among homosexual patients.

The infectious form of the parasite is the "mature cyst," which is resistant to the gastric and gastrointestinal (GI) secretions. The mature cyst can survive harsh environmental conditions and is resistant to the conventional chlorine used to purify drinking water.

Amebiasis is initiated by ingestion of the mature cyst from infected water or food. The disease is often asymptomatic; however, multiple manifestations may be seen throughout the body, including bloody diarrhea in a small percentage of patients. Diagnosis is confirmed by identification of the amebic trophozoites in the stool or by serological identification of ameba-specific antibodies, usually 7 days after the initial symptoms of amebiasis.

## Intestinal Amebiasis

Amebic invasion of the GI tract can result in different manifestations, each with its own radiological imaging features:

- *Ulcerative amebic rectocolitis (ambulatory dysentery)*: in 10 % of children, the trophozoites invade and penetrate the intestinal mucosa, resulting in intestinal erosions and bleeding. This is usually manifested as 4–6 episodes of bloody diarrhea per day without systemic manifestations or fever. Complications of ambulatory dysentery include anemia due to bloody diarrhea, intussusception, and/or rectal prolapse due to high-speed peristalsis.
- *Ameboma*: a granulomatous colonic lesion of ameba, with necrosis, edema, and inflammation, resembling a pseudotumor superimposed by secondary infection. It arises from the cecum or the ascending colon wall, measuring 5–30 cm. Ameboma is often solitary but can be multiple. Patients complain of bloody diarrhea, abdominal pain, and a colonic mass.
- *Amebic appendicitis*: cannot be differentiated from classic appendicitis, unless the patient's history of bloody diarrhea is known.
- *Fulminant colitis with toxic megacolon*: a rapidly progressing disease with up to 20 episodes of bloody diarrhea within 24 h. Patients present with abdominal pain, anorexia, fever, rapid pulse, hypovolemia, and intense, constant tenesmus. There is a high mortality rate, especially when massive thrombosis of the colonic wall venules and intestinal ischemia develop.
- *Chronic amebic colitis*: this term is used to describe patients with chronic, nonspecific abdominal pain with occasional *E. histolytica* evidence in the stool.

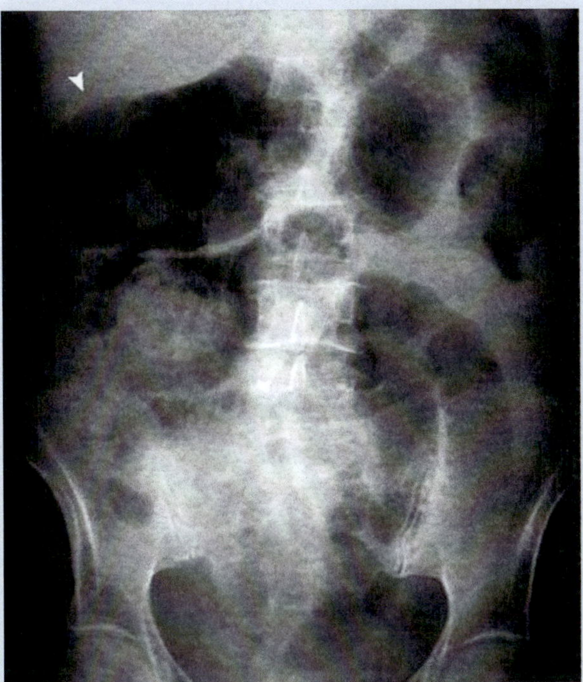

**Fig. 11.3.1** A plain abdominal radiograph of a patient with chronic amebic dysentery shows toxic colonic dilatation of the ascending and the transverse colon (*arrowhead*)

### Signs on Plain Abdominal Radiograph
Abdominal radiograph may show a dilated colon with loss of the haustrations (0.5 % of cases) (**Fig. 11.3.1**).

### Signs on Barium Enema
- *Ulcers*: seen as fine granular appearance of the mucosa with margin speculations. Deep ulcers penetrate the mucosa and result in "collar-button" ulcers.
- *Thumbprinting*: a term used to describe the shape of barium distribution inside the intestinal or colonic lumen due to edema. The barium will show filling defects at the mucosal edges as if a person's thumb has erased the barium from the edges (**Fig. 11.3.2**).
- *Conical cecum*: a term used to describe a rigid, ulcerated, and conical-shaped cecum. Conical cecum is often seen in intestinal tuberculosis, Crohn's disease, and amebiasis, because the cecum is affected in 90 % of cases (**Fig. 11.3.3**).
- *Ameboma*: seen as barium filling defect that resembles a carcinoma.

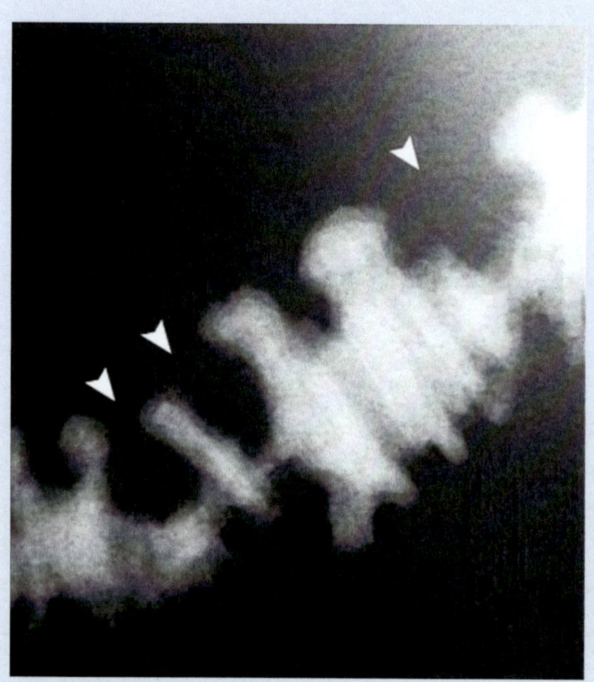

**Fig. 11.3.2** Intestinal barium CGI shows thumbprinting appearance (*arrowheads*)

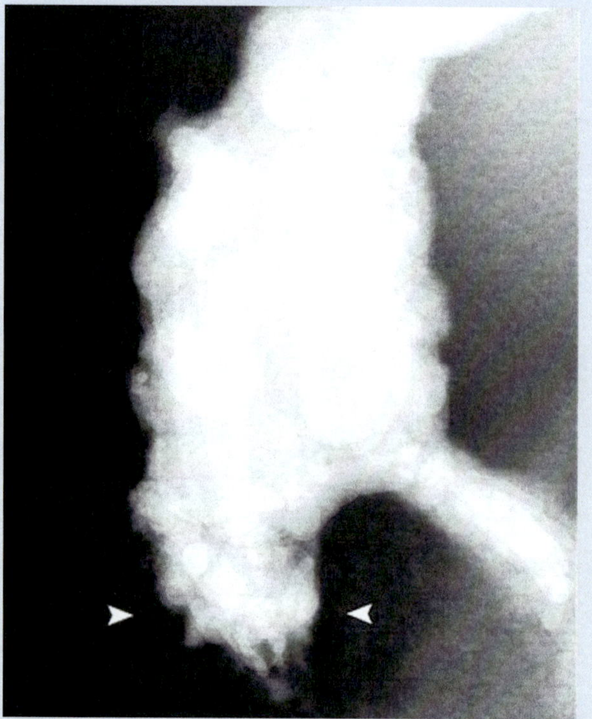

**Fig. 11.3.3** Intestinal barium CGI shows the classical appearance of conical cecum (*arrowheads*)

### Signs on CT

Colitis is seen as marked irregular thickening of the colonic wall, with enhancement after contrast administration.

## Hepatic Amebiasis

Occasionally, the amebic trophozoites can reach the liver via the portal system and form an abscess (30 % of cases). GI invasion is often seen in children, with a mortality rate of 1 %, while the formation of liver abscess is often seen in adults, with a mortality rate of 0.2–2 %.

Hepatic abscess may not be preceded by a history of diarrhea (59 % of cases). Patients often present with sudden onset of right hypochondriac pain radiating to the shoulder or the subscapular area. There is associated fever, anorexia, and vomiting, and the pain is exacerbated by deep inspiration or sitting in the right lateral decubitus position. The abscess is often seen in the right lobe of the liver. Differentiation between amebic and pyogenic hepatic abscess is important for proper patient management.

### Signs on Plain Chest Radiograph

Hepatic abscess may often reveal itself in the form of a raised right hemidiaphragm (■ Fig. 11.3.4).

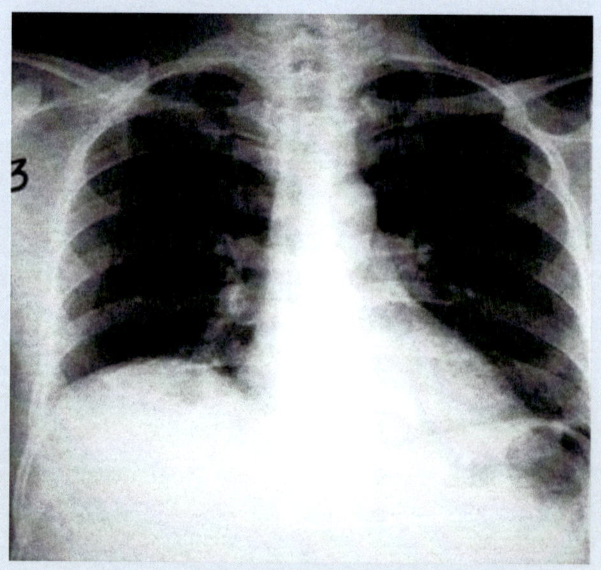


**Fig. 11.3.4** A plain chest radiograph shows a raised right diaphragm due to hepatic abscess

### Signs on US

Abscesses are seen as masses of heterogeneous echogenicity, with irregular wall and poor peripheral definition. Internal fluid-fluid level might be seen.

### Signs on CT

Hepatic abscesses can be either *pyogenic* (bacterial) or *amebic* (parasitic) in origin. It is often difficult to differentiate between amebic and pyogenic liver abscesses based on CT appearance alone, but some radiological clues may be of use:

- *Pyogenic abscess* can present without any signs of infection and shows uniform ring enhancement after contrast injection, air fluid level may be seen inside the abscess, and it shows microabscesses (satellite lesions), which are occasionally seen as hypodense lesions >2 cm around the main abscess. A pyogenic abscess classically reveals yellowish fluid after aspiration.
- *Amebic abscess* characteristically shows a halo of hypodensity surrounding the enhanced ring of the abscess, due to peripheral edema (◘ Fig. 11.3.5). After aspiration, an amebic abscess classically reveals brown fluid (*anchovy sauce appearance*), although it may be a pyogenic abscess mixed with hemorrhage from the needle. An acute amebic abscess can transform into a chronic abscess, which is characterized by fibrosis and hard mass formation that can be mistaken for hepatocellular carcinoma.

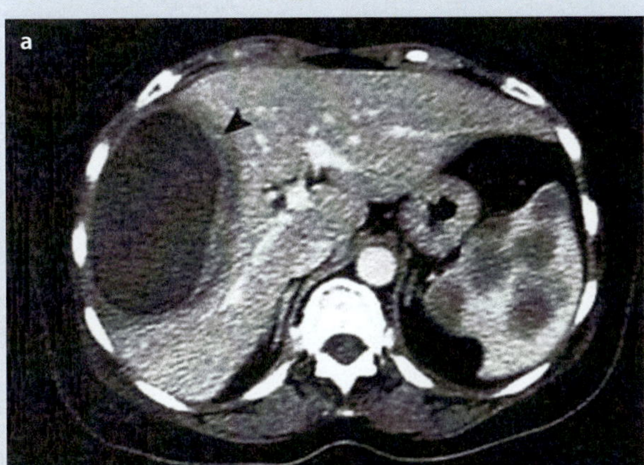

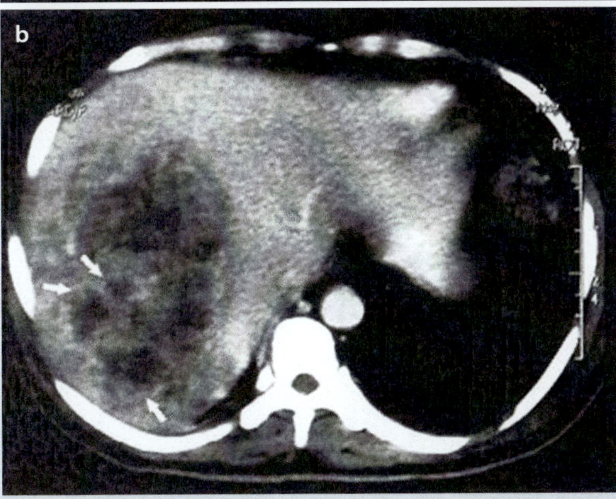

◘ **Fig. 11.3.5**  Axial hepatic postcontrast-enhanced CT images in two different patients with hepatic abscesses. In one patient (**a**), an amebic liver abscess is illustrated with its characteristic halo (*arrowhead*). Notice the multiple splenic microabscesses. In the other patient (**b**), a pyogenic liver abscess is demonstrated for comparison. Notice the lack of the surrounding halo, with the presence of multiple small satellite lesions (*arrows*)

## Differential Diagnoses and Related Diseases

*Meleney's synergistic gangrene* is a rare complication of progressive postoperative gangrene, which arises after empyema or intraperitoneal abscess drainage. This complication can arise due to *Staphylococcus aureus* infection or cutaneous amebiasis. Patients often present 10–14 days post empyema or intraperitoneal abscess drainage, with truncal ulcer and severe pain. Pathologically, the ulcer is sharply demarcated, with three zones of colors: an outer bright red zone, an inner raised purple zone, and a central zone of red granulation tissue obscured by yellowish exudates.

## Thoracic Amebiasis

Amebiasis from liver abscess may extend to the right lower lung lobes via invading the diaphragm. This rare complication is often seen in adults. Thoracic amebiasis is almost always secondary to amebic hepatic abscess. Empyema, pericarditis, and mediastinitis may occur due to amebic extension into the thoracic structures.

> **Signs on Plain Chest Radiograph**
> Chest radiograph often shows a raised right hemidiaphragm along with right basal pleural effusion, pneumonic patch, or atelectasis.

## Brain Amebiasis

Brain amebiasis is a rare complication seen in 1 % of patients with amebic dysentery. The parasites often reach the brain via the hematogenous route. Patients often present with convulsions, hemiplegia, meningitis, or cranial nerve lesions.

> **Signs on Brain CT**
> Amebic abscess is seen as a nonspecific parenchymal hypodense area with peripheral, uniform ring enhancement.

## Further Reading

Avron B, et al. Biochemistry of Entamoeba: a review. Cell Biochem Funct. 1988;6:71–86.

Cade D, et al. Amoebic perforation of the intestine in children. Br J Surg. 1974;61:159–61.

Davson J, et al. Diagnosis of Meleney's synergistic gangrene. Br J Surg. 1988;75:267–71.

Kimura K, et al. Amebiasis: modern diagnostic imaging with pathological and clinical correlation. Semin Roentgenol. 1997;32(4):250–75.

Yin LS, et al. Left lobe amoebic liver abscess mimicking a perforated gastric tumor. Eur J Radiol Extra. 2008;66:e25–7.

## 11.4  Leprosy (Hansen Disease)

Leprosy is a chronic, granulomatous, infectious disease that mainly affects the skin and the peripheral nerves and is caused by acid- and alcohol-fast bacilli *Mycobacterium leprae* (*M. leprae*).

*Leprosy* is divided into different clinical subtypes based on the capacity of the patient's immune system to resist the disease:

- *Indeterminate leprosy*: the initial form that either resolves spontaneously or progresses into the other forms according to the degree of cell-mediated immunity.
- *Tuberculoid leprosy* (*TL*): a form of leprosy that results from strong cell-mediated immune response to the disease. This type is characterized by the formation of multiple skin and nerve granulomas (tubercles), often restricted to a few locations. The granulomatous reaction in TL mimics tuberculosis but is non-caseating.
- *Borderline leprosy*: this form represents an intermediate state between the tuberculoid and the lepromatous forms of leprosy.
- *Lepromatous leprosy* (*LL*): this form results from low immunity of the infected host, resulting in widespread, extensive disease damage. The granulomatous reaction in LL is characterized by the formation of "lepromas," which are granuloma formations mediated by macrophages engulfing live bacteria (lepra cells).

The clinical features of leprosy are determined by the host response to *M. leprae*. Skin, nerves, eyes, mucosa, and bone may all be affected by leprosy. Laboratory results often show high erythrocyte sedimentation rate and increased finding of rheumatoid factor in LL (rheumatoid factor is positive in 58 % of cases).

Diagnosis of leprosy is established via clinical examination and identification of the acid- and alcohol-fast bacilli on skin or buccal mucosa smears stained by the Ziehl–Neelsen technique. Clinical diagnostic features of leprosy include skin lesions with definite sensory loss and thickened peripheral nerves.

### Skin Involvement

In TL, the early skin manifestation is hypopigmented macules or plaques. A macule is a localized area with textural or color change of the skin, while a plaque is a palpable, plateau-like elevation of skin >2 cm in size. TL is characterized by few skin lesions, which are often dry, scaly, and hairless.

In LL, widespread symmetrically distributed macules are often seen as early skin changes. The macules are poorly defined and show erythema (redness due to vascular dilatation). If the macules are untreated, dermal infiltration occurs, which causes skin thickening. When skin thickness occurs in

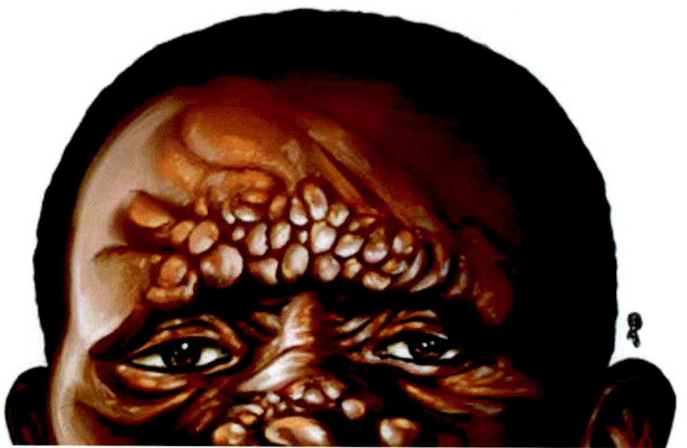

**Fig. 11.4.1**  Forehead skin thickening and plaques (leonine facies) with loss of the eyebrows (madarosis)

the face, it is called *leonine facies* (Fig. 11.4.1). The eyebrows and the eyelashes may be lost (*madarosis*). *Leprous alopecia* is characterized by scalp hair loss with preservation of the hair over the course of scalp arteries. Dystrophic nail changes, with development of peripheral edema of the legs and ankles, often occur. *Souza Campos nodule* is a rare form of TL seen in endemic areas of Brazil, where leprosy infection may infect patients during a kiss, and the highly resistant child develops a nodule at the site of the inoculation. *Lucio phenomenon* is a very rare reactional state of LL characterized by painful irregular skin patches that become purpuric and form bullae that break down, leaving widespread areas of ulceration. Healing is with scar formation. Lucio phenomenon arises due to cutaneous vasculitis.

### Nerve Involvement

Nerve involvement in leprosy affects sensory, motor, and autonomic peripheral nerves. The posterior tibial nerve is mostly affected, resulting in anesthesia of the soles and feet. Involvement of the peripheral autonomic fibers results in loss of skin sweating, with glove-and-stocking hypohidrosis, a situation similar to the changes seen in diabetic peripheral neuropathy. Loss of peripheral joint sensation causes repetitive trauma and osteomyelitis, later resulting in the development of Charcot's joint. Motor denervation of the hand causes progressive hand contracture deformity, known as "claw hand" (Fig. 11.4.2).

### Eye Involvement

Blindness may occur in up to 5.3 % of patients with leprosy, due to an inability to close the eyes normally (*lagophthalmos*), corneal ulceration, secondary cataract, and chronic iridocyclitis.

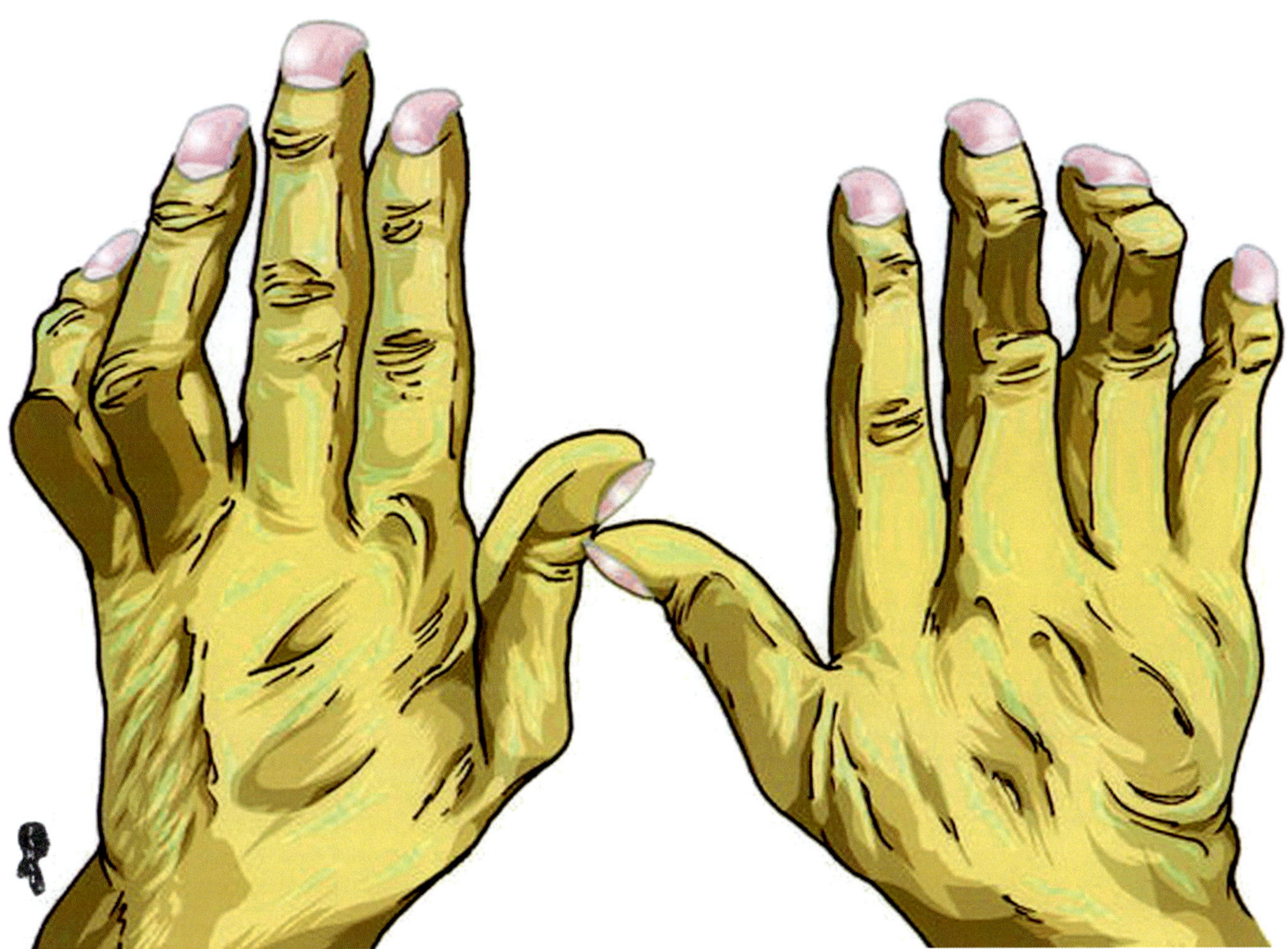

■ Fig. 11.4.2    Bilateral claw-hand deformities of leprosy

## Mucosal Involvement

Both the nasal and the oral mucosa may be affected by LL. Nasal mucosa involvement results in sneezing blood (epistaxis) due to ulceration and nasal stuffiness due to formation of polyps.

The oral mucosa is affected in TL and LL patients, who are often neglected and who receive delayed treatment. Oral mucosal lesions in LL include yellowish-white plaques, nodular infiltration of the tonsils, deep ulceration of the soft palate, and elongation of the uvula (■ Fig. 11.4.3).

## Bone Involvement

Bone involvement in leprosy may be seen due to reactional state arthritis (explained later), development of Charcot's joint due to peripheral neuropathy, osteomyelitis, or due to destruction of facial bones by leprosy. In osteomyelitis, the bacteria directly invade the articular bone and its bone marrow, causing infection and destruction of the joint. Up to 80 % of bone changes in leprosy are seen in the hands and feet.

*Facies leprosa* describes a triad of facial skull lesions that has been used by paleopathologists as a reliable marker for leprosy in ancient skeletal remains. The triad includes atrophy of the anterior nasal spine, atrophy and recession of the alveolar processes of the maxillae, and endonasal inflammatory changes (■ Fig. 11.4.4).

## Post-therapy Leprosy

When therapy is started to eliminate *M. leprae*, a cell-mediated autoimmunity may result which starts to fight both the bacteria and the normal cells, known as *reactional states*. Reactional states may also occur spontaneously, without treatment. The eyes, skin, nerves, and ears become swollen and painful. Reactional states are mainly divided into two types:

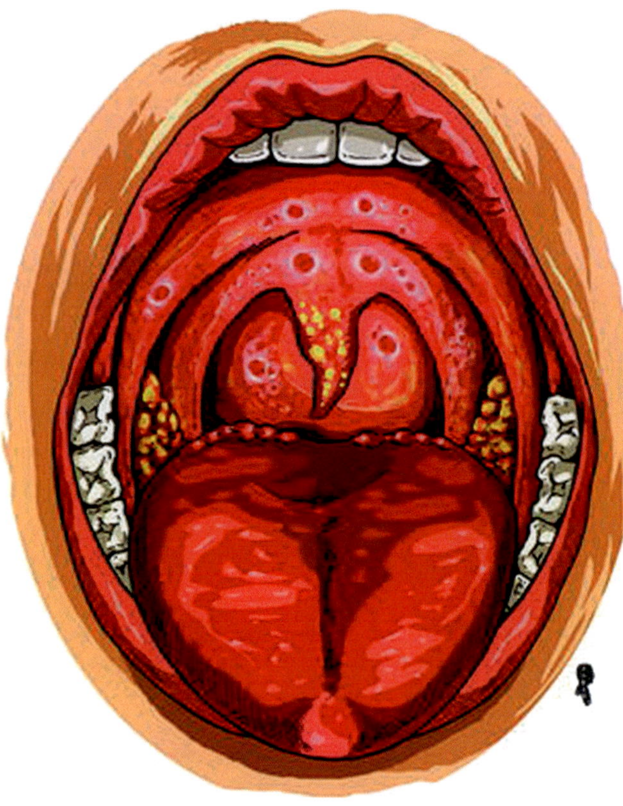



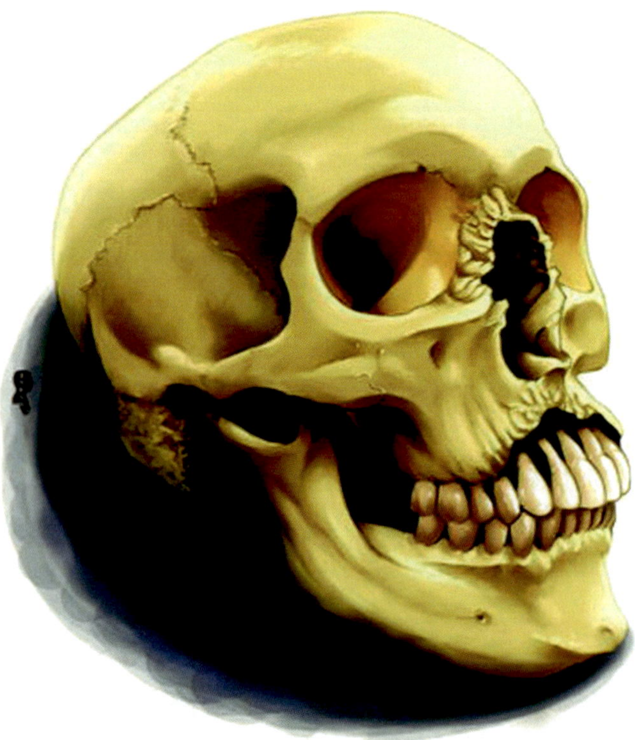

Fig. 11.4.4   Bony changes of facies leprosa. Notice the destruction of the nasal spine and the recession of the alveolar processes of the maxillae

— *Type 1 (reversal) reaction:* this type of reaction is seen in patients with BL (30 % of cases) and is characterized by skin and nerve inflammation, edema, and ulceration.
— *Type 2 reaction (erythema nodosum leprosum):* this type of reaction is seen mainly in LL (20 %) and TL (10 %). Symmetrical joint arthritis that involves small or large joints is a characteristic feature of patients with erythema nodosum leprosum (ENL). The arthritis can be monoarticular, oligoarticular, or polyarticular. The arthritis can be infective or sterile (reactive) arthritis. Reactive arthritis in leprosy has almost the typical clinical presentation as rheumatoid arthritis. In general, the severity of the arthritis parallels the severity of the ENL.

**Signs on Radiographs**
— In joint osteomyelitis, there is destruction of the juxta-articular bone, with joint collapse (■ Fig. 11.4.6).
— Diffuse osteoporosis.
— Joint destruction due to neuropathic arthropathy (Charcot's joint) (■ Fig. 11.4.5).
— The phalanges often show thinning of the bone with reduction in thickness, a finding that is usually called "sucked lollipop appearance" (■ Fig. 11.4.6).
— *Osteitis leprosum* are localized cortical bone erosions of the phalanges and metacarpals.
— Acroosteolysis (bone resorption) of the terminal phalangeal tufts (■ Fig. 11.4.6).
— Contracture of the hands, with soft-tissue swelling (claw-hand deformity).

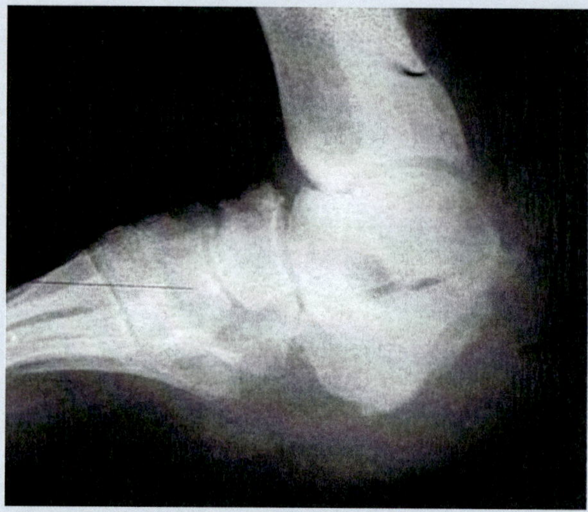

Fig. 11.4.5   A lateral ankle radiograph of a patient with leprosy shows severe calcaneus destruction

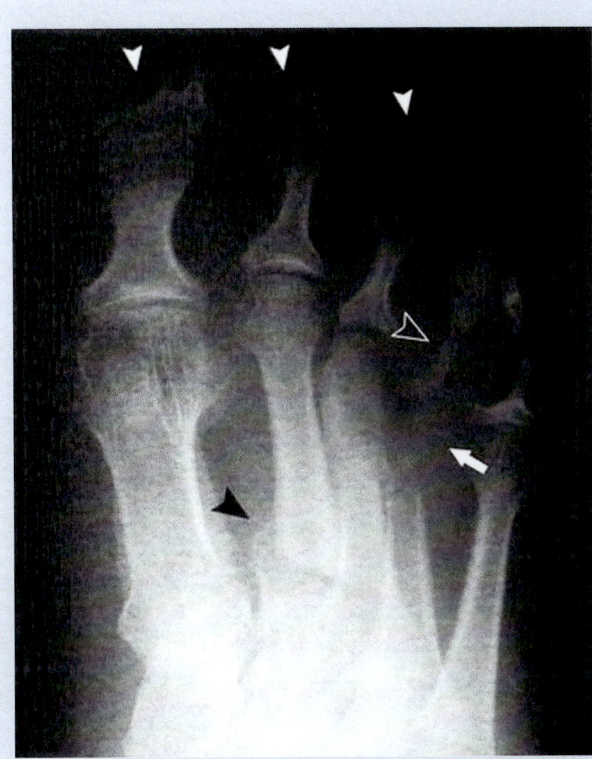



**◘ Fig. 11.4.6**  An anteroposterior radiograph of the forefoot of the other foot of the same patient shows acroosteolysis of the distal phalanges (*white arrowheads*), fracture of the second metatarsal diaphysis (*black arrowhead*), sucked lollipop appearance of the fourth phalange (*open arrowhead*), and cortical destruction of the fourth metatarsal head due to osteomyelitis (*arrow*)

## Further Reading


Boddingius J. Ultrastructural and histopathological studies on the blood-nerve barrier and perineural barrier in leprosy neuropathy. Acta Neuropathol. 1984;64:282–96.

David MS, et al. Oropharyngeal leprosy in art, history, and medicine. Oral Surg Oral Med Oral Pathol Oral Radiol Endod. 1999;87:463–70.

de Abreu MAMM, et al. The oral mucosa in paucibacillary leprosy: a clinical and histopathological study. Oral Surg Oral Med Oral Pathol Oral Radiol Endod. 2007;103:e48–52.

Gibson T. Bacterial infections: the arthritis of leprosy. Baillière's Clin Rheumatol. 1995;9(1):179–91.

Lupi O, et al. Tropical dermatology: bacterial tropical diseases. J Am Acad Dermatol. 2006a;54:559–78.

Paira SO, et al. The rheumatic manifestations of leprosy. Clin Rheumatol. 1991;10(3):274–6.

Rostom S, et al. Neurogenic osteoarthropathy in leprosy. Clin Rheumatol. 2007;26:2153–5.

Walker SL, et al. Leprosy. Clin Dermatol. 2007;25:165–72.


## 11.5  Toxoplasmosis

Toxoplasmosis is an opportunistic, protozoan infection of humans by *Toxoplasma gondii*. The name of the parasite is derived from the Greek word "toxon" meaning bow (the shape of the parasite) and "gondi," which is a local name for a desert rodent in North America that hosts this parasite.

The life cycle of *T. gondii* occurs commonly between cats and mice. The cat (definite host) harbors the parasite in its intestinal mucosa, where sexual reproduction occurs to produce the oocysts. The oocysts are passed through the cat feces into the soil. The oocysts mature into the infective form within the soil, depending on the temperature and other conditions. In the mouse, the sporozoites invade the intestinal mucosa and are distributed via the blood and lymphatics through the body. The cycle is completed when the cat ingests a mouse infected with the parasite.

Humans get *T. gondii* incidentally, as intermediate hosts, by ingestion of the oocyst in uncooked meat (pork mutton) or food contaminated with household cat feces. The transplacental route of infection from mother to fetus is also a common method of toxoplasmosis infection. Ingestion of uncooked meat is an important route of transmission worldwide. Cooking meats at high temperatures (>66 °C) or freezing the meat for 1 day is sufficient to kill the parasite. Fast food that is improperly grilled or barbecued may still be infective, as the parasite is not killed.

Pregnant women should avoid cats, as *toxoplasmosis* infection is one of the known infections that can pass through the placenta from the mother to her fetus, along with other infections, such as rubella, cytomegalovirus, and herpes simplex virus (collectively called the TORCH complex). Infection of the mother before pregnancy rarely results in the birth of a congenitally infected child. Half the women who are infected with *T. gondii* during pregnancy do not transmit the parasite to their fetus. Fetal infection commonly occurs in the third trimester. The effect on the fetus is more significant when transmission occurs in the first trimester. Diagnosis is confirmed by serological detection of *T. gondii* antibodies in the amniotic fluid.

Multiple manifestations are noticed in patients infected with toxoplasmosis, depending on host immunity. In immunocompetent patients, fever, hepatosplenomegaly, enlarged lymph nodes, and headache may be seen. In contrast, immunocompromised patients show more extensive clinical symptoms that include lymphadenitis, fever, myocarditis, rash, meningitis, pneumonia, and encephalitis (50 % of cases). Moreover, fundoscopic examination of the retina often reveals yellowish, cotton-like patches within the globe.

In immunocompromised patients, toxoplasmosis can cause rheumatic diseases such as acute myositis that resembles polymyositis or dermatomyositis due to direct infection of the muscles or due to autoimmune reaction affecting the muscles. Other rheumatic manifestations include fever and rheumatic-like arthritis of the small joints, with fever that resembles adult Still's disease and development of vasculitis and (rarely) Raynaud's phenomenon.

### Signs on US

In immunocompromised patients with toxoplasmosis, hepatosplenomegaly with retroperitoneal lymphadenopathy may be detected by ultrasound.

### Signs on Brain CT

- Toxoplasmosis commonly involves the basal ganglia, but other regions may be involved.
- In *congenital toxoplasmosis*, brain CT characteristically shows hydrocephalus, parenchymal atrophy, and multiple scattered parenchymal calcifications often found around the lateral ventricles and the basal ganglia (◘ Fig. 11.5.1). Hydrocephalus almost always arises due to aqueductal stenosis.
- Retinal calcifications may rarely be seen on CT in congenital toxoplasmosis due to retinochoroiditis (pathognomonic sign of ocular toxoplasmosis) (◘ Fig. 11.5.2).
- In immunocompromised patients, solitary or multiple hypodense lesions surrounded by vasogenic edema, with ring contrast enhancement, are often detected (◘ Fig. 11.5.3). Localization of the lesions in the basal ganglia is characteristic.
- *Asymmetric target sign* is a very characteristic sign of toxoplasmosis. There is an enhancing ring abscess that contains a similarly enhancing, eccentrically located nodule (◘ Fig. 11.5.4). It is found in 30 % of cases.
- A ringlike calcification may be seen in unenhanced images of treated toxoplasmosis lesions.
- Toxoplasmosis is often difficult to differentiate from lymphoma. The subcortical location of toxoplasmosis compared with the subependymal location of lymphoma and the involvement of the corpus callosum in lymphoma that is not often seen in toxoplasmosis are helpful differentiating clues. Also, lymphoma is usually hyperdense on nonenhanced CT images, while toxoplasmosis becomes hyperdense on nonenhanced images only when the lesion is hemorrhagic or calcified.

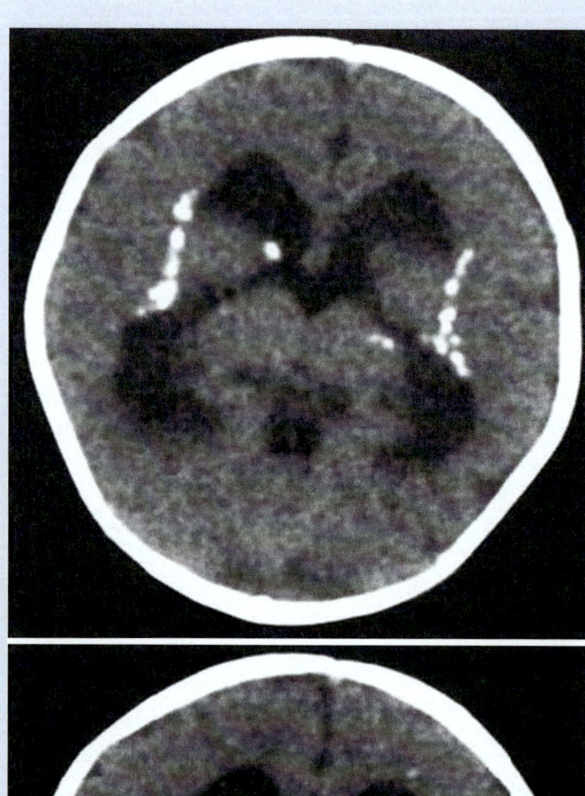
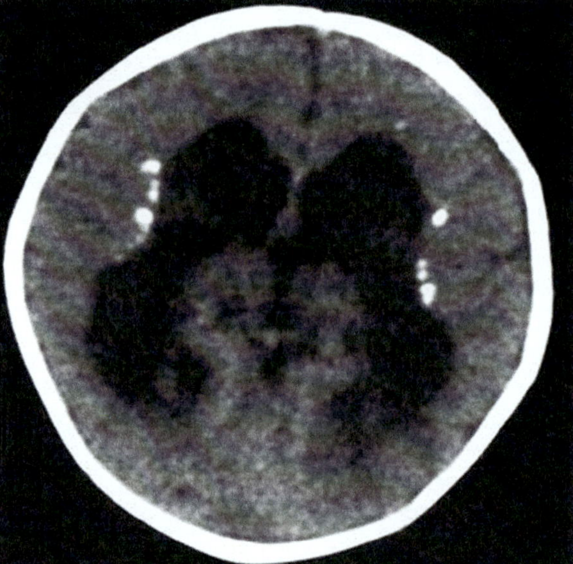

◘ **Fig. 11.5.1**    Axial nonenhanced sequential CT images of a child born with congenital toxoplasmosis show brain parenchymal atrophy, moderate ventricular system dilatation (hydrocephalus), and characteristic calcification along the ventricular edges

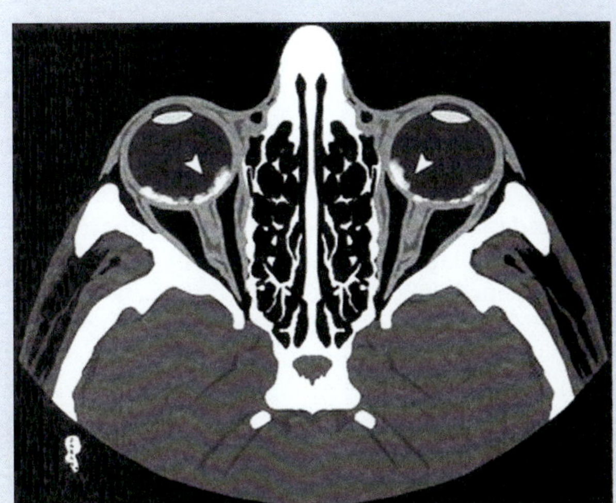

**Fig. 11.5.2** Axial orbital CT illustration shows bilateral retinal calcification as a rare manifestation of toxoplasmosis (*arrowheads*)

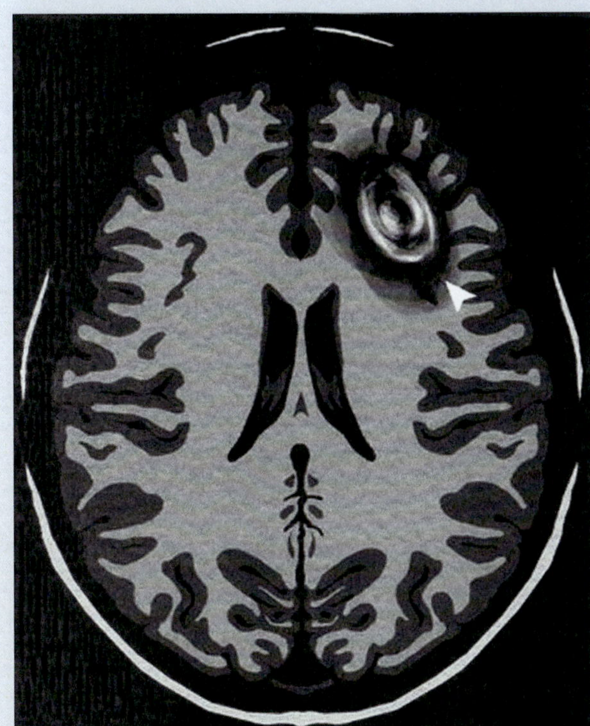

**Fig. 11.5.3** Axial T1W postcontrast MRI shows toxoplasmosis lesion seen in an immunocompromised patient as a rounded lesion with vasogenic edema and ring enhancement (*arrowhead*)

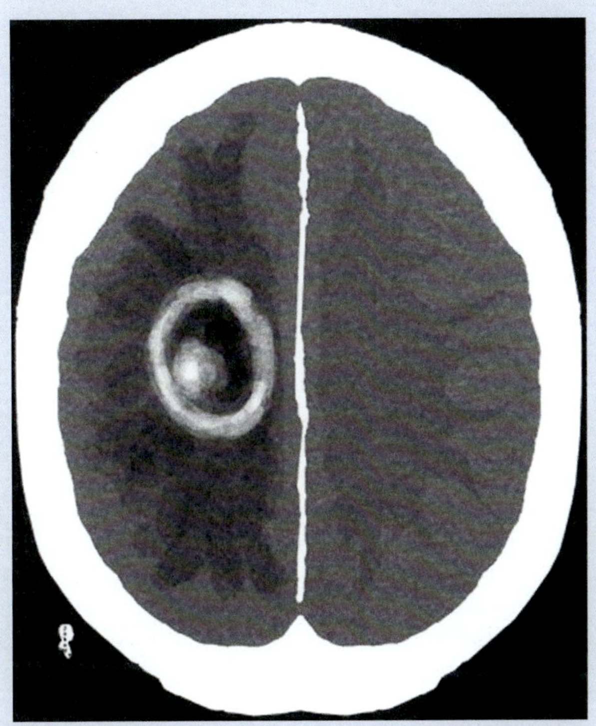

**Fig. 11.5.4** Axial postcontrast brain CT illustration demonstrates toxoplasmosis asymmetric target sign in the right centrum semiovale surrounded by vasogenic edema

## Further Reading

Alappat JP, et al. A case of cerebral toxoplasmosis. Neurol India. 2000;48:185–6.

Diebler C, et al. Congenital toxoplasmosis. Clinical and neuroradiological evaluation of the cerebral lesions. Neuroradiology. 1985;27:125–30.

Dunn IJ, et al. Toxoplasmosis. Semin Roentgenol. 1998a;33(1):81–5.

Mombró M, et al. Congenital toxoplasmosis: assessment of risk to newborns in confirmed and uncertain maternal infection. Eur J Pediatr. 2003;162:703–6.

Navia BA, et al. Cerebral toxoplasmosis complicating the acquired immune deficiency syndrome: clinical and neuropathological findings in 27 patients. Ann Neurol. 1986;19:224–38.

Palm C, et al. Diagnosis of cerebral toxoplasmosis by detection of Toxoplasma gondii tachyzoites in cerebrospinal fluid. J Neurol. 2008;255:939–41.

Peng SL. Rheumatic manifestations of parasitic diseases. Semin Arthritis Rheum. 2002a;31:228–47.

Singh S. Mother-to-child transmission and diagnosis of Toxoplasma gondii infection during pregnancy. Indian J Microbiol. 2003;21(2):69–76.

Surendrababu NRS, et al. Globe calcification in congenital toxoplasmosis. Indian J Pediatr. 2006;73(6):527–8.

Yanagisawa S, et al. Ocular toxoplasmosis in Brazilians living in Japan. Ann Opthalmol. 2002;34(1):54–7.

## 11.6    **Brucellosis (Malta Fever)**

Brucellosis, also known as "Malta fever," is a zoonotic disease caused by intracellular, gram-negative coccobacilli bacterium. Zoonosis is a term used to describe infections that are transmitted to humans from infected animals. The disease is named after the discoverer of the bacterium "David Bruce" in 1887. The name "Malta fever" is derived from the geographic endemic region where the fever is originally described.

Brucellosis is almost always transmitted to humans from infected animals. Different species of the bacteria are identified, and four species are responsible for most human infections: *Brucella melitensis* (found in sheep and goats), *Brucella abortus* (found in cattle), *Brucella suis* (found in swine), and *Brucella canis* (found in dogs). *B. melitensis* is the most common species infecting humans. The organism name is derived from *Melita* (honey), the Roman name for the Island of Malta.

Humans develop brucellosis after ingesting raw infected milk or dairy products such as cheese, yogurt, or ice cream prepared from unpasteurized milk. Camel milk is an important source of brucellosis infection in the Middle East and Mongolia.

For *B. melitensis*, a small infective dose of ten organisms is sufficient to initiate the disease. The incubation period is between 1 week and 10 months.

Brucellosis can infect any organ and may present with a variety of symptoms, depending on the infected organ. Patients typically present with a fever that can be acute (<2 months), subacute (2–12 months), or chronic (>1 year). The fever is typically normal during the early part of the day and rises during the night. Brucellosis is one of the common causes of pyrexia of unknown origin.

Other symptoms include influenza-like illness, sweating, malaise, myalgia, headaches, weight loss, lymphadenopathy, hepatosplenomegaly, and joint pain (arthralgia). Joint and back pain may be the first manifestations of brucellosis and is seen in up to 40 % of cases. Back pain arises either due to sacroiliitis or spondylitis. Peripheral arthritis is a common complaint and usually affects the knees, hips, and ankles.

Unilateral epididymo-orchitis is the most frequent complication affecting the genitourinary system.

The liver is commonly affected in brucellosis, and laboratory investigations often show liver enzyme abnormalities.

In 5–7 % of patients, the central nervous system is affected in the form of transient ischemic attacks, meningitis, encephalitis, and demyelinating diseases. Cranial nerves may be affected in neurobrucellosis, especially the optic, abducens, facial, and the cochlear branch of the vestibulocochlear nerve in the form of neuritis. Headache due to intracranial hypertension is a common symptom in neurobrucellosis. Diagnosis can be confirmed by identifying *Brucella* antibodies in the cerebrospinal fluid (CSF) or the serum. The organism is rarely isolated from the CSF.

The spine is commonly infected by brucellosis via hematogenous spread though the lumbar venous plexus. The lumbosacral region is the most frequently affected (60 %), followed by the thoracic region. Spondylodiscitis and vertebral osteomyelitis are common findings. Back pain and large joints arthralgia are described in up to 15 % of cases of chronic spinal brucellosis.

The skin is involved in 1–12 % of patients, mostly females, in the form of vasculitis or erythema nodosum. Up to 2 % of brucellosis deaths are attributed to *Brucella* endocarditis.

Brucellosis diagnosis is confirmed by demonstrating *Brucella*-specific antigens in the serum and blood culture (definite diagnosis) or by polymerase chain reaction performed on any clinical specimen.

**Signs on Plain Radiographs**
- Spondylitis often begins in the superior vertebral end plates. The organisms are located in the anterior part of the end plate, initiating epiphysitis. Erosion and destruction of the anterior-superior part of the end plates with new bone formation is a characteristic sign of vertebral brucellosis (*Pons' sign*) (□ Fig. 11.6.1).
- The healing process is marked by dense sclerosis, with the formation of anterior-superior end plate "parrot-peak" osteophytes.

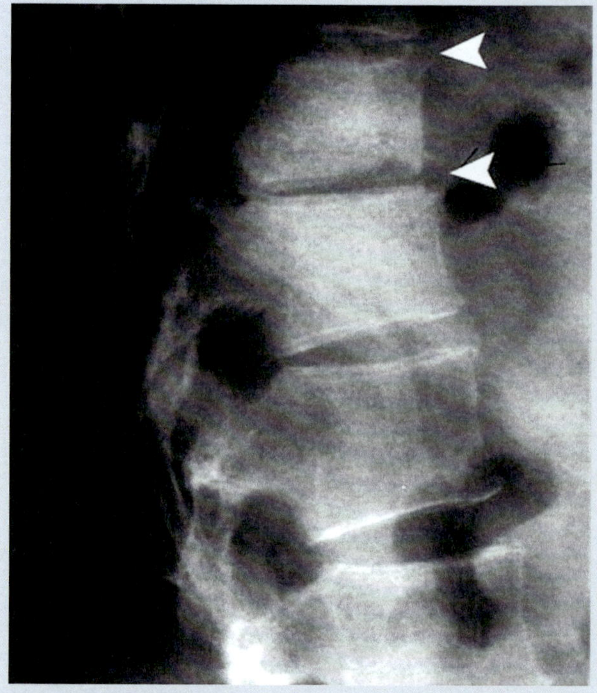

□ **Fig. 11.6.1**    Lateral plain radiograph of the lower thoracic vertebrae in a patient with brucellosis shows spondylitis affecting the anterior-superior and the anterior-inferior vertebral end plates (*arrowheads*)

## Signs on US
- Brucellosis epididymo-orchitis is seen as a focal, hypoechoic mass near the testes, with marginal flow signal on color flow Doppler sonography, reflecting hyperemia. The normal epididymis does not show high flow signal on color flow Doppler sonography.
- Hydrocele and scrotal skin thickening may be found.
- The resistance index may be reduced due to hyperemia, with low-resistance arterial flow pattern seen on pulsed Doppler sonography.

## Signs on MRI
- Signs of encephalitis or meningitis may be seen.
- Enhancement of the cranial nerves is detected when neuritis is suspected clinically.

*The main problem in diagnosing brucellosis of the spine is to differentiate it from tuberculosis (TB) of the spine. How can you differentiate between the two conditions?*
- Brucellosis commonly affects the lumbosacral vertebrae, while TB commonly affects the thoracic vertebrae.
- The vertebral height is preserved in brucellosis, while it is severely damaged in TB.
- The posterior elements and the epidural sac are usually spared in brucellosis, while they are affected in TB.

## Further Reading

Bayram MM, et al. Scrotal gray-scale and color Doppler sonographic findings in genitourinary brucellosis. J Clin Ultrasound. 1997;25:443–7.

Bilen S, et al. Four different clinical manifestations of neurobrucellosis. Eur J Intern Med. 2008;19:e75–7.

Estevão MHL, et al. Neurobrucellosis in children. Eur J Pediatr. 1995;154:120–2.

Glasgow MMS. Brucellosis of the spine. Br J Surg. 1976;63:283–8.

Guney F, et al. First case report of neurobrucellosis associated with hydrocephalus. Clin Neurol Neurosurg. 2008;110:739–42.

Jochem T, et al. Neurobrucellosis with thalamic infarction: a case report. Neurol Sci. 2008;29:481–3.

Koc Z, et al. Gonadal brucellosis abscess: imaging and clinical findings in 3 cases and review of the literature. J Clin Ultrasound. 2007;35:395–400.

Mantur BG, et al. Review of clinical and laboratory features of human brucellosis. Indian J Med Microbiol. 2007;25(3):188–202.

Mays SA. Lysis at the anterior vertebral body margin: evidence for brucellar spondylitis? Int J Osteoarchaeol. 2007;17:107–18.

Metin A, et al. Cutaneous findings encountered in brucellosis and review of the literature. Int J Dermatol. 2001;40:434–8.

Tali ET, et al. MRI of brucella polyneuritis in a child. Neuroradiology. 1996;38:S190–2.

## 11.7 Neurocysticercosis

Cysticercosis is a parasitic disease caused by human infection with *Taenia solium*, the pork tapeworm.

The definitive host of *T. solium* is the pig. The larvae are ingested by humans in improperly prepared, infected pork meat. After ingestion, the larvae attach themselves to the intestinal mucosa and develop into adult tapeworms in 5–12 weeks. The tapeworm eggs contain active embryos (oncospheres), which are excreted in the stool. Pigs ingest the infected stool, and the oncospheres are liberated into pigs' gastrointestinal tract, enter the mesenteric circulation, and develop into larvae in various tissues, completing the life cycle. Cysticercosis is endemic in parts of Asia, Thailand, India, Europe, and Latin America.

Cysticerci are found in various human tissues, but they have affinity for the central nervous system (neurocysticercosis). The clinical findings in neurocysticercosis are often nonspecific, and diagnosis is confirmed only by imaging and laboratory cerebrospinal fluid (CSF) studies. Patients commonly present with headaches, seizures (70%), and neurological deficits. Arachnoiditis, infarction, and obstruction of the ventricular system by intraventricular lesions or reactive ependymitis may occur.

Neurocysticercosis can be found within the brain parenchyma, within the arachnoid space, the intraventricular space, and (very rarely) within the spinal cord (<1% of cases).

Cisternal or subarachnoid cysticercosis is caused by two types of larval worms: *Cysticercus cellulosae* and *Cysticercus racemosus*. They are usually found in the basal cisterns, Sylvian fissures, or ventricles.

## Signs on Plain Radiographs
When the larval cysts are killed by the inflammatory reaction within muscles and subcutaneous tissues, calcification of the dead cysts is seen as ovoid flecks of calcification resembling grains of rice (rice grain calcification). These calcifications are characteristic of cysticercosis and usually parallel the long axis of the muscle.

The CT and MRI findings in neurocysticercosis mainly depend on the stage of the disease; four stages are recognized:
- *Stage 1 (vesicular stage)*: in this stage (□ Fig. 11.7.1), the cysticerci are viable, with immune tolerance. There is a cystic lesion in the brain with little or no sign of acute inflammation, because the cyst is able to escape the host's immune system surveillance. The cyst shows no contrast enhancement. A small eccentric nodule may be found within the cyst, which represents the parasite's head or scolex (□ Fig. 11.7.2). This is referred to as *hole-with-dot sign*, and it is almost a pathognomonic sign of neurocysticercosis. Single or multiple cysts may be found anywhere within the brain. Patients are often asymptomatic in this stage.
- *Stage 2 (colloidal stage)*: this stage develops after years, when the larvae start to die. The immune system starts an

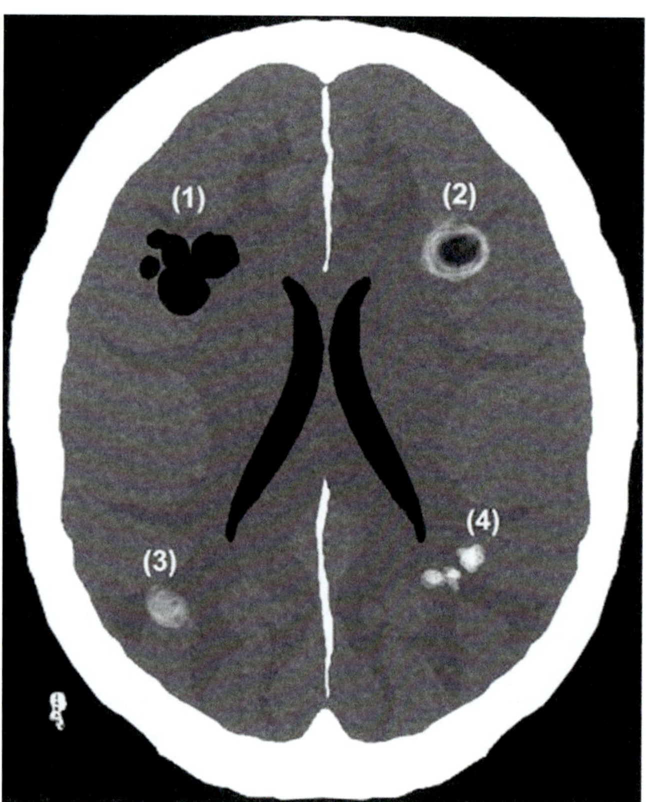

inflammatory response, and the fluid within the cyst becomes opaque. The cyst wall is thickened and shows contrast enhancement (■ Figs. 11.7.2 and 11.7.3). Edema around the lesions is demonstrated on T2W and FLAIR images.

— *Stage 3 (granular stage)*: in this stage, the colloid cyst is transformed into a nodular granuloma (■ Fig. 11.7.1). The lesion is nodular, with low T1/T2 signal intensities, surrounded by perifocal edema.

— *Stage 4 (calcified stage)*: in this stage, deposition of calcium occurs within the granuloma, and the lesion is calcified (■ Fig. 11.7.1). This stage is best demonstrated by CT.

— *Miliary neurocysticercosis*: this uncommon form of neurocysticercosis is characterized by small (3–5 mm), bilateral symmetrical nodular cystic parenchymal lesions with marked edema (■ Fig. 11.7.4). This form is often seen in children and young adults.

— *Racemose neurocysticercosis* is found in the subarachnoid space or the basal cisterns, with a similar signal and density to the CSF on MRI or CT, respectively. Racemose neurocysticercosis may manifest as a large lobulated (resembling bunch of grapes) cyst compressing the adjacent structures. It also frequently infiltrates the basal meninges, causing extensive meningitis and fibrosis. The cyst typically shows no scolex or contrast enhancement. The combination of a large lobulated cyst with no mural nodule inside it and enhanced basal meninges strongly suggests racemose neurocysticercosis, especially in endemic areas (■ Fig. 11.7.5).

■ **Fig. 11.7.1**  Axial brain CT illustration shows the four stages of neurocysticercosis: (*1*) vesicular stage, (*2*) colloidal stage, (*3*) granular stage, and (*4*) calcified stage

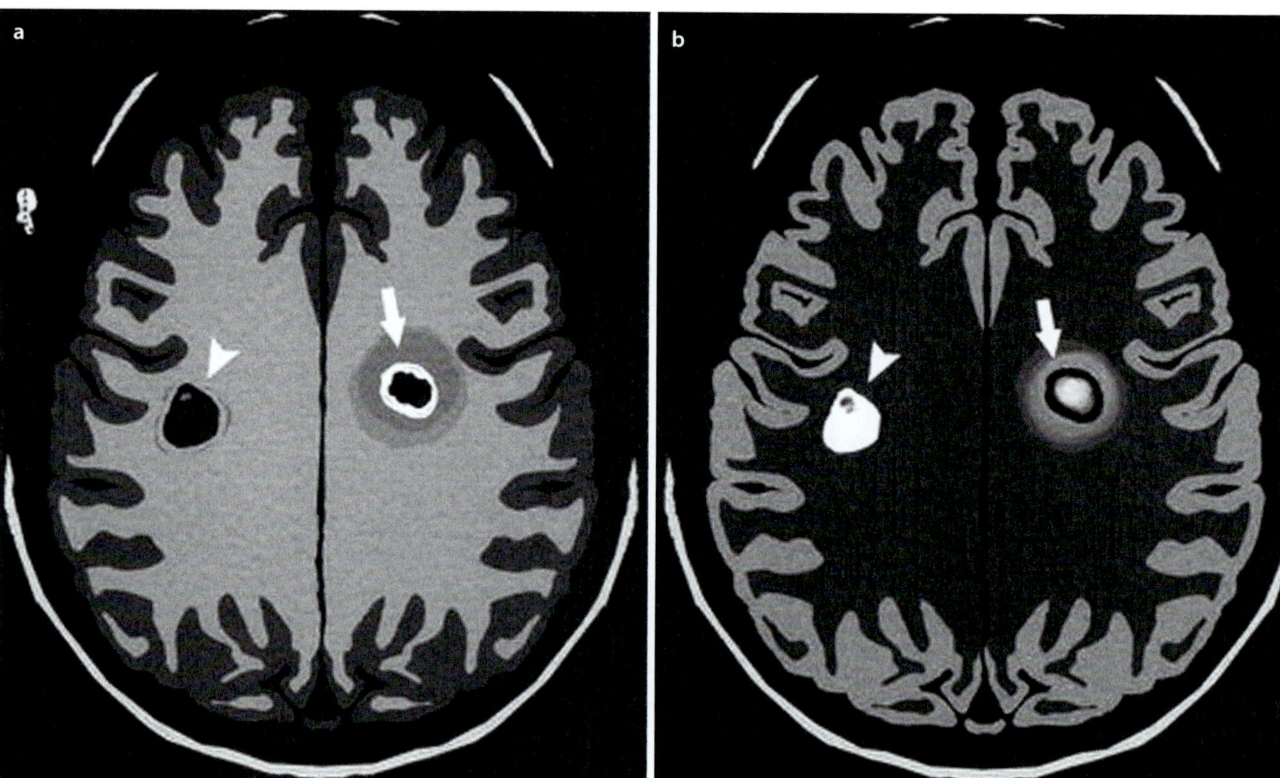

■ **Fig. 11.7.2**  Axial T1W postcontrast (**a**) and T2W (**b**) brain MR illustrations show different neurocysticercosis stages. In (**a**) and (**b**), the right cyst represents the vesicular stage, with eccentric scolex (*arrowheads*). The left cyst represents the colloidal stage, with rim contrast enhancement and edema around the cyst (*arrows*)

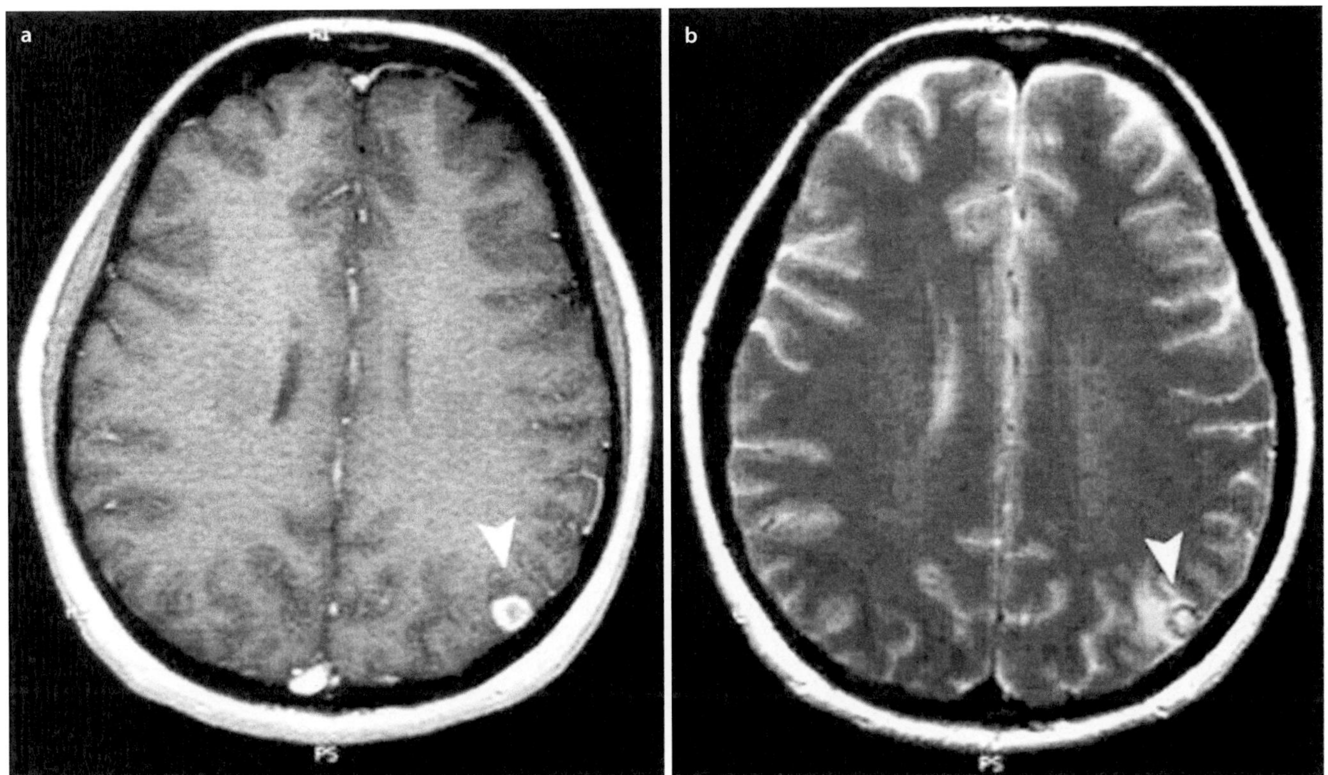

**Fig. 11.7.3** Axial T1W postcontrast (**a**) and T2W (**b**) brain MR images of colloidal stage neurocysticercosis (*arrowheads*)

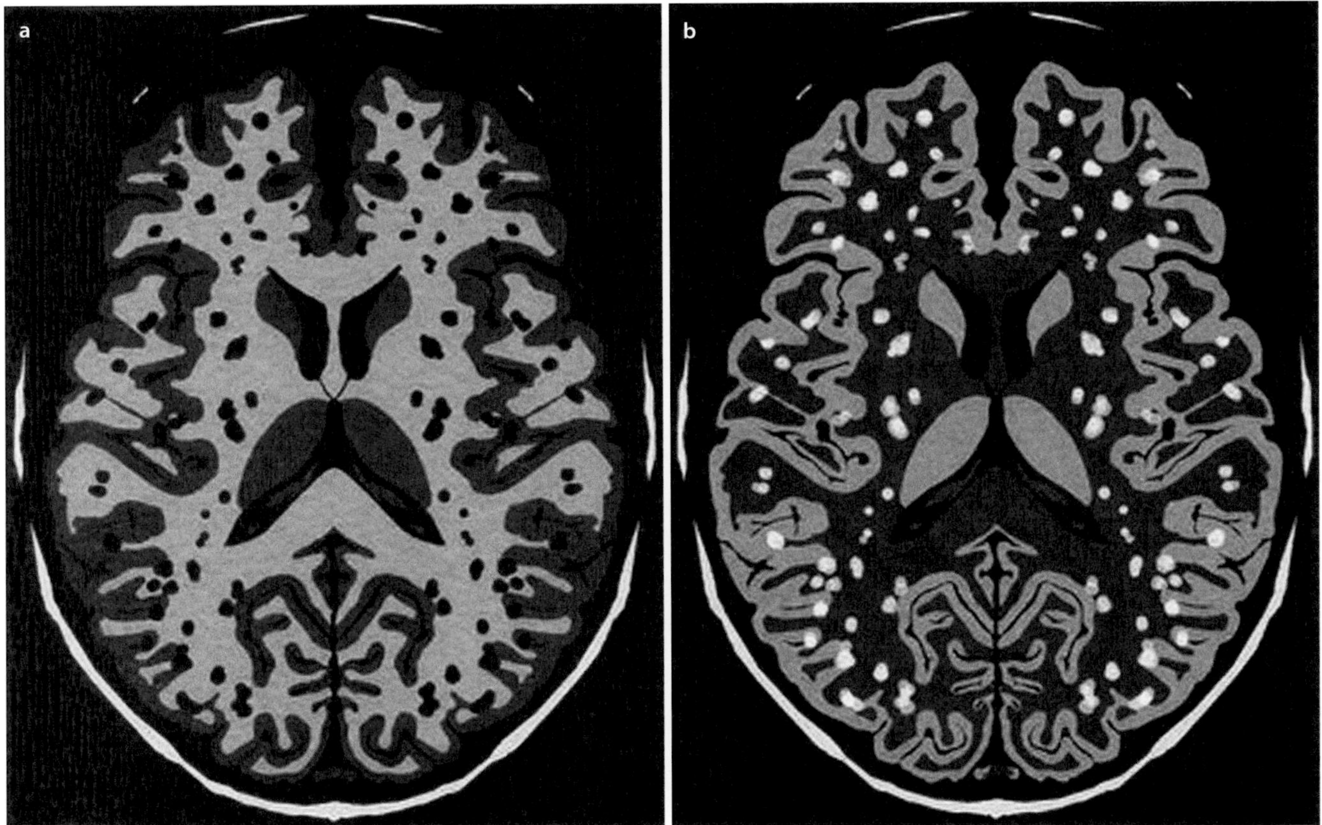

**Fig. 11.7.4** Axial T1W (**a**) and T2W (**b**) MR illustrations show the radiological appearance of miliary neurocysticercosis

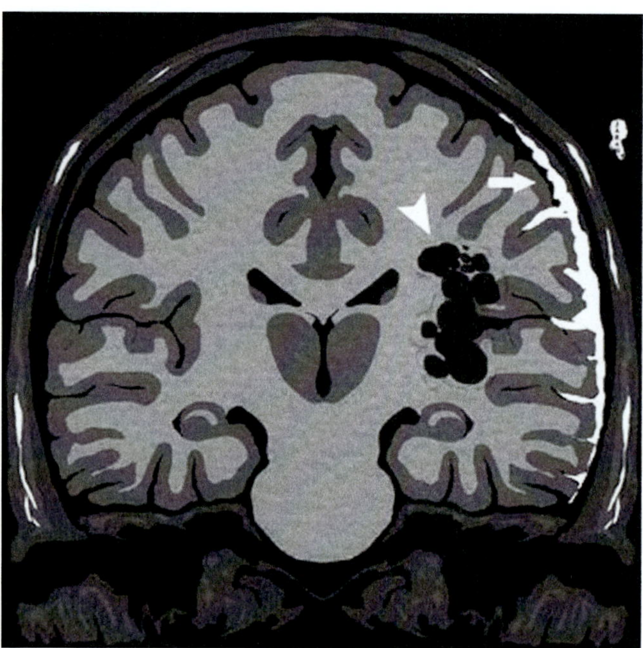

**Fig. 11.7.5** Coronal postcontrast T1W brain MR illustration demonstrates left lobulated cystic lesions within the Sylvian fissure (*arrowhead*), representing racemose neurocysticercosis with leptomeningitis ipsilaterally (*arrow*)

- *Intraventricular neurocysticercosis* is seen as intraventricular round lesions with signs of hydrocephalus due to ventricular obstruction.
- *Intraspinal neurocysticercosis* is seen on MRI as an intramedullary cystic mass with fluid signal with wall enhancement according to the stage. Serological testing of the CSF is helpful to establish the diagnosis.

### Further Reading

Chang KH, et al. MRI of CNS parasitic diseases. JMRI. 1998;8:297–307.

Dumas JL, et al. Parenchymal neurocysticercosis: follow-up and staging by MRI. Neuroradiology. 1997;39:12–8.

Palacios E, et al. Computed tomography and magnetic resonance imaging of neurocysticercosis. Semin Roentgenol. 1997;32(4):325–34.

Roche CJ, et al. Selections from the buffet of food signs in radiology. RadioGraphics. 2002;22:1369–84.

Ruiz-García M, et al. Neurocysticercosis in children. Clinical experience in 122 patients. Child's Nerv Syst. 1997;13: 608–12.

Yeh SJ, et al. Neurocysticercosis presenting with epilepsia partialis continua: a clinicopathologic report and literature review. J Formos Med Assoc. 2008;107(7):576–81.

### 11.8    Ascariasis

Worms, also known as "helminthes," are parasitic infections. Diagnosis is usually made by identifying the worm eggs in the stool.

Ascariasis is a parasitic disease that arises due to ingestion of food contaminated by the eggs of the roundworm (nematodes) *Ascaris lumbricoides*. Most patients are children between 1 and 15 years of age. Consuming uncooked vegetables and drinking polluted water from wells are important sources of ascariasis infection.

After ingestion of the eggs, the larvae hatch from the eggs before they reach the intestine, due to stimulation by gastric juices. The larvae penetrate the intestinal wall, enter the bloodstream, and travel via the portal venous or the lymphatic systems to the liver and then to the thoracic cavity. When they reach the lungs, the larvae grow and mature within the lung alveoli. When the worms are mature enough, they migrate from the lungs into the bronchi and from the trachea to the epiglottis, from where they are swallowed into the intestine for the second time. The matured larvae grow into adult worms in the intestine, especially the jejunum, and produce eggs that pass out in the feces. Up to 99 % of ascarids are found in the jejunum and ileum.

Most patients are asymptomatic, although severe ascariasis infection can cause abdominal cramps and malnutrition. The worms may also invade the gallbladder, appendix, liver, or bile duct. Ileocecal intestinal obstruction, ascending cholangitis, cholecystitis, appendicitis, and liver abscess are documented complications of ascariasis.

Respiratory symptoms in the form of fever, hemoptysis, cough, and pneumonia (*ascariasis pneumonia*) occur 5–26 days postinfection. The alveoli are filled with eosinophils and white blood cells attacking the larvae. Ascariasis is one of the most common causes of *Loffler's syndrome* (fever, systemic eosinophilia, asthma, cough with sputum, and signs of alveolar infiltration on chest radiograph). The adult worm can produce a neurotoxin that can result in neurological manifestations (*ascariasis encephalopathy*).

Diagnosis is made by identifying the *Ascaris* eggs in the feces and pronounced eosinophilia on complete blood count.

### Differential Diagnoses and Related Diseases

*Visceral larva migrans (VLM)* is a disease characterized by the invasion and residence of animal parasites in human tissues for a long time. The disease is often seen in children and often caused by *Toxocara canis* (from dogs) *and Toxocara cati* (from cats). Rarely, VLM can be caused by pig's roundworm, *Ascaris suum*, which is closely related to human roundworm, *Ascaris lumbricoides*.

> **Signs on Chest Radiograph**
> - Signs of patchy alveolar infiltration.
> - A pulmonary nodule can occur if the larvae form a granulomatous lesion when they die.

### Signs on Ultrasound

- In the gallbladder, the *Ascaris* worm is identified as a tubular structure with nondirectional movement causing a zigzag sign. The tubular structure has 3–4 parallel echogenic lines in longitudinal axis and a target sign in transverse axis.
- When the gallbladder is full of worms, echogenic, intraluminal, and spaghetti-like structures are seen.

### Signs on Barium Enteroclysis

- The ascarides are seen as long, tubular filling defects within the intestinal lumen in the jejunum or the ileum (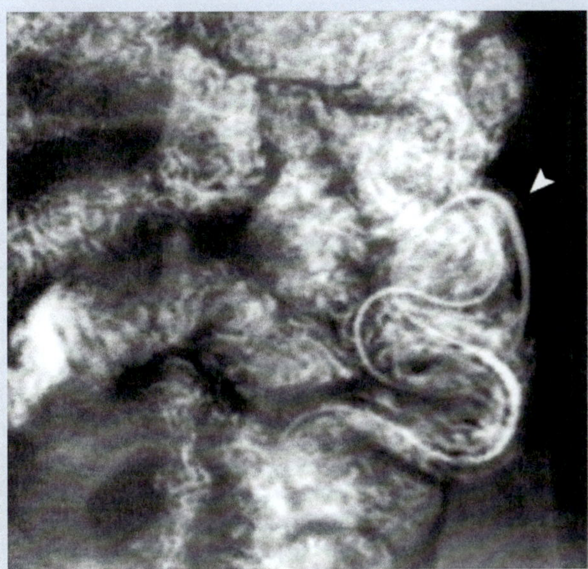 Fig. 11.8.1).
- The worm may ingest the barium, which will cause its gastrointestinal opacification, resulting in *double contrast* worm appearance around the barium (Fig. 11.8.1).

- In the gallbladder, the worms are seen as tubular, coiled soft-tissue structures within the gallbladder with no contrast enhancement. Speckles of curvilinear calcifications may be seen.

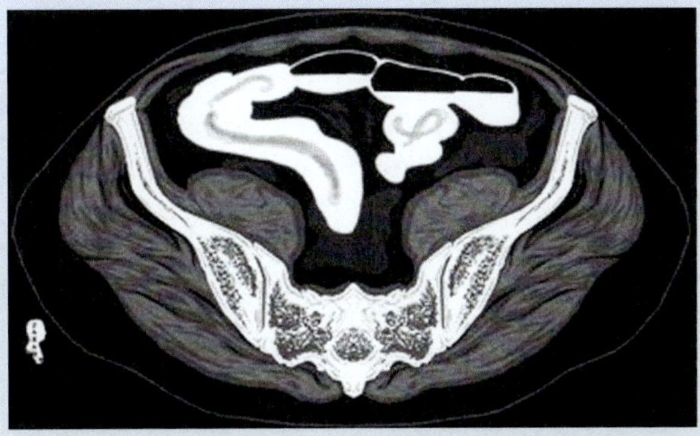

**Fig. 11.8.2**    Axial CT illustration demonstrates *Ascaris* worms within the intestinal bowel loops

**Fig. 11.8.1**    Barium enteroclysis radiograph of a patient with ascariasis shows a long, tubular filling defect in the jejunum, with a double contrast sign representing *Ascaris* worm with barium ingestion (*arrowhead*)

## Further Reading

Hayashi K, et al. Hepatic imaging studies on patients with visceral larva migrans due to probable Ascaris suum infections. Abdom Imaging. 1999;24:465–9.

Kakihara D, et al. Liver lesions of visceral larva migrans due to Ascaris suum infection: CT findings. Abdom Imaging. 2004;29:598–602.

Maheshwari PR. Gall bladder ascariasis. Clin Radiol Extra. 2004;59:8–10.

Ochoa B. Surgical complications of ascariasis. World J Surg. 1991;15:222–7.

Reeder MM. The radiological and ultrasound evaluation of ascariasis of the gastrointestinal, biliary, and respiratory tracts. Semin Roentgenol. 1998;33(1):57–78.

Robbani I, et al. Worms in liver abscess: extensive hepatobiliary ascariasis. Dig Liver Dis. 2008;40(12):962. doi:10.1016/j.dld.2008.03.008.

Sherman SC, et al. The CT diagnosis of ascariasis. J Emerg Med. 2005;28(4):471–2.

Slesak G, et al. Obstructive biliary ascariasis with cholangitis and hepatic abscess in Laos: a case report with gall bladder ultrasound video. J Infect. 2007;54:e233–5.

## 11.9    Guinea Worm Disease (Dracunculiasis)

Dracunculiasis is an infection of the body by *Dracunculus medinensis*, a tissue-invasive round worm (nematode).

The name "*medinensis*" is derived from the frequency of human guinea worm infestation near Medina, a city in Saudi Arabia. It is a disease that is seen in the Middle East, Asia, and Africa.

The parasite enters the body through drinking water infected with the larvae, which penetrate the intestine and

### Signs on CT

- On bowel oral contrast-enhanced CT, the worm is seen as a tubular filling defect within the bowel loops (Fig. 11.8.2). A thin enhanced line within the tubular defect can be seen representing contrast within the gastrointestinal tract of the worm due to contrast ingestion.

enter the bloodstream to lie deep within the subcutaneous tissues. The worm can grow under the skin up to 100 cm and usually exposes its uterus out of the host body through the skin to release its larvae into the water.

Patients infected with *D. medinensis* often present with allergic symptoms, nausea, and vomiting. Patients also present with skin blisters, sterile abscess, and (uncommonly) septic arthritis. The worm can be sensed under the skin within the abscess.

*D. medinensis* tends to migrate into the lower extremities, breast, and scrotum. Other sites in the body might be affected as well. It rarely affects the viscera.

The adult worm can directly invade any joint, resulting in monoarthritis. The knee is the most common joint involved, resulting in an intense destructive arthropathy (*Ibadan knee*). Other manifestations include sterile monoarthritis due to immune complexes, also commonly affecting the knee. The worm is often removed from the skin by driving a small stick under the part of the worm that is looped out of the skin, and the worm is slowly twisted to pull it out of the subcutaneous tissues (◘ Fig. 11.9.1).

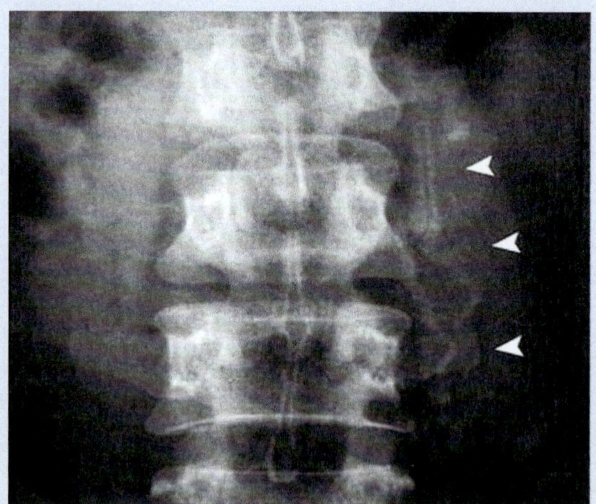

◘ **Fig. 11.9.2**   Anteroposterior plain radiograph of the thoracic spine shows linear, beaded, radio-opaque shadow in the left paraspinal region in a patient with dracunculiasis, representing a dead worm (*arrowheads*)

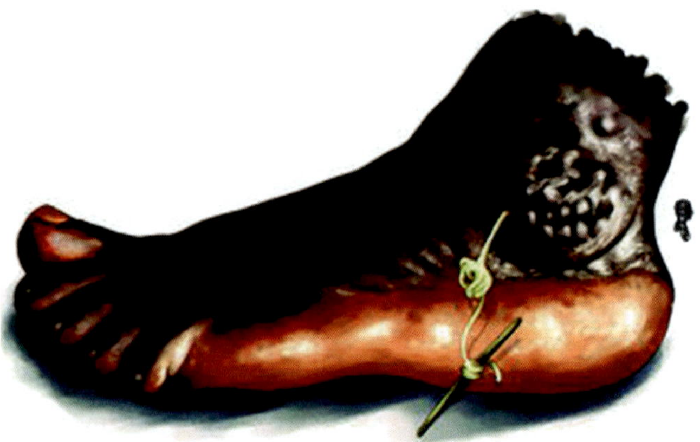

◘ **Fig. 11.9.1**   An illustration demonstrates the classical method of extracting the guinea worm from the body. The worm is wrapped around a stick and slowly pulled out. The worm can be very long, and the process of pulling the worm out may take days

### Signs on Radiograph

When the female worm dies, it will calcify, giving an intact, long, curvilinear, and beaded radio-opaque shadow in the radiograph, and this is diagnostic. No other parasite condition simulates this long, beaded full worm calcification within the muscles or the soft tissues in the body (◘ Figs. 11.9.2 and 11.9.3).

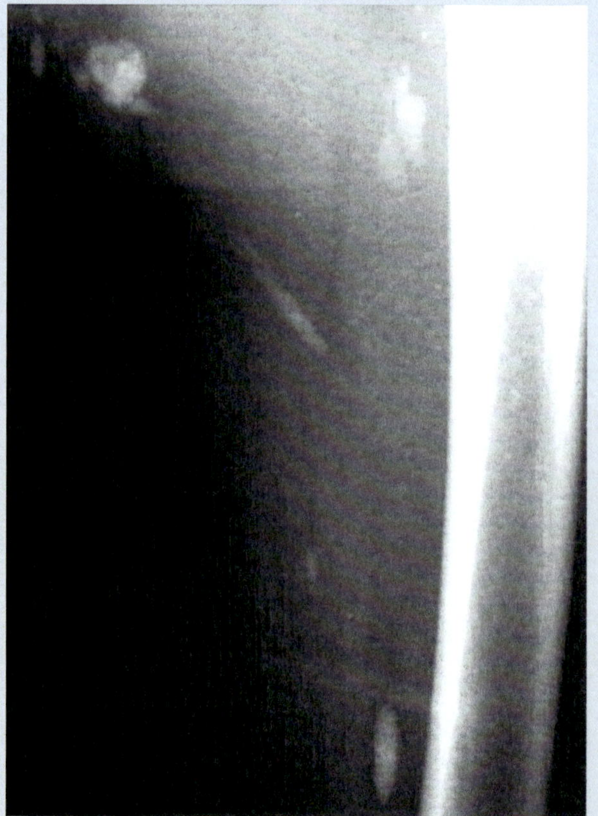

◘ **Fig. 11.9.3**   Plain radiograph of the soft tissue of the posterior thigh in the same patient shows multiple linear and rounded calcified lesions, representing dead intramuscular worms

## Further Reading

Iriemenam NC, et al. Dracunculiasis – the saddle is virtually ended. Parasitol Res. 2008;102:343–7.

Legmann P, et al. Epidural dracunculiasis. A rare cause of spinal cord compression. Neuroradiology. 1980;20:43–5.

Muller R. Dracunculiasis medinensis: diagnosis by indirect fluorescent antibody technique. Exp Parasitol. 1970;27:357–61.

Peng SL. Rheumatic manifestations of parasitic diseases. Semin Arthritis Rheum. 2002b;31:228–47.

Watts S. An ancient scourge: the end of dracunculiasis in Egypt. Soc Sci Med. 1998;46(7):811–9.

## 11.10 Hydatid Cyst (Echinococcosis)

Echinococcosis is a disease caused through infection from the human tapeworms *Echinococcus granulosus* and *Echinococcus multilocularis*. Each infection behaves in a different manner within the human body. *Echinococcus granulosus* produces cystic lesions within the body, while *Echinococcus multilocularis* produces tumor-like lesions.

### *Echinococcus granulosus* Disease

Infection with *E. granulosus* is found in the Middle East, Africa, Mediterranean countries, and Eastern Europe. The definitive hosts for the parasite are dogs and sheep. Humans are intermediate hosts who are infected with the parasite by ingesting food contaminated by the definitive hosts' feces or by direct contact with the definitive hosts.

After the parasite is ingested, the eggs hatch, and the embryos penetrate the intestinal mucosa, enter the portal circulation, and are carried to various organs. Any organ can be

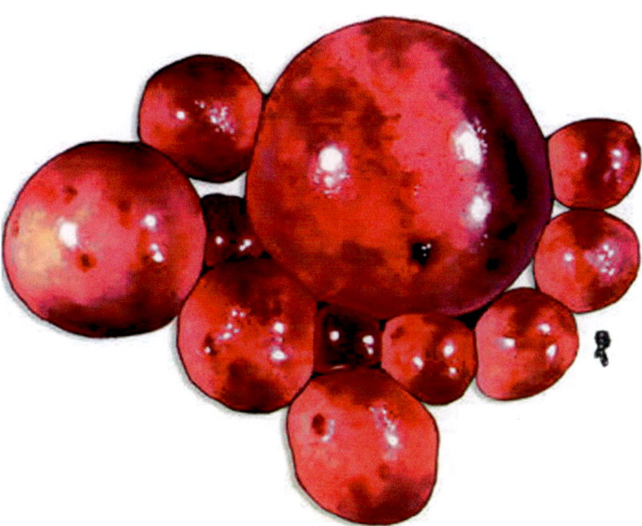

**Fig. 11.10.1** An illustration shows the gross pathological appearance of hydatid cysts

infected by *E. granulosus*, but the liver (75%) and lungs are considered the most common areas for hydatid cyst disease. The original cyst grows 2–3 cm per year; as the cyst enlarges, it starts to form internal daughter cysts ( Fig. 11.10.1).

Patients with *E. granulosus* infection are often asymptomatic, unless a cyst is ruptured. A ruptured cyst usually results in fever, pruritus, eosinophilia, and fatal anaphylactic shock.

### Grading of the Liver Lesions by *E. granulosus*

On the different radiological imaging modalities, different shapes of the hydatid cyst may be encountered. This is due to the fact that the cysts undergo different stages of life and death during the course of the disease ( Fig. 11.10.2).

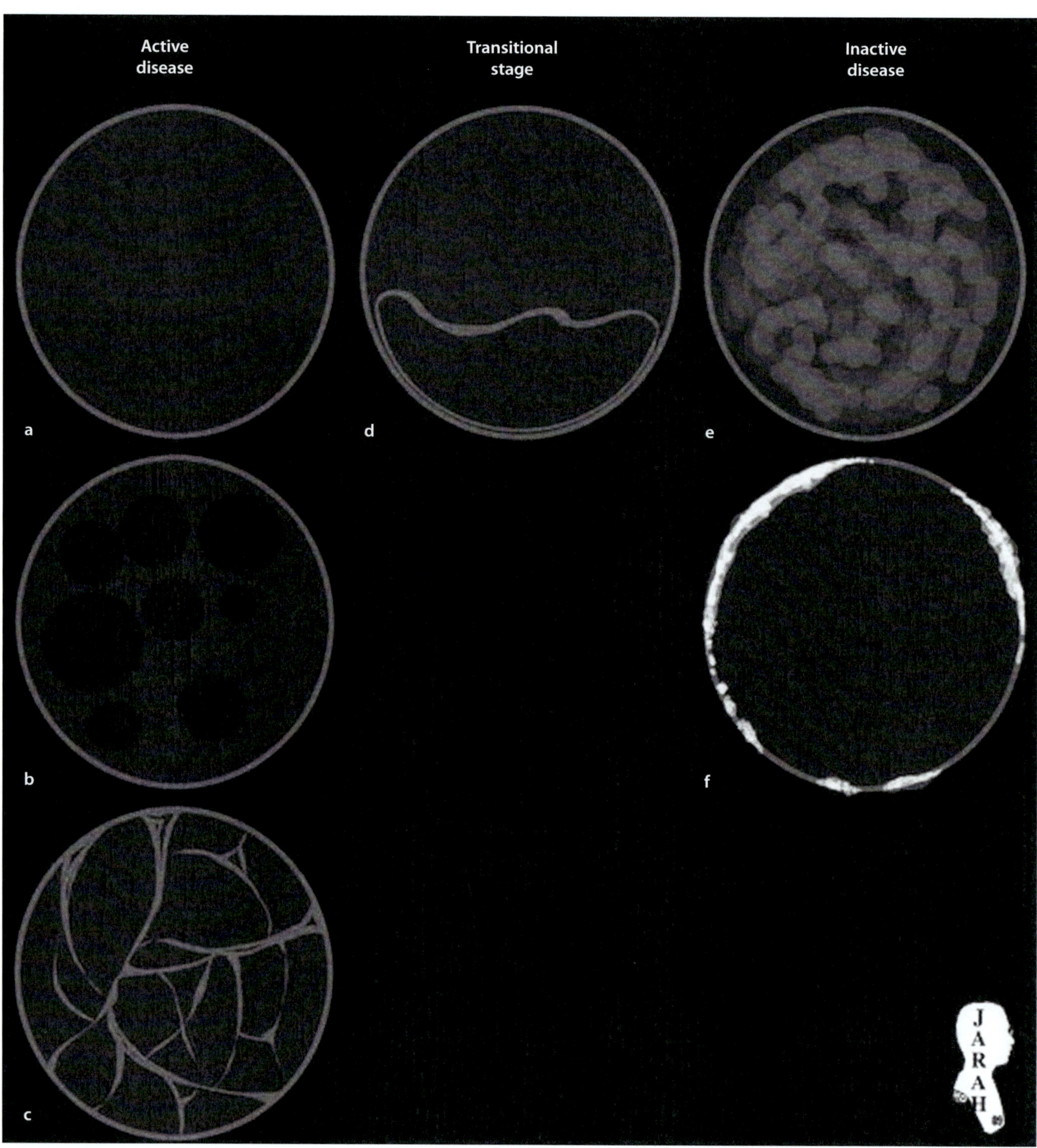



**Fig. 11.10.2**    An illustration shows the different stages of hydatid cysts that may be encountered during CT examination: (**a**) pure cystic form, (**b**) a cyst with multiple hypodense lesions within it, (**c**) a cyst with internal septations, (**d**) floating water lily sign, (**e**) ball of wool sign, and (**f**) calcified cystic wall

The hydatid cyst walls are composed of three layers. The first layer (pericyst) is made up of compressed host tissue and inflammatory cells. The second and the third walls are the true cyst walls. The second wall is an outer acellular layer (ectocyst), and the third is an inner cellular wall (endocyst). The daughter cysts arise from the endocyst wall.

– *Grade 1 lesion* (purely cystic lesions): This grade is seen on ultrasound, CT, or MRI as a pure cyst without internal inhomogeneities. This grade is explained by intact endocysts, and patients with grade 1 lesions benefit from percutaneous aspiration and scolicidal injection therapy.

### Signs on Chest Radiograph

Hydatid cyst lesions are seen as a well-circumscribed, round mass, with no internal texture (Figs. 11.10.2 and 11.10.3). It mimics a solid pulmonary mass and may lead to a false diagnosis of pulmonary tumor. Absence of symptoms and presence of other cystic lesions within the liver are important clues.

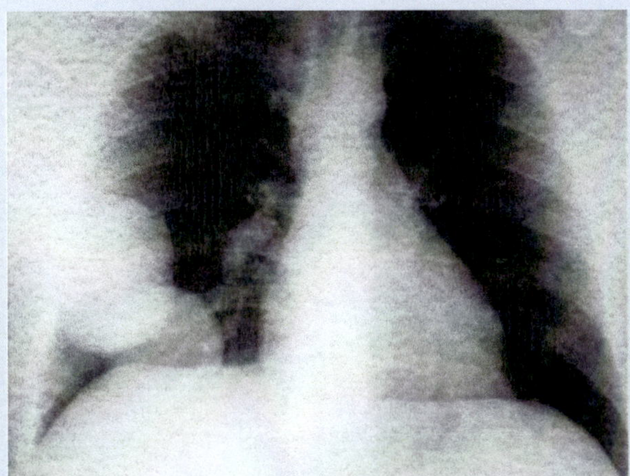

**Fig. 11.10.3** Posteroanterior plain chest radiograph shows two large masses located at the right middle and lower lung fields in a patient with hydatid liver disease. The masses represent intact hydatid cysts within the lung

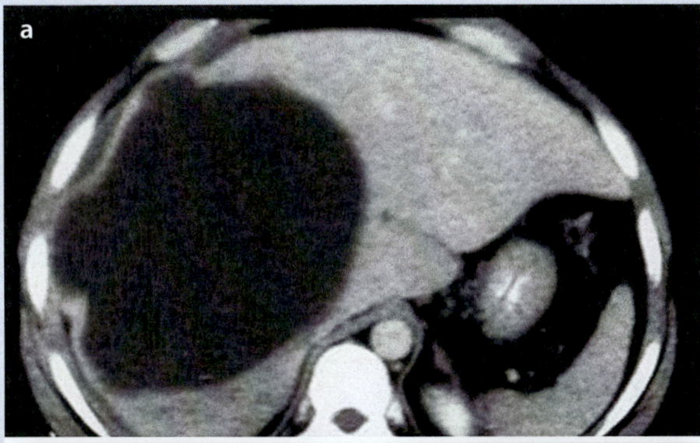

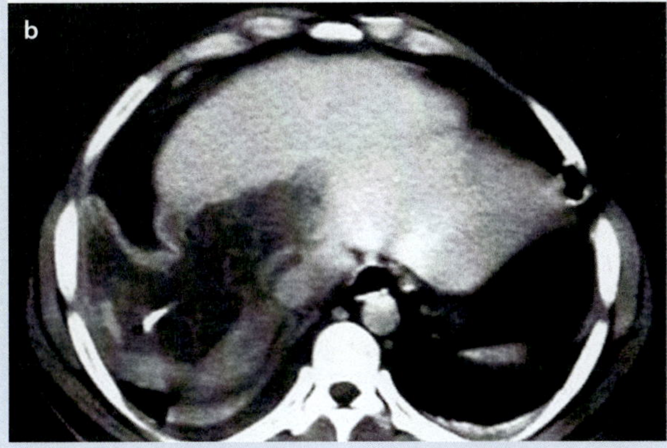

**Fig. 11.10.4** Axial abdominal CT images show a very large hydatid cyst that occupies almost the entire right lobe of the liver (**a**) and the cyst appearance after aspiration of the cyst contents (**b**)

### Signs on US

On ultrasound, the hydatid cyst shows a double wall (*double-line sign*). This is an important sign that differentiates a grade 1 hydatid cyst from a simple hepatic cyst, which shows a thin single wall.

### Signs on CT

The cyst appears as a simple cyst with no internal septations, densities, or contrast enhancement (Fig. 11.10.4).

— *Grade 2 lesions* (lesions with complex morphology with or without biliary dilatation around the lesion): This grade is characterized by the appearance of different intracystic textures. These textures arise due to previous rupture of an endocyst, with hydatid fluid leakage into the potential space between the endocysts and the pericyst. Later, this fluid causes different intracystic textures seen on ultrasound, CT, or MRI.

### Signs on US, CT, and MRI
- Internal septations with honeycomb-like appearance can be seen on ultrasound, CT, and MRI (Fig. 11.10.2).
- Small internal echoes may be seen on ultrasound, reflecting floating protoscoleces (*snowflakes sign*).
- The daughter cysts may be seen as multiple hypodense lesions, compared to the density of the original cyst on CT (Figs. 11.10.5 and 11.10.2).

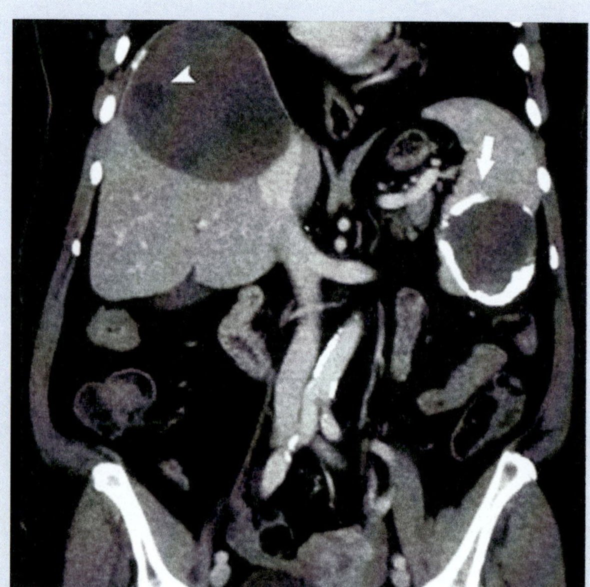

**Fig. 11.10.5** Coronal abdominal CT image in a patient with hepatic and splenic hydatid cyst shows hepatic hydatid cyst with internal hypodense lesions (*arrowheads*) and splenic hydatid cyst with calcified wall (*arrow*)

- *Grade 3 lesions* (lesions with intrabiliary rupture): Because the cyst is originally formed within the liver tissue, which in turn contains biliary canaliculi, cysto-biliary communication may occur as an uncommon complication. This grade is characterized by intrahepatic biliary dilatation with hydatid vesicle escape from the mother cyst into the biliary radicals, causing regional biliary obstruction (Fig. 11.10.6).
- *Grade 4 lesions*: This grade is characterized by rupture of the pericyst and the endocysts, with spillage of the cyst content into the neighboring organs or spaces. Leakages of the hydatid fluid into the peritoneum cause severe irritation and peritonitis. Later, peritoneal calcification arises (Fig. 11.10.7).

- *Grade 5 lesions*: This grade is characterized by death of the cyst (inactive disease). It is seen as collapse of the hydatid membrane (pericyst) over the residual endocysts. This is seen on plain radiographs, CT, and MRI as a thick wall plus an irregular, wavy, water-fluid level floating on top of the residual hydatid fluid.

This sign is known as the *floating water lily sign* (Figs. 11.10.8 and 11.10.2). Degeneration of cysts is seen as

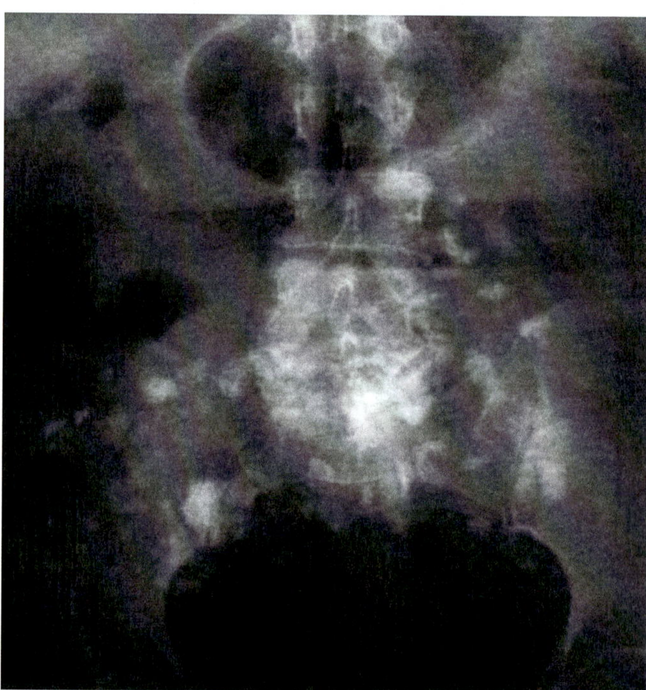

**Fig. 11.10.7** Plain abdominal radiograph in a patient with previous intraperitoneal ruptured hydatid cyst shows multiple calcifications involving the mesentery and the intraperitoneal structures

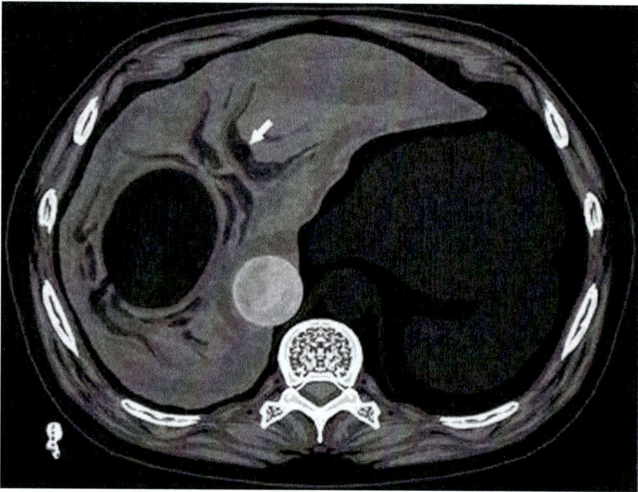

**Fig. 11.10.6** Axial CT illustration demonstrates grade 3 hydatid cyst disease. Notice the right lobe cyst with dilated biliary radicals around it, with an intrabiliary daughter cyst (*arrow*)

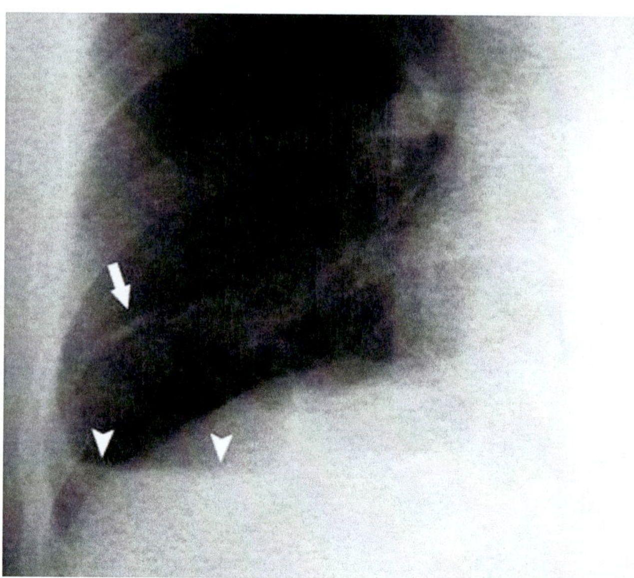

**Fig. 11.10.8** Posteroanterior plain chest radiograph shows ruptured hydatid cyst with floating water lily sign (*arrowheads*). Notice the cystic wall mimicking a cavity (*arrow*)

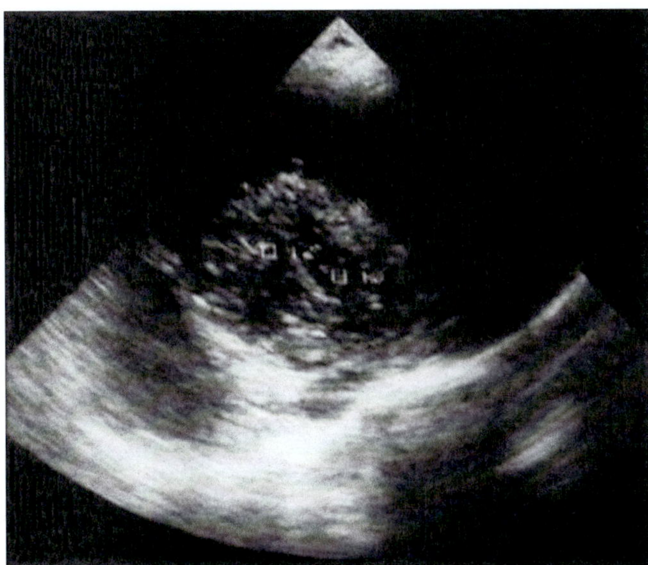



**Fig. 11.10.9** Ultrasound image of a liver hydatid cyst shows internal, multiple, solid-like lesions within the cyst (ball of wool sign)

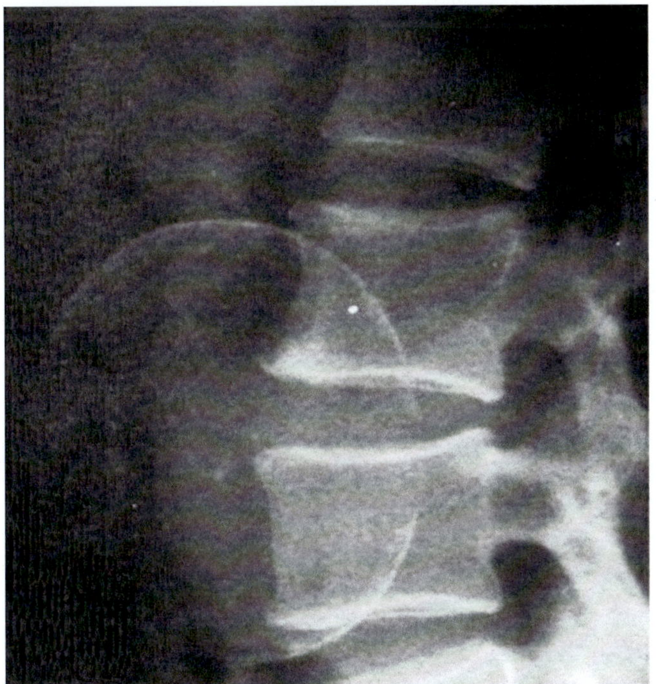

**Fig. 11.10.10** Lateral plain radiograph of the thoracic spine shows a calcified hydatid cyst in the paraspinal region

multiple, solid-like lesions within the mother cyst, resulting in a pseudotumor appearance on ultrasound or CT, known as the *ball of wool sign* (Figs. 11.10.9 and 11.10.2). Finally, circular or curvilinear calcification of the hydatid cyst wall is a sign of inactive disease (Figs. 11.10.10 and 11.10.2).

## Differential Diagnoses and Related Diseases

*Hepatic atrophy–hypertrophy complex* (*HAHC*): obstruction of a major hepatic or portal vein or biliary tree branch results

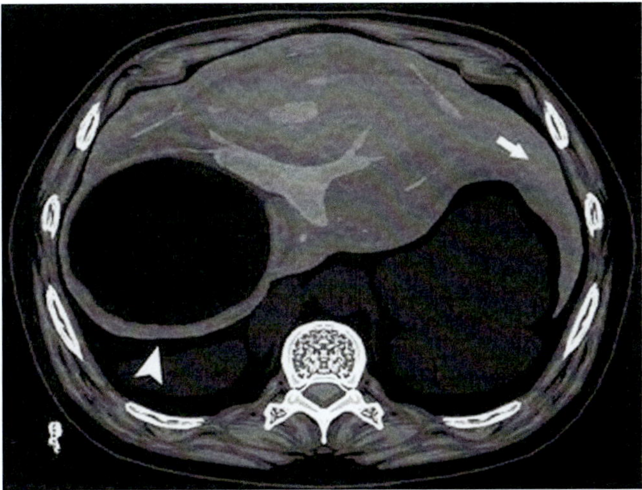

**Fig. 11.10.11** Axial CT illustration shows the hepatic atrophy–hypertrophy complex. Notice the large hydatid cyst occupying a large portion of the right lobe of the liver (*arrowhead*), with compensatory hypertrophy of the left liver lobe (*arrow*)

in atrophy of the hepatic segment supplied by this vein or biliary branch. As the liver has the ability to regenerate, compensatory hypertrophy of the liver is usually seen when a large segment of the liver parenchyma is atrophied. This phenomenon is known as the HAHC. HAHC may occur uncommonly as a complication of hydatid cyst disease, especially when the cyst occupies a large area within the right lobe of the liver. It is important for HAHC to be documented by the radiologist, because it informs the surgeon that the cyst is tightly involved with one or more of the portal triad structures or a major hepatic vein (Fig. 11.10.11).

*How does one differentiate between ruptured hydatid cyst and acute abscess?*

- The wall of the abscess is enhanced after contrast injection on CT, while the hydatid cyst wall will not enhance.
- The air–fluid level surface is straight in the abscess, while in the hydatid cyst, it has a wavy water surface due to the collapsed pericyst (floating water lily sign).

## *Echinococcus alveolaris* Disease

Infection with *E. multilocularis* is found in the United States, Canada, Japan, and Central and Northern Eurasia. The definitive hosts for *E. multilocularis* are foxes and rodents. Like *E. granulosus*, humans are intermediate hosts who are infected via ingesting food or water contaminated with the eggs or by direct contact with the definitive hosts.

In contrast to *E. granulosus*, *E. multilocularis* cysts are not confined within a pericyst layer and grow by external vesiculation. The cyst is small (1–10 mm in diameter) and forms multilocular alveolar cysts that resemble lung alveoli, hence the name *alveolaris*. The external parasitic proliferation initiates a fibroinflammatory response of the host within the affected organ, commonly the liver. This will later result in a fibrous, tumor-like lesion composed of *E. multilocularis* embedded in a keloid scar and necrotic liver tissue. Stenosis of the porta hepatic with the hepatic veins within the lesion is commonly found. When the lesion heals, multiple, punctuate calcifications arise within the lesion, which makes the lesion increasingly resemble a malignant hepatocellular carcinoma (HCC) or metastasis of the liver.

### Signs on US
In the liver, there are multiple echogenic nodules embedded within irregular and indistinct margins from the normal hepatic parenchyma (*hailstorm sign*).

### Signs on CT
- The liver often shows a hypodense mass with a "geographic map" appearance and inhomogeneous internal texture (◘ Fig. 11.10.12).
- Areas of punctuate calcifications within the lesions are very common in healed lesions (90 % of cases) (◘ Fig. 11.10.12).
- Unlike HCC, the lesion shows no enhancement or mild enhancement in the portal venous phase because of the fibrous stroma within the mass (characteristic and diagnostic).
- Areas of central liquefaction may be seen.
- There are no signs of retroperitoneal lymphadenopathy (another differentiating point from HCC).

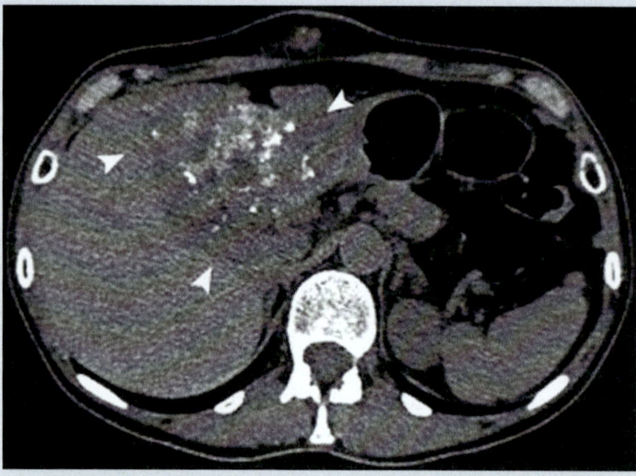

◘ **Fig. 11.10.12** Axial nonenhanced abdominal CT in a patient with *Echinococcus alveolaris* disease affecting the left lobe of the liver shows liver mass with geographic edges (*arrowheads*) and internal punctuated calcifications

### Signs on MRI
The scan shows an inhomogeneous mass with geographic margins and characteristically low T1 and low T2 signal intensities, with no enhancement or mild enhancement after contrast enhancement in the portal venous phase (◘ Fig. 11.10.13).

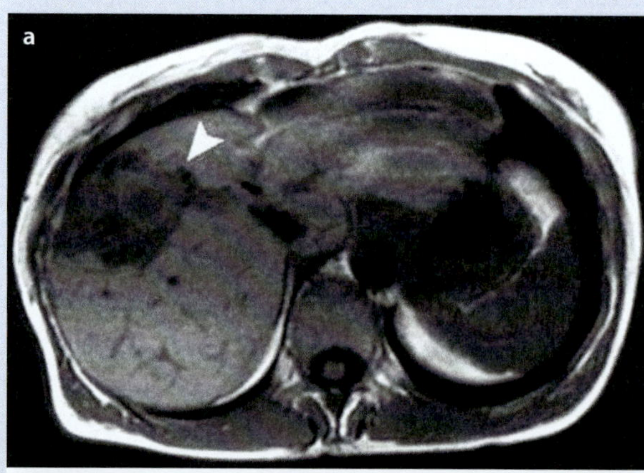

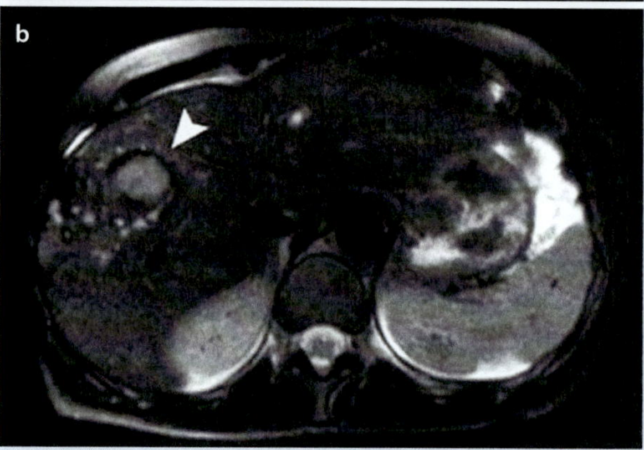

◘ **Fig. 11.10.13** Axial T1W (**a**) and T2W (**b**) nonenhanced MR images in a patient with *Echinococcus alveolaris* disease show a mass that resembles HCC (*arrowheads*), with multiple cystic lesions within the mass. Notice that the mass bulk is hypointense on T2W image (**b**) due to the fibrous (keloid) nature of the lesion

## Further Reading
Czermak BV, et al. Echinococcosis of the liver. Abdom Imaging. 2008;33:133–4.

Etlik Ö, et al. Contrast-enhanced CT and MRI findings of atypical hepatic Echinococcus alveolaris infestation. Pediatr Radiol. 2005;35:546–9.

Karabulut K, et al. Hepatic atrophy-hypertrophy complex due to Echinococcus granulosus. J Gastrointest Surg. 2006;10:407–12.

Katranci N, et al. Correlation CT MRI and histological findings of hepatic Echinococcus alveolaris: a case report. Comput Med Imaging Graph. 1999;23:155–9.

Rozanes I, et al. Grading of liver lesions caused by Echinococcus granulosus. Eur Radiol. 1993;3:429–33.

Sasaki F, et al. Alveolar echinococcosis of the liver in children. Pediatr Surg Int. 1994;9:32–4.

## 11.11 Chagas' Disease (American Trypanosoma)

Chagas' disease (CD) is an infectious, multisystemic disease caused by *Trypanosoma cruzi* (*T. cruzi*), a blood-borne flagellate. *T. cruzi* was first described in Brazil by Carlos Chagas, in

1909. The disease is one of the most common public health problems in South America from Texas to Argentina.

CD often affects children and young adults living in rural areas and mud huts. *T. cruzi* is transmitted to humans by the defecation of a vector bug known as the "kissing bug" (reduviid bug). The bite occurs around the face, often at night, and the parasite is found in the bug's feces. The bite can be painless or painful depending on the toxins found in the bug's saliva.

At the bite site, *T. cruzi* penetrates the skin and travels via the blood to the body organs. The parasite invades and enters the host cells, particularly the muscles, the glia, and the reticuloendothelial system. Multiplication occurs by binary fission until the cells rupture, and the parasite enters the blood or invades more tissues. At the site of multiplication, severe inflammatory reaction occurs with local lymphangitis, which is known as *chagoma*. Soon after that lymphatic spread to regional lymph nodes occurs, which is usually seen in the first 2 weeks postinfection.

Although the parasite can be found in any body tissue, *T. cruzi* often has a distinct predilection for striated and cardiac muscles, glial, and nerve cells.

There are four distinct phases of CD, each with its own pathological and radiological features.

## Acute Chagas' Disease

The main pathological process during this stage is chagoma affecting the heart and the central nervous system (CNS). The acute stage is frequently seen in neonates, although it may occur at any age.

After an incubation period of 2 weeks, patients often present with fever that can persist for months, malaise, loss of appetite (anorexia), vomiting, diarrhea, and muscle pain.

In the heart, there is severe lymphocytic myocarditis with focal areas of endocardium and epicardium inflammation, which leads to dilated cardiomyopathy and pericardial effusion. Hyaline necrosis of isolated myocardial fibers (*Magarinos–Torres' lesion*) is a characteristic feature of Chagas' myocarditis.

In the CNS, encephalitis or meningoencephalitis is often seen and may be the primary manifestation of CD. The trypanosomes may enter the conjunctiva in up to 50 % of patients, causing upper or lower eyelid edema, conjunctiva chemosis, and preauricular lymph nodes enlargement (*Romana's sign*).

Hepatosplenomegaly, and pneumonia when the trypanosoma affect the lungs, may be seen.

### ECG Abnormalities

The most common changes in electrocardiogram (ECG) are prolonged P-R interval, low voltage in an ECG rhythm showing electrical activity in the ventricles (QRS complex), and prolonged Q-T interval.





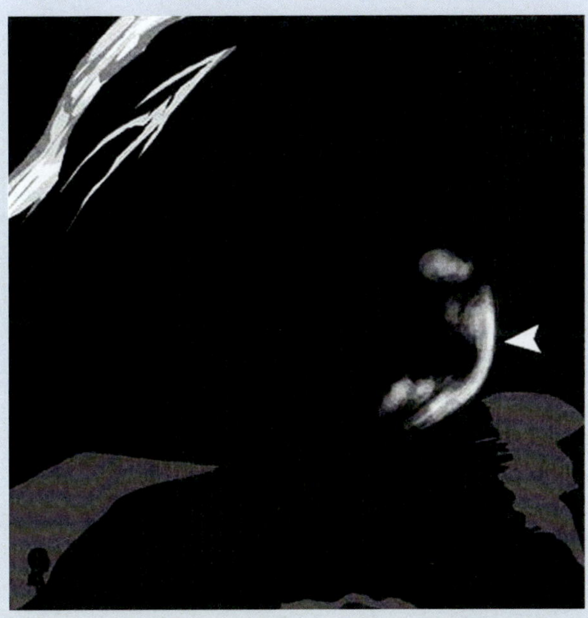

◘ **Fig. 11.11.1** Sagittal short-axis, T1W postcontrast cardiac MR illustration demonstrates the type of myocarditis enhancement seen in Chagas' disease (mid- to outer-wall enhancement) (*arrowhead*)

## Subacute Chagas' Disease

This stage is often seen in young adults, and the patient presents without any fever, with severe heart failure that does not respond to therapy.

## Latent Chagas' Disease

After the acute stage subsides, many patients completely recover, while others may pass into a latent or chronic stage. In this stage, 2–5 % of patients become symptomatic annually.

The number of ganglion cells in the Auerbach plexi in the gastrointestinal (GI) tract starts to diminish in this stage. All patients who recovered from the acute CD stage, or live in endemic areas, have a positive complement fixation test (*Machado–Guerreiro reaction*).

## Chronic Chagas' Disease

This stage develops after many years and is characterized by dilated cardiomyopathy, with esophageal and colonic dilatation. The main pathology is attributed to reduction in the motor ganglia of the GI tract, resulting in loss of motor function (aperistalsis), which results in dilatation and flaccidity of the affected organs.

In the esophagus, early stages are characterized by hypercontractility and hypertrophy of the circular smooth muscles. Later, denervation of the esophageal muscles results in marked esophageal dilatation. Food may become lodged in the esophagus. Carcinoma and esophageal abscess may develop in 7 % of patients with chronic CD.

In the colon, massive dilatation and chronic constipation is often seen. Sigmoid volvulus may occur in 10 % of patients.

> **Signs on Plain Chest Radiograph**
> - The dilated esophagus is seen as a mediastinal mass along the entire right side of the mediastinum with air or air–fluid level.
> - The heart is often dilated due to dilated cardiomyopathy of chronic CD.
> - Raised left hemidiaphragm due to splenic flexure dilatation may be found.

> **Signs on Barium Swallow and CT**
> - The esophagus is massively dilated (>7 cm), with bizarre, dysrhythmic contractions that mimic achalasia (◨ Fig. 11.11.2). Food may be found lodged within the esophagus.
> - On CT, megacolon with massive rectosigmoid dilatation is usually found.

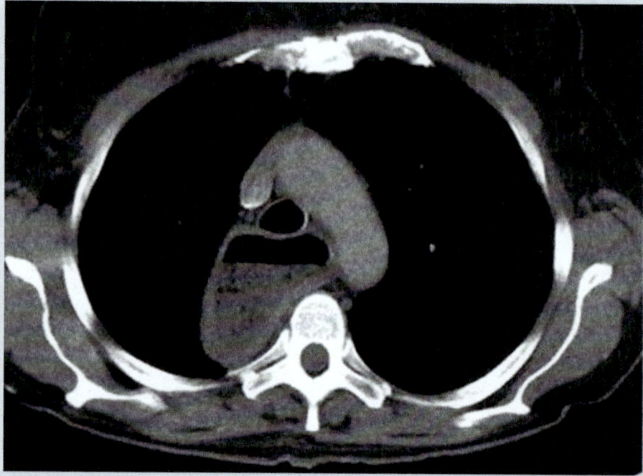

◨ **Fig. 11.11.2**   Axial thoracic CT in a patient with chronic Chagas' disease shows massive dilatation of the esophagus, with food lodged inside the esophagus, mimicking achalasia

## Further Reading

Barros MVL, et al. Doppler tissue imaging to access systolic function in Chagas' disease. Arq Bras Cardiol. 2003;80(1): 36–40.

de Souza AP, et al. Magnetic resonance imaging in experimental Chagas disease: a brief review of the utility of the method for monitoring right ventricular chamber dilatation. Parasitol Res. 2005;97:87–90.

Felippe L, et al. Radiological diagnosis of Chagas' disease (American trypanosomiasis). Semin Roentgenol. 1998; 33(1):26–46.

Ferreira-Santos R. Aperistalsis of the esophagus and colon (megaesophagus and megacolon) etiologically related to Chagas' disease. Am J Digest Dis New Ser. 1961;6(8):700–26.

Rochitte CE, et al. Myocardial delayed enhancement by magnetic resonance imaging in patients with Chagas' disease: a marker of disease severity. J Am Coll Cardiol. 2005;46:1553–58. Originally published online 22 Sep 2005. doi: 10.1016/j.jacc.2005.06.067.

## 11.12 Schistosomiasis (Bilharziasis)

Schistosomiasis is an infectious disease caused by freshwater *Schistosoma*. *Schistosoma* are flatworms that do not have a digestive tract and are commonly known as trematodes or blood flukes. Schistosomiasis is commonly known as "bilharziasis," after Bilharz, the discoverer of the parasite in 1815.

### *Schistosoma* Life Cycle

*Schistosoma* release their eggs in freshwater. Later, the eggs are hatched into larvae, which maturate in freshwater snails. After maturation, the mature larvae (cercariae) leave the snails and enter into humans by penetrating the exposed human skin in the freshwater. After skin penetration, the parasites travel within the lymphatic system through the thoracic duct to enter the circulation. The parasites lie in the lymphatic system for almost 21 days before they enter the hepatic portion of the portal venous system into the liver, where they further mature and mate. Depending on the type of the *Schistosoma*, the parasites migrate into the intestinal or the bladder venous system to lay their eggs. The adult worms are strictly intravenous and do not evoke the immune system, while both the cercariae and the eggs stimulate the immune system, resulting in the formation of granulomas around the eggs and the systemic cercariae, which will cause tissue fibrosis and calcification of the affected organ in advanced stages of the disease. Dead worms can be embolized almost anywhere within the body.

There are four types of *Schistosoma* worldwide:
- *Schistosoma japonicum* is found within eastern Asia, is located within the intestinal tract veins, and releases its eggs in the feces.
- *Schistosoma mansoni* is found within South America and Africa, is located within the intestinal tract veins, and releases its eggs in the feces.

- *Schistosoma haematobium* is found within Africa and the Middle East, is located within the bladder and ureters venules, and releases its eggs in the urine.
- *Schistosoma intercalatum* is found only in equatorial Africa and mainly affects the intestinal tract and the portal system.

The first symptom of the disease starts when patients develop itchy skin after larvae penetration, due to hypersensitivity reaction type 1 and type 4 (cercarial dermatitis or swimmer's urticaria). Weeks later, systemic manifestations like hematuria, fever, weight loss, diarrhea, and abdominal pain arise.

The living worm lives between 4 and 30 years. The living worm engulfs the red blood cells (RBCs) and excretes them as hemozoin, which is engulfed later by the macrophages. The other action by the living worm is laying eggs (ova). As the ova penetrate the wall of the intestine or the urinary bladder, they may cause chronic bleeding (resulting in anemia), be trapped in the wall of the organ, or enter the blood and circulate as emboli. The dead worms initiate a severe inflammatory reaction within the veins, causing thrombophlebitis, which can block the affected vein.

Diagnosis of schistosomiasis is confirmed by identifying the *Schistosoma* eggs in urine or feces and eosinophilia in the complete blood count (CBC).

The clinical and radiological manifestations of schistosomiasis can be classified according to the parasite type.

## Schistosomiasis by *S. japonicum*

*S. japonicum* lives in the mesenteric veins and mainly affects the liver, small bowel, and lungs. In the small bowel, the duodenum and the jejunum are mainly affected.

In the liver, the parasite eggs are deposited in the portal venules along the liver periphery. When the eggs die, fibrosis within the venules results in a polygonal network of periportal fibrosis that makes the liver look like a "turtle back" on gross appearance (◘ Fig. 11.12.1). The eggs are also deposited within the liver capsule, resulting in capsule thickening and fibrosis. There is a high incidence of liver carcinoma with *S. japonicum* infection.

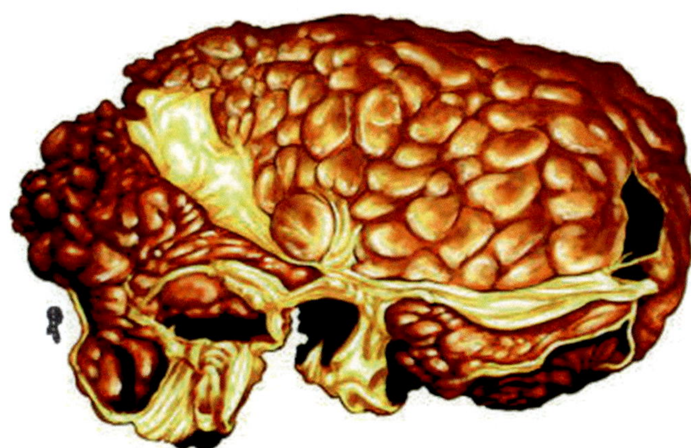

◘ **Fig. 11.12.1** An illustration demonstrates the gross turtleback appearance of *S. japonicum* liver schistosomiasis

### Signs on Ultrasound
The liver shows an internal echogenic polygonal network due to periportal fibrosis and calcification, which causes a "fish-scale" appearance (30 % of cases).

### Signs on Abdominal CT
There is internal periportal fibrosis (low-density bands) or calcification (high-density bands) within the liver parenchyma, along with liver contour irregularities (turtleback appearance) (◘ Fig. 11.12.2).

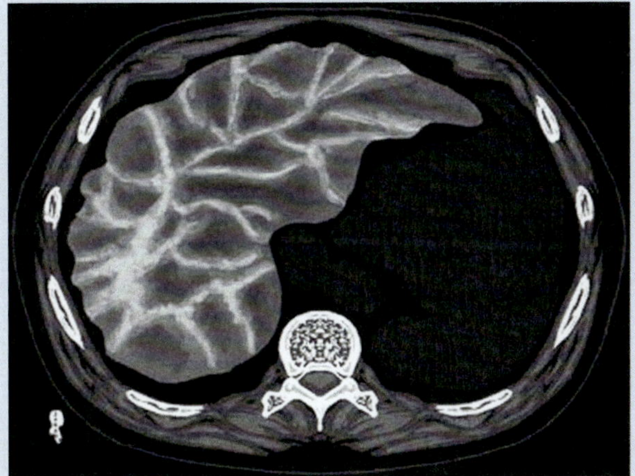

◘ **Fig. 11.12.2** Axial CT illustration of the liver in *S. japonicum* schistosomiasis demonstrates the internal periportal calcification and fibrosis causing the turtleback appearance

## Schistosomiasis by *S. mansoni*

*S. mansoni* mainly affects the liver, bowel, central nervous system, and lungs. In the bowel, the parasite causes granulomatous colitis, which causes loss of haustration and strictures later on, mimicking Crohn's disease. If the small intestine is affected, regional ileitis and protein-losing enteropathy may develop. In uncommon cases, when the calcification is so severe as to include all the layers of the colon wall, the ova start to accumulate freely within the peritoneal cavity outside the wall. This causes inflammation and fibrosis within the peritoneal cavity and the pericolic region, resulting in a pericolic mass that cannot be differentiated from carcinoma on imaging.

In the liver, the parasite deposits its eggs around the main portal vein at the liver hilum, later resulting in Symmers' pipestem fibrosis. *Symmers' pipestem fibrosis* is a condition that arises when egg granulomas aggregate around the portal vein, resulting in vascular fibrosis that causes obstruction of the small veins and presinusoidal cirrhosis. Portal hypertension (HTN), esophageal varices, and splenomegaly are common complications of this type of fibrosis.

In uncommon cases, *angiomatoid lesions* can develop within the liver. These angiomatoid lesions emerge as a secondary action taken by the body against severe fibrosis of the hepatic veins and portal HTN. The emergence of such lesions can be explained by the fact that in severe portal HTN, the blood within the veins cannot flow normally, which results in opening of sideway channels and collaterals to decrease liver congestion. This can result in angiomatoid formation of lesions (e.g., hemangiomas). These lesions seen in the liver represent a severe stage of portal HTN.

Splenomegaly in bilharziasis occurs at an early stage due to antigen stimulation, causing splenic parenchymal hyperplasia, and later in the course of the disease due to portal hypertension.

If eggs are embolized into the pulmonary vessels via the venous system, they damage the vascular wall by initiating an inflammatory reaction. The inflammatory reaction results in a characteristic "dumbbell" granuloma blocking the vessel or forms a pseudoaneurysm. Pulmonary hypertension may develop in advanced stages (20 % of cases). All *Schistosoma* species can affect the lungs.

Rheumatic manifestations are uncommonly seen with bilharziasis, resembling reactive arthritis or seronegative spondyloarthropathies and sacroiliitis. Rheumatoid-like disease affecting the metacarpophalangeal (MCP) and proximal interphalangeal (PIP) joints, wrists, ankles, and knees have been reported. Some of these manifestations are due to immune complexes or direct infection by the parasite.

In the central nervous system, *S. mansoni* produces conus medullaris thickening and arachnoiditis (*bilharzioma*).

### Signs on Plain Chest Radiograph
- Signs of pulmonary hypertension and enlarged pulmonary trunk in advanced stages.
- Localized bilharzias granulomas within the lung may be mistaken for a neoplastic nodule or mass.
- Calcification of the bowel walls may be seen (rarely) on plain radiographs (◨ Fig. 11.12.3).

### Signs on Ultrasound
- Hyperechoic lesions are noticed around the portal vein due to Symmers' pipestem fibrosis.
- Thrombosis of the portal vein may be seen as loss of Doppler signal flow within the portal main stem.
- Signs of liver cirrhosis and portal hypertension (e.g., splenomegaly).
- Gallbladder wall thickening is found in 80 % of cases.

### Signs on Abdominal CT
- The portal venous tracts are replaced by fibrous tissue, seen as low-attenuation bands or rings, with peripheral fibrosis radiating from the center of the liver around the main portal vein branches. Marked enhancement is noticed on postcontrast images.
- Shrunken liver, portal venous thrombosis, splenomegaly, and esophageal varices are commonly noticed (◨ Fig. 11.12.4).
- Splenic siderotic nodules (*Gamna–Gandy bodies*) are commonly seen within the enlarged spleen.

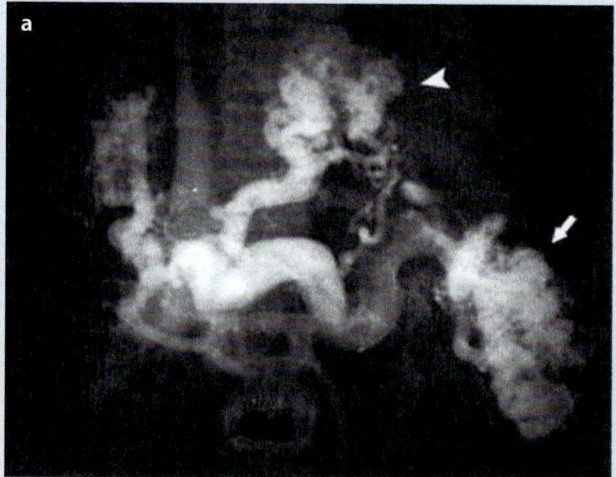

◨ **Fig. 11.12.4**   Portal cavography (**a**) and axial CT urography (**b**) in a patient with schistosomiasis and portal vein thrombosis shows a severely dilated portal vein, with development of esophageal varices (*arrowhead*) and splenic varices (*arrows*)

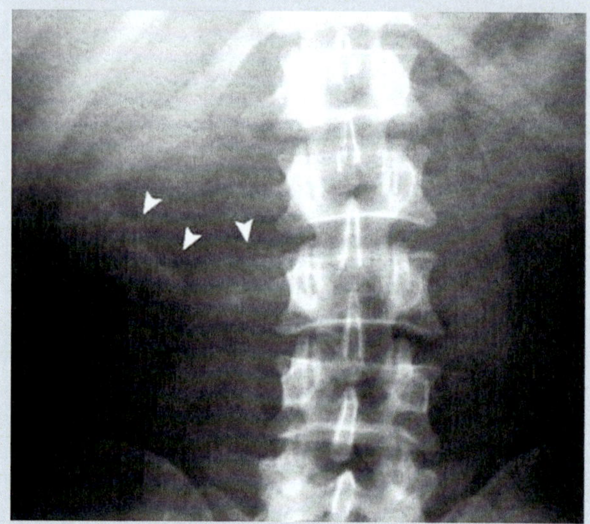

◨ **Fig. 11.12.3**   Plain abdominal radiograph shows calcification of the transverse colon walls in a patient with schistosomiasis (*arrowheads*)

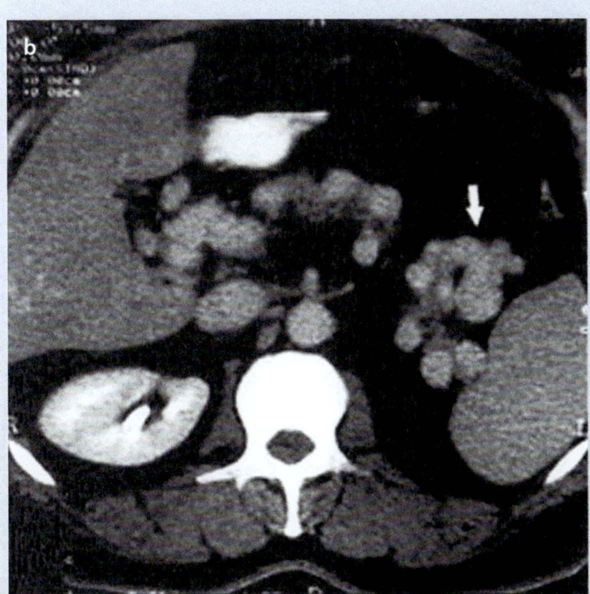



**Fig. 11.12.4**   (continued)

### Signs on Spinal Cord MRI
Bilharzioma is seen as localized conus medullaris thickening, with high signal intensity on T2W images and heterogeneous contrast enhancement postgadolinium injection (**Fig. 11.12.5**).

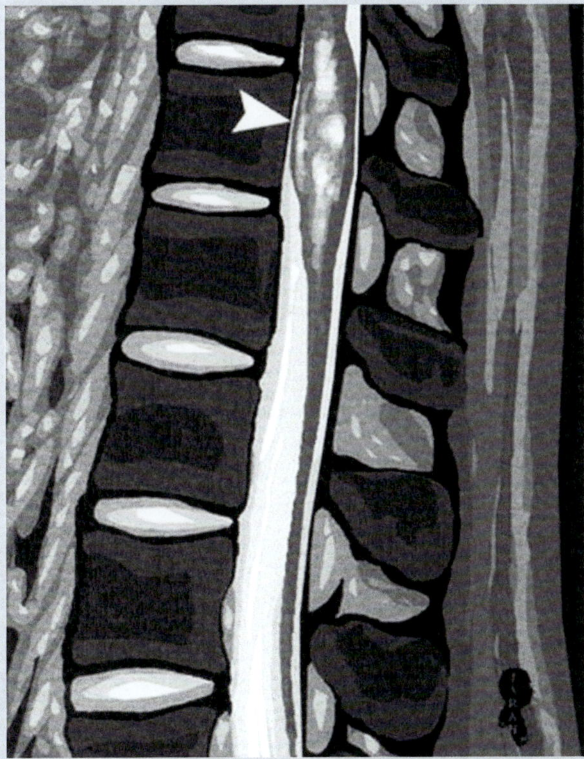

**Fig. 11.12.5**   Sagittal T2W lumbar MR illustration demonstrates enlarged conus medullaris with multiple high signal intensities representing bilharzioma (*arrowhead*)

## Schistosomiasis by *S. haematobium*

*S. haematobium* mainly affects the bladder and the ureters. The posterior part is the most vascular area of the bladder, and it is the area where most ova within the vesical veins are seen. *S. haematobium* lays more ova than *S. mansoni*. The eggs are trapped within the ureter and the bladder mucosa as they are carried by the urine to be excreted. The immune system surrounds the eggs and starts an aggressive granulomatous reaction that causes death and calcification of the eggs. As the disease advances, calcification can occur within the ureters, bladder, and seminal vesicles. When the ureters are calcified, obstructive uropathy and renal hydronephrosis may occur.

*Complications* of the ova within the bladder and intestinal walls are as follows:

— *Sandy patch* occurs when a huge number of ova die and calcify, causing the overlying mucosa to degenerate and atrophy.
— *Bilharzial polyp* occurs due to localized deposition of a huge number of ova, with hyperplasia of the wall. This is mainly seen in the intestine (*S. mansoni*).
— *Bilharzial ulcers* can arise due to penetration of huge numbers of ova, due to falling of the atrophic mucosa over a sandy patch lesion, or due to detachment of a bilharzial polyp.
— *Fibrosis* can arise as a consequence of chronic inflammation of the organ wall.
— *Urothilial changes* (only seen in the bladder) comprise a chronic reactive inflammatory disorder characterized by transitional epithelial hyperplasia in the form of nests called von Brunn's nests, due to an irritant (e.g., schistosomal ova). These nests may undergo central cystic degeneration, forming a condition called "cystitis cystica." The cystitis cystica transitional epithelium may undergo metaplasia into columnar mucin-secreting epithelium, causing another condition called "cystitis glandularis." The ova may cause squamous metaplasia of the transitional cell nest, causing leukoplakia, which may transform into dysplasia and carcinoma in situ. *Leukoplakia* is a thick, white patch of skin, commonly seen on the tongue, vulva, or the bladder. It is composed of thick layers of stratified epithelium with keratin, with chronic inflammation of the submucosa. Pathologically, it is explained by squamous metaplasia followed by cellular hyperplasia.

### Signs on Plain Abdominal Radiographs
— There is striking calcification of the ureters or the bladder (**Fig. 11.12.6**). The uniform and linear calcification of the schistosomiasis bladder is pathognomonic. In contrast, bladder calcification due to tuberculosis or radiation is often patchy and focal.
— Bilateral ureters calcification (**Fig. 11.12.6**) with hydronephrosis are a common finding.
— Calcification of the seminal vesicles, testes, and spermatic cords may be seen (**Fig. 11.12.7**).
— Fallopian tubes or cervical calcifications may occur in women.

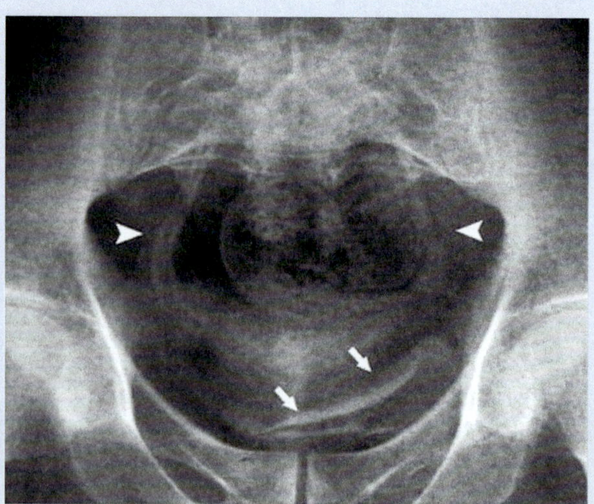

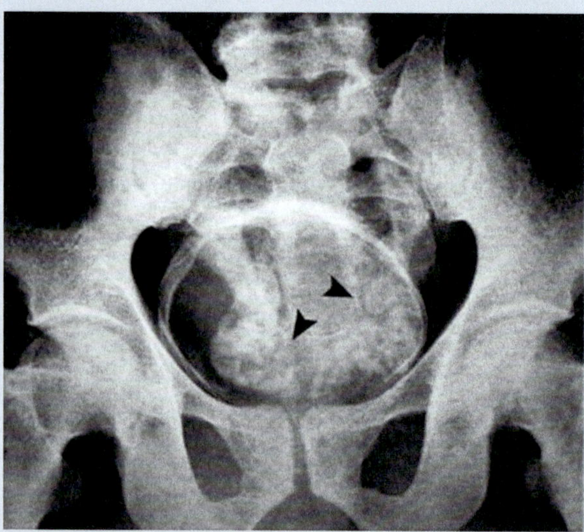

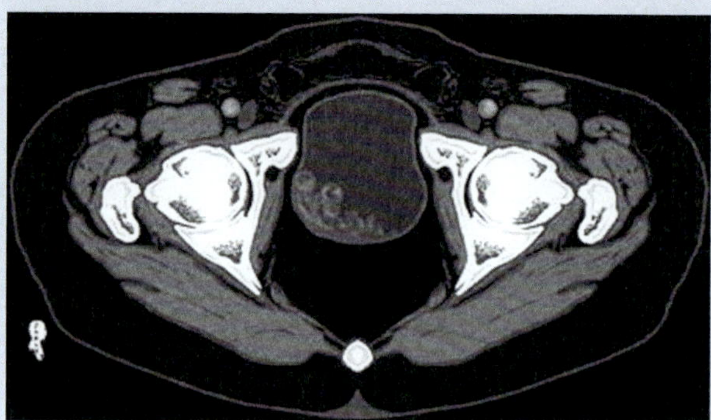

### Signs on CT and MRI

Cystitis cystica and cystitis glandularis are seen on MRI as hypervascular polypoid tissue with low T1 and T2 signal intensity, with central hyperintensity forming a branching pattern. The branching central areas show contrast enhancement. The muscular layer of the bladder should be intact and not disturbed or infiltrated, a characteristic feature that distinguishes cystitis cystica and cystitis glandularis from a real bladder tumor. On CT, the scan shows irregular bladder wall thickening and multiple polypoid masses arising, often from both the lateral walls of the bladder and the base of the trigone (◘ Fig. 11.12.8).

◘ **Fig. 11.12.6** Plain radiograph of the pelvis shows complete bilateral calcification of the ureters (*arrowheads*) and the bladder (*arrows*) in a patient with bilharziasis

◘ **Fig. 11.12.7** Plain radiograph of the pelvis shows complete calcification of the bladder with the seminal vesicles (*arrowheads*) in a patient with bilharziasis

◘ **Fig. 11.12.8** Axial postcontrast CT illustration of the pelvis shows multiple polypoid masses arising from the right lateral posterior wall of the bladder with contrast enhancement representing the radiological findings in cystitis cystica and cystitis glandularis

### Signs on Ultrasound

- Hyperechoic bladder wall, due to calcification.
- Bilateral, nonsymmetrical, hyperechoic dilated ureters are often seen.

### Signs on Intravenous Urography

- Bilateral ureteric dilatation with hydronephrosis is often seen.
- Marked bladder dilatation may be seen due to bladder neck stenosis and hypertrophy of the trigon. This finding is only reported in Egypt.

## *Differential* Diagnoses and Related Diseases

*Katayama syndrome* is a disease characterized by acute systemic immune reaction similar to the one seen in schistosomiasis patients but is not caused by mature worms or eggs. The patient typically has no immunity, presenting with skin redness and irritation or urticaria (swimmer's urticaria) after 1–2 days of swimming or washing in infected water. Weeks later, the affected patient often presents with fever, headaches, chills, lack of appetite (anorexia), and abdominal pain. Neck stiffness and coma may occur. CBC shows eosinophilia in almost 90 % of cases. Imaging investigations are often nonspecific. The disease is believed to be caused by eosinophil-mediated toxicity leading to vasculitis and small vessel thrombosis.

### Further Reading

Jauréguiberry S, et al. Neurological involvement during Katayama syndrome. Lancet Infect Dis. 2008;8(1):9–10.

Lee G, et al. Case report: cystitis glandularis mimics bladder tumor: a case report and diagnostic characteristics. Int Urol Nephrol. 2005;37:713–5.

Maia Jr ACM, et al. Spinal cord compression secondary to epidural bilharzioma: case report. J Neuroimaging. 2007;17:367–70.

Manzella A, et al. Schistosomiasis of the liver. Abdom Imaging. 2008;33:144–50.

Palmer PES. Schistosomiasis. Semin Roentgenol. 1998; 33(1):6–25.

Peng SL. Rheumatic manifestations of parasitic diseases. Semin Arthritis Rheum. 2002c;31:228–47.

Singh I, et al. Cystitis cystica glandularis masquerading as a bladder tumor. Int Urol Nephrol. 2001;33:635–6.

Wong-You-Cheong JJ, et al. Inflammatory and nonneoplastic bladder masses: radiologic-pathologic correlation. RadioGraphics. 2006;26:1847–68.

## 11.13 Tuberculosis

Tuberculosis (TB) is a multisystemic, granulomatous disease caused by the bacilli *Mycobacterium tuberculosis*. There are two main groups of gram-negative bacilli that infect humans: *Mycobacterium tuberculosis* and *Mycobacterium bovine*. *M. tuberculosis* is an infection from human to human. Humans are infected by inhalation (pulmonary TB), by ingesting infected food or drinks (tonsillar and intestinal TB), or by wound contamination (rare). *M. bovine*, on the other hand, infects humans who come into contact with an infected mastitis cow.

TB bacteria have a body composed of protein with an attached polysaccharide and a capsule composed of lipids. TB bacteria do not produce endotoxins and are noninvasive. When neutrophils engulf the TB bacilli, they do not digest the bacilli because neutrophils lack the enzyme lipase, which is necessary to dissolve the bacterial capsule. The bacteria remain alive within the neutrophils until the neutrophils die, when the bacteria are again released into the blood stream. The pathogenesis of TB is due to the antibody reaction evoked by the protein nature of the bacteria. The body produces antibodies against the bacteria antigen, resulting in a hypersensitivity reaction causing granulomas (tubercles).

*Tubercle (proliferative tissue reaction)* is the unit reaction of TB. It is grossly composed of a grayish nodule 1–2 mm in size. Microscopically, it is composed of caseating necrosis of epithelioid cells. The epithelioid cells can join together to form large cells with horseshoe-shaped peripheral nuclei, called Langerhans giant cells. A tubercle is a granuloma with a caseating center. An infected person becomes tuberculin test positive usually 1–2 months after initial exposure. The caseous lesion has three prognoses: it may heal, it may enlarge and spread to the lymphatic or the blood stream, or it may form a cavity.

Necrotic TB lesions are the result of hypersensitive immune reactions to the bacteria in different body systems (hypersensitivity necrosis) and ischemia, because granuloma does not form angiogenesis and the vessels within the area of the granuloma develop endarteritis obliterans due to the chronic inflammatory reaction (ischemic necrosis). *Exudative tissue reaction* is of a special type and is seen in TB when the inflammatory reaction affects serosal tissue. This reaction is characterized by serous fluid formation and a few epithelioid cells and macrophages.

As TB is a multisystemic disease, manifestations of TB are different from organ to organ, with many manifestations having characteristic radiological features that are best addressed separately.

### Pulmonary TB

Patients with pulmonary TB classically present with fever, weight loss, chills, night sweats, cough, and hemoptysis. Diagnosis is established by staining *M. Tuberculosis* with acid-fast bacilli stain. Laboratory investigations often show an elevated erythrocyte sedimentation rate (ESR), anemia, mild hyponatremia (43 %), moderate leukocytosis, and hypercalcemia (27 %).

In the lungs, there are four outcomes of TB infection:

- *TB clearance*: the disease is cleared from the body with dormant residuals, as long as the immune system is functioning properly.
- *Primary (acute) TB*: this type is usually seen in children with widespread disease and less tissue destruction. The rate of primary TB is 90 % and depends on the body's innate immunity and hypersensitivity. The infection in primary TB is called *primary complex*, composed of tuberculous focus, regional lymphangitis, and lymphadenitis. It can occur in the lung (by inhalation), the tonsils, or the intestine (by ingestion), or (rarely) in the spleen (by wound infection via hematogenous spread). Primary pulmonary TB is classically located in the apical segment of the lower lobes or middle lobes. When the lesion is healed, it results in a focal calcified lesion known as *Ghon focus*. Ghon focus is composed of multiple aggregated tubercles, with TB lymphangitis due to the spread of the bacteria in the nearby lymphatic vessels. The disease can spread from one region of the lung to another via the bronchi (bronchogenic spread). It generally heals without sequelae, with few cases of generalized spread.
- *Latent (chronic) infection*: a condition characterized by *M. tuberculosis* infection without any clinical signs of active disease. The patient is at risk of reactivation.
- *TB reactivation*: a situation where an old latent TB infection gets reactivated into an acute disease and mostly occurs in patients with low immunity, such as HIV patients, diabetics, or children. TB reactivation occurs in the lung apices; it is thought that this location is preferred by the bacilli due to the high oxygen tension or the low lymph flow at the lung apices. Cavity formation in the lung apices is seen in up to 40 % of reactivation TB patients.

**Signs on Chest Radiographs**

- Primary TB presents with a pneumonic patch in the middle or lower lobes, with ipsilateral hilar lymphadenopathy (◻ Fig. 11.13.1). When the TB pneumonic patch regresses and calcifies, it results in Ghon lesion.
- *Ranke's complex*: Ghon lesion with ipsilateral calcified hilar lymphadenopathy.
- *Tuberculoma*: a round, smoothly circumscribed pulmonary nodule (<3 cm) that usually contains central calcification. It is seen at the common areas of TB infection (upper lobes and apical segment of

lower lobes). The main differential diagnosis of tuberculoma is "pulmonary hamartoma," which has the same tuberculoma features, central popcorn calcifications, and occurs anywhere within the lungs. Tuberculoma is diagnosed by its features and locations.

— *Apical fibrosis* (*Simon's focus*): old TB in the lung apices may result in chronic granulomatous reaction that causes lung fibrosis (◘ Fig. 11.13.2). The term "old TB" should be used with caution, as the TB may be chronic but still active. "Stable TB disease" requires 6 months of unchanged radiological features to be acclaimed.

— TB reactivation is classically seen as lung apices cavitary lesions (40 %) or noncavitary lung infiltration (4–9 %). A TB cavity tends to have thick irregular walls (◘ Fig. 11.13.3), and air–fluid level may be seen (9–21 %). Superimposed infection of the cavity with fungi can result in fungal ball (mycetoma/aspergilloma) within the cavity (halo sign).

— *Cicatrization atelectasis*: atelectasis of the upper lobes due to previous fibrosis from TB infection, with retraction of the hilum upward.

— *Bronchiectasis* may occur in up to 87 % of patients due to bronchial wall and parenchymal destruction. Bronchiectasis is seen as focally dilated bronchi with honeycomb, cystic interstitial pattern.

— *Broncholithiasis* is an uncommon complication of TB characterized by the presence of calcified materials within the bronchial tree.

— Pleural calcification is often seen unilaterally, especially with previous empyema.

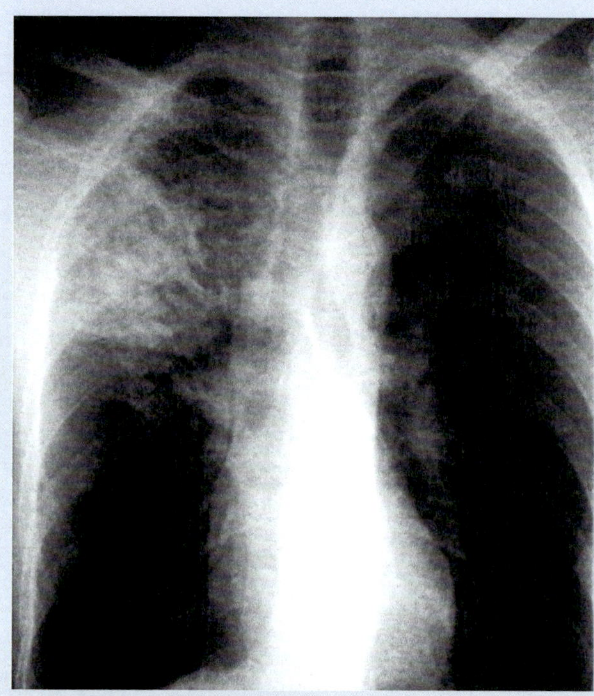

**Fig. 11.13.2**    Posteroanterior plain chest radiograph in a TB patient shows right apical fibrosis (Simon's focus)

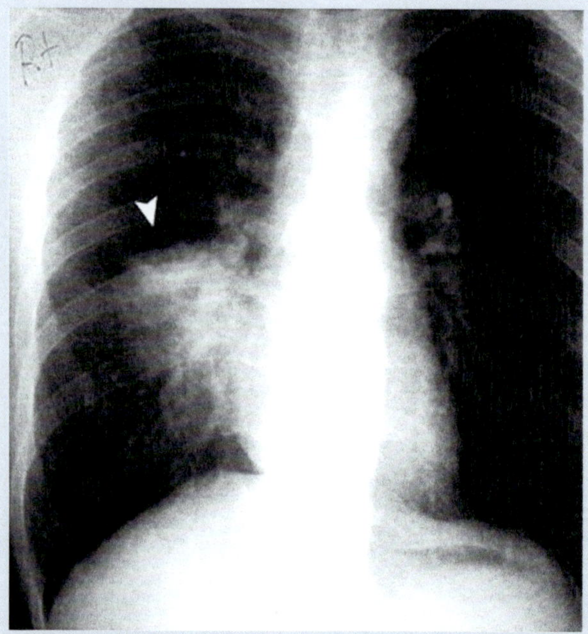

**Fig. 11.13.1**    Posteroanterior plain chest radiograph in a patient with primary TB shows a pneumonic patch in the right middle lung zone (*arrowhead*) with ipsilateral lymphadenopathy

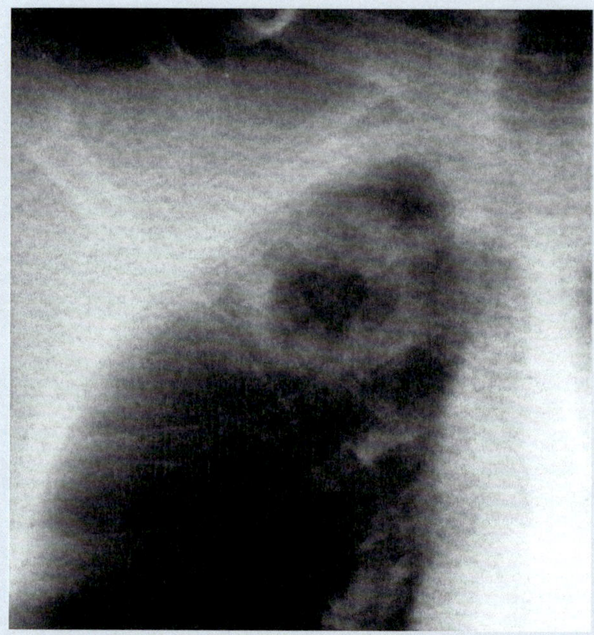

**Fig. 11.13.3**    Posteroanterior plain chest radiograph shows right apical TB cavity

### Signs on HRCT

- *Mycetoma* is seen as a fungal ball within a TB cavity at the lung apices in up to 55 % of patients (*halo sign*) (■ Fig. 11.13.4).
- *Tree-in-bud appearance* represents terminal bronchiole impaction with mucus, pus, or fluid, resulting in enhanced appearance of the normal branching bronchial tree that is normally invisible (■ Fig. 11.13.5). It is seen in diseases that affect the peripheral airways and cause material plugs deposition within them, such as TB, cystic fibrosis, and panbronchiolitis.

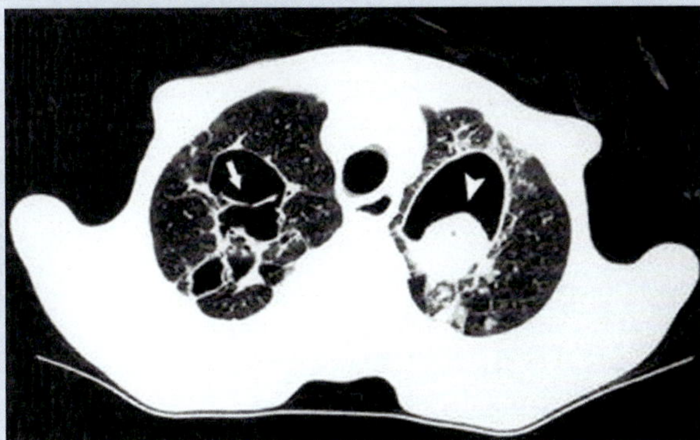

■ **Fig. 11.13.4** Axial lung window HRCT in a patient with TB shows apical left mycetoma with a halo sign (*arrowhead*) and marked bronchiectasis in the right lung (*arrow*)

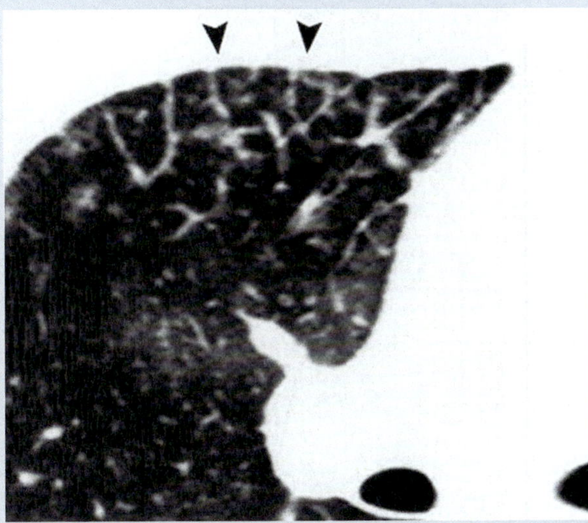

■ **Fig. 11.13.5** Axial lung window HRCT in a patient with TB shows peripheral tree-in-bud appearance (*arrowheads*)

### Signs on CT

*Rasmussen pulmonary aneurysm* is a rare phenomenon characterized by dilatation and weakening of the peripheral pulmonary artery wall from an adjacent TB cavity (■ Fig. 11.13.6). It is seen in up to 5 % of patients, and it may cause life-threatening hemoptysis. It is detected as TB inflammatory reaction or cavitary mass, with dilatation of the peripheral pulmonary artery adjacent to it.

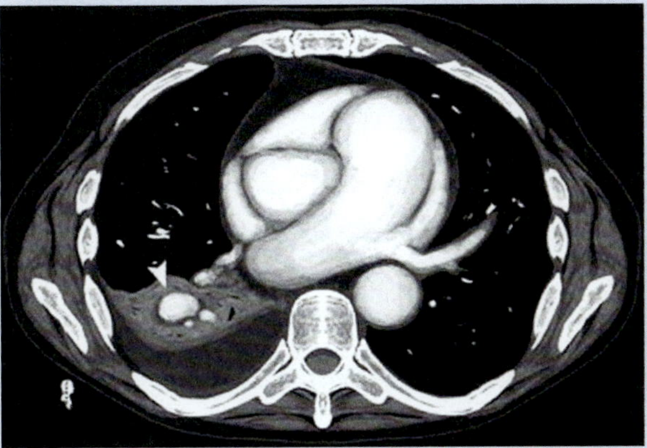

■ **Fig. 11.13.6** Axial postcontrast chest CT illustration demonstrates a mass of TB associated with dilated pulmonary vessels representing Rasmussen pulmonary aneurysm (*arrowhead*)

## Pleural TB

Pleural TB is the most common extrapulmonary manifestation of primary or reactivation TB, and it can alone be the only manifestation of primary TB.

The pleural fluid often contains granulomas and a few organisms. When the fluid contains pus, high protein content (>3 g/dL), and a large number of organisms, it is called *empyema*. Tuberculous empyema can be rarely caused by spinal TB draining into the pleural space via a sinus.

Patients with pleural TB present with pain during deep inspiration (pleuritic pain), fever, weight loss, and anorexia.

Chyliform (lymphatic) pleural effusion may occur in TB, with deposition of cholesterol within the pleural space. Fat–fluid or fat calcium level with calcified pleural margins may be seen on CT.

*Empyema necessitatis* is a rare situation that arises when the empyema spontaneously discharge through the parietal pleura into the chest wall, forming a subcutaneous abscess.

### Signs on Chest Radiograph and HRCT

- On plain radiograph, pleural effusion is seen as loss of the posterior and lateral costophrenic angles along with meniscus sign.
- Pleura thickening on CT is confirmed when the pleura is >2 mm in width.
- When the empyema calcifies, the CT scan shows empyema with calcified edges, a clinical condition called *fibrothorax* (◘ Fig. 11.13.7).
- Empyema necessitatis is detected as thickened pleural effusion with abscess formation that opens into the chest wall (◘ Fig. 11.13.8).

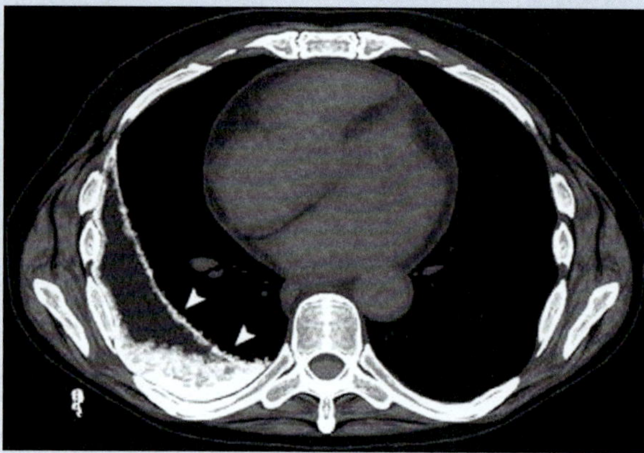

◘ **Fig. 11.13.7** Axial chest CT illustration demonstrates fibrothorax (*arrowheads*)

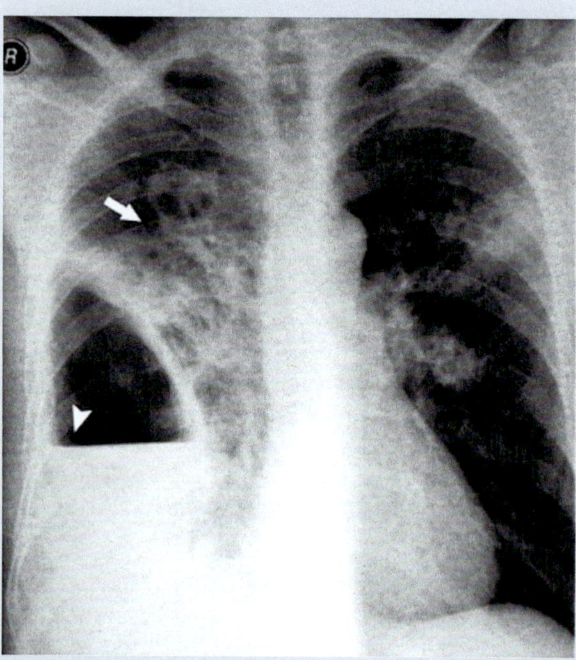

◘ **Fig. 11.13.8** Posteroanterior plain chest radiograph in a patient with old TB and chronic empyema that transformed into a lung abscess shows a huge right lung abscess (*arrowhead*) and bronchiectasis (*arrow*). The patient needed several pleural taps, and the abscess was beginning to open into the right lateral chest wall

## Miliary TB

Hematogenous spread of TB can be in small numbers causing no harm, moderate amount affecting one or two organs (isolated-organ TB), or in a diffuse large amount (miliary TB). In 5 % of primary TB patients, the infection is not contained within an organ and is disseminated into the bloodstream and the lymphatic system, resulting in miliary TB. The term "miliary" is given because the disseminated lesions (granulomas) are round and small, mimicking numerous millet seeds. Miliary TB in HIV patients arises when the CD4 count is <300/mL.

Miliary TB is divided into acute miliary TB or cryptic miliary TB. Acute miliary TB may be associated with hyponatremia, inappropriate secretion of antidiuretic hormone, or adrenal insufficiency. Cryptic miliary TB is characterized by silent TB foci that seed bacilli into the bloodstream from time to time; TB foci may be located within the lungs, kidneys, or lymph nodes.

### Signs on Chest Radiograph

- Miliary TB is seen as bilateral symmetrical interstitial nodular pattern (◘ Fig. 11.13.9). Absence of miliary pattern on chest radiograph does not rule out miliary TB.
- Bilateral pleural effusion may occur.

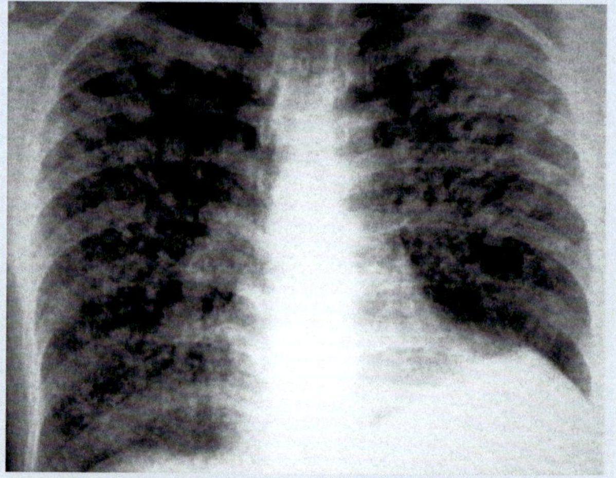

◘ **Fig. 11.13.9** Posteroanterior plain chest radiograph in a patient with miliary TB shows bilateral diffuse nodules in the lung fields representing miliary TB

### Signs on HRCT

Miliary TB shows multiple, bilateral small nodules (<3 cm in size) randomly distributed through the lungs (◘ Fig. 11.13.10).

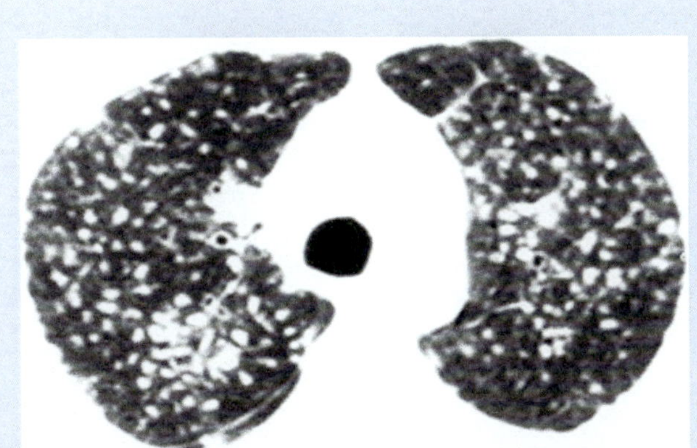



## Abdominal TB

Abdominal TB invades the abdomen, peritoneum, and pancreatobiliary system via hematogenous spread from a primary lung or reactivation TB or from swallowing infected milk. Although any structure can be involved, the ileocecal valve is the most frequently affected by granulomas, fibrosis, and later scarring.

Patients may present with fever, weight loss, diarrhea, and abdominal pain and distension. Duodenal TB may result in dyspepsia, while rectal TB may result in constipation (30 %) and passing fresh blood (hematochezia). Fistula-in-ano may arise due to anal TB. The chest radiograph may be normal in patients with abdominal TB in up to 60 % of cases.

TB peritonitis may develop causing ascites and omental and peritoneal thickening. TB peritonitis is divided into three forms: wet, fibrotic, and dry. Wet peritonitis is characterized by a large amount of viscous ascetic fluid (90 % of cases). Fibrotic peritonitis is characterized by large omental masses and intestinal adhesions, causing the omentum to form a hard mass on palpation. Dry or plastic peritonitis is characterized by fibrous peritoneal reaction, dens adhesions, and caseous nodules.

### Differential Diagnoses and Related Diseases

- *Bauhin's ileocecal valve syndrome* is a rare sporadic disease characterized by hypertrophic ileocecal valve in the absence of intestinal pathology. Patients classically present with vague abdominal pain, nausea, vomiting, diarrhea or constipation, and even active bleeding or melena. Differential diagnoses include TB, lymphoma, adenocarcinoma, and inflammatory bowel diseases.
- *Nonreactive TB* is a rare form of TB characterized by the formation large abscesses with large quantities of bacilli without granulomata. The abscesses may develop in the liver, lungs, or kidneys. Patients often present with fever, sepsis syndrome, and splenomegaly. This form of TB has been associated with AIDS, lymphoma, chronic steroid users, diabetics, and patients with hematological disorders.





## Hepatic TB

Hepatic TB is seen as a part of miliary TB and is characterized by hepatomegaly and liver failure. The bacilli reach the liver via hematogenous spread through the hepatic artery. TB can be one of the causes of hepatic peliosis.

*Hepatic peliosis* is a pathological condition characterized by segmentally or focally dilated liver sinusoids, with or without macroscopically visible blood-filled cysts formation, with no preferential location in the liver. The blood-filled cysts can be lined by hepatocytes (parenchymal type) or lined by endothelium and are based on aneurysmal dilatation of the central vein (phlebectatic type). Hepatic peliosis is caused by chronic wasting diseases like TB and malignancies, and it is also reported in long-term abuse of anabolic steroids or prolonged oral contraceptive use. Hepatic peliosis can be asymptomatic or causes liver failure, portal hypertension, or fatal intra-abdominal bleeding. Peliosis may also occur in the spleen, bone marrow, and lymph nodes.

### Signs on CT
- Liver tuberculomas are abscesses that are seen on CT as multiple, scattered, hypodense lesions through the liver, 1–3 cm in size (◘ Fig. 11.13.11).
- Large abscesses show ring enhancement after contrast injection.
- Hepatic peliosis has nonspecific features, and most reported features are variable. Histopathology is the definite diagnosing method. The most constant reported features are hypodense liver lesions that do not show mass effect over the adjacent vessels. The masses show a variable degree of enhancement, depending on the connection with the normal liver sinusoids. These masses represent areas of hepatic necrosis with internal hemorrhagic cysts formation.

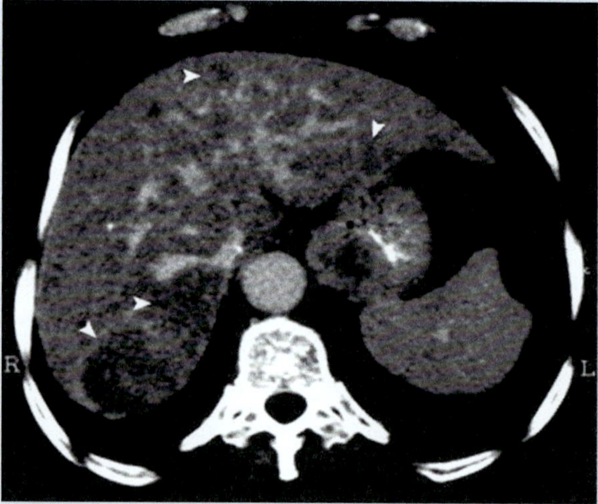

◘ **Fig. 11.13.11**   Axial abdominal-enhanced CT shows multiple hypodense lesions in a patient with liver TB representing tuberculomas (*arrowheads*)

### Signs on CT and MRI
- *Tuberculous meningitis*: there is thickening and enhancement of the meninges after contrast injection, along with signs of hydrocephalus due to basal meninges obstruction. Tuberculous meningitis usually occurs due to rupture of parenchymal granuloma into the subarachnoid space. Meningeal enhancement may persist for years after successful TB therapy.
- *Tuberculomas*: seen as multiple nodular, ring-enhancing lesions (<1 cm). Only active tuberculomas enhance with contrast, while nonactive tuberculomas will not enhance. Tuberculoma may show mass effect over the adjacent brain parenchyma.
- *Tuberculous abscess*: seen as a hypodense area surrounded by edema and uniform ring enhancement postcontrast injection (◘ Fig. 11.13.12).

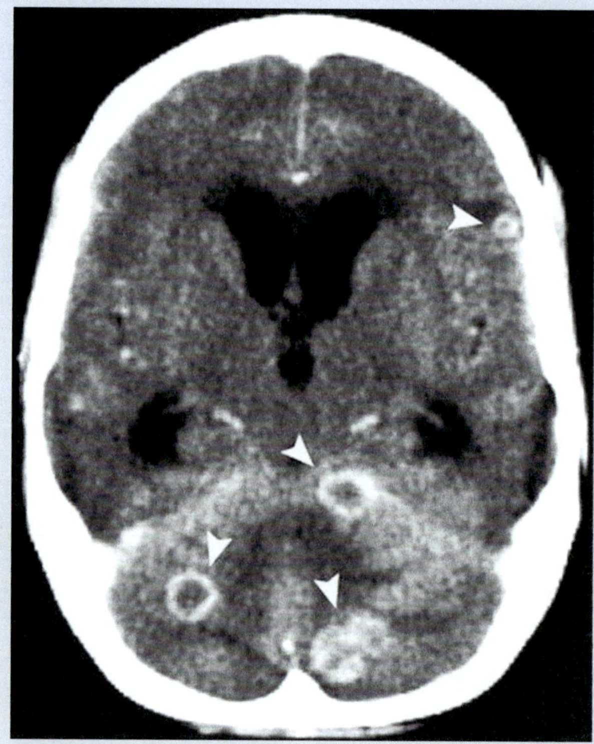

◘ **Fig. 11.13.12**   Axial postcontrast CT image shows multiple tuberculous abscesses in a patient with disseminated TB (*arrowheads*)

## Central Nervous System TB

Intracranial TB can occur without evidence of pulmonary TB. It occurs in 10 % of AIDS patients. Up to 60 % of patients with intracranial TB are younger than 20 years.

TB of the central nervous system may occur in the form of meningitis (often in children), abscess, tuberculomas, or spinal cord disease. Patients may present with seizures, cognitive changes, or neurological deficits.

## Genitourinary TB

Renal TB commonly occurs due to hematogenous spread of *M. tuberculosis* from adjacent primary focus, usually from the lungs. The urinary tract is infected in 15 % of patients.

In the kidneys, there are papillary lesions forming multiple granulomas and irregular renal cavities that may communicate with the calyces.

Patients classically present with burning micturation, frequent urination due to contracted bladder (29 %), renal colic (13 %), and (uncommonly) hematospermia. Patients with TB urinary symptoms do not respond to the usual antibiotics.

Epididymitis in males and tubo-ovarian abscess and infertility in females may be seen when the genital organs are infected with TB.

> **Signs on IVU**
> - There are strictures of the calyces and calcifications within the renal parenchyma (classic) (◘ Fig. 11.13.13).
> - The presence of psoas abscess supports the diagnosis of renal TB.
> - Ureteral strictures may present at the infundibulum, the ureteropelvic junction, or the distal ureters (sawtooth appearance). The ureter may become a straight rigid tube, known as *pipestem ureter*.
> - End-stage renal TB results in a small, shrunk, and fibrotic kidney with poor function and parenchymal calcifications (putty kidney).

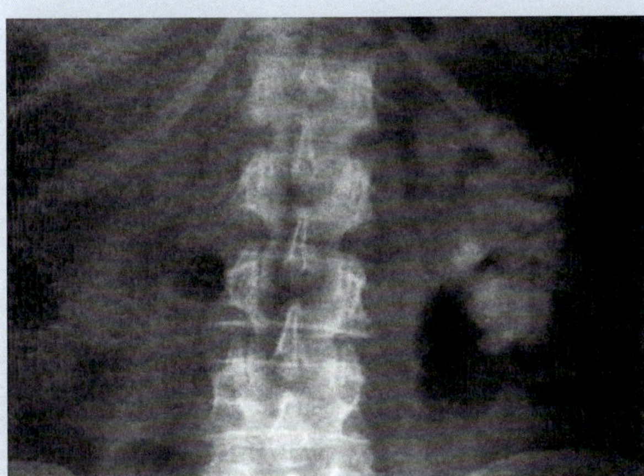

◘ **Fig. 11.13.13** Plain abdominal radiograph shows unilateral left renal parenchymal calcification in a patient with TB

> **Signs on CT**
> - Calcifications within the renal parenchyma are seen in up to 50 % of cases.
> - Fibrotic strictures of the infundibulum, renal pelvis, and ureters (diagnostic).
> - *Putty kidney* is a term used to describe end-stage TB kidney, characterized by a shrunken kidney with extensive calcification that is associated with autonephrectomy (◘ Fig. 11.13.14).
> - *Phantom calyx* is a kidney in which no collecting system element can be identified.

> - *Thimble bladder* is a very small bladder with reduced capacity due to thick extensive calcification of the bladder wall.

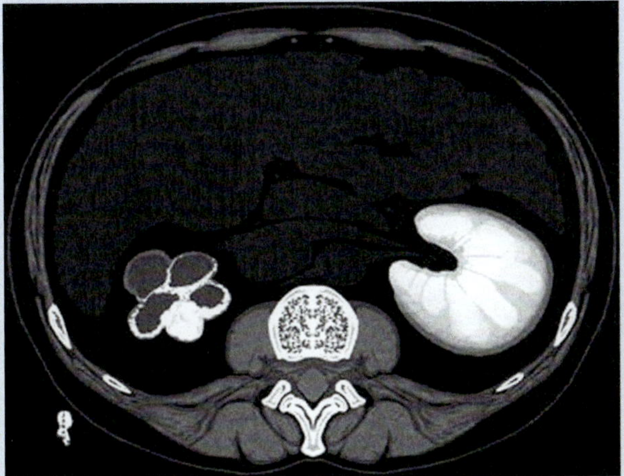

◘ **Fig. 11.13.14** Axial postcontrast abdominal CT illustration demonstrates right putty kidney

## Musculoskeletal TB

Musculoskeletal TB is an uncommon condition that occurs in 1–3 % of patients. *M. tuberculosis* often infects the musculoskeletal system via hematogenous spread.

Any bone can be affected, but the spine, hip, and knee are commonly affected, usually in young patients. Spinal TB is called *Pott's disease*, and it often affects the thoracic spine (50 % of cases). Pott's disease is characterized by kyphosis, cold abscess, and paraplegia. *Cold abscess* is a localized caseous collection that can be seen in the lymph nodes, TB of joints, and in Pott's disease. In Pott's disease, it occurs due to collapsed TB-infected vertebra with pus released into the adjacent paraspinal compartments. It can be seen as a retropharyngeal abscess (cervical Pott's disease), retrocardial abscess (thoracic Pott's disease), and psoas abscess (lumbar Pott's disease).

Patients often present with progressive focal back pain and muscle spasm. Neurological deficits, cauda equine compression syndrome, and paraplegia due to cord compression are uncommon neurological complications of Pott's disease. Paraplegia occurs in Pott's disease (10 % of cases) due to cord compression from a collapsed vertebra or due to spinal cord infarction from closed vessels due to endarteritis obliterans.

*Tuberculous arthritis* commonly affects one joint (monoarthritis). The hip or the knee joint is frequently affected. Patients present with progressive pain, swelling of the affected joint with loss of function due to septic arthritis, and synovial pannus formation.

*Spina ventosa* is a term used to describe a form of TB osteomyelitis where there is underlying bone destruction, overlying periosteal thickening, and fusiform expansion of the bone. Very rarely, TB osteomyelitis can result after vaccination with Bacille Calmette–Guérin (BCG) vaccine (*BCG osteomyelitis*). BCG vaccine is used for preventing TB in many areas of the world, and it is composed of a live attenuated strain of *Mycobacterium bovis*. BCG osteomyelitis usually arises in infants and children with low immunity, with a very low incidence (1 or 2 per several million vaccine recipients). Symptoms arise during a period ranging from a few months to 5 years postvaccination. The lesions occur in the epiphysis and metaphysis and may cross the growth plate. BCG osteomyelitis is radiographically identical to TB osteomyelitis. Diagnosis requires culture of the BCG strain for conformation.

## Differential Diagnoses and Related Diseases

*Mycobacterium marinum flexor tenosynovitis*: *M. marinum* is an atypical mycobacterial infection that inhabits saltwater fish and swimming pools. Patients are often infected with *M. marinum* after abrasions or puncture to the hand while working with aquariums. Lesions start to appear 2–4 weeks after inoculation in the form of focal tenosynovitis of the hand, usually with lymphadenopathy in the ipsilateral arm. Diagnosis is often delayed for months due to lack of clinical suspicion and is often mistaken for rheumatoid arthritis or gout arthropathy. Diagnosis is usually difficult and requires open surgical biopsy of the synovium with histological examination. Ziehl–Neelsen stain is often negative, and diagnosis is established by modified AFB (Fite) stain, which will stain the *M. marinum*. On MRI, there is flexor tenosynovitis with hypertrophied synovium und contrast enhancement similar to the image seen in chronic granulomatous diseases. Unlike acute purulent tenosynovitis, the bone and the underlying muscles are rarely affected (characteristic finding). Tenosynovitis with normal muscle and bone marrow signal on postcontrast MRI in a fisherman or a patient dealing with aquariums should bring *M. marinum* tenosynovitis to mind.

**Signs on Radiograph**
- Vertebral end plate irregularities with decreased high of the disk intervertebral space (■ Fig. 11.13.15). In contrast to Pott's disease, metastases destroy the vertebral bodies and spare the disk spaces, while in Pott's diseases both vertebral body destruction and intervertebral disk space reduction are found.
- *Step-off kyphosis*: there is loss of the anterior vertebral end plates with herniation of the intervertebral disk into the vertebral bodies, causing kyphosis.

- *Gibbus deformity* is referred to as destruction of multiple thoracic vertebrae, causing angular kyphosis.
- Paraspinal (cold abscess) and psoas abscesses may develop due to extension of the infection to the nearby structures.
- The affected joint in tuberculous arthritis shows soft-tissue mass swelling with loss of the joint surface definition (■ Fig. 11.13.16). Articular cartilage destruction and erosion are commonly seen.
- *Phemister's triad*: juxta-articular osteoporosis, gradual joint space narrowing, and peripheral osseous erosions. It suggests TB arthritis, but is not specific.
- *Spina ventosa* is typically seen in the short bones of the hands and feet as cyst-like cavities with expansion of the diaphyses and soft-tissue swelling (*TB dactylitis*).

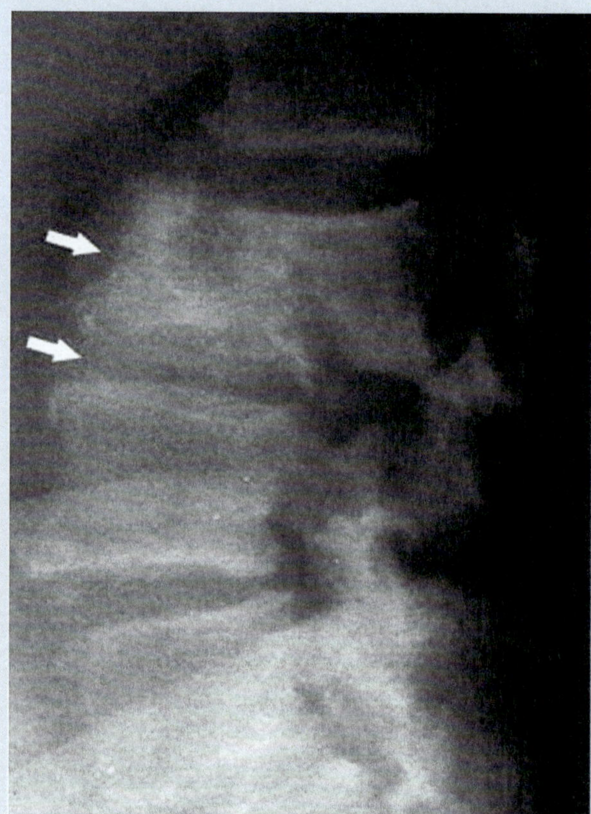

■ **Fig. 11.13.15**  Lateral plain radiograph of the thoracic spine in a patient with thoracic Pott's disease shows destruction of the vertebral body and narrowing of the intervertebral disk space (*arrows*)

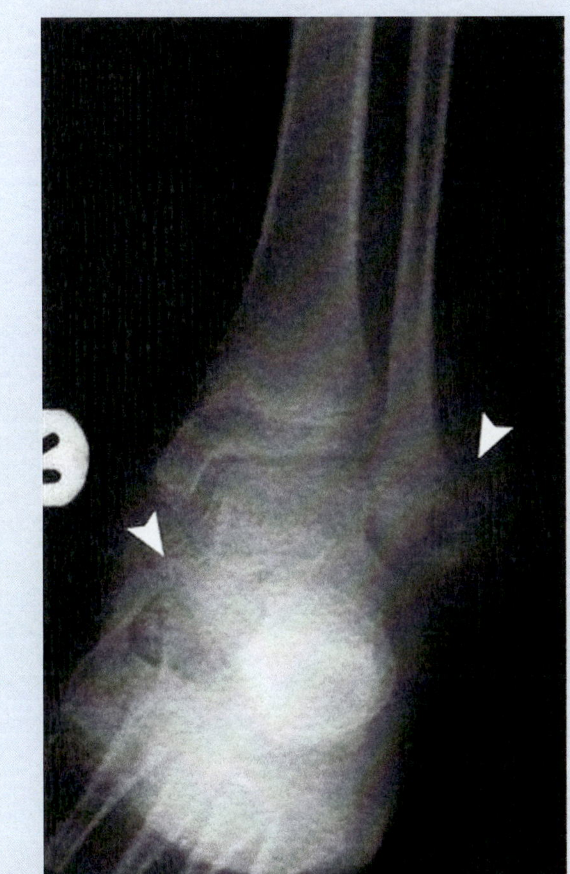

**Fig. 11.13.16** Plain radiograph of the ankle in a young patient with tuberculous arthritis shows lateral ankle soft-tissue swelling with bone destruction of the distal fibular epiphysis and the metatarsal bones, suggesting osteomyelitis (*arrowheads*)

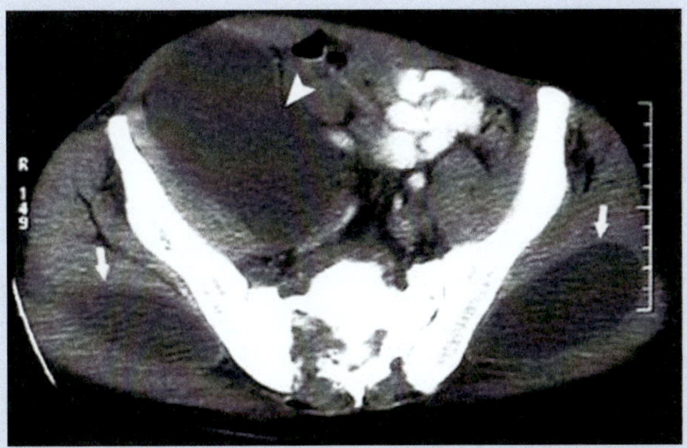

**Fig. 11.13.17** Axial pelvic CT in a patient with Pott's disease shows a large right psoas abscess (*arrowhead*), which drains into both gluteal muscles (*arrows*)

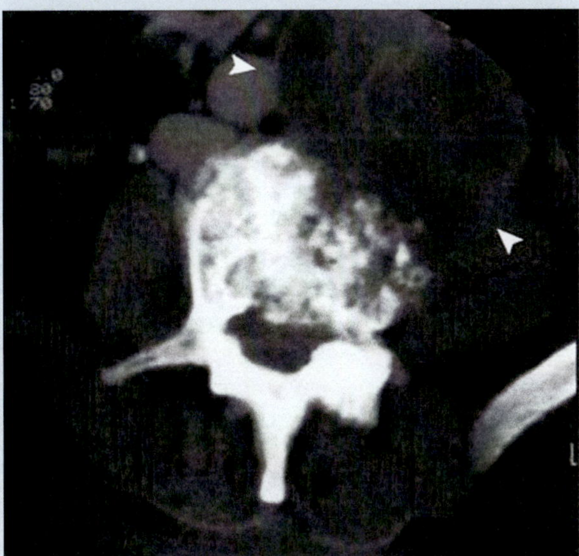

**Fig. 11.13.18** Axial nonenhanced vertebral CT shows vertebral destruction in a patient with Pott's disease, with left paraspinal cold abscess formation (*arrowheads*)

### Signs on CT

- Psoas abscess is seen as an enlarged psoas muscle with a hypodense center due to abscess formation (**Fig. 11.13.17**). Rim enhancement after contrast injection is typically seen.
- Paraspinal cold abscess is detected as abnormal fluid collection adjacent to vertebral destruction (**Fig. 11.13.18**).
- *Borrowing abscess* is a pathological situation characterized by tracts (sinuses) linking the infected vertebra with the peritoneal cavity. There may also be sinuses linking the infected vertebra with the muscles or the skin.
- Formation of an epidural abscess is the most feared complication of Pott's disease, and it develops in 10–47 % of patients.

## Tuberculous Lymphadenitis

Tuberculous lymphadenitis is a common cause of lymphadenopathy in primary TB patients. It may occur in the pulmonary hilar nodes, cervical lymph nodes (called *scrofula*), the mesenteric nodes, the para-aortic nodes, and the axillary and the inguinal nodes. *Tabes mesenterica* is a term used to describe primary TB lymphadenopathy of the mesentery.

Nodal infection arises from hematogenous or lymphatic TB dissemination. Clinical presentation depends on the lymph nodes affected. The affected nodes may erode into the adjacent organs, resulting in draining sinuses.

Tuberculous pericarditis that may lead to constrictive pericarditis may occur due to invasion of the pericardium from the adjacent tuberculous hilar lymphadenitis. It is a rare complication that may occur in 1% of cases. Also, direct bacilli invasion of the mediastinum from the adjacent hilar tuberculous lymphadenopathy may result in inflammation of the mediastinal structures (mediastinitis).

### Signs on Sonography and PD

- TB cervical lymphadenopathy shows different flow pattern signals on power Doppler sonography. The most frequent pattern is *hilar* flow, in which the flow signal branches from the hilus radially. The second pattern is *peripheral*, where the signal is spotted flowing along the periphery of the enlarged node. A mixed pattern between the hilar and the peripheral can be seen.
- Avascular nodes with no flow signal on PD may be seen and attributed to caseous necrosis within the nodes.

### Signs on CT

- Enlarged, circular nodes with a mean size of 20 mm. Calcification may be seen.
- Center caseation of the nodes is seen as low-attenuated center of the enlarged nodes (■ Fig. 11.13.19).
- After contrast administration, enhancement can be peripheral (characteristic of TB lymphadenopathy), homogeneous, or homogeneous mixed with peripheral enhancement.

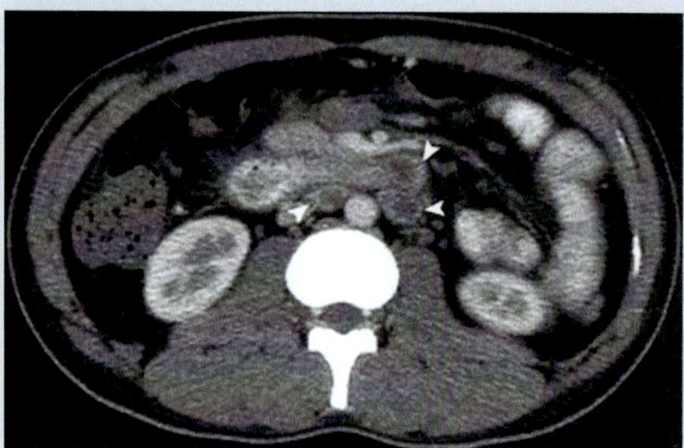

■ **Fig. 11.13.19** Axial abdominal postcontrast CT in a patient with TB shows enlarged para-aortic lymph nodes with a hypodense center (*arrowheads*)

## Dermatological TB

Cutaneous TB is generally classified into true cutaneous TB or tuberculid TB. In true cutaneous TB, also known as *tuberculous gumma*, multiple, painless cold abscesses form on the skin due to secondary metastasis of the bacteria from a primary focus via hematological routes. In contrast, tuberculid is a skin reaction to tuberculous lesions in other organs.

Tuberculous gumma is a very rare lesion, and it has been reported to occur in patients with no primary TB infection after trauma or venous blood test with a sterile needle, a phenomenon known as *pseudo-Köbner's phenomenon*. The lesion arises at the site of the trauma or the needle injection.

*Scrofuloderma* is an atypical dermatological manifestation of TB in tropical countries. Scrofula is a Latin word meaning "weal resistance to disease." Scrofuloderma arises due to infection of the skin with TB overlying another TB process, usually tuberculous lymphadenitis. It is commonly seen in the pediatric age group and typically located in the parotid, submandibular, supraclavicular, and lateral aspect of the neck regions (■ Fig. 11.13.20).

*Lupus vulgaris* is TB of the skin characterized by reddish-brown plaques located on the skin of the face and the neck. The term "lupus vulgaris" was given to the lesion because the skin looks as if the patient were attacked by a wolf (■ Fig. 11.13.21). The condition may transform into squamous cell carcinoma.

*Erythema induratum* (*Bazin's disease*) is a rare form of nodular vasculitis and lobular panniculitis (■ Fig. 11.13.22). The dermal lesions are typically seen in the legs. The lesions are caused by hypersensitivity reaction to the tubercle bacillus antigen. Patients with erythema induratum have a positive tuberculin skin test.

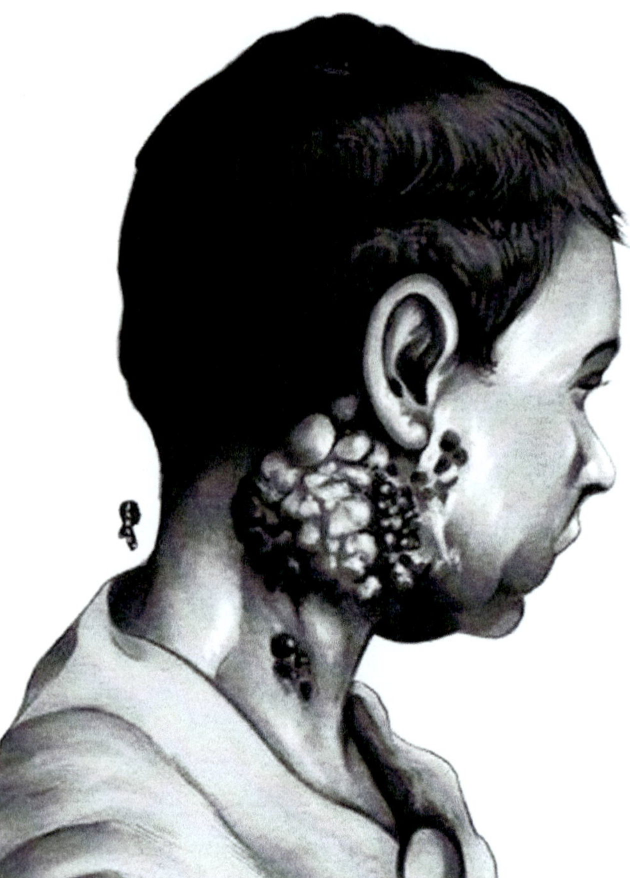

■ **Fig. 11.13.20** An illustration demonstrates scrofula at the lateral side of the neck

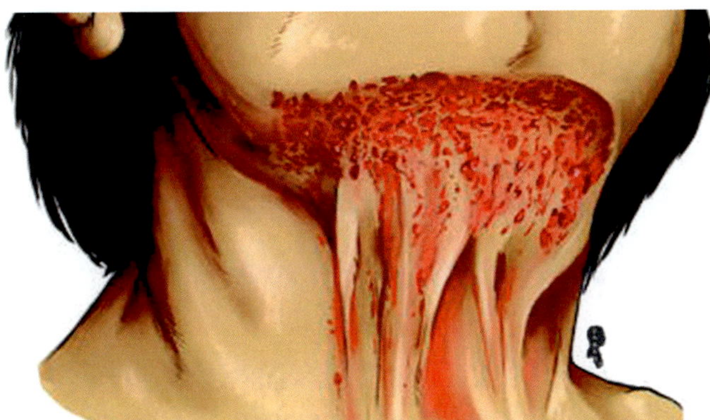

Fig. 11.13.21   An illustration demonstrates lupus vulgaris

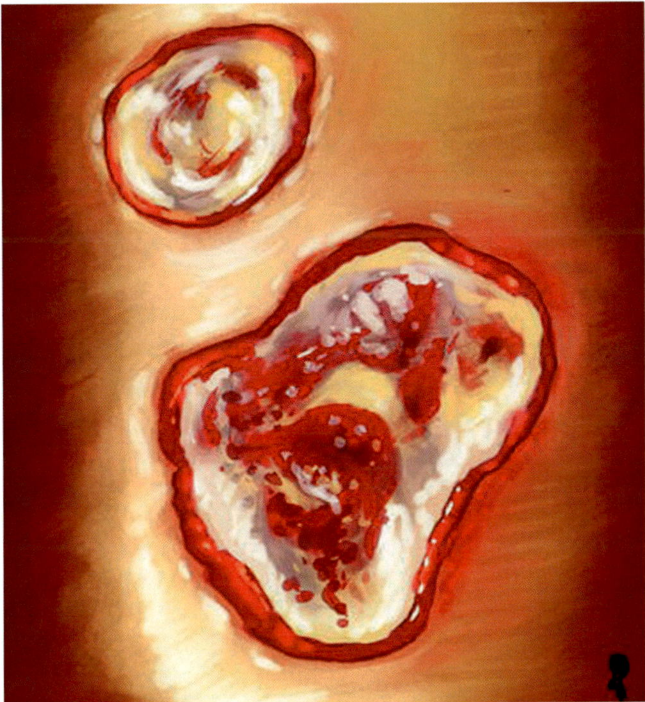

Fig. 11.13.22   An illustration demonstrates erythema induratum of Bazin

## Further Reading

Ahuja A, et al. Power Doppler sonography of cervical lymph-adenopathy. Clin Radiol. 2001;56:965–9.

Aslam N, et al. Pseudo-Koebner phenomenon: unusual manifestation of tuberculosis after venepuncture. Injury Extra. 2005;36:479–82.

Castaner E, et al. Congenital and acquired pulmonary artery anomalies in the adult: radiologic overview. RadioGraphics. 2006;26:349–71.

Dyer RB, et al. Classic signs in uroradiology. RadioGraphics. 2004;24:S247–80.

Funato M, et al. Refractory osteomyelitis caused by bacilli Calmette-Guérin vaccination: a case report. Diagn Microbiol Infect Dis. 2007;59:89–91.

Johnson MD, et al. Tuberculosis and HIV infection. Dis Mon. 2006;52:420–7.

Kanabar P. Tuberculosis of the lumbar spine. Indian J Orthop. 2005;39(2):18–89.

Kim HY, et al. Thoracic sequelae and complications of tuberculosis. RadioGraphics. 2001;21:839–60.

Lazarus AA, et al. Abdominal tuberculosis. Dis Mon. 2007a;53:32–8.

Lazarus AA, et al. Pleural tuberculosis. Dis Mon. 2007b;53:16–21.

Lazarus AA, et al. Tuberculous lymphadenitis. Dis Mon. 2007c;53:10–5.

Lee JJ, et al. High resolution chest CT in patients with pulmonary tuberculosis: characteristic findings before and after antituberculous therapy. Eur J Radiol. 2008;67:100–4.

Ludwig B, et al. Musculoskeletal tuberculosis. Dis Mon. 2007;53:39–45.

Lupi O, et al. Tropical dermatology: bacterial tropical diseases. J Am Acad Dermatol. 2006b;54:559–78.

Miller WT, et al. Tuberculosis in the normal host: radiological findings. Semin Roentgenol. 1993;28(2):109–18.

Myers JN, et al. Miliary, central nervous system, and genitourinary tuberculosis. Dis Mon. 2007;53:22–31.

Nesher E, et al. Bauhin's ileocecal valve syndrome – a rare cause for small-bowel obstruction: report of a case. Dis Colon Rectum. 2006;49:527–9.

Pereira JM, et al. Abdominal tuberculosis: imaging feature. Eur J Radiol. 2005;55:173–80.

Picard C, et al. Massive hemoptysis due to Rasmussen aneurysm: detection with helicoidal CT angiography and successful steel coil embolization. Intensive Care Med. 2003;29:1837–9.

Quast TM, et al. Pathogenesis and clinical manifestations of pulmonary tuberculosis. Dis Mon. 2006;52:413–9.

Rademarker M, et al. Erythema induratum (Bazin's disease). J Am Acad Dermatol. 1989;21:750–5.

Steinke K, et al. Unusual cross-sectional imaging findings in hepatic peliosis. Eur Radiol. 2003;13:1916–9.

Vidal D, et al. Tuberculous gumma following venepuncture. Br J Dermatol. 2001;144:601–3.

Wongworawat MD, et al. A prolonged case of Mycobacterium marinum flexor tenosynovitis: radiographic and histological correlation, and review of the literature. Skeletal Radiol. 2003;32:542–5.

Yun JS, et al. Latent tuberculosis infection. Dis Mon. 2006;52:441–5.

## 11.14 Typhoid Fever (Salmonellosis)

Typhoid fever (TF) is a disease caused by systemic infection with the bacterium *Salmonella typhi*. The occurrence of TF is high in developing countries due to poor sanitation.

Between 1900 and 1907, TF was notoriously linked to the name of an Irish cook in New York City named "Mary Mallon." Mallon, notoriously known as "typhoid Mary," was the first person defined as a "healthy carrier" of TF in the United States. Patients who are silent carriers of *S. typhi* can transmit the disease to other persons via feco-oral transmission. The carrier can transmit the bacteria by touching food or water with a dirty hand.

Typical manifestations of salmonellosis include fever, constipation during the first week of fever, diarrhea during the second week of fever, splenomegaly, rose spots, encephalopathy (*typhoid state*), leucopenia, and abdominal distension that may be complicated by intestinal perforation in the third week of fever (commonly in the terminal ileum). Typhoid encephalopathy typically occurs in the third week of fever.

Atypical manifestations of TF include psoas pyomyositis, splenic abscess, and (later) rupture, hepatic abscess, cerebellar ataxia, pneumonia, and vertebral osteomyelitis. These atypical manifestations are attributed to the bacteremia encountered during the first week of fever.

*Typhoid osteomyelitis* is a very rare complication of TF, with widespread bacteremia. It may develop years after the initial infection with a widespread disease. Usually, the patient does not show any spinal or skeletal involvement during the active intestinal disease. Patients with typhoid osteomyelitis often present with nonspecific lower back pain, without fever. A previous history of TF may be the only clue to the diagnosis of typhoid osteomyelitis. Raised erythrocyte sedimentation rate and positive blood cultures are found in 50–70 % of cases.

The liver manifestations of TF fall into three categories: asymptomatic patient, hepatomegaly with abnormal liver functions, and hepatic disease as the main manifestation of TF (*typhoid hepatitis*). On histopathology, the bacteria are found within the reticuloendothelial system, causing hyperplasia of the Kupffer cells (*typhoid nodules*).

Clinicopathologically, TF is diagnosed by a positive *Widal test*; however, a negative test result does not rule it out. The Widal test is only positive in the second week. Bacterial culture or isolation of the bacteria from the urine or the stools confirms the diagnosis of TF. Ultrasound is helpful in diagnosing TF within the first week, especially with high suspicion.

## Signs on CT

— Hepatic and splenic abscesses may be encountered on contrast-enhanced liver CT as multiple hypodense lesions, with characteristic rim enhancement within enlarged liver and spleen (◘ Fig. 11.14.1).

— Rarely, splenic infarction may be seen in cases of severe bacteremia as a hypodense area, commonly located at the periphery, with no contrast enhancement after contrast injection.

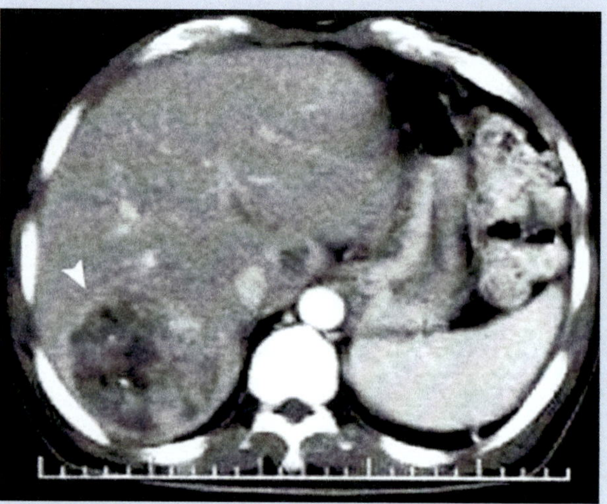

◘ **Fig. 11.14.1**   Axial postcontrast abdominal CT shows liver abscess developed in a patient after typhoid septicemia (*arrowhead*)

## Signs on US

— Hepatosplenomegaly may be present, especially during the second week.

— Uncommonly, splenic or hepatic abscesses may be found as multiple hypoechoic lesions.

— Increased bowel wall thickness is a common finding due to diarrhea and intestinal infection (commonly at the terminal ileum).

— Enlarged mesenteric lymph nodes with a diameter ranging from 8 to 34 mm.

— The gall bladder wall may be distended and thickened (>4 mm). Positive sonographic Murphy's sign plus increased vascular Doppler signal of the gallbladder wall indicate acute acalculous cholecystitis. In sonographic Murphy's sign, the probe has to be kept steady in the subcostal region in the right upper quadrant, and the patient must be asked to take a deep breath. If the patient stops breathing while the probe is still, then the sign is positive (exactly like the manual surgical Murphy's sign examination).

## Signs on Vertebral Plain Radiograph and MRI

— On plain radiographs, erosion of the vertebral end plates may be seen without evidence of diffuse vertebral destruction, according to the stage and severity of the osteomyelitis (◘ Fig. 11.14.2).

— On MRI, irregular end plates, erosions, vertebral disk infiltration, with high signal intensity on T2W images representing edema may be seen.

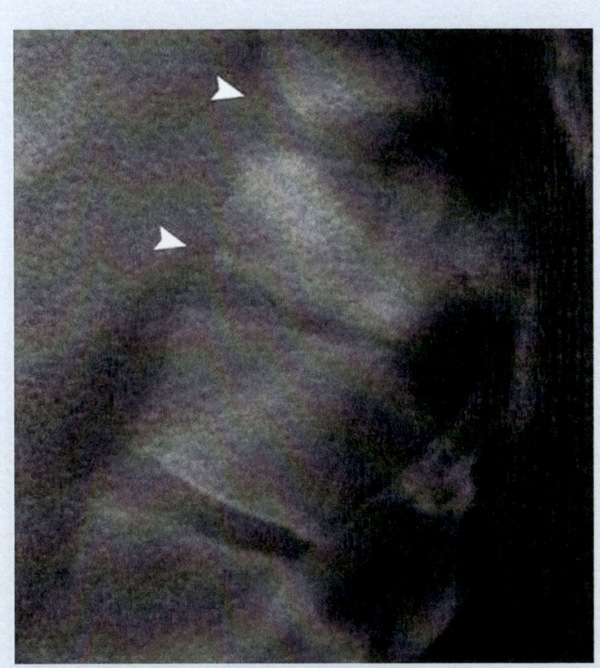



## Further Reading


Crichton EP, et al. Typhoid osteomyelitis of spine treated with chloramphenicol. Can Med Assoc J. 1953;69:529–30.

Dutta TK, et al. Atypical manifestations of typhoid fever. J Postgrad Med. 2001;47:248–51.

George P, et al. 2007. A sinister presentation of typhoid fever. Indian J Nephrol 17(4), 176–7.

Hart JL, et al. Life-threatening colonic haemorrhage in typhoid fever: successful angiographic localization and platinum microcoil embolization of several resources. Clin Radiol. 2008;63:727–30.

Karande SC, et al. Typhoid fever in a 7 month old infant. J Postgrad Med. 1995;41(4):108–9.

Khan FY, et al. Typhoid osteomyelitis of the lumbar spine. Hong Kong Med J. 2006;12:391–3.

Mateen MA, et al. Ultrasound in the diagnosis of typhoid fever. Indian J Pediatr. 2006;73(8):681–5.

Mehta LK, et al. Infarction of spleen in typhoid fever. Saudi Med J. 2007;28(2):271–2.

Mirsadraee M, et al. Typhoid myelopathy or typhoid hepatitis: a matter of debate. Indian J Med Microbiol. 2007;25(4):351–3.

Pandey A, et al. Typhoid sigmoid colon perforation in an 18-month-old boy. World J Pediatr. 2008;4(4):305–7.

Yüksel M, et al. Multiple splenic abscesses in a child as a complication of typhoid fever. Firat Tip Dergisi. 2005;10(2): 80–2.


## 11.15 Malaria

Malaria is a mosquito-borne disease, caused by the protozoan parasite *Plasmodium*. There are four main varieties of the genus *Plasmodium*: *P. falciparum, P. vivax, P. malariae,* and *P. ovale.*

Transmission of malaria is by the anopheline mosquito or occasionally by blood transfusion. The majority of the endemic areas are located within sub-Saharan Africa and Southeast Asia.

The clinical presentation of malaria is variable, ranging from a simple, mild flu-like illness to the full-blown disease of encephalopathy and intermittent fever. It must be on the list of differential diagnosis in any patient with unexplained symptoms returning from areas where malaria is endemic. Some patients possess immunity against malaria, especially people in endemic areas who have repeated infections or patients with hemoglobinopathies such as sickle cell disease and β-thalassemia.

Most mortality cases of malaria are related to the *P. falciparum* variant. The classical presentation is a febrile illness with cyclical fever, rigors, and chills; however, the disease is rarely present with its classical description. Additional symptoms include abdominal pain, vomiting, and mild diarrhea. The nonsevere malaria illness may be indistinguishable from any febrile illness caused by any infection. The severe form often presents with anemia, hypoglycemia, acidosis, and multisystemic manifestations.

The most common neurological symptom of *P. falciparum* encephalopathy is deep coma, which is defined as the inability to localize a painful stimulus in a patient with *P. falciparum* in whom other causes of encephalopathy have been excluded. Patients with *P. falciparum* coma typically have their eyes open, and seizures develop in approximately 70 % of cases. Sequelae of *P. falciparum* encephalopathy include hemiplegia (42 %), behavioral disorder (24 %), epilepsy (24 %), and blindness (8 %).

Respiratory abnormalities due to malaria have one or more of four abnormalities: deep, gasp-like breathing due to metabolic acidosis (*Kussmaul's breathing*), hyperventilation without acidosis, hypoventilation with nystagmus and excessive salivation due to status epilepticus, and periodic respiration associated with abnormalities in the papillary reflexes.

Anemia in malaria arises due to the parasitic infection of the red blood cells during the asexual life cycle, due to bone marrow suppression by the disease, or from iron deficiency due to poor intake. Hepatic disease with elevated liver enzymes is common due to the parasite cycle.

Rarely, malaria can cause rheumatic-like arthritis or polymyositis-like syndrome. The role of radiology in malaria is to monitor disease progression and therapy response or to detect complications. Diagnosis is essentially made by identifying the parasite by thick and thin blood films under microscopy.

## Differential Diagnoses and Related Diseases

*Hyperractive malarial splenomegaly (HMS) (tropical splenomegaly syndrome)* is a pathological condition characterized by splenomegaly due to disturbance in the T-lymphocyte control of the humoral response to recurrent malaria. HMS is recognized as a distinct entity from the splenic enlargement directly resulting from malarial parasitemia. Patients are typically young adults from a malarial area, presenting with persistent moderate to marked splenomegaly, which may be progressive or fluctuating in degree but does not spontaneously regress and which may at times give rise to severe pain. Laboratory investigations in HMS show pancytopenia with very high serum IgM levels and malaria antibody titers and an absence of malaria pigment in circulating erythrocytes, circulating monocytes, or tissue macrophages.

### Signs on Radiographs
Chest radiographs may show signs of bronchoalveolar edema or patchy pneumonic infiltrations.

### Signs on US
- Nonspecific splenomegaly is often found, while hepatomegaly is classically absent. However, absence of splenomegaly does not rule out malaria.
- Splenic infarction may be seen as a hypoechoic peripheral wedge-shaped area.
- Signs of portal hypertension may be seen in advanced liver disease.

### Signs on CT
- In the acute stage of the coma, profound brain edema with compressed ventricles is often found due to intraparenchymal inflammation.
- In the chronic stage, ventricular dilatation and brain parenchymal atrophy are commonly found.
- Severe brain edema may cause life-threatening brain herniation.

### Signs on MRI
MRI of reported cases of cerebral malaria show that cytotoxic edema often involves the centrum semiovale in a bilateral fashion and show cortical and subcortical ischemic lesions, central pontine myelinolysis, and myelinolysis of the upper medulla. *Central pontine myelinolysis*, or osmotic myelinolysis, is a disease characterized by focal demyelination in the middle of the pons, often seen as a consequence of excessively rapid correction of chronic hyponatremia. It is classically seen on MRI as a central area of high T2 signal intensity within the pons, sparing the periphery and the descending corticospinal tracts, with no enhancement or mass effect (◘ Fig. 11.15.1).

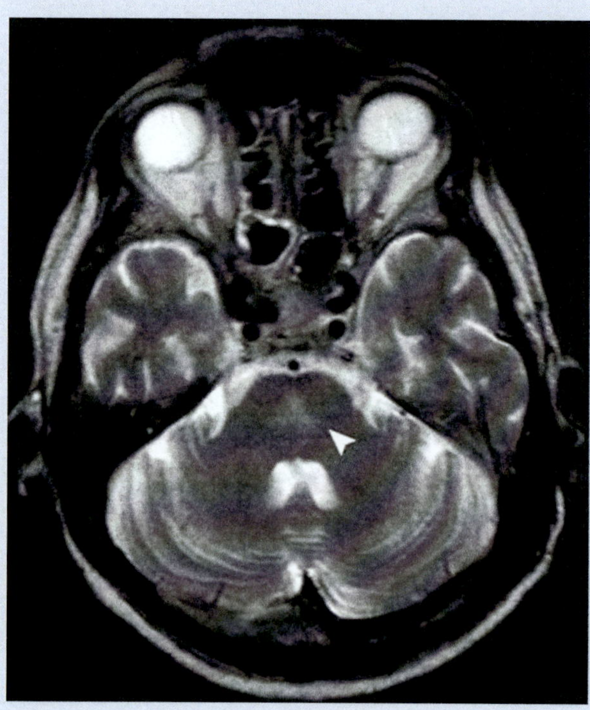

◘ **Fig. 11.15.1**   Axial T2W brain MRI shows central pontine high intensity signal in a patient with central pontine myelinolysis (*arrowhead*)

## Further Reading
Agrawal A, et al. Symmetric peripheral gangrene with mixed malaria. Indian J Pediatr. 2007;74:587–8.

Crane GG. Hyperactive malarious splenomegaly (tropical splenomegaly syndrome). Parasitol Today. 1986;2(1):4–9.

Dunn IJ, et al. Malaria. Semin Roentgenol. 1998b;33(1): 79–80.

Gamanagatti S, et al. MR imaging of cerebral malaria in a child. Eur J Radiol. 2006;60:46–7.

Idro R, et al. Pathogenesis, clinical features, and neurological outcomes of cerebral malaria. Lancet Neurol. 2005;4: 827–40.

Medana IM. Human cerebral malaria and the blood brain barrier. Int J Parasitol. 2006;36:555–68.

Peng SL. Rheumatic manifestations of parasitic diseases. Semin Arthritis Rheum. 2002d;31:228–47.

Richter J, et al. Is ultrasound a useful adjunct for assessing malaria patients? Parasitol Res. 2004;94:349–53.

## 11.16  Animal Bites and Stings

Animal bites and stings are uncommon medical conditions encountered in emergency rooms, but when encountered, they can present a life-threatening situation. In this topic, some of the most common animal bites are discussed, with radiological features that were occasionally reported in the radiological literature.

## Rabies

Rabies is a zoonotic disease arising due to human infection with the rabies virus, which is a single-stranded RNA virus that belongs to the genus *Lyssavirus* of the family *Rhabdoviridae*. The term rabies is derived from an old Indian root word *rabh*, meaning to make violent.

The rabies virus infects humans after a bite from an animal host, because the virus is abundant in high concentrations in the animal host's saliva. Almost any animal is capable of contracting rabies. The main hosts are foxes in Europe, raccoons in the United States, dogs in Asia, jackals in Africa, and vampire bats in Latin America.

The incubation period is typically 2–8 weeks, but it can be as long as 1 year (7 % of cases). There is no laboratory test to determine whether a person is infected with the rabies virus during the incubation period. Other modes of transmission are through inhalation and contact of infected saliva with an open wound or mucous membrane.

After the animal bite, the virus is introduced deep into the human soft tissues via the animal's saliva. The virus replicates in muscles and then starts its journey toward the central nervous system (CNS) through retrograde axoplasmic flow of approximately 12–24 mm per day. The virus enters the CNS via the dorsal spinal root ganglia and then propagates in a retrograde flow to the brain. The clinical manifestations start when the virus reaches the CNS.

In the CNS, rabies may present in one of two forms: encephalitic (furious) and paralytic (dumb). The encephalitic form is the classical form, which is characterized by fever, malaise, anorexia, hydrophobia (fear of water), aerophagia (swallowing too much air), hyperirritability, hyperactivity, seizures, and mood swings. In contrast, paralytic rabies has a clinical presentation that resembles Guillain–Barré syndrome with flaccidity and lack of hydrophobia and aerophagia. Both forms of the disease are fatal, and death is 100 % within 10 days of the onset of neurologic symptoms.

The rabies virus has an affinity to the gray matter. On histological examination of rabies specimens, neuronal *Negri bodies* are classically found. Negri bodies are eosinophilic cytoplasmic inclusions that contain the rabies virus in the neurons. They are commonly seen in the pyramidal cells of the hippocampus, cerebral cortex, and Purkinje cells.

### Signs on CT

A CT scan shows focal or diffuse hypodense areas involving the basal ganglia, periventricular white matter, brain stem, and hippocampus.

### Signs on MRI

- Bilateral high T1 and T2 signal intensities are seen in the basal ganglia, thalami, periventricular white matter, and the cervical spinal cord. The high T1 signal intensities are attributed to area of hemorrhage (■ Fig. 11.16.1a). The spinal cord may show signs of transverse myelitis or dorsal root ganglionitis (enhanced dorsal root after contrast injection).
- Moderate brachial plexus contrast enhancement ipsilateral to the site of the bite may be seen. This finding is due to neuronal inflammation in response to the presence of the rabies virus during its retrograde axoplasmic flow (■ Fig. 11.16.1b).
- MRI of the brain in a patient with the paralytic form may mimic the MRI of postvaccinial acute disseminated encephalomyelitis (ADEM). Rabies affects the gray matter, while ADEM predominantly affects the white matter.

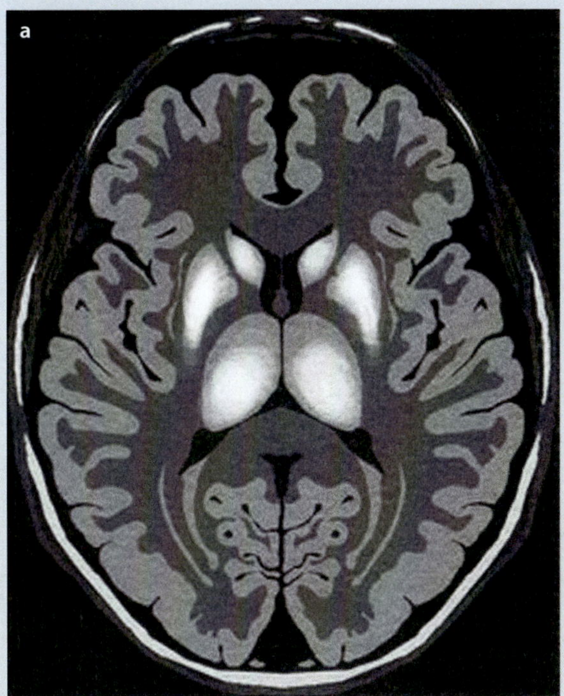


■ **Fig. 11.16.1** Axial FLAIR (**a**) and coronal T1W postcontrast brachial plexus MR illustrations show signs of rabies. In (**a**), the axial brain shows hyperintensity signal involving the basal ganglia and the thalami bilaterally in a symmetrical fashion. In (**b**), the brachial plexus illustration shows brachial plexus cords and roots enhancements

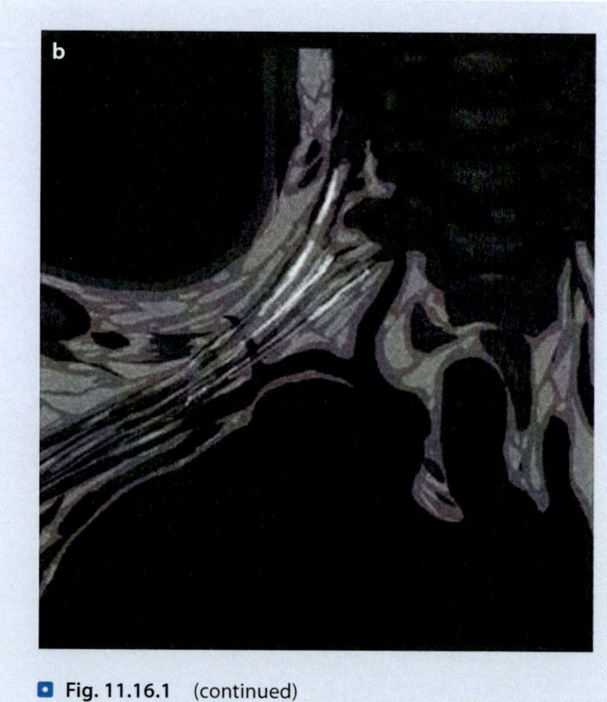

**◘ Fig. 11.16.1**   (continued)

## Viper Bite

Viperidae are a family of venomous snakes possessing long fangs that permit deep-tissue penetration and venom injection.

After a snake bite, vesicular and hemorrhagic reaction starts to develop from 8 to 24 h. Local manifestations include swelling, pain, and perhaps tissue necrosis. Systemic manifestations include faintness, weakness, hypotension, abnormal bleeding and clotting, hematuria, and renal failure. Most of the systemic manifestations of a viper bite are related to abnormal coagulopathy.

Snake venom enhances bleeding tendency due to blood depletion of fibrinogen and clotting factors V, VII, II, and XIII. Diffuse intravascular consumptive coagulopathy (DIC) with thrombosis of small and large vessels may occur. Uncommonly, a stroke may arise a after snake bite, which may be hemorrhagic in nature due to bleeding tendency or ischemic in nature due to thrombosis of the middle cerebral artery. Suspicion of stroke may be raised in a patient with drowsiness and altered consciousness after a snake bite.



## *Differential* Diagnoses and Related Diseases

*Kounis syndrome* is a disease characterized by development of angina pectoris after an allergic reaction (allergic angina pectoris). Kounis syndrome may develop in patients with snake bites due to immunological reaction and body hypersensitivity toward the snake venom.

## Hymenoptera Stings

Hymenoptera is a large group of membranous wing insects. There are three large families of stinging hymenoptera: *Vespidae* (wasps, yellow jackets, hornets), *Apidae* (honeybees and bumblebees), and *Formicidae* (stinging ants).

Insect stings cause localized or generalized reaction due to their venom. Localized reaction includes swelling, urticaria, and blister formation. Generalized reaction includes anaphylactic shock, which typically develops within 10 min, or is delayed for up to 5 h after the insect bite. Rare complications include rhabdomyolysis that induces renal failure, multisystem failure, nephrotic syndrome, and coagulopathy.

Necrotizing fasciitis (*flesh-eating disease*) is a rare complication of insect bites. It is a severe form of deep layer inflammation involving the skin and the subcutaneous tissues, commonly caused by group A *streptococcus* bacteria. Patients present with limb erythema, edema, crepitus, and pain out of proportion to the physical findings. Development of necrotizing fasciitis after an insect bite is attributed to superimposed infection of the bite site.

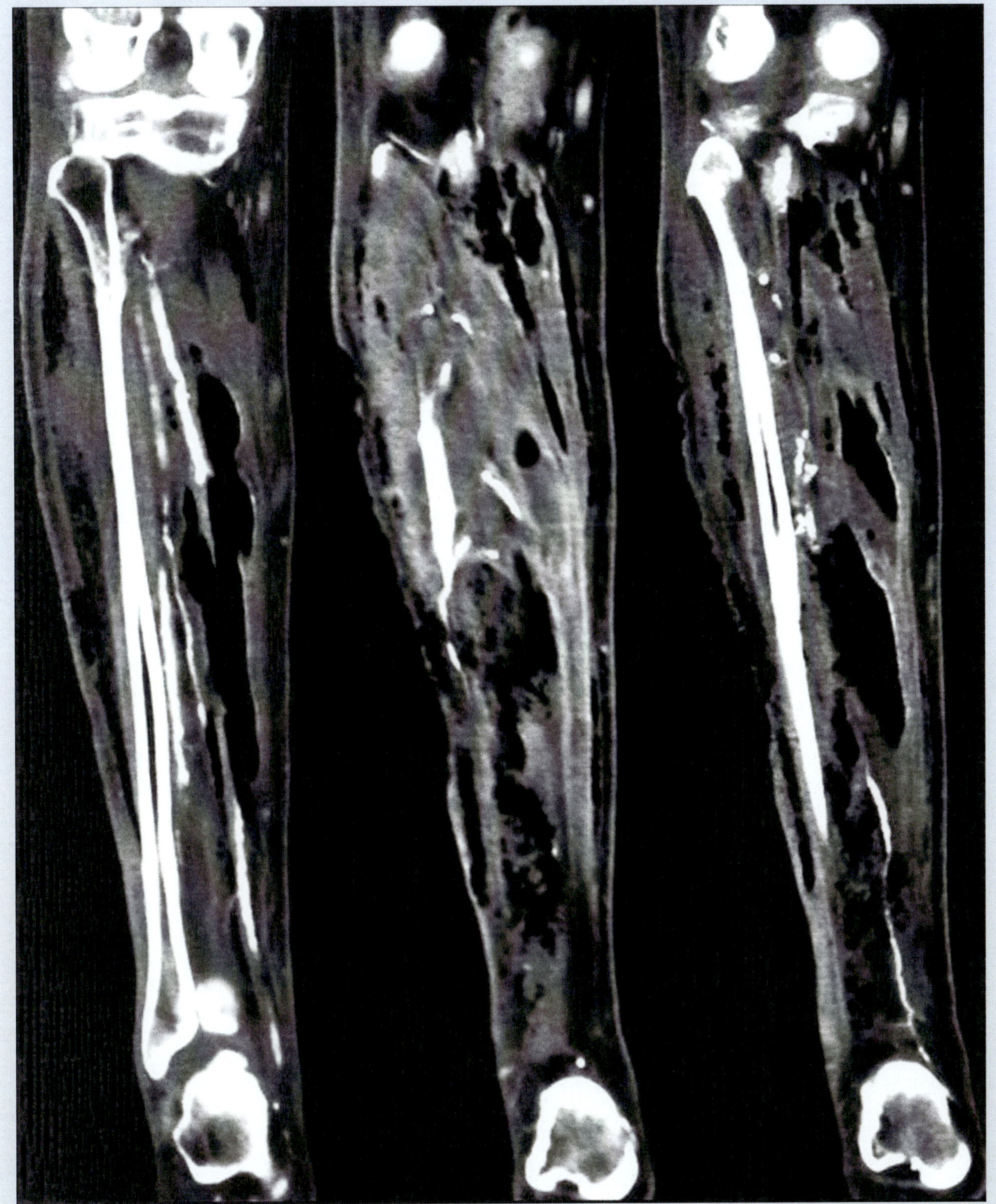

**Fig. 11.16.2** Coronal sequential leg CT images of a patient with necrotizing fasciitis. Notice the severe muscle necrosis and deep-tissue gas formation involving the soleus and the gastrocnemius muscles

## 11.17 Filariasis

Filariasis is an infectious disease of the lymphatic vessels and subcutaneous tissues caused by nematodes or filariae carried by mosquito vectors in endemic areas. Filariasis causes millions of people worldwide to suffer from skin purities, lymphedema and elephantiasis, and the cardinal manifestations and symptoms of this disease.

Filariae are very specific for their mammalian hosts and obligate intermediate vector species. Filariae include *Onchocerca volvulus* (river blindness disease), *Loa loa*, *Dipetalonema streptocerca*, *Mansonella perstans*, *Wuchereria bancrofti*, *Brugia malayi*, and *Mansonella ozzardi*.

The life cycles of all filariae are very similar; the cycle starts when the infective larvae are transmitted through the skin by the arthropod vector during a blood meal. The larvae then migrate to specific areas of the host's body, where they develop into adults and live for several years. For lymphatic filariae such as *W. bancrofti*, adults reside in the lymph nodes and lymph vessels. If both male and female adults are present, they will mate, and the females will release microfilariae. The microfilariae produced by the female worm will circulate in the blood, except for those of *O. volvulus* and of *M. streptocerca*, which will be found in the skin. During a subsequent blood meal, the microfilariae will be taken up by the arthropod, where they will transform into an infective filariform in 1–2 weeks.

### Further Reading

Awasthi M, et al. Imaging findings in Rabies encephalitis. Am J Neuroradiol. 2001;22:677–80.

Bashir R, et al. Cerebral infarction in a young female following snake bite. Stroke. 1985;16:328–30.

Dubinsky I. Rattlesnake bite in a patient with horse allergy and von Willebrand's disease: case report. Can Fam Physician. 1996;42:2207–11.

George P, et al. Wasp sting: an unusual fatal outcome. Saudi J Kidney Dis Transplant. 2008;19(6):969–72.

Hanchanale VS, et al. A costly sting! preputial gangrene following a wasp sting. Indian J Urol. 2006;22:370–1.

Loathamatas J, et al. MR imaging in human rabies. Am J Neuroradiol. 2003;24:1102–9.

Mani J, et al. Magnetic resonance imaging in rabies. Postgrad Med J. 2003;79:352–4.

Polo JM, et al. Aphasia in a farmer following viper bite. Lancet. 2002;359:2164.

Ryssel H, et al. Necrotizing fasciitis after a honey bee sting. Eur J Plast Surg. 2007;30:11–4.

Soufras GD, et al. Penicillin allergy in cancer patients manifesting as Kounis syndrome. Heart Vessels. 2005;20:159–63.

Takayama N. Rabies: a preventable but incurable disease. J Infect Chemother. 2008;14:8–14.

Tasic V. Nephrotic syndrome in a child after a bee sting. Pediatr Nephrol. 2000;15:245–7.

## 11.18 Most Common Infections Causing Human Filariasis

A. Cutaneous filariasis (mostly presents with skin purities, ulcers, and skin hypopigmentation)is subdivided into:
   1. *Onchocerca volvulus* (river blindness disease): it is located in Central Africa and South America; it causes subcutaneous nodules (onchocercomas), insomnia, fatigue, ocular complications, lymphedema, skin depigmentation (leopard skin), and severe pruritus and dermatitis. The intermediate vector is black flies (*Simulium*). Skin complications of *O. volvulus* infection also include acute and chronic papular onchodermatitis, lichenified onchodermatitis, skin atrophy, and onchocercoma, a freely mobile, painless, firm, 2–10 cm subcutaneous nodule located over a bony prominence. Ocular complications of *O. volvulus* infection include anterior uveitis, conjunctivitis, punctate keratitis, optic atrophy, glaucoma, iris atrophy, and cataracts.
   2. *Loa loa*: it is located in Africa and commonly causes allergic reaction and skin swelling. The intermediate vector is Tabanid flies (*Chrysops*). *Loa loa* infection presents with purities, arthralgia, fever, myalgias, regional lymphadenopathy, peripheral neuropathy, kidney glomerular disease, and lymphedema.
   3. Dipetalonema streptocerca: it is located in Central and West Africa; most cases are asymptomatic.
   4. *Mansonella perstans*: it is located in Central Africa, South America (Venezuela, Argentina, Guyana, and Amazonia); it infects both skin and pleura causing skin swelling and eosinophilia. The intermediate vector is biting midges (Culicoides).

B. Lymphatic filariasis (mostly present with lymphedema and scrotal swelling) is subdivided into:
   1. *Wuchereria bancrofti*: it is located in tropical Africa, Asia, and South Pacific regions. The intermediate vector is mosquitoes (*Mansonia, Anopheles, Aedes*). Acute scrotal manifestations of *W. bancrofti* infection include acute funiculitis, epididymitis, or orchitis. Microfilariae are difficult to show during the acute phase. Chronic manifestations of *W. bancrofti* infection include lymphadenopathy, hydrocele, chyluria, and lymphedema. After lymphatic obstruction, proliferative changes occur; the worms die and are absorbed or become calcified. The edema is soft at first but becomes fibrotic after the growth of connective tissue in the area. This advanced chronic disease, called "elephantiasis," develops in only a small percentage of highly reactive individuals who have been infected repeatedly for many years.
   2. *Brugia malayi*: it is located in South and East Asia and commonly associated with lymphangitis and elephantiasis.

C. Body cavity filariasis: include *Mansonella ozzardi* infection, which is located in Mexico, Panamá, Brazil, Colombia, and Argentina; it causes body itching and back pain. The intermediate vectors are black flies and midges.

Diagnosis of filariasis can be established by antigen microfilariae antigen detection with enzyme-linked immunosorbent assay (ELISA) or microfilarial detection in the peripheral blood during the early stages of lymphatic filariasis, even before clinical manifestations develop.

### Signs on Radiographs

Dead worms may calcify within the affected limb and appears on radiographs as linear or ringlike radio-opaque shadows (▣ Fig. 11.17.1).

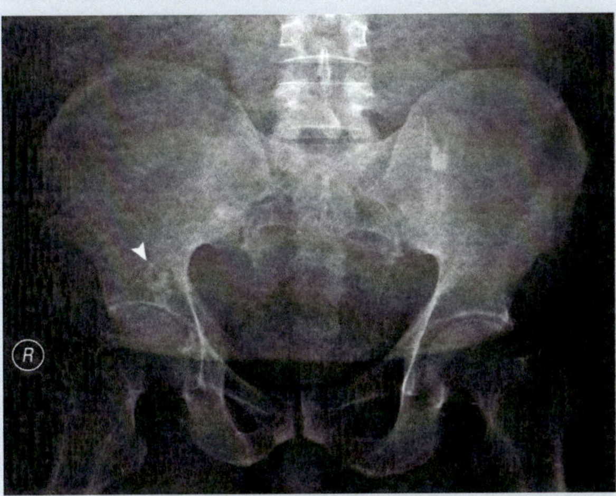

▣ **Fig. 11.17.1**  Anteroposterior plain radiograph the pelvis of a patient with filariasis shows ringlike radio-opaque calcification (*arrowhead*) at the right inguinal region, characteristic of dead worm

### Signs on US

1. In scrotal ultrasound examination, especially with *W. bancrofti* infection, movement of the adult filarial in the scrotal lymphatics as a constant thrashing movement is known as the "filarial dance sign." The filarial movement is described as "linear echogenic structures with persistent, random, almost tireless twirling movements." However, ultrasound is not useful in patients with filarial lymphedema because the adult worms are not present at this stage of the disease.
2. Scrotal ultrasound examination is not useful in patients with *B. malayi* infection because they do not involve the genitalia.
3. Affected limb musculoskeletal ultrasound will show the classical signs of lymphedema, characterized by loss of the normal fascial planes and the hyperechoic/hypoechoic, normal facial planes between the muscles and the fascia and replacement

by hyperechoic, hazy, diffuse texture of the hypodermis and the underlying structures due to lymphedema (▣ Fig. 11.17.2).

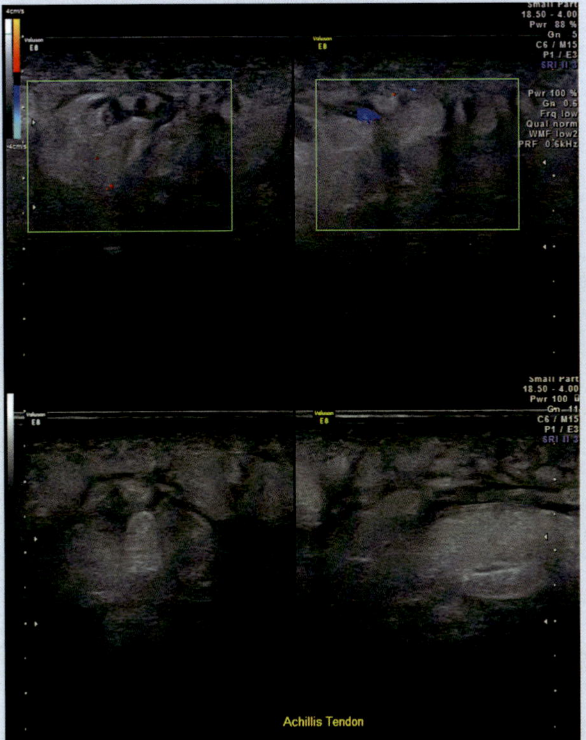


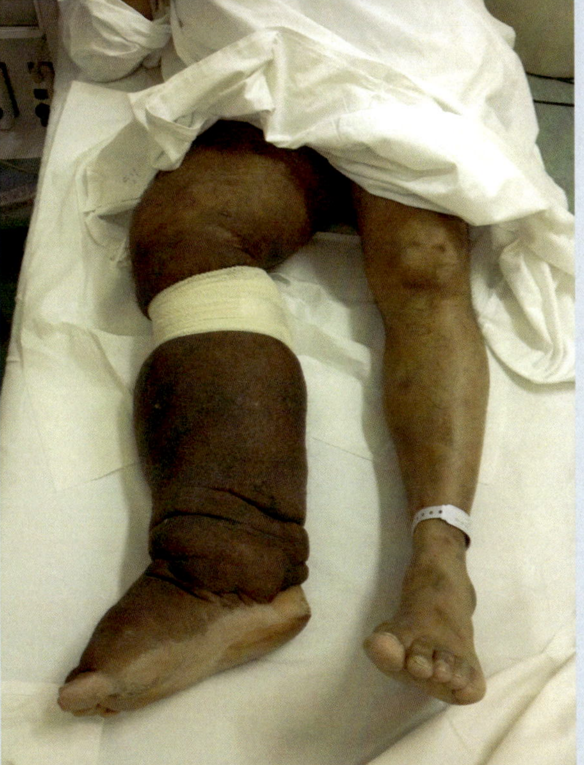

▣ **Fig. 11.17.2**  Ultrasound/Doppler images of the same patient in Fig. 11.17.2 show massive, right-sided lymphedema and skin changes of filariasis on the ultrasound images and the real photograph (lymphedema)

## Further Reading

Chaubal NG, et al. Dance of live adult filarial worms is a reliable sign of scrotal filarial infection. J Ultrasound Med. 2003;22:765–9.

Fonticiella M, et al. Congenital intracranial filariasis: a case report. Pediatr Radiol. 1995;25:171–2.

Melrose WD. Lymphatic filariasis: new insights into an old disease. Int J Parasitol. 2002;32:947–60.

Mendoza N, et al. Filariasis: diagnosis and treatment. Dermatol Ther. 2009;22:475–90.

Schick C, et al. Cystic lymph node enlargement of the neck: filariasis as a rare differential diagnosis in MRI. Eur Radiol. 2002;12:2349–51.

Shaw MTM, et al. A case of exposure to Bancroftian filariasis in a traveller to Thailand. Travel Med Infect Dis. 2006;4:290–3.

## 11.19 Fever of Unknown Origin

Fever of unknown origin (FUO) is defined as an illness of more than 3 weeks duration, with fever greater than 38.3 °C (101 °F) on several occasions, the cause of which was uncertain after 3 days of in-hospital investigation or three outpatients visits. FUO is divided clinically into four main categories:

1. Classical FUO
   - Fever ≥38.3 °C on several occasions
   - Duration ≥3 weeks
   - Diagnosis uncertain after 3 days despite appropriate in-hospital investigation or three outpatient visits
2. Nosocomial FUO
   - Hospitalized patients
   - Fever ≥38.3 °C on several occasions
   - Infection not present or incubating on admission
   - Diagnosis uncertain after 3 days despite appropriate investigations (including at least 48-h incubation of microbiological cultures)
3. Neutropenic FUO
   - Less than 500 neutrophils mm3
   - Fever ≥38.3 °C on several occasions
   - Diagnosis uncertain after 3 days despite appropriate investigations (including at least 48-h incubation of microbiological cultures)
4. HIV-associated FUO
   - Confirmed HIV infection
   - Fever ≥38.3 °C on several occasions
   - Duration of ≥4 weeks (outpatients), or ≥3 days in hospitalized patients
   - Diagnosis uncertain after 3 days despite appropriate investigations (including at least 48-h incubation of microbiological cultures)

FUO represents a major diagnostic challenge. Many investigators divide the diverse causes of FUO into five main categories:

1. Infections (the most common cause). Infections that causes FUO include:

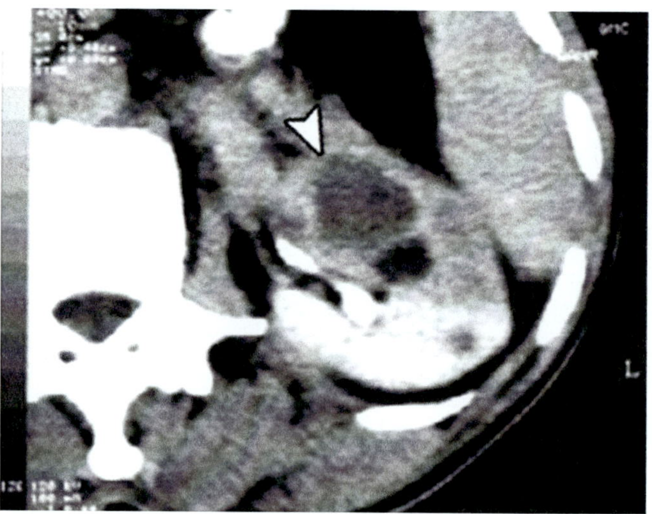

**Fig. 11.18.1**   Axial CT postcontrast of a patient with biopsy-proved renal malakoplakia show abscess formation with ring enhancement (*arrowhead*)

Bacteria: tuberculosis (most common), endocarditis pathogens, syphilis, *Yersinia* infection, cat scratch disease, tularemia, renal malakoplakia (an infectious condition caused by a monocytic-macrophagic bactericidal defect) (■ Fig. 11.18.1), Whipple's disease, and *Brucella* and Q fever (in Mediterranean countries and the Middle East)

Viruses: HIV infection, cytomegalovirus (CMV) infection, hepatitis C and B, Epstein–Barr virus (EBV), and Parvovirus B19

Fungi: histoplasmosis and other systemic fungal diseases

Parasites: toxoplasmosis, toxocara infection, and leishmania (in Mediterranean countries and the Middle East)

2. Neoplasms (2nd common cause)
   Neoplasms that cause FUO include lymphomas and Hodgkin's disease (57 % of cases), colon cancer, myelodysplastic disorders, leukemia, pancreatic cancer, renal cell carcinoma, sarcoma, and Pel–Ebstein fever (i.e., periodic fever associated with Hodgkin's disease)
3. Inflammatory conditions (3rd common cause): this group includes the following subgroups:
   Granulomatous diseases: sarcoidosis, Wegner's granulomatosis, giant cell arteritis (most common cause in patients >50 year), de Quervain's thyroiditis
   Autoimmune diseases: systemic lupus erythematosus, Felty's syndrome, and adult Still's disease
   Vasculitis: Takayasu arteritis, polyarteritis nodosa, and primary angiitis of the central nervous system
4. Rare and uncommon causes
   (a) Löffler's endocarditis
   (b) Cardiac myxoma (■ Fig. 11.18.2)
   (c) Castleman disease
   (d) Kikuchi's necrotizing lymphadenitis
   (e) Vitamin B12 deficiency
   (f) Occult hematoma (due to oral anticoagulant use)
   (g) Aortic dissection

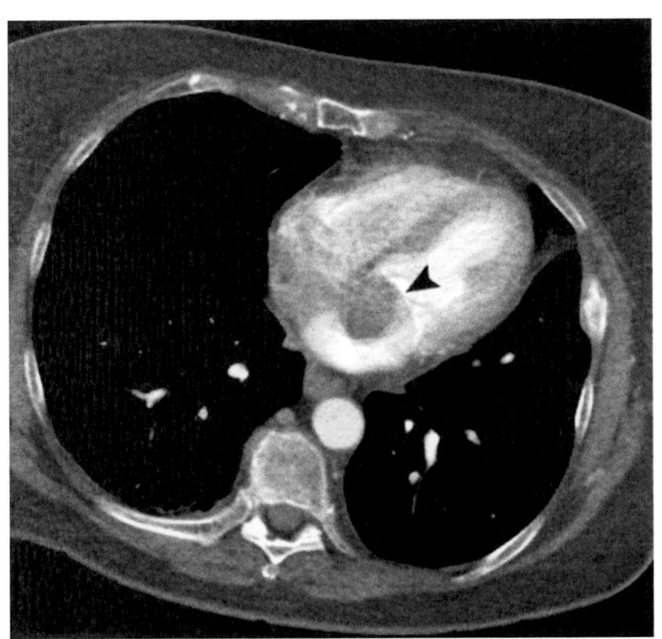

**Fig. 11.18.2** Axial cardiac CT with contrast of a patient with atrial myxoma (*arrowhead*) seen as a mass located typically in the atrial septum

(h)  Liver cirrhosis (cirrhotic fever)
(i)  Deep venous thrombosis and pulmonary embolism
(j)  Hyperthyroidism

Radiological workup investigations for a patient with FUO

1.  Ultrasound: To check for:
    (a)  de Quervain's thyroiditis
    (b)  Giant cell arteritis (temporal arteritis)
    (c)  Carotid Doppler: to exclude vasculitis
    (d)  DVT (leg Doppler): Before DVT can be considered as a possible cause of FUO, two findings must be present:
        1.  A positive venous duplex image for acute DVT
        2.  Fever resolution within 7 days of the initiation of anticoagulation therapy
2.  Contrast-enhanced CT (thorax/abdomen/pelvis): To check for:
    (a)  Lungs: Pneumonias (especially *Pneumocystis carinii* pneumonia), abscesses, and pulmonary embolism
    (b)  Heart: Cardiac myxoma, Löffler's endocarditis, valve vegetations (endocarditis)
    (c)  Abdomen: Abscesses and occult hematomas
    (d)  Lymph nodes: Lymphoma, Castleman disease, or inflammatory pseudotumor of the nodes
    (e)  Liver: Liver cirrhosis or liver inflammatory pseudotumor
    (f)  Arteries: Vasculitis (e.g., Takayasu arteritis) and pulmonary embolism
3.  MRA: To check for:
    (a)  Carotid/vertebral vasculitis
    (b)  Vertebral osteomyelitis

**Further Reading**

Chantal P, Bleeker-Rovers CP, et al. Fever of unknown origin. Semin Nucl Med. 2009b;39:81–7.

de Kleijn EMHA, et al. Fever of unknown origin: a new definition and proposal for diagnostic work-up. Eur J Intern Med. 2000;11:1–3.

Efstathiou SP, et al. Fever of unknown origin: discrimination between infectious and non-infectious causes. Eur J Intern Med. 2010;21:137–43.

Hahn PF, et al. Intraabdominal hematoma: the concentric-ring sign in MR imaging. AJR. 1987;148:115–9.

Knockaert DC, et al. Fever of unknown origin in adults: 40 years on. J Intern Med. 2003;253:263–75.

Wagner AD, et al. Standardised work-up programme for fever of unknown origin and contribution of magnetic resonance imaging for the diagnosis of hidden systemic vasculitis. Ann Rheum Dis. 2005;64:105–10.

# Occupational Medicine and Toxicology



© Springer International Publishing Switzerland 2017
J.A. Al-Tubaikh, *Internal Medicine*, DOI 10.1007/978-3-319-39747-4_12

## 12.1    Medications Toxicity

Toxicology is the study of the harmful effects of drugs, organic substances, and medication on the human body. Many medications and substance abuse can result in radiologic manifestations during imaging patients for a variety of conditions. Knowledge of the radiological signs of certain common medications and abused substances helps radiologists in the interpretation of these radiological abnormalities and artifacts when encountered incidentally. In this topic, selected medications and drugs which have well-recognized radiological signs are discussed and illustrated

## Antibiotics

Antibiotics abuse can kill the normal flora and cause pseudomembranous colitis in long-term use. *Pseudomembranous colitis* is a disease characterized by overgrowth of the organism *Clostridium difficile*, a colonic bacterium living as a part of the normal flora. The bacteria produce toxins that injure the intestinal mucosa and form a covering layer of exudates and necrotic cells from the intestinal mucosa; this layer impedes the intestinal absorption and leads to watery diarrhea. Pseudomembranous colitis may occur also with chemotherapy, abdominal surgery, and hypotensive episodes. Diagnosis is established by stool assay for *C. difficile*.

### Signs on CT

1. The most common sign of pseudomembranous colitis is circumferential or eccentric thickening of the colonic wall, typically more than 15 mm, while the normal colonic wall thickness in CT is 3 mm (*accordion sign*) (◘ Fig. 12.1.1). This sign however is not specific for pseudomembranous colitis, but characteristic.
2. Although colonic wall thickening can be seen in many inflammatory diseases, the colonic wall thickening in pseudomembranous colitis is generally greater than any other inflammatory disease.

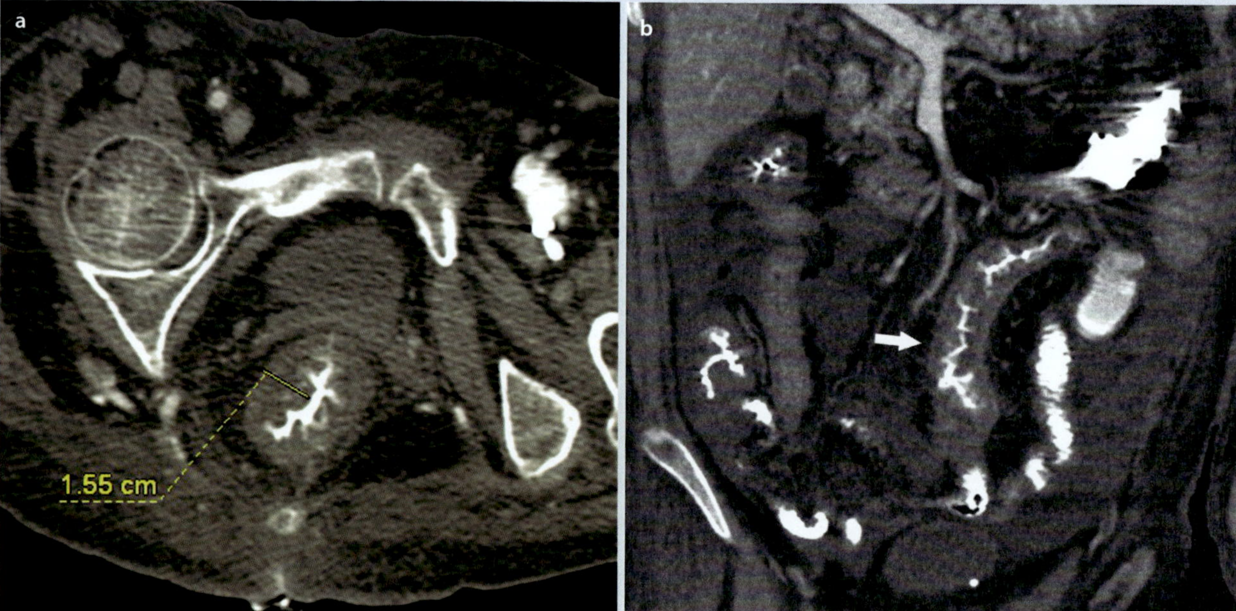


◘ **Fig. 12.1.1**    Axial (**a**) and coronal (**b**) CT images of a 72-year-old patient admitted to the hospital with repeated vomiting, weight loss, and watery diarrhea since 10 days, and she was treated with intravenous antibiotics for 5 days prior to the CT. The CT showed diffuse, concentric wall thickening (*15.5 mm max*) with diffuse haustral thickening (accordion sign; *arrow*) of the whole colon, characteristic of acute diffuse colitis (pseudomembranous colitis in conjunction with history of antibiotic use)

# Metformin (Glucophage, Oral Hypoglycemics)

Diabetes mellitus is treated with oral hypoglycemics and insulin, depending of the type of diabetes. The most commonly used oral hypoglycemic medications groups are sulfonylureas and biguanides.

Sulfonylureas are medications that increase insulin secretion and reduce peripheral resistance to insulin. An example of a sulfonylurea drug is gliclazide (*Diamicron*). Sulfonylureas causes inhibition of adenosine triphosphate (ATP)-sensitive potassium channels on the membrane of pancreatic beta cells, augmenting depolarization of the cell and enhancing the release of endogenous insulin. The main side effects of sulfonylureas include prolonged or recurrent hypoglycemia and weight gain.

Biguanides are medications that reduce glucose absorption, inhibit gluconeogenesis, and increase peripheral glucose utilization. An example of a biguanides drug is metformin (*Glucophage*). The main side effects of biguanides include gastrointestinal (GI) symptoms, anorexia, lactic acidosis, and maybe megaloblastic anemia. The GI symptoms of metformin include diarrhea, epigastric pain, and gastroparesis. Prolonged gastroparesis may predispose to the formation of gastric bezoars. *Gastric bezoar* is a rare condition characterized by foreign body mass formation within the stomach usually due to accumulation of indigested material in the form of masses or concretions. It usually forms from vegetable, fruits, or hair (in psychiatric patients) in patients with gastric emptying problems.

# Methotrexate

Methotrexate is a folate (vitamin B9)-antagonist used in the treatment of many malignant and inflammatory conditions such as leukemia, sarcomas, breast carcinoma, rheumatoid arthritis, and psoriasis. Routs of administration include oral, intravenous, intramuscular, and intrathecal routs.

Methotrexate toxicity is known to cause lung symptoms that include cough and dyspnea, fever, chills, malaise, and headache weeks after initiation of therapy. Other manifestations include peripheral eosinophilia (50 %), skin rash (17 %), pleural effusion, pulmonary fibrosis, hepatic steatosis, malabsorption and diarrhea, and hilar lymphadenopathy

Methotrexate lung-related changes may present with two rare manifestations: acute pleuritis (pleural chest pain with pleural effusion) or acute respiratory failure secondary to noncardiogenic edema (acute respiratory distress syndrome). Methotrexate can induce diffuse white matter lesions with demyelination and necrosis (leukoencephalopathy). *Disseminated necrotizing leukoencephalopathy* is a rare condition characterized by bilaterally symmetrical necrosis of the thalami and maybe other basal ganglia. Histopathologic features include multifocal, coalescing areas of coagulative necrosis with axonal swelling in the periventricular white matter.

## Signs on Radiographs

1. Noncardiogenic edema can be seen as bilateral diffuse alveolar shadows with normal-sized heart, typically starting from the periphery to the center. Pleural effusion with bilateral hilar lymphadenopathy may be seen.
2. Other rare pulmonary manifestation includes noncaseating granulomas. Pulmonary fibrosis may arise in chronic use.
3. Methotrexate can cause profound osteoporosis that can cause multiple insufficiency fractures.
4. Methotrexate use in children and adolescent may cause growth recovery lines (Harris lines). *Harris lines* are radiodense transverse lines that run parallel to the epiphyseal scar in the metaphysis (◘ Fig. 12.1.2). They represent periods of increased bone growth followed by periods of suppressed bone growth. These lines are usually seen in the distal femur or the proximal tibia. They are considered as normal variants in asymptomatic patients or patients without history of medication use. These lines must not be mistaken with stress fractures.
5. Other musculoskeletal features include metaphyseal corner fracture and ring epiphyses. These changes can be seen within 2 months after starting therapy.

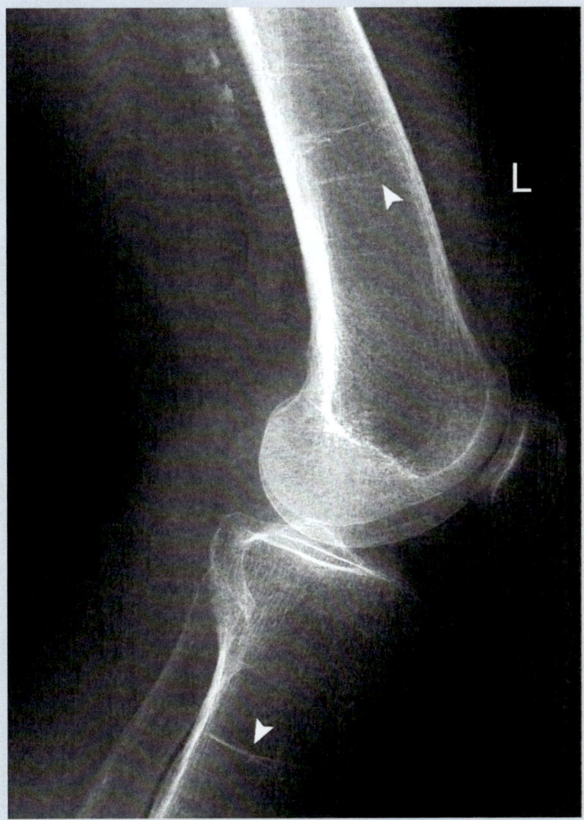


◘ **Fig. 12.1.2** Lateral plain radiograph of the knee that demonstrates Harris lines (*arrowheads*)

### Signs on US

Hepatic steatosis can be seen in long-term methotrexate use due to liver drug detoxifying injury.

### Signs on MRI

Acute necrotizing encephalopathy is classically seen as bilateral symmetrical thalamic high signal intensity lesions seen on T1W images with mixed high/low T2 signal intensity lesions due to necrosis and hemorrhage. DWI shows decreased signal in ADC map due to cytotoxic edema and hemorrhage. No contrast enhancement is typically seen (*due to ischemic nature of the injurious insult*).

## Hypervitaminosis A

Vitamin A is a fat-soluble vitamin primarily found in fish liver (*retinol*) and carrots (*β-carotene*). Vitamin A contains retinol esters; when the liver is saturated with vitamin A, retinol esters appear in the blood in toxic levels, causing different systemic manifestations.

*Hypervitaminosis A* is often seen in children and young adults treated with high doses of vitamin A (>100,000 IU per day). Also, vitamin A derivatives use during pregnancy can induce teratogenic effect (induce fetal malformations). Moreover, vitamin A can cause premature closure of the epiphyses in humans. The same condition can occur in calves, causing premature closure of their hind limb making their gait resemble that of hyena, a disease of calves known as *Hyena disease*.

Hypervitaminosis A targets mainly the central nervous system (*fatigue, irritability, hypersomnia, anorexia, and increased intracranial pressure and pseudotumor cerebri in children*), liver (*liver cirrhosis, jaundice, and hepatomegaly*), skin (*alopecia and skin peeling*), mucous membranes (*cheilitis and stomatitis*), and musculoskeletal system (*bone pain and unexplained swelling of extremities*). Diagnosis is confirmed by detecting high serum levels of retinol esters (>100 μg/dL). Radiologically, hypervitaminosis A causes diaphyseal periosteal reaction, which can mimics battered child syndrome.

*Battered child syndrome* (*child abuse*) refers to injuries sustained by a child as a result of physical abuse. The physical signs are arranged from internal injuries, cuts, burns or fractured bones. *Shaken baby syndrome* is another form of child abuse where the infant or the child presents with retinal hemorrhage, subdural or subarachnoid hemorrhage, with absence of external signs of physical abuse. It occurs due to shaking force inflicted to the baby by the abuser.

### Signs on Radiographs

1. Classically, chronic hypervitaminosis A shows osteoporosis, premature closure of physis, periosteal reaction, and cortical hyperostosis of the cranium and long bones. The periosteal reaction observed in long bones may mimic that reaction of Ewing's sarcoma, especially in young adults.
2. Typically, periosteal reaction due to vitamin A toxicity is seen in the diaphysis of the ulna and the metacarpals. Other sites affected include clavicles, tibia, and fibula.
3. Cervical osteophytes, syndesmophytes, and changes similar to ossification of posterior longitudinal ligament can be seen in long-term use of retinoic acid (vitamin A derivative), which is used to treat acne.
4. Battered child syndrome can be suspected radiologically by finding the following radiographic manifestations: cortical thickening without fractures or dislocations; metaphyseal fragments at the area where the periosteum joins the metaphysis in long bones due to old periosteal hematoma; single or multiple transverse fractures in the long bones, ribs, or humerus with different healing stages (*highly suspicious for child abuse*); diaphyseal spiral fractures, they result from twisting or torsion forces (*highly indicative of child abuse*); and scapular fractures in babies (*highly indicative for child abuse*).

### Signs on CT and MRI

1. In hypervitaminosis A, sutural diathesis and hyperostosis in association with signs of intracranial pressure and ventriculomegaly may be seen due to altered cerebrospinal fluid mechanics.
2. In shaken baby syndrome, unilateral or bilateral subdural hematomas are typically seen with signs of acute on top of old subdural hematoma may be seen due to recurrent abuse (◘ Fig. 12.1.3).

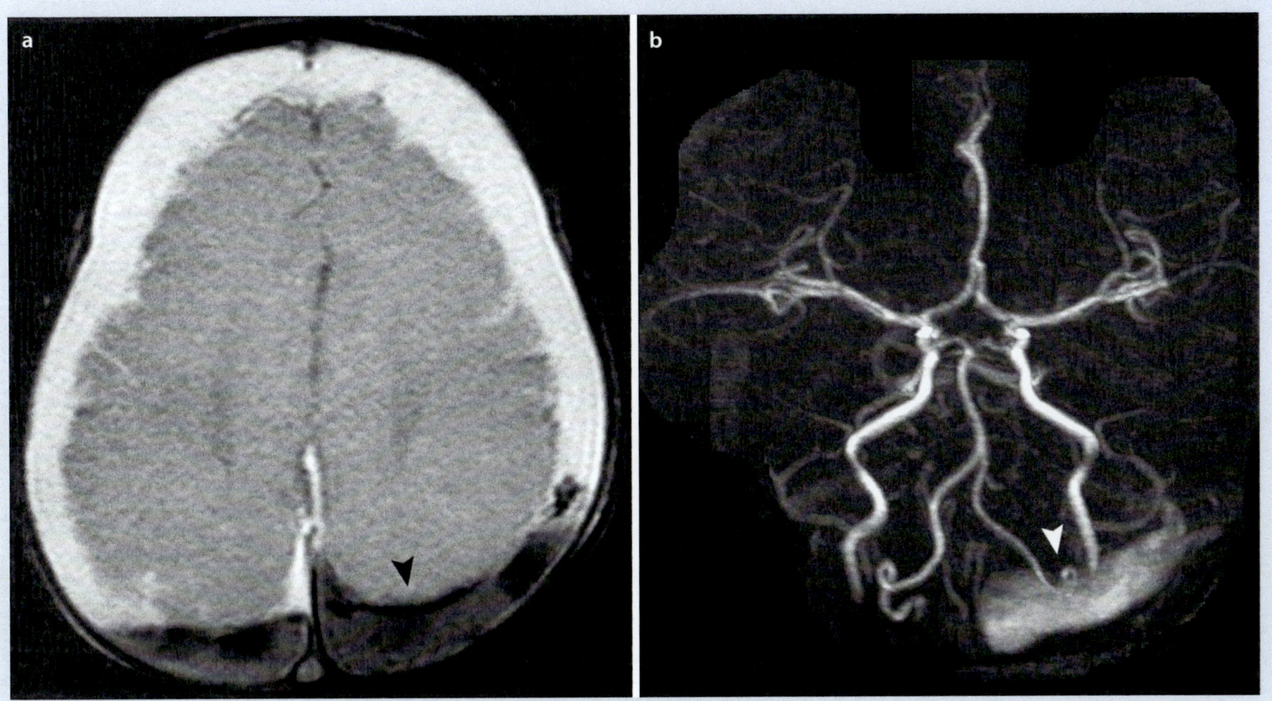



**Fig. 12.1.3**   Axial T* (**a**) and time-to-flight (TOF) angiographic MR images of an infant with bilateral subdural hematomas (*arrowheads*) due to child abuse (shaken baby syndrome); the infant stayed in the pediatric intensive care unit for 5 weeks before she died

## Anticonvulsants

Anticonvulsants are medications that prevent seizure incidence by raising seizure threshold or decrease the activity of epileptogenic foci in the brain. Most anticonvulsants act by decreasing levels of excitation neurotransmitters (e.g., glutamate) and increasing inhibitory neurotransmitters (e.g., *gamma-aminobutyric acid/GABA*). Examples of anticonvulsants include:

1. *Carbamazepine*: it decreases neuronal excitation by prolonging sodium ($Na^+$) channel activation. Carbamazepine toxicity includes cardiac toxicity, stupor, encephalopathy, and chorea. *Fetal carbamazepine syndrome* is a pathological condition that affects neonates in mothers treated with carbamazepine during pregnancy; features include nail hypoplasia, spinal dysraphism, congenital heart disease, microcephaly, tall forehead, malar hypoplasia, and micrognathia.

2. *Phenytoin*: like carbamazepine, it decreases neuronal excitation by prolonging sodium channels ($Na^+$) channel activation. Phenytoin toxicity includes cardiac toxicity (intravenous phenytoin mainly), gingival hyperplasia, ataxia, nystagmus, chorea, ophthalmoplegia, hypotension, and hirsutism. Phenytoin can cause immunodeficiency in children treated with phenytoin and infected with Epstein–Barr virus. *Fetal phenytoin syndrome* is a pathological condition that affects neonates in mothers treated with phenytoin during pregnancy; features include dwarfism, hypoplastic phalanges, nail hypoplasia, frontal bossing, tall forehead, maxillary hypoplasia, hirsutism, and microcephaly. Phenytoin can induce hypersensitivity syndrome characterized by lymphadenopathy and patchy alveolar infiltrations similar to Loeffler endocarditis. Lymphadenopathy due to phenytoin use is classified into four main categories: lymphatic hyperplasia, lymphatic hyperplasia that regresses after discontinuing the therapy (*pseudolymphoma*), lymphatic hyperplasia that regresses after discontinuing the therapy and then reemerge several months after (*pseudopseudolymphoma*), and true lymphoma (*Hodgkin's or non-Hodgkin's lymphoma*).

3. *Valproic acid*: it decreases neuronal excitation by prolonging sodium channels ($Na^+$) channel activation and increase GABA activity. Valproic acid toxicity can cause cardiac arrest in large doses, nausea, vomiting, cerebral edema, and rarely pancreatitis. Fetal valproate syndrome is a pathological condition that affects neonates in mothers treated with valproic acid during pregnancy; features include limb defects, spinal dysraphism, genital anomalies, cardiac anomalies, craniosynostosis (*trigonocephaly*), and tall forehead.

**Signs on Radiographs**

1. Up to one third of patients on phenytoin may show signs of osteopenia due to reduced calcium absorption from the intestines. Also, it can cause dental root abnormality and thickening of the diploic space (similar to acromegaly).
2. Phenytoin can cause thickening of the heel pad similar to that of acromegaly. On lateral plain radiographs, the soft-tissue density of the heel pad is >35 mm in diameter.
3. Patchy alveolar infiltrations with hilar lymphadenopathy may be seen rarely on chest radiographs due to hypersensitivity syndrome induced by phenytoin.

## Amiodarone Toxicity

Amiodarone is a class III antiarrhythmic agent used to control atrial and/or ventricular arrhythmia. Amiodarone is known to cause long-term complications that include pulmonary, endocrinal, ophthalmic, and hepatic manifestations.

Amiodarone can induce pulmonary toxicity found in the alveoli and the interstitial septae, inducing inflammatory reaction and fibrosis (13 % of patients using amiodarone). Patients present with nonspecific symptoms like fever, weight loss, cough, and dyspnea. The mechanism of amiodarone-induced pulmonary toxicity is presumed to be related to hypersensitivity pneumonitis or direct toxicity related to production of free radicals and phospholipidosis.

Amiodarone contains significant amount of iodine (37 % of its molecular weight), which can induce hyper- or hypothyroidism in patients using amiodarone (14–18 % of patients). The mechanism of amiodarone-induced hypothyroidism is thought to result from abnormal response of the thyroid to chronic high iodine load and then inability to resume normal thyroid function from the inhibitory effect of iodine uptake and hormone synthesis (*Wolff-Chaikoff effect*).

Amiodarone optic neuropathy is a very rare complication of amiodarone (0.36–2 % of patients using amiodarone for 5 years interval), and it mimics idiopathic anterior ischemic optic neuropathy (incidence is 0.3 % of population). Idiopathic anterior ischemic optic neuropathy is typically unilateral with visual loss that is not completely reversible. In contrast, amiodarone optic neuropathy is typically bilateral (*key feature of toxicity*) and visual loss is completely reversible

when the drug is discontinued. Amiodarone also can cause corneal microdeposits that can cause visual loss or blurry vision (10 % of patients).

Amiodarone hepatic toxicity has an incidence of 1 % in patients using amiodarone and is referred to as hepatic phospholipidosis. *Hepatic phospholipidosis*, also known as *pseudo-alcoholic liver disease*, is a condition characterized by accumulation of cytoplasmic phospholipid inclusions within macrophages, hepatic cells, and all body tissues as a cytotoxic effect of amiodarone and its metabolite desethylamiodarone. Liver histological characteristics of hepatic phospholipidosis include steatosis, necrosis, and cirrhosis. Patients may present with signs of hepatic liver dysfunction and hepatomegaly, with mild liver enzymes elevation.

Other manifestations of amiodarone toxicity include cutaneous photosensitivity, skin discoloration, vomiting, anorexia, and peripheral neuropathy.

**Signs on US**

Hepatic phospholipidosis is detected as highly echogenic liver due to steatosis, with or without signs of cirrhosis.

**Signs on Radiographs**

Amiodarone causes nonspecific patchy alveolar infiltrations, linear interstitial patterns, and reticular interstitial pattern due to fibrosing alveolitis.

**Signs on CT**

1. In lung HRCT, nonspecific features can be seen and include high-attenuation lung masses (e.g., 86–174 HU), pulmonary alveolar patchy infiltrations, thickening of the interstitial septae, pleural effusion, and subpleural high-attenuation deposits (◘ Fig. 12.1.4).
2. Hepatic phospholipidosis is typically detected as low-density liver due to steatosis, with or without signs of cirrhosis. Hepatomegaly may be seen.

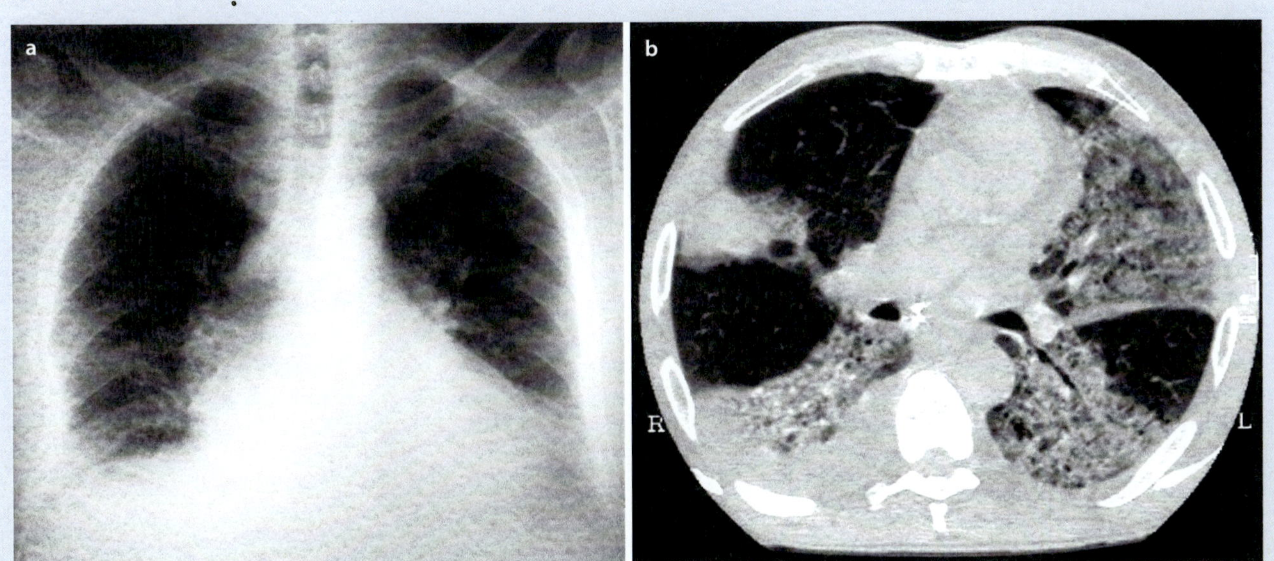



**Fig. 12.1.4** Posteroanterior chest radiograph (**a**) and axial pulmonary HRCT (**b**) of a patient with chronic amiodarone use shows extensive, patchy, lobular reticulo-interstitial lung disease reflecting "amiodarone-induced pulmonary fibrosis"

## Cyclosporine A

Cyclosporine A is a fungal metabolite that has the property of specifically and irreversibly inhibiting the induction of the cytotoxic effector and helper T cells without direct lymphocytotoxicity. It is one of the most commonly used drugs for transplantation rejection after steroids. Complications of cyclosporine include formation of pulmonary nodules (rarely), lymphadenopathy, hallucinations, and posttransplant lymphoproliferative disorder.

*Posttransplant lymphoproliferative disorder (PTLD)* has two different manifestation patterns: early and late. Early PTLD occurs within the 1st year after transplantation and is likely to regress after reduction in immunotherapy and less likely to result in disseminated lymphoma. Late PTLD, on the other hand, arises after 1 year posttransplantation and is associated with mortality in 70 % of cases due to disseminated lymphoma.

### Signs on MRI
1. Cyclosporine A toxicity causes reversible posterior leukoencephalopathy, which is seen as bilateral symmetrical occipital vasogenic edema that resolves when the drug is continued.
2. Abnormal high T2 signal intensity with contrast enhancement affecting the parietal cortex bilaterally has been reported in the literature to occur with cyclosporine toxicity.

## Glucocorticoids

Glucocorticoids are widely used, hormonal anti-inflammatory medications with wide adverse reactions. Glucocorticoids can induce pseudo-Cushing's disease features such as obesity, hirsutism, osteoporosis, avascular necrosis (due to fat emboli), lipomatosis, hypercalciuria, and nephrolithiasis.

### Signs on Radiographs
1. Bone osteoporosis is a well-known feature of long-term glucocorticoids use. The etiology of osteopenia is thought to be secondary to inhibition of osteoblastic activity and the effects of increased levels of parathyroid hormone, and negative nitrogen balance and loss of proteinaceous matrix of the bone.
2. Nephrocalcinosis is seen as patchy areas of calcifications at the renal shadows region on plain abdominal radiographs.
3. Avascular necrosis is detected through increased bone density (*due to ischemia which will affect the osteoclastic activity*), subchondral lucency (late finding), and maybe collapse of the articular surface.

### Signs on CT
Lipomatosis is seen as noncapsulated proliferation of fatty tissues. Classically, glucocorticoids-induced lipomatosis can be seen within the mediastinum, abdomen, or pelvis.

**Signs on MRI**

Avascular bone necrosis can be diagnosed early on MRI. Classically on post-contrast images, there is an outer low intensity line with an inner high intensity line seen in T2W sequence surrounding an area of low T1 and high T2 signal intensity within the affected epiphysis (*double shadow sign*). The high intensity line is believed to be caused by the zone of hyperemia. Double line sign is found in 80 % of cases of avascular necrosis.

## Gadolinium-Based Contrast Media

*Nephrogenic systemic fibrosis* (NSF) is an idiopathic, progressive systemic fibrosis that arises in patients with renal disease. Gadolinium (Gd)-based contrast media are responsible for development of NSF in renal disease patients performing contrast-enhanced MRI.

The clinical manifestations of NSF is divided into acute (<2 weeks after contrast exposure) and chronic (>2 weeks after contrast exposure). The early manifestations include limb pain (52 %), followed by pruritus (36 %), alopecia, swelling (25 %) of the hands and feet, paresthesias (24 %), burning skin sensation (16 %), abdominal pain, and diarrhea. The chronic manifestations include bilateral symmetrical plaques (58 %), papules (32 %), or nodules (17 %) of cutaneous and muscle hardening (mimicking scleroderma), with brownish hyperpigmentation involving predominantly the lower extremities (41 %). Other features include joint stiffness (34 %) and skin tightness (30 %). The arms and trunk are less frequently involved, and rarely yellowish scleral plaques formation has been reported.

NSF has been reported in association with gadodiamide (Omniscan, GE Healthcare), gadopentetate (Magnevist, Bayer Healthcare), gadoversetamide (OptiMARK, Mallinckrodt Inc.), and gadoterate meglumine (Dotarem – Guerbet SA). The United States Food and Drug Administration (FDA) issued a warning in June 2006 against the use of Gd-contrast in patients with moderate-to-severe reduction in glomerular filtration rate (<30 ml/min) and patients who have undergone liver transplantation. Also, the FDA warned that the use of 0.2–0.3 mmol/kg even in a single exposure carry a high risk of NSF development in patients with compromised glomerular filtration rate.

The definitive diagnosis of NSF is made by deep skin biopsy, which typically should include the entire dermis and subcutaneous fat to the level of the fascia, if possible. Histology shows extensive dermal fibrosis, with alteration of the normal pattern of collagen bundles with surrounding clefts and increased number of spindle cells which typically stain positive for CD34 and procollagen-1 surface markers.

**Signs on Radiographs**

Patients with chronic NSF may show diffuse osteopenia, joint contractures, and extensive intra- and periarticular soft-tissue calcification.

**Signs on CT and MRI**

1. Dural fibrosis with calcification has been reported to occur rarely in patients with chronic NSF in the presence of normal serum phosphorus levels.
2. Diffuse dural thickening and enhancement may be seen.

## Selected References

Brunner D, et al. CT of pseudomembranous colitis. Gastrointest Radiol. 1984;9:73–5.

Change PSM, et al. Amiodarone-induced hypothyroidism with EPO-resistant anemia in a patient with chronic renal failure. J Chin Med Assoc. 2008;71(11):576–8.

Chao CC, et al. Nephrogenic systemic fibrosis associated with gadolinium use. J Formos Med Assoc. 2008;107(3):270–4.

Cowper SE, et al. Clinical and histological findings in nephrogenic systemic fibrosis. Eur J Radiol. 2008;66:191–9.

Fishman EK, et al. Pseudomembranous colitis: CT evaluation of 26 cases. Radiology. 1991;180:57–60.

Foss C, et al. Gadolinium-associated nephrogenic systemic fibrosis in a 9-year-old boy. Pediatr Dermatol. 2009;26(5):579–82.

Glover SJ, et al. Ophthalmic findings in fetal anticonvulsant syndrome. Ophthalmology. 2002;209:942–7.

Horton KM, et al. CT evaluation of the colon: inflammatory diseases. Radiographics. 2000;20:399–418.

Leiner T, et al. Nephrogenic systemic fibrosis is not exclusively associated with gadodiamide. Eur Radiol. 2007;17:1921–3.

Lexa FJ. Drug-induced disorders of the central nervous system. Semin Roentgenol. 1995;30(1):7–17.

Neustadter LM, et al. Medication-induced changes of bones. Semin Roentgenol. 1995a;30(1):88–95.

Pace MT, et al. Cyclosporin A toxicity: MRI appearance of the brain. Pediatr Radiol. 1995;25:180–3.

Rothenberg AB, et al. Hypervitaminosis A-induced premature closure of epiphyses (physeal obliteration) in humans and calves (hyena disease): a historical review of the human and veterinary literature. Pediatr Radiol. 2007;37:1264–7.

Sharma P, et al. Toxic and acquired metabolic encephalopathies: MRI appearance. AJR Am J Roentgenol. 2009;193:879–86.

Siniakowicz RM, et al. Diagnosis of amiodarone pulmonary toxicity with high-resolution computerized tomographic scan. J Cardiovasc Electrophysiol. 2001;12:431–6.

Weigle JP, et al. Nephrogenic systemic fibrosis: chronic imaging findings and review of the medical literature. Skeletal Radiol. 2008;37:457–64.

Zelasko S, et al. CT and MR imaging of progressive dural involvement by nephrogenic systemic fibrosis. AJNR Am J Neuroradiol. 2008;29:1880–2.

## 12.2　**Drugs of Abuse**

### Cocaine and Heroin (Opioids)

Cocaine hydrochloride, or *benzoylmethylecgonine* ($C_{17}H_{21}NO_4$), is a naturally occurring alkaloid substance found in the leaves of the *Erythroxylum coca* plant. The plant is endogenous in South America, Mexico, Indonesia, and the West Indies.

Historically, cocaine has been ingested as part of popular wine (Vin Mariani) in 1863 marked by a chemist named Angelo Mariani. The cocaine was combined with alcohol forming a potently reinforcing compound (*Cocaethylene*). Also, cocaine was a part of the original 1886 Coca-cola recipe, which was initially sold as a medication. The drink was flavored using kola nuts, also acting as the beverage's source of caffeine.

The cocaine plant leaves are harvested and soaked with solvents such as kerosene until a thick pasty substance is isolated (cocaine paste). This paste, which contains 40–80 % cocaine, is treated with hydrochloride acid to form cocaine hydrochloride salt (cocaine powder). Because of its high melting point, cocaine hydrochloride cannot be smoked; the cocaine hydrochloride must be transformed into an alkaline form by mixing it with sodium bicarbonate before it can be smoked, a product known as "crack." The name *crack* is onomatopoeia for the sound the substance makes when it is heated. Crack is considered to be the most potent and most addictive form of cocaine because its effect can be obtained within seconds after inhalation.

### *Cocaine* Effect on Different Body Systems

1. *Central nervous system (CNS) effect*: cocaine blocks the reuptake of catecholamines and serotonin (*sympathomimetic*). The majority of cocaine effect on the nervous system is believed to be caused by excess brain dopamine. CNS symptoms include euphoria, increased self-confidence, disorientation, hyperthermia, hemorrhagic stroke, hypertension, cerebral vasculitis, and hallucination. Intracranial hemorrhage can occur in cocaine abusers even in the absence of predisposing lesion. Infarction in uncommon areas can occur after intravenous cocaine usage (e.g., central retinal artery). *Crack dancing* is a term used to describe choreoathetosis movement of the extremities associated with lip-smacking and repetitive eyeblink due to crack smoking. The effect is rarely seen to occur few minutes to hours after crack smoking. It is thought that crack dancing is due to supersensitivity to the effect of dopamine.

2. *Cardiovascular system effect*: because it is a sympathomimetic, cocaine can cause coronary artery spasm, myocardial ischemia and infarction, ventricular and supraventricular arrhythmias, cardiomyopathy, and aortic dissection.

3. *Renal system effect*: a rare condition that occurs after cocaine abuse characterized by rhabdomyolysis, hyperthermia, excited delirium, and acute renal failure due to myoglobinuria. This condition is referred to as "cocaine run amok syndrome."

4. *Respiratory system effect*: cocaine precipitates attacks of asthma, acute respiratory distress syndrome, pulmonary edema, and chronic obstructive airway disease.

Heroin, in contrast to cocaine, is another opioid that is administered by intravenous (IV) injections. Heroin smoking is an uncommon form of heroin abuse termed "chasing the dragon" in China since the 1920s to avoid the dangers of IV administration. A small quantity of powder is placed on aluminum foil, which is then heated underneath with a lighter or matches. The heroin liquefies into a reddish brown glob, which moves around on the foil and emits a white vapor. The glob or "dragon" is "chased" with the lighter underneath while the vapor is sucked through a straw or pipe. Patients with heroin inhalation present with motor restlessness, cerebellar signs, hypnotic paresis, and pyramidal and pseudobulbar signs.

Laboratory investigations to detect cocaine abuse uses detection of urinary benzoylecgonine level, which has an elimination half-life of 6 h (compared to cocaine elimination half-life of 1 h). Urine benzoylecgonine level can be positive up to 2 days after recent cocaine abuse. Ingestion of *Erythroxylum coca* tea can also result in positive urinary immunoassay for cocaine. Also, hair strand analysis for cocaine abuse can yield a positive result after 1 day after intranasal cocaine abuse. The advantage of hair testing is that the drug persists in hair for longer time intervals than they are present in urine and blood.

> **Signs on Radiographs**
>
> 1. *Body packing* is defined as smuggling drugs within the human body. Three major drugs type are smuggled with body packing (marijuana, heroin, and cocaine). Drug-filled packets in the intestine can be detected in plain abdominal radiographs. On plain radiographs, marijuana shows X-ray density more than stool, heroin has an air-stool X-ray density, and cocaine has an air X-ray density (◘ Fig. 12.2.1).
> 2. Bilateral diffuse pulmonary edema can be seen in cases of acute cocaine overdose. Smoking cracks has been linked to bilateral diffuse alveolar lung opacities due to pulmonary hemorrhage.

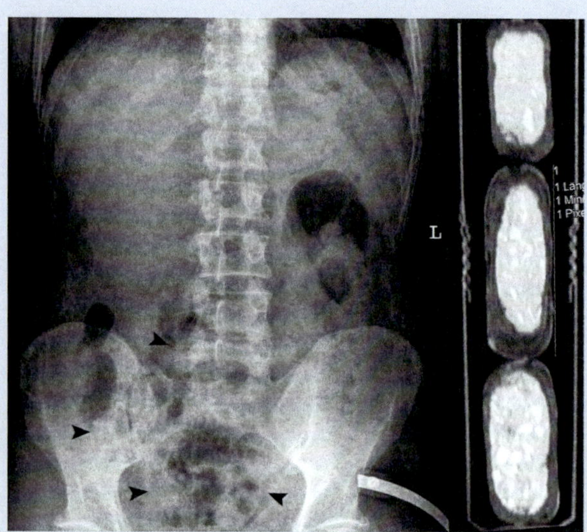



**Fig. 12.2.1** Anteroposterior plain abdominal radiograph that shows abnormal, radio-opaque shadows in the colon (*Arrowheads*), later was found to be marijuana packing in a drug smuggler's colon

### Signs on CT

The CT densities of body packing smuggling are as follows: marijuana shows a bone-like density (700 HU), heroin shows less than fat density (−520 HU), and cocaine shows less than fat density (−219 HU). Pneumoperitoneum or thickened peritoneum is a sign of perforation (*the most common complication of body packing smuggling*).

### Signs on MRI

1. Heroin inhalation can show characteristic features on MRI such as symmetric lesions affecting the posterior limb of the internal capsule; symmetric lesions involving the corticospinal tracts in pons, medial lemnisci and central tegmental tracts, making the findings mimic bearded (dentate nuclei) skull; and symmetric lesions involving the medial lemnisci and the spinothalamic tracts in the midbrain with sparing of the adjacent substantia nigra and red nuclei, making the image resemble bat-head staring at the viewer.
2. Involvement of the cerebellum and the posterior limb of the internal capsule, with sparing of the anterior limb, appear to be a characteristic finding of heroin inhalation.
3. Other MRI signs of heroin abuse include hypoxic brain injury, transverse myelitis, and brain abscess formation.

## Alcohol

Ethanol (*alcohol*) is a very common substance abuse around the world. Alcohol toxicity mainly affects the brain and the central and peripheral nervous systems.

Chronic alcoholics usually have both central nervous system neuronal loss and shrinkage. The brain weight is usually decreased on autopsy reports, with particular atrophy to the cerebellum. Moreover, reduced cerebral blood flow has been reported in alcoholic patients. Severe malnutrition and reduced glycogen stores are also common features in chronic alcohol abusers.

Chronic alcoholism is associated with hypertension, dilated cardiomyopathy (10 %), pancreatitis, liver cirrhosis, and fatty liver. Many other diseases and syndromes are almost strictly seen in patients with alcohol abuse.

*Alcoholic ketoacidosis* is a condition typically seen in chronic alcoholic characterized abdominal pain, metabolic acidosis, and vomiting. The body derives energy from burning fat because of the malnutrition and the reduced glycogen stores. Laboratory investigations show kenouria and high anion gap metabolic acidosis.

*Wernicke's encephalopathy* is a disease which arises due to thiamine deficiency (vitamin B1), causing confusion, ataxia, nystagmus, and ophthalmoplegia. Wernicke's encephalopathy is characterized by a triad of ophthalmoplegia, ataxia, and consciousness disturbances. It is most commonly seen in alcoholism, gastric diseases, hyperemesis, liver cirrhosis, and pregnancy. In Wernicke's encephalopathy, there is symmetric atrophy of the mammillary bodies, hypothalamus, periventricular white matter, and both thalami.

*Korsakoff syndrome* is considered as a chronic phase and a form of chronic complication of Wernicke's encephalopathy. Patients with Korsakoff syndrome present after an acute episode of Wernicke's encephalopathy with dense retrograde amnesia, temporospatial deterioration, confabulation, and emotional changes (e.g., apathy). Alcoholic amnesia has a more global state of mental functions impairment than Korsakoff syndrome.

*Marchiafava–Bignami disease* is a fatal complication of alcoholism characterized by degeneration and demyelination of the corpus callosum, mainly in the midportion. The disease has acute and chronic forms. The acute form is characterized by seizures, severe neurological disturbance, and coma. The chronic form is characterized by disconnection syndrome and progressive dementia.

*Alcoholic polyneuropathy* is a rare condition that arises due to severe vitamin $B_{12}$ deficiency. The condition is seen in less than 9 % of alcoholics with severe alcohol consumption (>100 g of alcohol/day). Up to 40 % of patients are asymptomatic; however, symptomatic patients show signs of muscle tenderness and dull aching and burning pain in the feet and legs. Other signs include hyperesthesia, hyperhidrosis of hands and feet, esophageal dysmotility, plantar foot ulcers (mainly 1st and 2nd metatarsal heads), and hoarseness due to cranial nerves palsies. The condition may be accompanied by Wernicke–Korsakoff syndrome.

### Signs on Brain CT and MRI

1. In *Wernicke's encephalopathy*, there is increase signal in T2W and FLAIR images in the periventricular area, mammillary bodies, periaqueductal gray (PAG) region, hypothalamus, both thalami, and the floor of the third ventricle (◘ Fig. 12.2.2). The affected structures may enhance after contrast administration. In chronic cases, mammillary bodies atrophy and third ventricle dilation are often seen.

2. In *Korsakoff syndrome*, atrophy and high T2 signal intensity lesions are noticed in the region of the mammillary bodies and the hippocampus.

3. In *Marchiafava–Bignami disease*, the corpus callosum is atrophied with areas of high T2 signal intensities and contrast enhancement. On CT, enlargement and hypodensity of the corpus callosum is often noticed.

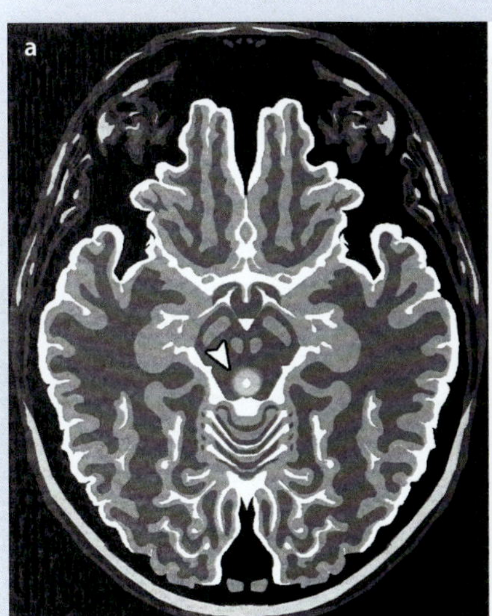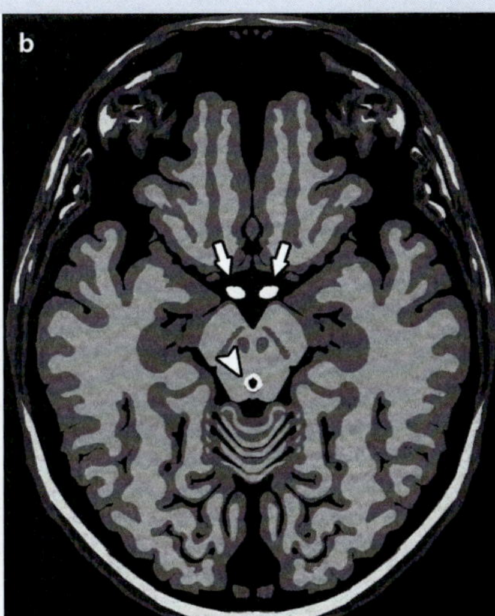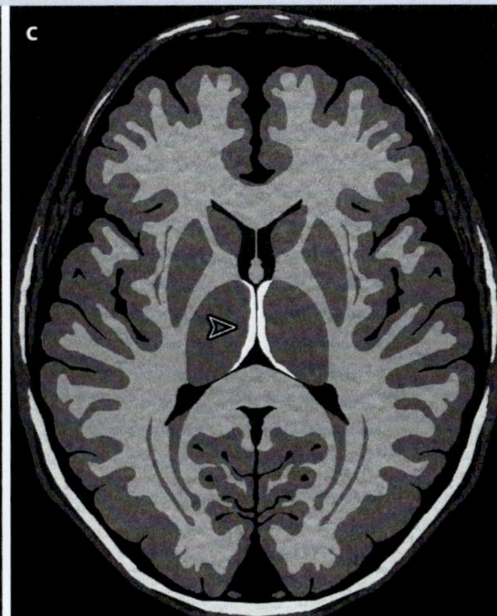

◘ **Fig. 12.2.2** Sequential MR illustrations that show the MR findings in Wernicke's encephalopathy demonstrated an edema with high T2 signal around the periaqueductal gray (PAG) in T2W image (*arrowhead* in **a**), high T1W, post-contrast enhancement around periaqueductal gray (PAG) (*arrowhead* in **b**), high T1W, post-contrast enhancement in the mammillary bodies bilaterally (*arrows* in **b**), and high T1W, post-contrast enhancement affecting the medial side of the thalamus bilaterally (*hollow arrowhead* in **c**)

## Toluene Toxicity

Toluene (*methylbenzene*) is an organic solvent commonly found in paints, glues, adhesives, inks, and cleaning liquids. It has a high potential for abuse, primarily by inhaling vapors from toluene-containing products (e.g., sprays). Chronic toluene abuse causes anion gap metabolic acidosis, renal tubular acidosis type 1, hyperchloremia, and diffuse demyelination and giant axonopathy in both the central and the peripheral nervous system. Clinical feature includes lack of smell (anosmia), personality changes, hearing loss, visual loss, and emotional instability.

### Sign on MRI

1. Mild to marked cerebral and cerebellar atrophy, with increased ventricular size due to parenchymal atrophy with high T2 signal intensity in the periventricular region.

2. There is marked low T2 signal intensity foci within the globus pallidus, putamen, caudate nuclei, red nuclei, thalami, and substantia nigra. This low T2 signal foci are believed to be due to iron deposition or due to direct effect of toluene.

3. Loss of the gray/white matter differentiation on T2W and FLAIR images can be seen.

4. Thin corpus callosum.

## Methanol Toxicity

Methanol (*wood alcohol*) is a clear colorless, flammable liquid with slight alcoholic odor. Methanol is used in industrial solvents such as aftershave, perfumes, cologne, antifreeze, and fuels (e.g., gasoline). Methanol toxicity occurs mainly through ingestion as a cheap substitution for ethanol.

Patients with methanol toxicity present 30–90 min after ingestion with blurred vision (snowstorm blindness) can progress to permanent blindness due to optic atrophy and demyelination. The blurry vision is due to formation of formate by hepatic methanol detoxification, which inhibits cytochrome oxidase in optic nerve. Other manifestations include abdominal pain, diarrhea, hemorrhagic gastritis, nausea, vomiting, seizures, and photophobia. Laboratory investigations show high anion gap metabolic acidosis.

> ### Signs on CT and MRI
> Methanol toxicity affects mainly the putamen, causing bilateral symmetrical putamen infarction and necrosis (low CT density/low T1 intensity lesions) or hemorrhage (high CT density/high T1 intensity lesions). Bilateral hemorrhagic or necrotic lesions confined mainly to the putamen are characteristic signs of methanol toxicity.

## Amphetamines Abuse

Amphetamines are synthetic agents with sympathomimetic properties on both central and peripheral nervous systems, since they simulate adrenalin effect on alpha ($\alpha$) and beta ($\beta$) receptors. Amphetamine abuse can be through oral ingestion or inhalation (smoked). Patients with amphetamine toxicity present with signs of increased sympathetic activity, causing chest pain, myocarditis, hypertension, delirium, hallucination, headache, rhabdomyolysis, stroke, and bilateral acute cortical necrosis.

*Bilateral acute cortical necrosis* (BACN) is a rare condition characterized by necrosis of the renal cortex with columns of Bertin, with sparing of the medulla and of a thin layer of subcapsular cortex. BACN is responsible for less than 1 % of renal failure causes. BACN can be seen also in patients with abruptio placenta, shock, viper bite, hemolytic uremic syndrome, renal transplant rejection, cocaine abuse, and acute pancreatitis.

Laboratory investigations show hyperkalemia (*due to hyperthermia and rhabdomyolysis*), myoglobinuria, and hypernatremia (due to dehydration). The condition is usually suspected with patients with severe oliguria or anuria (0–50 ml/24 h).

> ### Signs on Plain Radiograph
> Tram-track like or eggshell calcification (nephrocalcinosis) is a pathognomonic finding of old cortical necrosis.

> ### Signs on CT
> 1. In the complete form of BACN, there is lack of cortical enhancement bilaterally with preserved renal medullary enhancement (rim sign). A very thin layer of cortical enhancement can be also

seen. In the incomplete form of BACN, there is patchy enhancement of the renal cortices bilaterally with preserved renal medullary enhancement.
> 2. Brain CT may show intraparenchymal or subarachnoid hemorrhage.

## Marijuana

Marijuana (*Tetrahydrocannabinol*) is a psychoactive material from the flowers and leaves of the hemp plant *Cannabis sativa*. Marijuana has so many common street names such as dope, hashish, Panama red, pot, and weed.

Marijuana abuse causes alteration in sensation, perception, judgment, and psychomotor functions. Acute marijuana intoxication can induce acute psychosis and pneumomediastinum. When it is smokes, it takes 15 s for marijuana to reach the brain from the lungs, and the effect may last from 1 to 4 h. Chronic marijuana users may suffer from schizophrenia, abnormal sperm motility and morphology, and cancer of the mouth or tongue. In children, marijuana intoxication may induce coma.

Laboratory investigations show marijuana in urine in up to 3–8 weeks in chronic marijuana abusers and up to 3 days in sporadic users. False-positive urinary marijuana test can be caused by ingestion of ibuprofen, while false-negative urinary marijuana test can be caused by diuretic use.

## Butane Poisoning

Butane is a low molecular weight, volatile aliphatic hydrocarbon solvent usually found in spray and deodorant. Butane is abused through inhalation to achieve euphoric state, commonly among children and young adults (7–17 years).

Patients with butane inhalation often present with acute confusion state, cardiac arrhythmias, pulmonary edema, abdominal pain, ataxia, hallucinations, insomnia, and photophobia. Very few people may present with strange aroma or perioral "Huffler's rash."

*Sudden sniffing death syndrome* is a term used to describe deaths related to solvent abuse like butane. In butane inhalation, the myocardium is hypersensitized to epinephrine, so that any sudden stimulation or excitation of the used can result in cardiac arrhythmias that can cause cardiac arrest. Epinephrine is a contraindication in cases of cardiac arrests with butane or hydrocarbon solvent abuse.

A young patient with cardiac arrhythmia, strange odor, and central nervous system manifestations should be suspected to be poisoned by butane or other hydrocarbon solvents.

**Signs on MRI**

Patients with butane poisoning can show bilateral symmetrical thalamic lesions on T2W images mainly in the posterior thalamic regions (*pulvinar sign*) (◘ Fig. 12.2.3) that represent vasogenic edema without ischemic insult (*no contrast enhancement or diffusion restriction detected*).

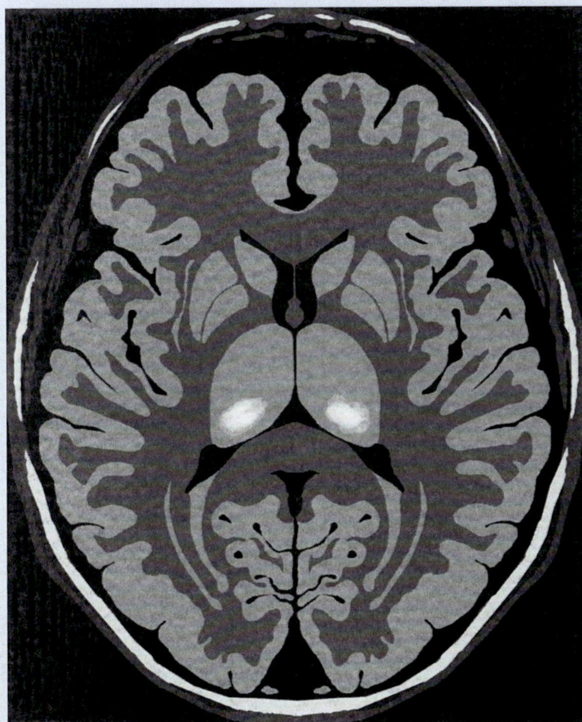

◘ **Fig. 12.2.3** FLAIR-T2W-MR image that demonstrates the "pulvinar sign" seen as bilaterally high signal intensities in the region of the pulvinar nucleus of the thalamus, the largest thalamic nuclei located posteriorly

## Selected References

Borsuzky S, et al. Confabulation in alcoholic Koraskoff patients. Neuropsychologia. 2008;46:3133–43.

Caparros-Lefebvre D, et al. Marchiafava-Bignami disease: use of contrast media in CT and MRI. Neuroradiology. 1994;36:509–11.

Catalano OA, et al. Contrast enhanced computer tomography of two cases of bilateral acute cortical necrosis, one of which related to amphetamine abuse. Emerg Radiol. 2005a;11:306–8.

Catalano OA, et al. Contrast enhanced computer tomography of two cases of bilateral acute cortical necrosis, one of which related to amphetamine abuse. Emerg Radiol. 2005b;11:306–8.

Goldstein RA, et al. Cocaine: history, social implications, and toxicity – a review. Dis Mon. 2009;55:6–38.

Harris D, et al. Butane encephalopathy. Emerg Med J. 2005;22:676–7.

Hergan K, et al. Drug smuggling by body packing: what radiologists should know about it. Eur Radiol. 2004;14:736–42.

Kamran S, et al. MRI in chronic toluene abuse: low signal in the cerebral cortex on T2-weighted images. Neuroradiology. 1998;40:519–21.

Kang SY, et al. Wernick's encephalopathy: unusual manifestation on MRI. J Neurol. 2005;252:1550–2.

Keogh CF, et al. Neuroimaging features of heroin inhalation toxicity: "Chasing the Dragon". AJR. 2003;180:847–50.

Kile SJ, et al. Bithalamic lesions of butane encephalopathy. Pediatr Neurol. 2006;35:439–41.

Lazarides SP, et al. Heroin induced osteopenia: a cause of bilateral insufficiency femoral neck fracture in a young adult. Eur J Orthop Surg Traumatol. 2005;15:322–5.

Leeds NE, et al. The radiology of drug addiction affecting the brain. Semin Roentgenol. 1983;18(3):227–33.

Otake S, et al. Marchiafava-Bignami disease: CT and MR findings. Eur Radiol. 1992;2:382–4.

Pagnan L, et al. Magnetic resonance imaging in a case of Wernick's encephalopathy. Eur Radiol. 1988;8:977–80.

Restrepo CS, et al. Pulmonary complications from cocaine and cocaine-based substances: imaging manifestations. Radiographics. 2007;27:941–56.

Rosenberg NL, et al. Toluene abuse causes diffuse central nervous system white matter changes. Ann Neurol. 1988;23:611–4.

Scardina GA. The effect of cigar smoking on the lingual microcirculation. Odontology. 2005;93:41–5.

Sefidbakht S, et al. Methanol poisoning: acute MR and CT findings in nine patients. Neuroradiology. 2007;49:427–35.

## 12.3 Gases, Inorganic, and Chemical Poisoning

### Arsenic Poisoning

Arsenic (As) is a natural earth crust element that is found in rocks and soil, foods (e.g., sea foods and shellfish), combustion of coals, fungicides, wood preservations, and galls and ceramics. Arsenic is present in two forms: organic (arsine) and inorganic (elemental arsenic and arsenite).

Arsenic binds to the globin portion of hemoglobin and impairs the cellular and mitochondrial respiration. Also, it inhibits the pyruvate dehydrogenase enzyme in Krebs cycle. Toxicity can arise via ingestion, inhalation, or through the skin. Arsenic gas is colorless and extremely toxic, with a garlic-like odor.

Acute arsenic poisoning is classically present within 30 min of absorption with a triad of abdominal pain, hematuria, and jaundice due to hepatitis; other acute symptoms include hypotension, vomiting, nonspecific headache, garlic-odor on the breath, and severe "cholera-like" diarrhea. In contrast, chronic arsenic poisoning presents with polyneuropathy affecting mostly the lower limbs, cortical atrophy, myocarditis and prolongs QT interval, hemorrhagic gastritis, exfoliative dermatitis, and hemolysis and pancytopenia. *Mees lines* are white lines seen on the nails suggestive of nail growth arrest from chronic arsenic poisoning. *Blackfoot disease* is a term used to describe dry foot gangrene due to atherosclerosis seen primary in endemic areas of chronic arsenicism on the south coast east of Taiwan. Diagnosis of arsenic poisoning is confirmed by detecting high arsine in blood (normal <7 μg/dL) and 24 h urine collection.

*Upward gaze-evoked nystagmus* (UGEN) is an uncommon condition reported with organoarsenic compound (*Diphenylarsenic acid*) poisoning characterized by nystagmus when the patient is asked to look upward due to gaze-holding failure, in association with cerebellar ataxia, involuntary movements (tremors and myoclonus), attention and memory deficits, and sleep disorders. However, ocular movements are intact (important clinical feature). UGEN is caused by bilateral damage to the oculomotor neural nuclei (of Cajal) in the midbrain, which has been reported with organoarsenic compounds poisoning such as diphenylarsenic acid.

> **Signs on MRI**
>
> In upward gaze-evoked nystagmus, MRI typically shows bilateral midbrain lesions involving the tegmentum, where the interstitial nucleus of Cajal lies (◘ Fig. 12.3.1).
>
> 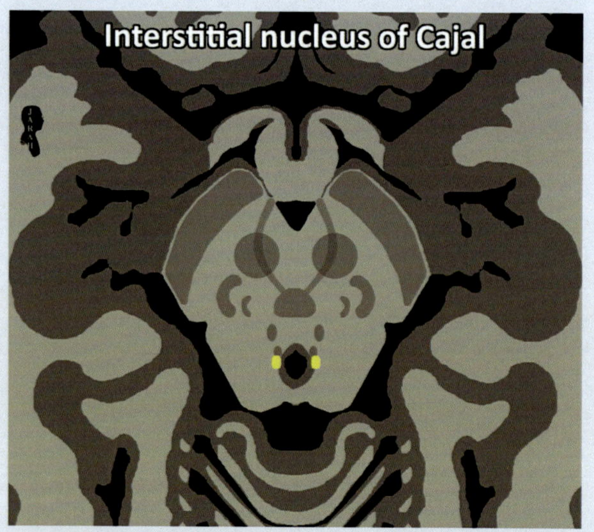
> 
>
> ◘ **Fig. 12.3.1** Axial T1W-MR illustration the demonstrates the normal location of the interstitial nucleus of Cajal on MRI (*yellow nuclei*)

## Mercury Poisoning

Mercury poisoning can be due to three main types: elemental, organic, and inorganic forms of mercury. Inhalation is the main route of mercury absorption of elemental mercury. Elemental mercury (*quicksilver*) is the only elemental metal that is a liquid at room temperature, and it is easily vaporized when spilled. Once it is in the bloodstream, it distributes to all tissues and can cross the placenta barrier and the blood–brain barrier.

Acute exposure to high elemental mercury vapor causes symptoms similar to those of metal fume fever. *Metal fume fever* is a viral-like occupational illness of welders characterized by fever, dyspnea, cough, chest pain, and diffuse muscle weakness. The disease is also known as "Monday morning fever" because symptoms often appear on Monday morning, when workers resume welding after a weekend off. The disease is caused by inhalation of metal fumes like zinc, iron, and copper. Patients with mercury poisoning present classically with a triad of intention tremor, erethism, and gingivitis. *Erethism* is a constellation of findings in mercury poisoning that include memory loss, insomnia, timidity, and sometimes delirium.

*Minamata disease* is a disease characterized by multiple neurological manifestations due to poisoning with methyl mercury (MeHg) or organic mercury. The disease is named after massive MeHg poisoning first reported in 1950s among residents living around Minamata Bay, a small inlet located in the southwestern coast of Kyushu island, Japan. The primary route of exposure to MeHg in this incident was the consumption of fish and shellfish contaminated with a high concentration of MeHg. The mercury resulted from the effluent of a new industrial plant that had been producing vinyl chloride, acetaldehyde, and its derivatives on a large scale.

Minamata disease has acute, chronic, and infantile forms. The acute form is characterized by bilateral symmetrical concentric constriction of visual fields with normal visual acuity and papillary reflexes, hearing loss, abnormalities in taste and smell, and psychiatric abnormalities. The chronic form is characterized by polyneuropathy and cerebellar ataxia due to cerebellar atrophy. The infantile form presents in the form of cerebral palsy due to extensive cerebral cortex spongiosis.

*Acrodynia*, also known as "pink disease," is a rare pediatric condition that arises due to chronic exposure to inorganic mercury (calomel) characterized by pink discoloration of the tips of fingers, toes, wrists, and ankles. Mercury poisoning can rarely cause brown-yellow discoloration of the lens due to direct deposits of mercury in the anterior capsule of the eye. Children with pink disease present with flushing, hypertension, excessive salivation, morbilliform rash, and desquamation of the palms and soles.

Diagnosis of mercury is confirmed by 24-h urine collection or measuring serum mercury level (normal <10 mg/L). Plasma elemental mercury half-life is about 60 days, and it is excreted mainly in the urine and feces.

> **Signs on CT and MRI**
>
> 1. Characteristically, cerebellar atrophy in Minamata disease affects mainly the middle and the inferior vermis.
> 2. The occipital cortex shows atrophy especially around the area of the calcarine sulcus.
> 3. Focal occipital lobe high T2 signal intensities can be found in the area of the striatal cortex.

# Chronic Beryllium Disease (Berylliosis)

Berylliosis is a multisystem disorder caused by exposure to dust or fumes of beryllium metal or salts. Beryllium is a metal that is usually mixed with copper to make alloys that are used in airplane landing gear, air conditioners, microwaves ovens, and electronics.

Acute beryllium disease is so rare, and the chronic form is the less rare form and the one usually seen. Chronic berylliosis is a granulomatous disease that affects the lungs, spleen, liver, lymph nodes, and bone marrow. It can also cause skin papules, hypercalcemia, and hypercalciuria. Onset of symptoms can occur months or years after exposure (up to 20 years). The most common symptom is exertional dyspnea; later core pulmonale and pulmonary hypertension may occur.

> **Signs in Radiograph**
> 1. The picture of this disease resembles the picture of sarcoidosis in chest radiograph. There will be diffuse interstitial nodular lung pattern with mild to moderate hilar lymphadenopathy.
> 2. Bilateral upper lobe fibrosis occurs in long-standing disease.

# Pneumoconiosis

Pneumoconiosis is a term used to describe a group of diseases caused by inhalation of *inorganic dust*. The most common inorganic dusts inhaled are silica dust (*Silicosis*), coal dust (*Coal worker's lung*), and asbestos.

*Silicosis* is a disease caused by inhalation of silica dust or silicon dioxide. Acute silicosis is called "silicoproteinosis" and is characterized by widespread consolidation with air bronchogram (*diffuse alveolar lung disease*).

*Coal worker's lung* (CPW) is a disease caused by inhalation of coal dust. *Erasmus syndrome* is a disease characterized by CWP in association with progressive systemic sclerosis (*scleroderma*). *Caplan's syndrome* (*rheumatoid pneumoconiosis*) is a rare disease that occurs due to formation of necrobiotic rheumatoid lung nodules on top of CWP. It is difficult to be distinguished from tuberculosis or other infective granulomas radiologically without a proper history.

> **Signs on Radiograph**
> 1. Silicosis produces interstitial nodular pattern with upper lobe predominance.
> 2. Hilar lymphadenopathy may be seen in silicosis. In 5 % of cases, pathognomonic peripheral calcification of the hilar lymph nodes can occur, which is classically described as "eggshell calcification pattern."

> 3. In minority cases of silicosis, parenchymal mass of fibrosis in the upper lobes occurs bilaterally, a condition known as *progressive massive fibrosis*.
> 4. In coal worker's lung, bilateral interstitial nodular pattern similar to silicosis is often seen. Key of differentiation is occupational history.

# Insecticides and Rodenticides Poisoning

Insecticides are compounds that are used to kill insects, whereas rodenticides are compounds used to kill rodents (e.g., mice). Different compounds of insecticides with different mechanisms of action are available commercially. Insecticides include organophosphate, carbamate, chlorinated hydrocarbons, pyrethrin, and DEET (*m-isomer of N,N-diethyl-3-methylbenzamide*). Rodenticides include superwarfarin, strychnine-containing compounds, phosphide, and barium.

Organophosphate and carbamate are insecticides used in agricultural and household purposes that work by inhibiting acetylcholinesterase (AChE). Inhibition of AChE results in accumulation of acetylcholine at synapses, causing overstimulation of the autonomic and somatic nervous system. Organophosphate can easily cross the blood–brain barrier (BBB), and it inhibits AChE irreversibly. In contrast, carbamate poorly penetrates the BBB and inhibits AChE reversibly.

Organophosphate and carbamate exposure can be through dermal, pulmonary, or gastrointestinal routs (e.g., *food contamination*). Patients with organophosphate or carbamate poisoning typically show clinical picture due to muscarinic receptors overstimulation that can be expressed by the mnemonic DUMBBELS (*d*iarrhea, *u*rinary incontinence, *m*iosis, *b*radycardia, *b*ronchospasm, *e*mesis, *l*acrimation, and *s*alivation). Stimulation of the nicotinic receptors at the neuromuscular junction results in muscle weakness, paralysis, and fasciculation. The CNS effect of organophosphate includes restlessness, seizures, and coma. Other features include acute pancreatitis and prolonged QT interval.

*Intermediate syndrome* is a term used to describe an uncommon condition that arises 24–96 h after the onset of organophosphate or nerve gas poisoning (e.g., *sarin*) characterized by diffuse muscle weakness that affects the neck muscles, extremities, diaphragm and respiratory muscles, and facial and ocular muscles due to multiple cranial nerve palsies. The condition is treated with pralidoxime. *Organophosphate-induced delay neuropathy* (OPIDN) is another uncommon delay complication of organophosphate poisoning characterized by symmetric lower limb pain, muscle cramps, gloves-and-stock paresthesia, and wasting of hand and peroneal muscles. If the condition is not well treated, spastic paresis affecting the spinal cord's long tracts may occur. OPIDN typically manifest 1–3 weeks after organophosphate exposure.

*Pyrethrum* is an insecticide made up of six active chemical called "pyrethrins," which is derived from dried flowers of Chrysanthemum cinerariifolium. Compounds such as pyrethrins are usually combined with synergistic compounds to inhibit the enzymatic degradation of the pyrethroids in insects. Pyrethrin compounds causes paralysis or "knockdown" effect on flying insects. Pyrethrins are divided into type I (*causes repetitive nerve axon discharge in insects*) and type II (*block inhibitory nervous system pathways by binding to GABA receptor-mediated chloride channels*).

Patients with pyrethrin toxicity presents with contact dermatitis, asthma, rhinitis, and cough when pyrethrins are inhaled. Ingestion of pyrethrins causes abdominal pain, diarrhea, and vomiting. Human exposure to pyrethrins type I cause increased body temperature and tremor, whereas human exposure to type II pyrethrins causes cutaneous burning sensation, chorea, vomiting, diarrhea, pronounced salivation, and seizures.

*DEET* is colorless liquid used as an insecticide against fleas, ticks, and mosquitoes. DEEt can be absorbed through the skin reaching peak blood level within 1–2 h. Half-life of DEET is 2.5 h and up to 10–15 % is excreted unchanged in the urine. Patients exposed to DEET can show seizures, acute manic psychosis, headache, ataxia, hemorrhagic bullae, contact dermatitis, and even coma.

*Strychnine* is a tasteless, odorless crystals used as rodenticides. Human exposure to strychnine can occur via cocaine abuse (mixed with cocaine), suicide attempts, or by accidental ingestion. Strychnine causes an increase in motor neuron stimulation via competing with the neurotransmitter glycine, especially in the brainstem and spinal cord. Strychnine toxicity is seen 15–30 min after exposure and is characterized by motor seizures while the patient is awake with no postictal phase, severe recurrent muscle contraction, trismus, and a twisted stretching of the facial muscles into a grimace (sardonic smile).

*Phosphide rodenticides* are rodenticides composed of zinc and aluminum phosphide. Phosphide rodenticides liberate phosphine gas when come in contact with weak acids. The phosphine gas gives the rat bait its characteristic fishy odor. Patients with phosphide rodenticides poisoning usually present with fatigue, headaches, dizziness, hypotension, fishy odor, pulmonary edema, hypocalcemia, and even coma and shock.

*Barium* is a compound that is used as a rodenticide, in manufacturing glass and ceramics, and extensively in radiological departments as a contrast material (barium sulfate). Barium can cause reduction in potassium ($K^+$) efflux from cells. Patients with barium toxicity presents with profound hypokalemia, muscle paralysis, abdominal pain, vomiting, and diarrhea. Moreover, barium has a direct stimulatory effect on skeletal and cardiac muscles, causing cardiac arrhythmias, rigidity, and muscle cramps. The condition is often treated by administration of magnesium or sodium sulfate, which can precipitate ingested barium as insoluble barium sulfate.



## Carbon Monoxide Poisoning

Carbon monoxide (CO) is a colorless odorless gas that arises from combustion of carbon-containing compounds such as burned fuel, cigarette smoking, faulty heating equipment (e.g., water heater), and pain stripper (e.g., methylene chloride). CO has a higher affinity to bind to hemoglobin and 200 times the affinity of oxygen for hemoglobin, resulting in the formation carboxyhemoglobin (COHb). COHb displaces the oxygen from hemoglobin, causing the main toxic effect of CO poisoning.

Patients with acute CO poisoning often present with cardiopulmonary arrest, ataxia, nystagmus, seizures, and coma. In contrast, patients who are exposed to mild to moderate levels of CO for a long time present with subacute or chronic CO poisoning, which is characterized by nonspecific symptoms such as headache, fatigue, and pulmonary symptoms. *Carbon monoxide-induced neuropsychiatric syndrome* (CO-DNS) is a condition seen in patients who recover from acute CO poisoning characterized by dementia, personality change, Parkinsonism, and rigidity. The condition is seen in 30 % of CO poisoning victims and may appear weeks to months after acute CO poisoning.

3. Chronic causes of CO poisoning classically shows bilateral symmetrical high signal intensity of the globus pallidus on T1W images, with or without contrast enhancement, associated with brain atrophy. However, the same sign has been reported to be seen in Wilson's disease, hepatic encephalopathy, and manganese poisoning (◘ Fig. 12.3.2).

brainstem injury, bilateral cerebellar lesions, and cerebral white matter demyelination.

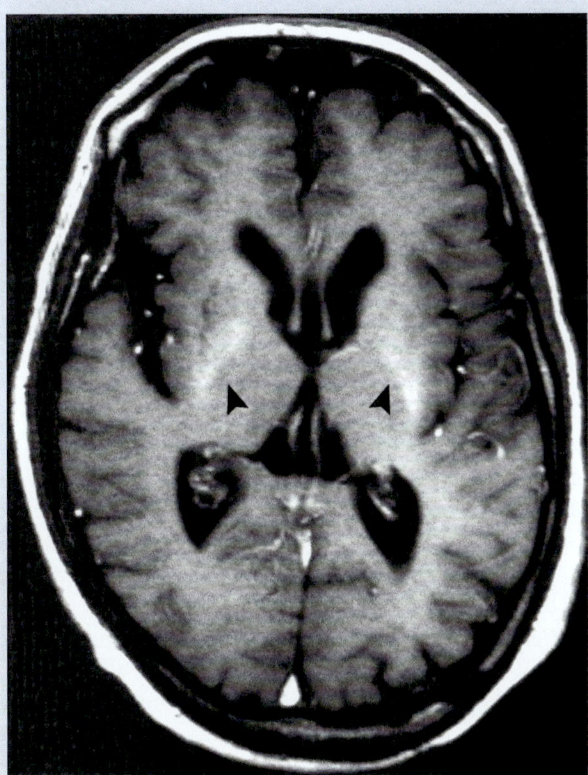

◘ **Fig. 12.3.2** Axial T1W, post-contrast image that shows enhancement of the globus pallidus bilaterally (*arrowheads*); this sign is seen most commonly in CNS poisoning diseases such as CO poisoning, manganese poisoning, cyanide poisoning, copper poisoning, and bilirubin poisoning

by poor response to levodopa and the presence of pyramidal signs (*discriminating it from classical Parkinson disease*). Laboratory investigations may show increased serum chromium levels.

> **Signs on MRI**
> There is bilateral symmetrical increase of T1 signal intensity on T1W images with or without contrast enhancement affecting the basal ganglia (◘ Fig. 12.3.2).

## Thallium Poisoning (Thallotoxicosis)

Thallium is a heavy metal that is toxic to humans and animals. Thallium is used as rodenticide and insecticide, in manufacturing optical lenses, imitation jewelry, and semiconductors. Also, thallium salts have been used for the treatment of syphilis, gonorrhea, tuberculosis, and fungal infections of the scalp. Thallium causes toxicity by substitution of potassium in Na-K-ATPase, as well as high affinity for the sulfhydryl or thiol group of mitochondrial membrane.

Acute thallium poisoning patients present with abdominal pain and diarrhea (day 1) and burning leg paresthesia and arthralgia (day 2–5). Dermatological manifestations (2–6 weeks) include skin rash, hair loss, hyperkeratosis, and Mees lines in nails. Neurological manifestations include muscle weakness, visual hallucinations, cranial nerve palsies, ataxia, tremor, and convulsions. *Encephalopathia thallica* is a term used to describe thallotoxicosis with nonspecific cognitive symptoms that include lack of derive, giddiness, memory impairment, and dementia. Other manifestations include cardiac failure and hypertension.

> **Signs on MRI**
> Patients with thallotoxicosis may show nonspecific signs of high T2 signal intensity brain lesions affecting the corpus striatum, thalamus, and/or hypothalamus.

## Manganese Poisoning

Manganese (Mn) poisoning occurs during inhalation of fume during welding. Welding is the process of joining metals by electrical arc or flames. Melting materials generates concentrated fumes containing high levels of manganese and several gaseous particles, of which 80–95 % can be inhaled by workers.

Chronic manganese poisoning causes distinctive syndrome characterized by Parkinsonism, severe dystonia (*Cock's gait*), psychiatric abnormalities, tinnitus, episodic vertigo, headache, diplopia, myoclonus, and maybe chorea. Parkinsonism due to manganese poisoning is characterized

## Methyl Bromide Poisoning

Methyl bromide ($CH_3Br$) is a highly volatile, odorless gas used in as insecticide and in refrigerators and as a fire extinguisher. Chronic exposure to methyl bromide is often through inhalation. Methyl bromide toxicity belongs to a group of diseases known as energy deprivation syndromes. *Energy deprivation syndromes* (EDS) are group of diseases (*toxic, genetic, and nutritional*) characterized by disturbance of the enzymes involved in metabolic pathways responsible for the generation of energy (e.g., glycolysis). Examples of EDS include Wernicke's encephalopathy (*nutritional EDS*), Leigh's disease (*genetic EDS*), methyl bromide toxicity (*toxic EDS*), metronidazole toxicity (*toxic EDS*), and 6-aminonicotinamide (*toxic EDS*).

Patients with acute methyl bromide toxicity usually present with nausea, vomiting, myalgia, visual disturbance, tremor, and myoclonus seizures. Chronic exposure to methyl bromide causes peripheral neuropathy, causing distal paresthesia, optic atrophy and loss of color vision, cerebellar atrophy, and psychiatric disorders.

> **Signs on MRI**
>
> Patients with methyl bromide can show bilateral symmetrical high T2 signal intensities involving the posterior pons, inferior colliculi, dentate nuclei, inferior olives, posterior putamen, subthalamic nuclei, and periaqueductal gray matter.

## Tattoos

Tattoos are ancient forms of permanent body ornamentation by using the human body as a canvas to draw different illustrations and symbols represents certain ideas. Today, tattoos become popular fashion accessories worldwide, especially for women (50 % of all tattoo customers).

Tattoos can induce skin burns when patients with tattoo on their skin are examined by MRI. It is believed that extremely dark tattoo ink contains a high concentration of iron oxide, and this ferrous pigment can become quite concentrated if sediment ink is used during the tattoo process. Iron oxide is both potentially magnetic and an electrical conductor; therefore, the heating during MRI could raise intracellular water temperature in the skin, resulting in a burn.

### Selected References

Bowler RM, et al. Parkinsonism due to manganese in a welder: Neurological and neuropsychological sequelae. Neurotoxicology. 2006;27:327–32.

Cooper DA, et al. Pneumoconiosis among workers in an antimony industry. AJR. 1968;103:495–508.

Ekino S, et al. Minamata disease revisited: an update on the acute and chronic manifestations of methyl mercury poisoning. J Neurol Sci. 2007;262:131–44.

Itoh K, et al. Cerebellar blood flow in the methylmercury poisoning (Minamata disease). Neuroradiology. 2001;43:279–84.

Josephs KA, et al. Neurologic manifestations in welders with pallidal MRI T1 hyperintensity. Neurology. 2005;64:2033–9.

Kenangil G, et al. Progressive motor syndrome in a welder with pallidal T1 hyperintensity on MRI: a two-year follow-up. Mov Disord. 2006;21(12):2197–262.

Korogi Y, et al. MR findings of Minamata disease – organic mercury poisoning. JMRI. 1998;8:308–16.

Kuczkowski KM. Lumbar tattoo, magnetic resonance imaging, and obstetric anesthesia: what do they have in common? J Anesth. 2007;21:293.

Lo CP, et al. Brain injury after acute carbon monoxide poisoning: early and late complications. AJR Am J Roentgenol. 2007;189:W205–11.

Matsumoto SC, et al. Minamata disease demonstrated by computed tomography. Neuroradiology. 1988;30:42–6.

Nakamagoe K, et al. Upward gaze-evoked nystagmus with organophosphate poisoning. Neurology. 2006;66:131–2.

Shila S, et al. Arsenic intoxication-induced reduction of glutathione level and of the activity of related enzymes in rat brain regions: reversal by DL-*a*-lipoic acid. Arch Toxicol. 2005;79:140–6.

Tsai YT, et al. Central nervous system effects in acute thallium poisoning. Neurotoxicology. 2006;27:291–5.

van der Linde AAA, et al. A previously healthy 11-year-old girl with behavioural disturbances, desquamation of the skin and loss of teeth. Eur J Pediatr. 2009;168:509–11.

## 12.4  Botanical, Environmental, and Organic Poisoning

## Hypersensitivity Lung Diseases (Hypersensitivity Pneumonitis)

Hypersensitivity lung diseases (HLD) are a group of diseases caused by inhalation of *organic dust*. HLD represent lung hypersensitivity to an inhaled allergen. Any allergen can cause this reaction in different individuals, and a specific condition is named after each allergen: mold hay (*farmer's lung*), pigeon's droppings (*pigeon's breeder lung*), moldy sugar cane (*bagassosis*), etc.

Patients with HLD usually present with dyspnea, cough, chills, and fever 4–6 h after the exposure to the allergen in the acute attacks. HLD diseases are not so common, with only 10 % of farmers having farmer's lung and only 15 % of pigeon breeders having pigeon's breeder lung. Medical and occupational history is very important to diagnose these conditions.

> **Signs in Radiograph and Chest CT**
>
> The radiograph and the HRCT of the chest of the hypersensitivity pneumonitis are usually normal; when radiographic abnormalities present, they are mostly diffuse bilateral nodular interstitial pattern due to diffuse interstitial granulomas.

Q: How can you differentiate between granulomas in sarcoidosis and hypersensitivity pneumonitis?

1. Pathologically, the sarcoid granulomas occur in the bronchial walls, while the granulomas of hypersensitivity pneumonitis occur in the alveolar walls.
2. Hilar lymphadenopathy, which is common in sarcoid, is rare in hypersensitivity pneumonitis.

## Cyanide Poisoning

Cyanide is an industrial toxic material that is used as a reagent in many industrial chemical processes such as fumigation, precious metal extraction, artificial nail glue remover (*Acetonitrile*), and photography. Cyanide often exists in salt forms such as sodium cyanide, potassium cyanide, and calcium cyanide. Cyanide poisoning often comes from ingesting high cyanide salts derived from botanical sources such as seeds of apple, pits of apricots ad peaches, bamboo sprouts, and cassava in Africa.

Cyanide exerts its toxic effect by inhibiting many mitochondrial enzymes, especially cytochrome c oxidase, inhibiting oxidative phosphorylation. Cells affected by cyanide are reverting to anaerobic metabolism to replenish energy, resulting in lactic acid build up (*lactic acidosis*). The characteristic effect of cyanide poisoning is hypoxia at the cellular level with intact oxygen delivery.

Patients with acute cyanide poisoning often present with headache, confusion, coma, seizures, hypotension, abdominal pain, and pulmonary edema. Death can occur within 30 min from ingestion of potassium cyanide in up to 95 % of cases. Chronic cyanide poisoning shows symptoms similar to Parkinson's disease.

Laboratory investigation classically shows increased oxygen saturation in venous blood on arterial blood gas (*arterialization of venous blood*) due to the inability of tissues to extract and use oxygen, lactic acidosis, and increased methemoglobin level. Diagnosis is confirmed by detecting high levels of cyanide in the serum (0.5–1.0 mg/L).

> **Signs on MRI**
> On brain contrast-enhanced images, acute cyanide poisoning has been reported to cause enhancement of the basal ganglia (caudate nuclei and putamen) bilaterally (◘ Fig. 12.3.2). The basal ganglia enhancement is presumed to be caused by neuronal necrosis.

## Botulism

Botulism is a paralytic disease caused by the neurotoxin of the gram-positive *Clostridium botulinum*, which causes muscle paralysis which typically involves muscles of the head, neck, and then chest (descending paralysis). The term botulism is derived from the Latin word *botulus*, meaning sausage-shaped. *C. botulinum* is found in soil, sea water, and air. It forms spores that are highly resistant for damage and can withstand boiling temperature of 100 °C for hours. The main action of *C. botulinum* involves inhibiting the release of acetylcholine from the presynaptic terminals, resulting in muscle paralysis.

**▪▪ Types of Botulism**

1. *Classic food-borne botulism* results from ingestion of food contaminated with preexisting neurotoxin (e.g., an expired canned food). Patients are present 6–8 h after neurotoxin ingestion with neurological signs that suggest cholinergic blockage such as visual disturbance, dysphagia, dysarthria, and dry mouth. Other symptoms include signs of food poisoning such as vomiting, nausea, and diarrhea. The main life threat is related to respiratory insufficiency.
2. *Infant botulism* (*<1 year*) results from ingestion of food contaminated with *C. botulinum* spores (e.g., raw honey). The spores proliferate in the GI tract producing neurotoxin, which is then absorbed systemically from the intestine. Infants with botulism present with constipation, hypotonia, weakness, and cranial nerve palsies manifesting as expressionless face, ptosis, ophthalmoparesis, and poor head control. Sudden onset of muscle weakness and regression of motor development in a previously healthy infant is characteristic of botulism. Other causes of infantile constipation include malnutrition, hypothyroidism, and adrenal insufficiency.
3. *Wound botulism*: results from wounds contaminated with *C. botulinum* spores.

> **Signs on Radiographs**
> Abdominal radiographs can show signs of bowel obstruction with retention of fecal material.

> **Signs on Barium Enema**
> Barium enema can show reduced peristalsis and barium retention in the bowel >2 days (normal barium is excreted within 24–48 h).

### Selected References

Diaz JH. Poisoning by herbs and plants: rapid toxidromic classification and diagnosis. Wilderness Environ Med. 2016;27(1):136–52.

Fernandes L, et al. Hypersensitivity pneumonitis in a housewife exposed to aspergillus flavus in poor living conditions: a case report. J Clin Diagn Res. 2016;10(1):OD16–7.

Fortin JL, et al. Cyanide poisoning and cardiac disorders: 161 cases. J Emerg Med. 2010;38(4):467–76.

Lacasse Y, et al. Diagnostic accuracy of transbronchial biopsy in acute farmer's lung disease. Chest. 1997;112(6):1459–65.

Millon L, et al. Aspergillus species recombinant antigens for serodiagnosis of farmer's lung disease. J Allergy Clin Immunol. 2012;130(3):803–5.e6.

Rosow LK, et al. Infant botulism: review and clinical update. Pediatr Neurol. 2015;52(5):487–92.

Zaknun JJ, et al. Cyanide-induced akinetic rigid syndrome: clinical, MRI, FDG-PET, b-CIT and HMPAO SPECT findings. Parkinsonism Relat Disord. 2005;11:125–9.

## 12.5  Drug-Induced Radiological Changes

This topic summarizes the common radiological features reported in the radiological literature regarding certain group of medications:

1. *Thalidomide*: it is a drug that is used as a sedative, to treat leprosy and to inhibit angiogenesis. Thalidomide acts on the mesoderm development, causing deficient bone formation. It can causes hemimelia of radius and thumb (radial ray deficiency) and even congenital absence of all four limbs (Amelia).
2. *Folic acid antagonist* (*e.g., methotrexate*): its use during pregnancy can cause absence of frontal bone and absence of lambdoid or coronal suture in the fetus.
3. *Prostaglandin E*: it is used to maintain patency of the ducts arteriosus in infants. It can cause cortical hyperostosis plus extensive diaphyseal cortical periosteal reaction seen in the ribs, clavicles, and long bones of extremities. This effect is usually noted after 1 month from starting therapy. Differential diagnoses include hypervitaminosis A, congenital syphilis, and battered child syndrome.
4. *Heparin*: heparin is a short-term medication used as an anticoagulant to treat thrombosis. The use of high doses of heparin (10,000 units)/day for more than 4 months can induce osteoporosis, hyperkalemia, and insufficiency fractures. On CT, multiple hyperdense lesions with or without intracutaneous air can be seen in the abdominal subcutaneous tissue due to subcutaneous heparin injections.
5. *Aluminum*: it is given to patients with dialysis to inhibit phosphate reabsorption, especially children with chronic renal failure. The use of aluminum can induce osteoporosis, osteomalacia, and hyperparathyroidism.
6. *Calcium gluconate*: it is medication that is often used in the neonatal period to address abnormalities in calcium metabolism. It can cause subcutaneous soft-tissue calcification.
7. *Hypervitaminosis D*: vitamin D toxicity (>100,000 IU per day) usually presents with fatigue, hypertension, diabetes insipidus-like symptoms (polyuria and polydypsia), hypercalcemia, and nephrocalcinosis. On radiographs, the most striking manifestation is large, amorphous clumps of soft-tissue calcification typically found around large joints, tendon, and bursae. Differential diagnosis includes tumoral calcinosis, hyperparathyroidism, and multiple myeloma.
8. *Warfarin* (*coumarin*): it is an anticoagulant that inhibits vitamin K-dependent clotting factors (factors II, VII, IX, and X) by the liver. Warfarin can cause bleeding diathesis, ecchymosis, mediastinal hemorrhage (rarely), acute interstitial nephritis, and skin necrosis in obese women (especially in the breast and buttocks). *Fetal warfarin syndrome* is a term used to describe the teratogenic effect of warfarin on fetus, especially when given within the first 3 months of life (6th to 9th weeks specifically). Fetal anomalies due to pregnancy warfarin use include prematurity, neonatal death, Dandy–Walker anomaly, cerebellar atrophy, encephalocele, agenesis of the corpus callosum, nasal cartilage hypoplasia, cardiac anomalies, shortened metacarpals, and nail hypoplasia. On plain radiographs, stippled epiphyses can be seen in neonates with fetal warfarin syndrome (differential diagnosis include chondrodysplasia punctate).
9. *Methysegide*: it is an ergot alkaloid drug used in the treatment of migraine headache. Ergot-derivative drugs are known to cause retroperitoneal fibrosis, as well as fibrosis of the pleura, pericarditis (constrictive type), heart valves, and great vessels. On radiographs, methysergide can cause unilateral or bilateral pleural effusions before developing lung fibrosis.
10. *Carmustine*: it is a nitrosourea frequently used in the treatment of CNS gliomas, melanoma, lymphoma, and GI malignancies. It can cause bilateral basal lung fibrosis and spontaneous pneumothorax.
11. *Gold salts*: they have been used in the treatment of rheumatoid arthritis and other inflammatory disorders. Gold salts rarely may induce hypersensitivity pneumonitis, causing lung fibrosis, eosinophilia (40 %), dermatitis, Crohn's-like disease, diarrhea, pancreatitis, and cryptogenic organizing pneumonia. On CT, gold salts cause high liver density on non-enhanced scan.
12. *Oxygen therapy*: 100 % oxygen is commonly used in the management of gas poisoning. Pulmonary toxicity due to oxygen therapy is dose related that arises 24–48 h after exposure. In the first stage of lung injury, the lung develops hyaline membrane, intra-alveolar hemorrhage, and capillary congestion. On radiographs, this stage may show patchy alveolar opacities or diffuse interstitial opacities. In the chronic phase of oxygen toxicity, proliferation of fibroblasts, pneumocytes type II, and lung fibrosis develops.
13. *Bromocriptine*: it is a dopamine agonist used in the long-term therapy of Parkinsonism. Bromocriptine may cause complications 1–2 years after therapy that include pleuritis, pleural fibrosis (2–5 % of patients), retroperitoneal fibrosis, and elevated eosinophils and lymphocytes count.
14. *Potassium chloride*: it can alter the gastric peristalsis and emptying forming congealed masses (bezoars) within the stomach.
15. *Oral contraceptives*: it can cause hepatic adenomas, focal nodular hyperplasia, hepatic peliosis, hepatic veno-occlusive disease (Budd–Chiari syndrome), vasculitis, and rarely hepatocellular carcinoma.
16. *NSAIDs*: nonsteroidal anti-inflammatory drugs (NSAIDs) are a class of medications characterized by antripyretic, analgesic, and anti-inflammatory action. NSAIDs are known to cause renal cortical necrosis and

drug-induced esophagitis. Drug-induced esophagitis (for any cause) affects usually the proximal to mid-third of the esophagus, sparing the distal esophageal third (almost pathognomonic). On CT, the esophagus wall diameter is thickened >5 mm (normal <5 mm) and shows submucosal enhancement. Uncommonly, esophageal septae may develop, which are seen on CT as soft-tissue thickening within the esophageal wall that gives the esophagus a "double lumen" appearance.

## Selected References

Berkovich GY, et al. CT findings in patients with esophagitis. AJR. 2000;175:1431–4.

Gatenby RA, et al. The radiology of drug-induced disorders in the gastrointestinal tract. Semin Roentgenol. 1995;30(1):62–76.

McCullough RW, et al. Pill-induced esophagitis complicated by multiple esophageal septa. Gastrointest Endosc. 2004;59(1):150–2.

Neustadter LM, et al. Medication-induced changes of bones. Semin Roentgenol. 1995b;30(1):88–95.

Oguz D, et al. Malformations due to warfarin: a case report. Int J Angiol. 2000;9:125–7.

Ramchandani P, et al. Radiology of drug-related genitourinary disease. Semin Roentgenol. 1995;30(1):77–87.

Young CA, et al. CT features of esophageal emergencies. Radiographics. 2008;28:1541–53.

# Chiropractic Medicine



© Springer International Publishing Switzerland 2017
J.A. Al-Tubaikh, *Internal Medicine*, DOI 10.1007/978-3-319-39747-4_13

## 13.1  The Human Fascia

Connective tissue makes up of about 16 % of the body's weight and stores about 25 % of body's total water content. Connective tissues are derived embryologically from the mesenchyme and forms the biological blocks of the skin, fascia, muscles, nerve sheaths, periosteum, aponeuroses, bones, ligaments, tendons, joint capsules, adipose tissues, blood vessels, and cartilage.

Fascia, an important form of the body's connective tissue, encloses body tissues up to the level of the smallest nerve and muscle fibers (e.g., epineurium). Each fascial layer is enclosed by another fascial layer, like a *plastic bag* within a bigger plastic bag. The human body is composed of many enclosed fluid systems like plastic bags. Since any pressure applied to a liquid-enclosed system at rest from a point will be transmitted equally within this system in all direction (Pascal's law), then we can say that an increased fluid pressure in one fascial compartment (plastic bag) can be transmitted to another fascial compartment, and vice versa.

The fascia is a continuous organ, and one can travel from any portion of the body to another and never leave the fascia. In the human body, four primary fascial layers are described:

1. *Pannicular fascia*: it makes the superficial body fascial layer and is derived from the somatic mesenchyme; it surrounds the entire body with the exception of its orifices such as the orbits, nasal passages, and the oral openings.
2. *Appedicular (axial) fascia*: like pannicular fascia, this fascia is also derived from somatic mesenchyme; it is fused to the panniculus peripherally and extends deep into the body forming the epimysium of skeletal muscle, the fascial layer that surrounds neurovascular bundles (e.g., the brachial plexus), the periosteum of bone, and the peritendon of the tendons.
3. *Meningeal fascia*: it makes the meninges (*pia, arachnoid, and dural layers*) that surrounds the central nervous system.
4. *Visceral fascia*: it forms the fascia that surrounds the viscera like the peritoneum, visceral pleura, perirenal (*Gerota's*) fascia, and cervical fascia that surrounds the pharynx and is attached to skull base. Visceral fascia also forms visceral ligaments (e.g., *ligament of Treitz*). Unlike ligaments in somatic tissue, visceral ligaments typically function to carry blood supply and innervations to an organ system or to loosely anchor an organ in the body cavity.

Fascia is a continuous structure, meaning that the skull's aponeurosis runs continuously up to the plantar fascia of the foot (fascial or meridian planes). If we think of the spine as a "bow," then the anterior fascial planes makes the "string" of that bow (bowstring theory). The anterior prevertebral fascia extends from the skull base, continues down into the clavicles, connects to the mediastinum and upper diaphragm, and follows the falciform; from the coronary ligaments of the liver, linea alba, umbilicus, median umbilical ligament of urachus, and investing fascia of the bladder to the pelvic diaphragm (perineum); and lastly from the pelvic diaphragm to the iliotibial band.

Fascia as a tissue poses unique characteristic in the form of deformation and elongation. Fascia can show both permanent (*viscous*) and temporary (*elstatic*) deformation; also, fascia can show permanent (*plastic*) elongation and contraction (*mechanical elongation*). Many of neurons, blood vessels, and lymphatic vessels travel within fascial planes and tunnels. Therefore, fascial disease such as fibrosis, contraction, and strains can cause musculoskeletal disorders due to exerting pulling tension on the joints, impeding the flow of the interstitial fluid, and impinging on nerves, vessels, and lymphatics.

Beside the mechanical injury, fascial disorder can arise from chemical injury. For example, dehydration causes fascia to shrink, irritating or compressing the sensory nerve fibers within it. Moreover, exogenous intake of corticosteroid or estrogen in the form of oral contraceptive interferes with/inhibits collagen synthesis. Women with chronic intake of oral contraceptive have a higher risk of lower back pain, bone fracture, persistent pelvic pain, and pelvic joint instability than normal women.

It is always wise to consider "neurovascular–lymphatic abnormality" in a patient with fascial disorder (e.g., regional fibrosis). There are many forms of free and encapsulated nerve endings found within the fascial layers that play different roles as "mechanoreceptors," such as:

(a) *Golgi receptors* (type Ib receptors) are located at the myotendinous junction, only responsive to muscular contraction, and have a role in striated muscles motor tonus control (*via inhibiting α-motor neurons*).
(b) *Pacini corpuscle* (type II receptors) are located at the myotendinous junction, responsive to "rapid" pressure change and vibration, and have a role in propioceptive feedback of the joints.
(c) *Ruffini corpuscle* (type II receptors) are located in the ligaments and dura matter, responsive to "sustained" pressure, and have a role in "sympathetic activity inhibition" of the joints.
(d) *Interstitial receptors* (type III, IV receptors) are located everywhere in the fascial layers (most abundant receptors), responsive to "sustained and rapid" pressure change, and have a role in vasodilation and plasma extravastion. These receptors are 50 % low threshold units (A-δ fibers) and 50 % high threshold units (C-fibers).

### Further Reading

Akeson W, et al. The connective tissue response to immobility: biochemical changes in periarticular connective tissue of the immobilized rabbit knee. Clin Orthop. 1973;93:356–61.

Cummings M, et al. Regional myofascial pain: diagnosis and management. Best Pract Res Clin Rheumatol. 2007;21(2): 367–87.

Dormus M, et al. The effects of single-dose dexamethasone on wound healing in rats. Anesth Analg. 2003;97:1377–80.

Elder CL, et al. A cyclooxygenase-2 inhibitor impairs ligament healing in the rat. Am J Sports Med. 2001;29(6): 801–5.

Hedley G. Notes on visceral adhesions as fascial pathology. J Bodyw Mov Ther. 2010;14:255–61.

Iwahashi M, et al. Mechanism of intervertebral disc degeneration caused by nicotine in rabbits to explicate intervertebral disc disorders caused by smoking. Spine. 2002;27(13):1396–401.

Murnaghan M, et al. Nonsteroidal anti-inflammatory drug-induced fracture non-union: an inhibition of angiogenesis? J Bone Joint Surg Am. 2006;88:140–7.

Myers TW. The "anatomy trains", part 2. J Bodyw Mov Ther. 1997a;1(3):135–45.

Myers TW. The "anatomy trains". J Bodyw Mov Ther. 1997b;1(2):91–101.

Schleip R. Fascial plasticity – a new neurobiological explanation: Part 1. J Bodyw Mov Ther. 2003a;7(1):11–1.

Schleip R. Fascial plasticity – a new neurobiological explanation: part 2. J Bodyw Mov Ther. 2003b;7(2):104–16.

Tozzi P, et al. Fascial release effects on patients with non-specific cervical or lumbar pain. J Bodyw Mov Ther. 2011;15:405–16.

Tozzi P. Selected fascial aspects of osteopathic practice. J Bodyw Mov Ther. 2012a;16:503–19.

Tozzi P. Selected fascial aspects of osteopathic practice. J Bodyw Mov Ther. 2012b;16:503–19.

## 13.2 Vertebral Malalignment (Subluxation) Syndromes

Malalignment syndrome, also known as "vertebral subluxation complex" (VSC), is a disorder characterized complex pathological processes that can be summarized as the following:

1. Vertebral joint articulation disturbance which can be due to ligamentous laxity, posttraumatic event, or due to degenerative changes (spondyloarthropathy). Vertebral malalignment commonly results in rotation of one vertebra over the other initially (◘ Fig. 13.2.1), which will progress if not corrected to retro- or anterolisthesis due to bilateral pedicular fracture (spondylosis).

2. Distortion of the pelvic ring associated with compensatory scoliosis of the lumbar vertebral column, which in turn causes compensatory distortion of the upper thoracic and cervical column. Rotational pelvic malalignment is detected in 80 % of cases, where the right or left pelvic bone rotates forward and the other usually compensates by rotating backward relative to the sacroiliac/coccygeal bone (◘ Fig. 13.2.2).

3. Compensatory changes in the soft-tissue structures resulting in uneven back muscles contraction, which predispose to chronic back pain and myofascial trigger points formation.

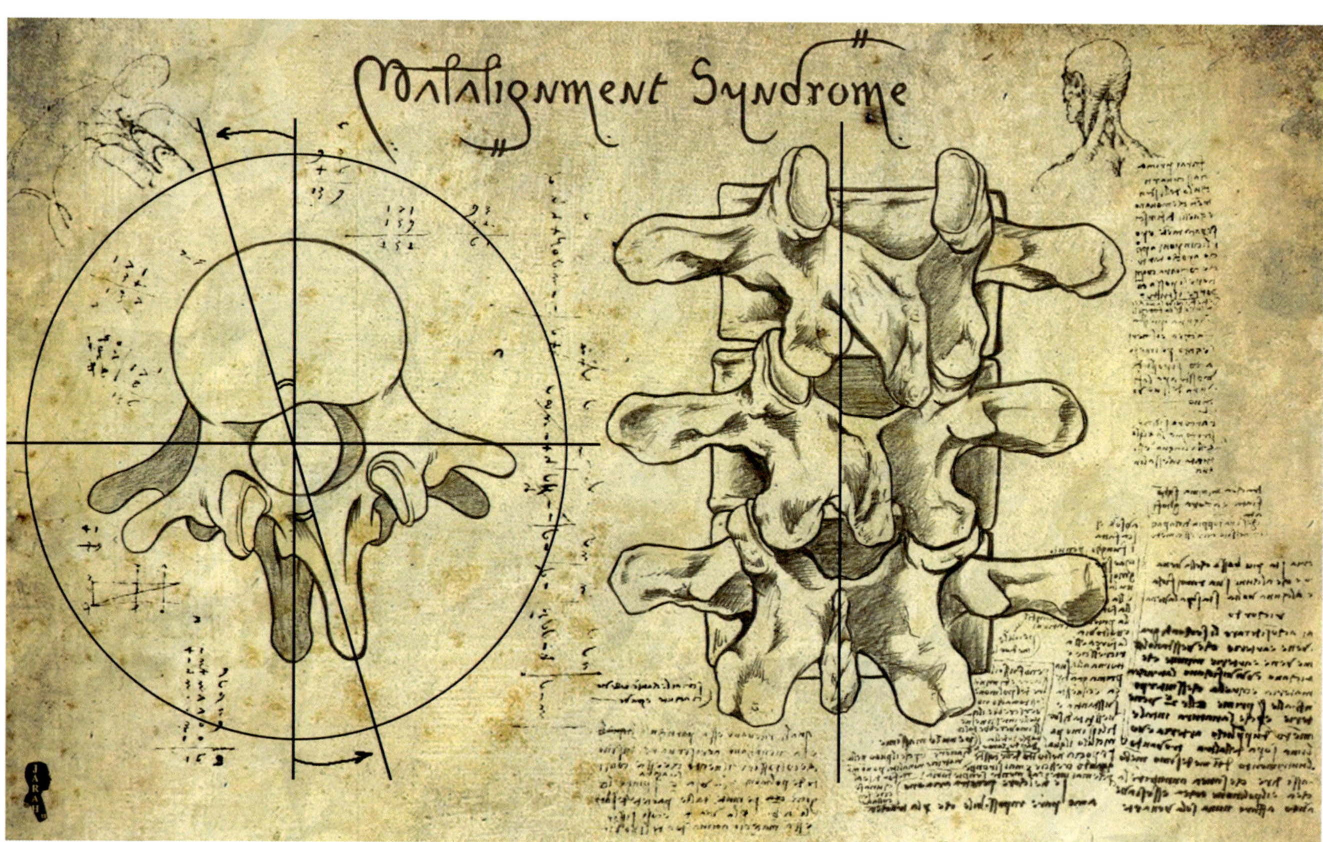


◘ Fig. 13.2.1    An illustration that demonstrates the rotational malalignment on axial and coronal planes

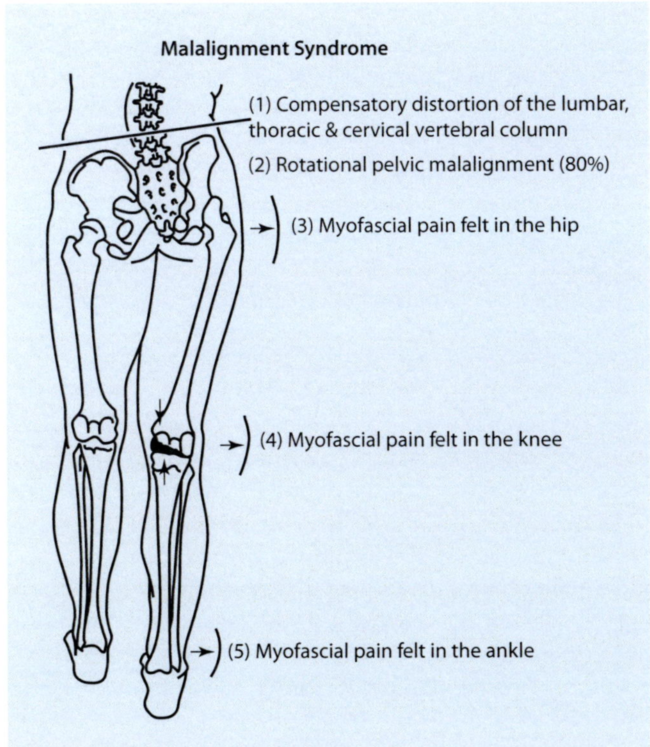



**Fig. 13.2.2** An illustration that demonstrates the complications of vertebral malalignment syndrome and its mechanical–pathological consequences

4. A long-standing vertebral malalignment causes intervertebral disk herniation disorder due to torsion of the annulus in a clockwise direction as a result of rotatory movement of one vertebra over the other (**Fig. 13.2.3**).

5. Uncommonly, vertebral malalignment can cause regional and distant somatovisceral dysfunction attributed to:
   (a) Spinal kinesiopathology: the spinal mechanics and motion irregularities resulted from pelvic obliquity can affect the genitourinary structures, for example.
   (b) Neuropathy: it is due to impingement or stretching of the nearby neural tissues.
   (c) Myopathy: it is due to myofascial trigger points formation in the regional muscular structures (see myofascial pain syndromes topic).
   (d) Inflammation: fascial tension that arises from rotatory vertebral malalignment impedes the interstitial and neurovascular–lymphatic flows, causing regional wastes accumulation, hypoxia, local inflammation, and edema.
   (e) Patho-anatomical changes: when all the past four components persists, local tissue degeneration occurs.

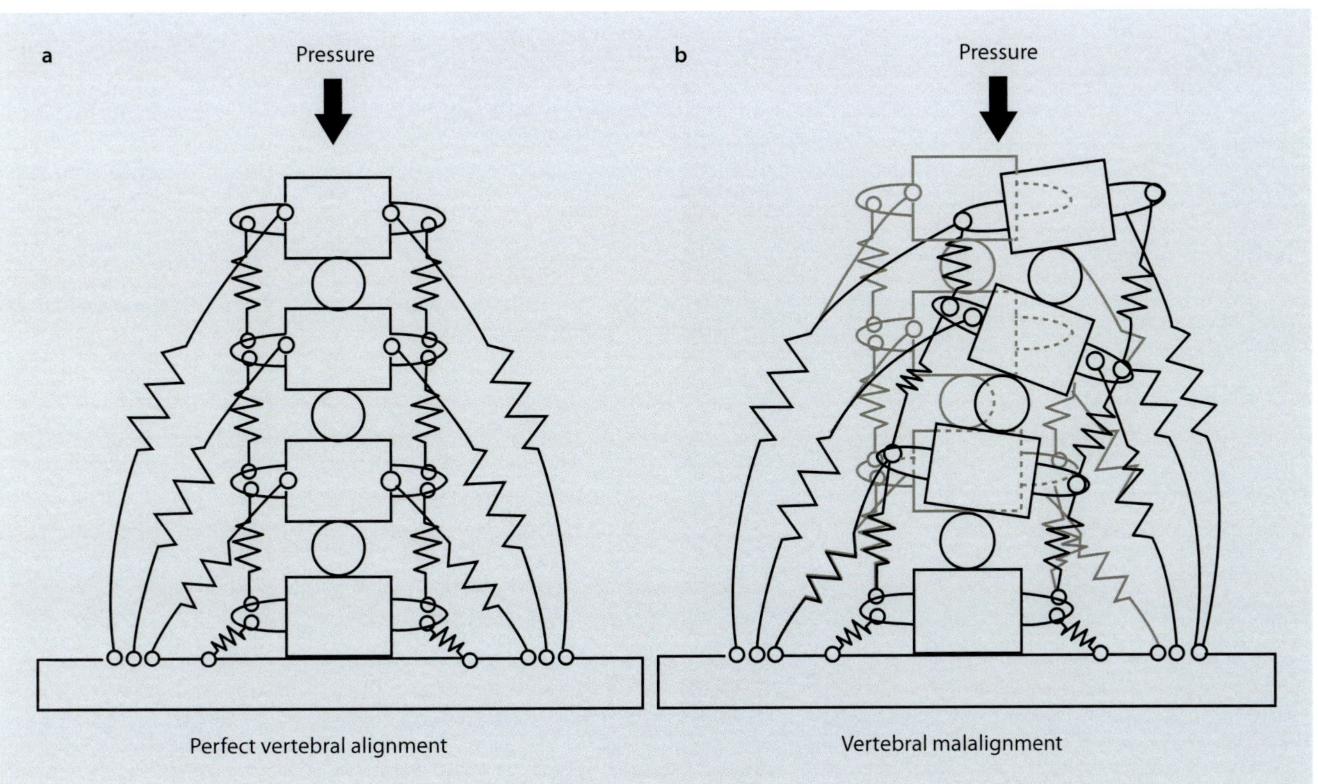



**Fig. 13.2.3** An illustration that demonstrates the effect of the vertebral malalignment over the intervertebral disks; in a perfect alignment (**a**), the pressure overload is equally distributed over the intervertebral disk volume. In contrast, a malaligned vertebra (**b**) will exert uneven pressure load over the intervertebral disk predisposing it for herniation or protrusion

## Anatomy

The vertebral column vertebrae are composed of two main segments: the vertebral body and the posterior arch. The posterior arch is the portion that extends posteriorly from the vertebral body and helps to formulate the vertebral foramen.

Each vertebra is articulated with each other by two joints: (1) fibrocartilaginous joint that lies in between the vertebral bodies (contains intervertebral disk) and (2) a synovial facet joint that exists between the vertebral arches. The fibrocartilaginous disk space dissipates forces that are transmitted along the vertebral column.

The vertebrae along the vertebral column are held in position via multiple ligamentous structures that include:
1. Anterior and posterior longitudinal ligaments: they run in an uninterrupted fashion along the anterior and posterior surfaces of the vertebral body, and they are highly innervated structures.
2. Ligamentum flavum: it attaches the vertebral laminae together.
3. Interspinous ligament: it attaches the superior and inferior portions of the spinous processes together.
4. Supraspinous ligament: it attaches the tips of the spinous processes together.
5. Intertransverse ligament: it attaches the transverse processes together.

A normal axial skeleton alignment is visualized in radiography as properly aligned pelvis, leg length is equal, and the spinouts processes are relatively straight, detected by a straight line that passes through all the spinous processes in anteroposterior radiograph (■ Fig. 13.2.4). Clinically, a normally aligned spine is characterized by equal length and tension in matching pairs of ligaments, muscles, and other soft tissues on the right and left sides of the human back. The past "ideal" description of the back is not applied, unfortunately, to many people, with up to 80 % of people "out of alignment" or "malaligned" by teens.

According to the chiropractic and osteopathic medical literature, up to 97 % of causes of lower back and leg pain are "mechanical" in origin, and only 23 % are due to degenerative changes such as spondyloarthropathies and herniated disk disease. In up to 2 % of cases, lower back pain can be due to visceral disease (e.g., pancreatitis, aortic dissection, etc.).

## Somatovisceral Malalignment Symptoms

As mentioned earlier, the vertebral malalignment syndrome can cause somatovisceral symptoms due to irritation of the spinal nerves exiting the neural foramina either by direct impingement or by the regional inflammation it produces. Many somatovisceral symptoms are known in the chiropractic and osteopathic medical literature to be directly or indirectly related to vertebral malalignment of a specific spinal segment because of the autonomic innervation emitted from that segment to visceral organs. Some of the common vertebral-origin symptoms include:

C1 (pituitary, scalp, brain vessels innervation): headache, tinnitus, insomnia, hypertension, and vertigo

C2 (optic, auditory, sinuses, mastoid, tongue innervation): chronic sinusitis, pain around the eyes, and hearing loss

C3 (facial skin innervation): occipital neuralgia (headache) and eczema (skin neurons irritation)

C4 (Eustachian tube innervation): hay fever, hearing loss, and otitis media

C5 (vocal cords innervation): hoarseness, laryngitis, and sore throat

C6 (neck muscles innervation): neck pain, shoulder pain, and chronic cough

C7 (thyroid, shoulder bursa innervation): thyroid conditions and shoulder bursitis

T1 (esophagus, trachea, upper limbs innervation): asthma, cough, apneas, and upper limb radiculopathy

T2 (coronary arteries innervation): functional heart diseases

T3 (lung, bronchial tree, heart innervation): bronchitis, pulmonary congestion, and pleurisy

T4 (GB, heart innervation): jaundice, GB disorders, and cardiac angina (T3–T7)

T5 (solar plexus, liver innervation): hypertension, arthritis, and liver disease

T6 (stomach innervation): gastroesophageal reflux disease, functional dyspepsia, and indigestion

T7 (pancreas, duodenum innervation): peptic ulcer and gastritis

T8 (spleen innervation): lowered immunity

T9 (adrenal innervation): allergies and hives

T10 (kidneys innervation): fatigue, nephritis, and renal arteriosclerosis

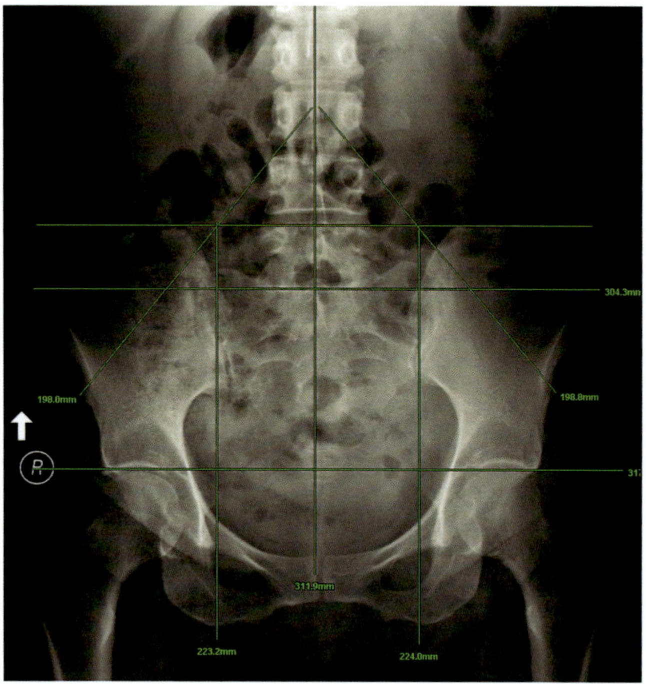


■ **Fig. 13.2.4**   An anteroposterior plain radiograph that demonstrates perfect alignment of the vertebral column in relation to the pelvis

T11 (kidneys, ureters, skin innervation): eczema, boils, and acne

L1 (colon, inguinal rings innervation): colitis, diarrhea, constipation, and hernias

L2 (abdomen, thighs innervation): cramps, difficulty in breathing, and minor varicose veins

L3 (genitalia, ureters, bladder, knees innervation): bladder disorders, painful menstruation, miscarriages, impotency, and knee trigger points

L4 (prostate, perineum, sciatic innervation): sciatica, back pain, and dysuria

L5 (lower legs, feet innervation): leg pain/cramps, cold feet, and weak ankles

Sacrum: buttock pain, back pain, and sacroiliitis

Coccyx: coccydynia and pudendal neuralgia

## 13.3    Imaging Signs

1. On plain radiographs, a normal vertebral alignment is detected by drawing a straight line overlying the spinous processes in anteroposterior (AP) radiographs of the cervical, thoracic, or lumbar vertebral column. Malalignment is simply detected as deviation of one or more spinous processes from the straight line alignment (◘ Figs. 13.2.5 and 13.2.6). The more the rotational malalignment, the more scoliosis or kyphosis detected in the radiograph.

2. On MRI, vertebral malalignment can be detected indirectly via observing the spinous process axis along the scan area on axial images. The spinous processes will show different axes in each vertebral segment on axial images (◘ Fig. 13.2.7).

## Further Reading

Bolton PS. Reflex effects of vertebral sublaxations: the peripheral nervous system. An update. J Manipulative Physiol Ther. 2000;23(2):101–3.

Good C. The sublaxation syndrome: a condition whose time has come? J Chiropr Humanit. 2004;11:38–43.

Harris JH. Malalignment: signs and significance. Eur J Radiol. 2002;42:92–9.

Husson JL, et al. The lumbar-pelvic-femoral complex: applications in hip pathology. Orthop Traumatol Surg Res. 2010;96S:S10–6.

Ratliff J, et al. Increased MRI signal intensity in association with myelopathy and cervical instability: case report and review of the literature. Surg Neurol. 2000;53:81–3.

Vernon H. Historical overview and update on sublaxation theories. J Chiropr Humanit. 2010;17(1):22–32.

## 13.4    Facet Joint Syndrome

Facet joint syndrome is a term used to describe pain originating from the facet joint, typically due to subluxation, nerve irritation, local inflammation, or degenerative changes and frictional spondyloarthritis.

## Basic Anatomy

Each spinal segment consists of a "three-joint complex" formed by an intervertebral disk with small, posterior, paired synovial facet joints. A disturbance in one element affects the other two elements of this triple joint complex. The facet joint is made of a superior articular process derived from

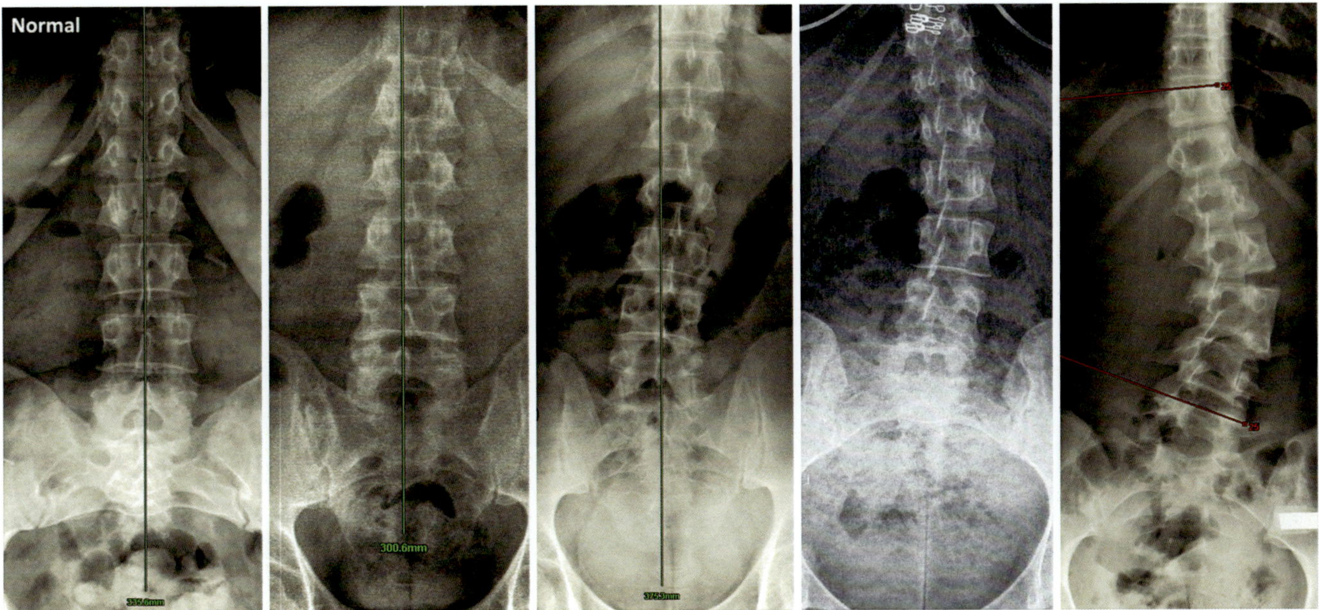


◘ Fig. 13.2.5   Sequential anteroposterior plain radiographs of the lumbar vertebral column of different patients demonstrating the progression of malalignment syndrome from normal (*left side*) to the extreme form of compensatory scoliosis (*right side*)

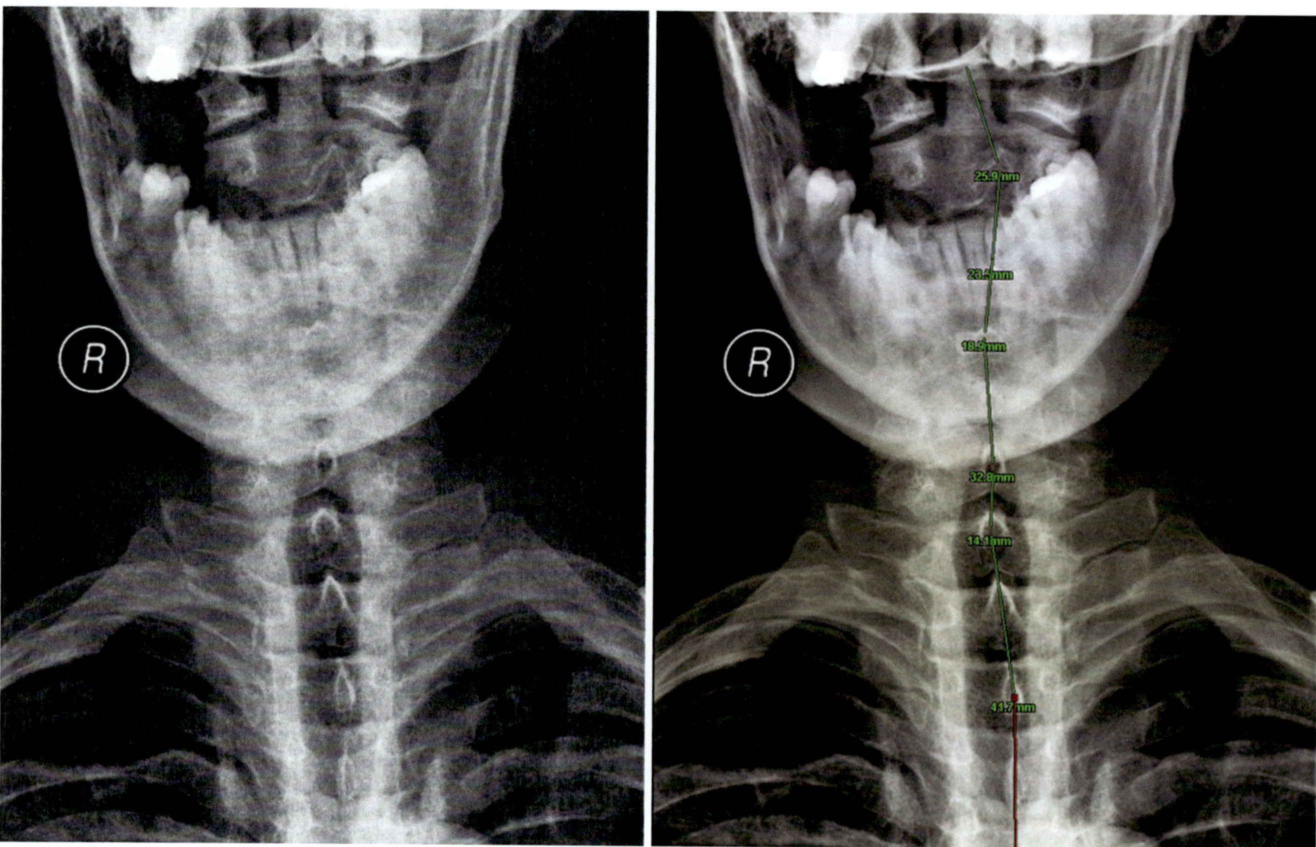

■ **Fig. 13.2.6** An example of anteroposterior plain radiograph of the neck in a patient presented with neck pain and posterior cranial headache; the plain radiograph shows uneven alignment of the cervical vertebrae detected by a line that joins between the spinous processes



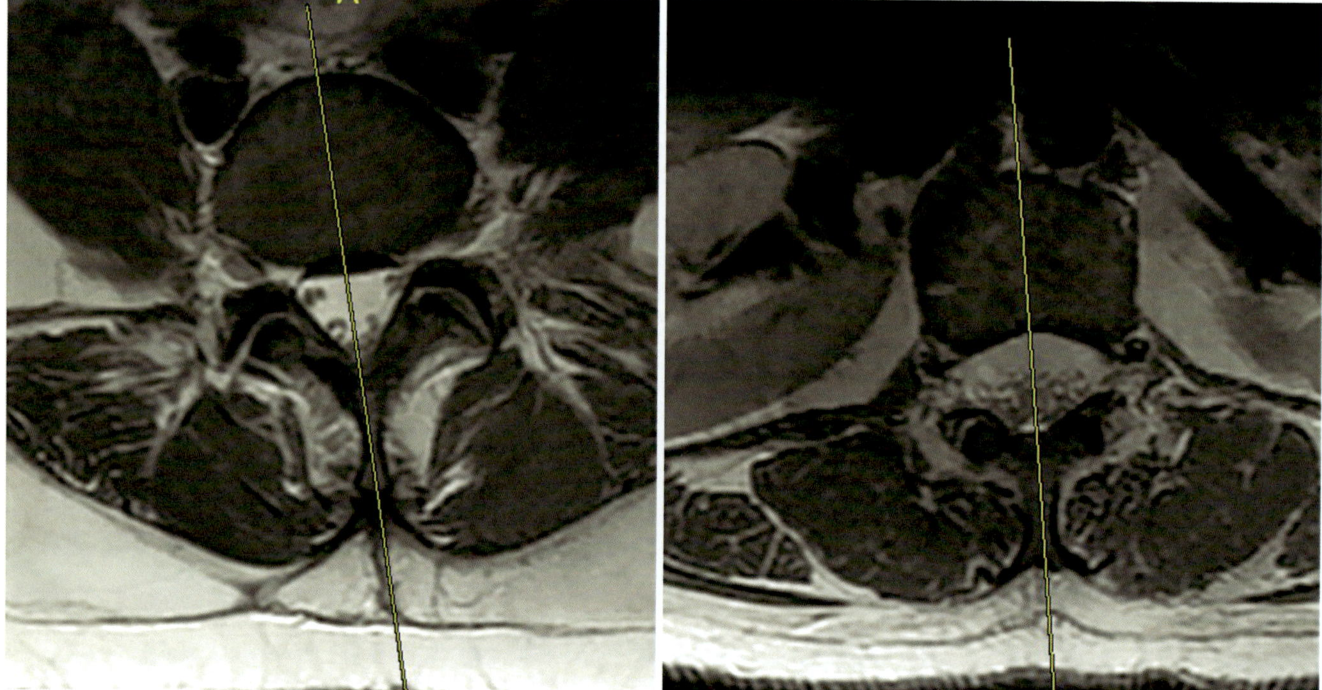

■ **Fig. 13.2.7** An example of MR images that indirectly show rotational malalignment in a patient presented for MR imaging to investigate lower back pain. The spinous process axis is deviated at the level of L4 vertebra (*left image*) and to a lesser degree at the level of L2 image (*right image*)

an inferior vertebra and faces dorsomedially, while the inferior articular process is derived from a superior vertebra and faces ventrolaterally. The facet joints are locked together during an attempted axial rotation of the spine. Also, the facet joint capsule has a role also in limiting excessive joint motion.

The healthy intervertebral disk dissipates its axial load uniformly across its endplates under compression and eccentric–compressive (e.g., compression and bending) loading conditions. Disk degeneration disturbs the "three-joint complex" allowing excessive facet joint motion to occur, which in turn assists in facet joint degeneration. The facet joint and the paraspinal muscles are supplied by proprioceptive nerve endings that help in analyzing the mechanical state of the facet joint each second by the central nervous system (position, tension, pressure, etc.).

## Pathophysiology

Spinal motions are governed by the orientation of the facet joints and the intervertebral disks, costal cage, and muscular and ligamentous attachments. The superior articular facets in the cervical, thoracic, and lumbar spine vary in their orientation, for example:

(a) Cervical vertebrae (C1–C7): the facets face posteriorly and superiorly at a 45° angle.
(b) Thoracic vertebrae (T1–T12): the facets face posteriorly and laterally in the vertical plane.
(c) Lumbar vertebrae (L1–L5): the facets face medially at 45° to the sagittal plane.

Asymmetry of facet orientation, also known as "facet tropism," can play a significant role in the production of faulty postural mechanics during activities of daily living, causing back and neck pain.

## 13.5 Imaging Signs

1. Wrap-around bumper sign: this is a sign described in CT, as a degenerated facet joint will show sclerosis and form an osteophyte along the capsular attachment of the facet joint, as an attempt to stabilize the degenerated joint (◘ Fig. 13.3.1).
2. Facet joint angle: this is calculated by drawing a straight line along the posterior aspect of the disk space at a given spinal level and another two lines bisecting each facet joint. A facet joint <77.9° has a double risk of developing degenerative spondylolisthesis compared with patients who have facet joint angle >77.9°. This angle is mostly described in thoracolumbar facet joints (◘ Fig. 13.3.2).
3. CT signs (Pathria's classification): facet joint arthropathy is graded on CT as grade 0 (normal), grade 1 (joint narrowing), grade 2 (sclerosis and hypertrophy), and grade 3 (severe sclerosis and osteophyte formation).
4. Facet joint effusion (MRI): it is normal to find 1–2 ml synovial fluid in facet joints on T2-weighted MT images, especially at the levels of L4–L5 vertebrae. A significant facet joint effusion is a sign of "spinal segmental instability" in up to 82 % of facet joint syndrome cases.
5. On radiography, the facet joint shows reduced joint space and sclerosis of the facet joint, typically detected on lateral radiographs (◘ Fig. 13.3.3).

### Further Reading

McLain RF. Mechanoreceptor endings in human cervical facet joints. Spine. 1994;19(5):495–501.
Silbergleit R, et al. Imaging-guided injection techniques with fluoroscopy and CT for spinal pain management. RadioGraphics. 2001;21:927–42.

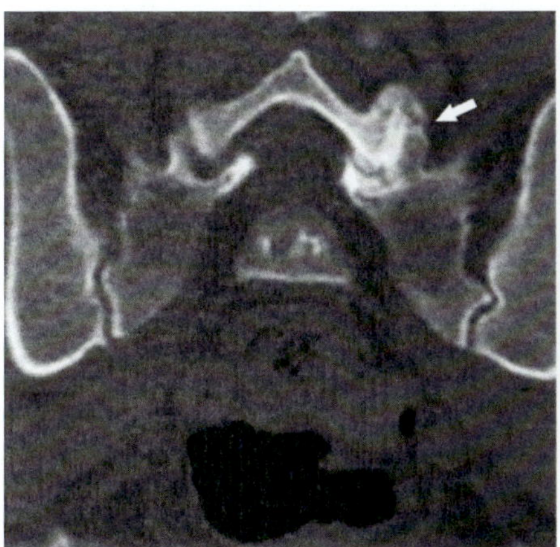
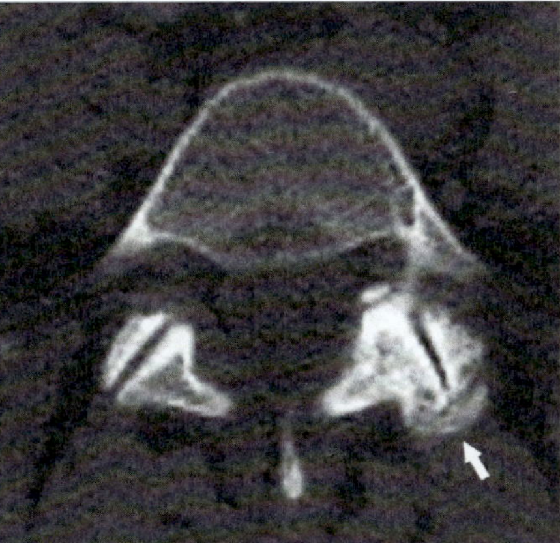
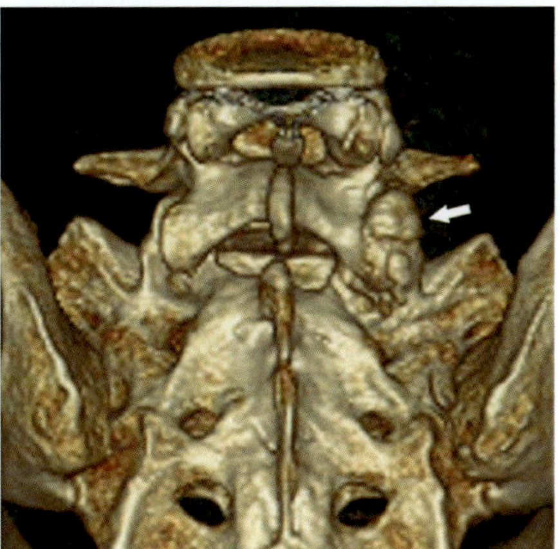

◘ **Fig. 13.3.1**  Multiple computed tomography (CT) images with 3D-reconstruction image that demonstrates the "wrap-around bumper sign" detected as halolike sclerosis wrapping around the left facet joint of L5/S1 vertebrae (*arrows*), with inner vacuum phenomenon detected as gas density in between the left facet joint space

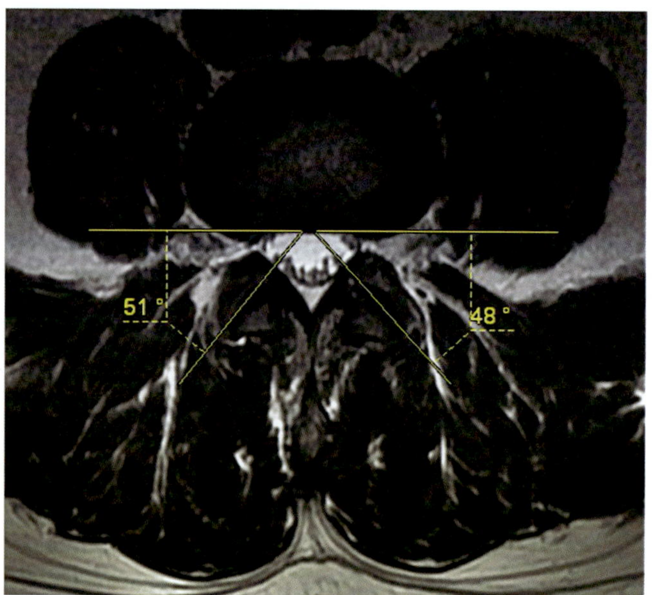

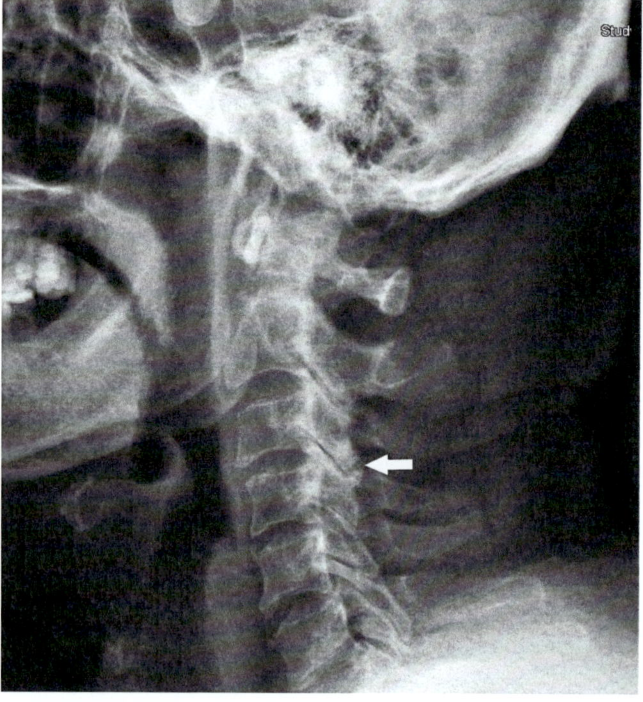

**Fig. 13.3.2** An axial MR image at the level of L4 vertebra demonstrates the measurements of the "facet joint angle" bilaterally

**Fig. 13.3.3** Lateral plain radiograph of a patient with neck pain shows facet joint spondyloarthropathy at the level of C3/C4 vertebrae (*arrow*)

Stone JA, et al. Treatment of facet and sacroiliac joint arthropathy: steroid injections and radiofrequency ablation. Tech Vasc Intervent Rad. 2009;12:22–32.

Varlotta GP, et al. The lumbar facet joint: a review of current knowledge: part 1: anatomy, biomechanics, and grading. Skeletal Radiol. 2011;40:13–23.

## 13.6 Myofascial Pain Syndrome

Myofascial pain syndrome is a term used to describe pain and maybe concomitant visceral dysfunction due to the presence of a "tight fascial–muscular band" within a muscle or muscle group that acts like a pain "trigger point," causing referred pain in another area. The area affected by this trigger point will show pain, decreased range of movement, muscular weakness, and often accompanied autonomic phenomenon. Predisposing factors for myofascial pain syndrome include:

1. Leg length discrepancy
2. Postural dysfunction and abnormalities (e.g., malalignment, scoliosis)
3. Endocrine disorders (e.g., hypothyroidism)

### Anatomy

To understand the muscle trigger point effect, it is crucial to understand the effect of fascia on the central nervous system. Stimulation of the fascial mechanoreceptors (Ruffini/Pacini corpuscles), like in tissue manipulation therapy, exerts effect on cortical system via the "proprioception pathway" transmitted via the spinal dorsal column–medial lemniscus system. This spinal effect will evoke an efferent response on skeletal muscles, causing change in their motor units tone. Stimulation of the fascial mechanoreceptors (A-δ and C-fibers), like in tissue manipulation therapy, exerts effect also on the autonomic nervous system. This autonomic effect will cause changes in local fascial capillary dynamics, intrafascial smooth muscles relaxation, and change in global muscle tone via hypothalamic tuning. The hypothalamus is tuned by the autonomic nervous system after stimulation of the fascial mechanoreceptors (A-δ and C-fibers), which will rust in change in global skeletal muscles tone. This effect seen in tissue manipulation therapy or deep tissue massage for skeletal muscles is also true for trigger points effect on the central nervous system. The former is a therapeutic effect, while the latter is a pathologic effect.

Another example of myofascial–nervous system interaction is seen in a technique known as "deep visceral massage," which targets tissue manipulation of the visceral fascia, which in turn stimulates the mechanoreceptors of the enteric system. Many of the sensory neurons of the enteric nervous system are mechanoreceptors, which – if activated – trigger important neuroendocrine changes. These include a change in the production of serotonin (an important cortical neurotransmitter, 90 % of which is created in the intestine) and histamine (which increases inflammatory processes).

The superficial fascia is perforated in multiple regions in the body by a triad of vein, artery, and nerve (unmyelinated autonomic nerves). Heine, a German researcher who has been involved in the study of acupuncture and other complimentary health disciplines, found that the majority (82 %) of these perforation points are topographically identical with the 361 classical acupuncture points in traditional Chinese acuncture, another proof of the myofascial–nervous system interaction.

A very interesting observation in the latest fascial physiology research correlates with the traditional Chinese medicine philosophy regarding the "Qi" energy. In Chinese medicine, Qi refers to movement or activity, not just any movement but the "proper" movement or activity of anything (e.g., human anatomy biomechanics). In Chinese medicine definition, Qi is the source of all movement in the body, protects the body, is connected to harmonious transformation (metabolism), retains the body's substances and organs, and warms the body. The "Qi" definition in Chinese medicine is the same definition of "fascia" in Western medicine, so we could say that fascia is the same as Qi. Moreover, the "meridian channels" that connect the Qi points in acupuncture in the meridian maps are almost the same paths of the "fascial planes" in anatomical illustrations.

## Pathophysiology

Fascia is an "electrical tissue" and considered the "largest sensory organ" in the body; also, it plays an important role in musculoskeletal biomechanics, peripheral motor coordination, proprioception, regulation of posture, and as a potential pain generator. Fascial restrictions can create abnormal strain patterns that can crowd or pull the osseous structures out of proper alignment, resulting in compression of joints producing pain and/or dysfunction (e.g., enthesitis). Moreover, neural and vascular structures can also become entrapped in these restrictions, causing neurologic symptoms, entrapment syndromes, veno-lymphatic stagnation and edema, or ischemic conditions.

The autonomic nervous system does not directly innervate the parenchymal cells, but it exerts its effect on the cells via mediating the chemical within the interstitial media (the extracellular fluid). If an injury is applied to the interstitial connective tissue (e.g., fascia), functional disturbance to the parenchymal cells homeostasis occurs and disease arises. For example, if a trauma is applied to the nerve fascia (e.g., the epineurium and perineurium), neurogenic inflammation arises which evoke nociception and possibly nerve trunk pain. Due to the bioelectric information capacity of the extracellular matrix (fascia), any situation that alters the electrical tone of the fascia can spread and be processed through the entire region, a potential by-product of cellular shock.

A myofascial trigger point pathophysiology can be summarized as the following:

1. Restricted movement: taut muscle bands lead to shortening of the muscles, which in turn leads to reduced mobility and articular dysfunction. Depending on the muscle involved, different symptoms can arise.
2. Vascular perfusion abnormality: if the taut bands compress the intra- or extra-muscular blood vessels, this leads to tissues ischemia, formation of edema, and trophic/metabolic changes (e.g., lactic acidosis within the muscle).

3. Neuromuscular entrapment: fascia contains many nerve fibers embedded within fascial tunnels (e.g., medial superior cluneal nerve tunnel). A tense muscle and fascial fibers can exert pressure over the surrounding nerve fibers, resulting in entrapment syndromes and variety of neurological symptoms.
4. Irritation of deep propioceptive and nociceptive nerve endings: connective tissue dysfunction alters the flow of impulses which come from the receptors which lie in the connective tissue of the muscle.
5. Metabolic abnormalities: fascial tension can disturb circulation in the interstitium, disturbing the cellular environment.
6. Breathing disorder: myofascial tension affects posture as well as abdominal and intrathoracic pressure.

To treat a myofascial trigger point, "myofascial release," a hands-on therapeutic technique is used to treat tightened fascia that facilitates a stretch into the restricted fascia. It is performed by a sustained pressure that is applied into the restricted tissue barrier; after 90–120 s, the tissue will undergo histological length changes, allowing the first release to be felt. The goal of myofascial release is to elongate and soften the connective tissue, creating permanent three-dimensional length and width (e.g., change the ground substance from a sol to a gel).

## Some Known Symptomatology of Myofascial Trigger Points Origin

Breast pain (mastalgia): pectoralis major and minor muscles.
Headache: temporalis, pterygoid, upper trapezius, and sternocleidomastoid muscles.
Lower back/SJ joint pain: pyramidalis, gluteus maximum, medius, and minimus muscles.
Inguinal pain: quadratus lumborum, Iliopsoas, and abdominal oblique muscles.
Pain during sitting: pyramidalis and obturator internus muscles.
Vulvar pain (vulvodynia): external anal sphincter.
Testicular pain (orchialgia): abdominal oblique, gluteus maximum, medius, and minimus muscles.
Penile pain: levator ani, bulbospongiosus, ischiospongiosus, and rectus abdominis muscles.
Prostate pain (prostatodynia): levator ani muscle.
Perianal pain: levator ani muscle.
Rectal pain (proctodynia): levator ani, coccygeus, and external anal sphincter muscles.
Sensation of a ball in the rectum: levator ani and obturator internus muscles.
Urethral syndrome: defined as urinary urgency, frequency, dysuria, and supravesical pain in the absence of any objective urological or laboratory findings. The disease arises due to spasm and myofascial triggers of the external urethral sphincter, obturator internus, and pyramidalis muscles (☐ Fig. 13.4.1).

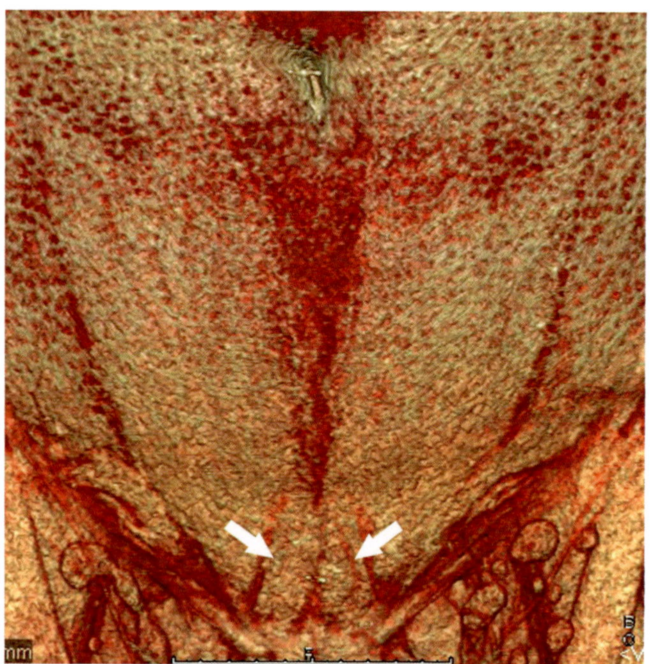

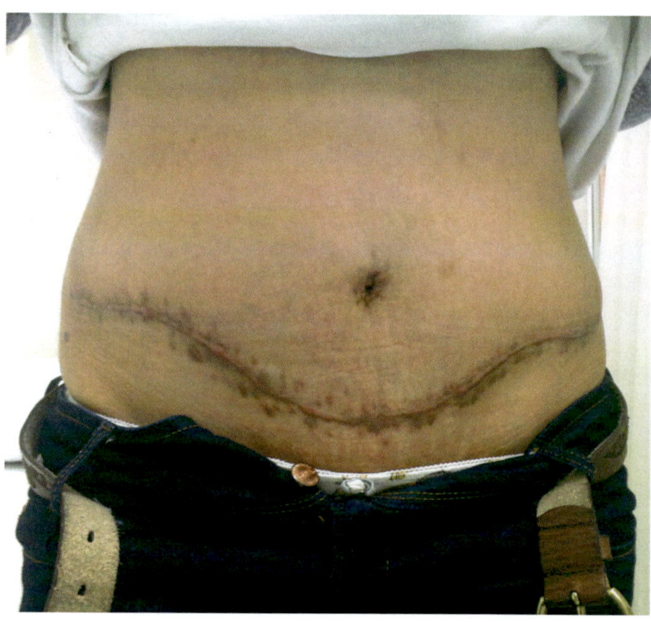



**Fig. 13.4.1** A computed tomography (CT) image with 3D reconstruction in coronal plane that demonstrates the pyramidal muscle (*arrows*), a common cause of suprapubic pain due to myofascial trigger point

**Fig. 13.4.2** A photograph of the patient's abdomen that shows the abdominoplasty keloidal scar extension

## 13.7    Imaging of a Case Study

A young 33-year-old female presented to our radiology department complaining of severe, intermittent, right-sided abdominal pain of the lower quadrant of stabbing nature with radiation downward to the thigh and upward to the breast. She had a history of abdominoplasty with a big scar in the abdomen that shows keloid changes ( Fig. 13.4.2). At first, my initial impression was that she is complaining of postoperative abdominal adhesions, adding to the fact that she has history of three caesarian section deliveries.

Computed tomography (CT) for her abdomen and pelvis did not show any intestinal adhesions; however, it showed recti muscle diathesis and a superficial fatty stranding around the scar ( Fig. 13.4.3a, b). MRI examination was done for her abdomen which showed enhancement of the scar at the region where anatomically the ilioinguinal and the iliohypogastric nerves are found ( Fig. 13.4.4). The diagnosis of suspected "abdominal cutaneous nerve entrapment syndrome" was finalized in the report as a high suspicion diagnosis that needs surgical conformation. A surgical exploration was done for the patient, and very thick nerves were found. A biopsy of these nerves was sent to the pathology lab which came back positive for fibrotic, hypertrophied nerves.

### Further Reading

Barnes MF. The basic science of myofascial release: morphologic change in connective tissue. J Bodyw Mov Ther. 1997;1(4):231–8.

Chang S. The meridian system and mechanism of acupuncture – a comparative review. Part 1: the meridian system. Taiwan J Obstet Gynecol. 2012;51:506–14.

Chang S. The meridian system and mechanism of acupuncture – a comparative review. Part 2: mechanism of acupuncture analgesia. Taiwan J Obstet Gynecol. 2013;52:14–24.

Dorsher PT, et al. Acupuncture for chronic pain. Techn Reg Anesth Pain Manag. 2011;15:55–63.

Finando S, et al. Fascia and the mechanism of acupuncture. J Bodyw Mov Ther. 2011;15:168–76.

Itza F, et al. Myofascial pain syndrome in the pelvic floor: a common urological condition. Actas Urol Esp. 2010;34(4):318–26.

Ivens D, et al. Abdominal cutaneous nerve entrapment syndrome after blunt abdominal trauma in an 11-year-old girl. J Pediatr Surg. 2008;43:E19–21.

Lindsetmo RO, et al. Chronic abdominal wall pain-A diagnostic challenge for the surgeon. Am J Surg. 2009;198:129–34.

Manni L, et al. Neurotrophins and acupuncture. Auton Neurosci Basic Clin. 2010;157:9–17.

Montenegro MLLS, et al. Abdominal myofascial pain syndrome must be considered in the differential diagnosis of chronic pelvic pain. Euro J Obstet Gynecol Reprod Biol. 2009;147:21–4.

Rahn DD, et al. Anterior abdominal wall nerve and vessel anatomy: clinical implications for gynecologic surgery. Am J Obstet Gynecol. 2010;202:234.e1–5.

Raj PP, et al. Myofascial pain syndrome and its treatment in low back pain. Semin Pain Med. 2004;2:167–74.

Zhao ZQ. Neural mechanism underlying acupuncture analgesia. Prog Neurobiol. 2008;85:355–75.

## 13.8    Spinal Transitional Zone Syndromes

The spinal transitional zone (STZ) is defined as the vertebral zone located between two adjacent spinal vertebrae with various differences in their "posterior element" orientation and

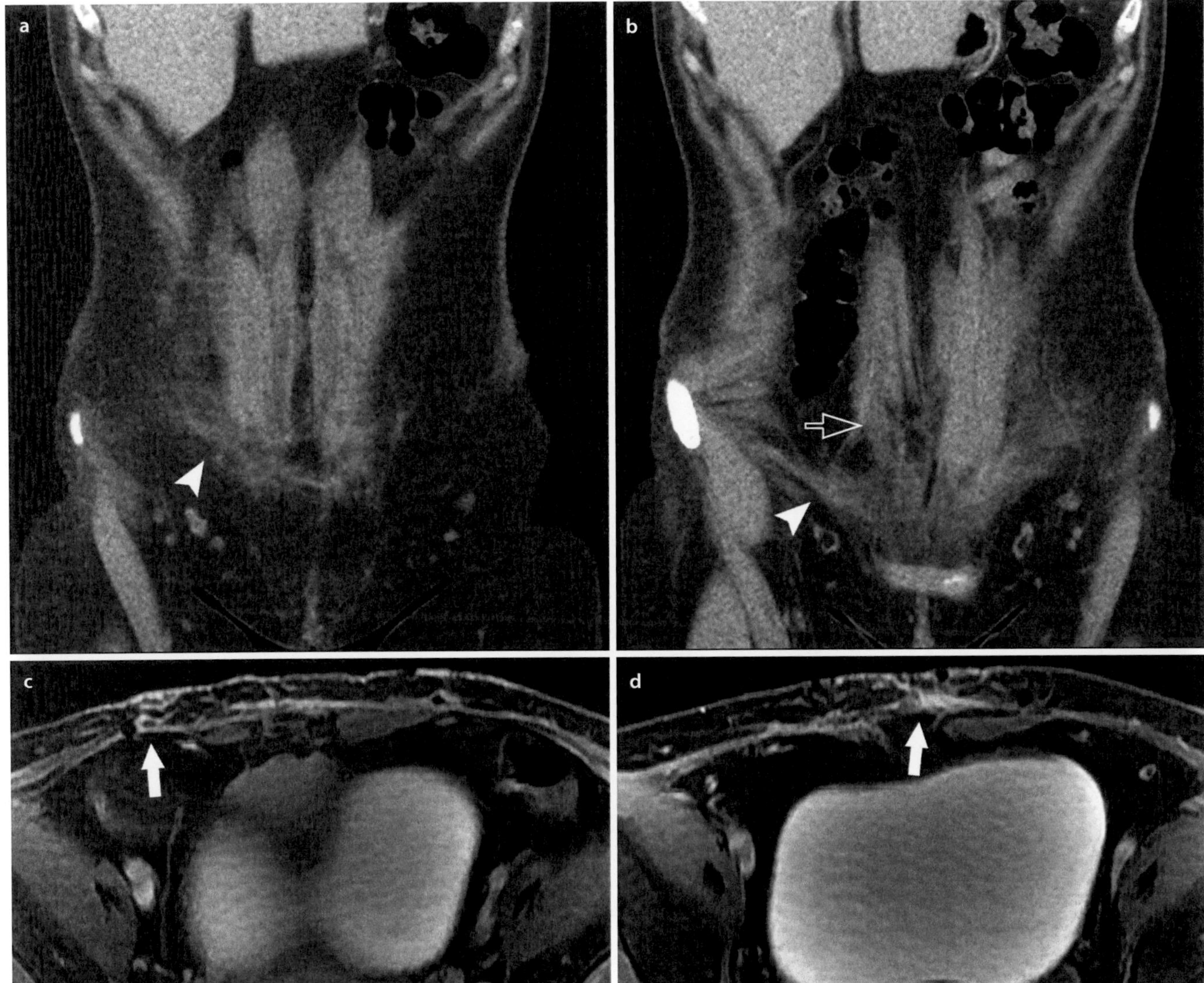

**Fig. 13.4.3**   Multiple CT images in coronal plane (**a**, **b**) and MR abdominal images in axial planes (**c**, **d**) of the patient; the myofascial scar is clearly seen as linear area of hyperdense fascia with fatty stranding (*arrowheads* in **a**, **b**). The right-sided rectal muscle show marked atrophy (*empty arrowhead* in **b**); on postcontrast MR images, the marked enhancement of the scar tissue is detected at the anatomical area of the ilioinguinal and the iliohypogastric neurovascular bundle; the diagnosis of suspected abdominal cutaneous nerve entrapment syndrome was made, which was confirmed by biopsy

differing degrees of mobility. A "transitional lumbosacral vertebra" is defined as a vertebra that shows elongation of its transverse process with variable degrees of fusion to the "first" sacral (S1) segment.

## Basic Anatomy

The spinal transitional zones (STZs) are prone to vertebral rotational malalignment (vertebral subluxation complex) with various subcutaneous fat, enthesis, and muscle (cellulo-teno-periosteo-myalgic) manifestations. Four vertebral transitional zones are described:

1. Cervico-occipital (CO) junctional zone
2. Cervicothoracic (CT) junctional zone
3. Thoracolumbar junctional zone
4. Lumbosacral (LS) junctional zone

## Pathophysiology

Malalignment/subluxation of the vertebrae in the STZs can result in somatovisceral symptoms according to the myotome/dermatome involved. STZ syndromes, elegantly described by the French osteopath Robert Maigne, are characterized by a triad (not necessary all three present together) of:

1. Cellulalgia: described clinically as painful, deep, burning-like subcutaneous tissue pain, swelling, and induration in all or part of the affected dermatome
2. Myalgia: described clinically as painful, taut bands of muscle fibers – trigger points – localized in some muscles of the affected myotome
3. Enthesitis: described clinically as hypersensitivity of the teno-periosteal insertions (entheses) of the affected sclerotome

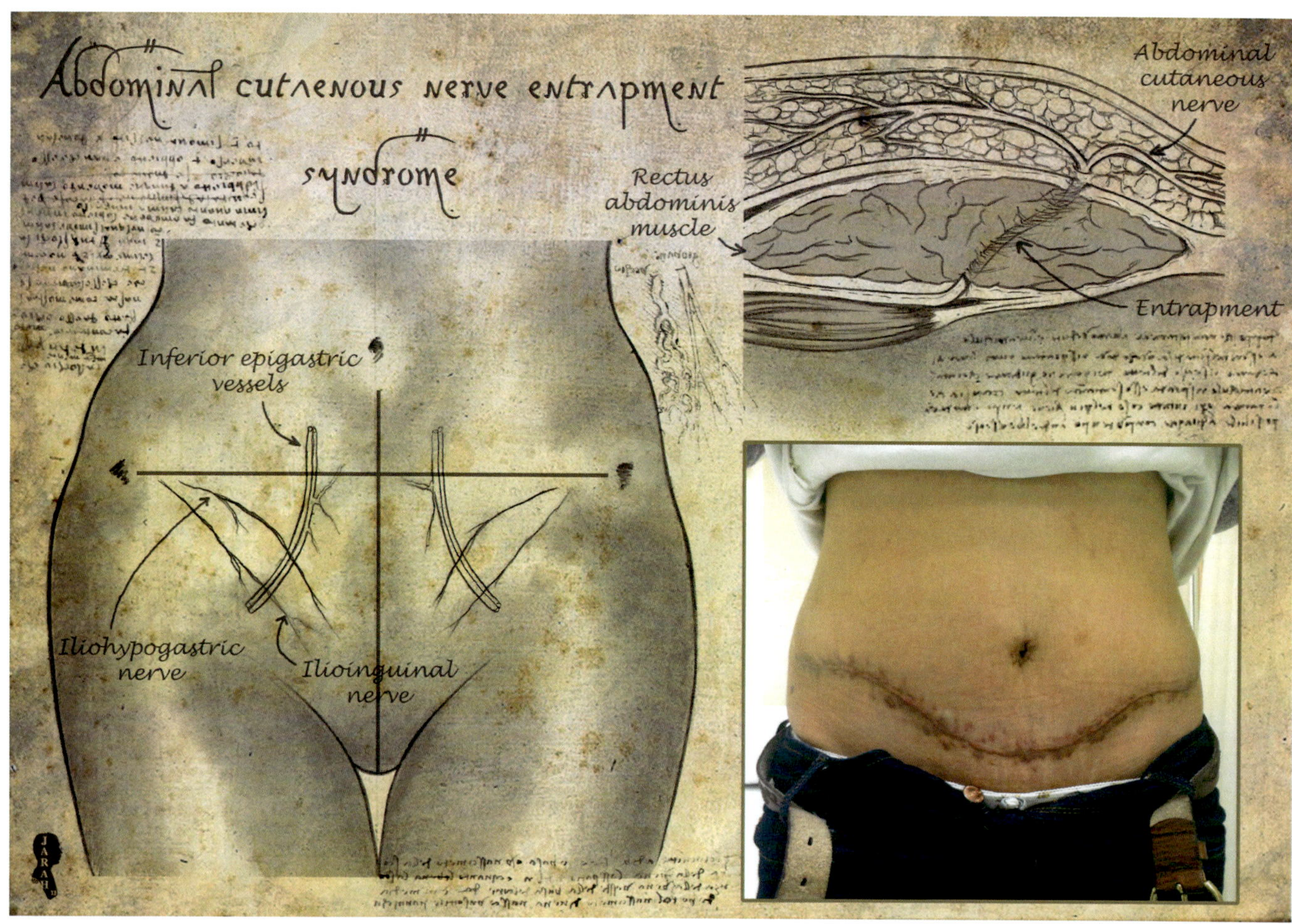


**Fig. 13.4.4** An illustration that demonstrates the anatomical site of the ilioinguinal and the iliohypogastric nerves and the entrapment process

According to Maigne and many other researchers in the osteopathic, chiropractic, and manipulative medicine field, four main STZs syndromes are recognized (**Fig. 13.5.1**):

### Cervico-Occipital Transitional Zone Syndrome

Cervico-occipital (CO) junction zone abnormality refers to the manifestations of vertebral subluxation complex that are detected mainly between the occipital skull base condyles and atlas (C1) vertebra. Beside C1 subluxation, other conditions that can cause CO junction zone abnormality include (a) atlanto-occipital assimilation (a condition characterized by fusion between the atlas and the skull base due to failure to segmentation of these two structures embryologically), (b) whiplash injury, (c) foramen magnum syndrome, (d) cervical torticollis, and (e) and basilar indentation (defined as displacement of the odontoid process into the foramen magnum).

Clinical manifestations of CO junction zone syndrome include:

1. Cervicogenic headache is defined as a headache that is caused by a lesion within the cervical spine or in the soft tissues of the neck detected by clinical, laboratory, and/or imaging evidence. Cervicogenic headache is the commonest manifestation of the CO subluxation and manifested typically as severe pain experienced in the occipital, hemicranial (migraine-like), or supraorbital region.

2. Trigeminal neuralgia arises typically due to indirect involvement of the "spinal trigeminal nucleus and tract." The trigemino-cervical nucleus is a region of the upper three cervical spinal cord (C1–C3) where sensory nerve fibers in the descending tract of the trigeminal nerve (trigeminal nucleus caudalis) are believed to interact with sensory fibers from the upper cervical roots. These functional convergences of upper cervical and trigeminal sensory pathways allow the bidirectional referral of painful sensations between the neck and trigeminal sensory receptive fields of the face and head.

### Cervicothoracic Transitional Zone Syndrome

Cervicothoracic (CT) junction zone syndrome refers to the manifestations of vertebral subluxation or facet joint abnormalities between C5–C6 and C6–C7 vertebrae. Clinical manifestations include one or all of the following features ipsilateral to the subluxation complex (**Fig. 13.5.2**):

1. Neck pain: due to myofascial trigger points in the neck muscles
2. Shoulder pain: due to involvement of the brachial plexus
3. Interscapular pain: due to vertebral malalignment, functional scoliosis, and/or thoracolumbar fascia tightness
4. Lateral elbow epicondylar pain: presents with tennis-elbow-like presentation (lateral epicondylitis)

nerve is known to carry visceral sympathetic fibers to the pelvic organs.

(c) Hip pain (56%): arises due to irritation/impingement of the "perforating lateral cutaneous branch" of T12–L1, which innervates the trochanteric region.

(d) Pubic pain (32%): due to irritation of the symphysis pubis, often unilateral to the vertebral subluxation site.

## 13.9  Imaging Signs

1. Most of radiographs in Maigne syndrome are normal; however, vertebral subluxation, degenerative changes, facet joints hypertrophy, or disk protrusion can be seen affecting the level of T12–L2 vertebrae, which can be diagnostic after excluding an organic cause of pain plus the classical distribution of symptoms (Fig. 13.5.4).

2. Atrophy and fatty degeneration of the paraspinal muscles with lack of other vertebral column pathology (e.g., normal vertebral disks MRI) is highly suggestive of Maigne syndrome because the main pathology is irritation of the dorsal spinal nerve ramus in the first place, which cannot be visualized in MRI directly yet.

3. In CT, Maigne syndrome can be suggested by a lesion affecting the intervertebral foramen, where the dorsal ramus exits. Other features on CT include facet joint spondylosis or hypertrophy, periarticular calcifications, and calcification of the ligamentum flavum at the level of T12–L2.

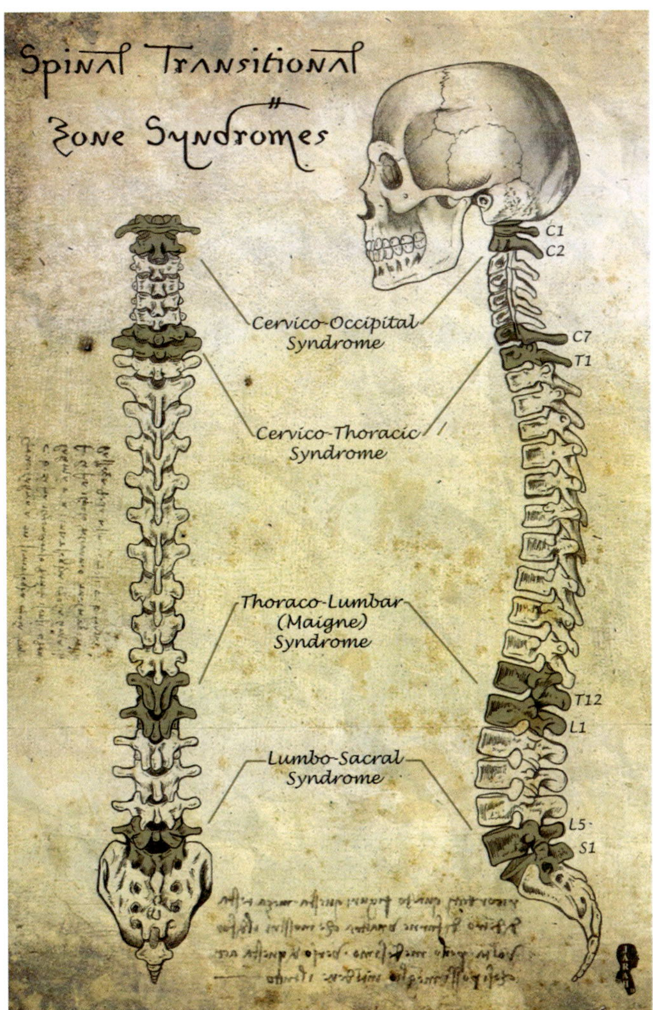


**Fig. 13.5.1**  An illustration that shows the four types of transitional zone syndromes according to Maigne and others

## Thoracolumbar Transitional Zone Syndrome

Thoracolumbar (TL) junction zone abnormality, also known as "Maigne syndrome," "Dorsal ramus syndrome," and "T12–L2 segmental vertebral cellulotenoperiosteomyalgic syndrome," refers to the manifestations of vertebral subluxation or facet joint abnormalities between T12 and L2 vertebrae. Manifestations of Maigne syndrome include (Fig. 13.5.3):

(a) Low back pain (97%): it arises due to irritation/impingement of the "dorsal" spinal nerve root ramus of T12–L1 (Iliohypogastric nerve), which supplies the superior gluteal and inferior lumbar subcutaneous tissues. Trigger points can be found within the rectus abdominis and the quadratus lumborum muscles. Back pain is the most common manifestation of Maigne syndrome.

(b) Lower abdominal visceral pain (60%): clinically can present with symptoms that mimic gynecological, testicular, renal colic, or irritable bowel syndrome such as bloating, constipation, and abdominal meteorism. These manifestations arise due to irritation/impingement of the "anterior" spinal nerve root ramus of T12–L1 (Iliohypogastric nerve). The iliohypogastric

## Lumbosacral Transitional Zone Syndrome

Lumbosacral transitional vertebra (LSTV) is a common finding in plain radiography of the general population reaching up to 20%. Two main lumbosacral transitional vertebrae are described:

(a) Lumbarization of S1 vertebra: described when the first sacral (S1) vertebra shows short transverse processes with an intervertebral disk between S1 and S2 vertebrae, resulting in S1 vertebra that mimics the lumbar vertebrae. On imaging, the patient will show 6 lumbar vertebrae rather than 5 (Figs. 13.5.5 and 13.5.6).

(b) Sacralization of L5 vertebra: described when the 5th lumbar (L5) vertebra shows short transverse processes with bilateral fusion of the L5 to the first (S1) sacral vertebra with no intervertebral disk in between the two vertebrae. On imaging, the patient will show 4 lumbar vertebrae rather than 5 (Fig. 13.5.7).

LSTV has been described with lower back pain since 1917 by Bertolotti, and it was referred to as "Bertolotti's syndrome" (e.g., lower back pain due to sacralization/lumbarization of L5–S1 vertebrae). The mechanisms of such the pain formation can be due to:

1. Abnormal L5–S1 biomechanics: LSTV predisposes to early L5–S1 spondyloarthropathy and intervertebral disk disease, causing uneven paraspinal muscle contraction

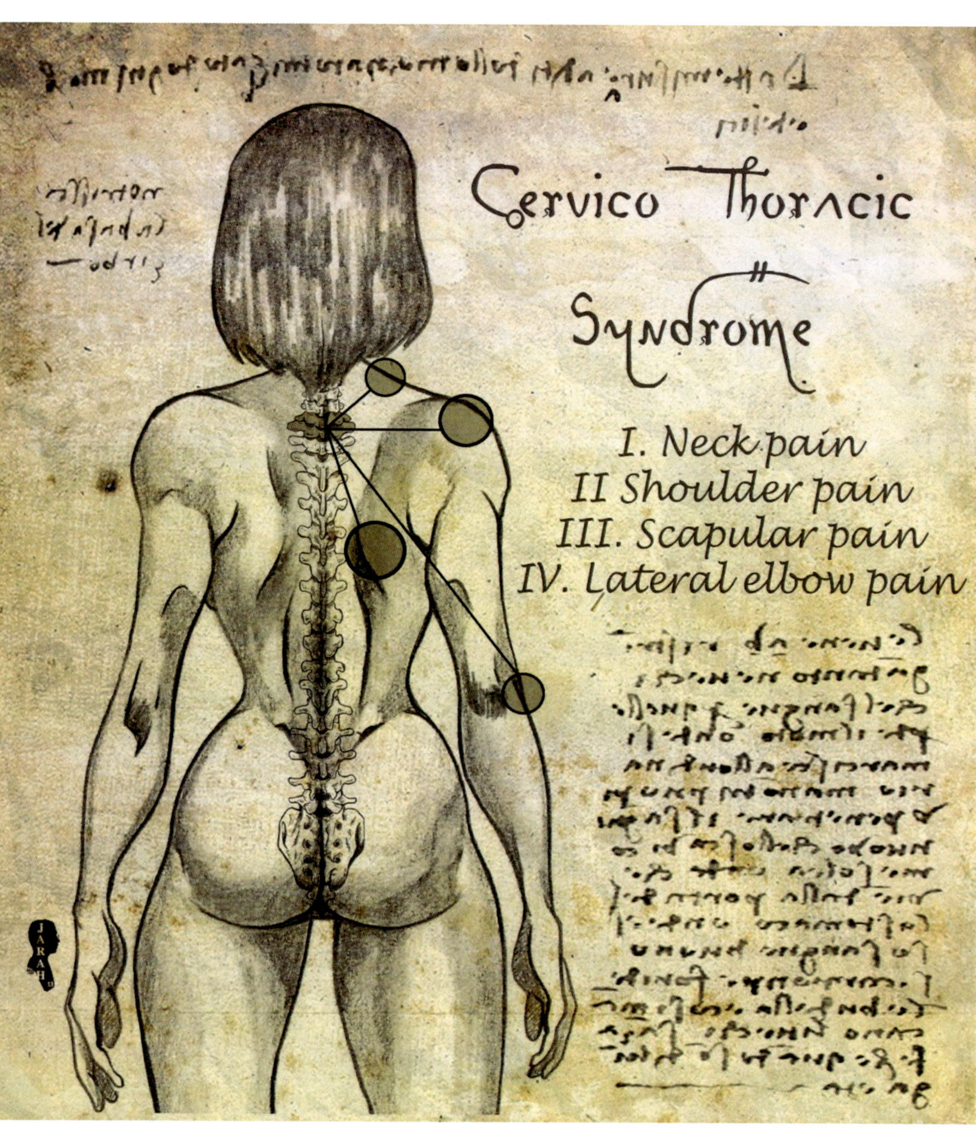



**Fig. 13.5.2** An illustration that shows the four types of cervicothoracic transitional zone syndrome clinical pain distributions

and formation of trigger points within the paraspinal and sacral muscle.

2. Far-out syndrome: described as a clinical condition where the L5 nerve is impinged "far-laterally" between the elongated transverse process of L5 and the ala of the sacrum. The condition was first described by Wiltse et al. (1984).

## 13.10 Imaging Signs

1. Lumbosacral transitional vertebrae (LSTV) have been classified by Castellvi (1984) into five main subtypes based on imaging features:
   LSTV type I: long, dysplastic transverse process >19 mm found unilaterally (Ia) or bilaterally (Ib) (**Fig. 13.5.8**)
   LSTV type II: large, squared transverse process with false joint formation (pseudoarthrosis) between the transverse process and the sacrum ala unilaterally (IIa) or bilaterally (IIb), forming incomplete lumbarization/sacralization (**Fig. 13.5.9**)
   LSTV type III: large, squared transverse process with complete fusion between the transverse process and the sacrum ala unilaterally (IIIa) or bilaterally (IIIb)
   LSTV type IV: mixed type (e.g., type IIIa on one side and type IIa on the other side)

2. Far-out syndrome can arise due to large osteophyte impinging on the L5 nerve, Castellvi type IIa LSTV, and impingement of the nerve inside a "lumbosacral tunnel" formed by the L5 vertebral body, the sacral ala, and the lumbosacral ligament.

## Further Reading


Bron JL, et al. The clinical significance of lumbosacral transitional anomalies. Acta Orthop Belg. 2007;73:687–95.

Castellvi AE, et al. Lumbosacral transitional vertebrae and their relationship with lumbar extradural defects. Spine. 1984;9:493–5.

Demondion X, et al. The posterior lumbar ramus: CT-anatomic correlation and propositions of new sites of infiltration. AJNR Am J Neuroradiol. 2005;26:706–10.

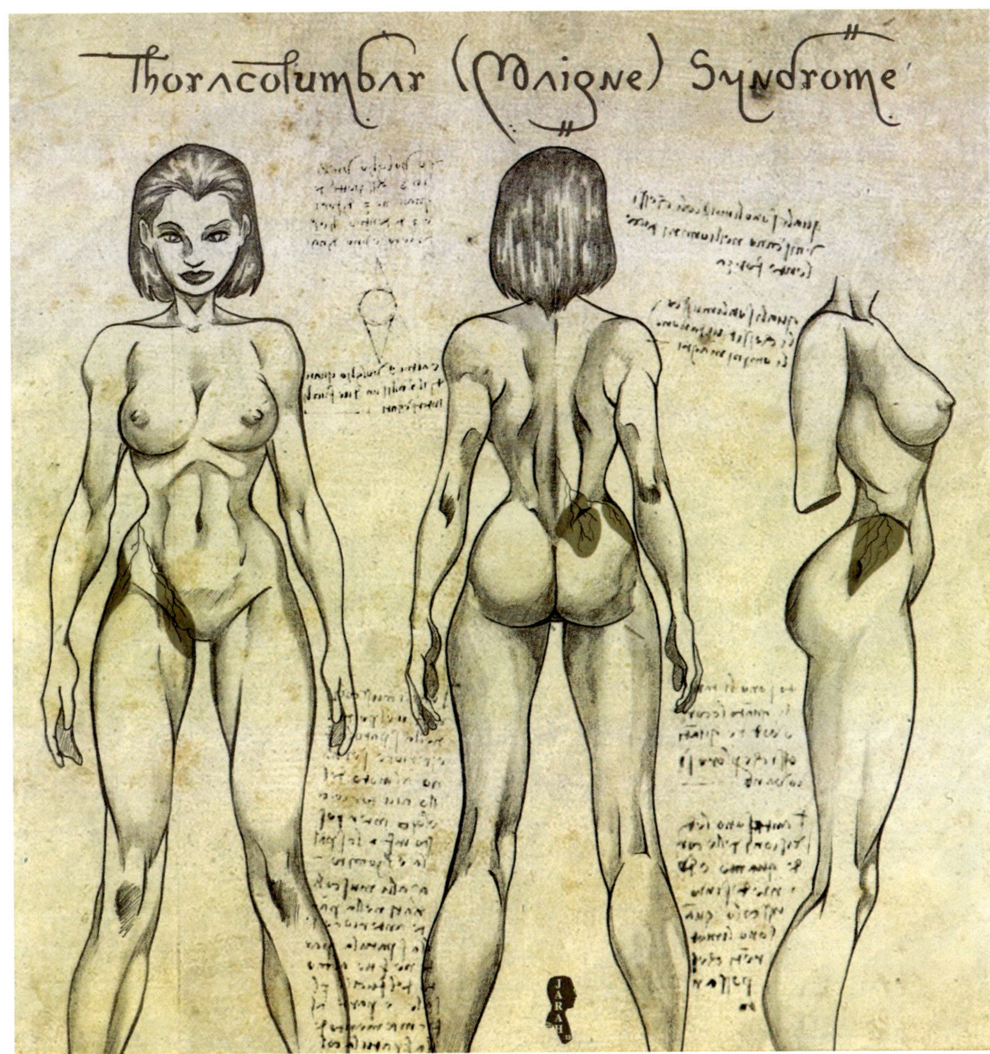



**Fig. 13.5.3** An illustration that shows the three clinical pain distributions of Maigne syndrome


Hughes RJ, et al. Imaging of lumbosacral transitional vertebrae. Clin Radiol. 2004a;59:984–91.

Hughes RJ, et al. Imaging of lumbosacral transitional vertebrae. Clin Radiol. 2004b;59:984–91.

Konin GP, et al. Lumbosacral transitional vertebrae: classification, imaging findings, and clinical relevance. AJNR Am J Neuroradiol. 2010;31:1778–86.

Wiltse LL, et al. Alar transverse process impingement of the L5 spinal nerve: the far-out syndrome. Spine. 1984;9: 31–41.


## 13.11 The Dentate Ligament–Cord Distortion Phenomenon

The dentate ligaments are small, triangular, 21-paired lateral bands of dural tissues representing extension of the spinal cord pia matter to the dural sheath and are located midway between the dorsal and ventral attachment of the spinal cord. They function as anchors that attach the spinal cord to the dura and keep it in a central position. These ligaments are found in the cervical, thoracic, and lumbar regions, and they are thicker in the cervical region than those ligaments seen in the thoracic and lumbar regions.

The first pair of the dentate ligaments is attached to the dura of the posterior fossa, attached to the foramen magnum, and located between the vertebral arteries anteriorly and the hypoglossal nerve posteriorly. The foramen magnum attachment is essential to prevent significant axial forces from neck flexion to be transmitted to the brainstem. The dentate ligaments serve a protective role for the central nervous system during normal spinal motion.

Human mesenchymal tissues, including the dentate ligaments, are affected by Davis's law which states that "soft tissue will model according to the imposed demand." This means that the ligament will hypertrophy or thickened if it is subjected to chronic stress load. Dysfunction of the dentate ligament can cause neurological dysfunction based on two main theories presented by Grostic (1988):

1. A vertebral malalignment of C2–C3 will exert abnormal traction forces over the dentate ligament at the spinal cord lateral sides. This ligamentous traction will exert force on both sides of the spinal cord, causing "flattening" of the spinal cord at its anterior–posterior sides (Poisson's

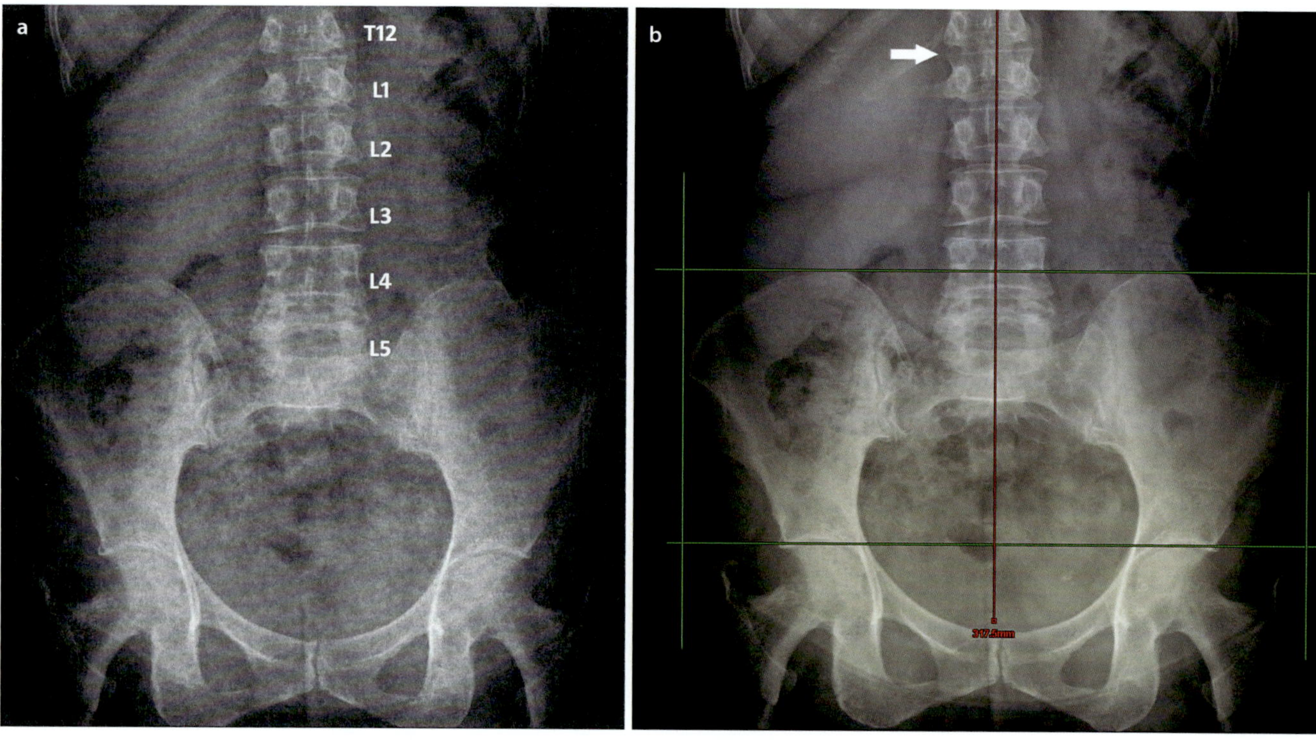

■ **Fig. 13.5.4**  Plain radiograph (**a** & **b**) of a patient who presented with right-sided lower back pain and inguinal pain; the radiograph shows slight, right-sided vertebral malalignment at the level of T12-L1 vertebrae (*arrow* in **b**)

■ **Fig. 13.5.5**  Plain radiograph of a patient who presented with chronic lower back pain; the plain abdominopelvic radiograph shows lumbarization of S1 vertebra

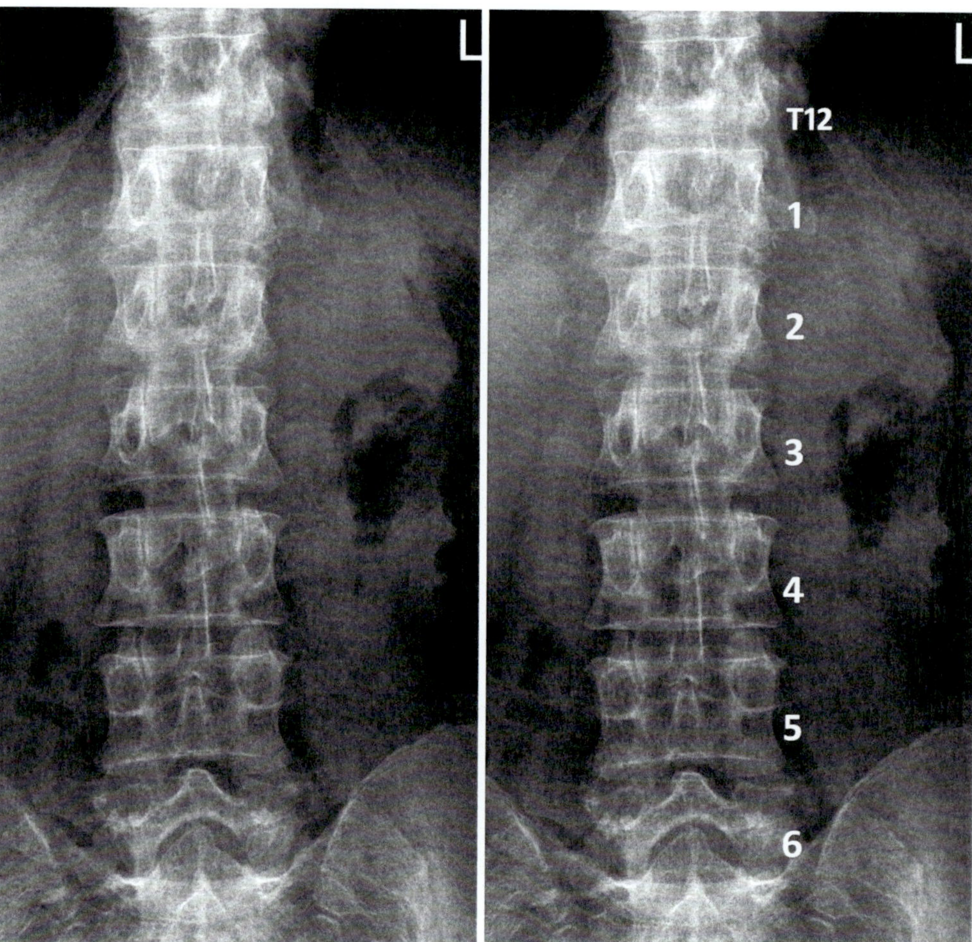

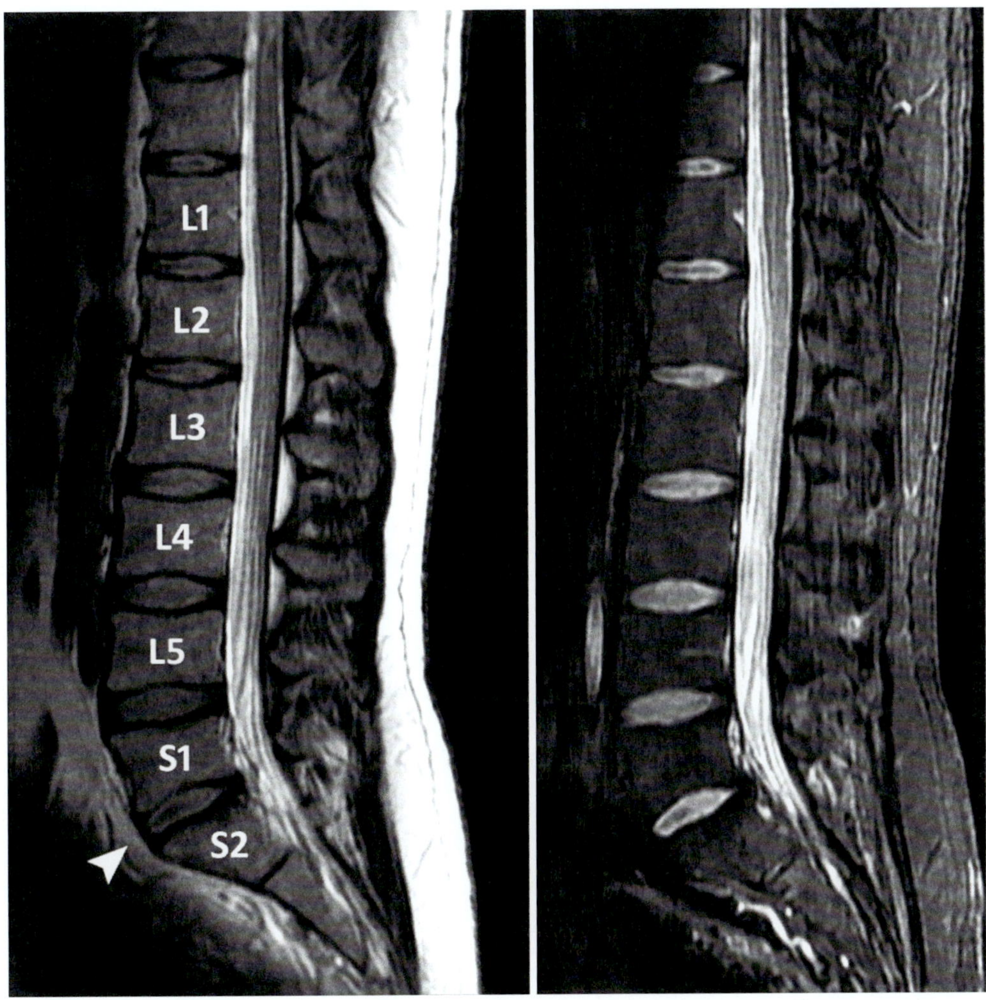

**Fig. 13.5.6** MR images of the same patient in **Fig. 13.5.5 shows clear, well-developed intervertebral disk that exists between S1 and S2 vertebrae due to lumbarization of S1 vertebra (*arrowhead*)



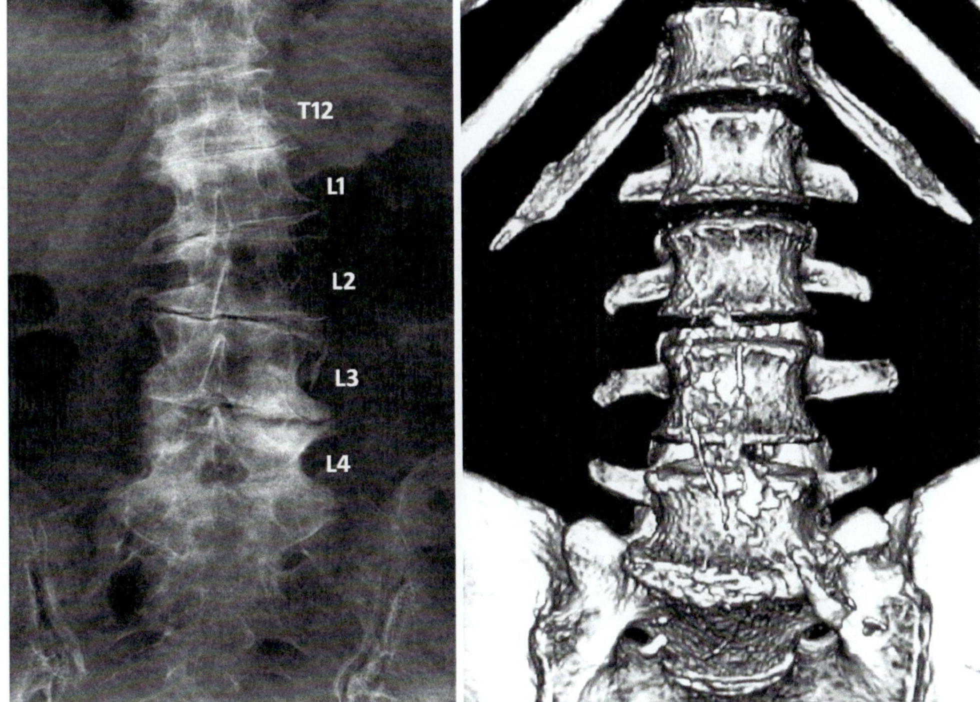

**Fig. 13.5.7** Plain radiograph and 3D-CT reconstructed image of a patient who presented with chronic lower back pain; the plain abdominopelvic radiograph and the CT show sacralization of L5 vertebra

effect). As an effect, the lateral spinal column (tracts) will be irritated (spinothalamic, anterior and posterior spinocerebellar, and maybe pyramidal tracts). The spinocerebellar tract is responsible for "muscle tone and joint position," while the spinothalamic tract is responsible for the "pain and temperature sensation."

In both tracts, the most lateral fibers innervate the most caudal structures (e.g., the most lateral fibers innervate the sacral region, while the most medial fibers innervate the cervical region). Chronic traction forces on the lateral tracts of the spinal cord can result in:

(a) Pelvic girdle and lower limb muscles hypertonicity and spasticity due to dorsal spinothalamic tract dysfunction, which in turn manifests as gait abnormality.

(b) Lower limbs pain and sciatica due to spinothalamic tract dysfunction.

(c) Amyotrophic lateral sclerosis-like presentation when the traction pressure over the spinal cord is chronic and severe enough to cause lateral spinal tracts degeneration.

2. The traction force exerted on the spinal cord veins by the hypertrophic dentate ligament causes collapse of the small radicular veins in the upper cervical cord, causing blood stasis and hypoxia in the spinal cord portions drained by these veins. The same pathological mechanism was reported in the literature in the pathogenesis of "Hirayama disease." Lower levels of hypoxia do not cut off the function of nerves, but increases their susceptibility to neurological dysfunction and hyperexcitability.

In patients with C2–C3 malalignment associated with neurological disturbances due to hypertrophic dentate ligament myelopathy, neck flexion should be avoided in the conservative treatment as it increased dural tension.

## 13.12 Imaging Signs

1. Chronic stress over the dentate ligament causes the ligament to become hypertrophic, cord-like in configuration. The spinal cord will be flattened in its anterior to posterior diameter, which may be associated with signal change reflecting degenerative myelopathy (Fig. 13.6.1).

2. Hirayama disease has been reported in the literature to be associated with severe spinal cord flattening, typically in the cervical region (Fig. 13.6.2). Flexion and extension MRI may show prominent peri-spinal vertebral veins due to varicosities.

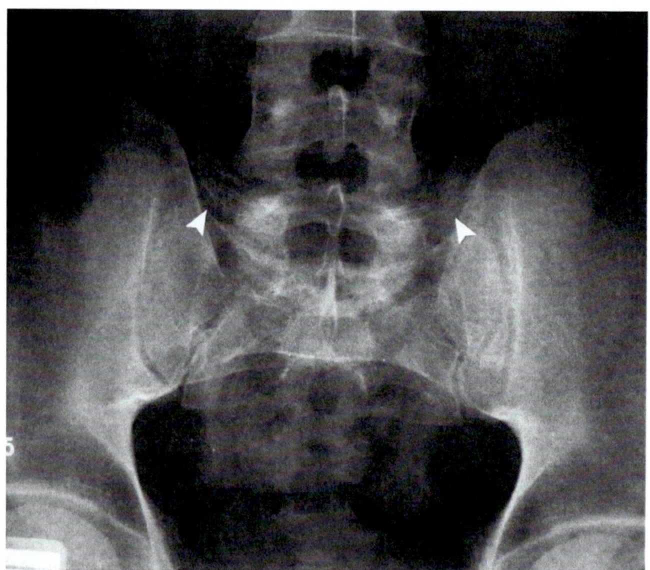

**Fig. 13.5.8**    Pelvic plain radiograph that demonstrates bilateral lumbosacral transitional vertebrae (Castellvi type I; *arrowheads*)

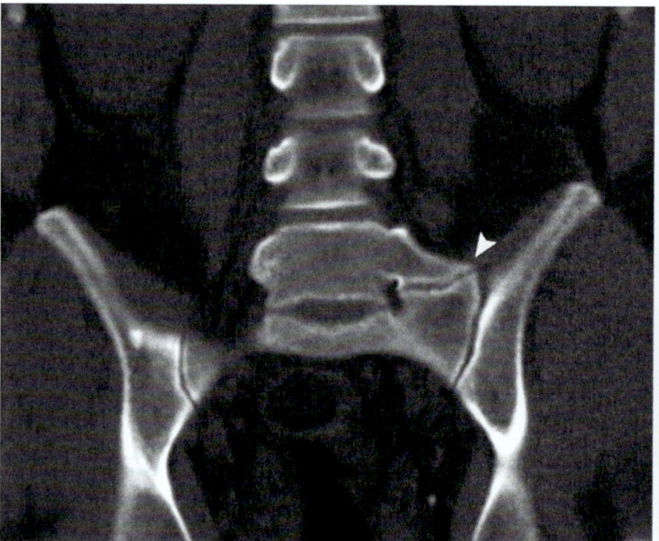
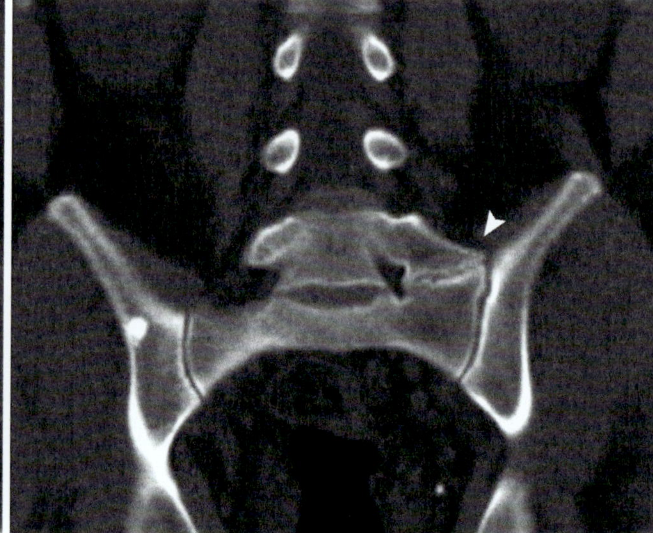

**Fig. 13.5.9**    Multilevel coronal, pelvic CT images that demonstrate lumbosacral transitional vertebra with formation of pseudoarthrosis between the left-sided transverse process and the sacral ala (Castellvi type II; *arrowhead*)

## Further Reading

Bedford PD, et al. Degeneration of the spinal cord associated with cervical spondylosis. Lancet. 1952;2:55–9.

Grostic DJ. Dentate ligament-cord distortion hypothesis. Chiropr Res J. 1988;1(1):47–55.

Harrison DE, et al. A review of biomechanics of the central nervous system – part II: spinal cord stresses from postural loads. J Manipulative Physiol Ther. 1999a;22(5):322–32.

Harrison DE, et al. A review of biomechanics of the central nervous system – part III: spinal cord stresses from postural loads and their neurologic effects. J Manipulative Physiol Ther. 1999b;22(6):399–410.

Khan EA. The role of the dentate ligament in the spinal cord compression and the syndrome of lateral sclerosis. J Neurosurg. 1947;4:191–9.

Kitajima M, et al. Familial amyloid polyneuropathy: hypertrophy of ligaments supporting the spinal cord. AJNR Am J Neuroradiol. 2004;25:1599–602.

Teng P. Myelographic identification of the dentate ligament. Radiology. 1960;74(6):944–6.

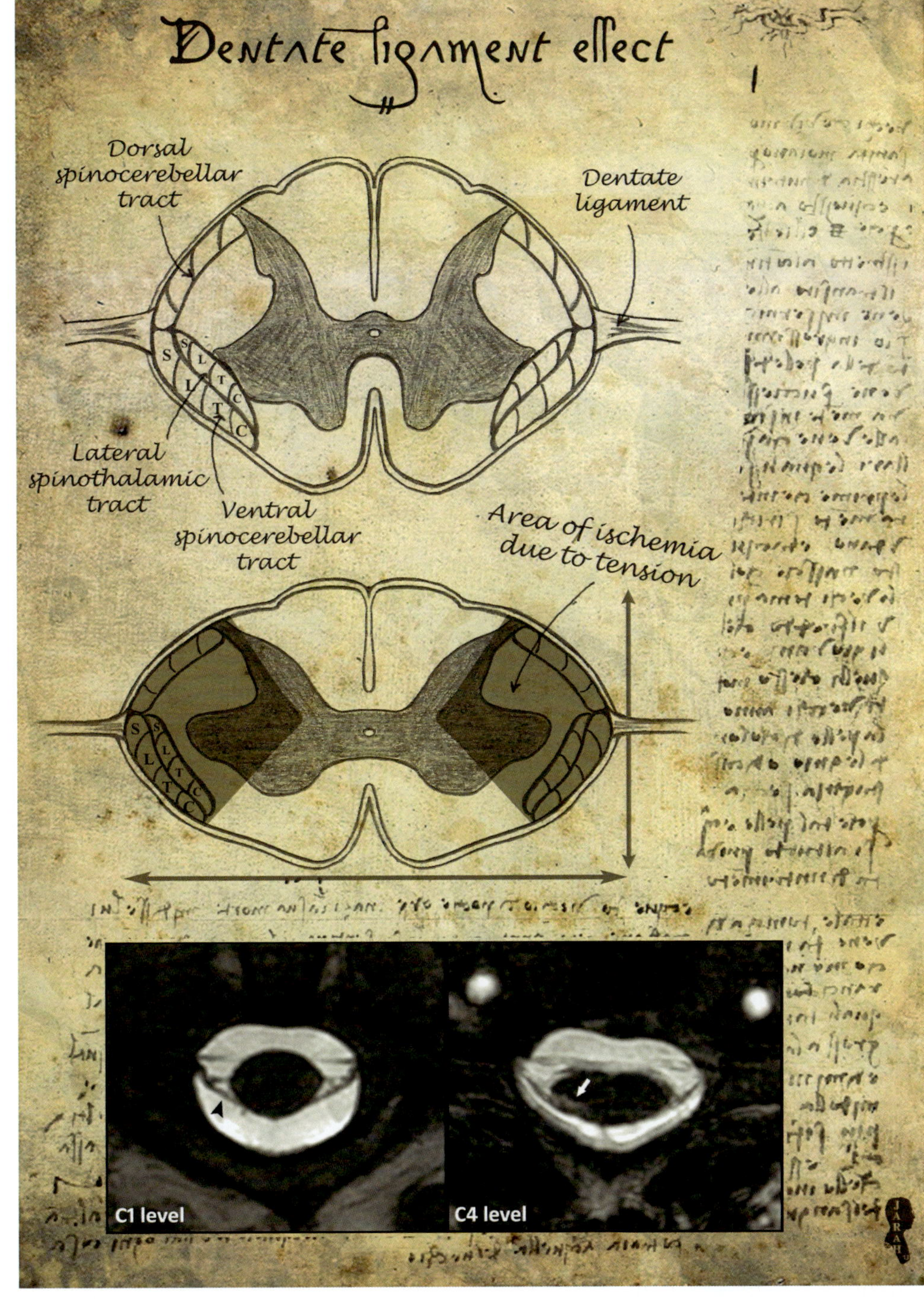



☐ **Fig. 13.6.1** An illustration that shows the effect of dentate ligament tension over the spinocerebellar and spinothalamic tracts; downward, axial 3D-CISS MR images of a patient who presented with sudden inability to walk associated with lower limb numbness. The MR image at C1 level shows normal spinal cord configuration, while the MR image at C4 level shows right-sided high signal intensity at the site of the ventral spinocerebellar tract (*arrow*), typically seen due to dentate ligament tension exerted over the spinal cord

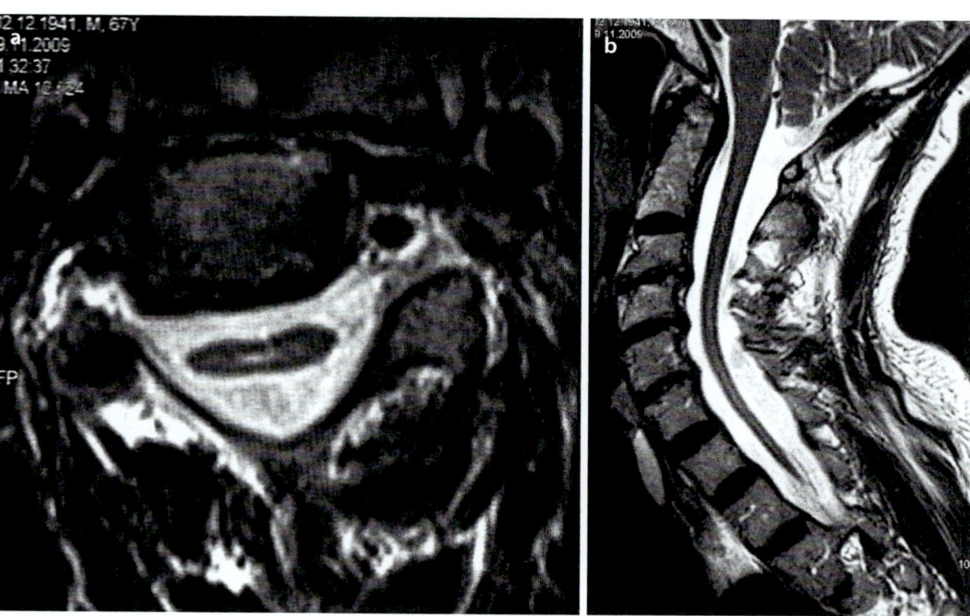

**◘ Fig. 13.6.2**  Axial and sagittal T2W-MR images of a patient with Hirayama disease showing marked flattening of the spinal cord (**a** & **b**); this patient presented clinically with unilateral atrophy, of the arm and forearm muscles a classical presentation of Hirayama disease

Tubbs RS, et al. The denticulate ligament: anatomy and functional significance. J Neurosurg (Spine2). 2001;94:271–5.
Wall EJ, et al. Experimental stretch neuropathy change in nerve conduction under tension. J Bone Joint Surg (Br). 1992;74(1):126–9.

## 13.13 Cervicogenic Headache

Cervicogenic headache is a term used by Sjaastad (1983) to define an intermittent, unilateral headache with associated symptoms typical to migraine often precipitated or aggravated by certain neck movements. Cervicogenic headache arises typically from subluxation or facet joint disease of the C2–C3 vertebrae. Typically, cervicogenic headache presents in: suboccipital, hemicranial, and supraorbital distribution. Cervicogenic headache is four times more common in women than men and up to 66% present with whiplash-associated disorder (WAD).

### Anatomy

Many investigators in the past such as Cyriax (1938), Kellgren (1939), and Kerr (1961) reported via human neurophysiological experiments that stimulation of facet joint, periosteum, ligaments, and paravertebral muscles are capable of generating pain that is different in characterization and topography than the classical nerve root dermatomal pain. All of the past spinal structures are supplied by the "dorsal rami" of the cervical spinal nerves, which are the source of cervicogenic headache due to their myofascial and subcutaneous neural supply.

### Pathophysiology

Many theories regarding headache arising from cervical origin exists, and they can be summarized as the following:

1. Myodural fibrous bridge tension: the dura matter in the posterior suboccipital region is attached to the "rectus capitis posterior minor (RCPM) muscle" by a fibrous band/bridge that is normally 13.6 mm in length and 1.1 mm in width according to the cadaveric dissections (**◘** Fig. 13.7.1). In cases of cervical vertebral subluxation, myofascial trigger point develops within the RCPM muscle, which will exert traction force on the pain-sensitive dura, causing dural inflammatory thickening and suboccipital pain (suboccipital headache). Other myodural bridges are detected between C1 and C2 vertebrae with the rectus capitis posterior major and obliquus capitis inferior muscles. The ventral dura is supplied by a sensory (nociceptive) nerve plexus that is derived from the "sinuvertebral nerve" and "the nerve plexus of the posterior longitudinal ligament." The dorsal dura is innervated from ventral dural plexi. The sinuvertebral nerve originates exclusively in the rami communicantes and has a "sympathetic component."

To further elaborate the myodural fibrous bridge tension in generating pain, it is wise to briefly discuss the dural system. The entire dural system is formed by a continuous, pain-sensitive membrane that starts covering the inner cranium and exiting the foramen magnum forming the spinal dura. The intracranial dural folds (e.g., falx and tentorial cerebelli) conduct the dural venous sinuses. The entire dural system has five main points of attachments that anchor the dura in proper position: (1) in front (the falx cerebri is anchored into the crista galli and clinoid processes, and it contains the superior sagittal sinus), (2) in the back (the falx cerebri is anchored into the foramen magnum and start from there to descend continuously forming the spinal dura. The spinal dura encloses the spinal cord, and the spinal cord is attached to the cervical dura via the dentate ligament), (3) laterally (the tentorial cerebelli are attached to the petrous bones bilaterally, and they contain the transverse sinuses and

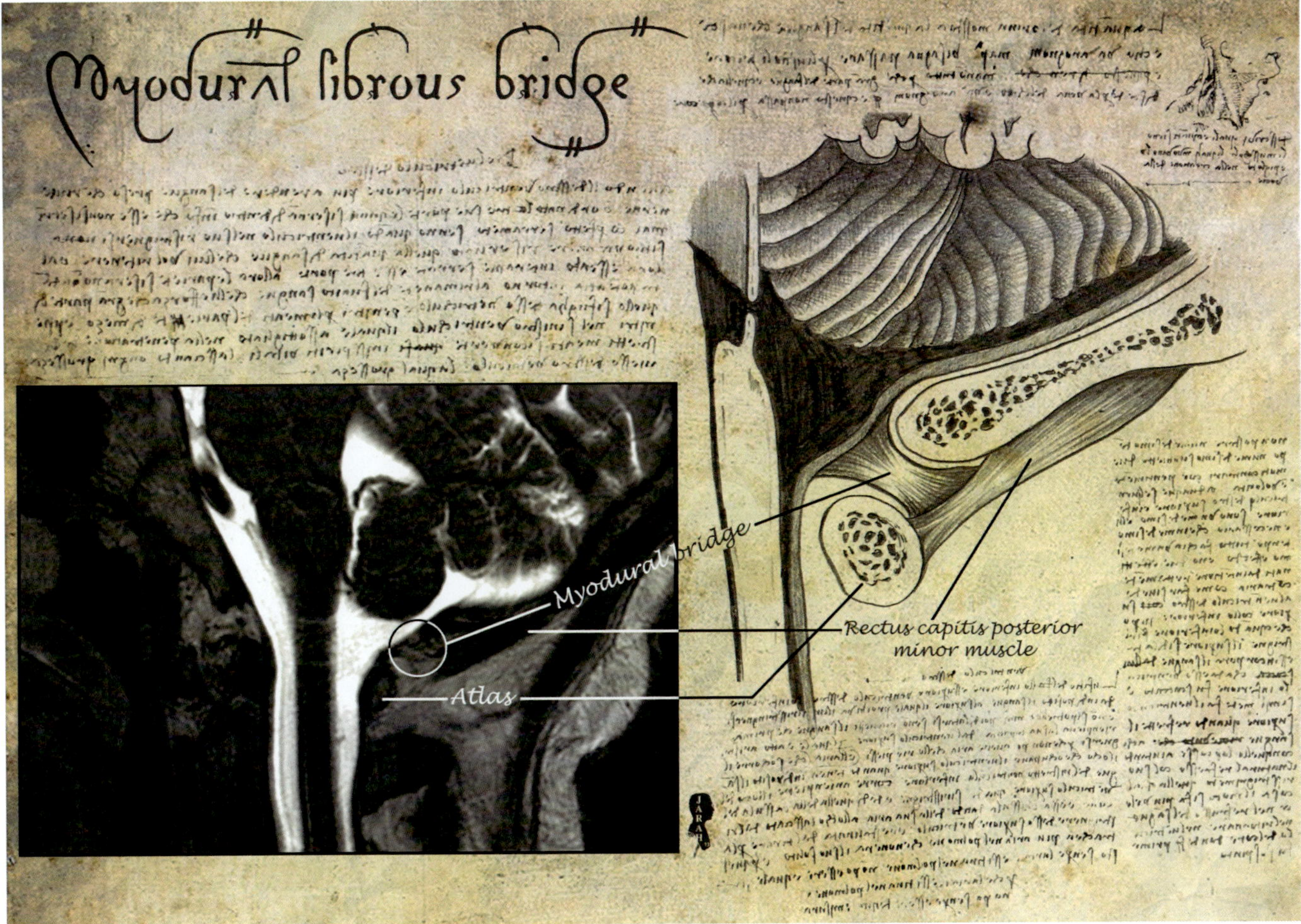



**Fig. 13.7.1** An illustration that shows the myodural fibrous bridge attaches between the dura matter and the rectus capitis posterior minor muscle with MR correlation (sagittal 3D-CISS sequence)

the confluence – torcular herophili), and (4) below (the spinal dura is anchored to the sacrum at "S1–S2" via the filum terminalis).

Dural tension at any of these points is capable of generating symptoms due to the pain-sensitive nature of the dura. For example, an occipito-atlantoaxial subluxation can create a cervical dural tension that radiates to the sacral region, causing sciatica-like pain (sciatica brachialis), while a sacroiliac instability can create a dural tension that radiates upward to the craniocervical region, generating suboccipital headache.

2. Trigeminal spinal nucleus involvement: the "spinal trigeminal tract" is defined as cells in the upper C1–C3 cervical spinal segments that receive pain and temperature fibers from the three divisions of the trigeminal nerve (ophthalmic, maxillary, and mandibular) plus nociceptive fibers from the face, upper neck, and throat. Nociceptive (pain) signals from the structure innervated by C1–C3 spinal levels (e.g., muscle, joints, ligaments, etc.) are capable of generating cervicogenic headache. Pain signals from the neck can evoke also other second-order nociceptive neurons within the spinal trigeminal tract (cross-sensitization phenomenon), resulting in trigeminal cephalgia or

trigeminal neuralgia associated with sympathetic symptoms due to concomitant cervical chain irritation (e.g., lacrimation, nasal congestion, erythema in the forehead, blurry vision, etc.).

3. Occipital (Arnold's) neuralgia: the greater occipital nerve supplying the suboccipital region receives neural supply from the dorsal ramus of C2–C3 spinal segments (**Fig. 13.7.2**). Vertebral malalignment of C2–C3 vertebrae can send nociceptive impulses through the dorsal ramus to the occipital nerve, resulting in "occipital neuralgia/headache" and tension within the occipitalis muscle (tension headache) (**Figs. 13.7.3 and 13.7.4**).

4. Neck–tongue syndrome: neck–tongue syndrome is disease characterized by the simultaneous occurrence of suboccipital pain associated with ipsilateral tongue numbness. The disease is caused by abnormal subluxation of the atlantoaxial joint that causes compression over the C2 ventral ramus and its ganglion. The tongue numbness doesn't originate from trigeminal lesion but originates from impaired deep proprioceptive afferents in the facial nerve fibers supplying the tongue due to the compression of the C2 ventral ramus.

**Fig. 13.7.2** An illustration that shows the anatomical course and origin of the greater occipital nerve

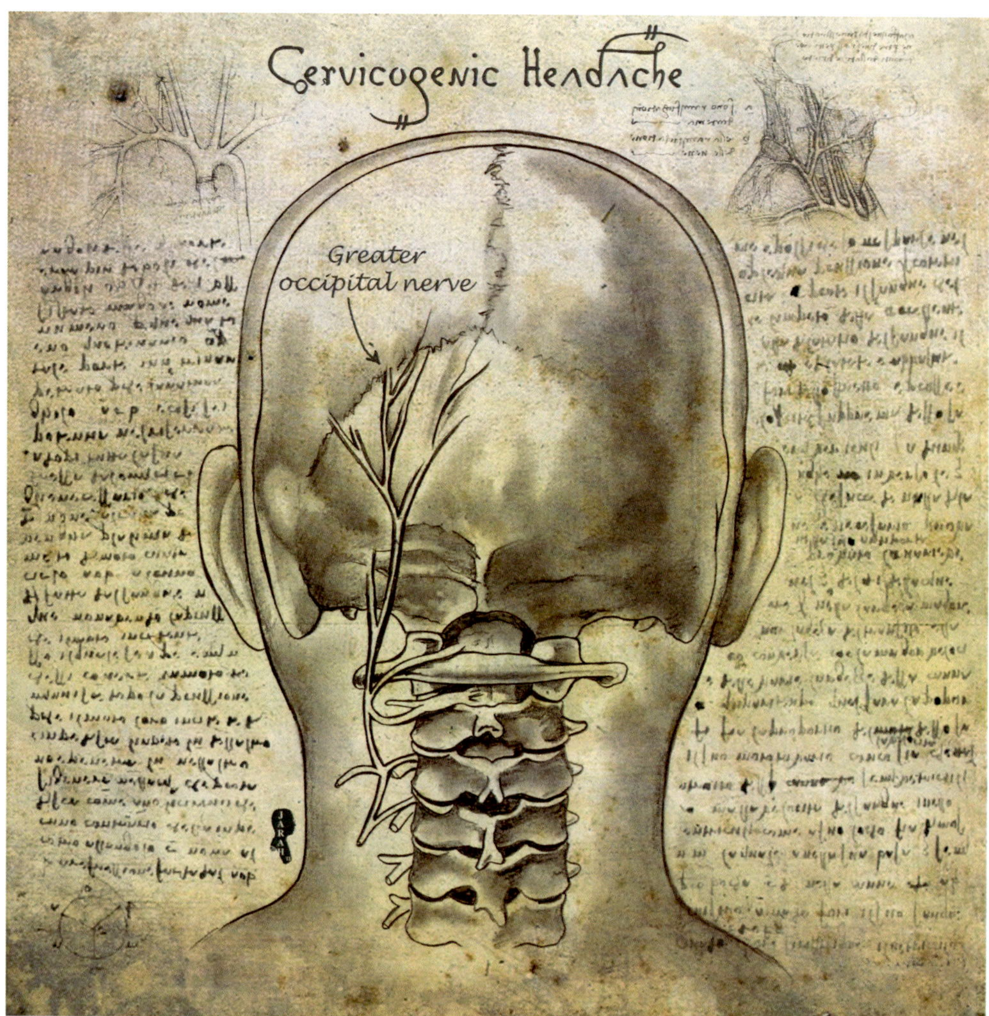


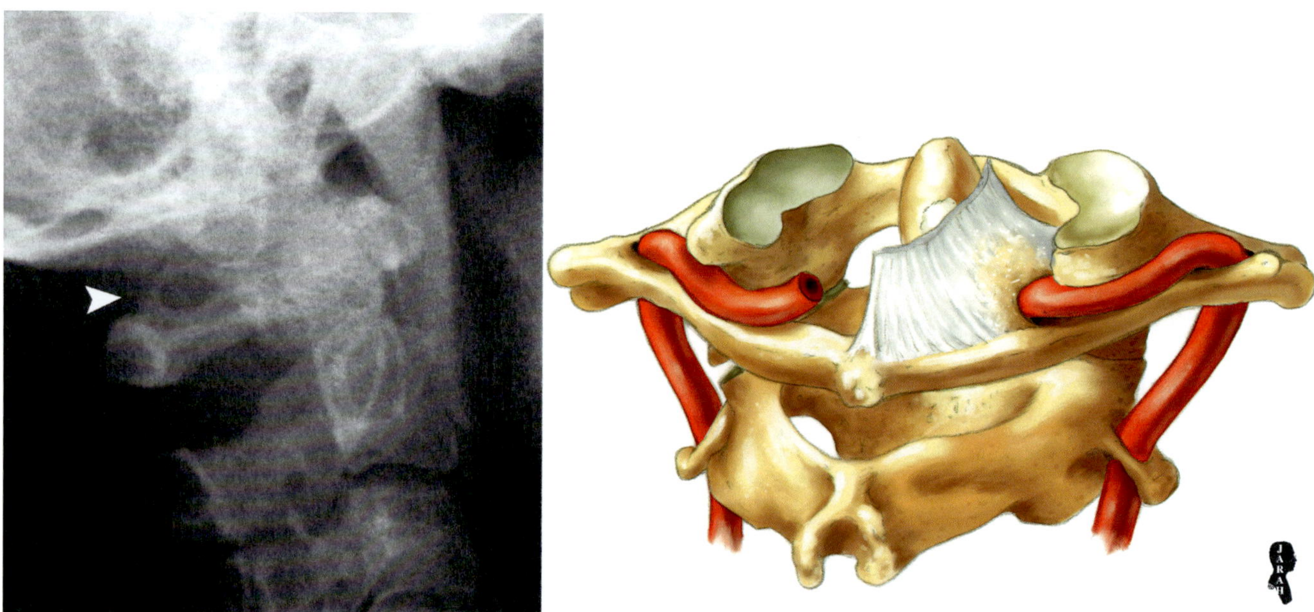

**Fig. 13.7.3** Lateral plain radiograph that demonstrates foramen arcuale (*arrowhead*), with an illustration that shows the calcification of the atlanto-occipital membrane surrounding the vertebral artery (from Al-Tubaikh JA. Congenital Diseases and syndromes – an illustrated radiological guide. 1st ed. Springer-Verlag; 2009. p. 147)

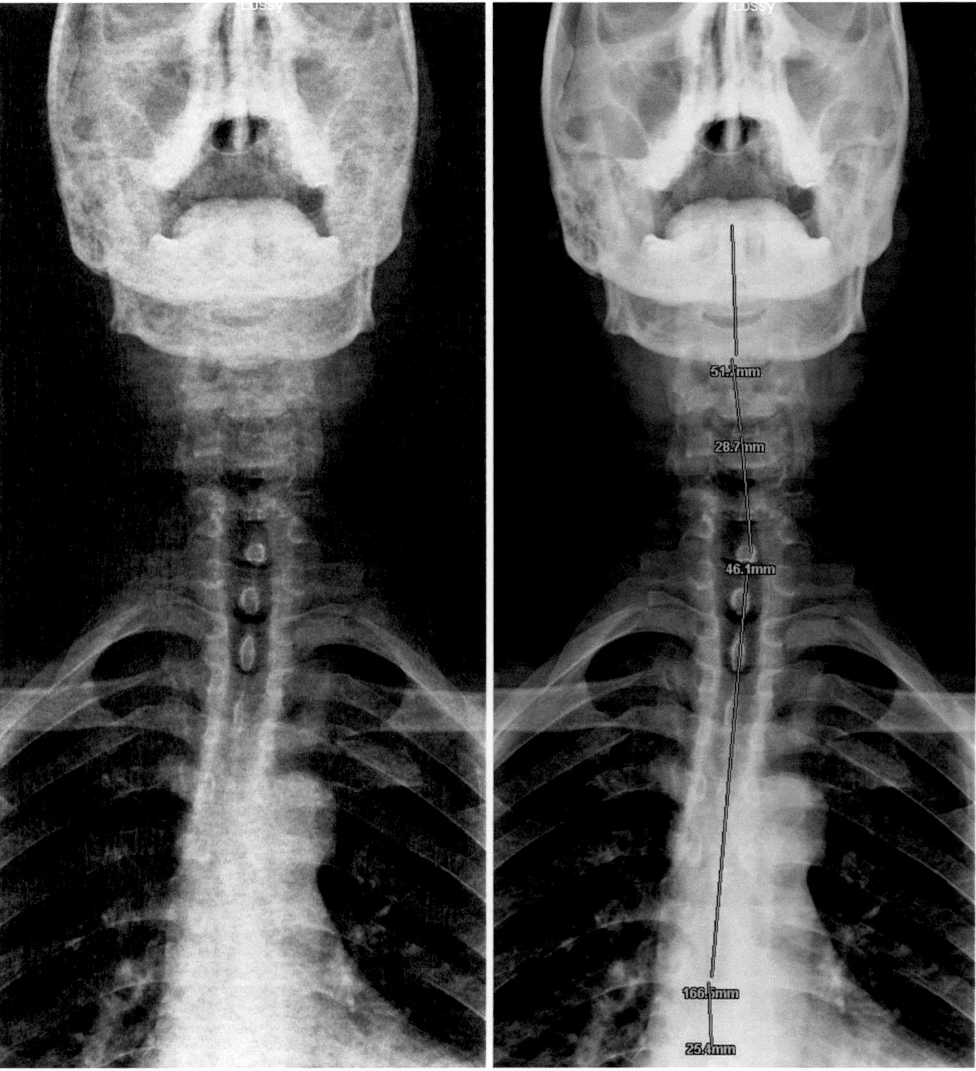

■ **Fig. 13.7.4** Nasium radiographic view of a patient presented with classical pain distribution of cervicogenic headache shows cervical vertebrae malalignment

5. Barré-Lieou syndrome: it is a disease characterized by headache, vasomotor disturbance, vertigo, and swallowing and phonation problems due to alteration of blood flow within the vertebral arteries as a consequence of compression and irritation of the sympathetic vertebral nerve plexus surrounding the vertebral arteries. Compression of the vertebral sympathetic nerve plexus occurs mainly within a calcified ligamentous border of the posterior atlanto-occipital membrane, also known as "foramen arcuale." This is one of the earliest theories of cervicogenic headache and vertigo and was reported in 1928 by J.A. Barré and his student Y. A. Lieou.

## 13.14 Imaging Signs

1. Cervicogenic headache can be suggested after excluding structural lesion in the brain in CT or MRI by anteroposterior cervical radiograph or "Nasium" view radiographs showing vertebral malalignment confined to the cervical vertebrae (most commonly in the C2–C4 region).

2. Foramen arcuale is detected as calcification of the ligamentous border of the posterior atlanto-occipital membrane on lateral radiographs as a normal variant, making a bony ring at the area where the vertebral artery travels through the posterior arch of atlas to enter the foramen magnum; the diagnosis of Barré-Lieou syndrome is a pure clinical diagnosis correlated with this innocent radiographic finding (in most cases).

## Further Reading

Al-Tubaikh JA. Congenital diseases and syndromes – an illustrated radiological guide. 1st ed. Springer-Verlag; 2009. p. 147.

Andary MT, et al. Neurogenic atrophy of suboccipital muscles after a cervical injury. A case study. Am J Phys Med Rehabil. 1998;77:545–9.

Barnsley L, et al. Whiplash injury. Pain. 1994;58(3):283–307.

Biondi DM. Cervicogenic headache: a review of diagnostic and treatment strategies. J Am Osteopath Assoc. 2005;105(4 Suppl 2):165–225.

Bogduk N. An anatomical basis for the neck-tongue syndrome. J Neurol Neurosurg Psychiatr. 1981;44(3): 202–8.

Bogduk N. The cervical-cranial connection. J Manipulative Physiol Ther. 1992;15(1):67–70.

Elliott J, et al. Fatty infiltration in the cervical extensor muscles in persistent whiplash-associated disorders. A magnetic resonance imaging analysis. Spine. 2006;31(22): E847–55.

Hack GD, et al. Anatomic relation between the rectus capitis posterior minor muscle and the dura matter. Spine. 1995;20(23):2454–86.

Lord SM, et al. Cervical synovial joints as sources of post-traumatic headache. J Musculoskeletal Pain. 1996;4(4): 81–94.

McPartland JM, et al. Chronic neck pain, standing balance, and suboccipital muscle atrophy – a pilot study. J Manipulative Physiol Ther. 1997;20(1):24–9.

Meloche JP, et al. Painful intervertebral dysfunction: Robert Maigne's original contribution to headache of cervical origin. Headache. 1993;33(6):328–34.

Nagasawa A, et al. A roentgenographic findings in the cervical spine in tension-type headache. Headache. 1993;33(2): 90–5.

Pfaffernath V, et al. Cervicogenic haeadche – the clinical picture, radiological findings and hypotheses on its pathophysiology. Headache. 1987;27(9):495–9.

Seletz E. Whiplash injuries. JAMA. 1958;168(13):1750–5.

Sjaastad O, et al. "Cervicogenic" headache. An hypothesis. Cephalalgia. 1983;3(4):249–56.

Sjaastad O, et al. Cervicogenic headache, C2 rhizopathy, and occipital neuralgia: a common connection? Cephalalgia. 1986;6(4):189–95.

Vernon H, et al. Cervicogenic dysfunction in muscle contraction headache and migraine. A descriptive study. J Manipulative Physiol Ther. 1992;15(7):418–29.


## 13.15 Cervicogenic Vertigo and Tinnitus

Dizziness is defined as a subjective sensation of postural instability or of illusory motion. In contrast, vertigo is a sensation of horizontal, vertical, or oblique illusory motion that is typically caused by vestibular system disturbance. Patients typically use the word "dizziness" to describe multiple conditions like vertigo, dysequilibrium, lightheadedness, spinning, giddiness, faintness, floating, feeling woozy, and many other sensations.

Tinnitus is defined as an auditory phantom sensation of ringing in the ears that is experienced in the absence of any external sound. The second largest cause of tinnitus, after insults to the cochlea, is putative abnormal activity in the somatosensory system resulting from head and neck injuries. Tinnitus is classified clinically as:

(a) Pulsatile tinnitus: the tinnitus follows the patient's pulse and is typically caused by vascular abnormality (e.g., glomus tympanicum tumor).

(b) Continuous tinnitus: the tinnitus forms a constant, non-relenting noise and is usually caused by neural insult to the ear (e.g., facial neuralgia).

## Anatomy

Balance is achieved via the interaction between complex sensorimotor systems that derives stabilizing sensory information from three main sensory stems:

1. The vestibular labyrinth sends sensory information regarding the head position in space.
2. Visual inputs sends sensory information regarding gaze orientation of the environment.
3. Somatosensory proprioception afferents send information regarding joint position sense and superficial sensation relayed in the spinal cord. It is believed that up to 90 % of the brain activity during standing and walking is attributed to balance control and proprioception. The facet joints in the cervical spines, especially the occipito-atlantoaxial facet joints, assume an important role in maintaining equilibrium. A disturbance in the occipito-atlantoaxial facet joint propioceptive afferents is capable of generating cervicogenic vertigo and nystagmus.

The sensory inputs from the vestibule and semicircular canals bilaterally are sent to the vestibular nuclei in the midbrain, which will be modulated by the "ponto-medullar reticular formation – PMRF." The PMRF modulates the vestibular inputs and sends them upward to the cerebellum, hypothalamus, and cerebral cortex. Vertigo results from sensory mismatch between what is received and what is optimal.

The reticular formation contains data bank information about the optimal perfect balance; any deviation of sensory imbalance from the optimal will result in reflex efferent inputs via:

(a) Vestibulo-ocular reflex is composed of projections from the vestibular nucleus to the oculomotor nerve, controlling muscle eye movement to stabilize gaze during head movement (e.g., to enable reading while walking). Abnormal vestibulo-ocular reflex results in the generation of "nystagmus."

(b) Vestibulo-spinal reflex is composed of projections from the vestibular nucleus to the spinal cord, controlling the neck, trunk, and lower limbs antigravity muscles.

(c) Vestibulo-autonomic reflex causes the unpleasant experiences that accompany vertigo (e.g., vomiting, nausea, vertigo).

Many causes of sudden falling, vertigo, and drop attacks are caused by vertebral artery insufficiency due to external compression that causes ischemia to the posterior fossa contents including the cerebellum. The total both vertebral arteries contribution to the cerebral circulation is (200 ml/min) compared to the contribution of both carotid arteries (800 ml/min). The vertebral artery is accompanied by sympathetic nerves along its course, and they arise from the stellate, the middle cervical, and the intermediate cervical ganglia. Dysautonomia in the head and neck can arise due to compression of these nerves by spondyloarthritic changes, especially in "joint of Luschka's disease."

Between the atlas and the axis, the vertebral arteries are directly covered by the obliquus capitis and the intertransversarii muscles, both which can cause external arterial compression during head movement. Atlantoaxial rotation of 30° can produce kinking of the contralateral vertebral artery at the C2 transverse foramen. Vertebrobasilar (bow hunter's) stroke can be caused by narrowing of the C2 transverse foramen with >45° atlantoaxial rotation in cases of atlantoaxial instability, paraspinal muscles tightness (myofascial triggers), and rarely by the presence of foramen arcuale.

Bow-hunter's stroke, also known as "rotational vertebral artery syndrome," is a rare symptomatic vertebrobasilar insufficiency presenting as dizziness, vertigo, syncope, nausea, or sensorimotor disturbance due to stenosis or occlusion of the vertebral artery (VA) upon head rotation. The extrinsic factors identified VA compression by osteophyte, cervical spondylosis, fibrous bands, cervical disk herniation, or VA stretching by intervertebral instability along the craniocervical axis.

## Pathophysiology

There are three main theories with clinical support that explains vertigo originated from the neck:

1. Cervico-ocular reflex: the vestibular system does not orient the head in relation to the body alone but receives information about the head position in space via the deep neck proprioceptors. A lesion to the C1–C3 vertebrae (e.g., whiplash injury) will overexcite the deep neck proprioceptors firing, which will cause abnormal firing reaching the vestibular nuclei in the brainstem, hypothalamus, and cerebellum; all of which at the end will result in vertigo sensation.
2. Cervical malalignment of C1–C2 vertebrae: it can cause myofascial trigger points in the obliquus capitis and the intertransversarii muscles, both of which can cause external arterial compression during head movement. Vertebral insufficiency will reduce the blood supply to the inner ear via the labyrinthine artery, causing ischemia and vertigo and tinnitus.
3. Cervical malalignment of C8–T3 vertebrae: it can exert pressure over the sympathetic chain, which in turn will disturb the sympathetic innervation of the iris. The iris sympathetic innervation is derived from the intermediolateral horn cells of T2–T3, sending fibers to the sympathetic chain, which then pass to the superior cervical ganglion traveling along with the carotid artery and then with the ophthalmic arteries, over the ciliary ganglion, but do not synapse here. Finally, fibers from the ciliary ganglion send sympathetic fibers via the nasociliary nerve to the dilator pupillae muscle in the eye, causing dilatation of the pupil (mydriasis) and blurry vision. This blurry vision can be described by some patients falsely as dizziness or vertigo.

## 13.16 Imaging Signs

1. On radiographs, cervicogenic vertigo can be suggested by the presence of cervical malalignment of the C1–C3 vertebrae in the absence of any other organic cause (◘ Figs. 13.8.1 and 13.8.2). Also, the most common clue of the vertebrobasilar insufficiency is the presence of cervical spins degenerative changes on lateral plain radiographs.
2. On Doppler sonography, vertebral insufficiency is detected when the vertebral artery segment (typically V2 and V1 segments) shows abnormal flow during a static and/or dynamic imaging (◘ Figs. 13.8.3 and 13.8.4). On both static and dynamic images, vertebral artery stenosis can be graded by the peak systolic velocity (PSV) as the following: < 50 % stenosis (PSV > 108 and <139 cm/s), 50–70 % stenosis (PSV >140 and <200 cm/s), and >70 % stenosis (PSV >210 cm/s).
3. For dynamic vertebral artery imaging, the patient is asked to rotate the head to the contralateral side with the neck extended and to keep the head in this position for at least 10 s. The difference in insonation angles between the two positions is kept less than a few degrees. Dynamic vertebral artery rotatory compression is diagnosed when "end-diastolic velocity (EDV)" is reduced to 10 cm/s or to zero during rotation (diagnostic finding). The normal vertebral artery end-diastolic flow velocity is 20–40 cm/s unilaterally or bilaterally.
4. On CT and MRI, the vertebral artery could be found impinged by an osteophyte within the vertebral canal on angiographic images. On chronic cases, signs of ischemic leukopathic changes might be detected on T2-weighted images in the brainstem and/or posterior fossa due to chronic vestibulobasilar insufficiency.

### Further Reading

Chen JJ, et al. Bow hunter's syndrome masquerading as definite Ménière's disease. Tzu Chi Med J. 2010;22(4): 219–24.

Fitz-Ritson D. Assessment of cervicogenic vertigo. J Manipulative Physiol Ther. 1991;14(3):193–8.

Fox MW, et al. Atlantolateral decompression of the atlantoaxial vertebral artery for symptomatic positional occlusion of the vertebral artery. Case Report J Neurosurg. 1995;83(4):737–40.

Haynes MJ, et al. Color Duplex sonographic findings in human vertebral arteries during cervical rotation. J Clin Ultrasound. 2001;29:14–24.

Haynes MJ, et al. Posterior pentacles and rotational stenosis of vertebral arteries. A pilot study using Doppler

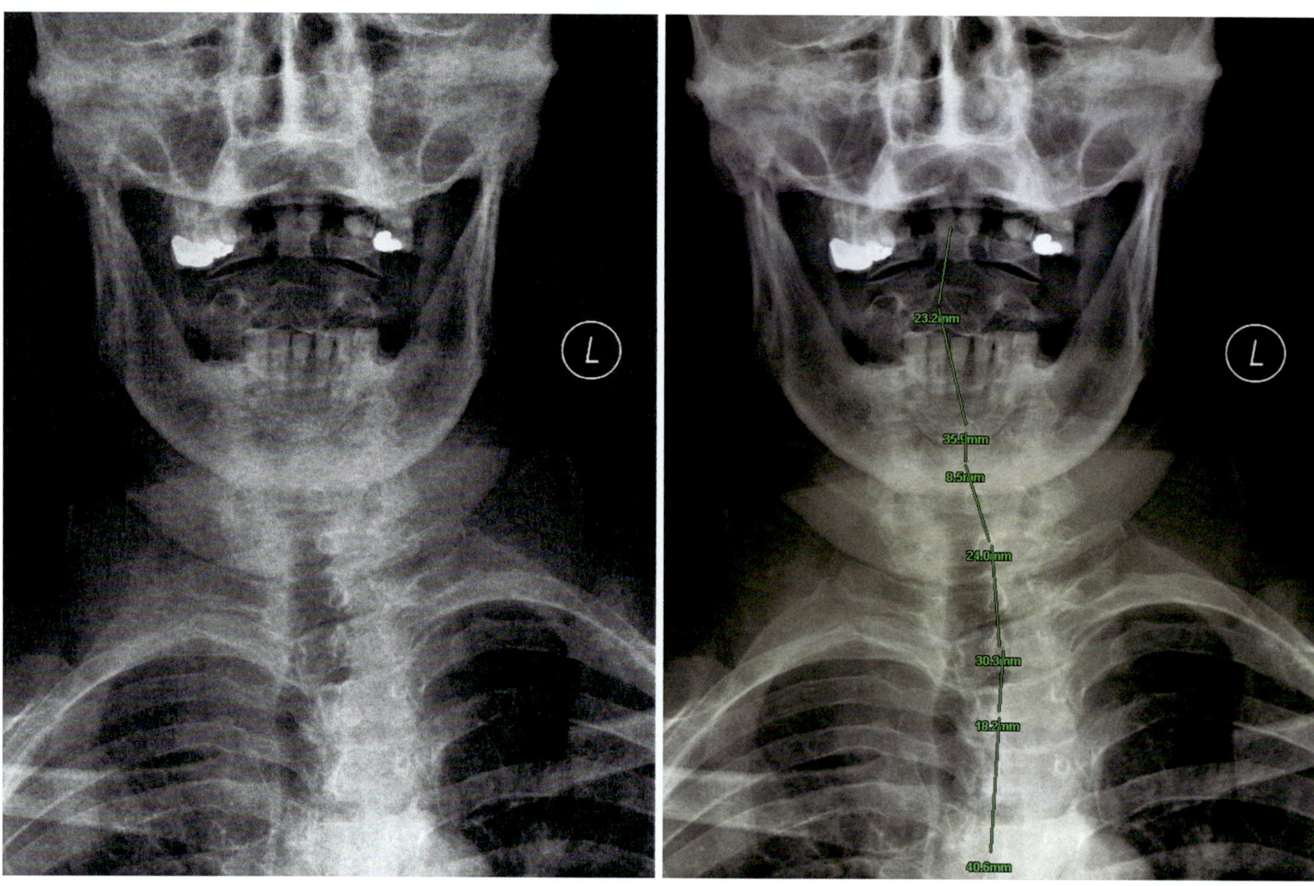



**Fig. 13.8.1**    Anteroposterior cervical radiograph of a patient presented with chronic dizziness and syncopal attacks. Significant cervical vertebrae malalignment, especially at C2–C3 vertebrae, is detected

ultrasound velocimetry and magnetic resonance angiography. J Manipulative Physiol Ther. 2005;28(5):323–9.

Iguchi Y, et al. Transcranial Doppler and Carotid Duplex Ultrasonography Findings in Bow Hunter's Syndrome. J Neuroimaging. 2006;16:278–80.

Kaute BB. The influence of atlas therapy on tinnitus. Int Tinnitus J. 1998;4(2):165–7.

Kessinger R, et al. Changes in visual acuity in patients receiving upper cervical specific chiropractic care. J Vertebral Sublaxat Res. 1998;2(1):43–9.

Kim ESH, et al. Radiologic importance of a high-resistive vertebral artery Doppler waveform on carotid duplex ultrasonography. J Ultrasound Med. 2010;29:1161–5.

Kim K, et al. Anterior vertebral artery decompression with an ultrasonic bone curette to treat bow hunter's syndrome. Acta Neurochir (Wien). 2008;150:301–3.

Kizilkilic O, et al. Color Doppler analysis of vertebral arteries. Correlative study with angiographic data. J Ultrasound Med. 2004;23:1483–91.

Mechler FP. Review of the anatomy, histology and clinical significances of the vertebral artery in health and disease. Chiropr Res J. 1988;1(2):17–33.

Moubayed SP, et al. Vertebrobasilar insufficiency presenting as isolated positional vertigo or dizziness: a double-blind retrospective cohort study. Laryngoscope. 2009;119:2071–6.

Murphy DJ. Whiplash and vision. Am J Clin Chiropr. 1999;9(2):16–7.

Ozdemir H, et al. Effects of cervical rotation on hemodynamics in vertebral arteries. J Diagnost Med Sonography. 2005;21:384–91.

Radtke A, et al. Migraine and Ménière's disease: is there a link? Neurology. 2002;59(11):1700–40.

Reker U. Function of proprioceptors of the cervical spine in the cervico-ocular reflex. HNO. 1985;33(9):426–9.

Sauvaget E, et al. Vertebrobasilar occlusive disorders presenting as sudden sensorineural hearing loss. Laryngoscope. 2004;114:327–32.

Selecki BR. The effect of rotation of the atlas on the axis: experimental work. Med J Austr. 1969;1(20):1012–5.

Strek P, et al. A possible correlation between vertebral artery insufficiency and degenerative changes in the cervical spine. Eur Arch Otorhinolaryngol. 1998;255:437–40.

Terrett AGJ, et al. The eye, the cervical spine, and spinal manipulative therapy: a review of the literature. Chiropr Tech. 1995;7(2):43–54.

van Norel GJ, et al. Drop attacks and instability of the degenerative cervical spine. J Bone Joint Surg (Br). 1996;78(4):495–6.

Yurdakul M, et al. Doppler criteria for identifying proximal vertebral artery stenosis of 50% or more. J Ultrasound Med. 2011;30:163–8.

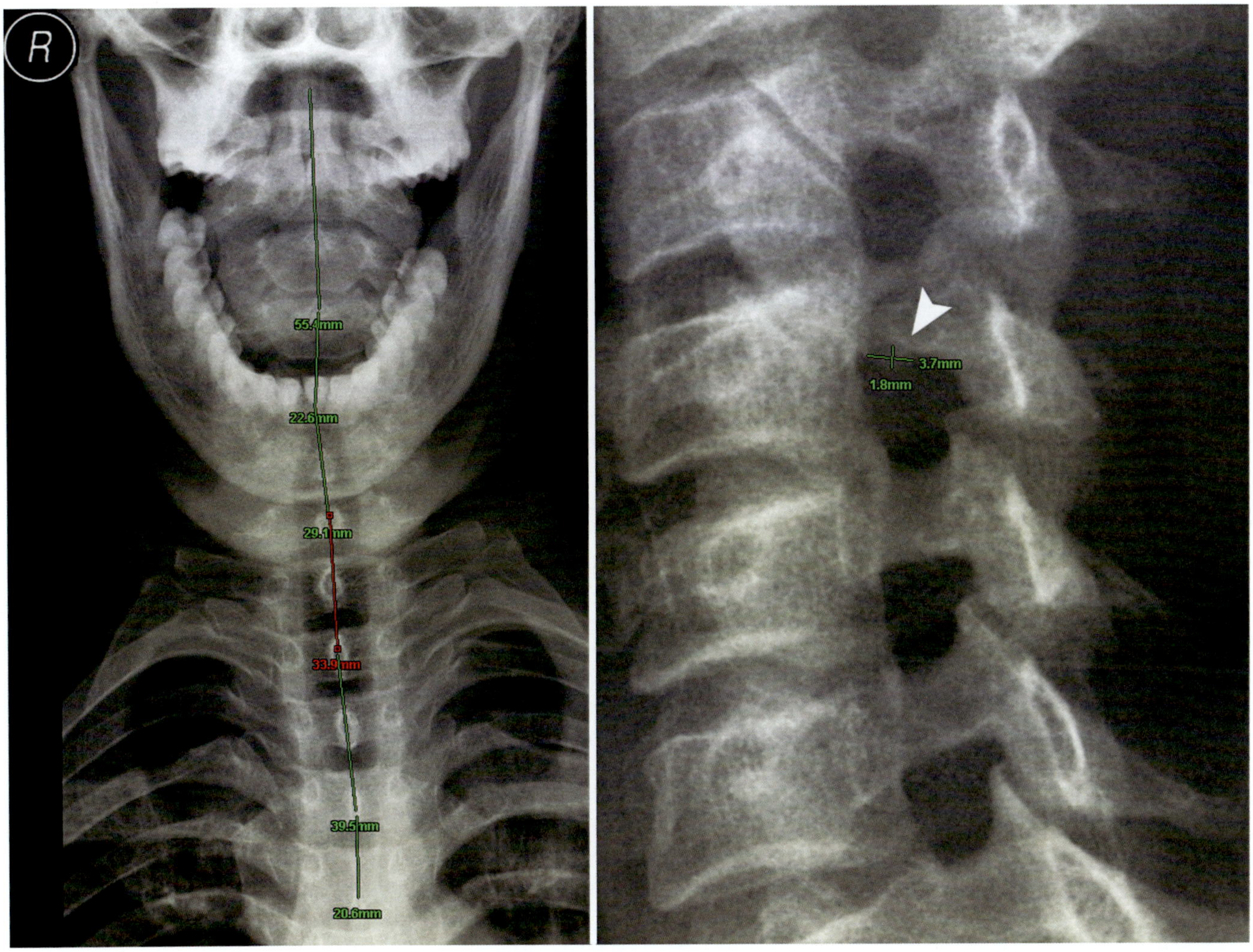

**Fig. 13.8.2**  Plain oblique radiograph of a patient who presented with attacks of vertigo as he/she moves head and neck in certain positions; the oblique radiograph showed an osteophyte in the right intervertebral foramen of C4–C5 level (*arrowhead*)

**Fig. 13.8.3**  Vertebral Doppler imaging of the same patient of  Fig. 13.8.2 shows mosaic phenomenon (aliasing artifact) at the V2 segment of the vertebral artery denoting blood flow turbulence (*arrowhead*), at the site where the right intervertebral foramen osteophyte at C4–C5 level was found on radiography

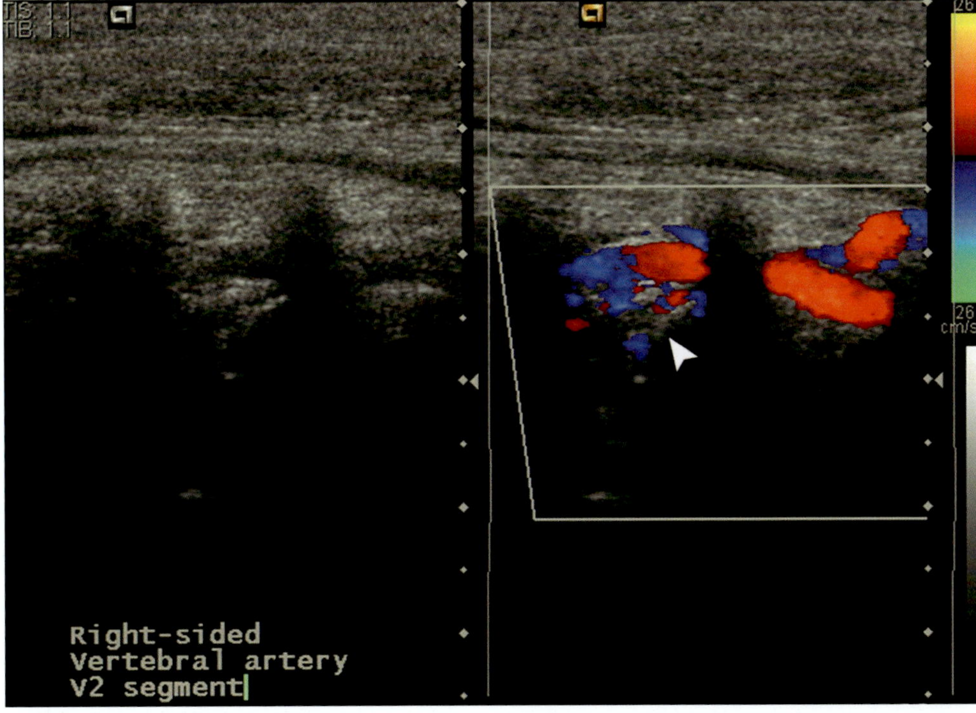

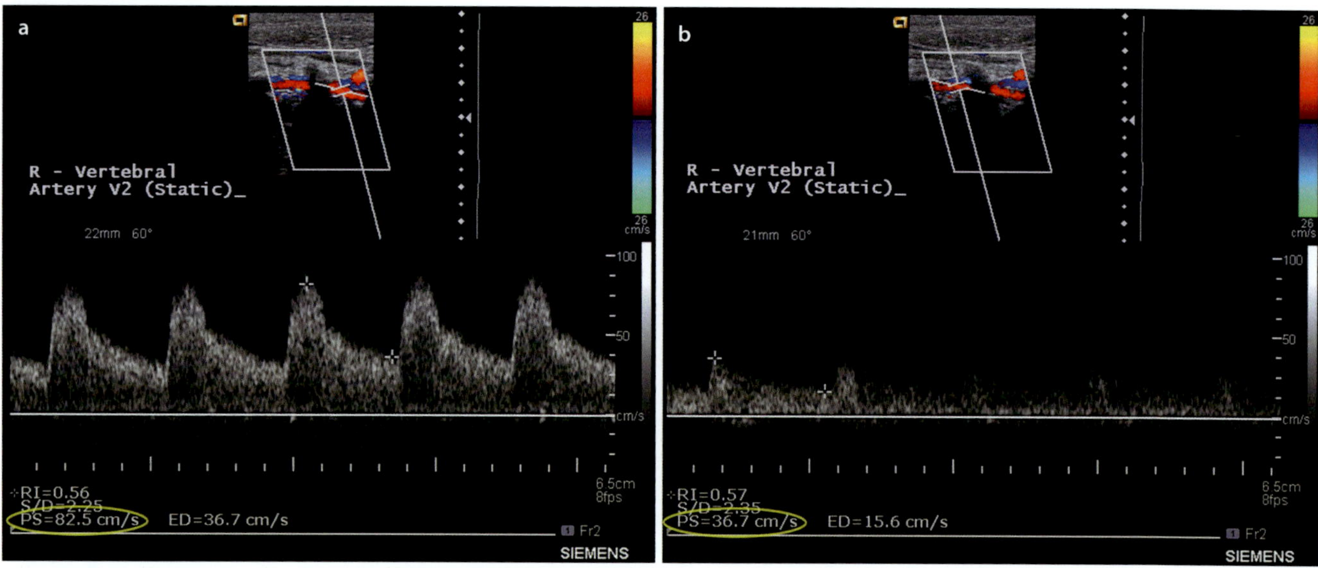

**Fig. 13.8.4**  Vertebral Doppler imaging of the same patient of  Figs. 13.8.2 and 13.8.3 shows marked reduction peak systolic velocity (almost 50 %) of the vertebral artery at the site of stenosis and distally (green circles in **a**, **b**). On dynamic images (not shown), the vertebral artery flow is markedly reduced

## 13.17 **Whiplash-Associated Disorder**

Whiplash-associated disorder (WAD) is a form of injury to the neck characterized by sudden acceleration and deceleration, which causes hyperextension and/or hyperflexion of the head and neck. WAD is commonly caused by vehicle accidents, sports injuries, high-speed rides like jet skis, and/or falls. WAD arises mainly due to ligamentous injury affecting the atlantoaxial and/or the cervical vertebral stability. Up to five of car occupants who attend a hospital after a crash have whiplash injury. While most patients recover from a relatively benign injury, around 25 % suffer prolonged morbidity.

### Basic Anatomy

The occipito-atlantoaxial joint is stabilized by (1) the alar ligaments, which have both atlantal and occipital attachments,(2) the transverse ligament, (3) the anterior atlanto-dental ligaments (part of the alar ligament), (4) the apical ligament of the dens, (5) the tectorial membrane, and (6) the ligamentum nuchae.

The "alar ligaments" are three strong, round band that arise from the tip of the dens and extends obliquely upward and laterally and insert into the medial side of the occipital condyles and atlas. The main function of the alar ligament is to control and limit axial rotation in the upper cervical spine, especially the occipito-atlantoaxial joint. The left alar ligament controls right axial rotation, and vice versa.

The "cruciate ligament" of the atlas is composed of two smaller bands known as the "transverse ligament" of the atlas and the "longitudinal bands." In contrast to the alar ligament, the transverse ligament's main function is to regulate and limit physiologic rotation between the atlas and the axis to protect the spinal cord from their rotation.

The "apical ligament of the dens" is a fibrous cord that extends from the tip of the dens to the anterior margin of the foramen magnum. The "tectorial membrane" is a strong, broad band that extends from the dorsal surface of the body of the axis and is considered as the cranial continuation of the "posterior longitudinal ligament." The "ligamentum nuchae" attaches from the crest of the occiput to the posterior tubercle of the atlas and the spinous processes of the cerebral vertebrae. The ligament functions as a stabilizer of the skull on the cervical spine.

### Pathophysiology

WAD is most commonly affects the occipito-atlantoaxial joint and the area around the cervical vertebrae C4 and C5. The injury is typically associated with injury to the alar ligament, the transverse ligament, and the anterior and posterior longitudinal ligaments. Other structures that can be injured, making this a severe injury, are the joint capsules, facet joints, and intervertebral disks. Muscles affected in whiplash injury include the sternocleidomastoid, scaleneus, and splenius cervicis muscles. In severe cases, muscle tears and chance fracture of the vertebrae can occur.

In acute whiplash injury, chiropractic and manual therapy is contraindicated since it can cause spinal cord transection in case of atlantoaxial instability or a fractured vertebra that went unnoticed. Patients with WAD typically present with:

(a) Headaches (82 %): the main generator of headache in WAD is the C2–C3 facet joint, and the headache can persist up to 2 years in 29–90 % of patients.

(b) Vertigo (50 %): due to cervical C2–C3 malalignment causing vertebrobasilar insufficiency.
(c) Cognitive disturbance (55 %).
(d) Neck pain (55 %): most commonly due to cervical facet joint malalignment.
(e) Visual disturbance (38 %).
(f) Low back pain (35 %).
(g) Interscapular pain (20 %), most commonly due to vertebral malalignment.

## 13.18 Imaging Signs

1. Imaging of whiplash injury sequel mainly should be established with MRI "15 days after the initial injury" to evaluate the alar and transverse ligament of the atlas and dens; another imaging "after 6 months" should be done to evaluate the appearance of posttraumatic syrinx. Posterior column soft tissue and bony injuries have been implicated as underlying the chronic pain of some whiplash sufferers. The scan coverage should be below the foramen magnum to the base of the dens axis (axial), anterior arch of the atlas to halfway through the spinal canal (coronal), and right to left occipital condyle (sagittal).
2. On plain radiographs, disturbance of the "George's line" representing cervical malalignment on lateral radiographs may be seen due to retrolisthesis/anterolisthesis development as a consequence of anterior/posterior longitudinal ligaments disruption.
3. On dynamic flexion/extension radiographs, the atlantodental interspace (a space between the dens and the posterior arch of the atlas) is normally up to 3 mm maximally in adults and <5 mm in children.

An atlantodental interspace of (7 mm) means "complete separation of the transverse ligament." An atlantodental interspace of 10–12 mm means "torn alar ligament."

4. On craniocervical junction MRI, imaging the craniocervical junction in proton density sequence (PD) without fat saturation shows signal change (high signal intensity within the ligaments rather than the normal black low signal), affecting the alar/transverse ligament (due to microtears and degeneration) and/or lateral displacement of the atlas.
5. On cervical spine MRI, spinal cord changes posttrauma can be summarized as the following: high T2 signal intensity within the cord (immediately after injury), retropharyngeal space edema may be detected in acute whiplash injury (up to 4 days after injury – ◘ Fig. 13.9.1), very high T2 signal intensity within the cord due to gliosis formation (3 months after injury), syrinx development (6 months after injury), and cyst formation within the spinal cord (1–2 years after injury).
6. Grading of whiplash injury in MRI (Quebec Task Force Classification).
   Grade 0: Low signal throughout the entire alar/transverse ligament (◘ Fig. 13.9.2)
   Grade 1: High signal in 1/3 or less of alar/transverse ligament
   Grade 2: High signal in 1/3–2/3 of alar/transverse ligament (significant)
   Grade 3: High signal in 2/3 or more of alar/transverse ligament (significant) (◘ Fig. 13.9.2)

### Further Reading

Bilkey WJ. Manual medicine approach to the cervical spine and whiplash injury. Phys Med Rehabil Clin North Am. 1996;7:749–59.

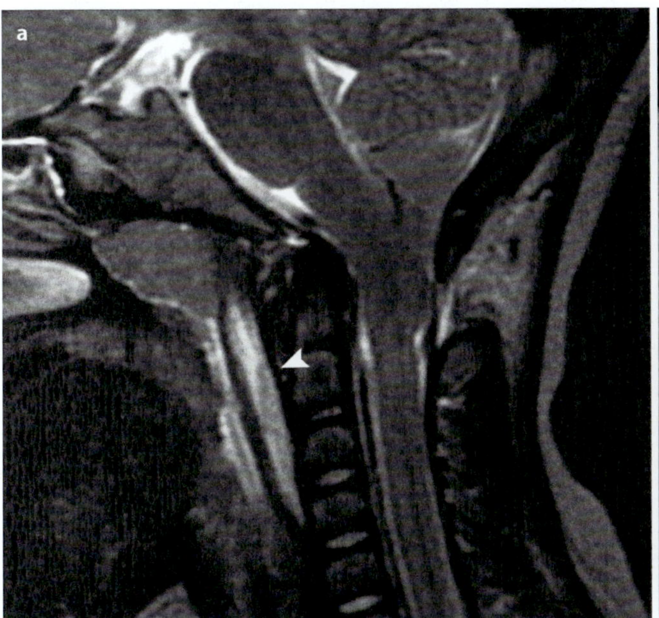
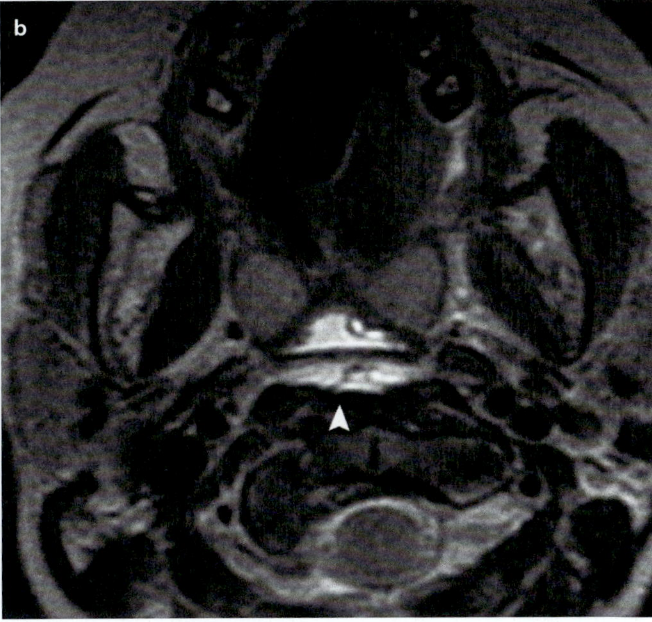

◘ **Fig. 13.9.1**   Sagittal (**a**) and axial (**b**) T2W-MR images of a patient with retropharyngeal edema (*arrowheads*)

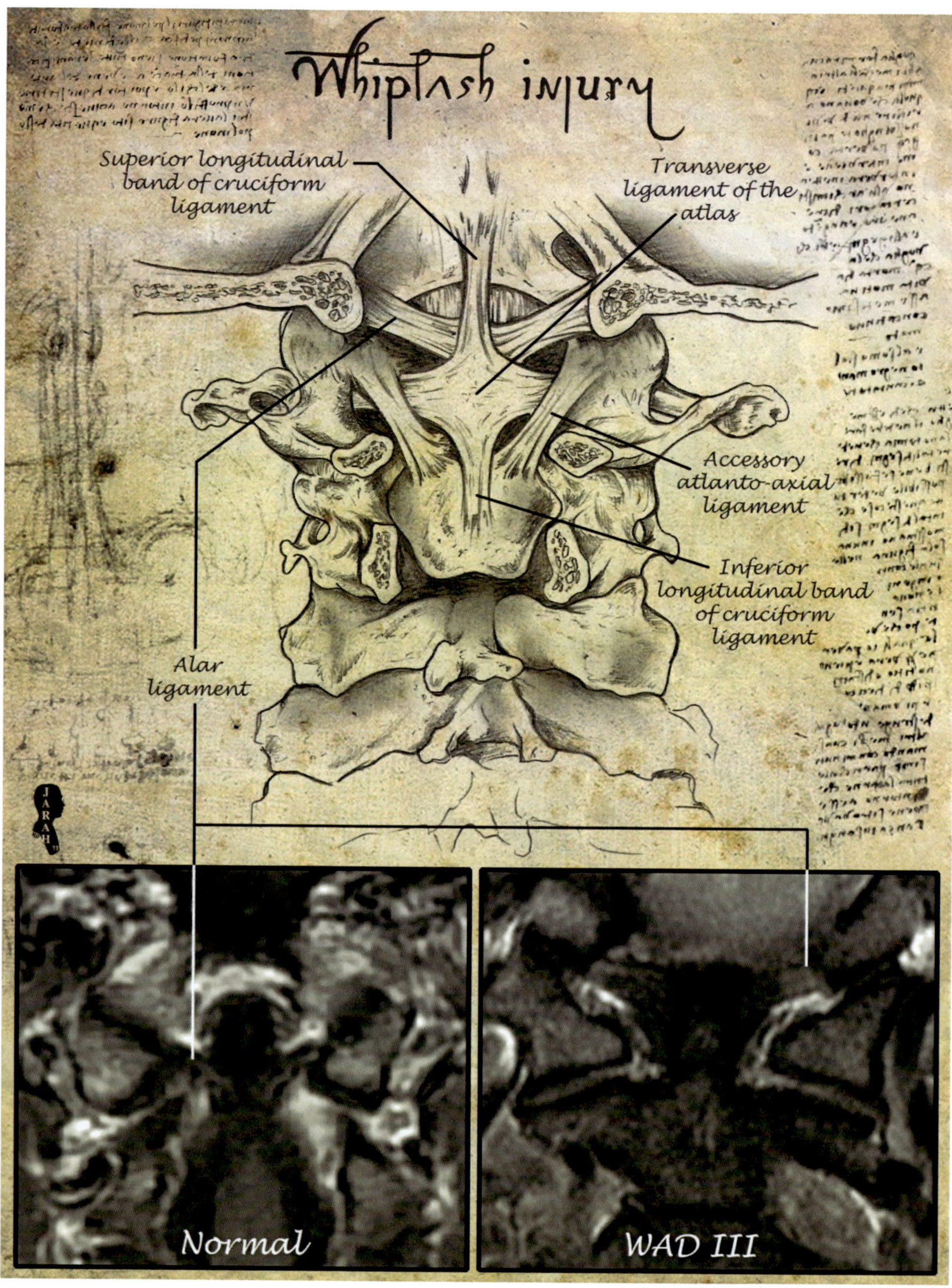



◻ **Fig. 13.9.2** An illustration that demonstrates the anatomy of the alar ligaments with normal and WAD III injury according to the Quebec Task Force Classification


Birnbaum K, et al. Functional cervical MRI within the scope of whiplash injuries: presentation of a new motion device for the cervical spine. Surg Radiol Anat. 2010;32:181–8.

Darian-Smith C. Synaptic plasticity, neurogenesis, and functional recovery after spinal cord injury. Neuroscientist. 2009;15:149–65.

Elliott J, et al. MRI study of the cross-sectional area for the cervical extensor musculature in patients with persistent whiplash associated disorders (WAD). Man Ther. 2008;13:258–65.

Fagerlund M, et al. MRI in acute phase of whiplash injury. Eur Radiol. 1995;5:297–301.

Freund P, et al. Tracking changes following spinal cord injury: insights from neuroimaging. Neuroscientist. 2013;19:116–28.

Hamid S, et al. Role of electrical stimulation for rehabilitation and regeneration after spinal cord injury. Eur Spine J. 2008;17:1256–69.

Krakenes J, et al. MRI assessment of the alar ligaments in the late stage of whiplash injury – a study of structural abnormalities and observer agreement. Neuroradiology. 2002;44:617–24.

Krisken K, et al. Upper cervical post X-ray reduction and its relashonship to symptomatic involvement and spinal stability. Chiropr Res J. 1997;4(1):10–7.

Vetti N, et al. MRI of the alar and transverse ligaments in whiplash-associated disorders (WAD) grades 1–2: high-signal changes by age, gender, event and time since trauma. Neuroradiology. 2009;51:227–35.

Vetti N, et al. MRI of the transverse and alar ligaments in rheumatoid arthritis: feasibility and relations to atlanto-axial subluxation and disease activity. Neuroradiology. 2010;52:215–23.

Voyvodic F, et al. MRI of car occupants with whiplash injury. Neuroradiology. 1997;39:35–40.

## 13.19 Thoracic Outlet Syndrome

Thoracic outlet syndrome (TOS) is a term used to suggest the presence of a disorder within the area of the thoracic outlet. TOS is a disease characterized by neuronal or vascular compression of the arm vessels or nerves as they exit from the thoracic outlet to the arm. The compression can be neuronal, venous, or arterial in origin.

### Basic Anatomy

The thoracic outlet (cervico-thoraco-brachial junction) is the space bounded by the upper part of the sternum, clavicle, first rib, and the first thoracic vertebra, and it is 10 cm wide. Centrally, it is limited by the trachea and esophagus. The thoracic outlet forms the communicating area at the base of the neck for the passage of blood vessels and nerves from mediastinum and neck to the axilla and into which the dome of the pleura rises upward. The vagus, phrenic nerves, sympathetic trunks, and thoracic duct also pass through the same openings.

The first rib is short, broad, has no angle, and attached to T1 vertebra only. It has a tubercle attaching the first head of the scalenus anterior muscle and a groove for the subclavian artery. The axillary artery starts on the lateral border of the first rib. The subclavius muscle is attached to its superior surface; this muscle may cause a minor role in TOS by depressing the clavicle and elevating the first rib, which can aid in narrowing the thoracic outlet where these vessels pass.

The thoracic outlet includes three spaces anatomically: (1) the interscalene triangle, (2) the costoclavicular space, and (3) the retropectoralis minor space (■ Fig. 13.10.1); these areas are the areas to look for vascular or arterial compression on imaging techniques (e.g., MRI):

(a) Interscalene space: it is the space where the subclavian artery and the three trunks of the brachial plexus are crossing through. Compression of the brachial plexus by the scalenus muscles is known as "scalenus anticus syndrome."

(b) Costoclavicular space: it is a space located between the clavicle anteriorly and the pectoralis minor posteriorly. It contains the subclavian vein, subclavian artery, and the three cords of the brachial plexus. Compression of the neurovascular bundle at this point is known as "costoclavicular syndrome." The costoclavicular space is the most common area for vascular compression, followed by the interscalene space.

(c) Retropectoralis minor space: it is limited anteriorly by the posterior boarder of the pectoralis minor muscle and posteriorly by the subscapularis muscle. It contains the subclavian vein, subclavian artery, and the three cords of the brachial plexus. Compression of the neurovascular bundle at this point is known as "pectoralis minor muscle syndrome."

### Pathophysiology

TOS can be caused by cervical rib, elongation of the seventh vertebra transverse process, fibrous band, posttraumatic fibrous scarring, and congenital muscular anomalies (e.g., scalenus minimus muscle).

The cervical rib is a normal variant that is found in 1–2 % of population, commonly females, and is found bilaterally in up to 50 % of cases. If cervical rib develops, the brachial plexus will come from C4–C8 rather than C5–T1. Only 5 % of patients with cervical rib will ever suffer from a thoracic outlet syndrome.

Patients with TOS typically present with a variety of symptoms that depends on the compression site: neural, arterial, or venous. The brachial plexus is involved in 98 % of

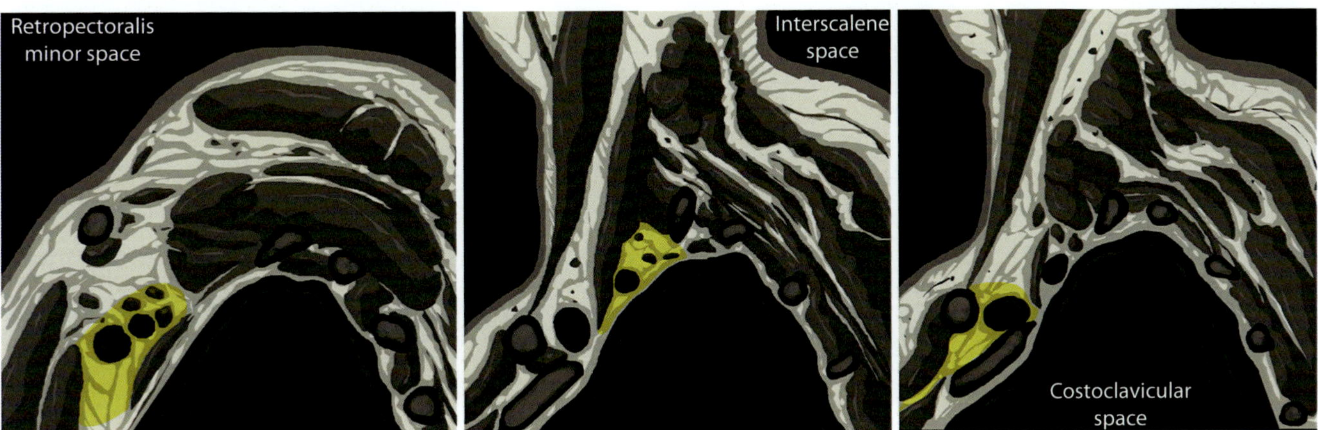


■ **Fig. 13.10.1**    An illustration that shows the interscalene triangle, the costoclavicular space, and the retropectoralis minor space

cases, the subclavian vein in 1.5%, and the artery in 0.5%. TOS symptoms are typically induced as the patient raises and sustains his/her arm. And many patients experience these symptoms at night. The disease is most commonly seen in females between 20 and 40 years of age. Symptoms depend on the compressed structure, such as:

1. Neurogenic symptoms (90%): results in pain, paresthesia, motor weakness, and cold arm after activities require prolonged arm elevation. Shoulder tip and back of the neck pain are frequently seen. Ulnar nerve compression causes numbness in the medial side of the arm and the ring and little fingers.
2. Arterial symptoms (10%): results in arterial claudication and distal microemboli, causing unilateral Raynaud's-like phenomenon.
3. Venous symptoms: results in arm swelling, cyanosis, limb swelling, and heaviness sensation. "Paget–Schroetter syndrome" is a disease caused by subclavian and axillary vein thrombosis due to effort, usually due to TOS.

## 13.20 Imaging Signs

1. On plain radiographs, look for elongated C7 vertebra, cervical rib or osteophytes, and degenerative changes of the clavicle (◘ Fig. 13.10.2).
2. On ultrasound, median nerve neuropathy can be detected by flattening of the nerve (>10 mm in diameter) and/or signal change of the nerve fiber. Normal nerves are fairly uniform, hyperechoic due to its sphingomyelin lipid content, reflecting their histological composition. On axial planes, US demonstrate nerves as honeycomb-like structures composed of hypoechoic spots (nerve fascicles) embedded in a hyperechoic fatty/myelin background (epineurium). On sagittal planes, nerves typically assume an elongated appearance with multiple hypoechoic parallel linear areas, which correspond to the neuronal fascicles that run longitudinally within the nerve, separated by hyperechoic bands, representing the myelin sheath. A diseased nerve will show loss of this texture with predominance "hypoechoic texture," representing diseased myelin and edema (◘ Fig. 13.10.3).
3. On Doppler sonography, the key Doppler findings in TOS are related to changes in the subclavian artery (SCA) Doppler wave spectrum during different maneuvers. Typically, there is narrowing, turbulence, and color aliasing in the SCA on (90° arm abduction), with complete absence of color flow on hyperabduction (120° arm abduction) (◘ Fig. 13.10.4). The normal velocities in

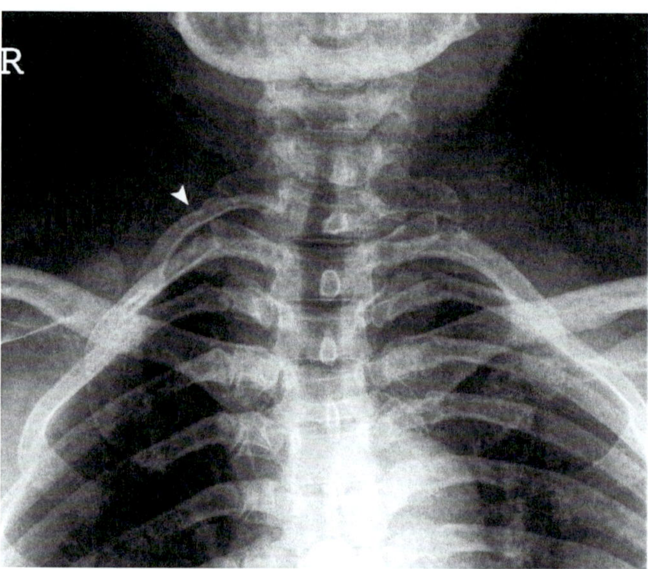

◘ **Fig. 13.10.2** Plain anteroposterior neck radiograph that shows right-sided accessory rib at C7–T1 vertebrae (*arrowhead*)

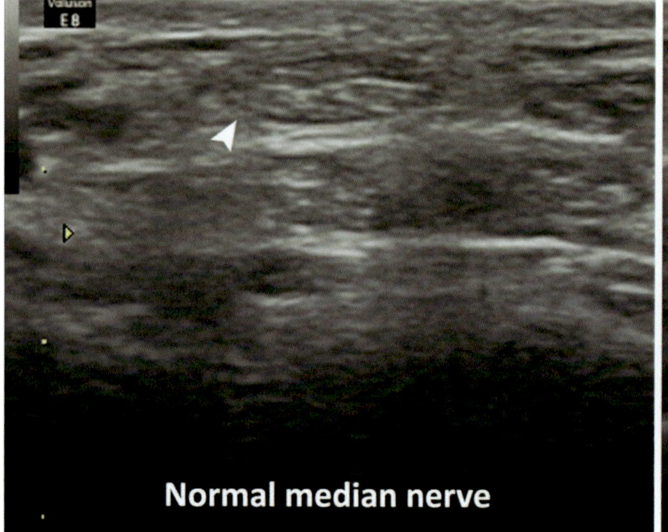


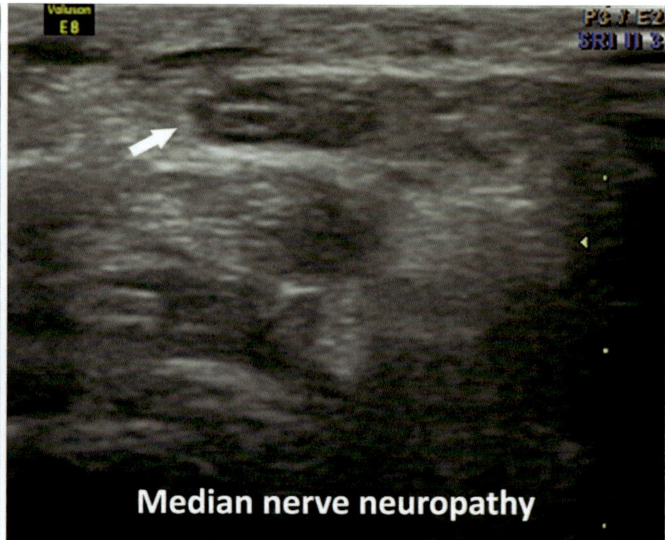


◘ **Fig. 13.10.3** Axial ultrasound images of a patient with normal, echogenic median nerve (*arrowhead*) and another patient with TOS presenting chronic, ischemic median nerve neuritis (*arrow*)

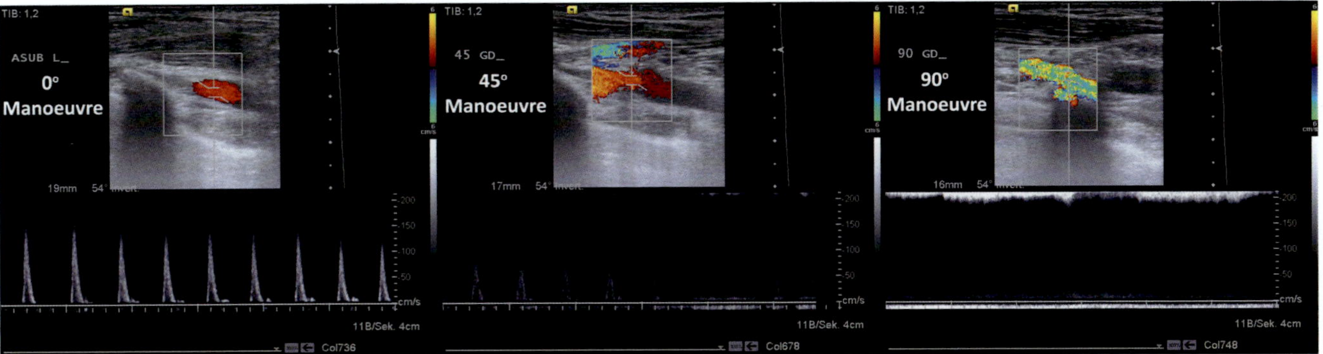

**Fig. 13.10.4** Multiple Doppler images of a patient with TOS. The patient was asked to keep his hand in a 0° abduction, 45° abduction, and 90° abduction. You can see how the flow within the subclavian artery is reduced in intensity until it is completely blocked in 90° abduction with aliasing artifact in the scan

the SCA in the neutral position are 50–100 cm/s; on abduction the velocities increased two to three times. Alterations in the flow of the subclavian artery and vein are seen when TOS present, such as cessation of the flow in the vein or increased flow velocity in the artery (>120 mm/s). The subclavian vein can show signs of compression and complete vascular signal loss on hyperabduction.

4. On CT, the patient is imaged with the arm on the side and then with elevated arm to produce the vascular stenosis. The contrast is injected into the opposite arm. Scan is started 15–20 s after a monophasic injection of 90 mL of contrast at the rate of 4 mL/s. Vascular compression is determined by showing filling defects or kinked subclavian vessels.

5. On MRI, the patient is imaged angiographically in the affected arm once with the arm on the side and then with elevated arm. Coils must be used to image area of interest (brachial plexus MRI technique). Look for all the three spaces; neurological compression is determined when the "fat around the brachial plexus is disappeared" and the brachial plexus are in contact with adjacent structures. The same principle can be applied to the subclavian artery, plus stenosis of its lumen. Assessment of TOS by MRI technique should look for stenosis on both normally positioned arm and raised arm images (dynamic imaging).

### Further Reading

Atasoy E. Thoracic outlet syndrome: anatomy. Hand Clin. 2004;20:7–14.

Bauwens F, et al. Thoracic outlet syndrome. Med Trends. 1990;5:252–7.

Demondion X, et al. Imaging assessment of thoracic outlet syndrome. RadioGraphics. 2006;26:1735–50.

Gunreben G, et al. Real-time sonography of acute and chronic muscle denenrvation. Muscle Nerve. 1991;14:654–64.

Maharaj D, et al. Paget von Schroetter syndrome secondary to exotic dancing: a case study. Int J Angiol. 2003;12:143–4.

Mautits NM, et al. Muscle ultrasound analysis: normal values and differentiation between myopathies and neuropathies. Ultrasound Med Biol. 2003;29(2):215–25.

Nichols H. Anatomic structures of the thoracic outlet. Clin Orthop Rel Res. 1986;207:13–20.

Ozcakar L, et al. Thoracic outlet syndrome, Paget-Schroetter syndrome and aberrant subclavian artery in a young man. Joint Bone Spine. 2066;73:469–71.

Pillen S, et al. Muscle ultrasound in neuromuscular disorder. Muscle Nerve. 2008;37:679–93.

Pillen S, et al. Skeletal muscle ultrasound: correlation between fibrous tissue and echo intensity. Ultrasound Med Biol. 2009;35(3):443–6.

## 13.21 Upper and Lower Crossed Syndromes

The upper and lower crossed syndromes are terms first mentioned by Vladimir Janda to describe a kinesiological abnormality of the skeleton characterized by tightened and weakened muscle groups in a crossed pattern around the shoulder (upper) and pelvis (lower), resulting in skeletal body distortion (◘ Fig. 13.11.1). Janda named this syndrome "crossed" because the weakened and shortened muscles are connected in the upper and lower body in a form of a cross. This condition is known in some literature as "Janda's syndrome."

1. Upper crossed syndrome: it is defined as imbalance between tightened muscles (upper trapezius, levator scapulae, pectoralis muscles) and weakened muscles (rhomboids, serratus anterior, middle and lower trapezius, and the deep neck flexors, especially the scalene muscles). This syndrome produces elevation and protraction of the shoulders, winging of the scapula, and protraction of the head.

   As a result of this atypical posture, there is overstress on the craniocervical junction, the C4–C5 and T4 vertebrae, and the shoulder due to altered motion of the glenohumeral joint. Manifestations of upper crossed syndrome include:

   (a) Pseudo-angina pectoris: due to excessive stress on the T4 spinal segment.

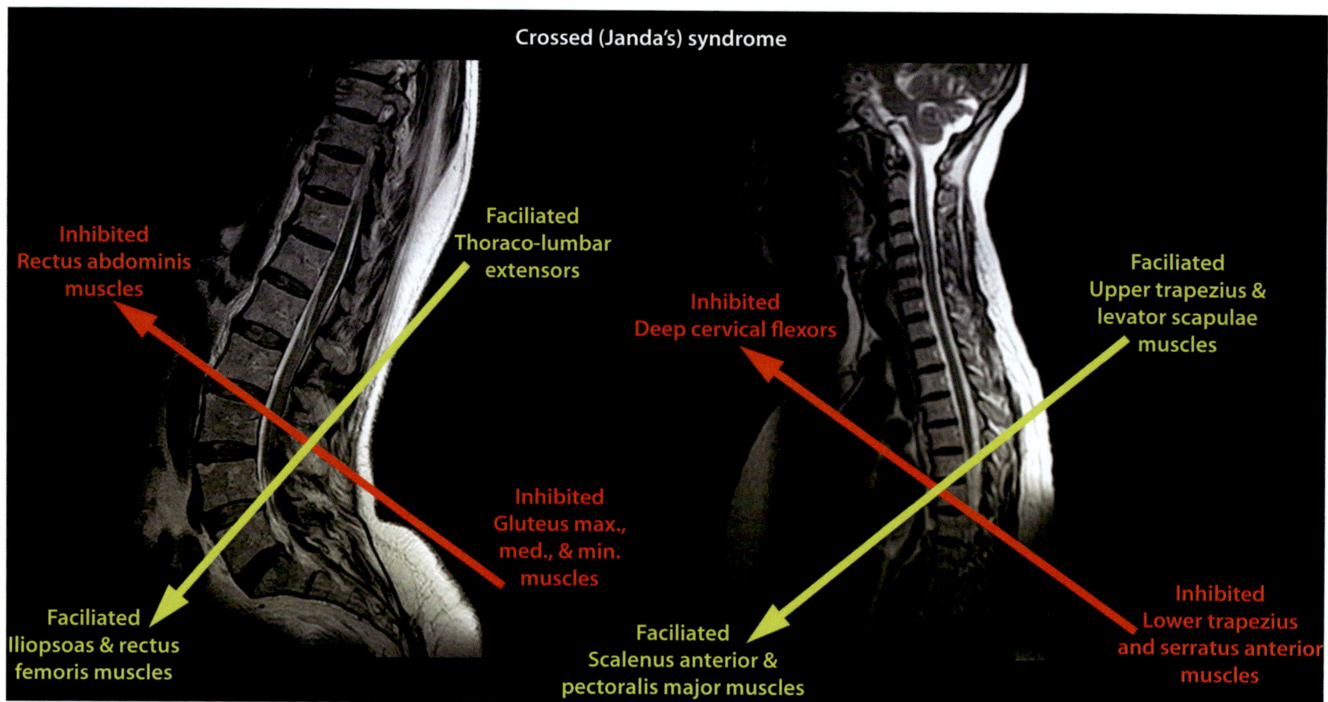


**Fig. 13.11.1**    Sagittal MR images of upper and lower body segments that demonstrate the muscle groups facilitated and inhibited in Janda's crossed syndrome

(b)  Shoulder impingement syndrome: the change of direction of the axis of the glenoid fossa will cause rotation and abduction of the shoulder blades. This will cause the levator scapulae and the upper trapezius to have additional muscle activity to stabilize the head of the humerus. This ends by increased and constant activity of the supraspinatus tendon, causing early degeneration of the muscle's tendon and "shoulder impingement syndrome."

(c)  Cervicogenic headache: the pathophysiology of the cervicogenic headache has also been associated with degenerative changes in the upper cervical spine. The most common origin of pain is typically in the upper cervical joints, namely, the occiput through C1 and the C1 and C2 spinal segments.

2.  Lower crossed syndrome: like upper crossed syndrome, the lower crossed syndrome arises due to contraction imbalance between tightened muscles (iliopsoas, quadratus lumborum, hamstrings, lumbar erectors, and piriformis muscles) against weakened muscles (rectus abdominis, gluteal, vastus medialis, vastus lateralis, and transverse abdominis muscles). This crossed muscle imbalance results in the pelvis tilting anteriorly, creating a hyperlordotic posture, predisposing the vertebral column to disk degeneration (especially L5–S1), facet joint malalignment, and subsequent lower back pain.

In Janda' s originally proposed pelvic crossed syndrome, the pelvis is more posterior, and this is associated with imbalanced co-activation of the trunk muscles with more dominant activity observed in the extensors, proposing this syndrome to be re-termed the "posterior pelvic crossed syndrome." Conversely, in the other broad group, the pelvis is postured more anteriorly, and this is associated with a predominant tendency to more axial flexor activity (anterior pelvic crossed syndrome).

### 13.22 Imaging Signs

1.  Upper crossed syndrome: lateral cervical radiographs can show degenerative changes of the atlantoaxial joint in patients who suffer from cervicogenic headache.
2.  Lower crossed syndrome: hyperlordosis (**Fig. 13.11.2**), due to facilitated iliopsoas muscle and weak gluteal muscles, is typically seen on radiographs and sagittal MR images as disturbed "sacral load line" (**Fig. 13.11.2a**) and increased "lumbosacral angle" (>30°). In many cases of patients with lower crossed syndrome coming for MRI to investigate lower back pain, thoracolumbar fascial edema is often detected in T2-weighted sagittal MR images as incidental finding (**Fig. 13.11.3**), reflecting the inflammation and ischemic changes the fascia suffers from due to the state continuous tension due to the abnormal biomechanics. A fascial edema in the thoracolumbar fascia can be a hint of lower crossed syndrome in a patient presenting with lower back pain, beside any other abnormality detected.

### Further Reading

Key J, et al. The Pelvic Crossed Syndromes: a reflection of imbalanced function in the myofascial envelope; a further

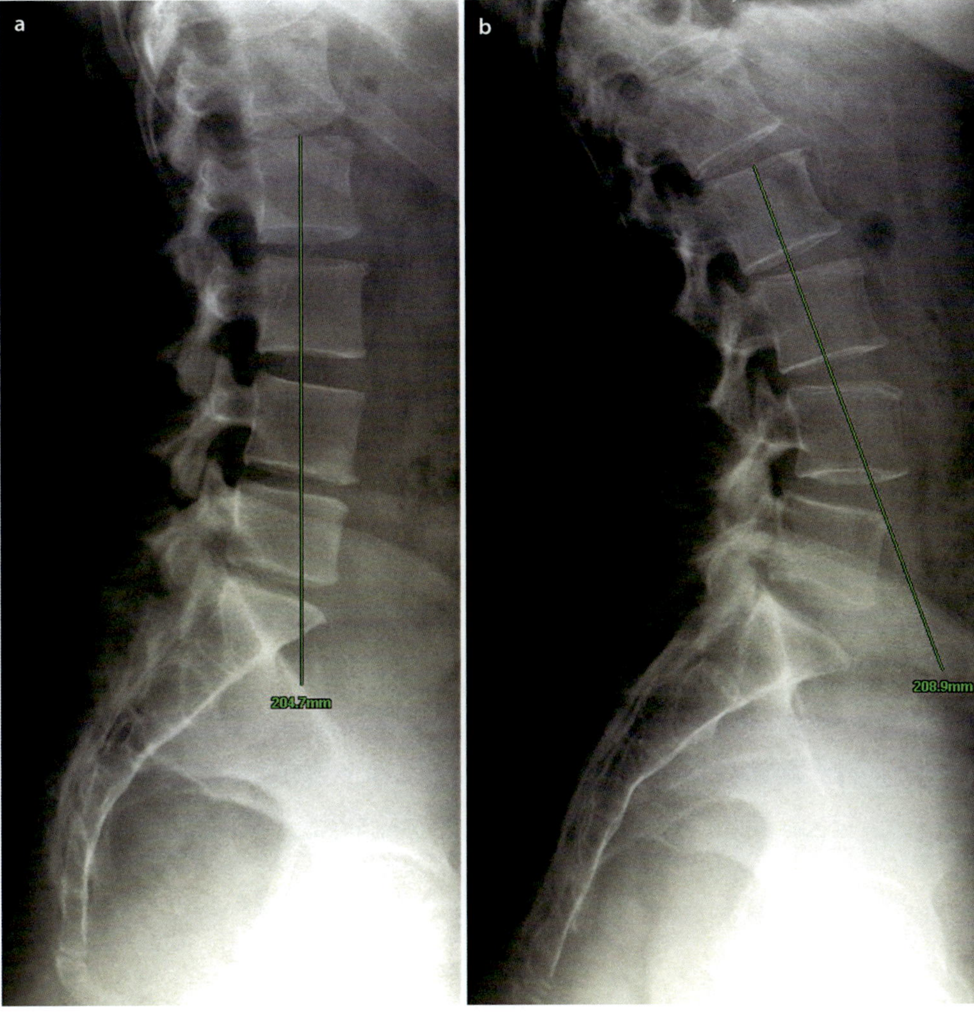

**Fig. 13.11.2** Lateral plain lumbar radiographs of two different patients: in (**a**), a normal "sacral load line" is demonstrated as a straight line drawn from the L2 or L3 vertebra that passes through the anterior segment of the sacral promontory and in (**b**), hyperlordosis demonstrated with line does not touch the sacral promontory

exploration of Janda's work. J Bodyw Mov Ther. 2010;14:299–301.

Moore MK, et al. Upper crossed syndrome and its relationship to cervicogenic headache. J Manipulative Physiol Ther. 2004;27(6):414–20.

## 13.23 Lumbago

Lumbago is a term used to describe a specific clinical condition characterized by:

1. "Sudden onset," severe, agonizing, lower back pain with a sudden "snap" feeling that occurs typically "immediately" after stressful physical activity. Lumbago is considered "acute sciatica" pain.
2. Pain that is aggravated by sitting and bending forwards, the latter even being impossible because the spine is held in the position of least pain by reflex spasm of the trunk muscles.
3. The pain is central and spreads bilaterally over the lower lumbar area and the buttocks. Although centralized in the lumbar and/or gluteal area, it spreads to the groin and abdomen, downwards to one or both legs as far as the ankles, or upwards in the trunk as far as the inferior aspect of the scapulae.
4. The pain can be aggravated by cough, deep, sneeze, and taking a deep breath.

Lumbago is typically caused by protrusion of the annular fibrosis (annular lumbago) or the nucleus pulposus herniation (nuclear lumbago), causing stretch tear of the posterior longitudinal ligament, a pressure exerted over the dura, and marked dural tension (**Fig. 13.12.1**). The pain experienced by lumbago arises mainly from dural tension, associated with pressure over the recurrent meningeal (sinuvertebral) nerve, which has an autonomic component to it.

Most patients with acute lumbago recover spontaneously and completely within 2–6 weeks. Recovery is possible because the tension in the posterior longitudinal ligament exerts counter pressure on the annular bulge, which moves gradually anteriorly, until compression of the dura mater ceases and symptoms disappear. However, since cartilage has little tendency to reunite, the intervertebral disk fragment that has moved backwards once will sooner or later move again, resulting in sciatica or chronic lumbago in some cases.

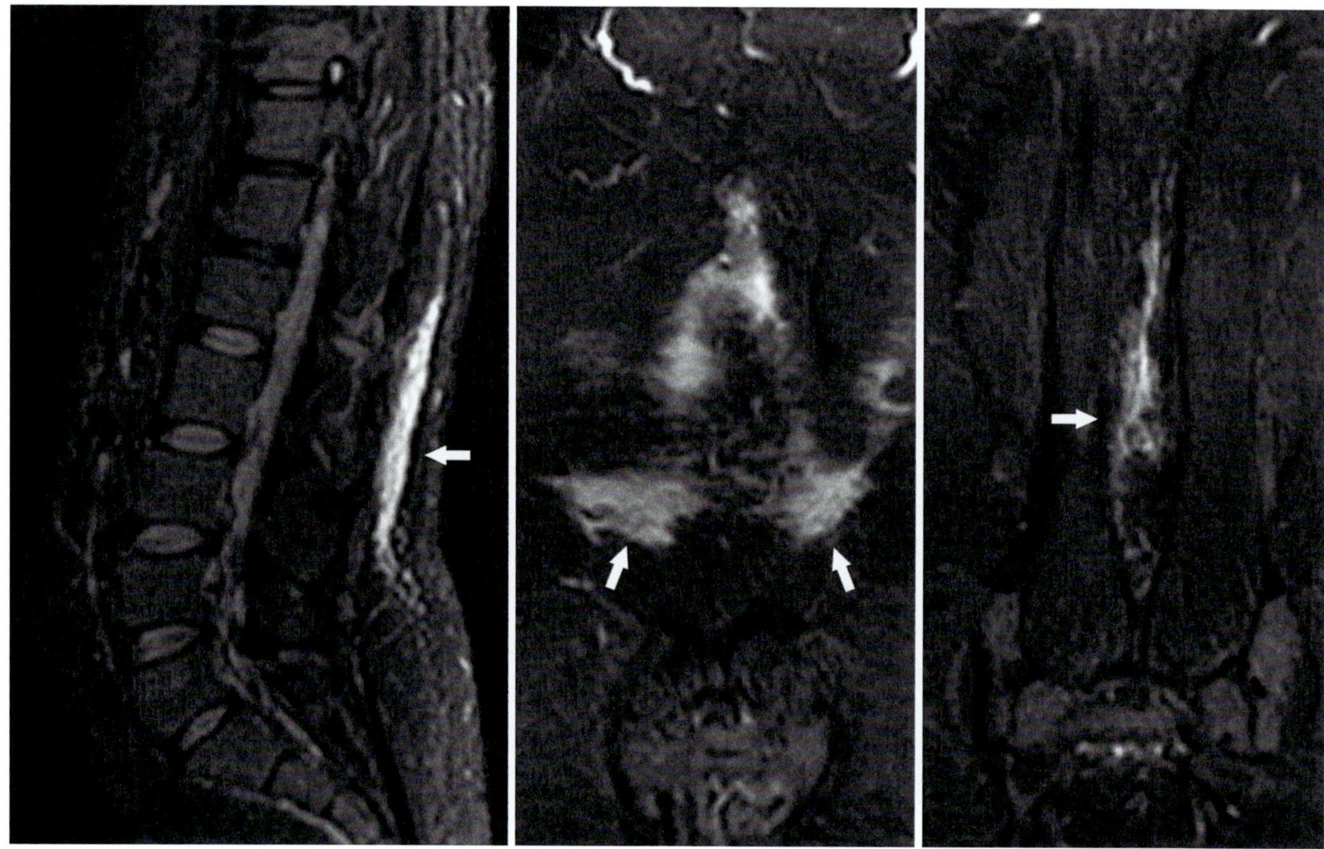



## 13.24 Imaging Signs

On MRI, annular lumbago will show posterolateral disk bulge that exerts pressure over the thecal dural sac without necessarily causing any spinal root or cauda equina compression associated with typical presentation of lumbago (□ Fig. 13.12.2). In nuclear lumbago, a posterior herniated disk is seen impinging the thecal dural sac. However, the MRI features can be also seen in nonspecific lower back pain. Therefore, the term lumbago with such radiological finding must be used in correlation with its strict clinical definition.

### Further Reading

Bashline SD, et al. Meningovertebral ligaments and their putative significance in low back pain. J Manipul Physiol Ther. 1996;19:592–956.

Takahashi H, et al. Inflammatory cytokines in the herniated disc of the lumbar spine. Spine. 1996;21:218–24.

Roberts S, et al. Mechanoreceptors in intervertebral discs. Morphology, distribution, and neuropeptides. Spine. 1995;20:2645–51.

Scapinelli R. Anatomical and radiologic studies on the lumbosacral meningovertebral ligaments of humans. J Spinal Disord. 1990;3:6–15.

Stankovic R, et al. Conservative treatment of acute low back pain; a prospective randomised trial: McKenzie method of treatment versus patient education in 'mini back school'. Spine. 1990;15:120–3.

Donelson R, et al. Centralization phenomenon; its usefulness in evaluating and treating referred pain. Spine. 1990;15: 211–3.

## 13.25 Shin Splint Syndrome

Shin splint syndrome is a term used to describe pain experienced on the anterior aspect of the leg. The pain is typically felt as diffuse tenderness along the posteromedial tibia in its middle to distal aspect. The underlying pathological process of shin splint includes multiple conditions with different pathologies; however, all present with shin splint or pain in the anterior aspect of the leg, such as:

1. Tibial stress syndrome: it is a condition typically seen in runners and is characterized by stress fracture of the tibia. The impact of running along with overpronation and poor support from the footwear creates pain on the anterior tibial surface.
2. Tibial periostitis: it is a condition characterized by tightened tibialis anterior, tibialis posterior, and soleus muscles with subsequent increase tension exerted on the tibial periosteum, resulting in "microtears" of the tibial periosteum as it starts to be pulled away from the bone.

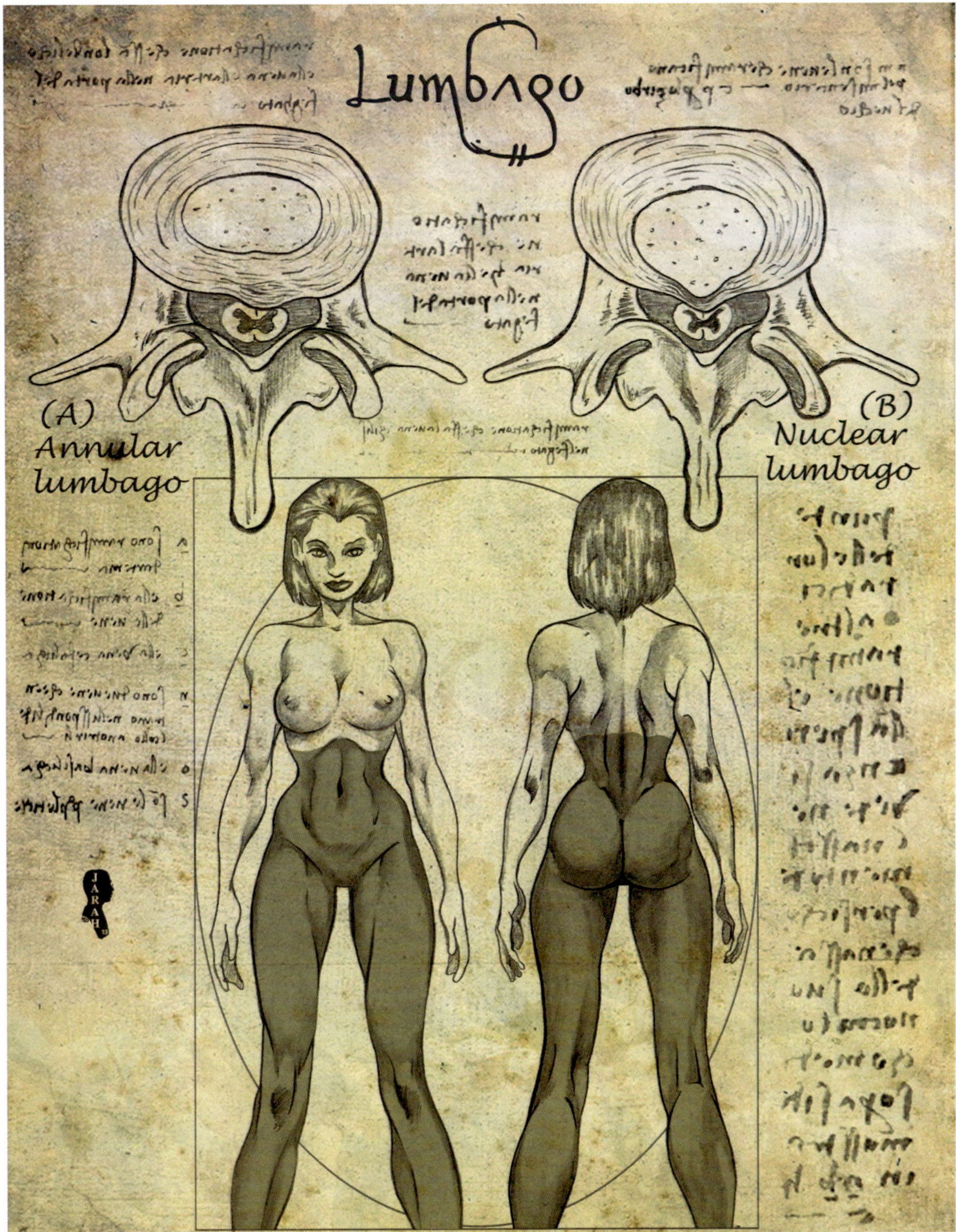



3. Acute anterior compartment syndrome: the term "compartment syndrome" denotes a clinical condition characterized by increased pressure within a confined fascial space (resting pressure postexercise >20 mmHg), causing decreased capillary blood flow below a level necessary for tissue viability, resulting in muscle ischemia, hypoxia, and maybe necrosis. Over 70 % of lower limbs acute compartment syndromes are due to fractures. When compartment syndrome affects the anterior compartment of the leg (contains tibialis anterior and peroneus muscles), it can present with shin splints.

4. Chronic anterior compartment syndrome: chronic compartment syndrome, also known as "exertional compartment syndrome," is a term used to describe a condition where the intramuscular pressure increases normally in patients with athletic activity and fail back to normal after cessation of the activities. These patients present with symptoms of acute compartment syndrome symptoms typically felt only after exercise. Muscle volume can increase up to 20 % of its resting size during exercise.

5. Short leg syndrome: the short leg will show pronation, which can present with shin splint presentation when the patient walks for a long time.

6. Femoral neuralgia: lumbar vertebral malalignment, disk herniation, or facet joint disease of the L3–L4 vertebrae results in irritation of the femoral nerve root, resulting in pain due to cellulagia along the anteromedial side of the knee, associated with trigger point formation within the vastus medialis muscle.

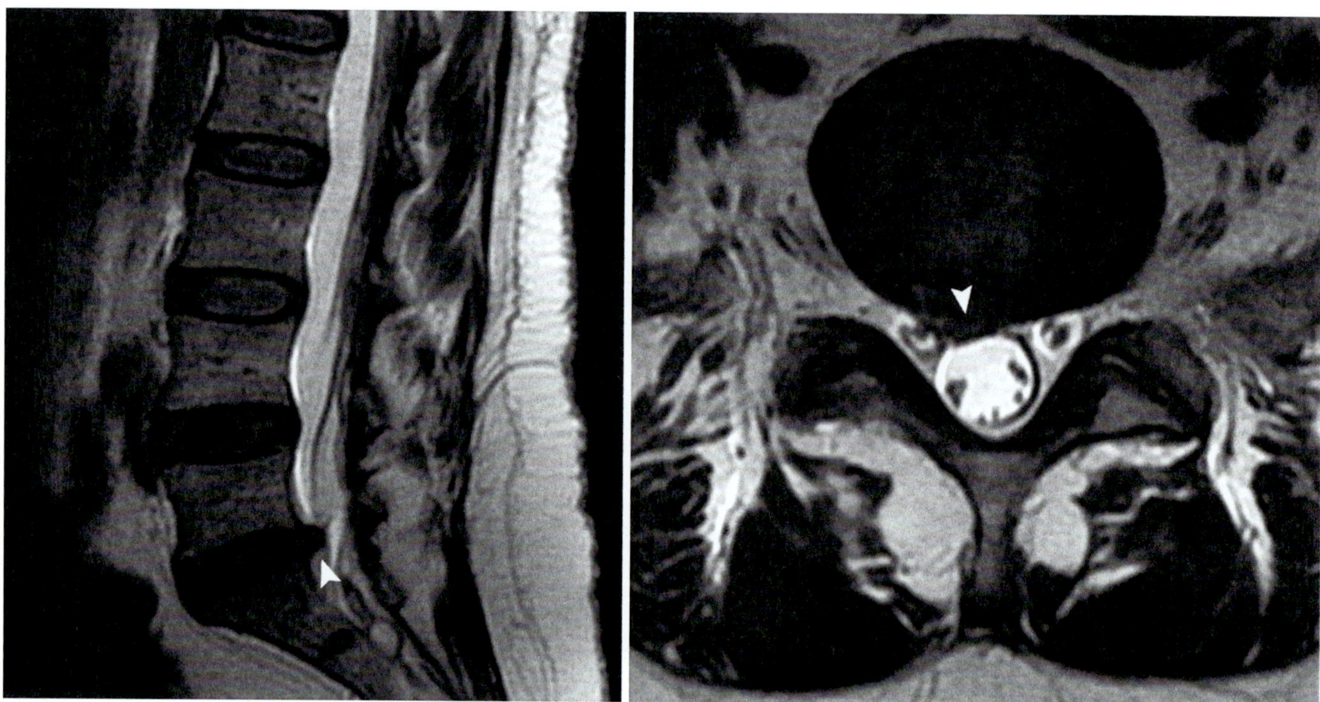

**Fig. 13.12.2** Sagittal and axial MR images of a patient who presented with a typical history of acute sciatic pain (Lumbago) showing focal disk protrusion that impinges over the thecal dural sac without spinal canal stenosis (*arrowheads*)

Femoral neuralgia can extend far distally up to the "anteromedial" side of the leg and ankle. In the leg, the pain is deep, internal, with nocturnal flaring (shin splint-like pain). In the thigh, the femoral nerve supplies the psoas, adductor, and quadriceps muscles. When the quadriceps muscle is involved, the patient cannot raise the heel from supine position.

7. Peroneal nerve entrapment (cross leg) syndrome: the common peroneal nerve is divided into medial and lateral branches at the level of the fibular neck, both exclusively sensory nerves. Entrapment of the superficial peroneal nerve (the lateral branch of the common peroneal nerve) will result in with "shin splint syndrome-like pain" with or without drop foot (in case of common peroneal nerve entrapment).

## 13.26 Imaging Signs

1. Tibial stress injury: bone marrow edema within the tibial shaft can be detected on proton density (PD) images with or without fracture line or gadolinium contrast enhancement.
2. Tibial periostitis: the MRI shows sign of periostitis along the tibia with muscle edema at the site of the tibial muscle attachment seen as linear (coronal) or circular (axial) high T2W, PDW signal intensity, and contract enhancement along the tibial shaft.
3. Leg compartment syndrome: affects mostly the anterior and the lateral compartment of the leg. On MRI, there is edema on T2W images and strong contrast

enhancement affecting a group of muscle within a compartment (characteristic) ( Fig. 13.13.1). The contrast enhancement can be seen affecting more the peripheral of the muscle, while the center is not well enhanced due to central muscle hypoxia/ischemia. The strong enhancement reflects disturbance of cell membrane permeability. To investigate exertional compartment syndrome, an MRI must be done immediately after exercise, which typically shows muscular hyperintensity and swelling within affected muscle compartment. On US, the affected compartment will show muscle enlargement (up to 20 % compared to the normal leg), hyperechogenicity due to myositis, and with loss of the normal myofascial planes due to muscle edema ( Fig. 13.13.2). No signs of vascular compromise in Doppler sonography are classically found on chronic compartment syndrome, while vascular compromise is found in acute compartment syndrome.

4. Femoral neuralgia: on MRI, the femoral nerve must be followed by its course in the pelvis (can be impinged/irritated in the pelvis by a ganglion cyst or colitis) and medially above the knee (pes anserinus tenosynovitis/bursitis may be found).
5. Perioneal nerve entrapment: on MRI, a lesion is typically found at the site of the "fibular neck" (where the peroneal nerve is found).

### Further Reading
Anderson MW, et al. Shin splints: MR appearance in a preliminary study. Radiology. 1997;204:177–08.

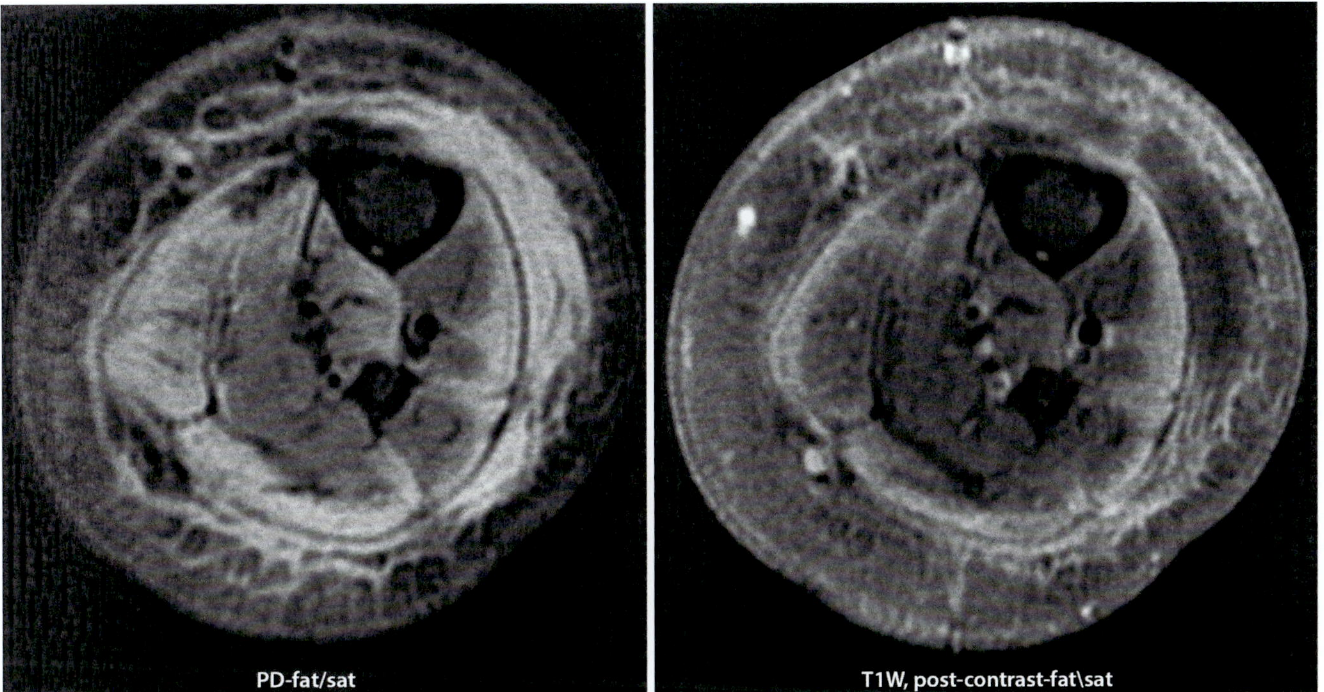



**Fig. 13.13.1** Axial MR-PD fat-sat and T1W post-contrast, fat-sat images that demonstrate the findings in leg compartment syndrome. Marked muscle edema is detected in PD image associated with fluid signal intensity in the facial planes and the subcutaneous tissue of the leg; on postcontrast images, significant contrast enhancement is detected in the affected planes due to hyperemia

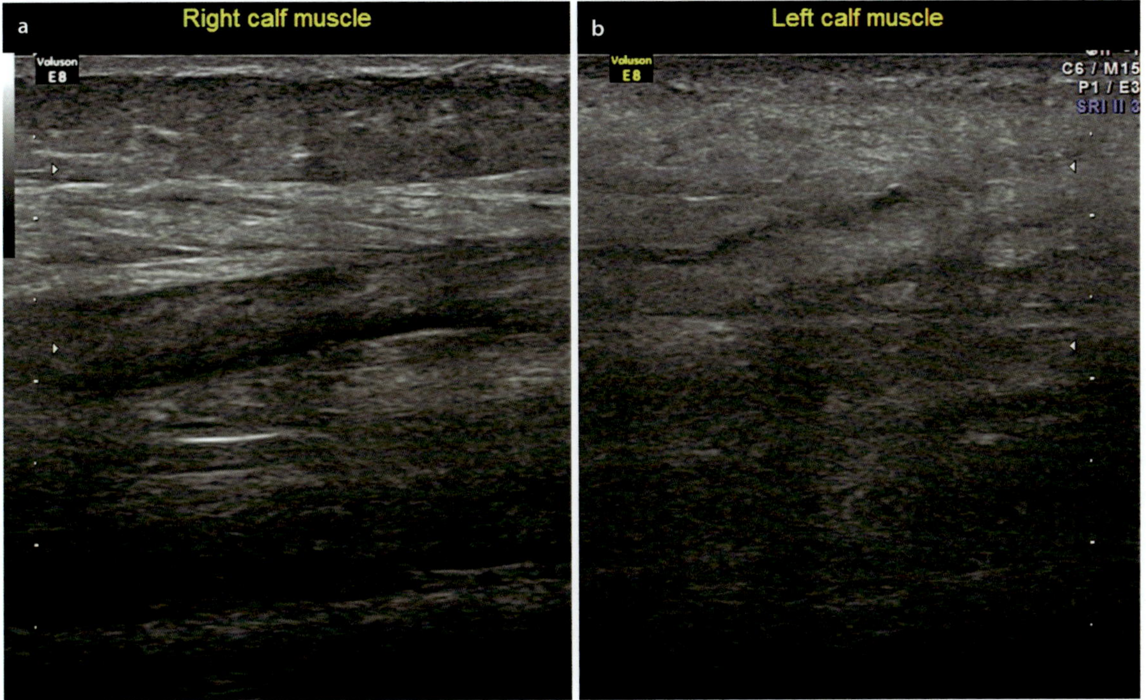



**Fig. 13.13.2** Sagittal ultrasound images of a patient with leg compartment syndrome (**b**) showing loss the normal myofascial planes on the left calf muscles due to edema compared to the opposite right calf muscles (**a**)

Crabtree M. Medial tibial stress syndrome – a case report. Int Emerg Nurs. 2009;17:233–6.

Gaeta M, et al. Diagnostic imaging in athletes with chronic lower leg pain. AJR. 2008;191:1412–9.

Gielen JL, et al. Chronic exertional compartment syndrome of the forearm in motocross racers: findings on MRI. Skeletal Radiol. 2009;38:1153–61.

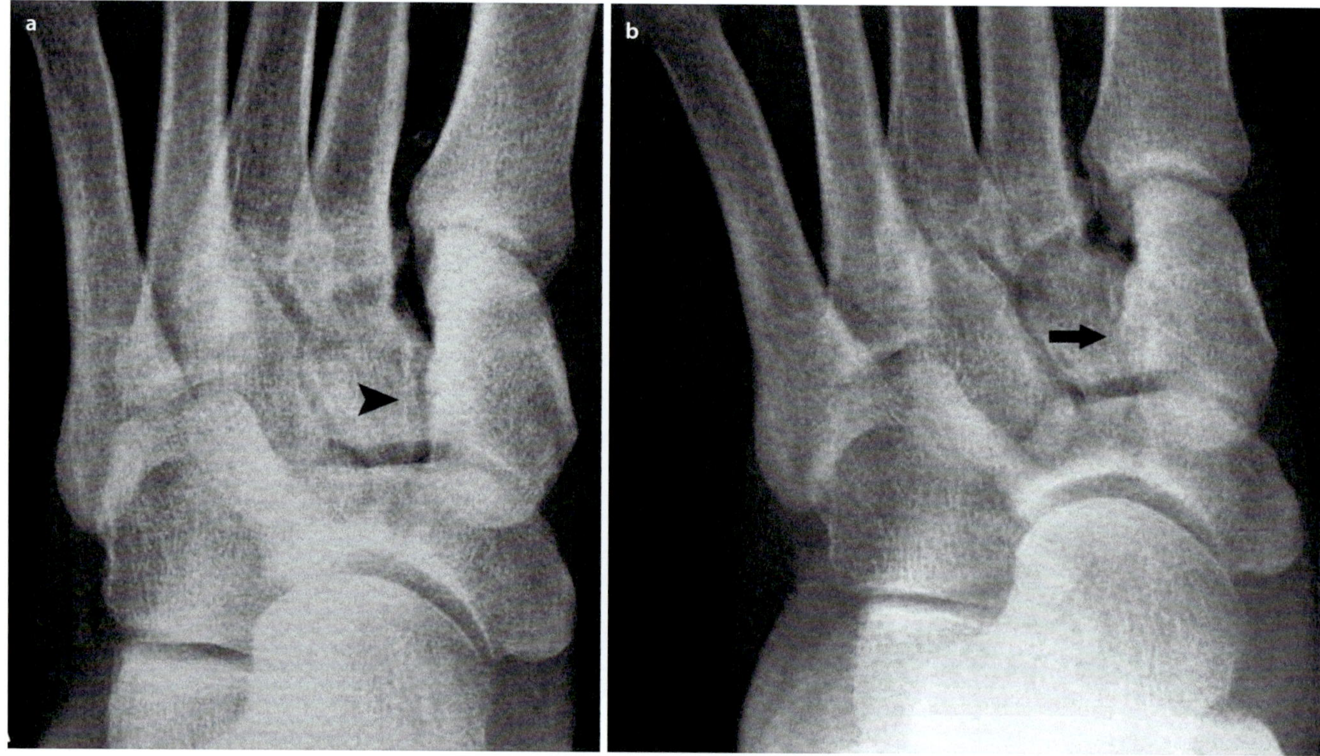



**Fig. 13.14.1**    Anteroposterior radiographs of a diabetic patient presented with pain in his mid-foot associated with clicking sensation. The patient is known to have Charcot's joint due to diabetic foot neuropathy. On (**a**), the radiograph shows a clear joint space between the cuboid and the cuneiform bones (*arrowhead*); on dynamic stress radiograph (**b**), the gap is closed (*arrow*), confirming the cuboid bone instability

Henry G, Chambers HG, et al. Medial tibial stress syndrome: evaluation and management. Oper Techn Sports Med. 1995;3(4):274–7.

Mattila KT, et al. Medial tibial pain: a dynamic contrast-enhanced MRI study. Magn Reson Imaging. 1999;17(7): 947–54.

Oaghino W, et al. Superficial peroneal nerve entrapment in a young athlete: the diagnostic contribution of magnetic resonance imaging. J Foot Ankle Surg. 1997;36(3): 170–2.

Sánchez-Márquez A, et al. Sport-related muscle injuries of the lower extremity: MR imaging appearance. Eur Radiol. 1999;9:1088–93.

Tucker AK. Chronic exertional compartment syndrome of the leg. Curr Rev Musculoskelet Med. 2010;3:32–7.

Verleisdonk EJMM, et al. The diagnostic value of MRI scans for the diagnosis of chronic exertional compartment syndrome of the lower leg. Skeletal Radiol. 2001;30:321–5.

Yu JS, et al. MR imaging of urgent inflammatory and infectious conditions affecting the soft tissues of the musculoskeletal system. Emerg Radiol. 2009;16:267–76.

## 13.27 Cuboid Syndrome

Cuboid syndrome is a term used to describe subluxation of the cuboid bone at the midfoot that occurs when a strong pull exerted by the tendon of the peroneus longus muscle causes rotation of the bone. This strong pull causes upward tilt of the lateral side and depression of the medial side, resulting in cuboid bone lock and pain sensation in the lateral side of the foot.

The cuboid is unique for the simple fact it is the only bone in the foot that articulates with both the tarsometatarsal joint (Lisfranc complex) and the midtarsal joint (Chopart's joint) and is the only bone linking the lateral column to the transverse plantar arch. The cuboid bone acts as a keystone of the lateral column and provides inherent stability to the foot.

A patient with cuboid syndrome will complain of lateral foot pain and weakness in the toe-off portion during the gait cycle. The cuboid syndrome is estimated to account for 4 % of athletes complaining of pain in the lateral midtarsal region. The condition seems to be more common in patients who have pronated feet (e.g., associated with short leg syndrome ipsilaterally). A pronated foot creates an unstable and hypermobile foot.

## 13.28 Imaging Signs

On normal foot radiographs, there are no visible abnormalities (Fig. 13.14.1a). However, when an image is stressed (a wedge is put under the fifth metatarsal and another radiograph is taken), the cuboid-fifth metatarsal joint shows widening or closure of the space gap between the cuboid and the cuneiform bones compared to the normal image, confirming the diagnosis (Fig. 13.14.1b).

## Further Reading

Blakeslee TJ, et al. Cuboid syndrome and the significance of midtarsal joint stability. J Am Podiat Med Assoc. 1987;77(12):638–42.

Helal B. Cubo-fifth metatarsal instability: a hitherto undescribed cause of pain in the outer border of the mid foot. Foot. 1991;1:7–9.

Patterson SM. Cuboid syndrome: a review of the literature. J Sports Sci Med. 2006;5:597–606.

Pet M. Cuboid subluxation in ballet dancers. Am J Sports Med. 1992;20(2):169–17.

Subotnick SI. Peroneal cuboid syndrome. J Am Podiat Med Assoc. 1989;79(8):413–4.

## 13.29 Scoliosis, Kyphosis, and Lordosis

Abnormal vertebral curves are direct result to the positioning of each vertebra relative to the others; this vertebral positioning often results from neuromuscular and myofascial imbalances that are holding the vertebrae out of alignment. Any kind of trauma, accident, or repeated bad posture can initiate this type of imbalance. Abnormal vertebral column curves can be divided into:

1. Scoliosis is defined as lateral curvature of the vertebral column. Scoliosis is classified according to age into: infantile (0–3 years), juvenile (3–10 years), adolescent (10–18 years), and adult (>18 years). Also, scoliosis can be classified according to the area involved (King's classification) into cervical (C1–C6), cervicothoracic (C7–T1), thoracic (T2–T12), thoracolumbar (T12–L1), lumbar (L2–L4), and lumbosacral (L5–S1). Moreover, scoliosis can be classified structurally into:

   (a) Congenital scoliosis arises due to actual deformities in the vertebrae, commonly due to genetic disorder (e.g., Charcot–Marie–Tooth disease). This type usually requires surgical intervention such as rods.

   (b) Functional scoliosis is a result of muscular imbalances such as hypertonicity of the quadratus lumborum, erector spinae, and transversospinalis muscle groups. Although muscular tension is a leading cause of functional scoliosis (e.g., malalignment syndrome) (◘ Fig. 13.15.1), minor structural abnormalities may also contribute to the imbalances like leg lengths (e.g., leg length discrepancy).

   (c) Rotoscoliosis is scoliosis with rotation of the vertebra in the axial plane (◘ Fig. 13.15.2).

   (d) Kyphoscoliosis scoliosis plus kyphosis.

   (e) S-shaped scoliosis is double lateral deviation of the vertebral column.

   (f) C-shaped scoliosis is single lateral curve of the vertebral column.

2. Kyphosis refers to the dorsal or posterior curvature seen in the "thoracic" vertebrae. Hyperkyphosis, also known as "humpback," is often seen in those who have a forward head position. A long-arc (arcuate) kyphosis can be seen in Scheuermann's disease, osteoporosis, and ankylosing spondylitis, while short-arc (angular) kyphosis can be seen in vertebral pathologic or compressive fractures and spondylitis. Normal vertebral kyphosis does not exceed (25–45°); any kyphosis exceeding this range is considered pathologic.

3. Lordosis is defined as a natural forward curvature of the spine. This curvature occurs in two areas of the body: the lumbar spine and the cervical spine. A "hyperlordosis" is defined as an accentuated curvature of either of these two areas. Lumbar hyperlordosis, also known as "sway back," can be seen with an anterior tilt in the pelvis and is often caused by tight low back and psoas major muscles. Poor posture and activities of daily living are major contributors of hyperlordosis.

Scoliosis, kyphosis, and hyperlordosis can result due to structural or functional disorders (e.g., tight back muscles, malalignment syndromes, joint displacement, structural defects, and genetic disorders). Muscular imbalances can create postural deviations that can result in impingements and compression discomforts. These imbalances end up causing other parts of the body to compensate to maintain balance.

According to the second law of Newton: "the net result of all the forces exerted on the body must equal zero"; as the body becomes out of balance from the proper posture, the muscles become engaged to maintain the new posture, canceling the imbalances in the pulling forces on the spine (compensation pattern); this compensating pattern causes some muscles of the pelvis and spine to become tight and short, whereas others are in a constant state of elongation.

Due to the continuous muscle tension imbalance, many patients with vertebral column distortion experience back pain. This pain can be explained by muscle hypoxia due to continuous tension state, trigger points formation, and pain that results from overstretch of Golgi tendon organ.

Golgi tendon organs (GTOs) are sensory nerve endings located in the muscle tendons. GTOs measure the degree of pull at the ends of the specific muscle fibers they are attached to. When the degree of pull or force increases, the GTOs send a signal to the reticular formation in the brainstem, which in turn sends an inhibitory signal back through the motor nerve to the bellies of the same muscle fibers; this causes them to relax to the degree of the increased force.

The muscle tone in the body (the tonus system) is a function of the Golgi tendon organs (GTOs) and the reticular formation in the brainstem. The "reticular formation – GTOs nervous system" is involved in the production and maintenance of neuromuscular tension, posture, and movement. Also, it plays a significant role in the accumulation and retention of chronic, excess muscle, and nerve tension.

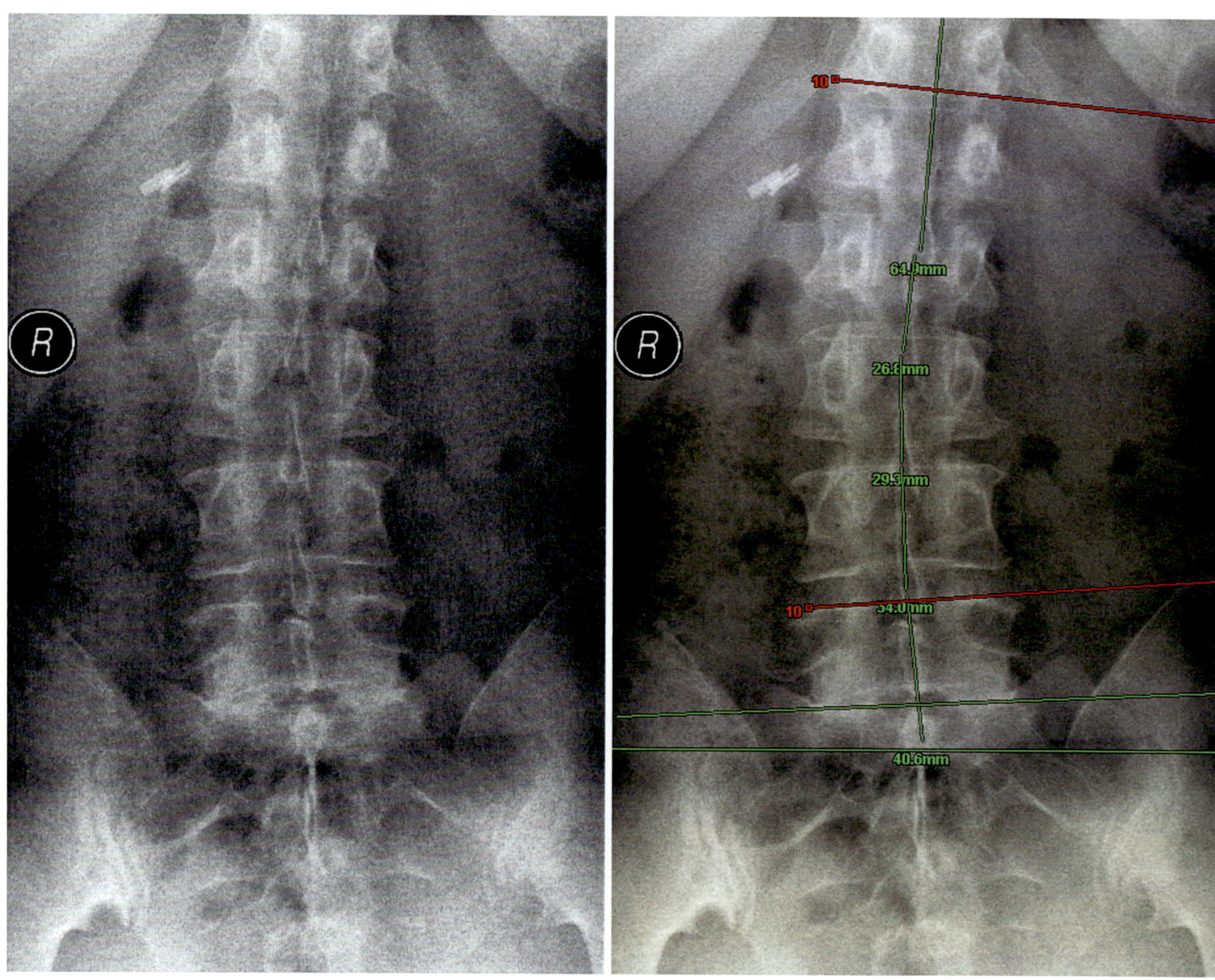



**Fig. 13.15.1**    Anteroposterior plain radiograph of the lumbar spine that shows functional scoliosis due to malalignment syndrome

## 13.30 Imaging Signs

1. The plain X-ray forms the basis of initial assessment of scoliosis apart from physical examination. It is inexpensive and readily available. It is also useful for curve monitoring. For congenital scoliosis, standing AP and lateral views of the whole spine are needed for the initial assessment. Lateral views allow assessment of the sagittal profile and also help diagnose any congenital deformity. Additional views include supine active bending films to assess curve flexibility and traction views in the neuromuscular or syndromic patient unable to actively bend. Hyperextension views can be used to assess flexibility in a kyphotic deformity. Other specialized views include the Ferguson view which allows assessment of the L5–S1 junction. In wheelchair-bound patients, sitting films will reveal pelvic obliquity and spinal deformity.

2. To measure the degree of scoliosis, you need first to determine the upper most and lower most apical vertebrae in the curvature. An "apical vertebra" is defined as "the most rotated vertebra in the curve, whose end plates are tilted into the concavity." To determine an apical vertebra in a scoliotic vertebral column, look for the upper most and lower most vertebrae in the curvature where their pedicles are "starting to rotate" from the midline ( Fig. 13.15.3).

3. Degree of vertebral rotation can be determined by Nash/Moe principle, which states that: "the more rotated the vertebra, the more the pedicle at the convexity passes towards and beyond the midline and the pedicle at the convexity disappear." It has 4 grades (1-IV).

4. After determining the apical vertebrae, the magnitude of the curve and its progression over time is measured by the "Cobb's angle," which is defined as "the angle measured between 2 apical vertebrae." Traditionally, Cobb's angle is measured between a line drawn along the upper end plate of the superior apical vertebra and another along the lower end plate of the inferior apical vertebra ( Fig. 13.15.3). Many of the radiographic workstations can determine Cobb's angle mathematically

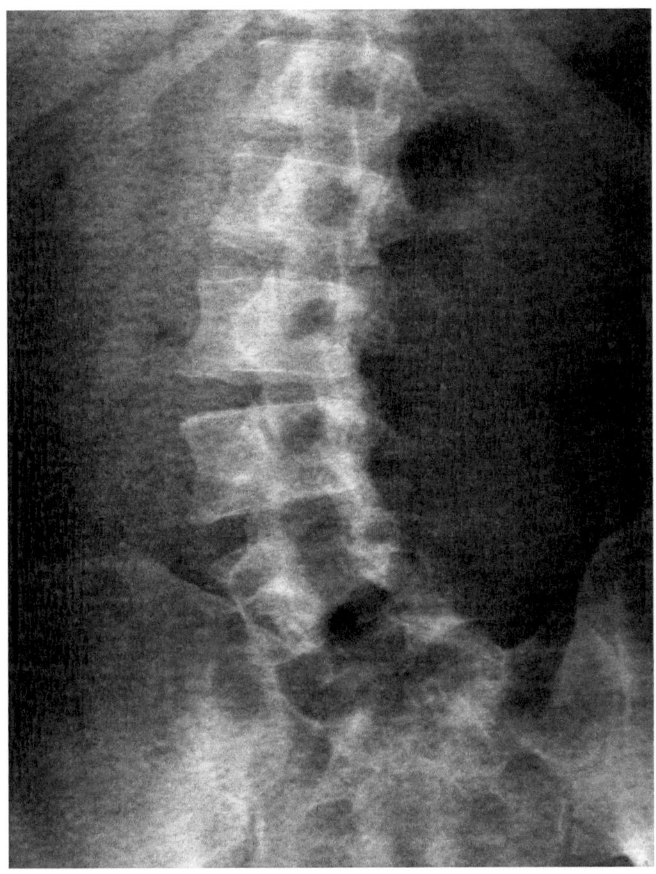

**Fig. 13.15.2** Anteroposterior plain radiograph of the lumbar spine that shows rotoscoliosis

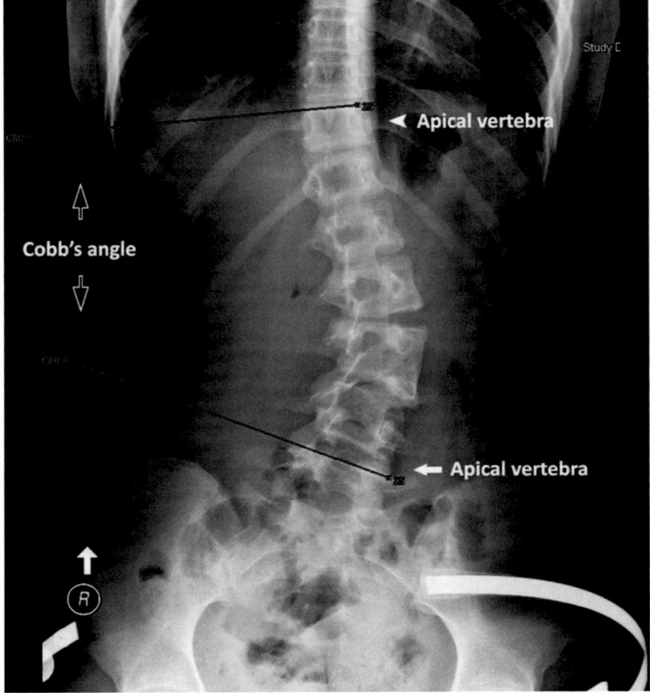


**Fig. 13.15.3** Anteroposterior plain radiograph of the lumbar spine that shows 25°, right-sided, C-shaped scoliosis demonstrating the upper apical vertebra (*solid arrowhead*), lower apical vertebra (*solid arrow*), and the Cobb's angle (*hollow arrowheads*)

simply by determining the upper and lower apical vertebrae by the user.

5. Risser's classification is a classification used to a measure of skeletal maturity and is commonly used in conjunction with scoliosis assessment in children and young adults for surgical or braces planning. It is measured from ossification of the iliac apophysis from front to back and graded 1–5. Risser 5 represents skeletal maturity. Risser's classification helps in determining the patient's management. For example, patients with scoliosis who want to use brace as a form of management need to have a scoliosis between 20° to 45°, no rigid hump, and their Risser's classification should not exceed 2. If their Risser's grade >2, then the scoliosis brace is not an option for therapy.

### Further Reading

Bergofsky EH, et al. Cardio-respiratory failure in kyphoscoliosis. Medicine. 1959;38:263–317.

Bradford DS, et al. Intraspinal abnormalities and congenital spine deformities: a radiographic and MRI study. J Pediatr Orthop. 1991;11:36–41.

Hefti FL, et al. The effect of the adolescent growth spurt on early posterior spinal fusion in infantile and juvenile idiopathic scoliosis. J Bone Joint Surg. 1983;65B:247–54.

Lonstein JE, et al. The prediction of curve progression in untreated idiopathic scoliosis during growth. J Bone Joint Surg. 1984;66A:1061–71.

Nash CL, et al. Risk of exposure to X-rays in patients undergoing long term treatment for scoliosis. J Bone Joint Surg. 1979;61A:371–80.

Nnadi C, et al. Scoliosis: a review. Paediatr Child Health. 2009;20(5):215–20.

Reem J, et al. Risser sign inter-rater and intra-rater agreement: is the Risser sign reliable? Skeletal Radiol. 2009;38:371–5.

Risser JC. The Iliac apophysis: an invaluable sign in the management of scoliosis. Clin Orthop. 1958;11:111–09.

## 13.31 Sacroiliac Joint Dysfunction

Sacroiliac joint (SIJ) dysfunction is a term used to describe pain evoked by subluxation of the sacroiliac joint, which can be occult radiographically and may be only visible through kinetic test

### Basic Anatomy

The sacroiliac joint represents a connection between the spine and the pelvis. The sacrum is wedge-shaped in both rostrocaudal and ventrodorsal dimensions; this keystone configuration functions with the many sacral ligaments to prevent displacement. The sacral articular surface is ear-shaped, concave, and lines by thick synovial membrane, while the iliac articular surface is convex, shows ridges, and lined by fibrocartilage.

The sacroiliac joint, pelvic ring, and the pelvic joints are inherently stable. However, both in vivo and in vitro kinematic studies have demonstrated various types of minor motion in the sacroiliac joints, such as gliding, rotation, tilting, nodding, and translation. None of the small movements of the sacroiliac joint is produced by active movements of the sacrum. The movements are indirectly imposed by gravity and muscles acting on trunk and lower limbs

The sacroiliac joint transmits forces from the vertebral column sideways into the pelvis and then to the lower limbs. Conversely, forces from the lower limbs can be transmitted through pelvis and sacrum to the vertebral column. During normal walk, the iliac bones move a very small movement along the SI joint from anterior to posterior with less than 4° rotation and less than 1.6 mm translation (medial motion).

## Pathophysiology

The sacroiliac joint motion is affected by motion of the spine, ilium, symphysis pubis, and hip joints. Asymmetric load transmission due to lumbar or thoracic malalignment or scoliosis can lead to adaptive pelvic motion that results in sacroiliac joint dysfunction/instability. Also, a disturbed muscle movement around the sacroiliac joint can lead to sacroiliac joint instability. The sacroiliac joint is 20 times more vulnerable to axial compression failure and twice as susceptible to axial torsion overloading than are the lumbar motion segments.

The sacroiliac joint is innervated posteriorly from L3 to S3 spinal roots, anteriorly from L2 to S2 spinal roots, and by branches from the superior gluteal and obturator nerves. The posterior sacroiliac joint ligament is innervated from the posterior ramus of S1 root. The fact that the joint capsule and the surrounding ligaments contain nociceptors suggests that the sacroiliac joint is a possible source of low back pain and also plays a role in somatic referred pain of variety of locations. Patient with sacroiliac joints dysfunction/instability present with (1) gluteal and low back pain, (2) pain on sitting, (3) sciatica, and (4) testicular or vulvar pain.

The sacroiliac joint is vulnerable for shear injury during walking; therefore, its stability is achieved via:

1. Form closure refers to joint surfaces that fit together perfectly and require no extra force to maintain stability. A disease that affects the articular surface (e.g., sacroiliitis) can disturb the joint stability.
2. Force closure refers to the external force that the joint requires to maintain stability, which includes the pelvic muscles and the surrounding ligaments. In cases of instability, the surrounding muscles will tighten as a protective mechanism to maintain stability, which results in pain and muscle spasm due to prolonged hypoxia. Important muscles for sacroiliac instability include gluteus muscles, hamstrings, rectus abdominis, hip external rotators, piriformis, obturator internus, iliopsoas muscles, latissimus dorsi, quadratus lumborum, and erector spinae muscles. The important ligaments for sacroiliac stability include (1) iliolumbar, lumbosacral, and anterior sacroiliac ligaments (anterior ligament group) and (2) interosseous, sacrotuberous, sacrospinous, and posterior sacroiliac ligaments (posterior ligament group).
3. Neural motor control refers to the sequencing and timing of muscle activation and release by neural firing that facilitates ease of load. Denervation for any reason can result in sacroiliac joint dysfunction (e.g., neuromuscular disorder, diabetes mellitus, etc.).
4. Thoracolumbar fascia is an important ligament for load transfer from the lower extremity through the pelvis, lumbar spine, and abdominals. There are several myofascial structures that influence movement and stability, the most notable of which are the latissimus dorsi via the thoracolumbar fascia, the gluteus maximus, and the piriformis. Abnormal tension within the thoracolumbar fascia, for whatever the cause, will extern negative effect on sacroiliac joint stability.

## 13.32 Imaging Signs

1. To assess the sacroiliac joint stability, it is essential to image the pelvis is static and stressed views. Some practitioners use fluoroscopy for dynamic assessment. To do it radiographically, an anteroposterior (AP) radiograph of the pelvis is imaged in static and dynamic states in standing position. The dynamic state can be done by making the patient carry equal weights in his both hands while standing or to image the patient in sitting position (SIJ stressed view). Normally balanced, aligned sacroiliac joints are detected radiographically by drawing a line from the umbilicus (L4 level) to the anterior superior iliac spine (ASIS) bilaterally. These two lines typically should be almost equal bilaterally. Also, the upper endplate of the first sacroiliac vertebra (S1), which is detected as the most radio-opaque line across the sacral base, should be straight when a perfect horizontal line is drawn above it, and another transverse line is drawn below it, making a perfect rectangle (◘ Fig. 13.16.1).
2. Oblique, uneven pelvis is detected radiographically by drawing a perfect horizontal line parallel to the sacral base (line A), with another perfect horizontal line below it as a reference (line B). Another two vertical lines are drawn intersecting both femoral heads, A line, and B line. An uneven, oblique pelvis is detected when an uneven rectangle appears (◘ Fig. 13.16.2).
   1. Iliac bone superior shear injury is detected radiographically on dynamic/stressed image when the iliac bone of the affected sacroiliac joint moves superiorly compared to the other side. This superior movement is seen as movement of the anterior superior iliac spine (ASIS) upward compared to the contralateral side.
   2. Iliac bone inferior shear injury is detected radiographically on dynamic/stressed image when the

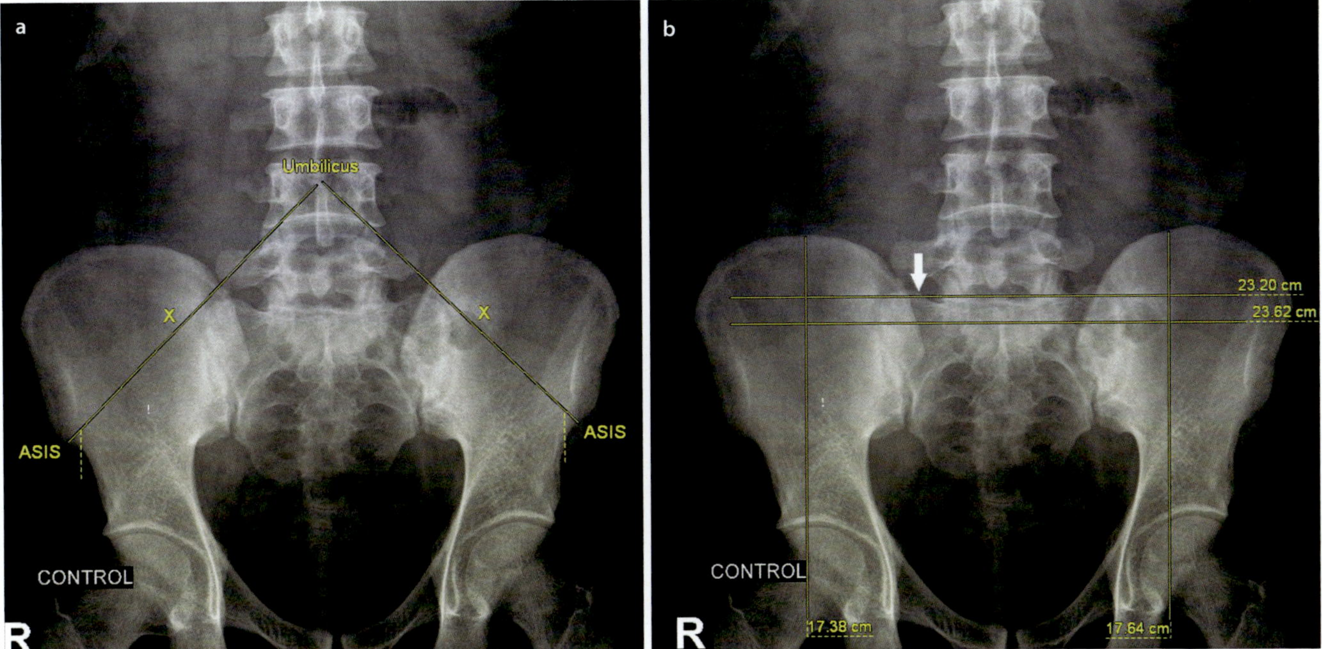



**Fig. 13.16.1** Standing anteroposterior radiograph of the lumbo-pelvic region demonstrates normal pelvic malalignment measured by 2 equal lines drawn from the L4 vertebra spinous process to the ASIS bilaterally (*X lines* in **a**) and a horizontal line that perfectly runs parallel to the superior end plate of S1 vertebra (*arrow* in **b**) and another line drawn below it making a perfect rectangle

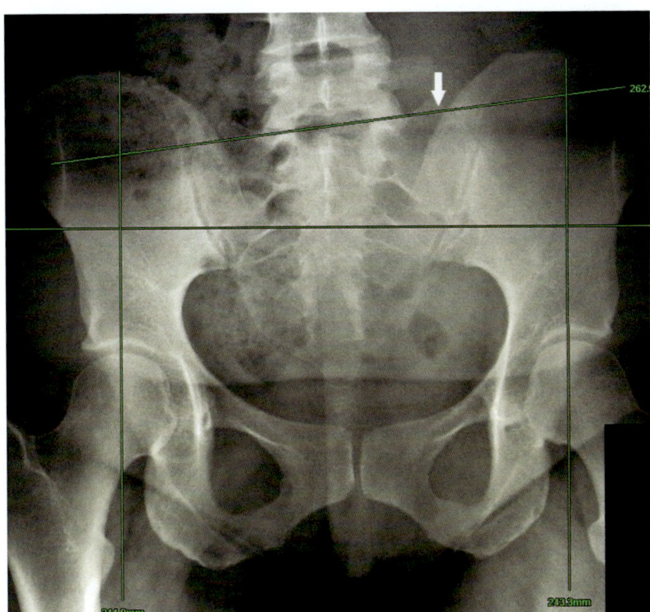

**Fig. 13.16.2** Standing anteroposterior radiograph of the lumbo-pelvic region demonstrates right-sided pelvic tilt with tilting of the horizontal line drawn over the endplate of S1 vertebra, causing an uneven rectangle (*arrow*)

iliac bone of the affected sacroiliac joint moves inferiorly compared to the other side (**Fig. 13.16.3**). This inferior movement is seen as movement of the anterior superior iliac spine (ASIS) downward compared to the contralateral side.

3. Somatic in-flare iliac dysfunction occurs when the iliac bone glides medially over the sacral articular surface and becomes restricted in this position. It is detected radiographically as drawing a line from the umbilicus (L4 level) to the ASIS (line X) bilaterally. The side affected will appear shorter (X – 1) compared to the contralateral side on dynamic/stressed image.

4. Somatic out-flare iliac dysfunction occurs when the iliac bone glides laterally over the sacral articular surface and becomes restricted in this position. It is detected radiographically as drawing a line from the umbilicus (L4 level) to the ASIS (line X) bilaterally. The side affected will appear longer (X + 1) compared to the contralateral side on dynamic/stressed image.

5. For superior pubic shear, the affected symphysis pubis side moves upward on stress images compared to the contralateral side on dynamic/stressed image.

6. For inferior pubic shear, the affected symphysis pubis side moves downward on stress images compared to the contralateral side on dynamic/stressed image.

7. Indirect instability signs are sclerosis and/or formation of gas within the sacroiliac joints or symphysis pubis articular surfaces, as the body starts to deposit more bone due to the continuous frictional load exerted on it (**Fig. 13.16.4**). Also, formation of osteophytes within the inferior border of the sacroiliac joints in association with inferior sacroiliac joints marginal sclerosis have been reported as secondary signs commonly associated with sacroiliac joint dysfunction/instability.

**Further Reading**

Bellamy N, et al. What do we know about the sacro-iliac joint? Semin Arthritis Rheum. 1983;12:282–313.

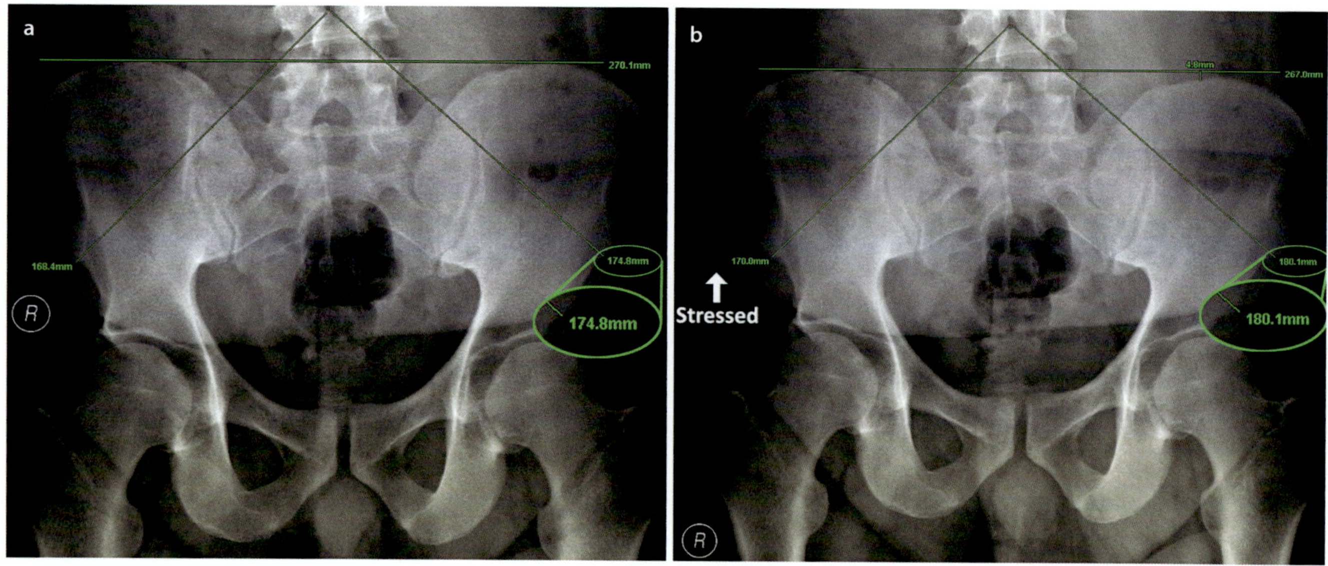



**Fig. 13.16.3**  Anteroposterior radiograph of the lumbo-pelvic region in static (**a**) and dynamic (**b**) stressed-standing views demonstrating "Iliac bone inferior shear injury"; in (**b**), the left iliac bone is mildly tilted downward after stressing the pelvic seen as 4.8 mm depression of the left iliac bone in (**b**) compared to static images in (**a**). Moreover, the line drawn from the L4 vertebra spinous process to the ASIS in the left side has elongated from 175 mm to 180 mm, while the right line changed from 168.4 mm to 170 mm only

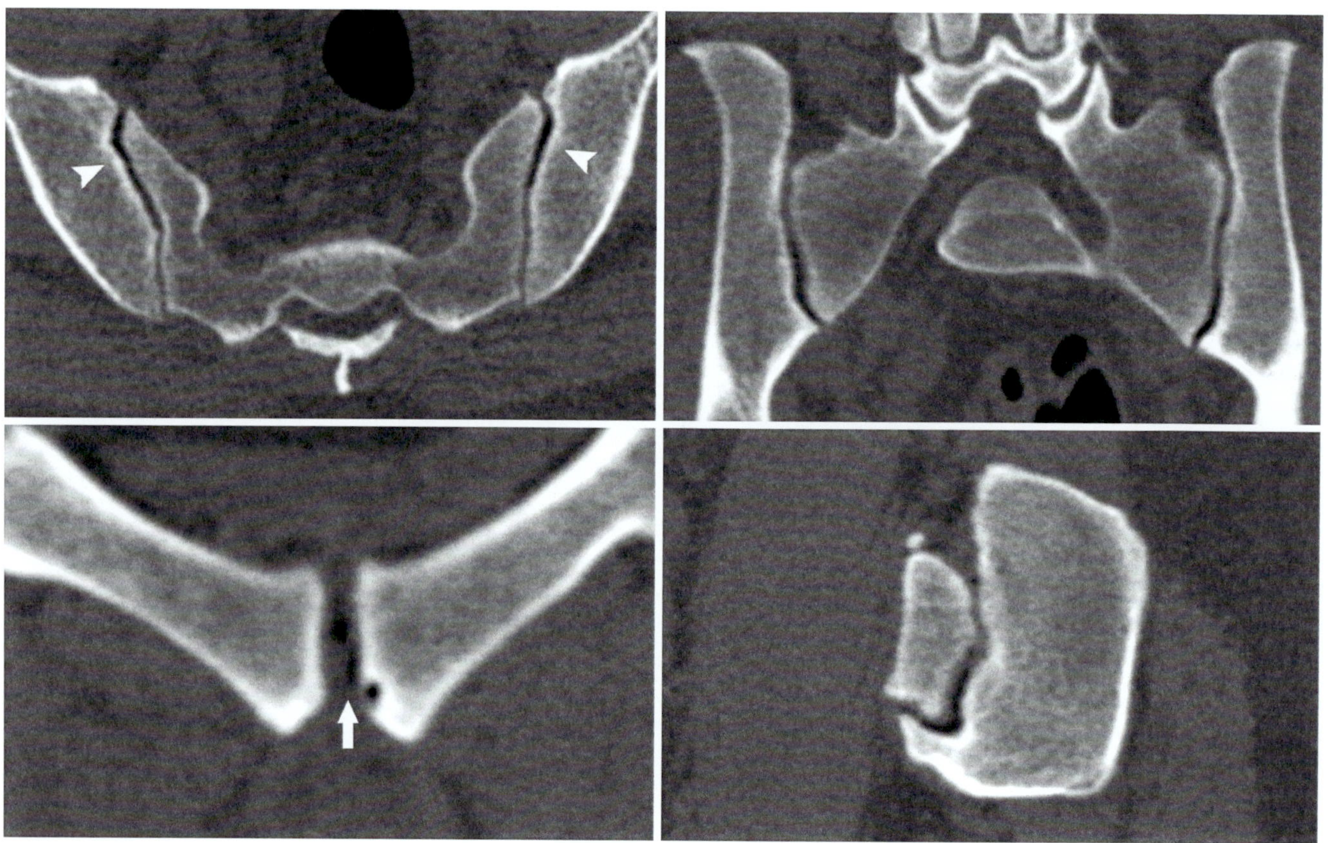

**Fig. 13.16.4**  Multiple CT images in different planes show gas (vacuum phenomenon) within the sacroiliac joint spaces (*arrowheads*) and the symphysis pubis (*arrow*)

Bowen V, et al. Macroscopic anatomy of the sacro-iliac joint from embryonic life until the eighth decade. Spine. 1981;6: 620–8.

Cooper RG, et al. Radiographic demonstration of paraspinal muscle wasting in patients with chronic low back pain. Br J Rheumatol. 1992;31(6):389–94.

DonTigny RL. Function and pathomechanics of the sacroiliac joint: a review. Phys Ther. 1985;65:35–44.

Fortin JD, et al. Can the sacroiliac joint cause sciatica? Pain Physician. 2003;6:269–71.

Fortin JD, et al. The Fortin Finger test: an indicator of sacroiliac pain. Am J Orthop. 1997;26:477–80.

Frost SL, et al. The sacroiliac joint: anatomy, physiology, and clinical significance. Pain Physician. 2006;9:61–8.

Grieve E. Mechanical dysfunction of the sacroiliac joint. Int Rehabil Med. 1982;5:46–52.

Grieve EFM. Mechanical dysfunction of the sacro-iliac joint. Int Rehabil Med. 1983;5:46–52.

Guglielmi G, et al. Imaging of the sacroiliac joint involvement in seronegative spondylarthropathies. Clin Rheumatol. 2009;28:1007–19.

Harmon D, et al. Ultrasound-guided sacroiliac joint jnjection technique. Pain Physician. 2008;11:543–7.

Irvin RE. Reduction of lumbar scoliosis by use of a heel lift to level the sacral base. J Am Osteopath Assoc. 1991;91(1):34–44.

Irvin RE. The origin and relief of common pain. J Back Musculoskelet Rehabil. 1998;11(2):89–130.

Lynch FW. The pelvic articulation during pregnancy, labor and the puerperium. X-Ray Study Surg Gynecol Obstet. 1920b;30:575–80.

Lynch FW. The pelvic articulations during pregnancy, labor and puerperium: an x-ray study. Surg Gynecol Obsrer. 1920a;30:575–80.

Prather H, et al. Sacroiliac joint pain. Dis Mon. 2004;50:670–83.

Sizer PS, et al. Disorders of the sacroiliac joint. Pain Pract. 2002;2(1):17–34.

Solonen KA. The sacroiliac joint in the light of anatomical, roentgenological and clinical studies. Acta Orthop Scand. 1957;27(Suppl):1–127.

Sturesson B, et al. A radiostereometric analysis of the movements of the sacroiliac joints in the reciprocal straddle position. Spine. 2000;25(2):214–7.

Sturesson B, et al. Movements of the sacroiliac joints. A roentgen stereophotogrammetric analysis. Spine. 1989;14(2):162–5.

Szadek KM, et al. Diagnostic validity of criteria for sacroiliac joint pain: a systematic review. J Pain. 2009;10(4):354–68.

Walker JM. The sacroiliac joint: a critical review. Phys Ther. 1992;72:903–16.

Weisl H. The movements of the sacroiliac joint. Acta Anat. 1955;23:80–90.

## 13.33 Psoas Syndrome

Psoas syndrome is a term used to describe chronic lower back pain involving the hip, leg, or thoracic regions that can often be traced to an iliopsoas muscle spasm. This syndrome develops as a result of chronic friction between the posterior aspect of the iliopsoas muscle and the protrusive cup overlapping the anterior rim of the acetabulum.

Malignant psoas syndrome, on the other hand, is a term used to describe a psoas muscle disease characterized by proximal lumbosacral plexopathy, painful fixed flexion of the ipsilateral hip, and radiological or pathological evidence of ipsilateral psoas major muscle malignant involvement (e.g., metastases).

### Basic Anatomy

The psoas muscle originates from the anterior surface of the transverse processes from L1 to L5, lateral boarder of the vertebral bodies and corresponding intervertebral disks of T12–L5. The iliacus muscle originates from the upper two thirds of the inner side of the ilium to the sacral wings and to the anterior sacroiliac, lumbosacral, and iliolumbar ligaments. Both the psoas and iliacus muscles fuse distally and are inserted to the lesser trochanter of the femur, creating the "iliopsoas muscle."

Just medial to the anterior–inferior iliac spine is the tendon of the psoas muscle, which at the level of the pelvic brim is surrounded by muscle fibers of the iliacus. The psoas tendon inserts onto the lesser trochanter of the femur. The muscle fibers of the iliacus extend distal to the lesser trochanter to insert onto the body of the femur in front of and below the lesser trochanter.

The psoas muscle neural supply is derived from L1 to L4 plexus, while the iliacus muscle neural supply is derived from L1 to L3 plus the femoral nerve. The iliopsoas muscle flexes the thigh and weakly rotates it laterally. It is the most active muscle in sitting up from supine posture and has a role in sacroiliac joint stability

Psoas muscle is the only muscle that attaches the lumbar spine to the femur, and it is considered primarily as a lumbar flexion. When the psoas muscle contracts, it draws the femur up toward the spine, assuming that the spine is more stabilized than the femur. If, however, the femur is more stabilized than the spine, the psoas then draws the spine toward the femur, causing the spine to flex forward (hyperlordosis).

### Pathophysiology

Prolonged sitting with hips acutely flexed causes the iliopsoas muscle to adaptively shorten. A pain from iliopsoas origin will mostly present at the insertion site on the lesser trochanter of the femur and on the anterior thigh and groin. Also, the so-called hip-click phenomenon is attributed to a hypertense psoas major muscle. The classic symptoms of an iliopsoas muscle spasm include (◘ Fig. 13.17.1):

1. Back pain: the pain is felt in the lower back and may radiate to groin.
2. Lumbar vertebral malalignment: the lumbar vertebra, starting from L2, will be shifted ipsilaterally to the side of the contracted muscle (◘ Fig. 13.17.1a).
3. Pelvic shift: the whole pelvis and sacrum will shift downward contralaterally (◘ Fig. 13.17.1b, d).

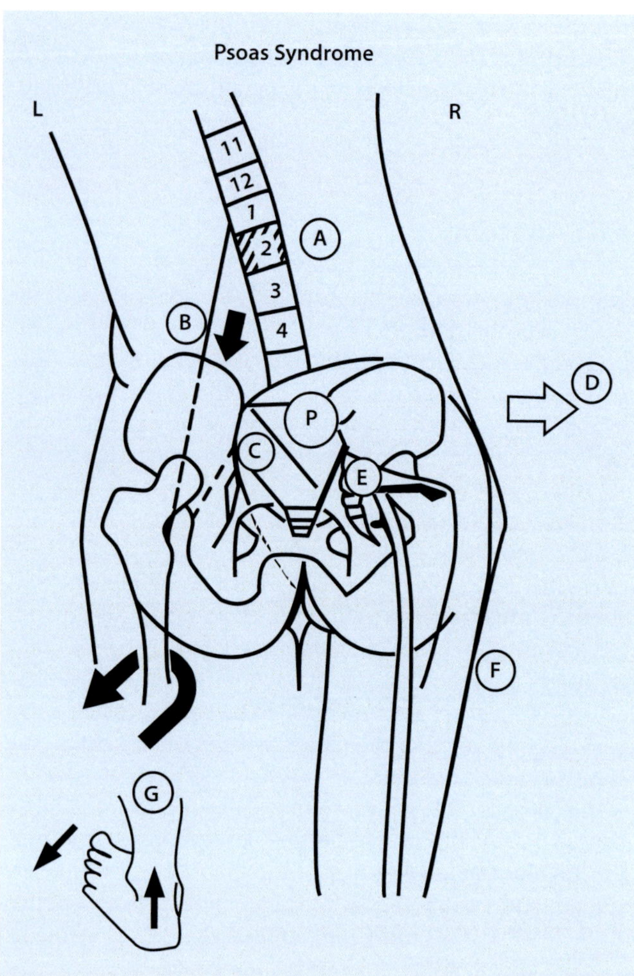





**Fig. 13.17.1**  An illustration that demonstrates the kinesiological findings of the psoas syndrome (refer to the text for the description of the letters)

4. Sacral rotation: the sacrum will rotate obliquely to the side of the contracted muscle (e.g., sacroiliac joint dysfunction) (■ Fig. 13.17.1c).
5. Piriformis muscle syndrome: the contralateral piriformis muscle will be under tension and strain from the pelvic shift created by the pelvic rotation, which will result in the development of classical piriformis syndrome (■ Fig. 13.17.1e). Moreover, whenever the sacroiliac joint is subluxated or under tension, its tension will be transferred to the piriformis syndrome. Symptoms include cramping pain in buttock due to sciatica (■ Fig. 13.17.1f), tight hamstrings, and pain with sitting.
6. Dyspnea: if the tension within the psoas syndrome transferred into the diaphragm, the myofascial layer covering both muscles can be thickened, limiting the movement of the diaphragm; this can result in shortness of breath and dyspnea.
7. Sexual dysfunction: tension over the inguinal fascia can arise from psoas muscle tension, resulting in damping the sexual enjoyment.
8. Foot pronation: the foot ipsilaterally will be pronated due to short leg syndrome (■ Fig. 13.17.1g).

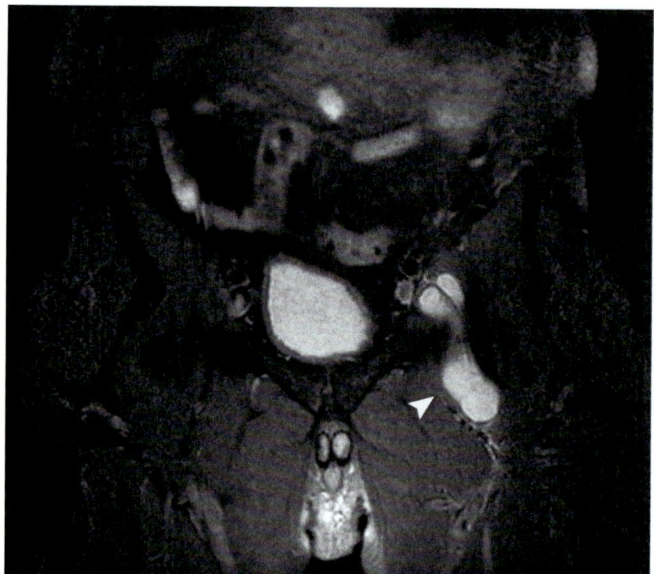

**Fig. 13.17.2**  Coronal PD-MR image that shows edema within the left iliopsoas bursa (*arrowhead*)

### 13.34 Imaging Signs

1. On radiograph or CT, the acetabulum may show osteophytes and osteoarthritic changes in psoas muscle syndrome (the area where the psoas tendon impingement occurs). On MRI, iliopsoas muscle bursitis can be seen as a fluid-filled structure surrounding the iliopsoas tendon associated with high T2-weighted signal intensity, usually with contrast enhancement (■ Fig. 13.17.2). In the literature, iliopsoas bursitis is also known as "internal snapping hip syndrome."
2. In malignant psoas syndrome, there is ipsilateral psoas major muscle malignant involvement (either direct metastasis or extranodal para-aortic extension) in any imaging modality.

### Further Reading
Agar M, et al. The management of malignant psoas syndrome: case reports and literature review. J Pain Symptom Manage. 2004;28:282–93.
Di Lorenzo L, et al. Psoas impingement syndrome in hip osteoarthritis. Joint Bone Spine. 2009;76:98.

### 13.35 Piriformis Muscle Syndrome

The piriformis muscle syndrome is a clinical condition characterized by impingement of the sciatic nerve by the piriformis muscle, resulting in a classical sciatica pain originating mainly from the pelvis. According to many authors, because of the lack of strict diagnostic criteria, piriformis syndrome is a controversial clinical entity and should be suspected as a part of the differential diagnosis in cases of low back and hip or thigh pain. Also, some authors consider piriformis syndrome as a diagnosis of exclusion in regard to sciatic and lower back pain.

## Basic Anatomy

The piriformis muscle arises from the anterior surface of sacrum between – and lateral to – anterior sacral foramen, capsule of sacroiliac articulation, margin of greater sciatic foramen, and sacrotuberous ligament. It exits the pelvis through the greater sciatic foramen to insert on the superior aspect of the greater trochanter of the femur. The piriformis is the only muscle that bridges the sacroiliac joint, and it is supplied by the sacral plexus (L4–S2).

The function of the piriformis changes depending on the position of the hip; this observation is important for understanding various examination findings. In extension, the piriformis externally rotates the hip, whereas in flexion, it becomes an abductor.

The sciatic nerve exits the pelvis via the sciatic foramen or notch. The piriformis muscle splits the sciatic foramen into the supra-piriformis foramen and the infra-piriformis foramen. The infra-piriformis foramen is triangular in shape and passing two neurovascular groups: the medial group includes the pudendal neurovascular bundle and the lateral group consists of the sciatic nerve, the inferior gluteal nerve, the posterior cutaneous nerve of the thigh, and the inferior gluteal vessels.

## Pathophysiology

The term "piriformis muscle syndrome" denotes impingement of the sciatic nerve by the piriformis muscle superiorly; this clinical situation is uncommon and occurs due to one of four main causes:

1. Hypertrophy of the piriformis muscle
2. Blunt trauma to the buttocks or sacroiliac region, with a hematoma formation at the region of the piriformis muscle compressing the muscle
3. Piriformis muscle spasm and tension, typically due to pelvic tilt, leg length discrepancy, or sacroiliac joint subluxation, causing trochanteric bursitis and myofascial trigger point formation within the piriformis muscle
4. Anomalous course of the sciatic nerve and/or one of its distal branches within the muscle (commonly the peroneal nerve)

Patients with piriformis muscle syndrome typically present with pain felt in the buttocks, over the sacroiliac region, lower back, and maybe radiation down to the leg along the sciatic nerve dermatomes. Gait abnormality increases pain due to piriformis muscle syndrome, especially if they result in increased internal rotation or adduction such as with a leg length discrepancy.

## 13.36 Imaging Signs

1. On plain radiography, the detection of pelvic tilt or leg length discrepancy can be suggestive of piriformis muscle tension or spasm, especially with a history that suggests piriformis muscle syndrome with lack of other differential diagnoses.
2. According to some investigators, (1) the normal MRI measurement of the piriformis muscle in axial sections is between 0.8 and 3.2 cm, and asymmetry of up to 8 mm can be normally seen without symptoms. A piriformis muscle with size >3.2 cm and asymmetry >8 mm in the absence of other causes explain the symptoms of the patient can be attributed to piriformis muscle abnormality (◘ Fig. 13.18.1).
3. Sacroiliac joint subluxation should be excluded by weight-bearing pelvic radiographs, since the piriformis muscle is abutting above the sacroiliac joint and is intimately related to abnormalities of the sacroiliac joint.

### Further Reading

Barton PM. Piriformis syndrome: a rational approach to management. Pain. 1991;47:345–52.

Byrd JWT. Piriformis syndrome. Oper Tech Sports Med. 2005;13:71–9.

Carare RO, et al. A unique variation of the sciatic nerve. Clin Anat. 2008;21:800–1.

Indrekvam K, et al. Piriformis muscle syndrome in 19 patients treated by tenotomy – a 1- to 16-year follow-up study. Int Orthop (SICOT). 2002;26:101–3.

Lee EY, et al. MRI of piriformis syndrome. AJR. 2004;183:63–4.

Pecina HI, et al. Surgical evaluation of magnetic resonance imaging findings in piriformis muscle syndrome. Skeletal Radiol. 2008;37:1019–23.

Rossi P, et al. Magnetic resonance imaging findings in Piriformis Syndrome: a case report. Arch Phys Med Rehabil. 2001;82:519–21.

Russell JM, et al. Magnetic resonance imaging of the sacral plexus and piriformis muscles. Skeletal Radiol. 2008;37:709–13.

Turtas S, et al. The piriformis syndrome: a case report of an unusual cause of sciatica. J Orthopaed Traumatol. 2006;7:97–9.

Windisch G, et al. Piriformis muscle: clinical anatomy and consideration of the piriformis syndrome. Surg Radiol Anat. 2007;29:37–45.

## 13.37 Coccydynia

Coccydynia (tailbone pain) is a disease characterized by pain in the posterior pelvis and the perineum due to a disease related to the coccyx. The word coccyx is a Latin word adopted from the Greek word "cuckoo," the birds' peak, and it has been called as the bone that resembles the bill of the cuckoo.

## Anatomy

The coccyx consists of three to five rudimentary, fused, triangular bones with the first coccygeal bone making the base and the last bone making the tip. The sacrococcygeal joint is

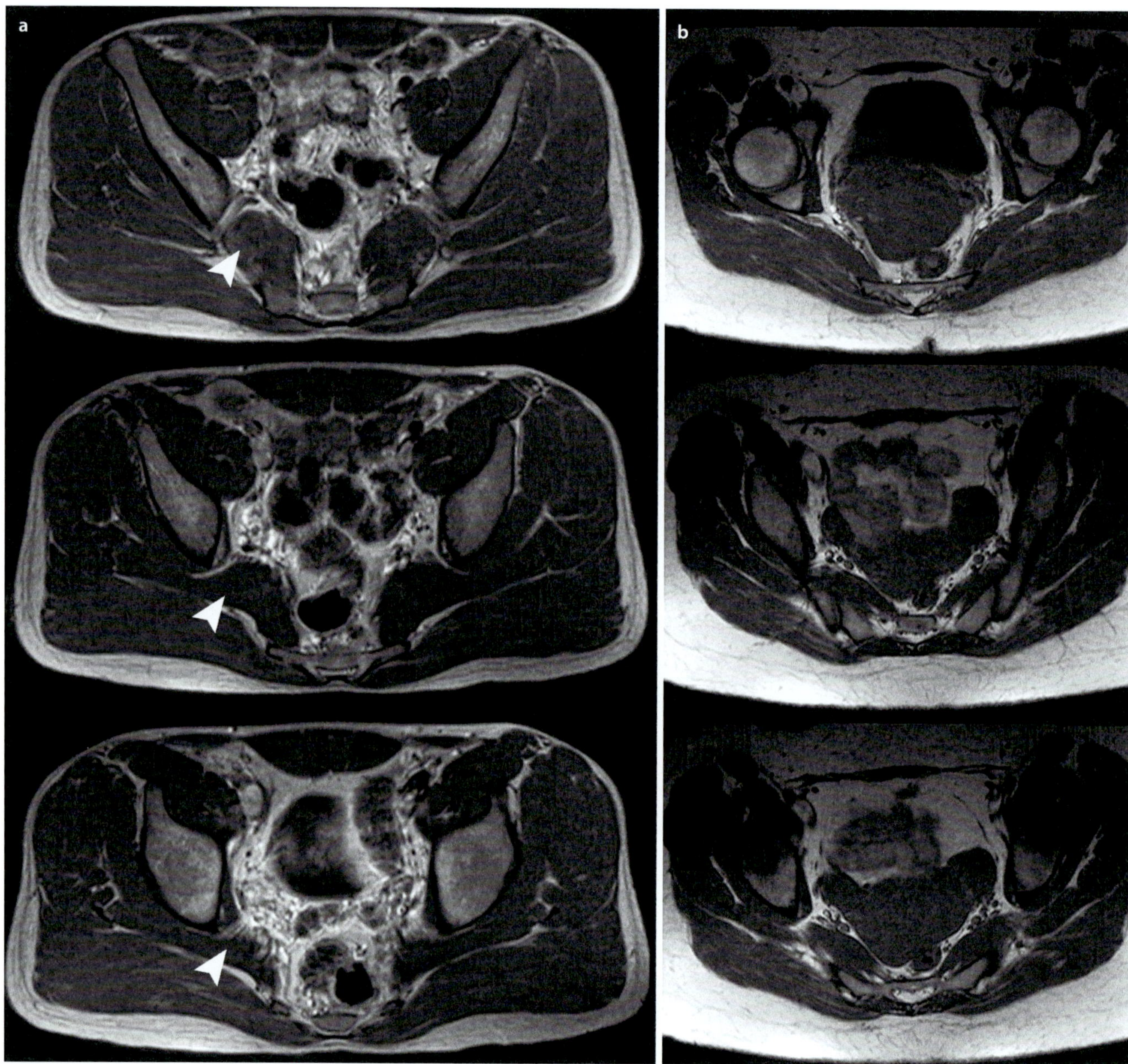

**Fig. 13.18.1** Sequential T1W-MR images of a patient with piriformis muscle syndrome (**a**), compared to a normal axial T1W-MR images of a normal patient. In (**a**), you can see clearly how the piriformis muscle bulk is hypertrophied compared to a normal person (**b**) (*arrowheads*). This patient was a professional Karate practitioner who presented to pain in the pelvis and the buttocks that increases in intensity, especially after excursive

a synovial joint that moves few degrees during walking. Most coccygeal vertebrae are fused at old age. Anatomical structures that are attached to the coccyx include:

1. Muscles: levator ani muscles, gluteus maximus muscle.
2. Ligaments: sacrospinous ligament, sacrotuberous ligament, anococcygeal ligament.
3. Dura: the distal dural attachment, the film terminalis, attaches to the periosteum of the first coccygeal vertebra (■ Fig. 13.19.1).
4. Nerves: the coccyx is innervated by the dorsal rami of S4 to S5 spinal segments, and the coccygeal nerve, emerging from the conus medullaris (S5). A sympathetic trunk is located anterior to the coccyx at variable positions between the sacrococcygeal junction and the tip of the coccyx, is known of "ganglion of impar," also known as "Walther ganglion."

5. Coccygeal body: it is composed of microscopic arteriovenous anastomoses, known in anatomy books as "glomus bodies." Glomus bodies are important for the control of local blood supply.

## Pathophysiology

According to the position of the coccyx, Postacchini and Massobrio described four different types:

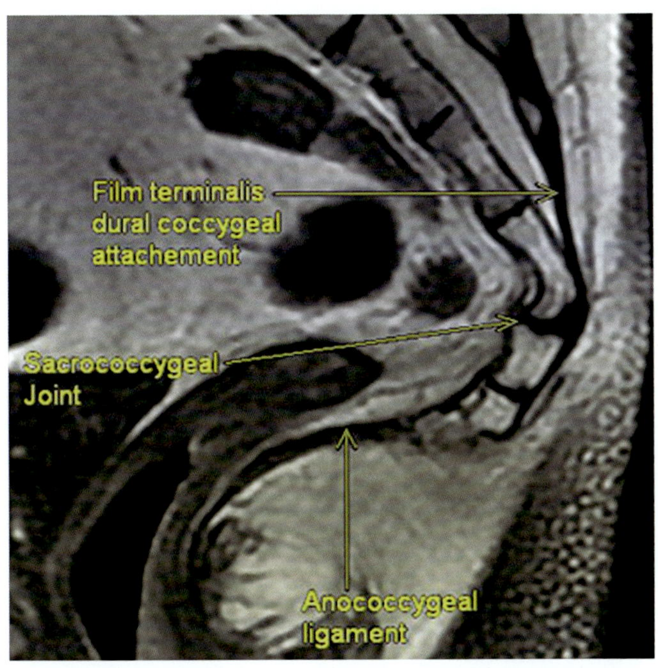



**Fig. 13.19.1** Sagittal T2W-MR image at the level of the coccyx demonstrating the dural attachment to the sacrococcygeal joint

Type I: the coccyx is curved slightly forward (68 %).

Type II: the curve of the coccyx is markedly pronounced and its apex points straight forward (18 %). This type predisposes to coccydynia.

Type III: the coccyx is angulated forward, not at the sacrococcygeal joint but between the 1st and 2nd or 2nd and 3rd segments (6 %). This type predisposes to coccydynia.

Type IV: the coccyx is subluxed anteriorly at the level of the sacrococcygeal joint or the first or second intercoccygeal joints (9 %). This type predisposes to coccydynia.

The most common causes of coccydynia are childbirth trauma, obesity, falling on the buttocks, and bad chair. Coccydynia can also result falsely from "referring pain to the coccyx," especially from a disk herniation at the level of L5 to S1 spinal segments (transitional zone syndrome type 4). Patients with coccydynia typically present with pain on sitting, pain felt in the gluteus maximus muscle on walking (severe cases). Classically, this pain is associated with sitting and is exacerbated when rising from a seated position.

## 13.38 Differential Diagnoses and Related Diseases

1. Proctalgia fugax is a condition characterized by perianal pain and pain on sitting that arises due to spasm of the internal anal sphincter muscle due to "sympathetic hyperstimulation." Many patients are associated with irritable bowel syndrome (52 %). A rare, autosomal dominant form of this condition exists in the medical literature known as "internal anal sphincter myopathy."

2. Levator ani syndrome, also known as "chronic proctalgia," is a condition characterized by perianal pain and pain on sitting that arises mainly due to spasm of the levator ani muscle or as a complication of previous sphincterectomy for anal fissure.

3. Pudendal neuralgia, also known as "Alcock's canal syndrome," is another perianal pain condition that arises mainly due to irritation of the pudendal nerve in the Alcock's canal. Pudendal nerve neuralgia can arise due to coccydynia since the coccyx is attached to sacrotuberous ligament, and sacrotuberous ligament is one of the boundaries of Alcock's canal. Pudendal neuralgia is characterized clinically by impotence, fecal incontinence, and orchialgia or proctalgia due to pudendal nerve entrapment. The syndrome is characterized by chronic burning pain in the perineal area; the pain is exacerbated by sitting and relieved by standing or walking.

## 13.39 Imaging Signs

1. Coccydynia is characterized radiographically by an anteriorly or posteriorly displaced coccyx due to sacrococcygeal joint instability (**Fig. 13.19.2**).

2. The diagnosis of coccygeal subluxation classically is achieved via taking lateral plain radiographs of the coccyx in standing and sitting positions. The normal coccyx shows minimal or no change in position. Quantifying the abnormal movement of the coccyx on radiography depends on three angles:
   A. Intercoccygeal angle is an angle created by a straight line from the first coccygeal vertebra and another line that runs tangential to the last coccygeal vertebra (**Fig. 13.19.3**). The intercoccygeal angle is pathologic if there is >48° angle difference detected between static and dynamic images.
   B. Sacrococcygeal angle is an angle created by a line drawn from the sacral promontory to the sacrococcygeal joint, with another line drawn from the sacrococcygeal joint that runs tangentially to the lower aspect of the pubic bone (**Fig. 13.19.4**). The sacrococcygeal angle is pathologic if there is >38° angle difference detected between static and dynamic images.
   C. Maigne's angle is an angle created by two lines drawn from the sacrococcygeal joint, one runs tangentially to the lower aspect of the pubic bone and another runs tangential to the last coccygeal vertebra (**Fig. 13.19.5**). The Maigne's angle is pathologic if there is >25° angle difference is detected between static & dynamic images.

3. On CT, coccydynia can be suggested by finding signs that show spondyloarthropathy affecting the sacrococcygeal joint, such as bony spurs, sacrococcygeal fusion, sacrococcygeal sacralization, and/or retroverted coccyx.

4. On MRI, signs of coccydynia include edema of the sacrococcygeal joint due to periosteal irritation (**Fig. 13.19.6**), or fracture of coccyx.

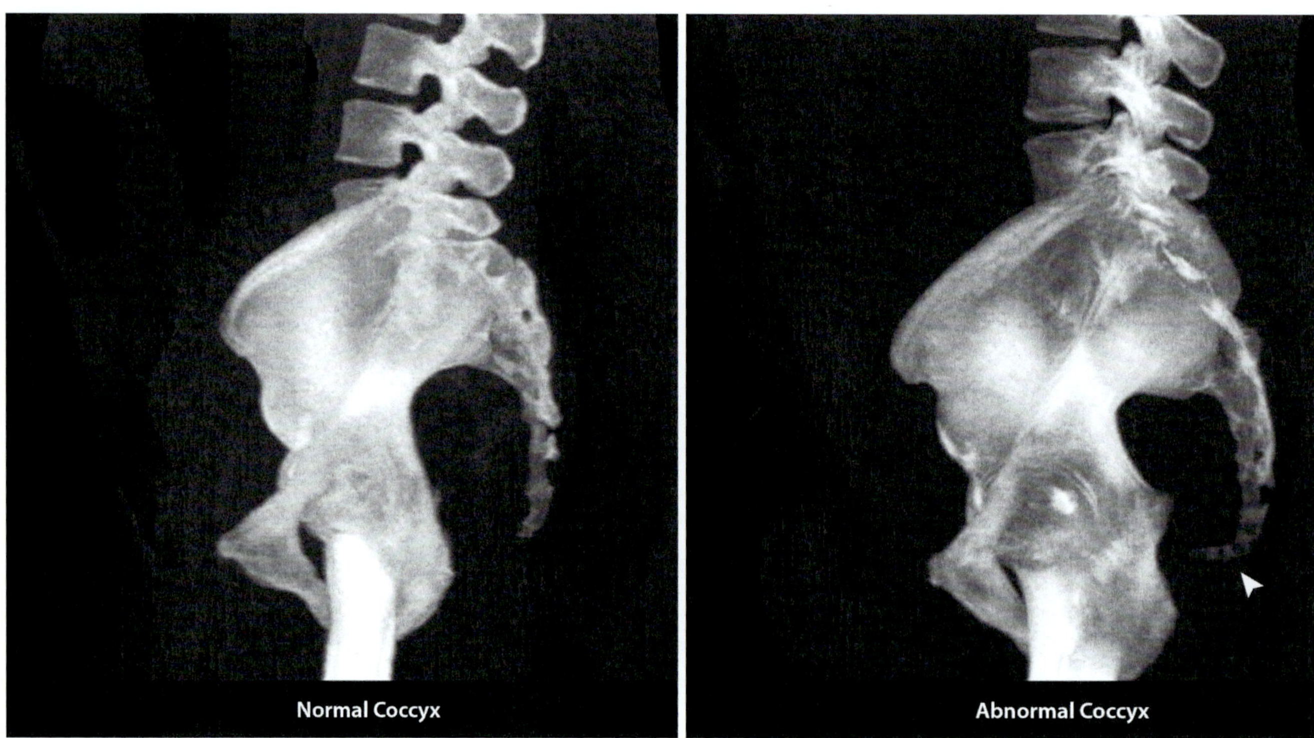



**Fig. 13.19.2**   Sagittal CT images of two different patients: one demonstrates a normal coccyx and another demonstrates a patient presented with coccydynia showing abnormally, anteriorly displaced coccyx (*arrowhead*)

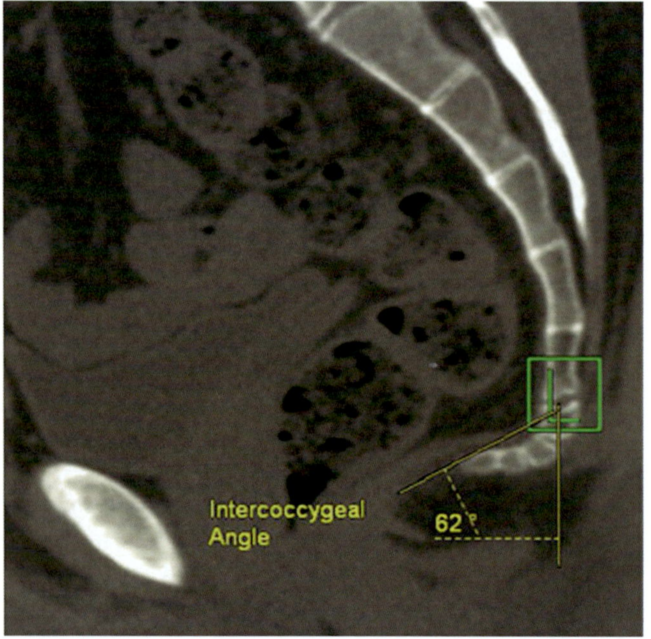



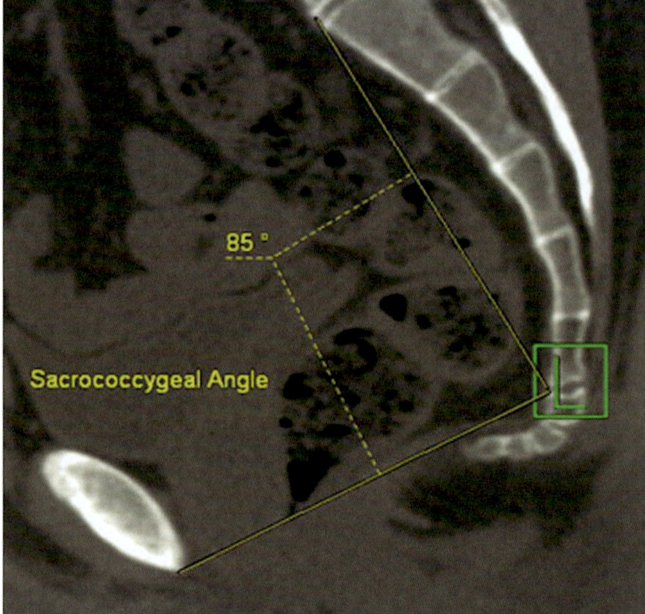



**Fig. 13.19.3**   Sagittal CT image that demonstrates the "intercoccygeal angle"

**Fig. 13.19.4**   Sagittal CT image that demonstrates the "sacrococcygeal angle"

5. Pudendal neuralgia can be diagnosed by MRI when there is a lesion found within the Alcock's canal (**Fig. 13.19.7**), or atrophy and fatty infiltration of the internal oblique muscle is found, denoting pudendal neuropathy.

6. Proctalgia fugax can be suggested in MRI when there is circumferential thickening of the internal anal sphincter >2 mm.

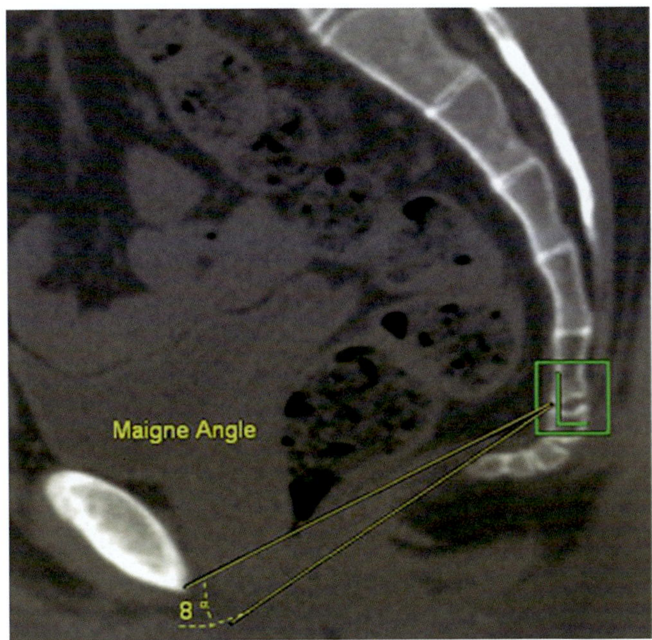


■ **Fig. 13.19.5**  Sagittal CT image that demonstrates the "Maigne's angle"

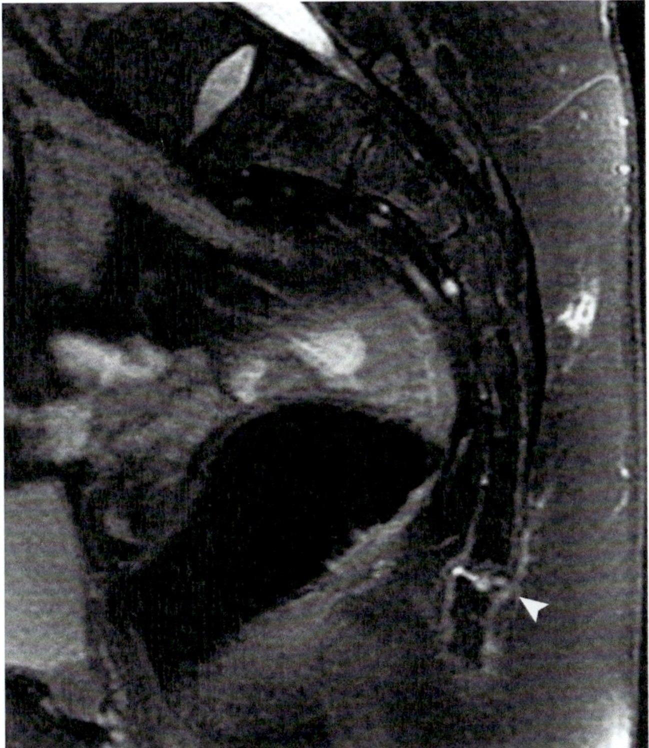

■ **Fig. 13.19.6**  Sagittal PDW-MR image at the level of the coccyx demonstrating edema within the sacrococcygeal joint with edema of the overlying periosteum (arrowhead)

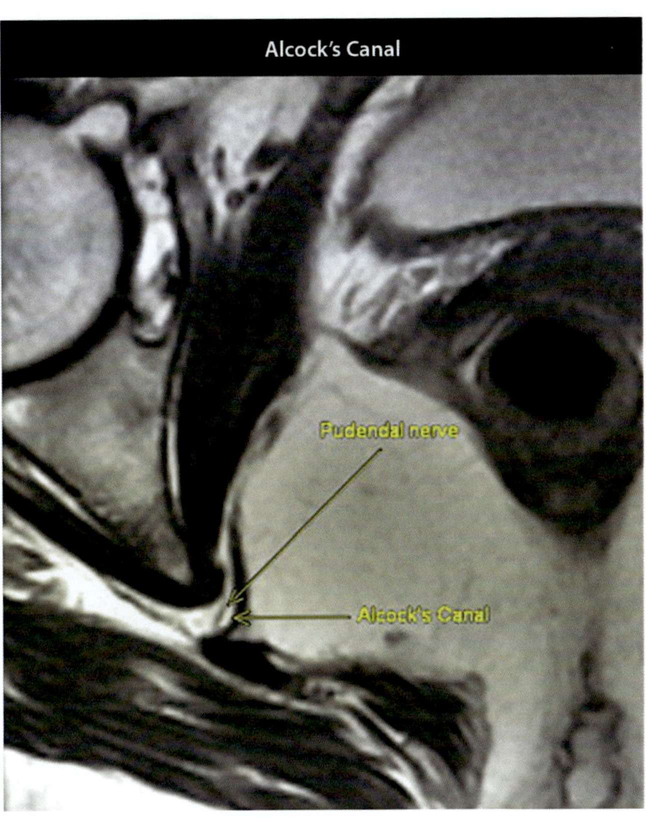


■ **Fig. 13.19.7**  Axial T2W-MR image that demonstrates the boundaries of Alcock's canal

## Further Reading

Cebesoy O, et al. Coccygectomy for coccygodynia: do we really have to wait? Injury. Int J Care Injured. 2007;38:1183–8.

Kennedy AM, et al. MRI of the female pelvis. Semin Ultrasound CT MRI. 1999;20(4):214–30.

Maigne JY, et al. Causes and mechanisms of common coccydynia. Spine. 2000;25(23):3072–9.

Woon JTK, et al. Clinical anatomy of the coccyx: a systematic review. Clin Anat. 2012;25:158–67.

Woon JTK, et al. CT morphology and morphometry of the normal adult coccyx. Eur Spine J. 2013;22:863–70.

Mouhsine E, et al. Posttraumatic coccygeal instability. Spine J. 2006;6:544–9.

Patel N, et al. Anatomy and imaging of the normal meninges. Semin Ultrasound CT MRI. 2009;30:559–64.

Trouvin AP, et al. Role for magnetic resonance imaging in coccydynia with sacrococcygeal dislocation. Joint Bone Spine. 2013;80:214–6.

Diel J, et al. The sacrum: pathologic spectrum, multi-modality imaging, and subspecialty approach. RadioGraphics. 2001;21:83–104.

Patel R, et al. Coccydynia. Curr Rev Musculoskelet Med. 2008;1:223–6.

# Energy Medicine






© Springer International Publishing Switzerland 2017
J.A. Al-Tubaikh, *Internal Medicine*, DOI 10.1007/978-3-319-39747-4_14

## 14.1   Microcurrent Therapy

Microcurrent therapy is a form of therapy that uses Galvanic, direct current (DC) with low amperage (<1000 µA) and low frequency (0.5–100 Hz) for healing purposes. Microcurrent therapy simply produces electrical signals like those naturally produced in the body during repair and healing process.

Electric current is defined as the *flow of charged particles, mostly electrons.* When the current flows in "one direction," it is called direct current (DC). In contrast, when the flow is "back and forth," it is called alternating current (AC). As a general rule, DC heals, while AC inhibits.

The human body works via DC electricity, which is in the range of pico-ampere (*Trillionths*), nano-ampere (*Billionths*), and micro-ampere (*Millionths*). DC microcurrents are essential part of any "healing process" in the body, according to the work of *Robert O. Becker* – a famous American orthopedic surgeon who is considered the father of electromedicine due to his famous work on salamanders – published in his book *The Body Electric.*

Microcurrent therapy follows the same physiological mechanisms of action as acupuncture and neural therapy after Huneke. Acupuncture and microcurrent healing follow the theory of *Rudolf Arndt* (1835–1900) and *Hugo Schulz* (1853–1932), also known as the *Arndt–Schulz law,* which states that weak electrical stimuli increase physiological activities and strong electrical stimuli inhibit physiological activities.

In 1965, *Melzack* and *Wall* described the "gait theory" of pain, which states that "Both sensory and pain signals are competing to access the brain via the spinal horn dorsal horns. Sensory neurons are faster than pain neurons, and when sensory neurons are activated, they will block the pain signals." The gait theory resulted in the formation of "transcutaneous neurostimulation (TENS)" devices.

## Basic Electrical Healing Physiology

Trauma and cellular injury manifest themselves as a dysfunction of the autonomic homeostasis. Most research data on pain management and therapy suggests that chronic pain originates from the autonomic nervous system.

It has been shown that injured areas are more electroconductive than the surrounding skin due to the formation of what is known as healing microcurrents. Therefore, any physical disorder which increases autonomic activity can be measured at specific points using a point-specific probe, which is the basis of many acupuncture-based diagnostic devices.

According to *Jerry Tennant,* an American ophthalmologist from Texas and a pioneer in the field of electric and quantum medicine, disorders can be viewed as lack of energy (*voltage*) or excess energy (*voltage*) within the injured tissue; correcting the electrical status of the injured tissue results in *immediate* pain relief.

Acute injuries generally cause the injured tissue to have a combination of abnormally high and abnormally low resistances. Basic physics teaches that electricity flows toward the path of least resistance. Therefore, endogenous bioelectricity avoids areas of high resistance (*inflamed areas*) and takes the easiest path, generally around the injured tissues. *Robert O. Becker* discovered through his studies on salamanders that healing takes place in the body via initiating "DC current" at the damaged tissues; he called them "healing biocurrents" (◘ Fig. 14.1.1).

When there is damage to a tissue, the adenosine triphosphate (ATP) is reduced, impairing the cellular membrane sodium–potassium pump. The dysfunction cellular membrane and the localized edema increase the tissue's electrical resistance compared to the normal tissues surrounding them. Moreover, an abnormal electrical current and magnetic field are created due to leakage of the intracellular ions and disruption of the sodium–potassium



◘ **Fig. 14.1.1**   An illustration that demonstrates the healing biocurrents

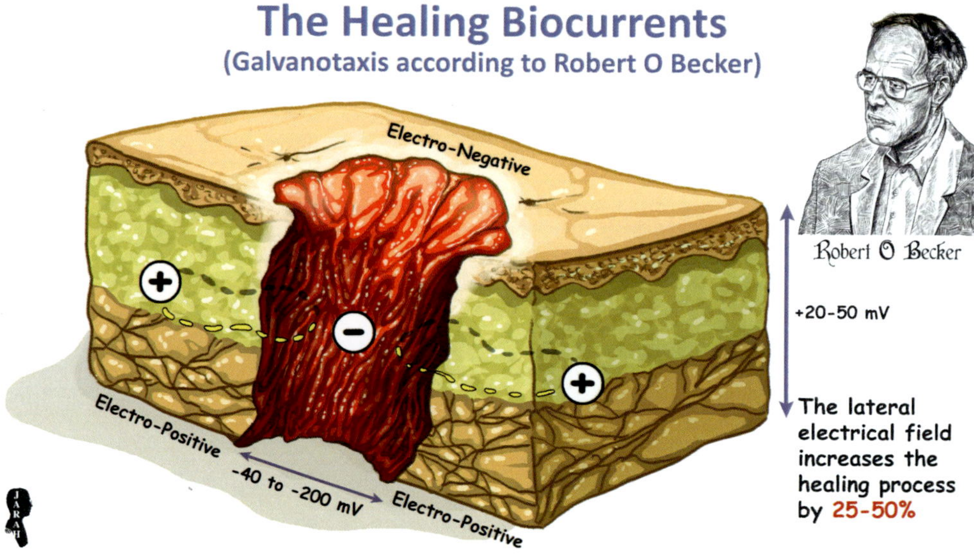

# Quantum Therapies

These therapies depends heavily on the <u>Frequency</u> & the <u>Waveform</u> … one principle with only the method of delivery changes

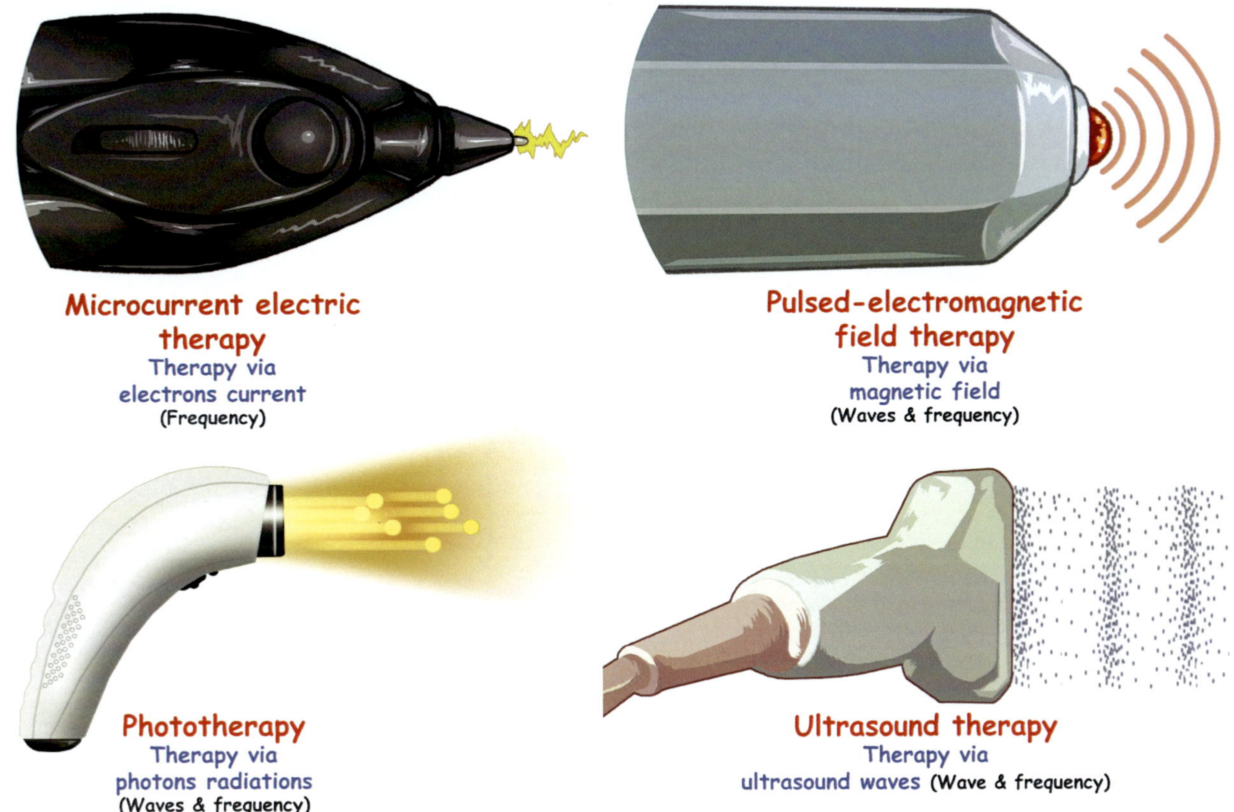


**Fig. 14.1.2** An illustration that demonstrates the quantum therapies and their mode of energy wave delivery

pump; this abnormal electrical current is known as the "current of injury," and it is perceived as pain.

According to *Jerry Tennant*, in order to overcome this electrical resistance and initiate healing process, the surrounding tissues have to increase the "voltage" of the electrical current they supply to (−50 mV), so healing can be initiated. Without such voltage, the current produced will not be a constant DC, which is the basic current required for healing the tissues.

## Microcurrent Therapy Benefits

Microcurrent therapy delivers a DC in the range of normal body healing DC, which is like an external intervention for the injured tissue. If constant DC with high voltage (−50 mV) is not supplied, the acute insult will progress into a chronic insult. In quantum medicine teachings, your drug is the "frequency" you send, and your vehicle of delivery is the "wave" (*electrical, magnetic, ultrasonic, or photonic*) (**Fig. 14.1.2**). Some of these waves match the waves produced by hormones and other metabolic messengers, which will initiate the normal cascade of cellular functions (*similar to tuning a radio toward a specific channel*). It is important to mention here that these waves have to be in a specific range; otherwise, the cells will not respond. The cellular endogenous reaction to external vibration (e.g., *resonance*) is "windowed" for biological systems like the *endocrine, immune, and neural* systems. This means that there is a frequency "window" or "range," called *Adey's window*, at which the effect occurs; below or above this window, no biological reaction will be seen. The established benefits of microcurrent therapy in the literature are summarized as follows:

1. It treats myofascial trigger points efficiently and easily.
2. Microcurrent supplies electrons, which accelerate ATP production by 300–500 %.
3. It boosts protein synthesis by 70 %.
4. It accelerates healing of acute injuries by 200 %.
5. It reduces inflammatory cytokines in the blood.
6. It softens scars and swellings (*will drain within minutes if the correct frequency is applied*).

## Microcurrent Therapy Healing Mechanisms

Microcurrents accelerate healing (*work as a catalyst*) via the following suggested mechanisms:

1. *Accelerate inflammatory response*: in contrast to steroids and nonsteroidal anti-inflammatory drugs, which suppress

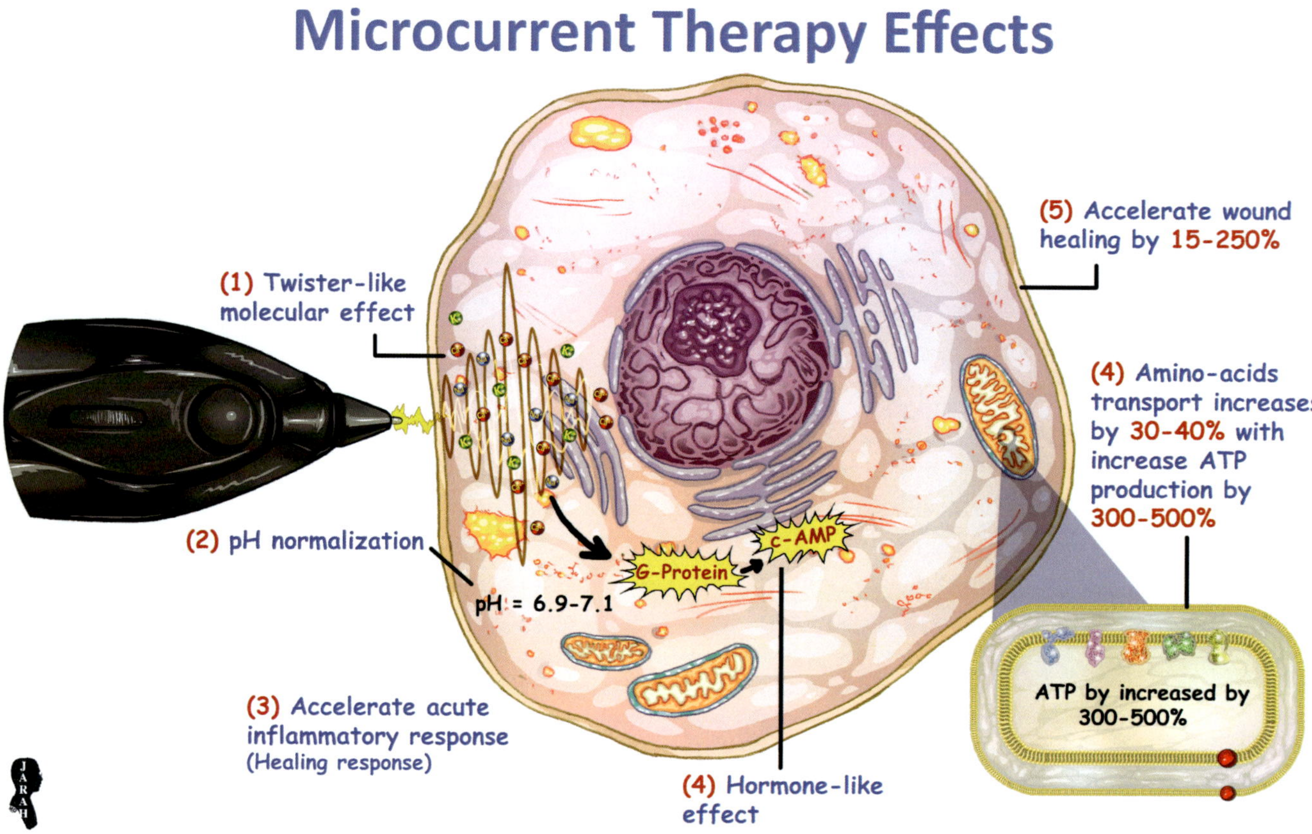

# Microcurrent Therapy Effects



**Fig. 14.1.3**    An illustration that demonstrates the metabolic effects of microcurrent therapy

inflammatory mediators, microcurrents *accelerate* the inflammatory response, which results in healing, since acute inflammatory response is part of healing. Acceleration of the acute inflammatory response presents the inflammatory reaction from going into sideways that can lead to prolongation of the inflammatory response leading to chronic inflammation.

2. *The tsunami effect*: microcurrents applied to the tissues change polarity from positive to negative, which will exert an oscillo/torsional response (**Fig. 14.1.3**); this response causes twister-like effect on the molecular composition of the tissues and increases their kinetic energy, which will increase the probability that a specific chemical group of substrates interacts with their enzymes, accelerating the metabolic processes.

3. *pH normalization*: it is well known that acidity causes pain by evoking the C-fibers and the Aδ fibers in the extracellular matrix. Microcurrents, like any electrical current, are associated with electromagnetic field; this electromagnetic field exerts a direct effect on charged molecules like hydrogen protons ($H^+$), causing their redistribution (*diffusion*) from their area of high concentration distributing them almost equally through the injured tissue, normalizing their pH effect (**Fig. 14.1.3**).

4. *Hormonelike effect*: microcurrents have been proven to exert "hormonelike effects" via electrical activation of the "cell membrane G protein" (**Fig. 14.1.3**) that will influence the formation of the second messenger cyclic adenosine monophosphate (cAMP), which in turn has a direct effect on cell-specific activities, including cellular repair processes. cAMP is the second messenger created during hormone stimulation, which causes opening of the voltage-gated channels in the Aδ and C-fiber neurons, causing washing out of their wastes products, causing analgesia.

5. *Metabolic challenge*: microcurrents cause repeated cell membrane depolarization activity, which requires subsequent membrane repolarization; this requires additional energy ATP production, increasing the cellular metabolism to meet the new demand.

6. *ATP replenishment*: the energy used by human cells requires the hydrolysis of 200–300 mol of ATP everyday. Thus, each ATP molecule is recycled 2000–3000 times during a single day. Since ATP can't be stored, then its consumption must closely follow its synthesis.

ATP is created from ADP via two main mechanisms in the cells: phosphorylation (*by adding a phosphate group to a protein or a small molecule*) and chemiosmosis (*via pumping $H^+$ within the electron transport chain ATPase in the inner mitochondrial membrane*).

In 1983, Cheng et al. showed that microcurrent stimulation increases adenosine triphosphate (ATP) generation at

500 µA by 500 % and increases amino acid transport by 30–40 % above control levels ( Fig. 14.1.3). Also, another study showed that microcurrent stimulation between 300 and 700 µA increases wound healing by 150–250 % when used as 2-h session per day for 6 weeks.

Microcurrents are believed to increase ATP synthesis via electrolysis of water within the body at the positive electrode (*anode*), which will migrate through the cell into the mitochondria, used as a substrate to generate ATP via chemiosmosis. The abundance of ATP within the cells will result in muscle contraction, protein biosynthesis, nerve transmission, and active transport of wastes and substrates across the cellular membrane.

## Microcurrent Healing Cases

The author has been using quantum therapies for private use and on a narrow scale on patients in the hospital for the past 3 years, using microcurrent devices, pulsed electromagnetic field devices, ultrasonic devices, and phototherapeutic devices. For microcurrent therapy, the author uses the Tennant's Biomodulator®, the Dolphin Neurostim®, and the Acutron®.

My aim in this chapter is to present to the clinicians reading these pages a relatively new kind of therapy that has been approved worldwide, but still its uses are limited due to the technicality of the devices, ignorance of their existence, plus the cost sometimes. I sincerely hope that in the future, quantum medicine thrives and it takes its proper place in the hospitals and medical clinics.

### ▪▪ Case 1

A 62-year-old female patient with "trigger finger," also known as sclerosing tenosynovitis, was treated with microcurrent therapy. Sclerosing tenosynovitis typically arises due to reduction in the formation of the lubricating synovial fluid around the tendons, causing continuous friction between the tendon and its sheath, which will eventually cause adhesions and limited movement.

Microcurrents cause vasodilation in the treated region; providing heat is a common practice in osteoarthritis and frozen shoulder cases (adhesive capsulitis) because heat causes vasodilation, which will increase oxygen and nutrient delivery to the diseased area assisting in accelerating healing process.

In  Fig. 14.1.4, the patient was treated within 5 min by microcurrents (Dolphin Neurostim®), which caused marked gush of blood at the treated region in the thermal images (hyperemia) and resolution of the mild cyanosis seen at the middle finger (arrows and arrowheads) prior to the therapy session.

### ▪▪ Case 2

A 55-year-old female patient with "plantar fasciitis" was treated by microcurrents (Tennant Biomodulator®); the edema within the subcutaneous tissue over the plantar area showed mild reduction in signal intensity on the PDW-MR images, and the patient reported moderate reduction in pain after 1-h session ( Fig. 14.1.5).

### ▪▪ Case 3

A 28-year-old female patient with "rheumatoid arthritis" presented with painful right shoulder. Musculoskeletal ultrasound revealed supraspinatus inflammation detected as high power Doppler (PD) signal, a technique used to detect hyperemia in the inflamed tissues. The patient was treated by microcurrents (Tennant Biomodulator®) for 1-h session. Ultrasound images after the session showed no PD signal, with pain reduction to almost 80 % reported by the patient( Fig. 14.1.6).

## 14.2 Pulsed Electromagnetic Field Therapy

Magnetism is a force created in the space around "*moving charged*" particles (e.g., *electrons*). The space by which this magnetic force exists is known as "magnetic field." In contrast, electric field is defined as the field created by a "*charged particle*," without motion (static field); magnetic field is the field created by a "moving charged particle," while electromagnetic field is the field created by an "*accelerated charged particle*."

In biology, the movement of electrolytes ($Na^+$, $K^+$, $Cl^-$, $Ca^{2+}$, etc.) in the blood or tissues creates a very weak magnetic field. This biological magnetic field interacts with the Earth's magnetic field (0.5 G), which forms the background field covering the entire planet. In the cell, multiple ions ($Na^+$, $K^+$, $Cl^-$, *etc.*) move in and out of the cell membrane. The movement of these charged molecules creates weak electric current. Any electric current has a magnetic field perpendicular to it (Faraday's law); and any magnetic field has a "frequency."

Magnetism and electricity are interrelated phenomena; this means that a moving electrical charge (e.g., electrons) in an electrical wire, for example, is capable of creating a magnetic field perpendicular in orientation to the electrical flow direction. In the same logic, a magnetic field that varies in time (e.g., pulsed) induces the flow of electric current (Faraday's law of induction). Based on the last fact, human body movements or exercise generates electricity within the body's neurons and muscles due to movement of the blood and fluid electrolytes within the Earth's external magnetic field. This human's magnetic field has a frequency of 0–10 Hz, which is very important for cellular function.

Research in magnetic field therapy is divided into two main areas: pulsed bioelectric magnetic therapy (electrical magnets) and fixed magnetic therapy (permanent magnets). A fixed magnet emits magnetic field *only*, while pulsed electromagnetic apparatus emits both *electric* and *magnetic* fields.

The body's own biomagnetic fields have both time-varied (frequency) and direct-current (DC) components. In living system, a "static magnetic field" is negligible because everything from molecule to organelle is in motion. Endogenous magnetic fields generated by muscle contraction, nerve impulse, or piezoelectric bony force are short and generated in a pulse fashion (pulsed magnetic field – PEMF). The human magnetic field arises from three main interlocked

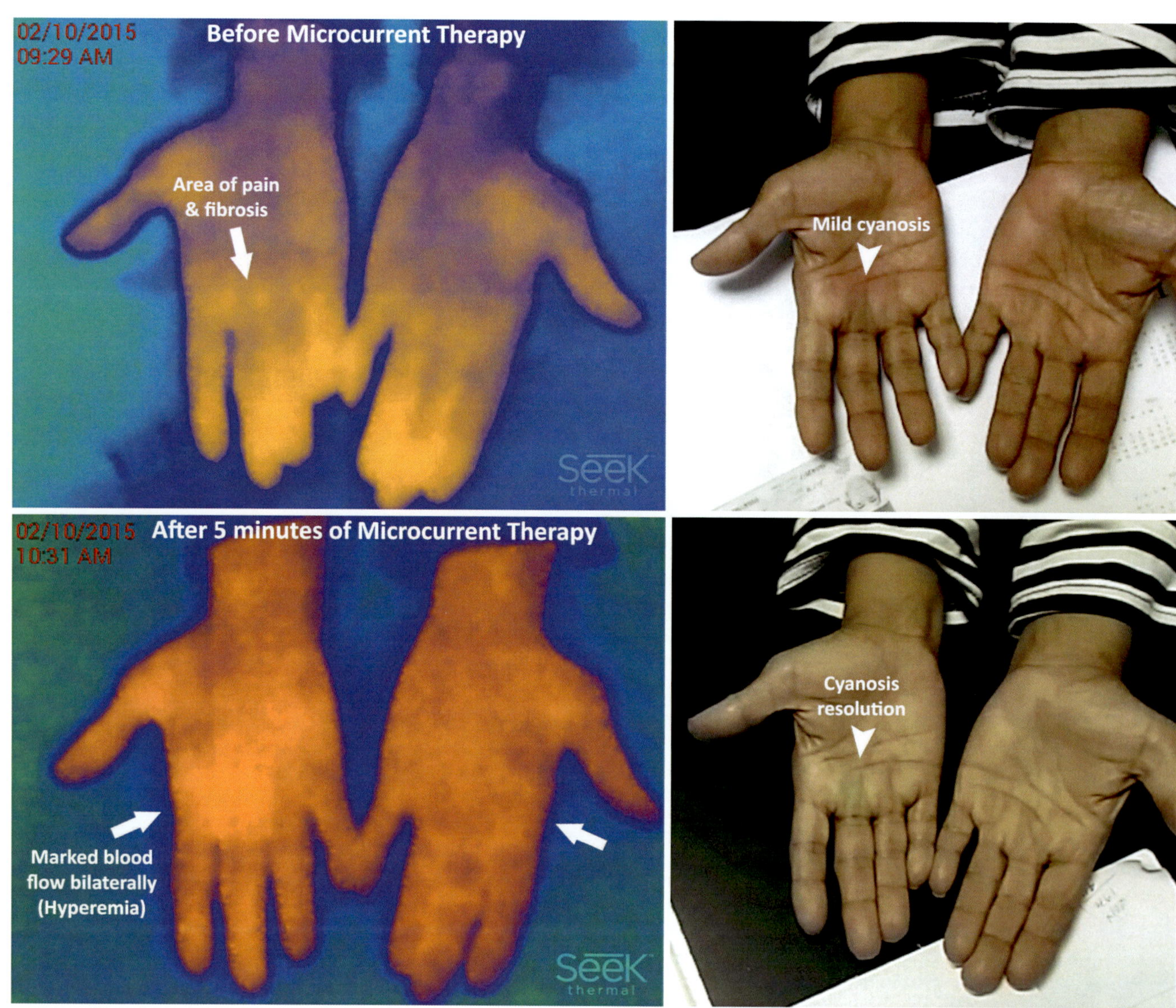


**Fig. 14.1.4**    Thermogenic and photographic images of a patient treated with microcurrent therapy for trigger finger (Read the text for details)

systems: the heart (circulatory system), the myofascial planes (acupuncture system), and the nervous system.

## Pulsed Electromagnetic Fields (PEMFs)

Pulsing a wave means that the signal is *on* for a brief period, then *off*, then on, then off, etc. Pulsing is independent of the frequency, which is equivalent to a note in music. Speaking musically, the "on, off, on, off" aspect of the wave could also be regarded as note, rest, note, rest, etc. The movement of the electromagnetic (EM) radiation in the body translates into ion transport, increase in blood and lymph flow, and more. Any frequency can be pulsed. PEMF induces therapeutic results, which is why it is used in therapy.

Piezoelectric effect is the phenomenon observed when a material produces electrical polarization due to *mechanical* stress. Many biological tissues are piezoelectric such as the skin, bone, tendons, dentin, ivory bone, aorta, trachea, intes-

tine, and nucleic acids. In contrast, pyroelectric effect is the phenomenon when a material produces electrical polarization when it is *heated*. All pyroelectric materials are piezoelectric (*but the converse is not true*).

Since bone has a piezoelectric effect, bone growth is induced by electrical current within the bone matrix induced by stress. This effect has been reported by many investigators as a mean to treat osteoporosis. Pulsed electromagnetic fields, often with magnetic coils, have a history of success with various structural injuries in the body, including spinal cord injuries, edema from ankle sprains, migraine headaches, and whiplash.

## Pulsed Electromagnetic Fields (PEMFs) and Body Metabolism

PEMF therapy is a form of therapy which consists of a mat or a device connected to a small electrical unit that generates a pulsed magnetic field. PEMF is used by many German clinics

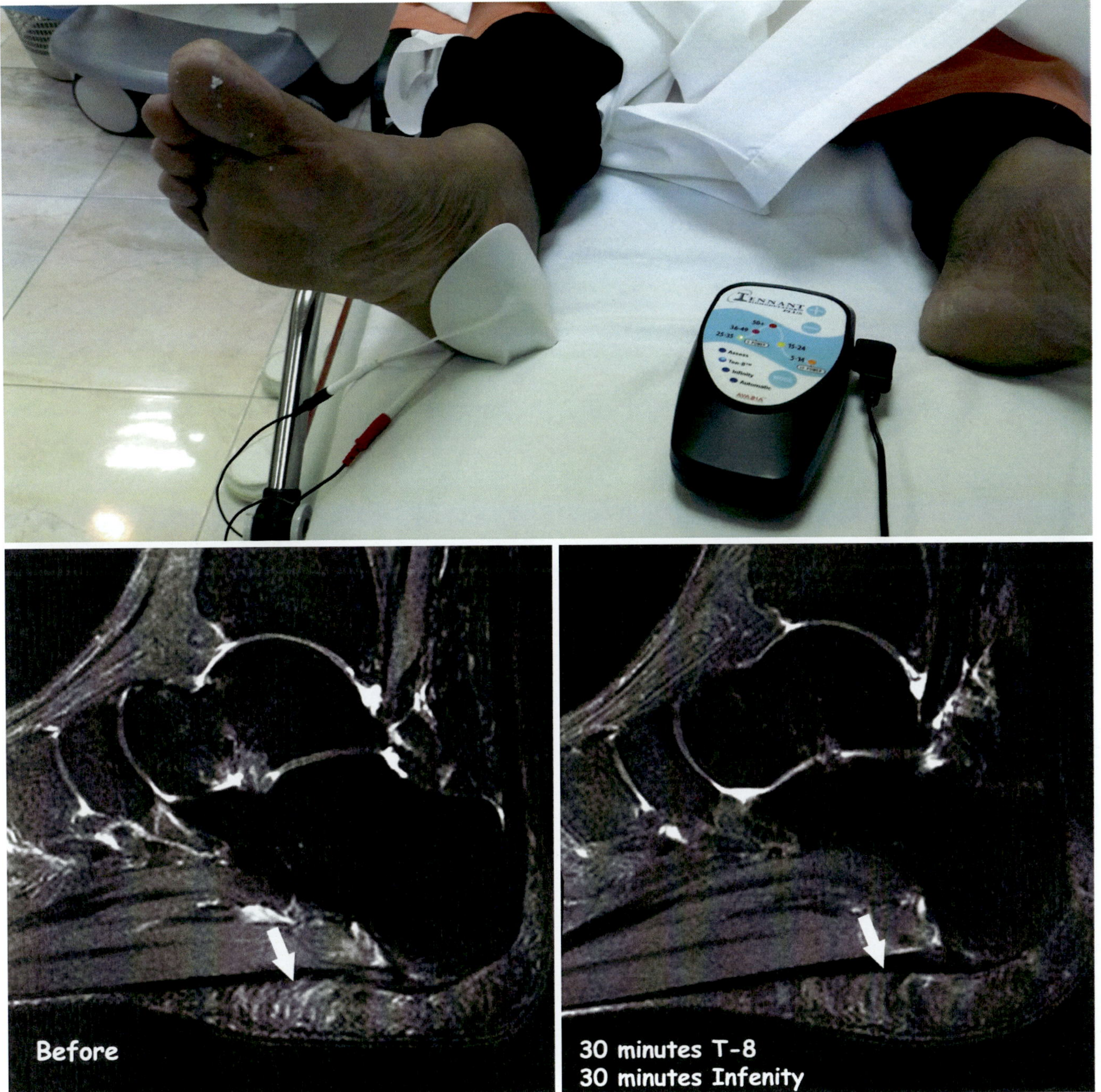



❑ **Fig. 14.1.5** Sagittal PDW-MR and photographic images of a patient treated with microcurrent therapy for plantar fasciitis (Read the text for details)

to treat many disorders, including cancer. Healthy cells in the tissue have a voltage difference between the inner and outer membrane referred to as the "membrane resting potential" that ranges from −70 to −80 mV. This causes a steady flow of ions through its voltage-dependent ion channels.

The living cells can be considered as "small batteries," where their charge is located in the "cellular membrane voltage," also known as "transmembrane potential (TMP)," which is typically equal to −70 to −90 mV. This electric current in the cell membrane has a perpendicular magnetic field component, which has a frequency of 62–78 MHz. The highest membrane potential is found in neurons (−90 mV) and cardiac cells (−120 mV).

The human magnetic field is created by all the cells and is typically hardly detected because their vectors are not in one alignment. In magnetic resonance imaging, the human's magnetic field of the cells is made in one alignment, making it easier to image the magnetic field of the cells, a common knowledge for any radiologist.

There are three main magnetic fields that affect the human cells, generated internally and externally: (1) the brain magnetic field (80 % created by neurons), (2) the heart

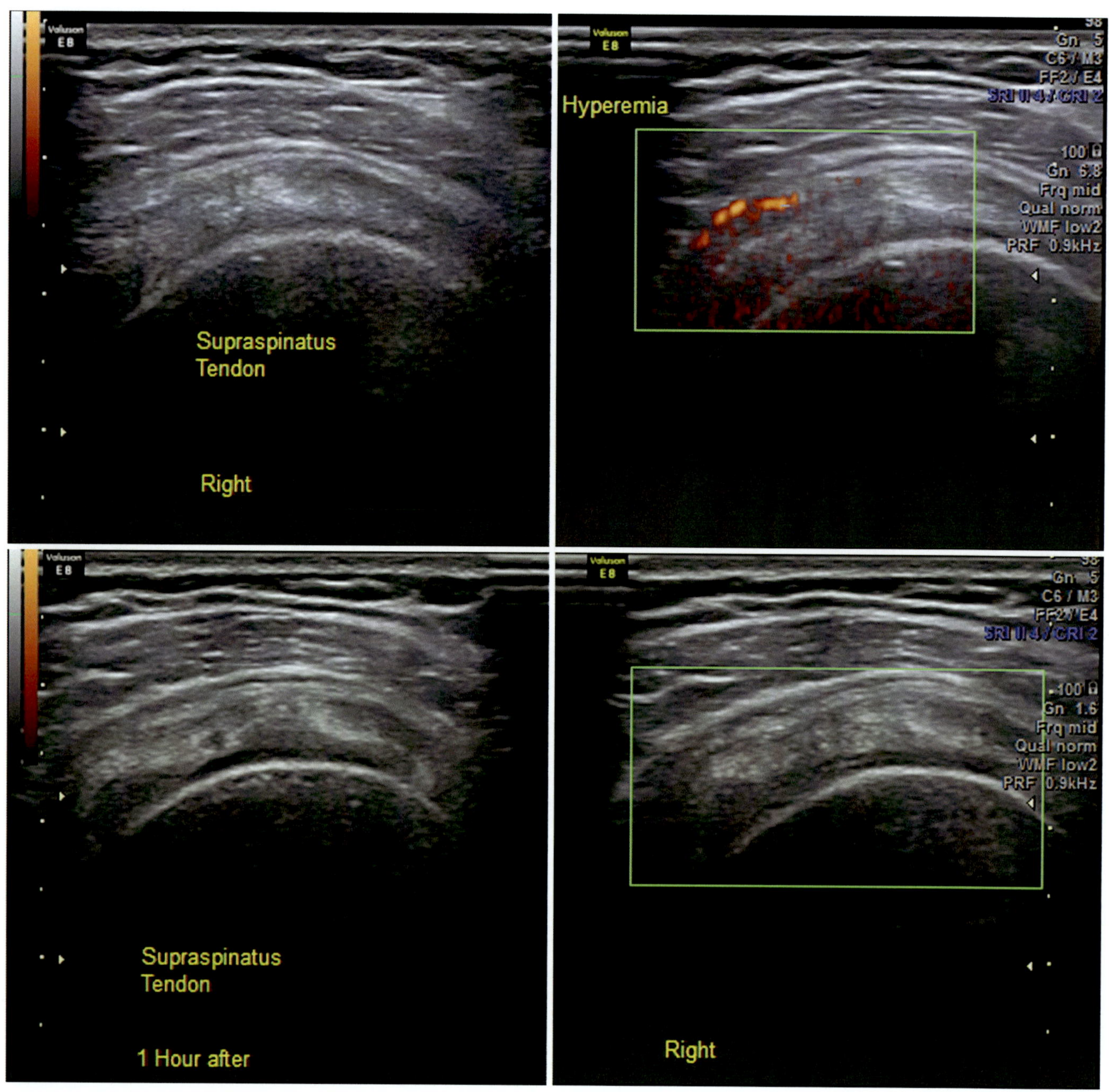


**Fig. 14.1.6** Coronal ultrasound images of the supraspinatus tendon of a patient treated with microcurrent therapy for supraspinatus tendinopathy (Read the text for details)

magnetic field, (3) and the Earth's magnetic field (also known as Schumann's resonance = 7.83 Hz). These three magnetic fields affect the "body metabolism" in regard to adenosine triphosphate (ATP) production, oxygen delivery, waste removal, nutrient absorption, and immune cell function. PEMFs can affect body metabolism via the following, scientifically proven mechanisms:

1. *Recharging the cell membrane voltage*: In physics, when you place an atom in a magnetic field and you start to increase the magnetic field flux strength, the electron speed of the that atom will either increase or decrease depending on the *direction* of the applied magnetic field (polarity principle). According to the effect wanted, either "north" or "south" poles are used to move the electrons of the body cells.

According to *Robert O. Becker* and *Jerry Tennant*, the proteins embedded within the cell membrane work as diodes, permitting current to flow in one direction only (**Fig. 14.2.1**). The exposure of the cells to magnetic field causes the electrons within the cell membrane to move in one direction, recharging the TMP of the cell membrane. Increasing the cell membrane TMP results in increasing the activity of the sodium/potassium ($Na^+/K^+$) pump, which is essential for the cell health and balance. According to *Albert Szent-Györgi*, the Nobel Prize Laureate in Physiology or Medicine in 1937, cell health is directly proportional to the sodium–potassium pump activity and inversely proportional to the cell membrane voltage (TMP).

2. *Nitric oxide induction*: Magnetic fields increase the motion of electrolytes and ions in the body's fluids, which will increase their charge by 500 %!! For example, the pulsed magnetic field causes the shift of intracellular ionized calcium ions ($Ca^{2+}$) to move along the direction of the field (Fig. 14.2.2). The movement of ionized calcium ions ($Ca^{2+}$) will facilitate their kinetic binding with a protein called "calmodulin" (CaM). The calcium/calmodulin ($Ca^{2+}$/CaM) complex activates the "nitric oxide synthase (NOS)" in endothelial cells (eNOS), immune cells (iNOS), and neurons (nNOS), which will result in vasodilation and anti-inflammatory action.

3. *Analgesia*: Neurons have a TMP that ranges from −70 to −80 mV. Action potential and nerve signaling arise when the resting membrane potential of neurons is raised (e.g., from −80 to −65 mV). In neurons, pain signals arise when the axonal membrane potential decreases (e.g., +10 mV).

   When a resting cell voltage raises from −70 to −50 mV, for example, the cell is called "depolarized," and ionized calcium ($Ca^{2+}$) and sodium ($Na^+$) will start to influx intracellularly from the extracellular fluid.

   PEMFs can result in analgesia by the following suggested mechanism: PEMFs lower the axonal membrane potential (voltage) from −70 to −90 mV, causing neuronal "hyperpolarization." When a pain signal is generated, it will typically raise the voltage from −70 to +10 mV, for example; however, when the neuron is hyperpolarized, the membrane potential will be lowered from +10 to −30 mV, which is insufficient to generate a pain signal by releasing neurotransmitters into the synaptic cleft; therefore, the pain signal is "blocked."

4. *Anti-inflammatory effect*: When a cell is injured, its TMP is raised (e.g., degenerative and immunocompromised cells have TMP of −30 mV, and fibrotic cells have a TMP of −15 mV). As the cellular TMP rises, inflammatory cytokines are released, causing inflammation as a desperate attempt from the body to heal. PEMFs "recharge" the cellular membrane voltage, resulting in stopping the inflammatory cytokine release. Any cell in the body works optimally with a cellular membrane voltage of −70 mV, and as the cell is damaged, up to 80 % of its cellular membrane voltage is lost. To recharge the cells, "electrons" have to be supplied via antioxidant substances (e.g., *vitamin E*) or electronic devices.

5. *Electroporation*: PEMF exposure of the cell membrane during pulses induces a phenomenon known in biophysics as "electroporation." Electroporation is defined as *a significant increase in the electrical conductivity and permeability of the cell plasma membrane caused by an externally applied electromagnetic field*. The energy required for energy-mediated molecular transport is typically provided by ATP molecules; however, it can also be

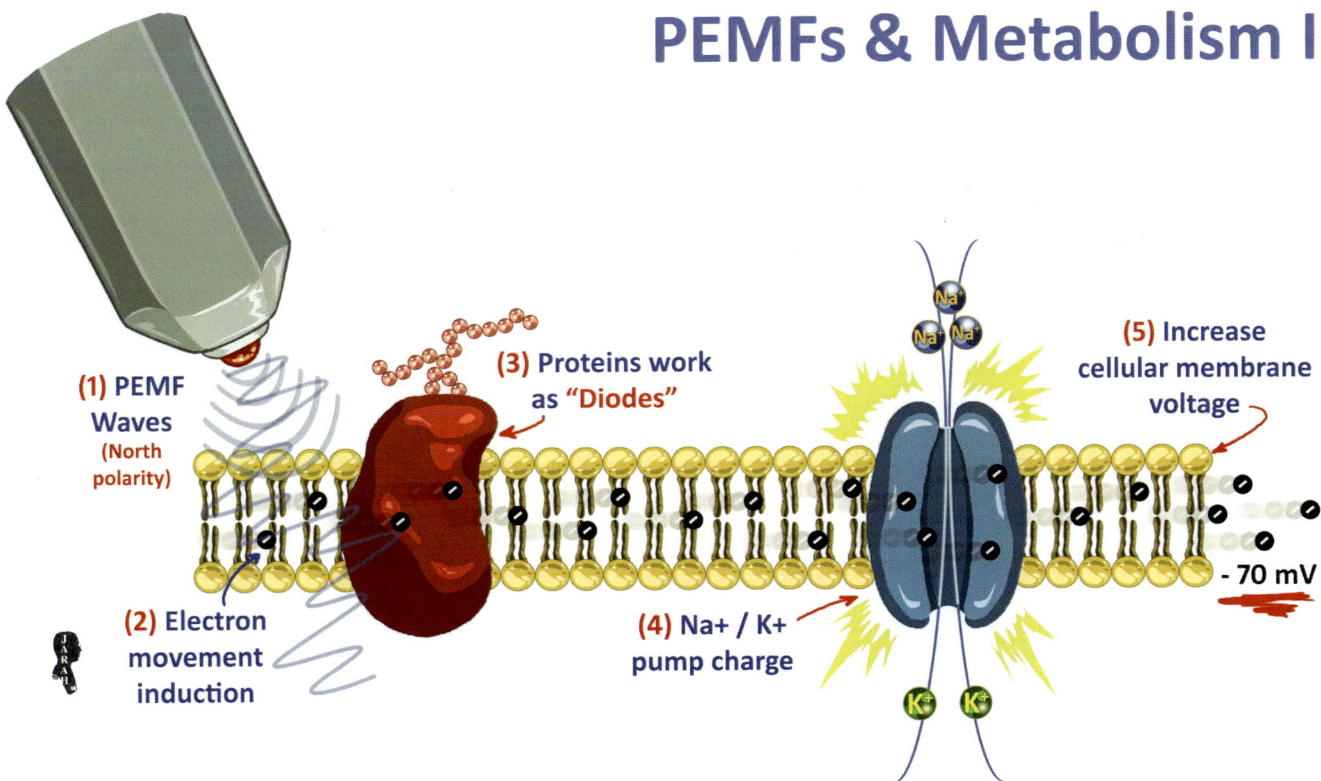


**Fig. 14.2.1** An illustration that demonstrates the effect of PEMFs on cell membrane proteins, which works as diodes permitting the flow of electrons in one direction; the flow of electrons will charge the sodium/potassium pump, increasing the resting membrane potential

# PEMFs & Metabolism II

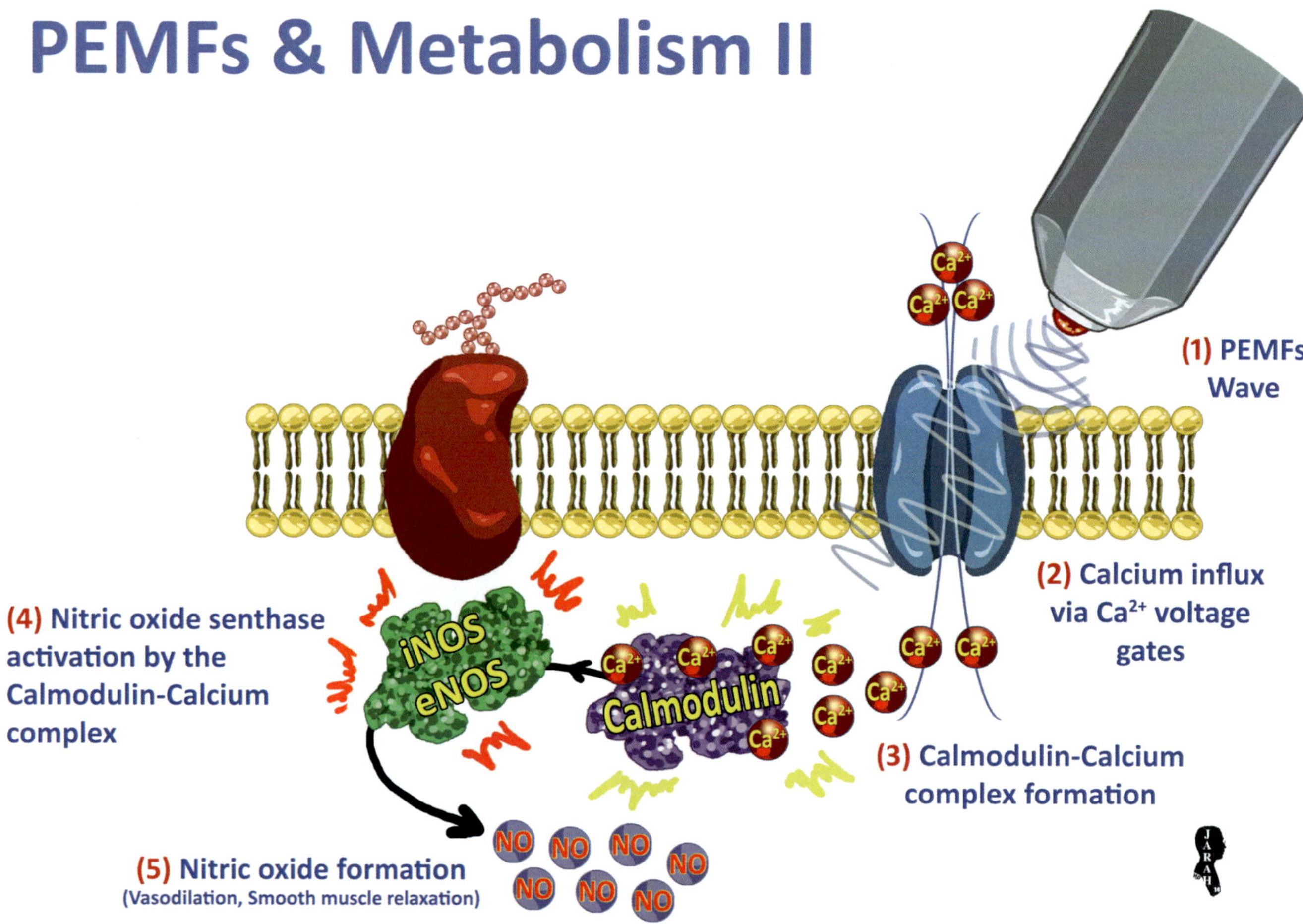



**Fig. 14.2.2** An illustration that demonstrates the effect of PEMFs over the calcium channels, facilitating the formation of nitric oxide via the activation of intracellular ionized calcium, inducing the enzyme "nitric oxide synthase" (iNOS)

provided by electromagnetic field or photons absorbed by the cell. Therefore, when the cells are exposed to high EMFs or electrification, their active channels will absorb this energy and open the cells, making the cells "leaky." This leakage can cause harmful substances to enter the cells (e.g., *microbes*), especially if the patient's blood contains toxins or bacteremia.

Electroporation allows cellular introduction of large and highly charged molecules which would NEVER passively diffuse across the hydrophobic bilayer core (**Fig. 14.2.3**). This electroporation effect increases (1) transmembrane potential (TMP); (2) electron transport through the membrane, hence increasing the membrane potential; and (3) free radical scavenging, which all are significantly important for antiaging and treating chronic diseases including cancer.

During electroporation, the lipid molecules are not chemically altered but simply shift position, opening up pores which act as the conductive pathway through the bilayer as it is filled with water. PEMF therapy can increase the effectiveness of antioxidants 100-fold!

6. *Increases blood oxygenation* (*Hall effect*): In red blood cells (RBCs), hemoglobin is composed of an iron atom surrounded by four heme molecules. Each heme molecule has a pair of free electrons (eight electrons total). Each electron will bind to an oxygen atom; therefore, a hemoglobin molecule is able to carry eight oxygen atoms in total. However, not every hemoglobin molecule carries eight oxygen molecules, and in cases of electromagnetic field (EMF) toxicity, medications, and acidity, the RBCs will clump or stack together (rouleaux phenomenon), further reducing the oxygen capacity. External field application increases the electrostatic charge outside the RBCs causing them to repel each other (**Fig. 14.2.4**), removing the clumping and stacking; this in turn will increase the chance of blood oxygenation (Hall effect).

7. *Increases brain function*: In 1952, the physicist *Winfried Otto Schumann* discovered that the space between the Earth crest at sea level and the conductive ionosphere sky level acts like a resonant cavity for

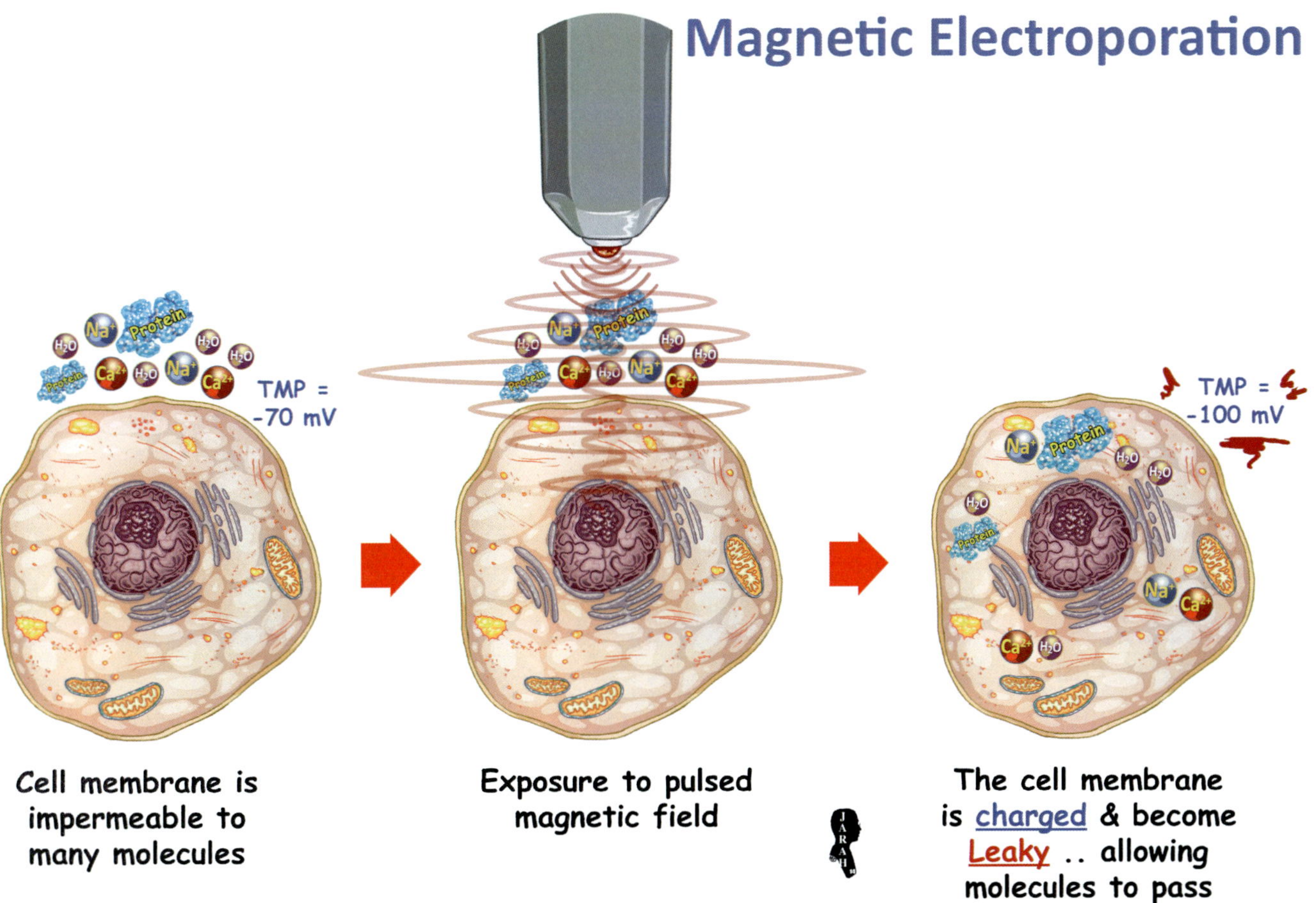


**Fig. 14.2.3** An illustration that demonstrates the cellular "electroporation" phenomenon created by PEMF exposure

vibrations in the "extremely low frequencies (ELFs)" band, which include Earth's magnetic field (7.83 Hz). Interestingly, the same frequency (7.83 Hz) is used by the brain's hippocampus (in the temporal lobe) in many animals for "maze navigation"! Humans and animals have been found to have natural magnetite (iron crystals) in the brain and other tissues that sense magnetic field changes. Shielding humans from earth magnetic field creates "circadian rhythm desynchronization."

## PEMF Therapy Healing Cases

The author has been using PEMF therapy in private practice for some patients with a variety of clinical conditions. For pulsed electromagnetic field (PEMF) devices, the author uses the Tennant's Biotransducer®, the Magnetic Field System (MAS) mat®, and the SOTA Magnetic Pulser MP6®.

Like in the chapter of microcurrent therapy, my aim is to demonstrate for the reader some cases that have been imaged by me before and after as a personal interest, documenting therapeutic effect of these therapies detected in radiological

modalities, which is compatible with many documented effects reported in the medical literature.

### Case 1

A 72-year-old male patient with history of diabetes mellitus and hepatitis C presented with severe right knee osteoarthritis. The patient was informed that the only solution for his pain is knee replacement surgery; however, because of his multiple medical problems, he was sent home on oral analgesics only. The patient was offered to try PEMF therapy free of charge. He used to come for 30 min to the hospital daily for a PEMF therapy session. The device used was "Tennant Biotransducer®," manufactured by Avazzia and distributed from Texas, in United States, by Senergy Medical Group (**Fig. 14.2.5**).

A magnetic resonance image of the knee was performed to assess the degree of damage in the knee, which revealed marked bone marrow edema in the medial femoral condyle, grade VI chondropathy of the knee joints, and severe osteoarthritic bony changes and geode formation in the tibial plateau bilaterally (**Fig. 14.2.6a**). After 2 months of daily 30-min PEMF session, marked pain relief was reported by the patient, with significant reduction in the bone marrow

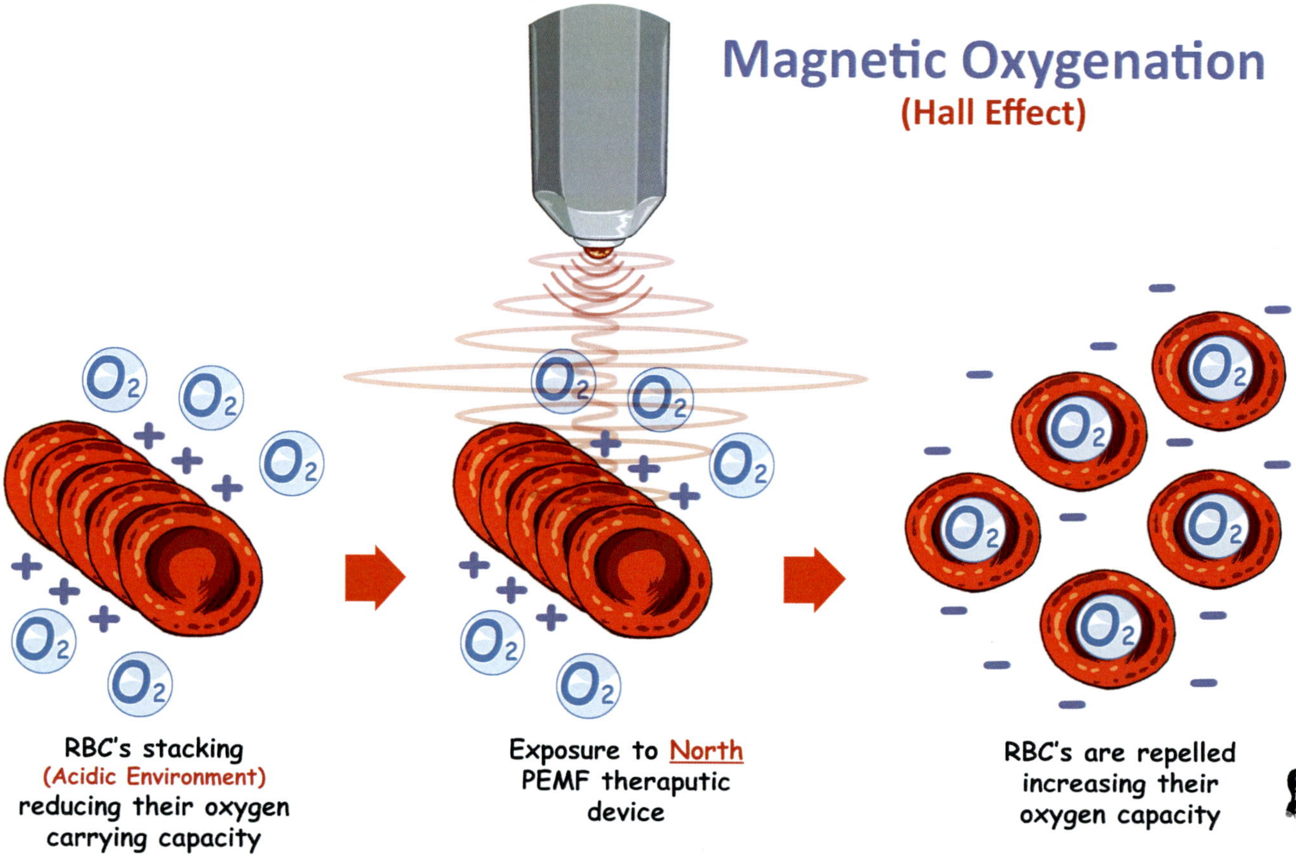

# Magnetic Oxygenation
## (Hall Effect)



**Fig. 14.2.4** An illustration that demonstrates the RBC "Hall effect" phenomenon created by PEMF exposure

edema detected in MRI examination performed after 2 months ( Fig. 14.2.6b).

The PEMF probe was placed mainly on the medial femoral condyle, where the maximum area of pain was. Imaging the knee before and after a regular PEMF session in thermal imaging camera ( Fig. 14.2.7) showed significant increase in blood content in the knee. The blood gushing in the knee after the PEMF session confirms the Hall effect; and as any medical student known in pathology lectures, more blood to the wound equals faster healing process.

### ▪▪ Case 2

A 51-year-old female nurse in radiology department complains of posterior ankle pain at the site of Achilles tendon attachment since 2 months. The patient was imaged in MRI and was found to have bone marrow edema at the attachment of the Achilles tendon into the calcaneus. A 30-min PEMF therapeutic session by Tennant's Biotransducer® was done for her, and she was imaged after the session; the MR images showed significant bone marrow edema changes, and the patient reported up to 60 % pain resolution ( Fig. 14.2.8).

### ▪▪ Case 3

A 73-year-old Kuwaiti female patient with history of previous brain strokes, left knee replacement, diabetes mellitus, mild Parkinsonism, and hypertension. The patient had a

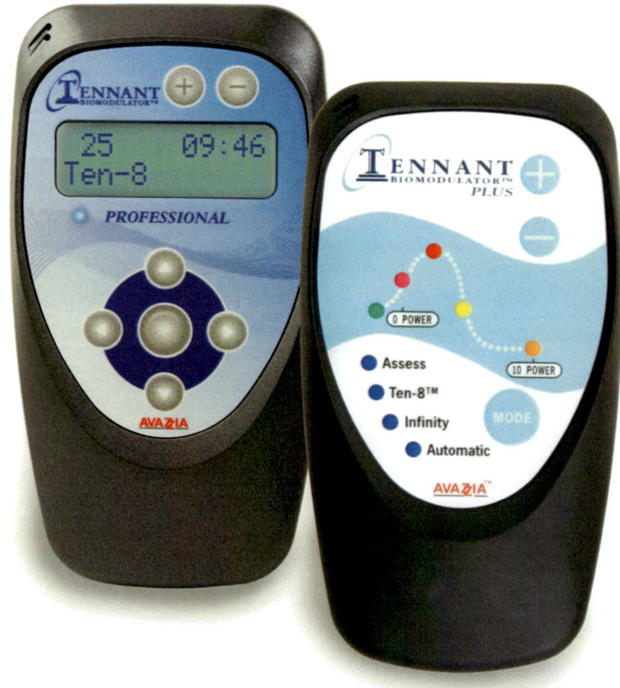


**Fig. 14.2.5** Images of Tennant Biomodulator® devices (Plus and Pro) (Manufactured by Avazzia; Texas, USA; distributed by Senergy Medical Group; Texas, USA)

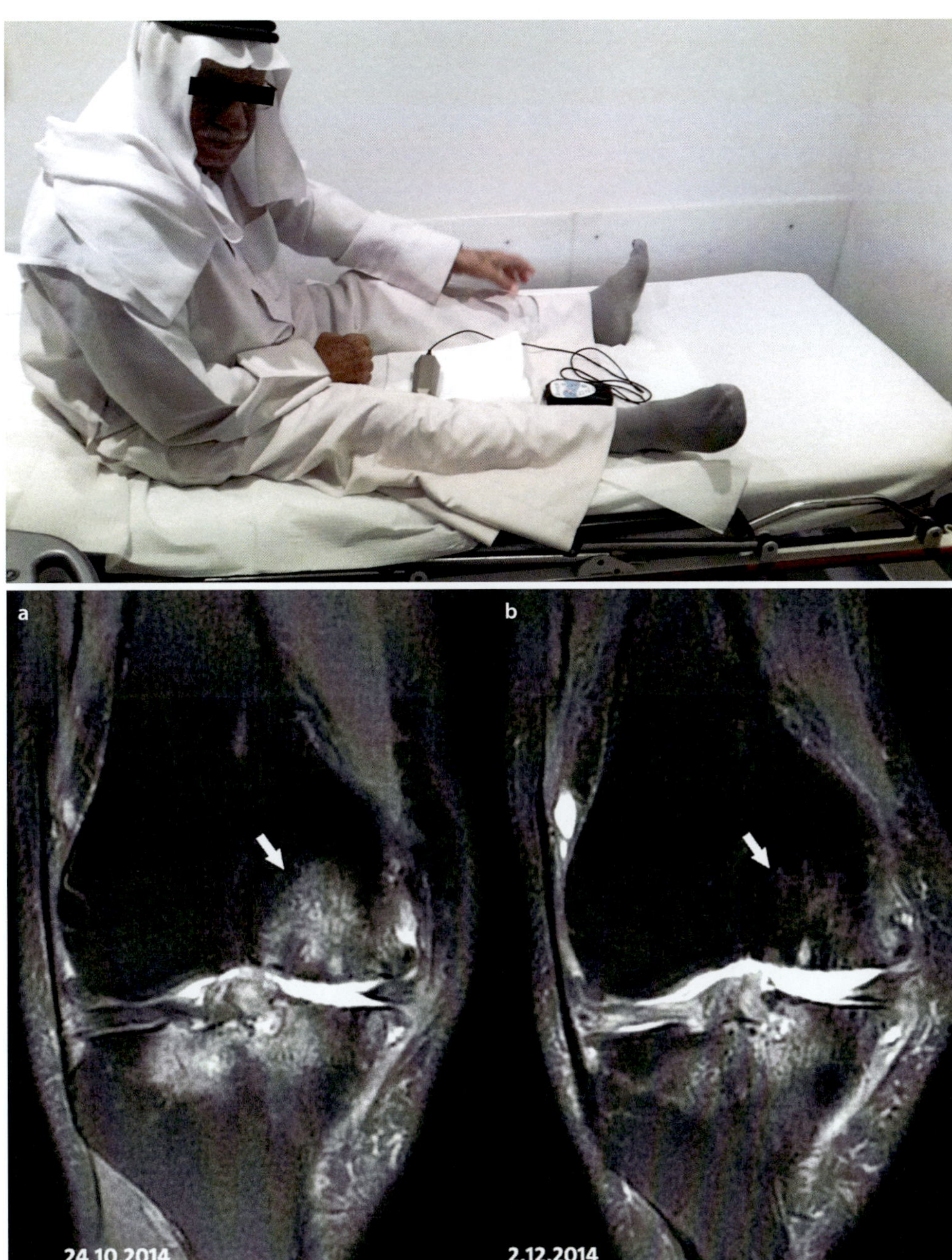

**◘ Fig. 14.2.6** MR-PDW images of the right knee of a 72-year-old patient with osteoarthritis; the first MR image was taken in October 24, 2014 (**a**) that shows marked bone marrow edema and osteoarthritic changes. After 2 months of PEMF therapy (**b**), the bone marrow edema in the medial femoral condyle (*arrow* in **a**, **b**) shows significant resolution, compared to the tibia, which was not exposed to the PEMF probe as the pain was concentrated more in the area of the medial femoral condyle, which was the only area treated locally by PEMF therapy



fall on her knees, and her X-rays show left comminuted tibial fracture (◘ Fig. 14.2.9). Due to her multiple risk factors and her old age, plus the patient on anticoagulant therapy, no invasive intervention was decided by her treating physicians. The only thing they can do for the time being is to put her knee on a cast and hope that the bone will heal itself within 3–4 months, according to the orthopedic surgeon.

I started the patient on organic silica to accelerate the bone formation based on the work of the French, Nobel Prize nominee *Louis Kervran* (biological transmutation) and PEMF therapy using *SOTA Magnetic* Pulser MP6®

(◘ Fig. 14.2.10). I advised the family to use it for 30 min maximum, four to five times per day, with at least 1-h break in between sessions.

The result can be seen on the X-rays (◘ Fig. 14.2.9), which showed the initial comminuted fracture and how the fracture space started to become more and more blurry with time, denoting the formation of callus. The orthopedic surgeon told the family that he was expecting a full healing within 3–4 months. With such X-ray findings, the healing is faster than what he anticipated, and he believes that within 1 and half month, the callus formation will be complete.

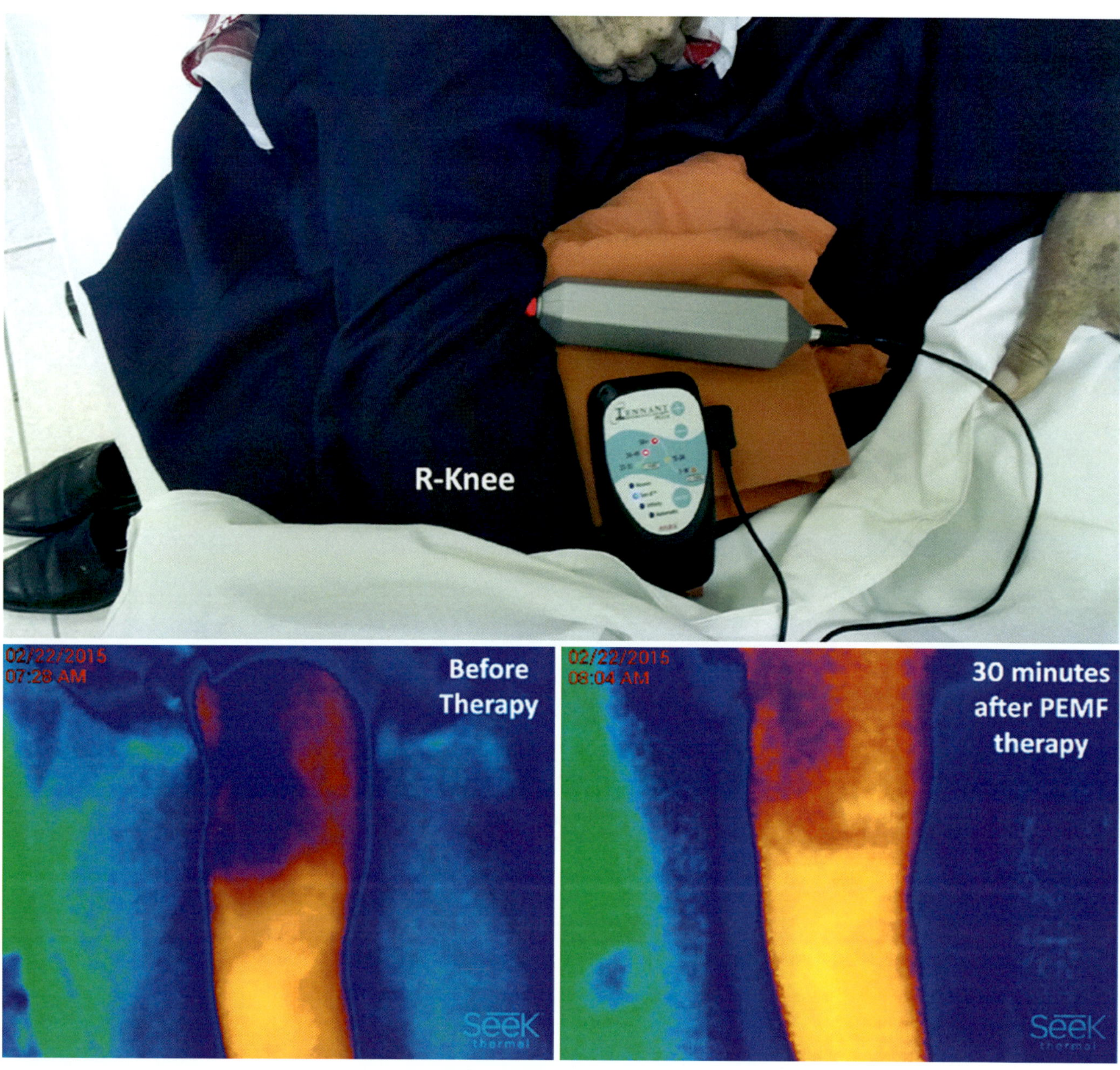


**Fig. 14.2.7** Thermal images taken for the same patient in Fig. 14.6 that shows significant blood gush into the knee after 30 min of PEMF therapy session (*yellow hue*), especially at the area treated (where the PEMF probe was)

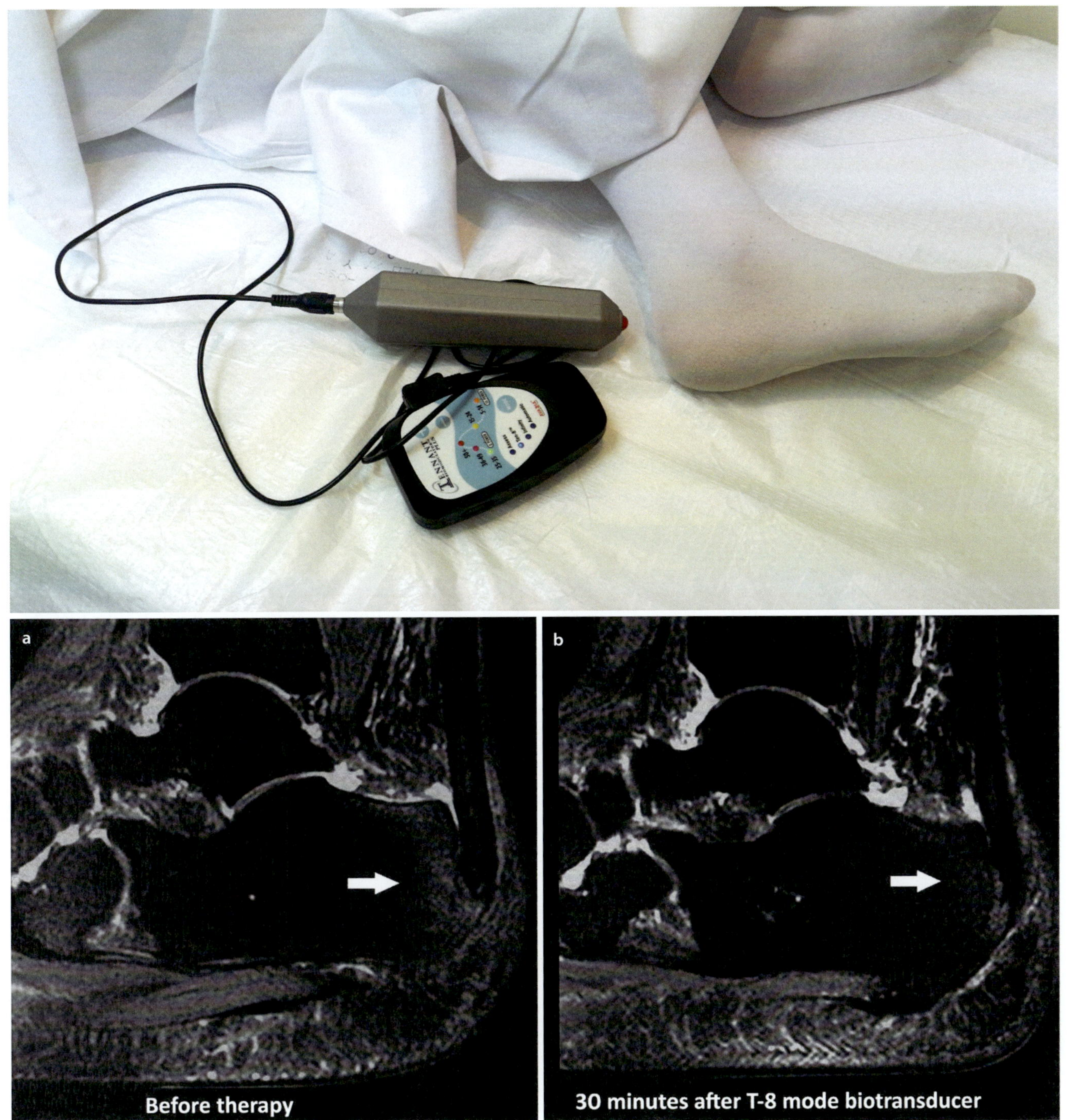



**Fig. 14.2.8** MR-PDW images of the calcaneus of a nurse patient; the bone marrow edema (*arrow* in **a**) showed significant reduction after 30 min of PEMF therapeutic session (*arrow* in **b**)

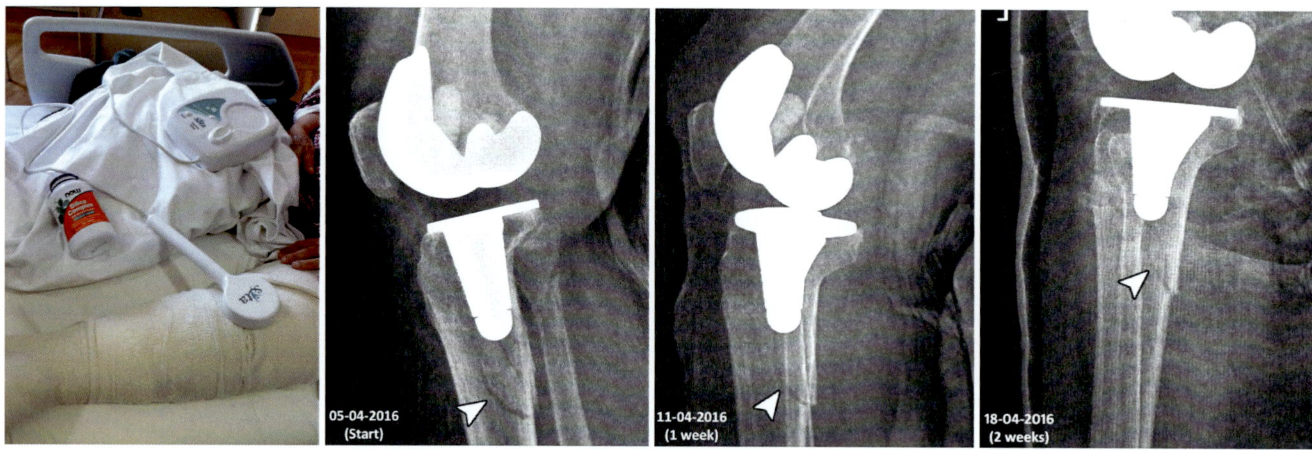



**Fig. 14.2.9**   Serial lateral knee radiographs that show tibial plateau fractures (*arrowheads*) and their progression within the first week and the second week after PEMF therapy with organic silica. No other medical therapy was given to the patient except the plaster cast

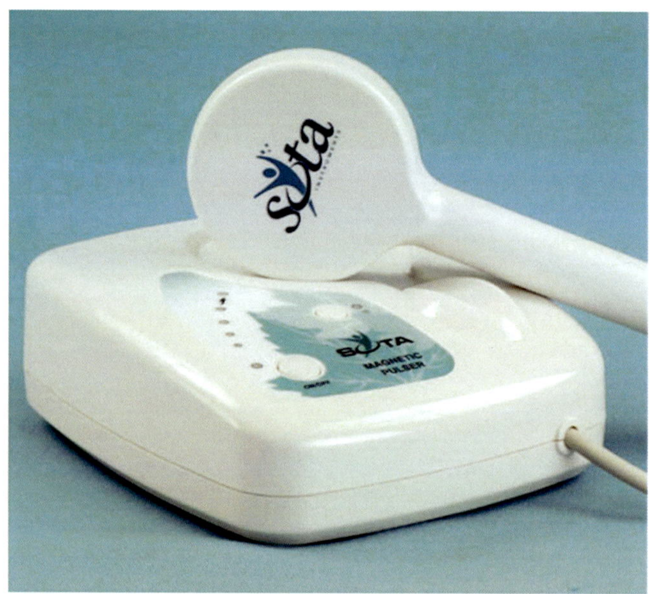

**Fig. 14.2.10**   Image of SOTA Magnetic Pulser MP6® (manufactured by SOTA Instruments Inc.; Canada)

## Further Reading

### Microcurrent Therapy

Tennant J. Healing is voltage. The handbook. 3rd ed. CreateSpace Independent Publishing Platform; 2010.

McMakin C. Microcurrent treatment of myofascial pain in the head, neck, and face. Top Clini Chiropr. 1998;5(1):29–35.

McMakin CR. Microcurrent therapy: a novel treatment method for chronic low back myofascial pain. J Bodywork Movement Ther. 2004;8:143–53.

Mercola JM, et al. The basis for microcurrent electrical therapy in conventional medical practice. J Adv Med. 1995;8(2):107–20.

Braddock M, et al. Current therapies for wound healing: electrical stimulation, biological therapeutics, and the potential for gene therapy. Int J Dermatol. 1999;38:808–17.

Rossen JS. Microcurrent stimulation – why it is replacing many other forms of electrical therapy. Am Chiropractor. 1989;3:78–89.

Wieder DL. Microcurrent therapy; wave of the future? Rehab Manag. 1991;4(2):34–5.

Tan G, et al. Electromedicine. Efficacy of microcurrent electrical stimulation on pain severity, psychological distress, and disability. Am J Pain Manage. 2000;10(1): 35–44.

Blackiston DJ, et al. Bioelectric controls of cell proliferation: Ion channels, membrane voltage and the cell cycle. Cell Cycle. 2009;8(21):3519–28.

Cho MR. A review of electrocoupling mechanisms mediating facilitated wound healing. IEEE Trans Plasma Sci. 2002;30:1504–15.

Chang PC, et al. Galvanotropic and galvanotaxic responses of corneal endothelial cells. J Formos Med Assoc. 1996;95:623–7.

Hotary KB, et al. Endogenous electrical currents and the resultant voltage gradients in the chick embryo. Dev Biol. 1990;140:149–60.

Borgens RB. What is the role of naturally produced electric current in vertebrate regeneration and healing? Int Rev Cytol. 1982;76:245–98.

Cheng N, et al. The effects of electric currents on ATP generation, protein synthesis, and membrane transport in rat skin. Clin Orthop Relat Res. 1982;171:264–72.

### Pulsed Electromagnetic Fields Therapy

Adey WR. Biological effects of electromagnetic fields. J Cell Biochem. 1993;51:410–6.

Adey WR. Tissue interactions with non-ionizing electromagnetic fields. Physiol Rev. 1981;61:435–514.

Pall ML. Electromagnetic fields act via activation of voltage-gated calcium channels to produce beneficial or adverse effects. J Cell Mol Med. 2013;17(8):958–65.

Markov MS. Pulsed electromagnetic field therapy history, state of the art and future. Environmentalist. 2007a;27(4):465–75.

Markov MS. Effects of electromagnetic fields on biological systems. Electromagn Biol Med. 2013;32(2):121–2.

Markov MS. Magnetic field therapy: a review. Electromagn Biol Med. 2007b;26(1):1–23.

Ganesan K, et al. Low frequency pulsed electromagnetic field – a viable alternative therapy for arthritis. Indian J Exp Biol. 2009;47:939–48.

Funk RHW, et al. Electromagnetic effects – from cell biology to medicine. Prog Histochem Cytochem. 2009;43:177–264.

Raylman RR, et al. Exposure to strong static magnetic field slows the growth of human cancer cells In vitro. Bioelectromagnetics. 1996;17:358–63.

Bagnato GL, et al. Pulsed electromagnetic fields in knee osteoarthritis: a double blind, placebo-controlled, randomized clinical trial. Rheumatology (Oxford). 2016;55(4):755–62.

Jacobson JI. A look at the possible mechanism and potential of magnetotherapy. J Theor Biol. 1991;149:97–119.

Trostel TC, et al. Effects of picoTesla electromagnetic field treatment on wound healing in rats. Am J Vet Res. 2003;64:845–54.

Kirschvink JL, et al. Magnetite in human tissues: a mechanism for the biological effects of weak ELF magnetic fields. Bioelectromagnetics Suppl. 1992;1:101–13.

Challis LJ. Mechanisms for interaction between RF fields and biological tissue. Bioelectromagnetics Suppl. 2005;7:S98–106.

Walleczek J. Electromagnetic field effects on cells of the immune system: the role of calcium signaling. FASEB J. 1992;6:3177–85.

Glaser R. Current concepts of the interaction of weak electromagnetic fields with cells. Bioelectrochem Bioenergetics. 1992;27:255–68.

# Index



© Springer International Publishing Switzerland 2017
J.A. Al-Tubaikh, *Internal Medicine*, DOI 10.1007/978-3-319-39747-4